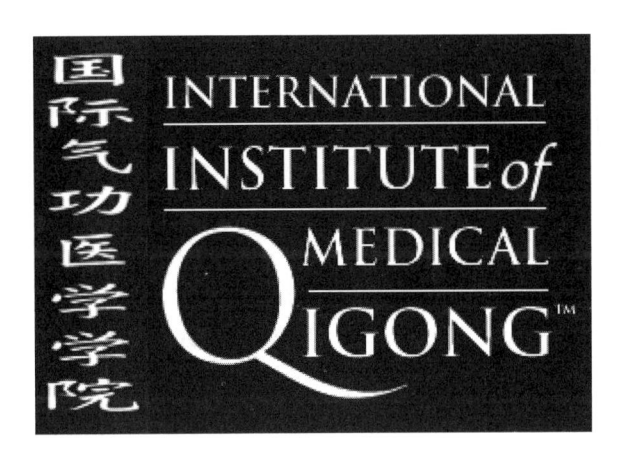

**QIGONG THERAPY
VOLUME 1**

ENERGETIC ANATOMY
AND PHYSIOLOGY

PROFESSOR JERRY ALAN JOHNSON, PH.D., D.T.C.M., D.M.Q. (CHINA)

EDITED BY

L. FRANCESCA FERRARI, L.AC., D.T.C.M., D.M.Q. (CHINA)

GIDEON B. ENZ, D.M.Q. (CHINA)

SUZANNE B. FRIEDMAN, L.AC., D.M.Q. (CHINA)

First published in March 2002 by:
The International Institute of Medical Qigong
P.O. Box 52144
Pacific Grove, CA 93950
U.S.A.

© 2005   Professor Jerry Alan Johnson, Ph.D., D.T.C.M., D.M.Q. (China)

All rights reserved under the International and Pan-American copyright conventions. No part of this publication may be reproduced, stored in a retrieval system, or transmitted in any form or by any means, electronic, mechanical, photocopying, recording or otherwise, without the prior written permission of the publisher (The International Institute of Medical Qigong). Reviewers may quote brief passages.

ISBN# 1-885246-28-5
Printed in the United States of America.

Disclaimer:
Qigong medicine is not intended to replace orthodox medicine, but rather to complement it. The meditations, practices, techniques and prescriptions described herein are currently practiced in the government hospitals, Medical Universities and clinics of The Peoples Republic of China. These techniques can be very powerful and may in some cases be too mentally and physically demanding for some individuals. The readers should therefore use their own discretion and consult a doctor of Medical Qigong therapy, an acupuncturist, medical doctor, or mental health professional before engaging in these exercises and meditations. The author, the International Institute of Medical Qigong, and the publishers are neither liable or responsible to any person or entity with respect to any loss or damage caused, or alleged to be caused, directly or indirectly by reading or following the instructions for any condition, or interpreting information provided in this text. The treatments mentioned in this book are not meant to be used as symptomatic prescriptions. The treatment of specific organs, channels, channel points, and prescriptions must always be selected based on a thorough understanding of the origin of the patient's disease. If an ailment is severe, or if symptoms persist, please consult a medical professional immediately.

Throughout the text I will suggest that the doctor prescribe herbs for certain conditions along with Medical Qigong therapy. The Medical Qigong Treatments and Homework Prescription Exercises and Meditations assigned to patients sometimes require herbal prescriptions, as well as regulation of the patient's diet and living environment. Herbal prescriptions will vary according to the patient's constitution, condition and specific illness, and must be prescribed only by a doctor or herbalist qualified to prescribe Chinese medical herbs. Each state in the U.S. has its own regulations and restrictions. Therefore, it is advisable for the reader to consult his or her own state medical board regarding the legalities and liabilities of the techniques described in this text.

Throughout the text I have used the term *doctor* when referring to professional practitioners of Traditional Chinese Medicine, as well as to those who use energetic medicine to treat patients. The word "doctor" means "to teach." I believe that the foremost duty of any doctor of medicine (Western or Chinese) should be as educator, to teach his or her patients the knowledge and skills for the prevention and treatment of disease and injury. Currently, the official title *Doctor of Medical Qigong Therapy* is only licensed by The People's Republic of China.

Table of Contents

Foreword XIV

Preface XIX

Acknowledgments XXIII

Introduction XXVII

Section I
Foundations of Chinese Energetic Medicine 1

Chapter 1 Introduction to Medical Qigong 3
- Understanding the Concept of Qi 4
- The Five Realms of Energy 4
- Defining the Energy of Yin and Yang 6
- The History of Qigong and Chinese Medicine 7
- History of Ancient Chinese Shaman Doctors: Wu Yi 14
- Qigong of the Imperial College 23
- Three Main Schools of Qigong 25
- Medical Qigong Defined 27
- Medical Qigong Training in China 28
- Medical Qigong Examination and Clinical Qualifications in China 30
- Medical Qigong Training in the U. S. 32
- Medical Qigong Training in T.C.M. Colleges 32
- Traditional Chinese Medicine and Medical Qigong Therapy 32
- Acupuncture 34
- Herbology 37
- Chinese Massage Therapy 39
- Medical Qigong Therapy 41

Chapter 2 Understanding Ancient Chinese Metaphysics 45
- Introduction 45
- The Energetic Formation of the Universe 46
- The Dao: Divine 46
- The Wuji: Infinite Space 48
- Taiji: Supreme Ultimate 51
- Bagua: Eight Trigrams 53
- The Wu Xing: Five Elements 55
- The Physical, Energetic and Spiritual Worlds 56
- Energetic Formation of the Human Body 59
- The Dao: Divine 59
- Shen Ling: Supernatural Spirit 59
- Shen Xian: Eternal Soul 60
- Zhi Yi Tian: Will and Intent of Heaven 63
- Yuan Shen: Human Soul 64
- Shen Zhi: Acquired Spirit 65
- The Three Bodies 67
- Overview 68

- Energetic Embryological Development 70
- Interactions of Essence, Energy and Spirit 70
- Daoist Perspectives on Early Embryological Development 72
- Understanding Fetal Toxins 73
- The Body's Developmental Sequence 73
- The Five Elemental Jing Formations 74
- The Ten Lunar Months of Creation 79
- Month One 80
- Month Two 83
- Month Three 84
- Month Four 85
- Month Five 86
- Month Six 87
- Month Seven 88
- Month Eight 90
- Month Nine 91
- Month Ten 92
- Postnatal Energy Development 93
- Congenital or Acquired Disorders 95
- Prenatal and Postnatal Energetic Patterns 95
- Conception and the Prenatal Ancestral Traits 96
- Birth and the Postnatal Energetic Patterns 98
- Ancient Daoist Archetypes of the Human Soul 99
- The Ethereal Soul and Corporeal Soul 100
- The Hun: Three Ethereal Souls 100
- Tai Guan, Shang Ling, and Yu Jing 101
- The Po: The Seven Corporeal Souls 107
- The Death Roots of the Womb 116
- The Final Exit of the Human Soul 116
- Overview 118

Chapter 3 Tissue Formation and Development 121
- Fascial Development and Energy Flow 121
- The Three Types of Body Classifications of Ancient China 122
- Yin and Yang Structural Formation 122
- Yin and Yang Anatomical Aspects 123
- The Body's Five Elements 125
- Congenital Constitutions 126
- Classification of the Five Element Physical Constitutions 127
- The Wood Constitution 128
- The Fire Constitution 131
- The Earth Constitution 133
- The Metal Constitution 135
- The Water Constitution 137
- Combined Constitutions 139
- Personality Constitutions of the Eight Extraordinary Vessels 139
- Yin and Yang and the Yao Image 142
- Ancient Daoist Prenatal and Postnatal Yao Formations 143
- Yao Image and Physical Anatomy 144
- Identifying Introverted and Extroverted Structures 147
- Congenital and Acquired Cellular Patterns 149
- Summary 150

Table of Contents

Chapter 4 The Five Energies of the Human Body 151
- Cellular Vibration and the Five Energies of the Human Body 152
- Sound Energy Resonances 153
- Sound Energy and the Human Body 155
- Light Energy 165
- Projecting Colored Light 172
- Magnetic Energy 177
- Magnetic Fields and the Body 177
- Heat 180
- Electricity 182
- The Body's Piezoelectric Qualities 183

Chapter 5 The Taiji Pole and Three Dantians 185
- The Taiji Pole 185
- The Taiji Pole and the Chakra System 191
- Introduction to the Chakras 193
- Yin and Yang and the Seven Internal Chakras 193
- Awakening The Seven Internal Chakras 194
- First Chakra 195
- Second Chakra 197
- Third Chakra 198
- Fourth Chakra 199
- Fifth Chakra 200
- Sixth Chakra 201
- Seventh Chakra 202
- Awakening The External Chakras 203
- The Eighth Chakra 203
- The Ninth Chakra 205
- The Twelve Chakra Gates and The Three Dantians 206
- Energetic Function 206
- The Bottom Chakra Gate 207
- The Second Chakra and Gates 207
- The Third Chakra and Gates 207
- The Fourth Chakra and Gates 208
- The Fifth Chakra and Gates 208
- The Sixth Chakra and Gates 208
- The Upper Chakra Gate 208
- Precautions 208
- The Twelve Earthly Branches and the Twelve Chakra Gates 208
- Reconstructing The Chakra Gates 209
- Energizing The Chakras Through The Twelve Gates 210
- The Three Dantians 211
- Outer and Inner Alchemy 212
- The Lower Field of Cinnabar: Xia Dantian 213
- The Middle Field of Cinnabar: Zhong Dantian 219
- The Upper Field of Cinnabar: Shang Dantian 225
- The Energetic Functions of the Three Dantians 233
- The Dantian's Yin and Yang Energetic Chambers 235
- The Doctor's Projected Aura Fields and the Three Dantians 236
- The Moveable Bones of the Three Dantians 237

Chapter 6 The Eight Extraordinary Vessels 239
- The Eight Extraordinary Vessels 239
- Energetic Embryology 240
- The Function of the Eight Extraordinary Vessels 242
- The Eight Extraordinary Vessels and Medical Qigong Therapy 244
- Clinical Manifestation and Use 244
- Energetic Functions 245
- The Eight Extraordinary Vessels and The Eight Confluent Points 245
- Eight Confluent Points 247
- Governing and Conception Vessels: Ren and Du Mai 248
- The Governing Vessel: Du Mei 249
- The Conception Vessel: Ren Mai 253
- Thrusting and Belt Vessels: Chong and Dai Mai 257
- The Thrusting Vessels: Chong Mai 257
- The Belt Vessel: Dai Mai 261
- Yin and Yang Heel Vessels: Qiao Vessels 264
- The Yin Heel Vessels: Yin Qiao Mai 265
- The Yang Heel Vessels: Yang Qiao Mai 268
- Yin and Yang Linking Vessels: Wei Vessels 271
- The Yin Linking Vessel: Yin Wei Mai 271
- The Yang Linking Vessels: Yang Wei Mai 274
- Summary of Eight Extraordinary Vessels 276

Chapter 7 The Six Extraordinary Organs 279
- Introduction 279
- Functions of the Six Extraordinary Organs 280
- The Eight Extraordinary Vessels and the Six Extraordinary Organs 281
- The Uterus: Bao 282
- Function of the Uterus 282
- The Uterus as the Heart of the Lower Dantian 284
- The Uterus and Daoist Mysticism 285
- The Brain: Nao 285
- The Brain as the Sea of Marrow 285
- The Brain and Daoist Mysticism 286
- Western Medical Viewpoint 286
- Brain-Wave Patterns 288
- Science, the Brain and Memory 289
- Chinese Energetic Medicine 290
- Pathology of the Brain 291
- The Brain Detects Emitted Qi 291
- Scientific Controls 292
- The Gall Bladder: Dan 293
- Function of the Gall Bladder 294
- The Gall Bladder and Daoist Mysticism 295
- The Marrow: Sui 295
- The Marrow and Jing 295
- The Marrow and Daoist Mysticism 296
- Pathology of the Marrow 296
- The Bones: Gu 296
- Bones and Marrow 298
- Bones and Daoist Mysticism 298
- Bones Produce Piezoelectric Charges 298

Table of Contents

Western Medical Perspective	298
Pathology of the Bones	299
The Blood Vessels: Mai	299
Qi and Blood	300
The Energetic Channels and Streams of the Blood Vessels	300
The Energetic Pathways of the Blood Vessels	301
Function of the Blood Vessels	302
The Blood Vessels and Ancient Daoist Mysticism	302
Pathology of the Blood Vessels	303
Western Medical Perspective	303

Chapter 8 The Twelve Primary Organs, Channels and Collaterals ... 307

The Internal Organs and Chinese Internal Medicine	307
Energetic Anatomy	308
Energetic Physiology	308
Introduction to Channels	314
Classification of Channels	315
The Channels' Relationship to Qi and Blood	319
Function of the Channels	321
Centrifugal and Centripetal Energy Flow	322
Internal and External Channel Flow	322
Hun and Po Channel Influence	323
The Gall Bladder: Dan	324
Chinese Character for the Gall Bladder: Dan	324
The Gall Bladder in Chinese Medicine	324
The Gall Bladder Channels	325
Channels' Energy Flow	325
The Influence of Climate	327
The Influence of Taste, Color, and Sound	327
Gall Bladder Pathology	327
T.C.M. Patterns of Disharmony	327
The Gallbladder in Western Medicine	328
Common Disorders of the Gall Bladder	329
The Liver: Gan	330
Chinese Character for the Liver: Gan	330
The Yin and Yang of the Liver	330
The Liver's Wood Jing Formation	330
The Liver in Chinese Medicine	331
The Liver Channels	336
Channels' Energy Flow	336
The Influence of Climate	337
The Influence of Taste, Color, and Sound	337
Liver Pathology	337
T.C.M. Patterns of Disharmony	338
The Liver in Western Medicine	341
Anatomy of the Liver	342
Physiology of the Liver	344
Common Disorders of the Liver	345
The Lungs: Fei	347
Chinese Character for the Lung: Fei	347
The Yin and Yang of the Lungs	347
The Lungs' Metal Jing Formation	347

THE LUNGS IN CHINESE MEDICINE	347
THE LUNG CHANNELS	353
CHANNELS' ENERGY FLOW	353
THE INFLUENCE OF CLIMATE	353
THE INFLUENCE OF TASTE, COLOR, AND SOUND	353
LUNG PATHOLOGY	353
T.C.M. PATTERNS OF DISHARMONY	355
ANATOMY OF THE RESPIRATORY SYSTEM	357
THE LUNGS IN WESTERN MEDICINE	360
BLOOD SUPPLY TO THE LUNGS	361
RESPIRATION	361
DIAPHRAGMATIC AND COSTAL BREATHING	362
RESPIRATORY VOLUMES	362
RESPIRATORY CAPACITIES	362
COMMON DISORDERS OF THE LUNGS AND RESPIRATORY SYSTEM	363
THE LARGE INTESTINE: DA CHANG	364
CHINESE CHARACTER FOR LARGE INTESTINE: DA CHANG	364
THE LARGE INTESTINE IN CHINESE MEDICINE	364
THE LARGE INTESTINE CHANNELS	366
CHANNELS' ENERGY FLOW	366
THE INFLUENCE OF CLIMATE	366
THE INFLUENCE OF TASTE, COLOR, AND SOUND	366
LARGE INTESTINE PATHOLOGY	366
T.C.M. PATTERNS OF DISHARMONY	366
THE LARGE INTESTINE IN WESTERN MEDICINE	369
THE STOMACH: WEI	372
CHINESE CHARACTER FOR THE STOMACH: WEI	372
THE STOMACH IN CHINESE MEDICINE	372
THE STOMACH CHANNELS	373
CHANNELS' ENERGY FLOW	375
THE INFLUENCE OF CLIMATE	375
THE INFLUENCE OF TASTE, COLOR, AND SOUND	375
STOMACH PATHOLOGY	375
T.C.M. PATTERNS OF DISHARMONY	376
THE STOMACH IN WESTERN MEDICINE	377
THE SPLEEN: PI	379
CHINESE CHARACTER FOR THE SPLEEN: PI	379
THE YIN AND YANG OF THE SPLEEN	380
THE SPLEEN'S EARTH JING FORMATION	380
THE SPLEEN IN CHINESE MEDICINE	380
THE SPLEEN CHANNELS	383
CHANNELS' ENERGY FLOW	385
THE INFLUENCE OF CLIMATE	385
THE INFLUENCE OF TASTE, COLOR, AND SOUND	385
SPLEEN PATHOLOGY	385
T.C.M. PATTERNS OF DISHARMONY	385
THE SPLEEN IN WESTERN MEDICINE	388
COMMON DISORDERS OF THE SPLEEN.	390
THE HEART: XIN	391
CHINESE CHARACTER FOR HEART: XIN	391
THE YIN AND YANG OF THE HEART	391

Table of Contents

The Heart's Fire Jing Formation	391
The Heart in Ancient Chinese Medicine	392
The Heart in Chinese Medicine	392
The Heart Channels	395
Channels' Energy Flow	397
The Influence of Climate	397
The Influence of Taste, Color, and Sound	397
Heart Pathology	397
T.C.M. Patterns of Disharmony	398
The Heart in Western Medicine	400
Anatomy of the Heart	402
The Four Chambers of the Heart	402
The Heartbeat: Cardiac Cycle	403
The Heart's Electrical System	404
Common Disorders of the Heart	404
The Small Intestine: Xiao Chang	405
Chinese Character for Small Intestine: Xiao Chang	405
The Small Intestine in Chinese Medicine	405
The Small Intestine Channels	406
Channels' Energy Flow	408
The Influence of Food Temperature	408
The Influence of Taste, Color, and Sound	408
Small Intestine Pathology	408
T.C.M. Patterns of Disharmony	408
The Small Intestine in Western Medicine	410
The Urinary Bladder: Pang Guang	412
Chinese Character for Urinary Bladder: Pang Guang	412
The Urinary Bladder in Chinese Medicine	412
The Urinary Bladder Channels	413
Channels' Energy Flow	415
The Influence of Climate	415
The Influence of Taste, Color, and Sound	415
Bladder Pathology	415
T.C.M. Patterns of Disharmony	415
The Urinary Bladder in Western Medicine	416
The Kidney: Shen	418
Chinese Character for the Kidney: Shen	418
The Yin and Yang of the Kidneys	418
The Kidney's Water Jing Formation	419
The Kidneys in Ancient Chinese Medicine	420
The Kidneys in Chinese Medicine	420
The Kidney Channels	426
Channels' Energetic Flow	426
The Influence of Climate	426
The Influence of Taste, Color, and Sound	426
Kidney Pathology	427
T.C.M. Patterns of Disharmony	427
The Kidneys in Western Medicine	428
Pericardium: Xin Zhu	433
Chinese Character for Pericardium: Xin Zhu	433
The Pericardium in Chinese Medicine	434
The Pericardium Channels	435

CHANNELS' ENERGY FLOW	435
THE INFLUENCE OF CLIMATE	437
THE INFLUENCE OF TASTE, COLOR, AND SOUND	437
PERICARDIUM PATHOLOGY	437
T.C.M. PATTERNS OF DISHARMONY	437
THE PERICARDIUM IN WESTERN MEDICINE	438
TRIPLE BURNERS: SAN JIAO	439
CHINESE CHARACTER FOR TRIPLE BURNERS: SAN JIAO	439
THE TRIPLE BURNERS IN ANCIENT CHINESE MEDICINE	439
THE TRIPLE BURNERS IN CHINESE MEDICINE	439
THE TRIPLE BURNER CHANNELS	441
CHANNELS' ENERGY FLOW	442
THE ENERGETIC ANATOMY OF THE TRIPLE BURNERS	442
THE BODY'S TRUE FIRE	444
THE INFLUENCE OF CLIMATE	446
THE INFLUENCE OF TASTE, COLOR, AND SOUND	446
TRIPLE BURNER PATHOLOGY	446
T.C.M. PATTERNS OF DISHARMONY	446
THE TRIPLE BURNERS IN WESTERN MEDICINE	447
UNDERSTANDING INTERNAL ORGAN PATHOLOGY	448
UNDERSTANDING CHANNEL PATHOLOGY	448
THE ANCIENT DAOIST SHAMAN'S TWELVE INTERNAL ORGANS	451

CHAPTER 9 THE CONNECTING VESSELS, DIVERGENT CHANNELS, MUSCLE AND TENDON CHANNELS AND SKIN ZONES 453

THE FIFTEEN CONNECTING VESSELS: LUO MAI	453
ORIGIN OF NAME	453
ENERGETIC ANATOMY	454
EMBRYOLOGICAL FUNCTION	454
TRANSVERSE AND LONGITUDINAL LUO	454
ENERGETIC FUNCTION	454
THE TWELVE DIVERGENT CHANNELS: JING BIE	459
ORIGIN OF NAME	459
ENERGETIC ANATOMY	459
EMBRYOLOGICAL FUNCTION	460
ENERGETIC FUNCTION	461
YIN AND YANG	461
THE TWELVE MUSCLE AND TENDON CHANNELS: JING JIN	464
ORIGIN OF NAME	464
EMBRYOLOGICAL DEVELOPMENT	465
ENERGETIC FORMATION	465
YIN AND YANG	465
CLINICAL APPLICATION	465
THE SKIN ZONES: PI FU	470
ORIGIN OF NAME	470
ENERGETIC FUNCTION	470
PATHOLOGICAL SYMPTOMS	471
THE CONNECTIVE TISSUE OF THE TWELVE SKIN ZONES	473
CLINICAL DIAGNOSIS AND THE TWELVE SKIN ZONES	473
CHANNEL AND COLLATERAL THERAPY	475
CONTROLLING QI EXTENSION THROUGH THE CHANNELS	475
THE DEPTH OF THE BODY'S ENERGETIC CHANNEL FLOW	476

Chapter 10 The Body's Energetic Points 477
- Introduction to Energetic Points 477
- Historical Use of Energetic Points 477
- The Three Energetic Levels of Points 479
- The Formation of Energetic Points 479
- Scientific Research of Acupoints 480
- The Four Categories of Energetic Points 480
- The Two Gates of Energetic Points 481
- The Three Functions of Energetic Points 481
- Centrifugal and Centripetal Energy Flow 484
- Point Names 484
- Classification of Energetic Points 484
- Summary of Points 492

Appendix 1 Chronology of Chinese Dynasties 493
- Introduction 493
- China's Pre-Dynasty Myths 493
- The Three Rulers Period 493
- Dynasties of China 493

Appendix 2 Medical Qigong Instruction 495
- Introduction 495
- Medical Qigong Classes 495
- Medical Qigong in T.C.M. Colleges 495
- The International Institute of Medical Qigong in Pacific Grove, Ca. 496
- Master of Medical Qigong Graduating Classes 497
- Doctor of Medical Qigong Graduating Classes 498
- Medical Qigong Classes at the Five Branches T.C.M. College in California 501
- the Medical Qigong Clinic at the Five Branches Institute T.C.M. College 501
- Medical Qigong Classes at the Academy For Five Element Acupuncture, in Florida ... 502
- The Medical Qigong Clinic at the Academy For Five Element Acupuncture 503
- The Medical Qigong Classes and Clinic at the Acupuncture and Integrative Medicine College, in Berkeley, Ca. 504
- Two Year - 200 Hour Medical Qigong Practitioner (M.Q.P.) Course 505
- Three Year - 500 Hour Medical Qigong Therapist (M.Q.T.) Course 506
- Changing Times in China for Medical Qigong Therapy 507
- The Medical Qigong Clinic at Xi Yuan Hospital in Beijing, China 508
- The Hai Dian University of Traditional Chinese Medicine in Beijing, China 509

Glossary of Terms 511

Bibliography 543

Clinic Protocol References 561

About the Author 577
- Medical Background 578
- Martial Arts Background 582
- Daoist Background 583
- Author and Publisher: 584

The International Institute of Medical Qigong Academic Directory ... 587
Faculty of the International Institute of Medical Qigong ... 587
The International Institute of Medical Qigong - California ... 589
The International Institute of Medical Qigong - Florida ... 591
The International Institute of Medical Qigong - Pennsylvania ... 591
The International Institute of Medical Qigong - Tennessee ... 592
The International Institute of Medical Qigong - Texas ... 592
The International Institute of Medical Qigong - Washington ... 592

International Branches ... 593
The International Institute of Medical Qigong - Belgium ... 593
The International Institute of Medical Qigong - Bosnia ... 593
The International Institute of Medical Qigong - Canada ... 593
The International Institute of Medical Qigong - Central America ... 594
The International Institute of Medical Qigong - Ireland ... 594
The International Institute of Medical Qigong - Isreal ... 594
The International Institute of Medical Qigong - Sweden ... 595
The International Institute of Medical Qigong - United Kingdom ... 595

The International Institute of Medical Qigong Clinical Directory ... 597
Arizona ... 597
California ... 597
Florida ... 600
Illinois ... 600
Pennsylvania ... 600
Tennessee ... 600
Texas ... 601
New York ... 601
Washington ... 601
Wisconsin ... 601

International Clinical Directory ... 602
Bermuda ... 602
Canada ... 602
Ireland ... 602
Israel ... 602
Sweden ... 602

CHINESE MEDICAL QIGONG COMPANION VIDEO OR DVD-R SERIES 603
    VIDEO OR DVD-R #1: GATHERING ENERGY FROM HEAVEN AND EARTH 603
    VIDEO OR DVD-R #2: STATIONARY AND DYNAMIC MEDICAL QIGONG POSTURE TRAINING 603
    VIDEO OR DVD-R #3: TREATING PATIENTS WITH MEDICAL QIGONG THERAPY (#1) 604
    VIDEO OR DVD-R #4: TREATING PATIENTS WITH MEDICAL QIGONG THERAPY (#2) 604
    VIDEO OR DVD-R #5: MEDICAL QIGONG ENERGY TECHNIQUES AND QI EMITTING METHODS 605
    VIDEO OR DVD-R #6: MEDICAL QIGONG INVISIBLE NEEDLE TECHNIQUE, FIVE ELEMENT QIGONG
        MASSAGE AND ENERGETIC POINT THERAPY 605
    VIDEO OR DVD-R #7: MEDICAL QIGONG HEALING SOUND THERAPY AND PRESCRIPTIONS 606
    VIDEO OR DVD-R #8: TREATMENT OF INTERNAL ORGAN DISEASES WITH MEDICAL QIGONG 606
    VIDEO OR DVD-R #9: TREATMENT OF CYSTS, TUMORS AND CANCER WITH MEDICAL QIGONG
        THERAPY 607
    VIDEO OR DVD-R #10: SOUL RETRIEVAL 607
    CHI KUNG: THE HEALING WORKOUT VIDEO 608
    TAI CHI: THE EMPOWERING WORKOUT VIDEO 608
    TAI CHI MEDITATION CASSETTE #1: LIFE FORCE BREATHING 609
    TAI CHI MEDITATION CASSETTE #2: EIGHT DIRECTION PERCEPTION 609
    MEDICAL QIGONG VIDEO OR DVD-R #11: MEDICAL QIGONG FOR UNDERSTANDING, PREVENTING AND
        TREATING BREAST DISEASE 609

MEDICAL QIGONG THERAPY FOR CANCER DVD-R SERIES 610
    DVD-R #12: HOUSTON CANCER SEMINAR #1 - INTRODUCTION TO MEDICAL QIGONG THERAPY AND
        CANCER TREATMENT: SETTING A CLINICAL FOUNDATION 610
    DVD-R #13: HOUSTON CANCER SEMINAR #2 - AN ENERGETIC APPROACH TO ONCOLOGY 611
    DVD-R #14: HOUSTON CANCER SEMINAR #3 - .. MEDICAL QIGONG TREATMENT PROTOCOLS USED FOR
        BREAST, CERVICAL, PROSTATE, OVARIAN, AND UTERINE CANCER 611
    DVD-R #15: HOUSTON CANCER SEMINAR #4 - MEDICAL QIGONG TREATMENT PROTOCOLS USED FOR
        BRAIN, SKIN, AND BONE CANCER, LEUKEMIA, MALIGNANT LYMPHOMA, AND MULTIPLE MYELO-
        MAS 612
    DVD-R #16: HOUSTON CANCER SEMINAR #5 - MEDICAL QIGONG CANCER PRESCRIPTION EXERCISES
        AND MEDITATIONS 612
    DVD-R #17: HOUSTON CANCER SEMINAR #6 - MEDICAL QIGONG TREATMENT PROTOCOLS USED FOR
        RADIATION AND CHEMOTHERAPY 613

Foreword

Despite the many wonderful advances in modern scientific medicine, human beings continue to become ill. Many chronic diseases such as diabetes, asthma, other allergic disorders, heart disease and cancer are increasing in frequency, and it is clear that medical intervention alone is not sufficient to help protect and maintain human health.

Alongside its great traditions of herbal medicine, acupuncture and remedial massage, Chinese traditional medical culture has long studied and practised the science of health preservation. This subject is concerned with how we can lead our daily life in such a way as to build and protect our own health, by attending to our dietary, sleeping, emotional, exercise and sexual habits. As a dedicated follower of recent research into these fields, I am continually astonished by how frequently studies confirm what was known so many hundreds of years ago. In dietary practice, for example, health preservation taught moderation in overall consumption, the importance of eating vegetables at every meal, the use of only small amounts of meat, and the value of plentiful tea drinking and regular but small amounts of alcohol. All of these have been demonstrated in the last few years to have a major impact on health.

The practise of Qigong belongs to this science of health preservation. There are numerous methods of practice but most share in common the principles of softness and relaxation of the body, calming of the mind and breath, and directing of the mind, usually with the aim of healing the whole organism. The practice of Qigong combines some of the benefits of physical exercise with what is known in modern medicine as psychoneuroimmunology – the application of the mind to treat disease and promote good health. It is increasingly understood, and evidenced by research, that the power of the directed mind to heal is a potent tool, and it would be fair to say that the long Chinese tradition of Qigong practice embodies the most sophisticated knowledge of this method available in the world today.

Furthermore, once a person has developed substantial experience in working with the energy within their own body and mind, they can learn to direct it outwards with the aim of healing others. Whilst this form of healing has existed in every human culture throughout history, it normally appears as either a more or less random ability in a unique individual, or is associated with intense religious belief. Neither of these approach energy healing as an objective phenomenon that can be cultivated by all of us if we practise assiduously under the guidance of an experienced teacher.

As always in life, who we turn to when we want to learn something can have a crucial influence on the outcome. Dr. Jerry Alan Johnson is an outstanding teacher and practitioner of Medical Qigong. He combines a most thorough grounding in the tradition (having studied and practised extensively in China) with the more Western skills of clear and methodical explanation. Added to this, his great passion for the subject and his ability to work with intense dedication has enabled him to produce what can only be called a masterwork. Nothing else published in English begins to compare with *Chinese Medical Qigong Therapy*.

Peter Deadman, Lic.Ac.
Founder of The Journal of Chinese Medicine,
Brighton, England
Author of *A Manual of Acupuncture*

Foreword

This massive compendium on Qigong therapy is a veritable encyclopedia on the subject. Dr. Jerry Alan Johnson's textbooks, well recognized and greatly revered, are in many ways the professional standard. Unlike many Traditional Chinese Medicine works, they also include numerous selections on the mind and emotional states, as well as on spiritual aspects of the practice, such as the soul and spirit, the stars, magical diagrams, and the *Yi Jing*.

They are a valuable resource on Qigong therapy and practice, and contain information on numerous issues and problems. The scope is admirable, the execution with its many illustrations highly recommendable. These volumes are a treasure trove and serve well as a reference work for students and practitioners.

Livia Kohn, Ph.D.,
Professor of Religion and East Asian Studies
Boston University, United States
Author of *Taoist Meditation and Longevity Techniques; Early Chinese Mysticism; The Taoist Experience: An Anthology; Laughing at the Tao; Lao-tzu and the Tao-te-ching; God of the Dao*

Foreword

In 1994, I was honored to write the Preface for the two volumes of *The Essence of Internal Martial Arts*, which was published in France by Chariot d'Or. The Preface emphasized the originality of the explicit nature of these two incredible works by Dr. Jerry Alan Johnson, which have now become the primary reference material used in the domain of the internal martial arts, within Chinese Kung Fu.

Today, I salute the publication of a *magnus opus*, with an exhaustive description of Chinese Medical Qigong Therapy. These volumes are a statement of the energetic treatments and clinical protocols which have found great hope in both curative and palliative Qigong. One would have expected such publications from Chinese experts, and yet to this day, no work of such amplitude has ever come forth, neither in China nor in the West.

Professor Jerry Alan Johnson's merit is to have brought forth the most complete traditional and particularly Daoist methods of Medical Qigong Therapy. This largely surpasses the structure of the simple outline of gymnastic health exercises, fully expanding toward the fields of physiology, psychology, and spirituality.

In addition, all of the therapeutic aspects of Medical Qigong are also evoked with respect to the particular needs of the practitioners of this discipline. We can add that the theoretical aspects of these works go largely beyond the simple framework of Traditional Chinese Medicine, reaching the esoteric, metaphysical and spiritual roots of this art.

Professor Gérard Edde, Ph.D.
Director of Daoist Studies,
L'Institut Dragon Celeste, France
Author of *Contes du Tao Sauvage; Le Chemin du Tao; Tao et Santé; Santé et Méditation dans l'énergétique Chinoise; Digiponcture Taoiste; Qigong de la Régénértion des Moelles; La Medicina Ayurvedica; Chakras y Salud: La Medicina Tantrica de los Centros de Energia*

Foreword

There are a number of excellent books on various aspects and methods of Qigong. However, there has not been, in English, a comprehensive exploration of Medical Qigong. Dr. Johnson has created a breakthrough work on Medical Qigong, which is a clear and useful revelation of the Medical Qigong curriculum at the Hai Dian University Medical Qigong College of Beijing, China, and an excellent synthesis of Medical Qigong theory from throughout China. This textbook will very likely remain the definitive compendium of Medical Qigong in the West for many years, and become the foundation from which the field of Medical Qigong will evolve in Western society.

Roger Jahnke, O.M.D.
Chair, Department of Medical Qigong
Santa Barbara College of Oriental Medicine
Author of *The Healer Within: The Four Essential Self-Care Methods For Creating Optimal Health, The Healing Promise of Qi*

Preface

As we enter the new millennium, a new era of medical therapy is beginning to blossom. According to a 1993 study published in the *New England Journal of Medicine,* alternative medicine was capturing an estimated $14 billion in out-of-pocket health care revenues from Americans each year. By 1997, the *Journal of American Medical Association* reported that the figure had more then doubled. What this trend means in real terms, is that despite the historical lack of official recognition by the American Medical Association, despite the lack of endorsement and coverage by Medicare and the majority of health insurance plans, people, in ever increasing numbers, are going to acupuncturists, energetic healers, herbalists, chiropractors, massage therapists, ayurvedic specialists, homeopathic doctors, and other traditional "healers" to meet some portion of their health care needs.

This growth of public reliance on alternative medicine has caused the Western medical establishment to sit up and take notice. In fact, some of the most vocal proponents of combining alternative medical traditions with Western medicine are medical doctors. Visionary physicians such as Deepak Chopra, Andrew Weil, Larry Dossey, Dean Ornish, and Bernie Seigel have led the way toward creating a new climate of respect for ancient medical philosophies and modalities. They have pioneered the advent in the West of health care facilities where Western medical and alternative health modalities are available under the same roof, with the goal of providing patients with the best of both worlds. This combination of ancient and modern medical traditions has been dubbed *integrative* or *complementary* medicine.

In assessing the full implications of this unlikely marriage, one must understand the differences between conventional Western medicine and traditional Eastern medicine in their approach to health and healing.

Contemporary Western medicine grew out of the scientific revolution of the seventeenth century. The philosophy of science, rooted in Aristotle's "empirical materialism," was given a new spin by the French mathematician, Descartes. Viewing reality as that which could be substantiated materially, Descartes applied an analytical reductionist logic to penetrating the secrets of nature, including biology. These views were echoed in the physics of Sir Isaac Newton, applying a linear cause-and-effect model to explain the workings of a material universe.

Man was seen as being separate from nature, mind was seen as separate from body, and all of these processes, in nature and in humans, were seen as similar to the workings of a machine composed of discreet parts. Mechanical laws were seen to govern all processes. Structure determines function; therefore, the physician's role developed into that of a mechanic: repairing, removing, transplanting, and replacing broken down-parts. Diseases had isolated causes, which needed to be removed from the rest of the parts. Because of this approach, Western medicine has the most highly developed pharmaceuticals to kill specific organisms and the finest surgical procedures in the world today.

By contrast, Eastern medicine grew out of the empirical observation of nature, beginning at least 4,700 years ago. Asian philosophy, from the Vedas of India to the Yellow Emperor of China, views reality as an interdependent whole. This "pre-scientific" understanding parallels to the broader view of modern quantum physics and general systems theory. Rather than limiting reality to that which is material, the Eastern philosophers recognized the interdependence of mind and body, the nonlinear nature of time and space, and the interweaving patterns of relationship between humanity and nature; in fact, they believed, we are nature. Anatomy, the study of human structure, takes a back seat to physiology, the study of human function. Thus, the Chinese formulated a general systems theory, in which the patterns of change that exist in nature are the same patterns that govern human biology, wherein function is viewed from a holographic perspective, and each part reflects the whole. Rather than being fixed and stable, the whole is in a dynamic process of constant change. For the whole to function harmoniously, every part must remain in balance. Therefore, the role of the Eastern physician is more similar to a gardener, following the patterns of change, diagnosing functional disharmony and restoring overall balance. Because of this approach, Oriental medicine has some of the most highly developed procedures for preventative medicine and for treating chronic diseases in the world today.

Western medical science, with its fundamental distrust of subjective diagnostic reliability, has progressed toward developing more and more expensive high-tech laboratory tests and diagnostic equipment. Thus we have the modern miracles of x-rays, MRI's, and ultrasound. Eastern medicine, trusting in human capacity, has progressed in a low-tech direction toward ever deeper training of the physician's sensory and spiritual diagnostic tools. Thus, we have the miracles of pulse diagnosis, tongue reading, and Qigong hand scanning.

With such fundamental divergencies in philosophy and technique, it is almost inconceivable that these two medical systems could ever operate together in the same setting. The fact is that they do function together, and quite effectively, too. Ironically, we can thank Mao Zedong for the union of these two unlikely bedfellows.

Recognizing that there were far too few Western trained physicians and nurses to meet the primary health care needs of China's vast population, from the outset of his leadership Mao advocated the systemization of Traditional Chinese Medicine (TCM), and advocated its implementation alongside Western medicine in China's hospitals and clinics. The results of this integration have been astonishing, as witnessed in the effective use of acupuncture anesthesia during surgery.

Nonetheless, in his efforts to create a "modern" Chinese medicine, Mao shunned some of the traditional theoretical aspects of Chinese medicine, such as the concept of Qi, which he considered feudalistic and counterrevolutionary. For this reason, he actively discouraged Medical Qigong practice as superstitious. It was not until the end of the Cultural Revolution in 1975 that Qigong reclaimed its rightful place as one of the major branches of Chinese medicine.

During Chairman Mao's reign, a high party official in Beijing was suffering from an "incurable" disease. Both Western medicine and TCM had failed to alleviate his suffering. In desperation, he went to one of the few Medical Qigong clinics operating in the country and was cured. The official then lent his support to the promotion of Medical Qigong for the benefit of the Chinese people. Before long, there were hundreds of Medical Qigong hospitals and clinics throughout China.

Thereafter, Qigong experienced an unprecedented growth in China, and became available to the general populace for the first time in history. Qigong was taught in the public education system, beginning at the elementary school level. Qigong departments were added to large urban hospitals. Colleges of Traditional Chinese Medicine developed and established sound Medical Qigong training programs. According to a recent survey, one third of the population of Beijing, China's capital city, practiced Qigong daily.

It has taken acupuncture and Chinese herbology nearly 20 years to develop into a respected profession in the United States. When the first edition of this book went to press in March of 2000, 37 states had legislation licensing professional acupuncture practice, with an additional 10 states in which legislation had recently been introduced.

Medical Qigong, however, is still at the very early stages of public recognition, understanding, and acceptance. Traditional Chinese Medicine schools around the United States, as well as independent Medical Qigong masters, are only now beginning to establish comprehensive Medical Qigong training programs.

Traditional Chinese Medicine (T.C.M.) is divided into four main branches: acupuncture, herbs and diet, massage therapy, and Medical Qigong. It is important for T.C.M. practitioners to have exposure to all four branches to be able to understand the relative strengths and limitations of their particular field of expertise, so that they will be able to select the most effective and appropriate treatment modality for their patients. Until very recently, most schools in America have been relatively unaware of the extent to which Medical Qigong therapy has developed in China, and have failed to present Medical Qigong as a significant part of their training programs for students of Oriental medicine.

This five volume Medical Qigong textbook series contains information on how to effectively diagnose and treat patients with Medical Qigong therapy, as set forth by the Hai Dian Medical Qigong College of Beijing. At one time in China, the Medical College at the Hai Dian University was recognized as one of the top leading Medical Qigong colleges in Beijing. By the end of 1999, however, many of the Medical Qigong colleges and universities had been closed due to the political actions of the Falun Gong organization.

Although these five textbooks have been primarily written for students and practitioners of Chinese medicine, it is also my hope that Western medical professionals and other alternative healers will benefit from the information contained herein, and that it may serve to enrich their clinical practice.

I have done my best to present the esoteric knowledge and wisdom of this ancient Chinese art of healing as it was passed onto me personally by several of my respected teachers, to whom I owe undying gratitude. Qigong has survived nearly five thousand years of growth and refinement and is now available to you, the reader, for your own personal and professional benefit. I sincerely hope that these five textbooks may serve to further bridge the partnership between Eastern and Western medicine, and that all humanity benefit from the interchange between these two great schools of healing. It is my hope and dream that all healers, both Western and alternative, return to the "heart" of medicine, and that each doctor may view the patient as a complete energetic integration of body, mind, emotion, and spirit. May we all support each other's skills and methods of alleviating our patients' suffering.

Jerry Alan Johnson, Ph.D., D.T.C.M., D.M.Q. (China)
Pacific Grove, California
March, 2005

When the spiritual powers are passed on and transmitted they can no longer turn back; and when they turn back they cannot be transmitted, and then their moving powers are lost to the universe. In order to fulfill destiny man should go beyond that which is near at hand and consider it as trifling.

One should make public upon tablets of jade that which was hidden and concealed in treasuries and storehouses, to study it from early dawn until night, and thus make known the precious mechanism of the universe.

Huang Di Nei Jing
(The Yellow Emperor's Canon of Internal Medicine)

Acknowledgments

I would like to express my sincere gratitude to my many friends and colleagues who helped encourage and support me in writing this textbook series: Dermot O'Connor Dip.Ac., M.P.N.L.P., M.M.Q.; Jan Eeckhout, D.O., M.M.Q., M.T.C.M., Ba Fysiother.; Vic Wouters, Msc. Fysiother., M.M.Q., M.T.C.M.; Roger Jahnke, O.M.D.; Hu Jiting, D.T.C.M.; Zhang Jingchuan, D.T.C.M.; Xu Zhuoqun, D.T.C.M.; Guo Xianhe, D.T.C.M.; Wan Taowang, D.M.Q.; William H. Lewington, L.Ac., M.M.Q.; Adam Atman, L.Ac. M.M.Q.; Tim M. Haun, D.C.; Kerrean D. Smith; Geoffrey Greenspahn M.M.Q.; Michael Winn; Mark Johnson; and my good friend Joseph Crandall.

I am also indebted to Dr. Pang Donghui, the Executive Deputy President of the Hai Dian Qigong College of Beijing, China, and to Li Fudong, D.M.Q. the university's chief director of Medical Qigong Science, and his assistants, Lu Guohong, D.M.Q. and Niu Yuhua, D.M.Q. for their constant support and encouragement, and for sharing their innermost secrets on Medical Qigong therapy.

I am very grateful to Professor Teng Yingbo, D.M.Q., president and secretary general of the Beijing Western District Qigong Science and Traditional Chinese Medicine Research Institute, for his constant support and openness in sharing the wealth of knowledge contained with the Institute's clinical modalities.

A special thanks to Doctor Bi Yongsheng, D.M.Q.; Yu Wenping, D.M.Q.; and the Shandong Provincial Qigong Association for their wealth of knowledge and enthusiastic support in sharing their clinical Qigong modalities, and to Dr. He Sihai, D.M.Q., of the Zhe Jiang Qigong Hospital for his openness and kindness in sharing his knowledge.

A special thanks to Qigong Grandmaster Zheng Zhanding, D.M.Q., for being my mentor, taking me under his powerful wing, and teaching me advanced clinical modalities of energetic diagnosis and treatment therapies.

A special thanks to Medical Qigong Master Yu Yan Min for teaching me advanced esoteric sound therapy, and for supporting and encouraging my energetic and healing practice.

A special thanks to Qigong and Taiji Master Shifu Zhang Yufei for teaching, supporting, and encouraging my energetic and healing practice.

I am also indebted to Professor Zang Lu and doctors Xu Hongtao, D.M.Q.; Ren Shuntu, D.M.Q.; Xu Zongwei, D.M.Q.; and the directors, teachers, interpreters and staff at the Xi Yuan Hospital of Traditional Chinese Medicine for their time, effort, knowledge and support.

I am very grateful to Sun Shuchun, D.T.C.M., the assistant professor and dean of the Beijing Academy of Acupuncture, Orthopedics, and Traumatology and the Hu Guo Si Hospital of Traditional Chinese Medicine for their time, effort, knowledge and support.

I would like to thank Professor Meng Xiantong and Tara Peng, D.M.Q., of the Beijing Chengjian Integrated Traditional Chinese Medicine and Western Medical Experts Clinic for sharing their knowledge of advanced clinical modalities, and for opening my eyes to the "ancient" world of esoteric medicine.

I am very grateful to Madame Wang Yan of the Beijing International Acupuncture Training Center, the Acupuncture Institute of China Academy of Traditional Chinese Medicine, and the World Health Organization Collaborating Center for Traditional Medicine for their years of support and for believing in me.

I would also like to thank President Yue Licui, D.T.C.M., of the World Academic Society of Medical Qigong and all my friends and colleagues at the Beijing College of Traditional Chinese Medicine for their years of help and support.

A special thanks to the Five Branches Institute, College and Clinic of Traditional Chinese Medicine in Santa Cruz, California, for having the faith and intuitive foresight in establishing the first 200 hour Medical Qigong Practitioner (M.Q.P.) program and Medical Qigong Clinic in the United States. Also, a special thanks to Five Branches President and CEO Ron Zaidman, M.B.A., M.T.C.M., and the Academic Dean and Clinical Medical Director Dr. Joanna Zhao L.Ac., Dipl. Ac. (NCCA), D.T.C.M. (China) for their never ending support. A special thanks to the Associate Dean of Medical Qigong Science Jean Vlamynck, M.M.Q., M.T.C.M., L.Ac., for her undying help and assistance in maintaining the high standards and clinical integrity of all the Medical Qigong classes.

A special thanks to the Academy For Five Element Acupuncture, College and Clinic of Traditional Chinese Medicine in Hallandale, Florida, for establishing the first 500 hour Medical Qigong Therapist (M.Q.T.) intensive program in the United States. Also, a special thanks to the Academy's president and Clinical Director Dorit Reznek, M.Ac., A.P., M.Q.T. for her never-ending support in establishing the Medical Qigong clinic, and to Lisa Van Ostrand, M.M.Q. for her help and assistance in maintaining the high standards and clinical integrity of all the Medical Qigong classes.

A special thanks to the Medical Qigong college at the He Nan University of Traditional Chinese Medicine in Zheng Zhou China, for establishing the first Chinese-American Overseas Medical Qigong University program in the United States via the International Institute of Medical Qigong. Also, special thanks to Professor Lu Shi Cai for his never-ending support in integrating the I.I.M.Q.'s Medical Qigong programs at the He Nan University, and for his assistance in maintaining the high standards and clinical integrity of all the Medical Qigong classes.

A special thanks to Peter Deadman, Lic. Ac., of the Journal of Chinese Medicine, in England, for writing the Foreward and for supporting and encouraging this work.

A special thanks to Stephanie Taylor, M.D., Ph.D., M.M.Q., whose encouragement and support has enabled Chinese Medical Qigong therapy to expand far into the terrain of conventional Western medicine, bridging the gap between these two schools with complementary modalities of healing.

A special thanks to Jason Gill, L.Ac., for his unselfish heart of giving and his invaluable help and technical input on Traditional Chinese Medicine, and his own personal experiences with Medical Qigong therapy.

A special thanks to Kenneth M. Sancier, Ph.D., and the Qigong Institute of Menlo Park, CA. Dr. Sancier's extensive research in Medical Qigong therapy, and the validity of its effect as a clinical modality is a true gift to future health practitioners. Dr. Sancier is also a council board member of the World Academic Society of Medical Qigong, sanctioned in Beijing, China.

A special thanks to Richard H. Lee. and the China Healthways Institute of San Clemente, CA. Mr. Lee has performed extensive research and scientific investigations into Medical Qigong therapy and infrasonic resonation, as well as the validity of its effect as a clinical modality. Mr. Lee is also a council board member of the World Academic Society of Medical Qigong, sanctioned in Beijing, China.

A special thanks to Dr. Ted J. Cibik, N.D., D.M.Q., and Dr. Suzanne B. Friedman, L.Ac., D.M.Q., for their invaluable contributions to the Nutrition and Diet recommendations mentioned in the Oncology section of this textbook series.

I greatly appreciate the assistance of Robert Collier, Jed Friedland, Stephanie Hensey, Terri Vandercook, and Rose Mary Stewart, M.M.Q., who spent many painstaking hours typing and deciphering my personal notes and course manuals. I would especially like to thank Madeleine H. Howell, M.F.T., M.M.Q., Jampa Mackenzie Stewart, D.O.M., L.Ac., Marlene Merritt L.Ac., Gaeir L. Dietrich, Leela Marcum, M.M.Q., M Ed.,

ACKNOWLEDGEMENTS

and Jean Vlamynck, M.M.Q., M.T.C.M., L.Ac., for their invaluable help and contribution in editing this textbook series.

A special thanks to Dr. Michele A. Katsabekis, D.M.Q., for her constant support and painstaking hours of research. Her quest for the latest medical knowledge and clinical modalities has elevated this textbook series to a higher academic level.

Special thanks to the Mao Shan Monastery of Jiang Su Province, for sharing their wealth of knowledge. I would like to especially thank Abbot Cao Dao Zhang for his assistance in gathering ancient Daoist esoteric knowledge; to Fa Shi He Yu Hong, for sharing privileged information on esoteric Shengong training and exorcism. Special thanks to my teacher, Master Min Xian, a powerful Jing Shi and master of the talisman. Special thanks to Yue Shi Min Guan and Professor Pan Yi De for sharing ancient Mao Shan Daoist history and esoteric Qigong.

Special thanks to the Longhu Shan Monastery of Jiang Xi Province, for sharing their wealth of knowledge. I would like to especially thank senior Abbot Zhang Jing Tao, the 65th Celestial Master, for his assistance in gathering ancient Daoist esoteric knowledge; and to my teacher, Grand Master Qiu Yusong of the Celestial Masters Mansion, for sharing the skills of creating talismans and invocations to bind evil spirits. He is a powerful exorcist and has been a guiding light in my spiritual growth. A special thanks to Master Zeng Guang Liang for sharing with me the most ancient skills of Long Hu Shan Daoism.

A special thanks to my good friend and Daoist brother, Father Michael Saso, for his invaluable contribution, encouragement and support. His years to intense study as a Professor and true scholar of ancient Daoist traditions helped enhance this textbook series.

A special thanks to my Daoist brother, Professor Gerard Edde, Ph.D., for his invaluable contribution, encouragement, and support.

A special thanks to Tomo. Y., Robert Blaisdell, and Jason Morissette for their excellent artwork and graphics.

A special thanks to Y. S. Lim for his many painstaking hours of translating ancient Chinese Medical texts, which enabled me to draw from more comprehensive and clinical resources.

A special thanks to Daniel Burton-Rose for his many painstaking hours of translating ancient Chinese medical and Daoist texts, which enabled me to draw from more comprehensive resources. Also, special thanks to Daoist Master Chang Jiun Li for his assistance in deciphering and expounding on several esoteric Daoist texts.

A special thanks to Dr. Bernard Shannon, D.M.Q. and Professor Ma of the Defense Language Institute, in Monterey California for their many painstaking hours of providing translations and information on specific ancient Chinese medical texts. As a youth, Professor Ma served as a librarian in Beijing, China, and had access to the imperial library which contained several ancient unpublished medical texts. These texts were later destroyed by the Red Guard during the Cultural Revolution. Professor Ma's insight contributed extensive knowledge to the historical understanding of ancient Chinese medicine written in this textbook.

A special thanks to Madhu Nair and Tomoko Koga for their many painstaking hours of translating ancient Japanese Medical texts, which enabled me to draw from additional sources of ancient Chinese clinical records.

A special thanks to Jody Thomas Ho for his many painstaking hours of translating the French versions of ancient Chinese Medical texts, which also enabled me to draw from more comprehensive and clinical resources.

An additional thanks to Wendy Ferrari, B.A., C.N.A for her many hours of French translations.

I am grateful to Willis Campbell and Niki Norrell, L.Ac., Dipl.Ac. (NCCA), M.T.C.M. for taking several of the photos depicted in Volume 1, Chaper 1.

A special thanks to Tony Duarte for his outstanding digital photo-graphics of several of the Medical Qigong exercise prescriptions, as depicted in Volume 2, Chapter 16 and Volume 5, Chapter 63.

A special thanks to Dr. L. Francesca Ferrari, L.Ac., D.T.C.M., D.M.Q., clinical instructor at the Five Branches Institute, College and Clinic of TCM, as the senior editor of this manuscripts for publication, for her invaluable contribution on the indexing and herbal prescriptions written in the oncology section of this textbook series. Her keen eye for detail and constant encouragement to re-write, explain, and expound on the contents within this textbook has resulted in a more comprehensive resource for future Medical Qigong students and Western medical professionals.

A special thanks to assistant editor Dr. Gideon B. Enz, D.M.Q., for his invaluable contributions in the editing of this manuscript for publication. His personal insights in the Qi Deviation, Twelve Chakra Gates, Seven Chakra Systems and Six Transportations of Shen sections of this textbook series greatly enhanced the depth of information. Additionally, his input on Western medicine as well as personal spiritual insights and information on intuitive clinical diagnosis further enriched this textbook series, allowing future generations the gift of privileged "hidden" knowledge.

A special thanks to assistant editor Dr. Suzanne B. Friedman, L.Ac., D.M.Q., Chair of the Medical Qigong Science Department at the Acupuncture and Integrative Medicine College in Berkeley, California, for her invaluable contribution, encouragement and support in preparing the editing of this manuscript for publication.

A special thanks to Irene Morris for her excellent work on designing the front and back cover of these five textbooks, and for encouraging the production of this voluminous work.

Above all, I would like to express my love, gratitude, and respect to my parents Antoinette and Lt. Cdr. (Rt.) Perry E. J. Johnson for their years of love, understanding, and encouragement. They have equally been my support and light in this present journey.

Finally, to my three beautiful daughters: Laura Marie, Leah Ann, and Hannah Daniel, whom I will always love and forever be honored and proud to be called their father.

Introduction

The following research presented in these five Medical Qigong textbooks has taken me a lifetime of study and investigation. This exploration into Chinese energetic medicine includes knowledge gathered from my personal clinical observations here in the United States, as well as from treating patients in several of the People's Republic of China's Medical universities, hospitals, and clinics in Beijing.

In my life I have been fortunate enough to be introduced to several unique teachers, and have been honored to apprentice with several gifted masters of the "hidden" knowledge concealed within the obscure veil of Chinese esoteric medicine (including powerful healers from both Taiwan and the People's Republic of China). After procuring several out-of-print texts written in the 1800's by Jesuit priests on the subject of ancient Chinese metaphysical sorcery and Daoist mysticism, my understanding of Chinese energetic medicine broadened enormously. Initially, all of the missing pieces slowly began to fit together, revealing a multidimensional form of healing based on the microcosm and macrocosm of energetic and spiritual cause and effect.

The primary goal in releasing this esoteric knowledge to the public is twofold: first, to return to the Chinese people the lost riches of their ancient culture; and second, to provide an accurate historical foundation for modern energetic medicine, which has been lost or removed from current T.C.M. colleges and universities.

It has long been said that, "The proper study of Chinese medicine involves the study of its ancient history." The development of Traditional Chinese Medicine originated not only from generations of refined skills and sciences, but also from its ancient culture and beliefs. In their most early stages, the knowledge of science and magic were indistinguishable, and it was difficult to differentiate between them. Chinese medicine, as an applied science, has an ancient history submerged in energetic magic and Daoist shamanism. There is an old expression, "the only difference between "occult magic" and "science" is time." After centuries of extensive energetic study, the founders of ancient Chinese medicine made immense contributions to the scientific fields of clinical medicine, pharmacology, and chemistry.

The ancient Chinese approach in explaining medical concepts is generally expressed through a three dimensional convergence, seeing the physical body as an energetic hologram and observing the physical, mental, emotional, energetic, and spiritual aspects of the tissues. By stimulating any one of these five energetic matrices, a Qigong doctor can affect the other four and influence the body to initiate either health or disease. Diagnosis and treatment is therefore approached in a nonlinear progression, working holographically towards the health and healing of the multidimensional person. Western Medicine, however, is taught to view the physical body on a two dimensional level, as a completed progression of cause and effect, separating the reactions of the tissues from the effects of the mind and emotions, as well as from universal and environmental influences. Though this attitude is gradually changing within the Western scientific and medical community, this change has been slow to reach the population at large.

In order to help the Western mind understand Chinese energetic medicine, this five volume Medical Qigong textbook series was written with the goal of comprehensive instruction combined with practical clinical application of Chinese energetic medicine. It embraces the concepts of both Traditional Chinese Medicine, in particular Chinese Medical Qigong therapy, as well as the study of ancient Chinese medicine as found in energetic Daoist shamanism.

The understanding of Chinese energetic medicine in the West has been hampered by the lack of accessibility to the "ancient" knowledge that has been handed down from master to student through centuries of secrecy. Through gross manipulation of source materials, the history and theory of "modern" Traditional Chinese Medicine was rewritten to reflect the interests of the Communist Party. Therefore, edited versions subjected to the censorship of metaphysical ideas due to political influence, and the "cleaning up" for scientific respectability have been introduced to the public as the acceptable norm. The primary purpose of writing this five volume textbook is to "reinstate" the energetic and spiritual dimensions innate within ancient pre-communist Chinese energetic medicine.

This entire Medical Qigong textbook series provides a basic understanding of the complex energetic structure, theory and practical application of ancient Chinese energetic medicine:

- Volume 1 contains the study of the ancient Chinese approach to Energetic Anatomy and Physiology.
- Volume 2 contains the ancient Chinese system of esoteric Energetic Alchemy and Dao Yin Therapy used to establish a foundation for energetic medicine, as well as an in-depth study of Qi Deviations and ancient Daoist Mysticism.
- Volume 3 contains several different energetic approaches to Medical Qigong Diagnosis and advanced Clinical Treatment Principles and Clinical Protocols.
- Volume 4 introduces the reader to Medical Qigong Prescription Exercises and Meditations, the Treatment of Internal Organ Diseases, Pediatrics, Geriatrics, Gynecology, Neurology and Energetic Psychology.
- In Volume 5 introduces the reader to specific techniques, applications and research collected from various doctors and clinics throughout China which implement Medical Qigong therapy as an effective and complementary clinical modality in the treatment of cancer patients.

Ancient Chinese medical terminology is extremely subjective and metaphoric, and is used to describe the many aspects of the human body through physical, mental, emotional, energetic, and spiritual domains of existence. Many technical terms in Traditional Chinese Medicine have numerous meanings, depending on the context of the subject and from which discipline they stem (Daoist or Buddhist). Much of the obscure terminology existing in Chinese medicine comes directly from ancient shamanistic sources. These terminologies can sometimes be extremely vague in their explanations, yet deeply profound in their true meanings.

Throughout these textbooks, I have chosen to periodically use the term "divine" when expressing the energy of the Dao, or of God. This will help the reader comprehend the original context in which the terminology arose.

Also, for clarity, the Chinese terms in this book are capitalized along with the English words for which ancient Chinese medicine, as well as Traditional Chinese Medicine, assigns a special meaning. Such words include, but are not limited to, the following: Gall Bladder, Small Intestine, Spleen, Pericardium, Bladder, Liver, etc. When you see words such as Blood, Heart, and Marrow capitalized, assume that their meaning differs from that ascribed by Western medicine. In Traditional Chinese Medicine, the word Marrow, for instance, does not refer only to bone marrow as it is traditionally recognized in the West, but rather describes the substance which is the common matrix of bones, bone marrow, the brain, and spinal cord. Non-capitalized terms retain their traditional Western meanings.

Historically, many of the terms used to describe the Daoist natural forces of nature (existing within Heaven, Earth, and Man) were personalized and referred to as "gods" or "spirits" by "Religious Daoism" in order to compete with the colorful deities imported by the Buddhists into China from India. Therefore, when reading this textbook, the reader should not become confused or alarmed by certain terminologies describing "deities" which govern specific energetic principles. For example, when reading the section on the Human Soul, the title "Lords of the Three Dantians" implies the fact that the soul has three primary, separate, yet interconnected energetic properties rooted and sustained within each of the Three Dantians.

In China, many of the Medical Qigong doctors and masters with whom I have trained asked me to keep these advanced energetic and spiritual theories in confidence for fear of governmental reprisal. Currently, due to the Chinese government's response to the Falun Gong association's activities, many of the Medical Qigong colleges and clinics have been closed. Therefore, I have decided to openly share these ancient energetic theories concerning the interactions of the body, mind, spirit, soul, and divine, without revealing my sources.

Finally, within this five Medical Qigong textbook series, I have included years of extensive research from several sources:
- Ancient Daoist energetic medicine and advanced spiritual disciplines of the *Beiji* (Northern Pole Star) Daoist sect, from Wu-Dang Shan Daoist teachings; *Lung Hu* (Dragon-Tiger) Daoist sect, from the Zhengyi Celestial Master Daoism; and Shangqing (Highest Purity) Daoist sect, from the Mao Shan Thunder Magic Daoism (of which I am an 80th generation disciple).
- Ancient Buddhist energetic medicine and advanced spiritual disciplines from Shaolin Monastery teachings, Tantric Buddhism, and Orthodox Buddhism.
- Ancient Tibetan Buddhist energetic medicine and advanced spiritual disciplines from several Tibetan Monastery teachings, including the Tibetan Tantric, and Tibetan Bon shamanic traditions.

To quote one of my teachers, "Sanjiao gui yi - the three teachings make a whole person." Meaning that through exposure to the esoteric knowledge contained within all three energetic and spiritual sources, the individual can become a more complete human being.

In writing and presenting these five Chinese Medical Qigong volumes to the public, I hope to condense the diverse fields of ancient Asian energetic healing into a comprehensive medical compendium for the Western mind. With this goal in mind, I have found it necessary to repeat certain sections in order to emphasize important information for increased comprehension.

Jerry Alan Johnson, Ph.D., D.T.C.M., D.M.Q. (China)
Pacific Grove, California
March, 2005

xxx

Section I
Foundations of Chinese Energetic Medicine

Chapter 1
Introduction to Medical Qigong

More than 5000 years ago, the ancient Chinese masters of esoteric healing came to the understanding that everything is composed of the same energetic substance, which they called Qi (pronounced "chee"). These ancient masters observed that there is a oneness and wholeness in all existence and that everything is energetically interconnected as one body.

Traditional Chinese Medicine is primarily based on the understanding of the transformations of Qi. The ancient Chinese believed that all transformations happened under the influence of Qi. The birth, aging and death of all things within Heaven and Earth, including wind, clouds, thunder, rain, water, mountains, forests, deserts, oceans, humans, animals and insects are caused by and formed out of Qi. Although energy may appear to take on many different forms, all things in nature and, in fact, all things in the universe are intrinsically woven together so that we are, quite literally, all symbiotically one with the universe through the system of Qi.

Qi is vibrating in constant energetic motion within all things. It is the catalyst for everything to relate and interrelate within the universe. The ancient Chinese believed that the Qi of Yin and Yang fulfills the "Great Void" (Wuji), enveloping all things and leaving nothing outside its boundary.

In modern times, the laws of physics have demonstrated that matter and energy are interchangeable and that matter is simply another form of energy. Matter is constantly vibrating in the form of particles or wave forms; it is constantly changing, either affecting or interacting with energy. Energy is inherent in the living human body, and the human body is sustained by energy (Figure 1.1).

The ancient Chinese mastered specific tech-

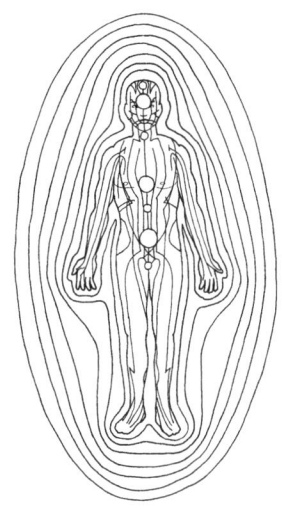

Figure 1.1. The body's Qi rises from the tissues to form the external Wei Qi fields.

niques to balance the body's energy (Qi) in order to live in harmony with the environmental (Earthly) Qi, as well as the universal (Heavenly) Qi. Traditional Chinese Medicine maintains that when living things start to lose their Qi, they lose their vitality. An ancient Chinese saying states, "Life comes into beginning because Qi is amassed; when Qi is scattered, the person dies."

Qi is stored within the body in the form of energetic pools, creating the energetic matrix of the internal organs. From these internal pools, the body's life-force energy flows in the form of rivers and streams. These energetic rivers and streams form the body's vessels, channels, and collateral systems.

The most ancient character for Qi appeared on the Shang Dynasty (1600-1028 B.C.) oracle bones, and on the Zhou Dynasty (1028-221 B.C.) bronze inscriptions as three horizontal lines (similar to the modern Chinese character used for the num-

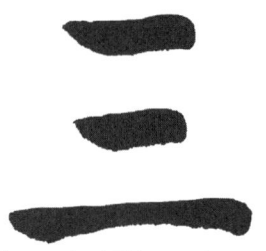

Figure 1.2. The ancient Chinese character for "Qi," depicting mist that rises from the earth to form clouds

ber three). According to Chinese medical researchers Zhang Yu Huan and Ken Rose, in their book, *A Brief History of Qi*, the most ancient Chinese character for Qi originally depicted "mist that rises from the earth to form the clouds." This ideographic form of Qi was retained until the early Western Zhou Dynasty (1066-770 B.C.) (Figure 1.2). The character was also used to indicate heat waves that rise from the heated surface of the earth and later used to describe exhaled breath that can be seen on a cold day.

Understanding the Concept of Qi

While the concept of Qi may seem complicated, it is actually quite simple. Matter progresses to energy and energy to spirit, and vice-versa. Qi is considered the medium, or bridge, between matter and spirit. Qi has mass, the same way that smoke or vapor has mass. Qi as energy can manifest within the body through three primary levels:

- **Physically as Matter:** Energetically manifesting through the body's cells and tissues in the form of Jing, Marrow, Blood, and Body Fluid.
- **Energetically as Resonant Vibrations:** Energetically manifesting through heat, sound, light, and electromagnetic fields.
- **Spiritually as Divine Light:** Energetically manifesting through subtle vibrations which extend through infinite space (Wuji) to the Dao (Figure 1.3).

Through observation and study, Chinese Qigong (pronounced "chee-gung") masters discovered that each internal organ within the human body has a different function and a different speed of energetic vibration. By tracing the energetic pathways of Qi through each internal organ, and observing its affects on bodily functions, the Chinese developed the basic theories upon which Traditional Chinese medical practice was founded. For thousands of years, Chinese medicine has successfully cured serious illnesses by stimulating the body's Qi in very specific ways.

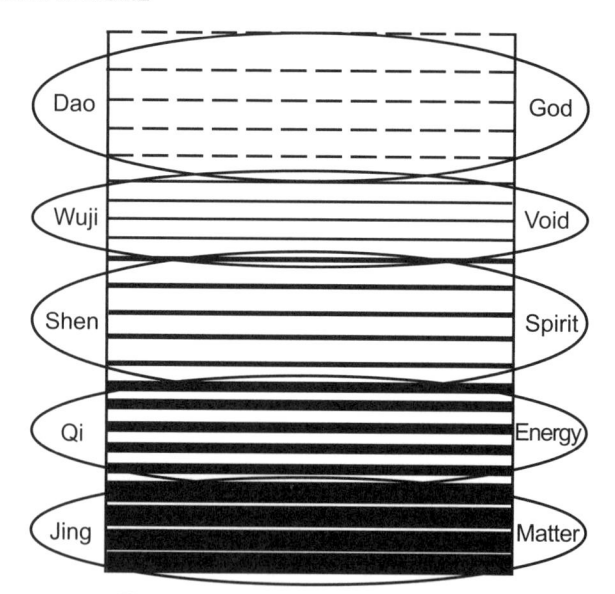

Figure 1.3. The Five Energetic Fields

Through the study and practice of Qigong, one can cultivate an awareness of Qi and its individual pathways, and can learn to influence and even control its energetic power. Medical Qigong practitioners use these skills to heal and strengthen the immune system and to improve the function of various organ systems within the body. In the year 2000, China Healthways International estimated that in Beijing alone more than 1.3 million people practiced some form of Qigong every day; and in China as a whole, around 80 million people practiced the art of Qigong.

The Five Realms of Energy

The nature of energetic fields is still considered mysterious by most modern scientists. According to modern physics, energetic fields are more fundamental than matter. Energetic fields cannot be explained in terms of matter; rather, matter is explained in terms of the energy within the fields.

The ancient Chinese masters observed that Qi can be divided into five separate realms, manifesting in various forms of matter and energy: mineral, plant, animal, human, and divine. Each energetic "form" draws from the energetic realm of the next, resonating and interacting with the divine through the form's relationship within the Wuji (infinite space). With each increase in vibrational frequency, there is a corresponding increase in consciousness and level of awareness. The five realms or manifestations of matter and energy are described as follows (Figure 1.4):

1. **The Realm of Minerals** is considered the lowest (densest and slowest) form of energetic vibration. The disintegration or division of the mineral's particles combine with the elements of air and water to form the Earth's soil. Every particle in the soil still retains the original primordial energy force of the mineral, which interacts with the energy of the divine.

2. **The Realm of Plants** is considered the next higher form of energetic vibration. All of the Earth's vegetation (trees, bushes, flowers, herbs, plants) absorb a part of its life-energy from the minerals' energetic field, increasing and multiplying its energetic potential. The plant's energetic field is considered the next ascension in energetic evolution towards the divine energetic field.

3. **The Realm of Animals** is considered the next higher form of energetic vibration. The animal consumes and absorbs energy from the plant's energetic field, further increasing and multiplying its own energetic potential, thus bringing it one step closer towards the divine energetic field.

4. **The Realm of Humanity** is considered the second highest form of energetic vibration. Humanity stands between Heaven and Earth, partaking in all of the energetic fields (from Earth: the mineral, plant, animal and human; from Heavens: the divine). Through diet, Qigong practice, prayer, and meditation, humans can further refine and enhance their energetic potential.

5. **The Realm of the Divine** is the highest vibrational expression of energy known. As it envelops and becomes active within the human body, it further increases and multiplies the body's energetic potential, allowing humanity to attain divine consciousness.

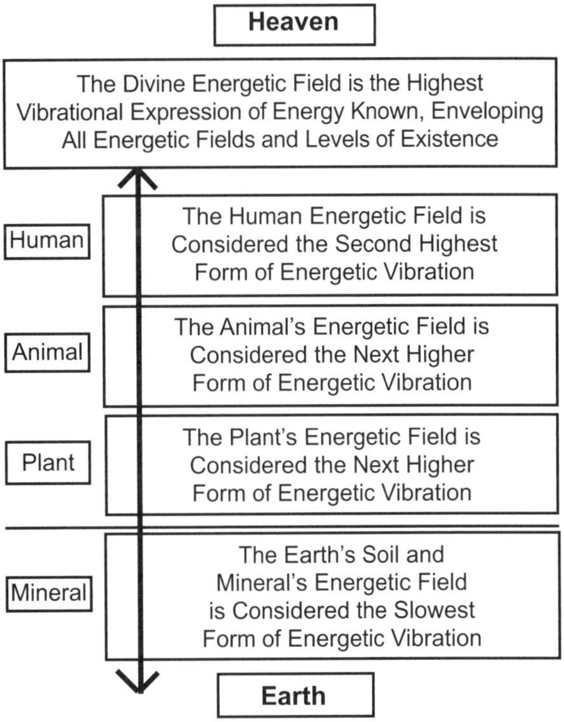

Figure 1.4. The Five Dominions of Qi

All of these energetic fields originate from one source, and thus contain the vibrational resonance of the one divine life-force. Knowing this, it is possible to enhance the nutritional value of what we eat with an attitude of deep respect for the plants and animals that give their life-force energy for our consumption. The blessing of food, and preparing food with a loving attitude, allows for the absorption of not only the vitamins and minerals contained therein, but also the absorption of the higher vibrations of the one divine energy inherent in all things. This is why many ancient cultures, often referred to as "primitive," prayed before hunting so that the animal spirit would willingly give its body and life-force energy for sacrifice. Prayers were also given after the kill to free the animal's spirit so that it could return to the divine.

Once individuals become aware of the divine energetic field, they begin to experience the refined vibrational energy fields of minerals, plants, animals, and human beings. This increased awareness of the divine life-force energy strengthens the awareness of one's own energetic fields and that

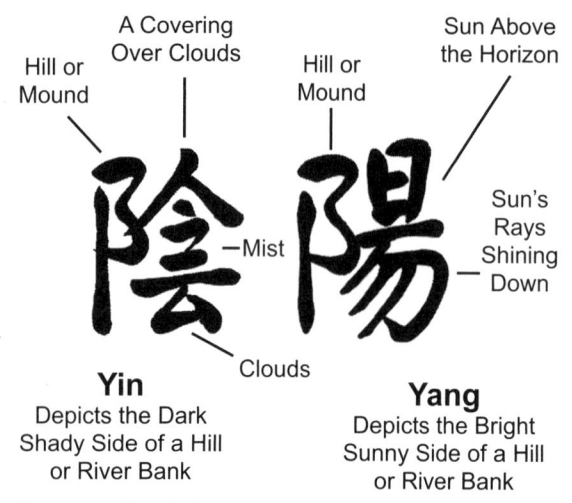

Figure 1.5. The Chinese characters for "Yin" and "Yang"

of others. This in turn can deepen the conscious and unconscious energetic connections between ourselves and minerals, plants, animals, other humans, or the divine. There is an old Buddhist saying that states, "Consciousness sleeps in minerals, dreams in plants, begins to stir in animals, and has the potential to be fully awaken in humanity."

DEFINING THE ENERGY OF YIN AND YANG

Each of the five energetic fields can be further divided into aspects of Yin and Yang. In Traditional Chinese Medicine, the theory of Yin and Yang energy represents the duality of balance and harmony within the body, as well as within the universe. Earth energy is Yin, while Heaven energy is Yang.

The Chinese ideogram of Yin depicts the dark, shady side of a hill or river bank; Yang depicts the bright, sunny side of a hill or river bank (Figure 1.5). Yin exists within Yang, and Yang exists within Yin. Yang manifests as active, creative, masculine, hot, hard, light, Heaven, white and bright. Yin manifests as passive, receptive, feminine, cold, soft, dark, Earth, black and shadow.

Yin is dependent on Yang, and Yang is dependent on Yin. Thus, all things have a Yin and Yang aspect, which can be further subdivided into Yin and Yang. Yin and Yang mutually create each other, control each other, consume each other and

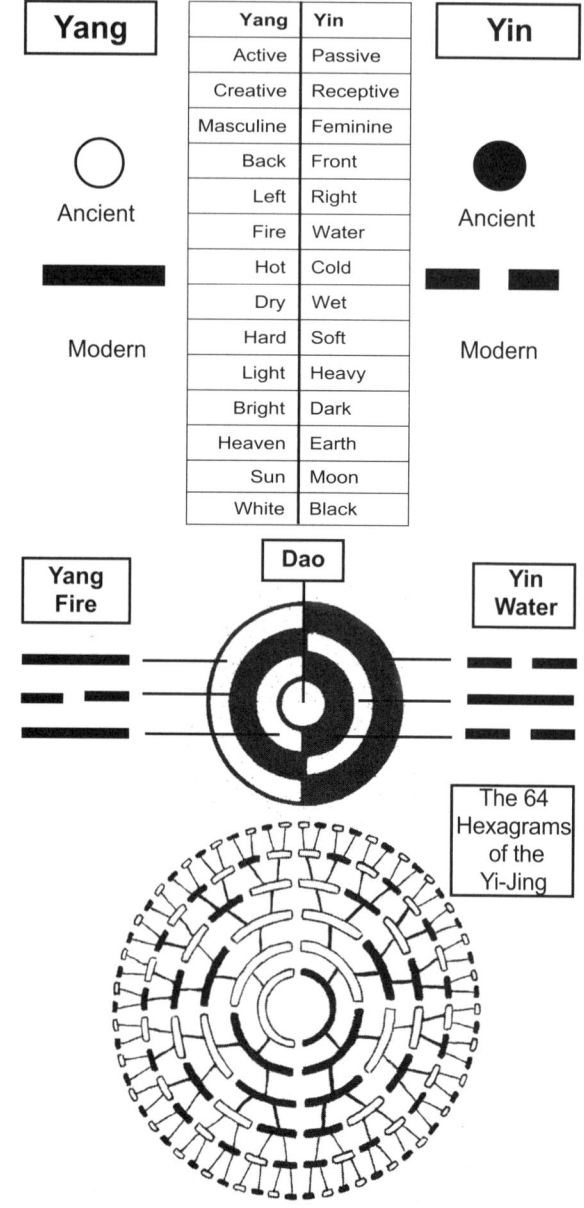

Yang	Yin
Active	Passive
Creative	Receptive
Masculine	Feminine
Back	Front
Left	Right
Fire	Water
Hot	Cold
Dry	Wet
Hard	Soft
Light	Heavy
Bright	Dark
Heaven	Earth
Sun	Moon
White	Black

Figure 1.6. The table above shows the ancient Chinese Yang (Heaven) and Yin (Earth) symbols: Yang is represented by white, and Yin is represented by black. The center of the circle represents the Eternal Dao within the Wuji.

Yin and Yang give birth to the Elements of Fire and Water, which give birth to four phases of universal energy (Great Yang, Lesser Yang, Great Yin and Lesser Yin). The four phases the energy create the Bagua (Eight Trigrams) which transform into the 64 Hexagrams of the Yi-Jing.

transform each other. This dynamic balance of Yin and Yang constantly changes and transforms the body's life-force energy.

In ancient Daoism, the Dao creates Yin and Yang, which in turn give birth to further subdivisions of Yin and Yang, manifesting as four phases of universal energy (Great Yang, Lesser Yang, Great Yin and Lesser Yin). These four phases of universal energy form the energetic bases of the Prenatal and Postnatal transformations, manifested in the form of eight energetic actions. The eight energetic actions (also known as the Bagua Trigrams) act as a template for all creation and can further be manifested through the ever-changing energetic form of the 64 Hexagrams of the Yi-Jing (I-Ching) (Figure 1.6).

The later symbol for Yin and Yang (which became popular in the Song Dynasty) still expresses the energetic concept of the Dao transforming into Yin and Yang. However, unless an individual has received competent instruction, the subtleties are easy to overlook (Figure 1.7).

Successful practitioners who train and master the art of balancing the body's Yin-Yang energies were considered "Tian Shen" or "Xian," meaning "immortals." They were able to harmonize the body with the mind, the mind with the will, the will with the breath, the breath with the spirit, the spirit with motion, and finally, motion with the surrounding environment (Earth), the universe (Heaven), and the divine (Dao).

THE HISTORY OF QIGONG AND CHINESE MEDICINE

Energetic medicine developed in China over a span of thousands of years. Although the art and clinical skill of Chinese Medical Qigong is considered an integral and critical component of modern Traditional Chinese Medicine, its historical origin can be traced back further than the invention of written language.

In ancient China, energetic medicine and all forms of healing were the exclusive domain of the tribal shamans. Qigong was then known by other names, for example *Xingqi* (aiding the flow of Qi),

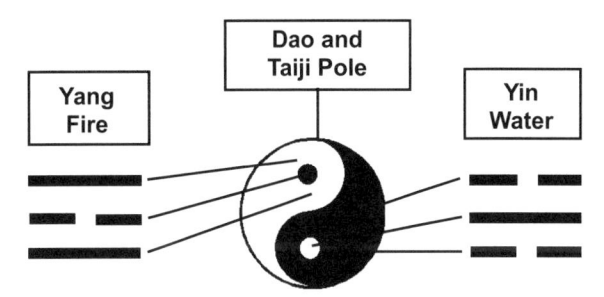

Figure 1.7. The table above shows the Song Dynasty's Yin and Yang symbol (960-1279 A.D.): the Yang is represented by white and the Yin is represented by black. Here, the concept of the Dao and the Eternal Soul which reside within Taiji Pole has been transformed to the image of the inverted "S," melding both the Yang and the Yin energies.

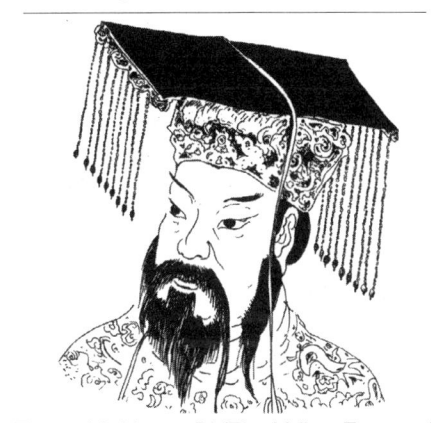

Figure 1.8. Huang Di (The Yellow Emperor)

Tuna (exhalation and inhalation), and *Daoyin* (harmonizing the body, breath and mind through moving the limbs and torso).

According to tradition, the origination of Daoist Magic, esoteric Qigong practices, and acupuncture has always been linked to Huang Di (the Yellow Emperor), whose surname was Gongsun (also called Xuanyuanshi after Xuanyuan Hill, the place of his birth). The Yellow Emperor ruled over a confederation of tribal clans in northern China from approximately 2696-2598 B.C. (Figure 1.8). The Yellow Emperor is said to have practiced Qigong breathing exercises and meditations, internal alchemy, herbology, and sexual alchemy, and lived to the age of 111 years old. Huang Di's discourses on health and longevity with his chief medical advisors Qi Bo and Lei Gong were eventually compiled and recorded in twelve scrolls during the Warring States period. This work is known as the *Huangdi Neijing* (Yellow Emperor's Cannon of Internal Medicine). According to the *Biographies of the Immortals*, written in the Han Dynasty, the Yellow Emperor had magical powers to control and order about various deities and spirit entities.

THE ZHOU DYNASTY (1028-221 B.C.)

During the Zhou Dynasty (1028-221 B.C.), the ancient book of divination known as the Yi-Jing (I-Ching), or Book of Changes arrived publicly, became the theoretical basis for Qigong training. In ancient China, there was no clear separation between the study of medicine and the study of divination. Heaven's Qi related to the study of Chinese Astrology, Earth's Qi related to the study of Feng Shui, and Man's Qi related to the study of the Yi-Jing. The Yi-Jing was originally titled Zhouyi (the Zhou Changes) and represents the foundation of Chinese culture, influencing the basic concepts of Traditional Chinese Medicine. It is rooted in the interaction of the Prenatal Bagua and Postnatal Bagua (see Chapter 2).

The ancient Chinese believed that there was a unique energetic and spiritual connection between an individual's birth and the eight energetic fields manifesting within the eight directions of the Bagua (Figure 1.9). So important was this energetic relationship that the famous Han physician Sun Simao once said, "You cannot master medicine until you have studied the Yi-Jing." In fact, according to medical historian Yang Li, no doctor in Chinese medical history has ever studied the *Huangdi Neijing* (Yellow Emperor's Cannon of Internal Medicine) without consulting the *Yi-Jing* (Book of Changes).

During the Spring and Autumn (770-476 B.C.) and Warring States (475-221 B.C.) Periods, ancient China experienced an unprecedented academic and literary phenomenon known as the "contention of 100 schools of thought." This movement helped to further spread the development and refinement of Qigong. At this point in time, Qigong had already developed through its embryonic stage of being utilized for ancient rituals of worship, the development of hunting skills, and ceremonial dance.

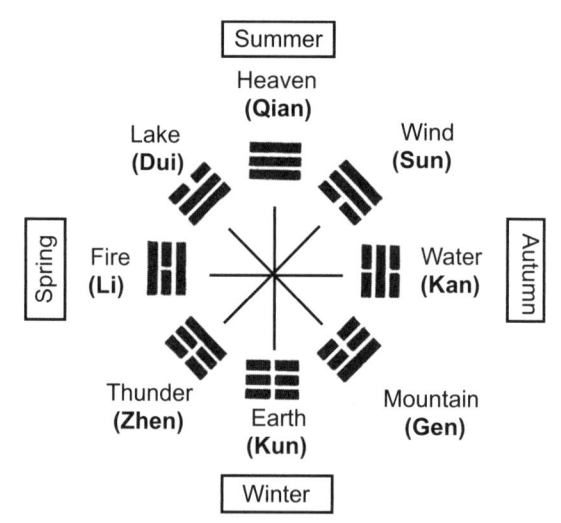

Figure 1.9. The Eight Energetic Fields Manifesting Within the Eight Directions of the Prenatal Bagua

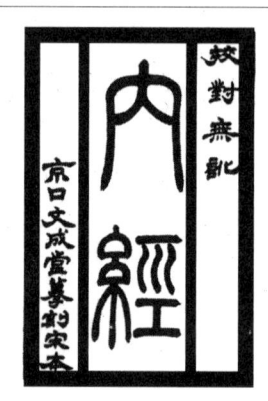

Figure 1.10. The Title Page of the *Huangdi Neijing* (Yellow Emperor's Canon of Internal Medicine)

The ancient Chinese began to extensively apply Qigong in the practice of medicine, and the first monograph combining both Qigong and medicine was written during the Warring States period in the *Huangdi Neijing* (Yellow Emperor's Cannon of Internal Medicine). In the twelve scrolls were listed five therapeutic methods, the nine needles application, herbal decoctions, moxibustion, stone needling, massage and Dao Yin training (in which Qigong is included). Also included within the twelve scrolls are basic theories and methods for applying Qigong training for health care (Figure 1.10).

CHAPTER 1: INTRODUCTION TO MEDICAL QIGONG

The *Huangdi Neijing* represents the first time in China's history that Qigong is introduced in a systematic and theoretical format. During this time period, many famous philosophers such as Laozi and Zhuangzi (the forefathers of Daoism), as well as Confucius, were all publicly recognized as great Qigong masters. According to the *Shi Ji* (Records of the Historian), the great physician Bian Que used Dao Yin and massage in treating diseases.

During the Warring States period, Laozi (Old Sage), to whom the *Daodejing* (The Way and Its Power) is attributed, was regarded as the preeminent Daoist philosopher. Therefore, the Daoists during this time period were known as Huang Lao Dao (The Way of the Yellow Emperor and the Old Sage).

Additionally, during the early years of the Warring States period, records of Qigong training methods and theory were compiled in the *Xing Qi Yu Pei Ming* (Jade Pendant Inscriptions of Qigong), and the *Zhou Yi Can Tong Qi* (Analogs of Principles of Changes Formulated in the Zhou Dynasty).

THE QIN DYNASTY (221-206 B.C.)

During this time period, the Qin Prime Minister Lu Buwei, compiled a text entitled *Spring and Autumn Book of Lu*. In this text, Lu Buwei compiled many of the ancient Daoist practices of "The Harmony of Heaven and Man," discoursing the effects of seasonal changes and other natural forces on the human body. The ancient Daoist book, *The Way of Cultivating Life*, which contains Dao Yin training, diet regulation, and sexual practices, became codified during this time.

THE WESTERN HAN DYNASTY AND EASTERN HAN DYNASTIES (206 B.C.-220 A.D.)

Many of the earliest known Medical Qigong prescription exercises were derived from martial applications and the movements of animals. In 1972, archaeologists began excavating the Mawangdui Han Dynasty tombs (206 B.C.-220 A.D.) in Hunan Province, and in one of the coffins uncovered a silk relic that portrayed drawings of Dao Yin postures (also known as the *Dao Yin Tu*) dating prior to the third century B.C.

This silk scroll is considered the first complete

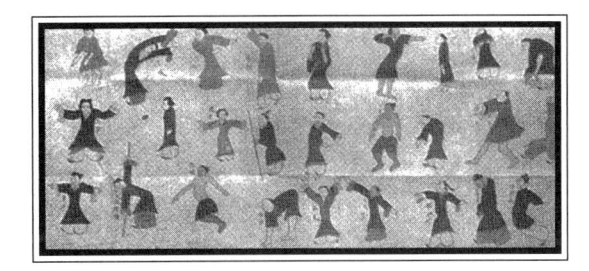

Figure 1.11. The *Dao Yin Tu* postures from the King Ma Tomb

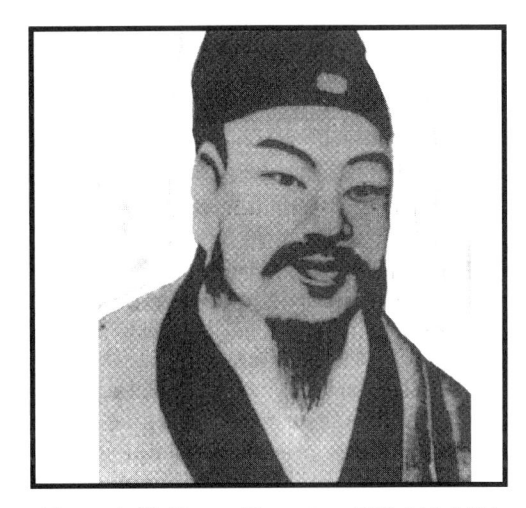

Figure 1.12. Zhang Zhongjing (150-210 A.D.)

set of Qigong movements, and is commonly known as the "Dao Yin Breathing Drawings of the Han Dynasty." Contained in these forty-four ancient Qigong Classic illustrations are descriptions of postural movements and the names of the diseases that they treat. Over half of these illustrated postures are of animal movements (Figure 1.11).

During the Han Dynasty, one famous physician named Zhang Zhongjing mentioned in his book *Jin Kui Yao Lue* (Synopsis of Prescriptions of the Golden Chamber), that Dao Yin, Tuna (exhalation and inhalation), massage, acupuncture and moxibustion should be used to purge the body's channels, regulate the Yin and Yang, and treat illnesses (Figure 1.12).

Also during the Han Dynasty, the great physician and Daoist alchemist Hua Tuo (Figure 1.13) created a set of systematic Dao Yin physical training known as the *Wuqinxi* (Five Animal Play). These five exercises mimic the various movements and gestures of the Deer, Bird, Ape, Tiger, and Bear (Figure 1.14). The initial goal of these five exercises is to help the practitioner improve his or her health and counteract disease by opening the channels in order to cultivate Essence (Jing), Energy (Qi) and Spirit (Shen). Each of the Five Animals relate to a specific internal organ, for example:

- **The Deer Form:** stimulates and strengthens the function of the Liver and Gall Bladder, stretches and strengthens the legs, spine and waist, and helps improve flexibility
- **The Bird Form:** stimulates and strengthens the function of the Heart and Small Intestine, improves balance, opens the joints, relieves congestion and helps cool the body
- **The Ape Form:** stimulates and strengthens the function of the Spleen and Stomach
- **The Tiger Form:** stimulates and strengthens the function of the Lungs and Large Intestine
- **The Bear Form:** stimulates and strengthens the function of the Kidneys and Urinary Bladder, develops rooted power, strengthens the Bones, and helps warm the body

During the end of the Han Dynasty, the Daoist adept Wei Boyang wrote the classic *Zan Dong Ji* (The Union of Three Equations), in which he discusses the inner alchemy of Qigong Breathing, Qi

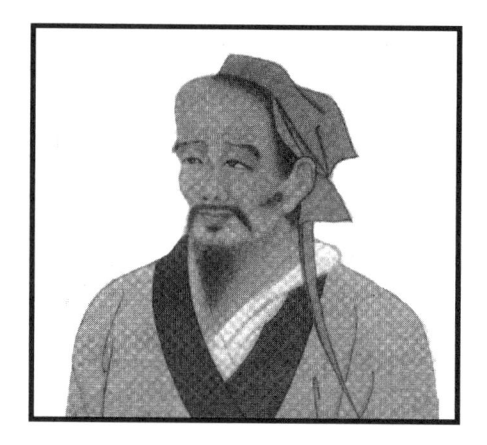

Figure 1.13. Hua Tuo (110-207 A.D.)

Transformation, and the Dual Cultivation of Sexual Practices. The *Tai Ping Jing* (Classic of Great Peace), also during this period, summarized many of the traditional Daoist teachings from the Huang Lao lineage.

THE THREE KINGDOMS PERIOD (220-280 A.D.)

During the Three Kingdoms period, many people practiced Qigong, including several famous scholars, physicians and alchemists. Ji Kang (224-263 A.D.), both a famous scholar and musician during the Wei Dynasty (220-265 A.D.), wrote the *Yang Sheng Lun* (On Health Preservation) and *Da Nan Yang Sheng Lun* (On Difficulties of Health Preservation) which described various Qigong exercises used for healing.

Deer   Bird   Ape   Tiger   Bear

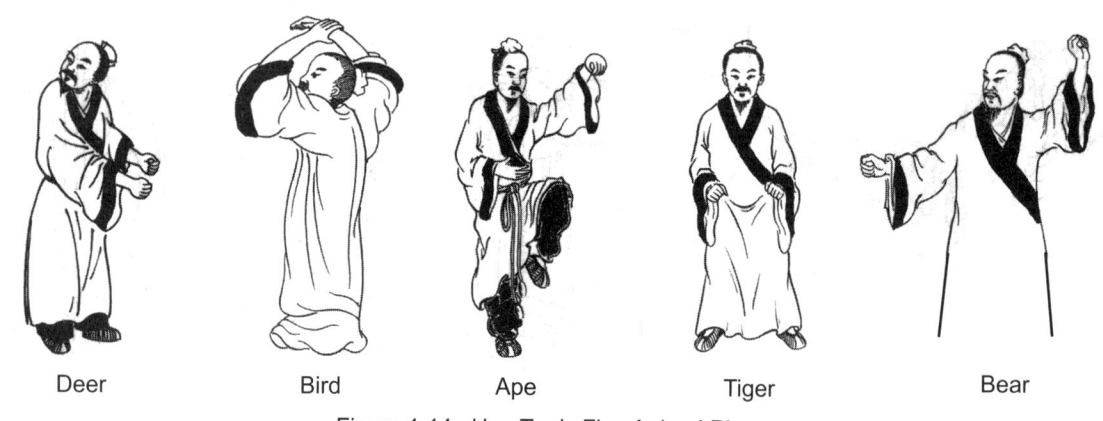

Figure 1.14. Hua Tuo's Five Animal Play

During the Jin Dynasty (265-420 A.D.)

The important Daoist text, *Huang Ting Jing* (Yellow Court Classics) was published during the Jin Dynasty, and caused the Nei Dan (Internal Elixir) School of thought to become the prevalent basis for all Qigong training. This text thoroughly explained the key components of Daoist practice, including the skill of gathering Internal Energy, as well as the regulation of the Three Dantians.

Ge Hong (284-364 A.D.), another noted Daoist scholar, physician, and alchemist from the Eastern Jin Dynasty, wrote a milestone compendium of Daoist theory and practice. In his book *Bao Pu Zi* (He Who Embraces the Uncarved Block), Ge Hong detailed techniques for developing physical longevity (using static Qigong exercises to cultivate Jing and Qi), and spiritual immortality. This text is still regarded today as one of the most influential texts used in the development of Qigong practice (Figure 1.15).

The Northern and Southern Dynasty Period (386-588 A.D.)

Tao Hongjing (456-536 A.D.), a noted Daoist scholar and physician in the Southern Dynasty, compiled the ancient Daoist Qigong book, *Yang Xing Yan Ming Lu* (The Record of Cultivating One's Nature and Longevity). It was during this period that the famous Daoist Qigong monograph *Huang Ting Nei Jing* (Classic on Cultivation of the Internal Essence) and an important Daoist Qigong reference book, *Huang Hai Jing* (Cultivation of the Sea of Essence) were compiled.

During the Southern Liang Dynasty (520-556 A.D.), the Indian Buddhist monk Da Mo (Bodhidharma) came to China teaching an unorthodox style of Tantric Buddhism. In 527 A.D., Da Mo traveled to the Shaolin temple of the Song Mountain, in Henan province. It was at the Shaolin monastery that the famous Muscle/Tendon Changing and Marrow/Brain Washing Qigong Exercises were created.

The Sui Dynasty and Tang Dynasties (581-907 A.D.)

By the time of the Sui and Tang Dynasties, Qigong was extensively utilized in clinical application, including Laozi Qi Massage and various

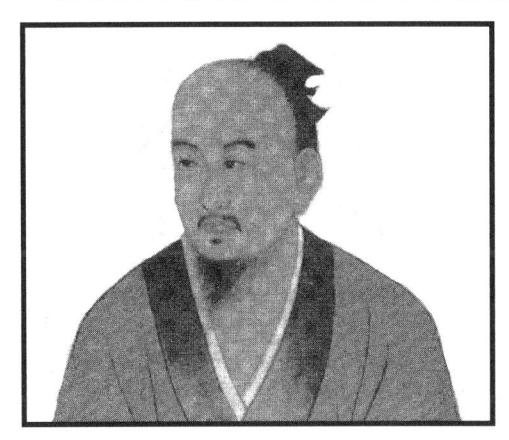

Figure 1.15. Ge Hong (281-341 A.D.)

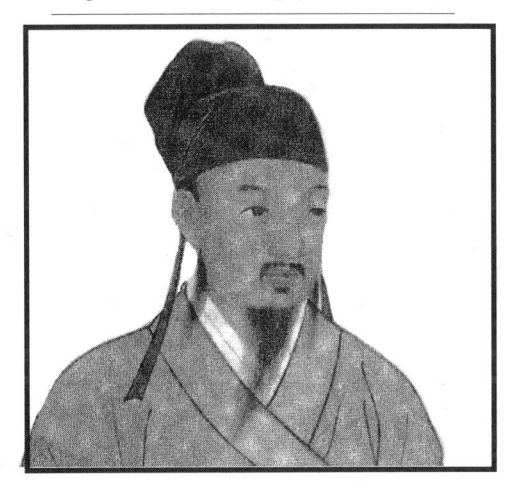

Figure 1.16. Sun Si Miao (590-682 A.D.)

Qigong prescription exercises. Because of their effectiveness as powerful healing modalities, three medical classics were written recording these ancient Qigong protocols. The three books that included detailed Qigong training methods were: *Zhu Bing Yuan Hou Lun* (General Treatise on the Causes and Symptoms of Disease), *Bei Ji Qian Jin Yao Fang* (One Thousand Prescriptions for Emergency Cases), and *Wai Tai Mi Yao* (The Medical Secrets of an Official).

The most famous physician and Daoist alchemist during the Tang Dynasty (618-907 A.D.), was Sun Simiao (Figure 1.16). A prolific author, clinician, and Daoist alchemist, he contributed much to the promotion of Chinese medicine and Qigong training. Although the first acupuncture charts were believed to be produced during the Han Dynasty (206 B.C.-220 A.D.), Sun Simiao is credited with drawing the first charts of the anterior, posterior, and lateral views of the body. These charts showed the Twelve Primary Channels in Five Element colors, with the Extraordinary Vessels drawn in a sixth color. This anatomical format is still being used today in all T.C.M. universities, colleges and clinics around the world. Sun Simiao is also credited with the introduction of the system of proportional measurement (called "cun"), which allows for accurate location of the channel points.

During this time period, another physician named Chao Yuan Fang (Figure 1.17), included in his book, *Zhu Bing Yuan Hou Lum* (A General Treatise on the Causes and Symptoms of Diseases), 250 ways of enhancing the body's internal and external flow of energy with various forms of Qigong.

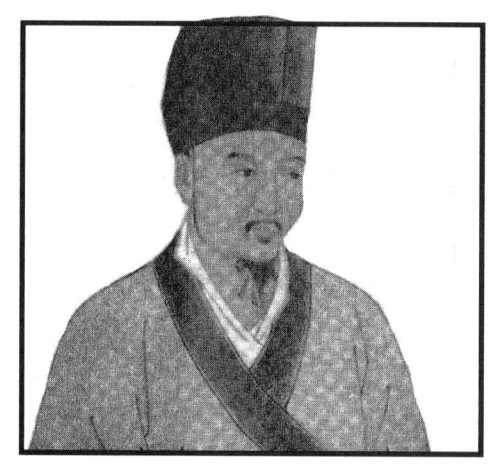

Figure 1.17. Chao Yuan Fang (550-630 A.D.)

THE SONG, JIN, AND YUAN DYNASTIES (960-1368 A.D.)

During the Song, Jin, and Yuan Dynasties, there was an upsurge of interest in Daoist *Nei Dan* (Internal Alchemy), which is used as an integral part of Qigong exercises. Greater developments of fitness-oriented Qigong emerged as people began to pay special attention the health and healing benefits of Qigong exercises and meditations. Su Shi (1037-1101 A.D.), a famous writer of the Northern Song Dynasty (960-1127 A.D.), enthusiastically promoted the health healing effects of Qigong. Even today his ideas continue to influence the practice of Medical Qigong.

Also during this time period, a philosopher of the Northern Song Dynasty named Zhou Dunyi (1017-1073 A.D.), and a philosopher of the Southern Song Dynasty named Zhu Xi (1130-1200 A.D.), developed Neo-Confucian-based Qigong. This Qigong system advocated the "Quiescence" theory of meditation and the study of the *Tai Ji Tu Shuo* (The Teaching of the Taiji Symbol).

Among the many Daoist masters whose works served to promote Qigong during this time period, was Zhang Boduan. His writings incorporated lucid explanations of advanced Daoist principles from the *Quan Zhen* (Complete Reality) School of Daoism. Among his writings, the most famous of his works are, *The Secret of the Opening the Passes, The Four-Hundred Character Treatise on the Golden Elixir,* and *Understanding Reality.*

THE MING DYNASTY AND QING (MANCHU) DYNASTIES (1368-1911)

During the Ming and Qing Dynasties, Qigong was extensively adopted by all physicians for the treatment of disease and health maintenance. In the early Ming Dynasty (1368-1644 A.D.), discussions on the effects and proper applications of Qigong were found in two medical textbooks. One textbook was written by Wang Lu entitled *Yi Jing Su Hui Ji* (Recall of Medical Classic), the other was written by Wan Jin entitled *Wan Mi Zhai Yi Shu Shi Zhong* (Ten Medical Books of Wan Mi Zhai).

During the Ming Dynasty, the great physician and Qigong master Li Shizhen (1518-1593 A.D.) extensively combined the use of Qigong with his clinical treatments.

In the Qing Dynasty (1644-1911 A.D.), Dao Yin techniques were extensively mentioned in the famous medical opus known as *Gu Jin Shu Ji Cheng* (Collected Ancient and Modern Books), written by Chen Menglei. Also during the Qing Dynasty, in *Zhang Shi Yi Tong* (Zhang's Medical Experience) compiled by the famous physician Zhang Lu, discussed Qi Deviations for the first time in Chinese history.

THE REPUBLIC OF CHINA (1912-1949 A.D.)

During the Republic of China, China suffered from the effects of foreign invasion, as well as from corrupt imperialistic powers. The confusion and infighting between warlords wreaked havoc throughout the country, causing a halt in the development of both Qigong and Chinese Medicine.

THE PEOPLE'S REPUBLIC OF CHINA (1949 A.D.-PRESENT)

In 1953, Liu Guizhen compiled the *Qigong Liao Fa Shi Jian* (Application of Qigong to Medical Practice), and the term "Qigong for Health" became popular among the Chinese people. In 1955, the first Qigong sanitarium was created in the city of Tangshan, introducing Qigong Therapy to the public. By 1956, Qigong workshops were established in Tangshan and Beidaihe in order to foster a select group of Qigong professionals. As a result, several institutes and clinics sprang up throughout the country. Qigong Therapy won the support of the government, and in October of 1959, the First National Qigong Experience Exchange Conference sponsored by the Ministry of Public Health for the People's Republic of China was held in Beidaihe. Participants came from 64 Medical colleges and institutes, and 17 different provinces.

From 1966-1976, during the Great Proletarian Cultural Revolution, Chairman Mao Zedong dispersed the Red Guard to enforce the "Out with the Old in with the New" policy. During that time period, Chinese martial arts and Qigong training were strictly forbidden. Most practitioners either fled to Taiwan, went "underground" (denying any specific training or skill), or were sent to "reeducation" camps. Chairman Mao also issued a decree that all doctors of Chinese medicine should now study Western Medicine, and the practice of Chinese medicine was forbidden.

With fewer than 30,000 trained Western physicians in all of China, however, the Chinese were suddenly faced with a new problem. Lines of patients waiting for treatment at the various hospitals literally extended for miles. Doctors, constantly working seven days a week, were utterly exhausted. The state of medical care in China had now evolved into a serious health crisis.

During that time, one of Chairman Mao's cabinet members became sick with cancer (leukemia) and could not be healed by the Western medical protocols. He learned of a Qigong master hiding out in Beijing, and there he sought help and treatment. Within three months the cabinet member was completely healed. He reluctantly reported what had transpired to Chairman Mao, and that the healing had occurred not through Western Medicine, but through Qigong therapy and herbs. Noting the current health crisis, Chairman Mao reevaluated his policy and restriction of Chinese medicine, and initiated the widespread training of "barefoot doctors" of Traditional Chinese Medicine.

Immediately thereafter, the Chinese government began to focus attention on resurrecting the ancient treasure of Chinese medicine. Hospitals and clinics of Traditional Chinese Medicine once again began to flourish throughout China. In order to combat the current health crisis, the new government policy required every patient with a chronic health condition to be given a hospital pass. Each hospital pass consisted of a sheet of paper with 30 squares, each square represented a space for 30 wood-block chopped signatures.

Taiji and Qigong instructors were positioned in each park, and offered free instruction to the public. After each lesson, the master would chop the participant's hospital pass. In order to return to the hospital, the patient was required to have his or her sheet of paper completed with 30 individual chops from either the Qigong or Taiji master. Within a very short time, the health crisis was solved. This is why by the 1970's there were millions of people practicing Taijiquan and Qigong in parks throughout China.

In 1978, extensive research on Qigong was conducted using modern scientific techniques and equipment in Beijing and Shanghai. By 1998, there were several experimental bases established in Beijing, Nanjing, and Guangzhou for specific research into the energetic potential of Qigong training. At that time, Qigong was applied and studied in medicine, nuclear physics, industry, agriculture, engineering, and sports. Encouraging results were achieved in each of these fields. The Chinese government became extremely concerned about the future development of Medical Qigong and sought to promote it as a viable clinical modality.

In 1999, the study of Qigong took a sudden change in formal development. Due to the political antics of the fanatical Falun Gong "Qigong" organization, the Chinese government put a sudden halt to any and all Qigong practices. In the middle of the night, armed guards entered the various Medical Qigong colleges, laboratories, and clinics, removed all of the scientific equipment, and chained and padlocked the doors. Some Qigong doctors and instructors were held and interrogated, and several Medical Qigong hospitals and clinics throughout China were closed. All of Qigong practice groups were dispersed. Even individuals practicing in the various parks were ordered to disband and the leaders were taken in for questioning.

As of 2004, only two Medical Qigong organizations are recognized by the People's Republic of China, and are allowed to work in the government-sponsored hospitals and clinics. These two organizations are the China Medical Qigong Association and the World Association of Medical Qigong. Additionally, most of the doctors from both organizations are formal members of the World Academic Society of Medical Qigong.

To date, many of the Medical Qigong application and prescription exercises that were taught to the author and were normally implemented in the Medical Qigong hospitals are no longer being taught to the public, or utilized in the various clinics.

HISTORY OF ANCIENT CHINESE SHAMAN DOCTORS: WU YI

It is important for the reader to understand that the ancient roots of Chinese energetic medicine originated within the mystical realm of ancient Chinese shamanism. These shamans were known as Wu Yi, and were highly respected in the community. The Wu Yi were consulted regarding medical ailments, problems in relationships, spiritual disharmonies, and various occult practices.

The Wu Yi understood that the birth, existence, transformation, and death of everything in the universe happened under the influence of the energetic transformations of Qi. The major philosophical and spiritual basis for all Traditional Chinese Medicine owes its existence to shamanistic Daoism.

According to ancient Chinese belief, the founder of esoteric shamanistic Daoism (or Magical Daoism) was not Laozi (whose original name was Li Er), the keeper of the archives in the Zhou Court, but the Yellow Emperor (Huang Di), who was believed to live in China as early as 3,000 B.C. It is known by many ancient historians that the Yellow Emperor's Daoists Shengong and Qigong magical practices were legendary.

At the time of Laozi's birth (in the state of Chu) during the Qin Dynasty (221-206 B.C.), the reigning Emperor Qin Shi Huang was already a strong devotee of Daoist shamanistic magic. By the time Laozi was born, most of the ancient energetic practices became commingled with the sage's teachings.

The Chinese character Wu translates as "magician or sorcerer." In ancient China there were two characters used to represent the Wu, one was used for men and the other for women.

- **The Female Wu (Xi):** Before 1,000 B.C., the majority of "Wu" were predominantly female. The ideograph consists of the character "Gong" (work) surrounded by two characters "Ren" (man or person). The upper horizontal stroke can also be translated as "above," or "Heaven;" while the lower horizontal stroke can be translated as "below," or "Earth." A complete translation can therefore be explained as "working to connect the energetic power of the unseen spirits within Heaven and Earth" (Figure 1.18).

  The female Wu were directed to perform exorcisms annually, at specific times, while using specific fragrances to wash their bodies. In times of drought, the Wu priestesses (representing the Yin or feminine aspect of the Universal Order, to which clouds and rain belong) performed dances or offered specific prayers at the altars during the sacrifice for rain. In times of disaster and great calamity in the kingdom, the female Wu would entreat celestial immortals with chants and wailing, expressing the peoples' grief and distress. Additionally, whenever the emperor's consort paid a visit of condolence, the female Wu would walk before her with the female "Jian" (invokers or conjurers, also

known the Imperial Seers).
- **The Male Wu:** The male ideograph for Wu included the extra character "Jian" (meaning to "see") towards the right side of the ideograph, and depicted clairvoyant "seeing" (Figure 1.19). In ancient China, the male priest represented the Yang or masculine aspect of the Universal Order, to which the source of light, lucidity and brightness belong.

The male Wu's responsibility was to turn his attention towards the sacrifices and to invite spiritual immortals, calling and gathering them from the six directions of Heaven and Earth before the altar. In the winter (when spiritual entities dominate the Earth), the male Wu were responsible for purging and exorcising evil from the imperial halls. In the spring, the male Wu were responsible for calling celestial immortals for the prosperity of agriculture, averting demons or evil, and warding off disease. Additionally, whenever the emperor paid a visit of condolence, the male Wu would walk before him with the male "Jian" (invokers or conjurers, also known the Imperial Seers). It was not until the Han Dynasty (206 B.C. - 220 A.D.) that the terminology Wu Jian was later used to denote the combined metaphysical functions of both the Wu and the Jian.

During the later Zhou Dynasty (1028-221 B.C.) the character "Yi" (doctor of medicine) was sometimes used or substituted for "Wu" (magician or sorcerer) in order to denote specific clinical applications. At that time, the ancient Chinese character for doctor of medicine (Yi), originally used the radical "Wu" as its bottom ideograph. Later, the bottom ideograph was substituted for the radical "Jiu" which translates as "a bottle of wine," denoting the medical application of herbs.

The Chinese character for doctor of medicine (Yi) is divided into three parts. The top left ideograph translates as, "to treat disease," and depicts a box or quiver containing arrows. Some historians have speculated that the quiver full of arrows was used to preform an ancient type of minor surgery or acupuncture; others speculate that the arrows represented certain spiritual powers and were used to drive off evil influences, as well as heal diseases.

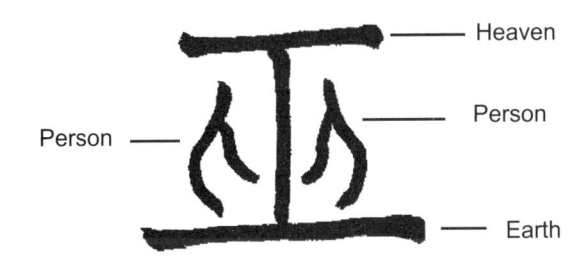

Figure 1.18. The ancient Chinese character "Wu," Female Shaman (sometimes known as a "Xi")

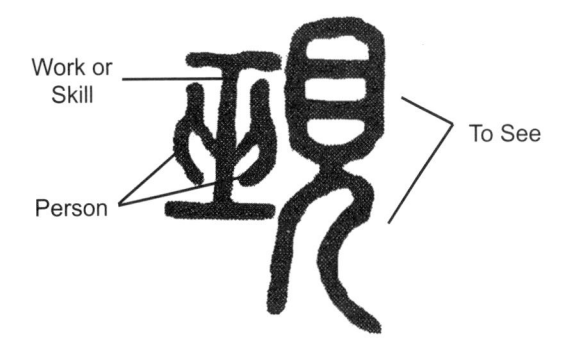

Figure 1.19. The ancient Chinese character "Wu," Male Shaman

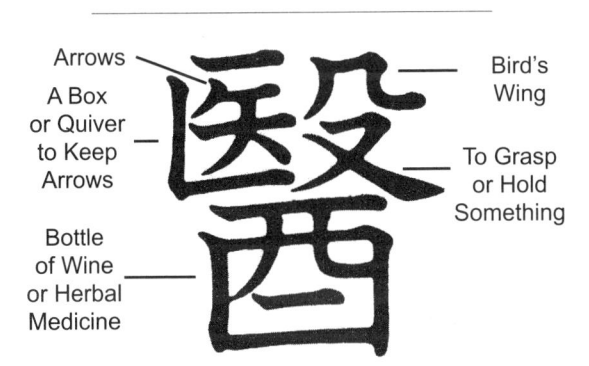

Figure 1.20. The Chinese character "Yi," Doctor

The top right ideograph depicts a bird's wing, and below is the image of a right hand, raised as if "to hold" or "to grasp something." Together, the image depicts a seat or table and something being held in the right hand to make quick actions. The bottom ideograph "Jiu" translates as "a bottle of wine." Certain historians speculate that the wine was used as an herbal medicine to anesthetize the patient before treatment, or to sterilize a wound (Figure 1.20).

Duties of the Wu Yi Doctors

- Conjuring Spirits and Removing Malevolent Spirits
- Spirit Travel and Dream Interpretation
- Reading Omens
- Rainmaking
- Healing
- Celestial Divination

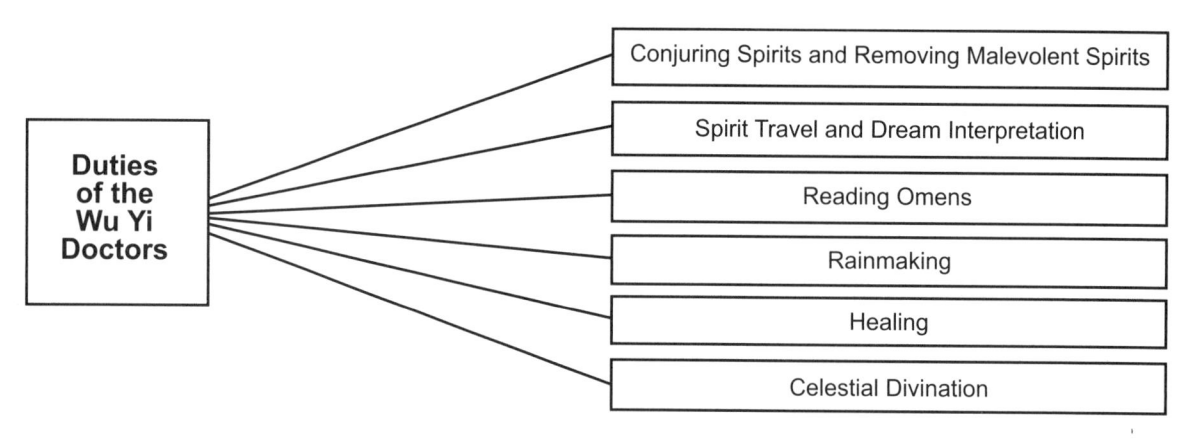

Figure 1.21. The Six Primary Duties of the Wu Yi Doctors

The ancient sorcerer/doctors (known as Wu Yi) were believed to possess special magical powers. They relied on their ability to cultivate the fundamental energetic forces of nature for healing, spinning webs of intrigue, secrecy and magic into every aspect of China's ancient culture. By controlling and utilizing Qi, the Wu Yi doctor could communicate with the energetic forces of supernatural beings. Invisible spirits could be contacted, demons could be exorcized, and various diseases could be treated. These ancient masters of supernatural energy were reported to be able to fly into the sky, journey underground, converse with animals, initiate the dance of power to conjure spiritual entities, control the power of the elements, possess extensive knowledge of herbs, and to excel in numerous other healing arts.

In order to initiate control over the Qi of nature and to intercede between their human patients and the supernatural world, the Wu Yi doctors would use magical chants and incantations, herbal formulas, Qi and Shen emission, massage, point stimulation, various elaborate rituals, dancing, and healing prayers. These ancient doctors also utilized the power of the spoken word in conjunction with strong imagination, visualization and powerful affirmation in order to perform their magical medicine.

When treating patients, in order to diagnose the root cause of the patient's disease, the Wu Yi doctors were able to journey into the energetic spiritual world through prayer and movement. One of the ministers of the Yellow Emperor (the founder of Chinese medicine) was a Wu Yi doctor named Zhu You. Zhu You practiced an ancient form of Qi emission combined with sacred prayer while treating his patients. So effective was this method of treatment that the *Yellow Emperor's Classic of Internal Medicine* states that in ancient times most illnesses were treated according to Zhu You's healing methods. Practitioners of this method were known as professional "prayer healers," and were once widespread throughout ancient China.

During the Shang Dynasty (1600 - 1028 B.C.), the Wu Yi doctors rose to prominence, holding high social positions as oracles, sages, and judges. Oracle records inscribed on the back of tortoise shells and the leg bones of oxen explained how ancient kings and emperors of the Shang dynasty invoked the power of Heaven before embarking on journeys, hunting, building projects, royal burials and warfare. The oracle bones made a clear distinction between the "Spirits of Heaven" who control the weather, the "Spirits of Earth" who control nature, and the "Immortal Spirits" or "Demons" of the afterlife who control illness and the suffering of humanity.

Evidence from the oracle records suggests that these powerful Wu Yi sorcerers were influential in counseling kings and emperors, who were themselves reluctant to follow any military strategy without the advice of these powerful spiritual guides. Since the emperors were known as the "Sons of Heaven," and the Wu Yi doctors were the standing messengers between the mysterious realms of Heaven and Earth, the Wu Yi doctors wielded enormous social and political power. Many of the fundamental notions about the origin and treatment of disease in Traditional Chinese Medicine stemmed from the spiritual insights gathered by the Wu Yi doctors who worked as advisers, diviners and healers.

DUTIES OF THE WU YI DOCTORS

During the Zhou Dynasty (1028-221 B.C.), the special duties of the Wu Yi doctors were specifically detailed, and any failure to perform an assigned task was often punishable by death. The six primary duties of the Wu Yi doctor were as follows: conjuring spirits and removing malevolent spirits, spirit travel and dream interpretation, reading omens, rainmaking, healing, and celestial divination (Figure 1.21):

1. **Conjuring Spirits and Removing Malevolent Spirits:** This energetic skill required the Wu Yi doctor to either invite spiritual deities and immortals into the mortal realm to ask for knowledge, or to ask that they temporarily stay as a protector (Figure 1.22). Additionally, the Wu Yi doctor was sometimes summoned to remove malevolent spirits. The ancient Chinese believed that spirit beings could be summoned, controlled and dispatched to carry out tasks; or when needed, a spirit could be expelled by a qualified individual such as a Wu Yi doctor.

- **Conjuring Spiritual Deities and Immortals:** The Wu Yi doctor would perform either an evocation, invocation or necromancy to connect with the spirit world.

    An evocation is the skill of conjuring a spiritual entity from another plane of existence, causing it to manifest as a visible entity in either the energetic plane or the physical plane. When evoked, the spiritual entities were brought into the presence of the Wu Yi doctor (never within his or her body) where they could be observed and communicated with. The spiritual entities summoned in an evocation were not dead (necromancy), but existed within other spiritual dimensions.

    An invocation occurs by allowing a benign spiritual entity to inhabit the body and speak through the Wu Yi doctor. The power and prestige of the Wu Yi largely depended on the number of spirits he or she could voluntarily incarnate and control within the body. This was sometimes achieved through the aide of magical songs, incantations, dances, drumming, and psychedelic herbs and mushrooms. Specific dances for spiritual visitation were commonly performed before entering into a trance to allow a spiritual entity to enter the

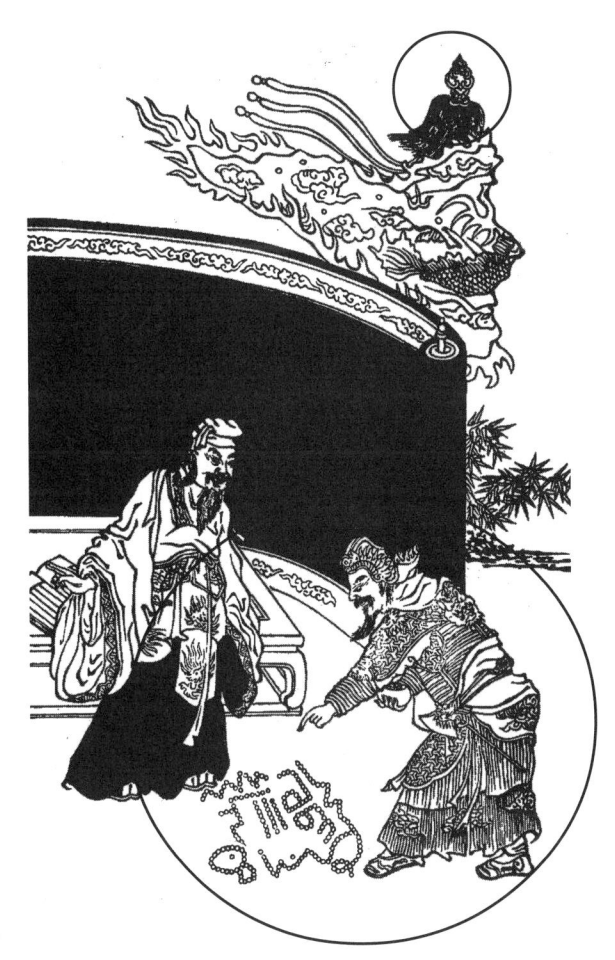

Figure 1.22. Spirit beings could be summoned, controlled, ordered, and dispatched by the Wu Yi.

Combined Circular "Tread" Pattern of "Terrestrial Regulation"

Earth is Expressed Through the Mystic Spiral of the Three Complete Circular Rotations

Big Dipper "Flight" Pattern of "Celestial Rules"

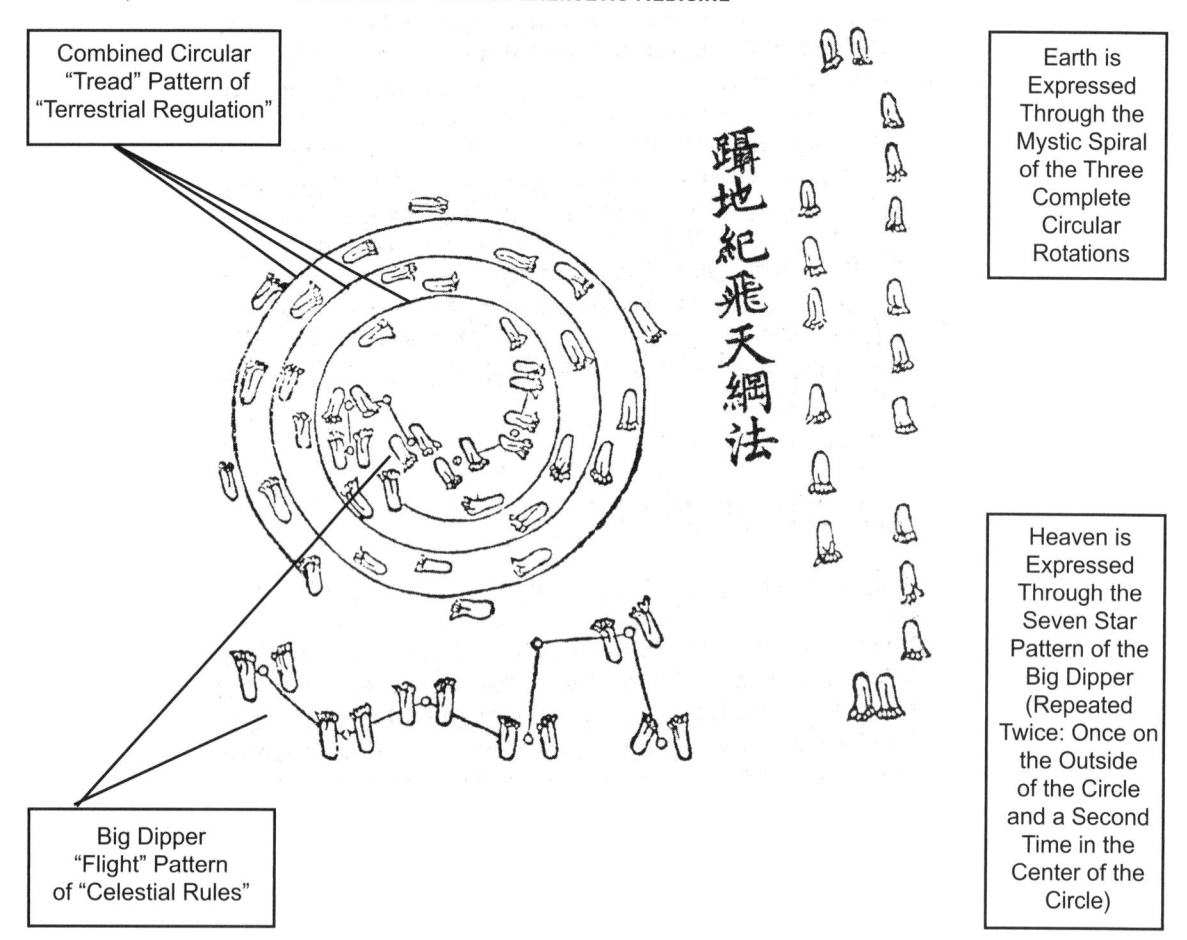

Heaven is Expressed Through the Seven Star Pattern of the Big Dipper (Repeated Twice: Once on the Outside of the Circle and a Second Time in the Center of the Circle)

蹋地紀飛天網法

Figure 1.23. The "Dance of Wu," is used for invocation. This pattern, originally used to demonstrate the energetic and spiritual union of Heaven and Earth, shows the combined circular "Tread" pattern of "Terrestrial Regulation" and the Big Dipper "Flight" pattern of "Celestial Rules."

Wu Yi doctor's body (Figure 1.23). Sometimes sand, flower or ash writing divination was employed while the Wu Yi was in this trance state. "Channeling" is but one example of an invocation used to bring a foreign intelligence into the body.

Necromancy is the skill of calling forth spirits of the dead for revealing past, present and future events. A "medium" is an example of an individual skilled in contacting the dead.

- **Removing Malevolent Spirits:** The removal of spiritual entities sometimes required the use of powerful incantations (Mantras), Hand Seals (Mudras), talismans and other magical implements (Figure 1.24). "Holy Water," fire, incense, and "Bagua Mirrors" were all used to combat destructive spiritual forces.

Sometimes after a malevolent spirit had been bound, it was transported and contained within a cave. The cave was then sealed and a "talisman of containment" was written and placed at the entrance of the cave.

2. **Spirit Travel and Dream Interpretation:** This energetic skill required the Wu Yi doctor to transcend his or her normal conscious perceptions and senses to observe and communicate with the spiritual Yin world. This was known in ancient times as having "Yin eyes." Indi-

viduals who possessed "Yin eyes" were able to see and talk to the spirits of the dead. The Wu Yi doctor was occasionally required to administer "soul retrieval" to recover life-force or soul qualities that had been damaged, lost, stolen or were otherwise trapped within the Spirit World.

- The Wu Yi doctor was required to spirit travel into the celestial realms of the cosmos, and to commune with the deities and immortals dwelling within the constellations. Other times, the Wu Yi doctor's journey into the spiritual world required him or her to travel underground and enter into the underworld in order to rescue souls of the dead who had been abducted by malevolent spirits. Specific rites were performed to free them from the negative influences that had ensnared them, and to support and guide them through the "Celestial Gate of Life."
- In ancient China, dreams were considered the carriers of omens, and the Daoist shamanic doctor was considered a "dream master," who could not only interpret these subconscious messages (akin to modern psychology), but could also travel into the dream world (lucid dreaming) to communicate with the spirit realm. When a Wu Yi doctor consulted a tortoise shell about a particular dream, it had to be interpreted first thing in the morning or by the next evening (after sundown the divination had passed beyond the boundaries of the rituals).

The ancient Chinese also understood the principle of antithetical (reverse) dream interpretation, in which the true meaning of a individual's dream is sometimes just the opposite of what the images would normally suggest. It was considered "the dream life inverting the waking life."

3. **Reading Omens:** this energetic skill required the Wu Yi doctor to observe and interpret the changes in the Earth (Feng Shui), and predict whether the courses of events were auspicious or destructive. The ancient Chinese believed that one's destiny could be revealed in omens.

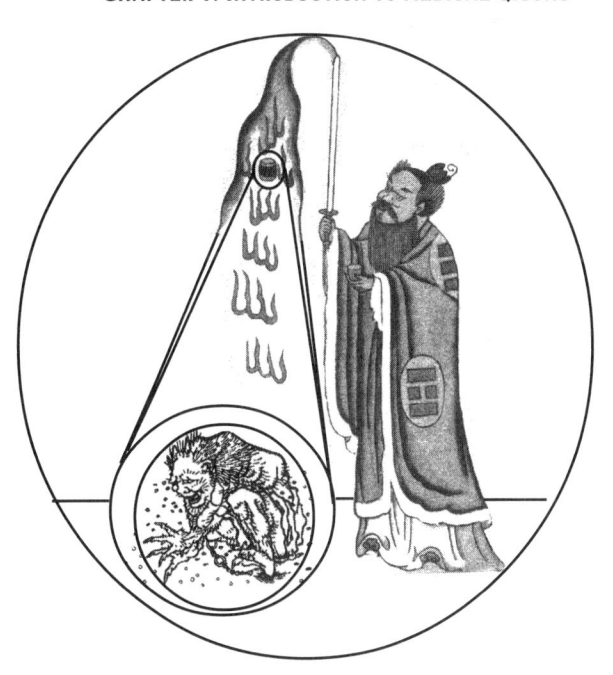

Figure 1.24. A Wu Yi removing a malevolent spirit

Omens were seen as meaningful because they had been specifically arranged for an individual by "higher" forces, and because everything within the cosmos (the energetic natures of Heaven, Earth and Man) was influenced through the Dao. It was also believed that spirits communicated through signs and symbols encountered in daily life.

Auguries were used in the form of the examination of tea leaves and oracle bones (heating tortoise shells or ox shoulders), and the examination of celestial changes, cloud formations, weather conditions, sounds of water, and dreams. An augury is something that serves as a sign of future happenings. It is the skill of reading divinations from auspicious events or omens and interpreting these energetic patterns in the context of human destiny. An augury is an ancient practice that observes a particular energetic pattern at a precise moment in time, revealing the deeper nature of the universe and its manifest design.

The skill of reading omens set the foundation for divination in ancient China, thereby establishing an interest in the study of the Yi-Jing (Book of Changes) (Figure 1.25). The most common questions requiring the Wu Yi doctors' omen reading skills involved matters of sacrifice, war, hunting, trips and future weather conditions.

- **Tortoise Shell Divination:** Tortoise shells were commonly used as tools of divination (Figure 1.26). It was believed that the tortoise was an ordained animal, capable of acting as an oracle. The top of the tortoise shell is round, representing Heaven; the bottom of the tortoise shell is square and flat, representing Earth. Together, both parts of the tortoise shell represent a microcosm of life as a whole. The tortoise shells were heated until they cracked. Each of the cracks were then interpreted by the Wu Yi doctors according to the trigram patterns recorded in the Yi-Jing.

The ancient Chinese used four primary types of divination for revealing future events. These included the study of motion or impressions created within energetic manifestations of the Heavens, Earth, water and fire, described as follows (Figure 1.27):

- **Geomancy (The Study of the Earth):** This type of divination reveals the future according to the motion or impressions created within the Earth. This study includes sudden changes occurring within the ground, trembling noises, swelling and ground elevation, fissures, landslides, pits and other impressions suddenly created. Earthquakes generally revealed impending bloodshed, the destruction of crops, famine, plague and other evils, depending on the types of buildings that were destroyed and other circumstances (structures of tombs moving, etc.).

- **Aeromancy (The Study of the Winds):** This type of divination reveals the future according to the motion or impressions created within the air and wind. This study includes sudden changes occurring within the directions of the wind, mist and cloud formations.

Clouds were considered highly significant when they appear near the sun or moon, or

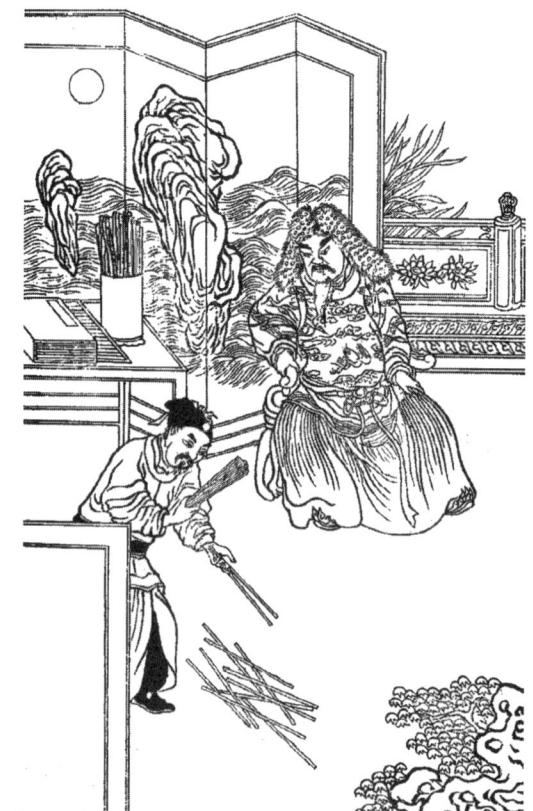

Figure 1.25. A Wu Yi was skilled in the art of reading omens. Yarrow sticks were commonly used as oracles. Fifty sections of yarrow stems were laid out according to the correspondences of Heaven, Earth, and Man. The odd and even residues of whole or broken stems were then formed into trigrams and subsequently expanded into the specific hexagrams of the Yi-Jing.

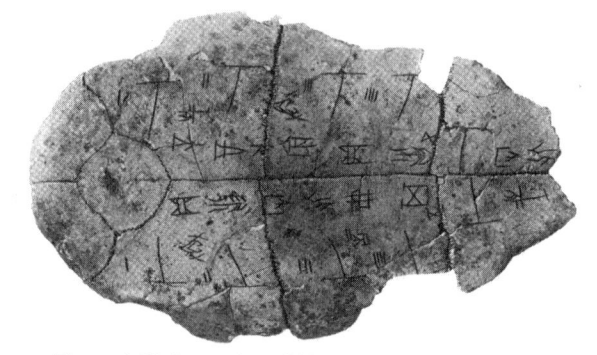

Figure 1.26. In ancient China, tortoise shells were used as an augury for divination, each crack represented a specific energetic change or an approaching form of destiny.

in the shape of halos. Also noted were clouds bursting open, clouds displaying the formation of armies, dense clouds that cover the sky without shedding a drop of rain, as well as specific visions created within mist (fog) and clouds.

Careful attention was placed on the formation, movement and colors of mist and dew appearing at sunrise and sunset. Certain types of dew were considered very auspicious and were sometimes called "sweet dew," "celestial wine," or "honey dew" because they always represented luxurious growth and abundance.

Rainbows were considered to be like the wind, composed of both Yang and Yin, and an excellent means of investigating the will of the Dao. Their colors and times of appearance were intensely studied. Pail rainbows, for example, were always considered unfavorable omens.

- **Hydromancy (The Study of Water):** This type of divination reveals the future of things according to the motion or impressions created within water. This study includes sudden changes occurring within the directions of the water, aquatic ebbing and flowing, increases and depressions, colors and specific visions created within water. If, for example, a brook or well suddenly dried up or changed its water color (especially if it became as red as blood or so foul that fish died), it was particularly considered an ill omen. However, if the water should suddenly become clear and clean, it was considered an auspicious omen. Additionally, gales and typhoons, as well as excessive rainfall which destroyed crops and caused floods were considered ill omens.
- **Pyromancy (The Study of Fire):** This type of divination reveals the future according to the motion or impressions created within fire. This study includes sudden changes occurring within the directions of the fire or its smoke, specific sounds, colors, motions or patterns created within the fire or from its ashes, and specific visions created within the flames.

4. **Rainmaking:** This energetic skill required the Wu Yi doctor to summon and control the foundational powers within the universe. By con-

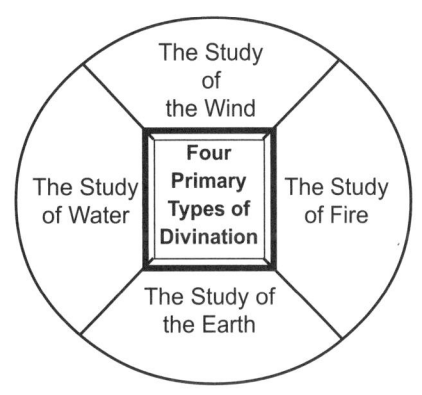

Figure 1.27. The ancient Chinese used four primary types of divinations for revealing future events.

trolling the ancient powers of the Bagua, the Wu Yi doctor could summon and control the four powers of Heaven: clouds, mist and rain, fire, and thunder; and the four powers of Earth: soil, mountains, water and wind. One important power needed to ensure the kingdom's survival was the ability to create rain, avoiding drought and famine. The ancient Chinese believed that clouds and mist (fog) float between Heaven and Earth, and are the vapor of the Dao. They therefore saw clouds, mist and dew as containing the "essence of the primordial vapor of the Dao," and sought to join with the Dao in order to summon or create rain. There were two approaches to rainmaking:

- In the first approach, the "elements" of the clouds and rain were summoned. A very powerful Wu Yi doctor could call down thunder, rain or even snow, and create rain clouds out of a clear sky. A less powerful Wu Yi doctor had to call in existing clouds and rain from a nearby area.
- In the second approach, the Wu Yi doctor would petition a spiritual deity or immortal, asking and "persuading" the celestial powers to send rain.

5. **Healing:** This energetic skill required the Wu Yi doctor to treat and cure diseases. Healing was divided into three main approaches: healing the physical body, healing the mental and emotional body, and healing the spiritual body.

- **Healing the Physical Body:** This energetic skill required the Wu Yi doctor to use various types of herbal medicine, Medical Qigong, acupuncture, massage and dietetics. For the Wu Yi doctor, herbs were associated with specific elemental energies and spiritual natures. The qualities of the herbs' elemental energies and spiritual natures were assimilated through drinking infusions in teas, soups or wines; eating the herbs in either raw or cooked form; or by burning them and inhaling the smoke.
- **Healing the Mental and Emotional Body:** This energetic skill required the Wu Yi doctor to use emotional counseling skills, usually based on the patient's spiritual belief system.
- **Healing the Spiritual Body:** This energetic skill required the Wu Yi doctor to use various types of rituals to access the patient's spiritual state. The ancient Chinese believed that occasionally illness was a result of malevolent spirits invading the body. In some instances black sorcerers and magicians were hired to harm people by inflicting illness. To combat such unethical energetic practices, the Wu Yi doctors would use powerful incantations, hand seals, and talismans. It is also believed that fragments of the oracle Bones were sometimes shaped into needles and used to perform acupuncture for the treatment of demonic possession by stimulating the thirteen "Ghost Points" (currently used in acupuncture clinics for the treatment of mental illness).

6. **Celestial Divination:** This energetic skill required the Wu Yi doctor to observe and decipher the changes in Heaven. The Wu Yi doctor possessed the ability to predict the course of events and whether they were auspicious or destructive (astrology of prediction), or predict the course of a disease (astrology of diagnosis). The ancient Chinese believed that peace and prosperity lay in following the "Will of Heaven," and that the phenomena occurring within the macrocosm of Heaven had parallels occurring within the microcosm of Man.

The official observation of nature was a statutory obligation in ancient China. Records gathered during the Han Dynasty (206 B.C.-220 A.D.) and mentioned in the *Shu King* (Canon of History), categorize celestial divination into three primary observations: divinations of the sky, divinations of the sun and moon, and divinations of the stars and planets. These three types of celestial divinations are described as follows (Figure 1.28):

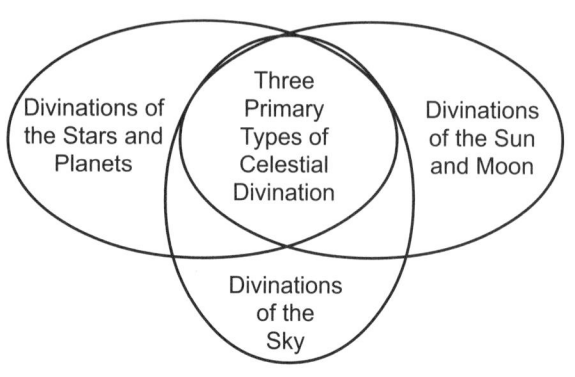

Figure 1.28. The ancient Chinese used three primary types of celestial divinations for revealing future events.

- **Divinations of the Sky:** In order to derive messages from the sky, the ancient Wu Yi studied strange or sudden changes occurring within the sky, such as changes in sky color, blood colored streams of light, voices resounding in the wind or air, thunder and lightning. Thunder was always considered to be an auspicious phenomenon, unless it occurred without rain. Lightening (called the "fire of heaven"), was considered to be an instrument of the Dao, and was commonly believed to strike demons, evil men, and other objects.

    The Wu Yi believed that hail was produced when Yang and Yin collide; and hail was therefore thought to be an inauspicious omen. The predictions of the evil derived from hail would differ according to the specific season in which it fell.

- **Divinations of the Sun and Moon:** In order to derive messages from the sun and moon, the ancient Wu Yi studied energetic changes occurring during the times of an eclipse, the appearance of strange or sudden spots or protuberances on the sun or moon, specific colors of the haloes or circles around the moon,

CHAPTER 1: INTRODUCTION TO MEDICAL QIGONG

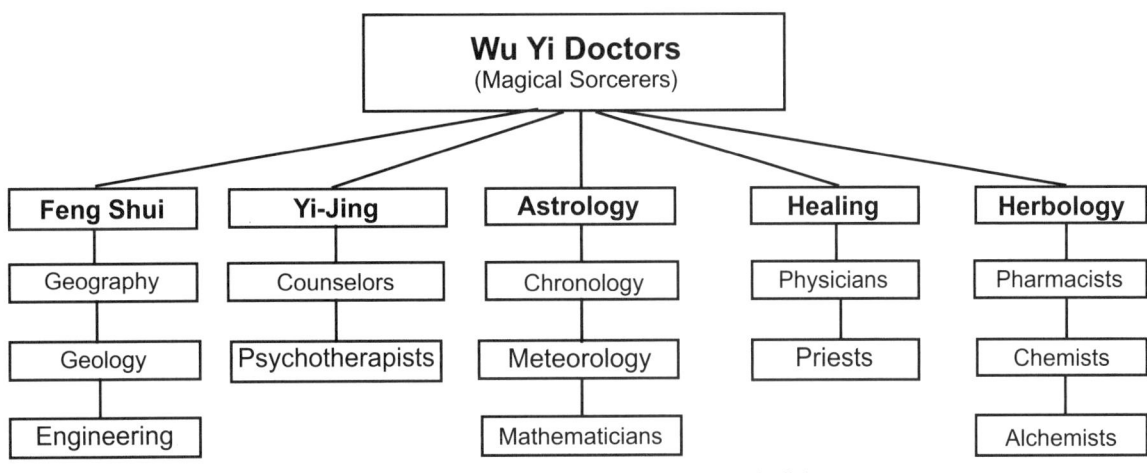

Figure 1.29. The Progression of Ancient Medicine

and strange colorations surrounding these illuminations.

- **Divinations of the Stars and Planets:** In order to derive messages from the stars and planets, the ancient Wu Yi studied changes in the aspects and brightness of the stars and planets, their conjunctions with the sun and moon, their position in the Heavens at the times of an eclipse, and circles occurring around the stars. Also important were subtle vibrations such as musical tunes and other sounds that were believed to be emitted by the stars and planets, the movements of comets through the constellations, falling stars, and meteor showers.

THE EVOLUTION OF CHINESE MEDICINE

As the Chinese civilization continued to expand, the theories and practice of medicine became more refined, formalized and recorded. The primary structure of Chinese medicine was organized to reflect the energetic harmony and influential interactions between the energies of Heaven, Earth and Man. This evolution transformed the healing arts developed by the Wu Yi doctors into the various intellectual sciences and artisan skills. No longer considered primitive magical sorcerers, the Wu Yi doctors became established in the new scientific world as alchemists, astronomers, chemists, physicians, pharmacists, counselors, engineers, and mathematicians, etc. (Figure 1.29).

QIGONG OF THE IMPERIAL COLLEGE

Throughout China's vast medical history, therapeutic categories and specialties were classified into separate divisions or medical departments, also known as "classes of mastery." The following is a brief synopsis of seven major changes occurring within the various medical departments of China's Imperial Colleges (Figure 1.30):

1. **Zhou Dynasty (1028-221 B.C.):** This was the first Imperial Dynasty to organize clinical medicine into separate divisions or medical departments.
2. **Northern Wei Dynasty of the Six Dynasties Period (386 A.D.-533 A.D.):** The Imperial Medical Colleges maintained four departments: Internal and External Medicine (surgery, traumatology, dermatology and antiseptic techniques); Acupuncture and Moxibustion; Massage and Tissue Manipulation; and Demonology.
3. **Tang Dynasty (618-907 A.D.):** The Imperial Medical Colleges maintained four departments: Medicine (Herbs and Diet); Acupuncture and Moxibustion; Massage and Tissue Manipulation; and Charms and Incantations.
4. **Song Dynasty (960-1279 A.D.):** The Imperial Medical Colleges maintained nine departments: Internal Medicine; War Wounds; Ophthalmology; Pediatrics; Obstetrics and Wind Diseases (including stroke); Fractures, Abscesses and Ulcers; Diseases of the Mouth, Teeth and Throat; Acupuncture and Moxibus-

VOLUME 1, SECTION 1: FOUNDATIONS OF CHINESE ENERGETIC MEDICINE

1. Zhou Dynasty (1028-221 B.C.):	First Imperial Dynasty to organize clinical medicine into separate divisions or medical departments
2. Northern Wei Dynasty of the Six Dynasties Period (386 A.D.-533 A.D.):	Four Departments: Internal and External Medicine; Acupuncture and Moxibustion; Massage and Tissue Manipulation; and Demonology
3. Tang Dynasty (618-907 A.D.):	Four Departments: Herbs and Diet; Acupuncture and Moxibustion; Massage and Tissue Manipulation; Charms and Incantations
4. Song Dynasty (960-1279 A.D.):	Nine Departments: Internal Medicine; War Wounds; Ophthalmology; Pediatrics; Obstetrics and Wind Diseases; Fractures, Abscesses and Ulcers; Diseases of the Mouth, Teeth and Throat; Acupuncture and Moxibustion; and Written Incantations
5. Yuan Dynasty (1279-1368 A.D.):	Thirteen Departments: Internal Medicine; War Wounds; Orthopedics and Bone Setting; Ophthalmology; Pediatrics; Obstetrics; Wind Disease; Mouth and Teeth Disease; Nose and Throat Disease; Miscellaneous Diseases; Needling Therapy and Moxibustion; Supplications; and Incantations
6. Ming Dynasty (1368-1644 A.D.):	Thirteen Departments: Internal Medicine; War Wounds; Orthopedics and Bone Setting; Carbuncles and Ulcers; Ophthalmology; Pediatrics and Gynecology; Obstetrics; Febrile Diseases; Diseases of the Mouth and Teeth; Diseases of the Nose and Throat; Massage and Tissue Manipulation; Acupuncture and Moxibustion; Prayers and Supplications
7. Qing Dynasty (1644-1911 A.D.):	Nine Departments: Internal Medicine; Orthopedics and Bone Setting; Ulcers and Abscesses; Ophthalmology; Pediatrics; Gynecology; Febrile Diseases; Diseases of the Mouth, Teeth and Throat; Acupuncture and Moxibustion
8. The Peoples Republic of China (1949 A.D. -Present):	Western Medicine: This system of medicine contains several branches, including Internal Medicine; Orthopedics; Oncology; Ophthalmology; Obstetrics; Pediatrics; Gynecology; Neurology, Geriatrics, etc.)
	Traditional Chinese Medicine: This system of medicine contains four main branches: Acupuncture; Herbology and Dietetics; Massage and Medical Qigong Therapy

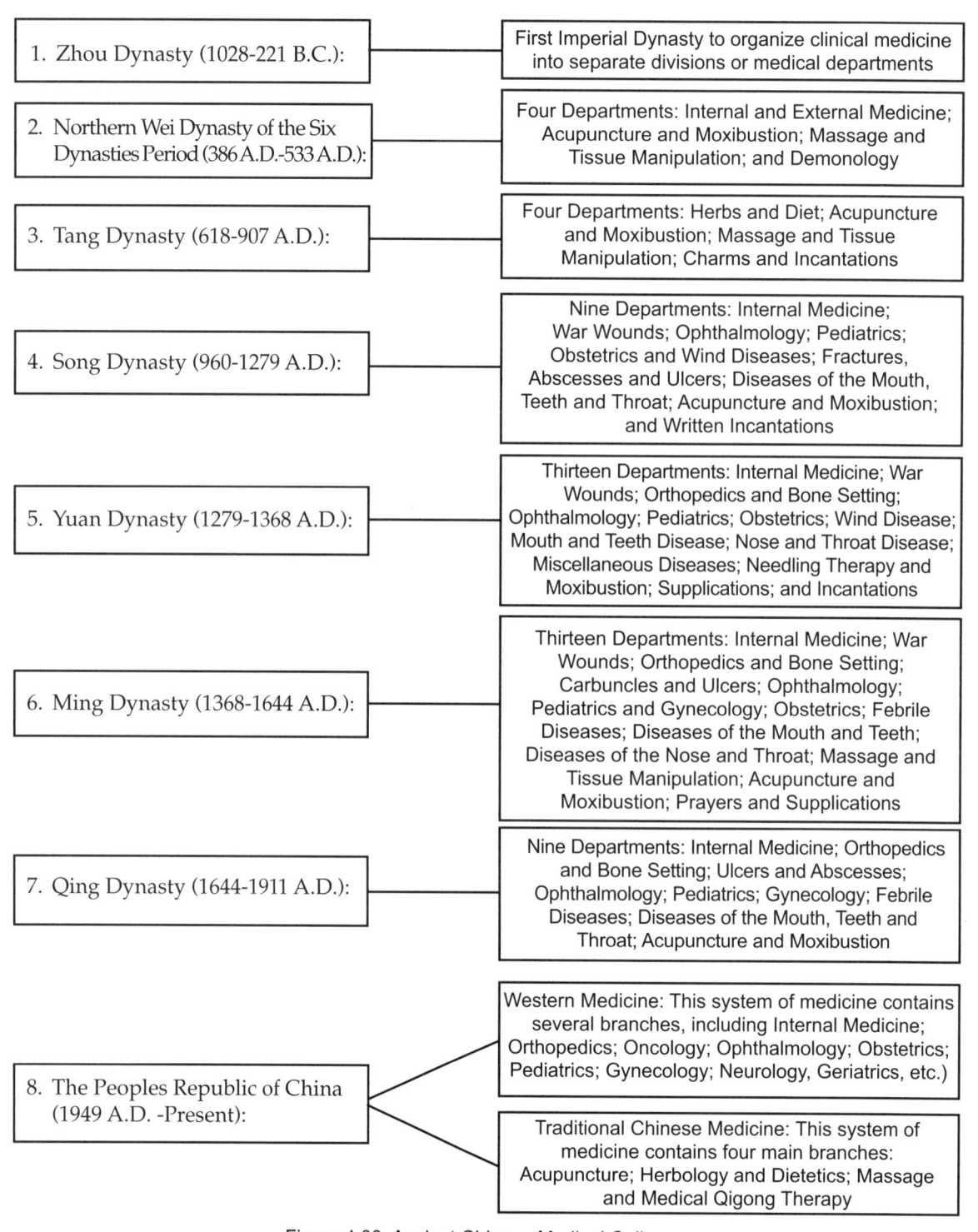

Figure 1.30. Ancient Chinese Medical Colleges

tion; and Written Incantations.
5. **Yuan Dynasty (1279-1368 A.D.):** The Imperial Medical Colleges maintained thirteen departments: Internal Medicine; War Wounds; Orthopedics and Bone Setting; Ophthalmology; Pediatrics; Obstetrics; Wind Diseases (including stroke); Diseases of the Mouth and Teeth; Diseases of the Nose and Throat; Miscellaneous Diseases; Acupuncture and Moxibustion; Prayers and Supplications; and Incantations.
6. **Ming Dynasty (1368-1644 A.D.):** The Imperial Medical Colleges maintained thirteen departments: Internal Medicine; War Wounds; Orthopedics and Bone Setting; Carbuncles and Ulcers; Ophthalmology; Pediatrics and Gynecology; Obstetrics; Febrile Diseases; Diseases of the Mouth and Teeth; Diseases of the Nose and Throat; Massage and Tissue Manipulation; Acupuncture and Moxibustion; Prayers and Supplications.
7. **Qing Dynasty (1644-1911 A.D.):** The Imperial Medical Colleges maintained nine departments: Internal Medicine; Orthopedics and Bone Setting; Ulcers and Abscesses; Ophthalmology; Pediatrics; Gynecology; Febrile Diseases; Diseases of the Mouth, Teeth and Throat; Acupuncture and Moxibustion.
8. **The Peoples Republic of China (1949 A.D.-Present):** Medical Colleges are now divided into two main tracks, each containing several departments: Western Medicine and Traditional Chinese Medicine, briefly described as follows:
- Western Medicine: this system of medicine contains several branches, including Internal Medicine; Orthopedics; Oncology; Ophthalmology; Obstetrics; Pediatrics; Gynecology; Neurology, Geriatrics, etc.)
- Traditional Chinese Medicine: this system of medicine contains four main branches: Acupuncture (including needling, cupping, bloodletting, moxa burning, and magnet healing); Herbology and Dietetics (including nutritional education; teas and soups; tinctures and wines; oils, balms, and liniments; and compresses, powders, and pills); Massage Therapy (including scraping therapy, tissue manipulation and traumatology, bone setting, visceral manipulation and channel point therapy); and Medical Qigong Therapy (including Qi emission, prescription exercises and meditations, Qigong massage, sound therapy, and invisible needle therapy).

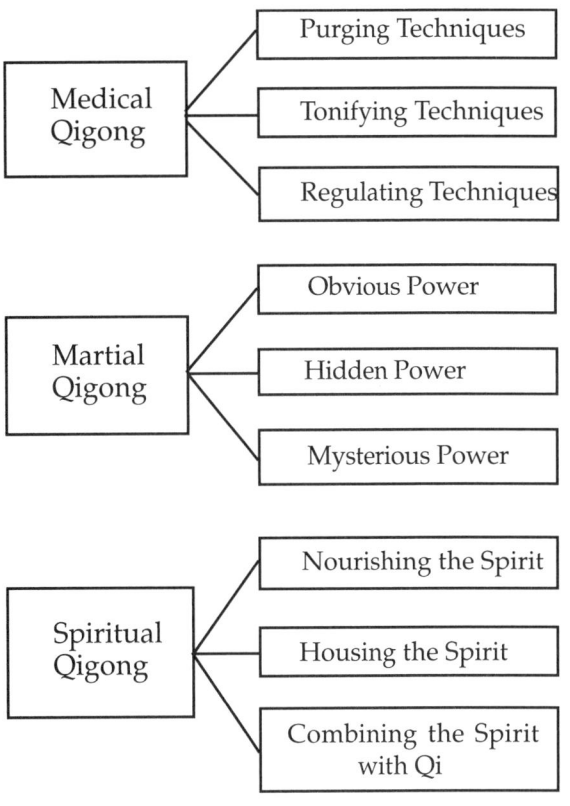

Figure 1.31. The Three Different Schools of Qigong

THREE MAIN SCHOOLS OF QIGONG

The term "Qigong" first appeared in the Jin Dynasty (265-420 A.D.) in a Daoist text entitled *"Records of the Clear Mirror of Religion"* by Xu Xun. Qi means "life-force energy" and Gong means "skill." Qigong is therefore the skillful practice of applying life-force energy. In modern China, Qigong practice is divided into three main schools: medical, martial, and spiritual. The three schools are all based on the same philosophical system and share many of the same meditations and techniques. They differ primarily in focus. Students choose a specific school based on how they want to apply their Qigong training (Figure 1.31). Briefly, each

Qigong school focuses on one of the following specialties:

1. **The Medical Qigong Schools:** These schools train doctors and healers in special Qigong methods for health maintenance and longevity, disease prevention, and the diagnosis and treatment of diseases and disorders. The three primary modalities of Medical Qigong therapy are described as follows (Figure 1.32):
   - **Purging Techniques:** Used to detoxify the body of pathogens
   - **Tonifying Techniques:** Used to strengthen the body's internal organs and organ systems
   - **Regulating Techniques:** Used to balance the body's internal Essence (Jing), Energy (Qi) and Spirit (Shen)

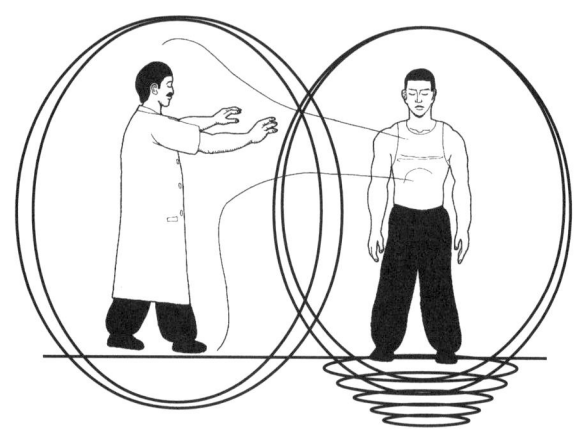

Figure 1.32. Medical Qigong Schools Focus on Purgation, Tonification and Regulation.

2. **The Martial Qigong Schools:** These schools train warriors in specific strength, power, speed and endurance techniques needed for performing martial arts combat. The three primary stages of Martial Qigong applications include Nei Gong (Internal Skill), Qi Gong (Energy Skill) and Shen Gong (Spirit Skill) training, described as follows (Figure 1.33):
   - **Clear or Obvious Power (Ming Jing):** These specific techniques emphasize the training and conditioning of the muscles, strengthening the bone structure, and increasing the individual's overall stamina and root. This stage also includes such techniques as conditioning the body (arms, hands, legs, torso and head) to strengthen and toughen the tissues.
   - **Hidden or Secret Power (An Jing):** These specific techniques emphasize stretching and twisting the tendons and ligaments (known as Reeling and Pulling the Silk) to cultivate resonant vibration within the body for striking and issuing power.
   - **Changing or Transforming Power (Hua Jing):** These specific techniques emphasize the training and conditioning of the individual's mind and spirit. The focus in Hua Jing training is placed on acquiring and developing the individual's Yi (imagination and intention) and Zhi (will power), needed to energetically project and utilize the power of the Shen (Spirit).

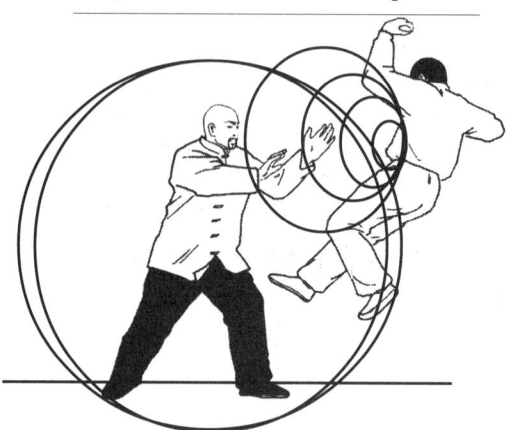

Figure 1.33. Martial Qigong Schools Focus on Building Speed, Endurance, Strength and Power.

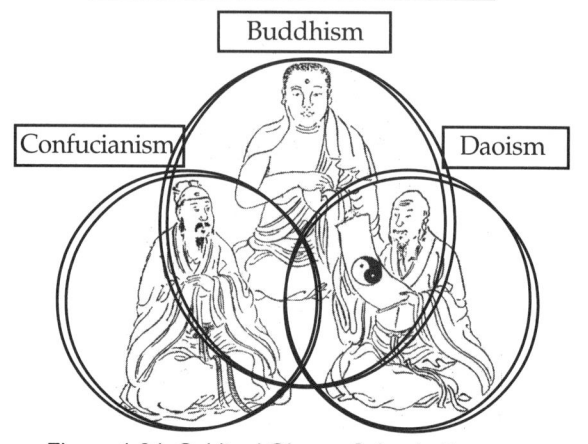

Figure 1.34. Spiritual Qigong Schools Focus on Spiritual Transformation and Enlightenment.

3. **The Spiritual Qigong Schools:** These schools train priests who seek spiritual transformation and enlightenment (known as Shen Ming or Spiritual Brightness). In China, the three primary spiritual schools, Daoism, Buddhism, and Confucianism, each have their own unique energetic approaches and Shengong techniques. These Shengong techniques include meditations for fusing, as well as releasing, the individual's Eternal Soul (Shen Xian) by cultivating the internal energy of his or her Wu Jing Shen (Five Essence Spirits). When the Original Spirit (Yuan Shen) is fully developed, the individual acquires certain extraordinary powers and abilities, such as spirit travel and soul travel. The goal, is to achieve transformation and a state of enlightenment, and the student must take care not to be led astray by the glamor of extra powers. The three primary techniques of Spiritual Qigong training include the following (Figure 1.34):

- **Nourishing the Spirit (Shen):** These specific techniques emphasize strengthening and refining the power of the individual's Yuan Shen.
- **Housing the Shen:** These specific techniques emphasize disciplining the thoughts and emotions. This helps to relax and tranquilize the individual's Yuan Shen, and to increase receptivity to divine energy and guidance.
- **Combining the Shen with the Qi:** These specific techniques emphasize the coordination of the breath and intention for directing the Yuan Shen to guide the body's life-force energy.

Qigong training involves all of the individual's physical senses. Concentration is focused on the development of the individual's faculties of imagination, visualization, hearing, smelling, tasting, touching, in addition to breathing, muscle relaxation and proper posture. Massage and movement are also used to develop and control the body's intrinsic energy. Studying Qigong requires not only comprehending the immeasurable wisdom gathered for medical, martial, or spiritual development, but also studying the ancient Chinese culture inherent within these systems.

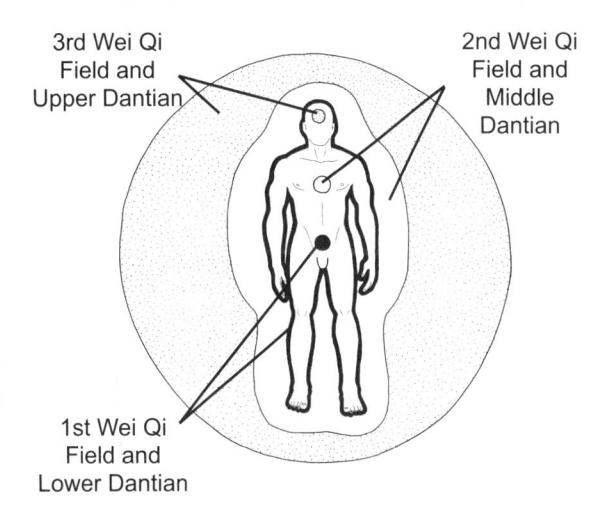

Figure 1.35. The Three External Wei Qi Fields

MEDICAL QIGONG DEFINED

All living bodies generate an external field of energy called Wei Qi (pronounced "whey chee"), which translates as "protective energy." The definition of Wei Qi in Medical Qigong is slightly different than that of Traditional Chinese Medicine (T.C.M.). In classical T.C.M. texts, the Wei Qi field is seen to be limited to the surface of the body, circulating within the tendon and muscle tissues. In Medical Qigong, however, the Wei Qi field also includes the three external layers of the body's auric and subtle energy fields (Figure 1.35). These energetic fields originate from each of the internal organs and radiate outside the body through the external tissues. The body's Lower Dantian is responsible for sustaining the power of the first Wei Qi field. The Middle Dantian is responsible for sustaining the power of the second Wei Qi field, and the Upper Dantian is responsible for sustaining the power of the third Wei Qi field (see Chapter 5). The Wei Qi fields completely surround and protect the body's tissues from the external invasion of pathogens while constantly communicating and interacting with the subtle universal and environmental energetic fields.

The body's Wei Qi fields can be strengthened through the proper intake of food, air, drink, sleep, prayer and meditation. Consequently, the Wei Qi field will also diminish and weaken due to an insufficient intake of food, air, drink, sleep, prayer and meditation. In the clinic, in order to protect themselves, Medical Qigong doctors will occasionally visualize specific colors, lights and sounds in order to fortify their Wei Qi field.

Both internal and external pathogenic factors affect the structural formation of the Wei Qi. Internal pathogenic factors include suppressed emotional influences such as anger and grief from emotional traumas. External pathogenic factors include exposure to adverse environmental influences, especially when they are extreme (such as Cold, Damp, Dry, Heat, Fire, or Wind). Physical traumas can also affect the Wei Qi field.

Any negative interchange affects the Wei Qi by literally creating holes within the matrix of the individual's external energetic fields. Without proper attention, these holes leave the body vulnerable to invasion, and disease can begin to take root. Strong emotions, in the form of toxic energy, become trapped within the body's tissues when one suppresses or does not integrate feelings. These unprocessed emotions block the natural flow of Qi, thus creating stagnant pools of toxic energy within the body.

Medical Qigong consists of specific techniques that use the knowledge of the body's internal and external energy fields to purge, tonify, and balance these energies. Medical Qigong therapy offers patients a safe and effective way to rid themselves of toxic pathogens and years of painful emotions that can otherwise cause mental and physical illness. This therapy combines breathing techniques with movement, creative visualization, and spiritual intent to improve health, personal power, and control over one's own life.

Medical Qigong Training in China

According to Professor Zhou Qianchuan, Qigong master and doctor of Traditional Chinese Medicine, all of the most famous Chinese doctors of acupuncture and moxibustion, herbal medicine, bone setting and massage therapy either practiced Qigong themselves or incorporated Qigong into their clinical practices (Figure 1.36).

There were numerous colleges of Traditional Chinese Medicine throughout China that focused

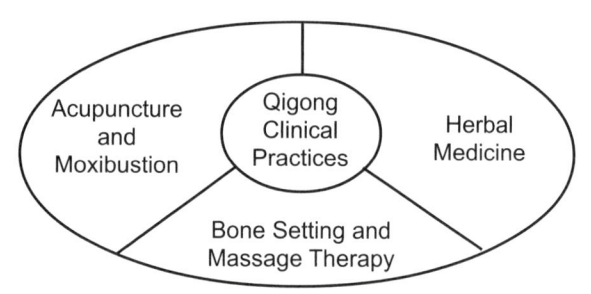

Figure 1.36. Qigong as a Foundation for all Chinese Clinical Practices.

on Medical Qigong training until the year 1999. The majority of these schools supported the scientific study and expansion of Medical Qigong applications and Traditional Chinese Medicine treatments.

Major Traditional Chinese Medical colleges in China offered comprehensive, government-sponsored, three-year programs in Medical Qigong therapy. Programs included classes, labs, and seminars on Traditional Chinese Medical theory. These studies included the foundations of Chinese medicine for internal diseases according to the *Huangdi Neijing* (Yellow Emperor's Inner Canon): *Ling Shu* (Magical Pivot) and *Su Wen* (Essential Questions), and the *Nanjing* (Canon of Perplexities). The Medical Qigong classes also included energetic anatomy and physiology, diagnosis and symptomatology, energetic psychology, Qigong pathology, Medical Qigong therapy, as well as a survey of other related medical modalities. These other related modalities included herbal medicine, acupuncture therapy, and Chinese massage. Classes of Western anatomy and physiology, Western internal diseases, and health and recovery were also required (Figure 1.37).

As part of the certification program, three to five training hours per day were required in addition to the standard six-day-a-week classroom curriculum. Course content, personal mastery of energy extension, and diagnostic techniques were rigorously tested each week. Upon completing the required courses and passing the final exams, the student received a certificate of completion. Next, a six-month to one-year internship was required at a program-affiliated hospital or clinic. Upon successful completion of this internship, the new

CHAPTER 1: INTRODUCTION TO MEDICAL QIGONG

Foundations of Chinese Medicine for Internal Diseases	Huangdi Neijing (Yellow Emperor's Inner Canon): Ling Shu: Magical Pivot / Su Wen: Essential Questions
	Nanjing: Canon of Perplexities
Energetic Anatomy and Physiology	Energetic Embryological Development
	Internal Organs, Channels and Points
	Interactions of Matter, Energy and Spirit
	Five Energies of the Human Body
Diagnosis and Symptomatology	Differential Diagnosis of Energetic Principles
	Clinical Examination and Diagnosis
Energetic Psychology	Differentiation of Psycho-Emotional Disorders
	Soul Retrieval
Qigong Pathology	Jing, Qi and Shen Disorders
	Qi Deviations and Dao Yin Therapy
Herbal Medicine, Massage Therapy and Acupuncture Therapy	Distance Qi Emission Therapy
Medical Qigong Therapy	Self-Regulation Prescription Therapy
	Qigong Massage Therapy
	Healing Sound Therapy
	Invisible Needle Therapy
Western Anatomy and Physiology	Histology, Signs and Symptoms
Western Internal Diseases	Pharmaceutical Terminology

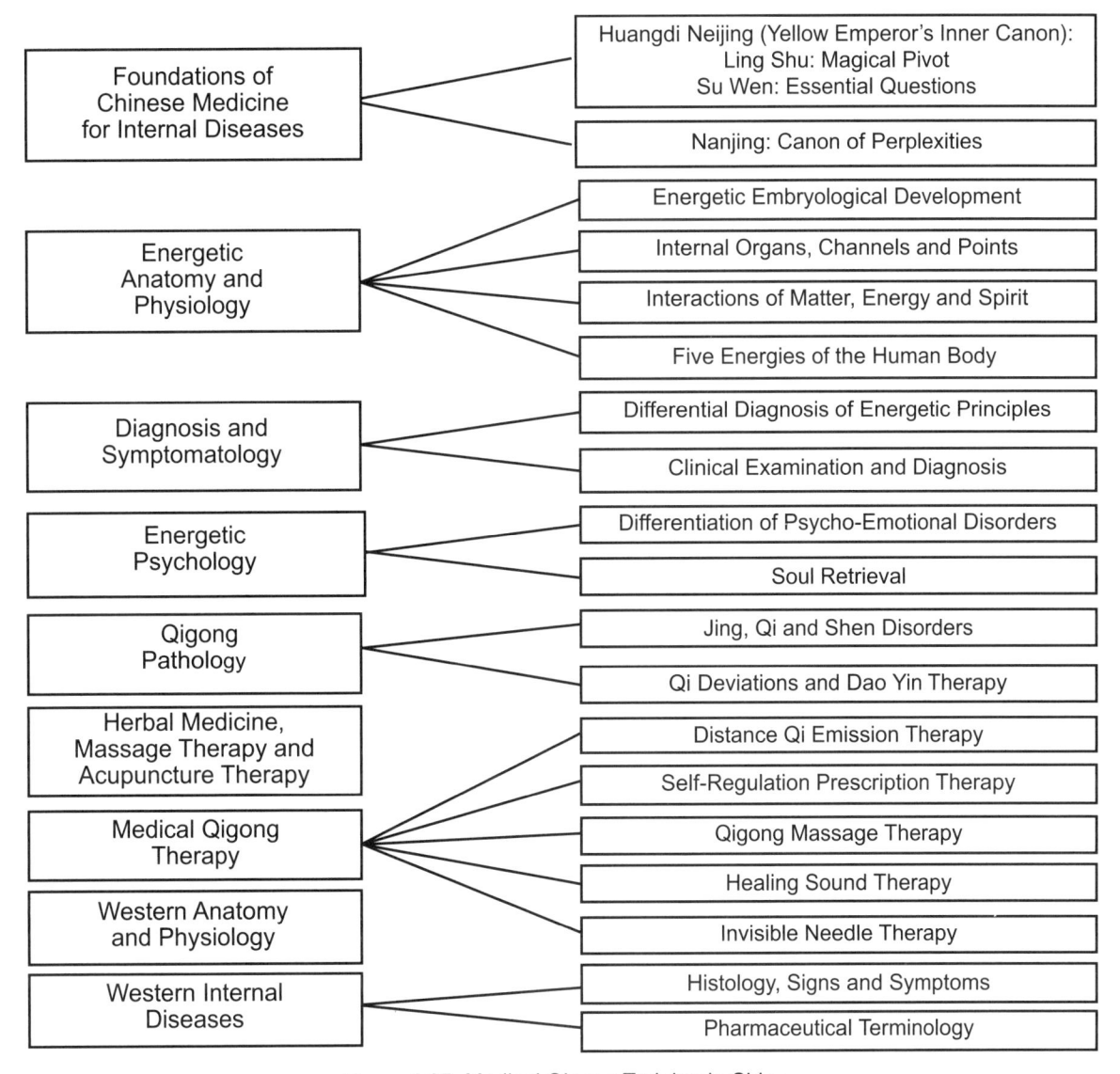

Figure 1.37. Medical Qigong Training in China

intern is licensed by the People's Republic of China's Ministry of Health, as a Doctor of Traditional Chinese Medicine specializing in Medical Qigong Therapy.

Each internship program was assigned a separate wing in select Chinese hospitals. Both inpatient and outpatient facilities were available to the public. Each wing had specific approaches to healing a patient, and its own unique set of ground rules for diagnosis and treatment.

FIVE CLINICAL POSTS OF CHINESE MEDICINE

After graduating from a local medical university, a student can progress through five separate positions of clinical rank. These five distinct levels represent the clinical "pecking order" within each branch of Traditional Chinese Medicine in China today. The five distinct clinical positions are described as follows:

- **Intern Doctor:** The first position is that of an "Interning Doctor," whereby the intern is re-

sponsible for refining his or her treatment skills under the strict guidance of a qualified, seasoned doctor.
- **Doctor:** The second position is that of a "Doctor," who is responsible for the treatment of all clinic patients. The doctor positions are generally filled by T.C.M. medical college graduates who have spent a minimum of three years in clinical internship and practice.
- **Doctor in Charge (Clinic Director):** The next level is called a "Clinic Director" or "Doctor In-Charge," and denotes a senior position within the clinic. The Doctor In-Charge is responsible for the supervision of all the doctors and the interns. This position is usually obtained only after spending a minimum of five years in the hospital as an active clinical doctor.
- **Vice-Chief Doctor (Associate Professor):** The next position is that of a "Vice-Chief Doctor" or "Associate Professor," who has the responsibility of overseeing the Doctors In-Charge, as well as teaching, treating, and training other doctors. This position is usually obtained after spending a minimum of five to six years in the clinic as a Doctor In-Charge.
- **Chief Doctor (Professor):** The highest position in the hospital is called a "Chief Doctor," or "Professor." This position is responsible for overseeing the Vice-Chief Doctors, as well as publishing researched studies in order to pass on clinical knowledge to future generations. This position is usually obtained after a minimum of five to six years as a Vice-Chief Doctor and publishing several researched clinical records.

The licensing is reviewed and issued by the People's Republic of China's Ministry of Health. The doctor's skills are tested through oral, written, and practical examinations and a license is issued accordingly. In China, currently there are four divisions of training available for a Doctor of Traditional Chinese Medicine (D.T.C.M.). These four divisions are described as follows (Figure 1.38).

1. **Doctor of Acupuncture Therapy (D.Ac.):** Specializes in the five main modalities of Chinese acupuncture: needle insertion, cupping, bloodletting, moxa burning, and magnet healing.

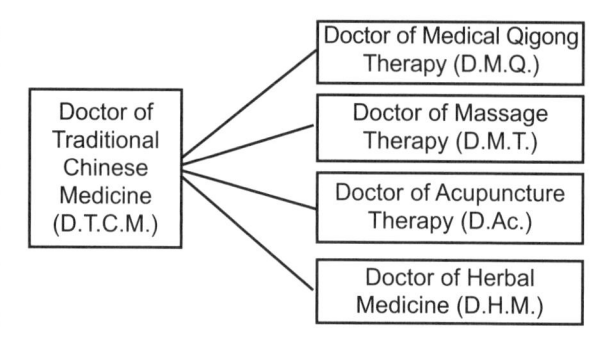

Figure 1.38. The Five Types of Doctors in Traditional Chinese Medicine

2. **Doctor of Herbal Medicine (D.H.M.):** Specializes in the five main modalities of Chinese herbology: nutritional education; formulating and prescribing teas and soups; tinctures and wines; oils, balms, and liniments; and compresses, powders and pills.
3. **Doctor of Massage Therapy (D.M.T.):** Specializes in the five main modalities of Chinese Massage and tissue alignment: Jie Gu-bone setting, Tui Na-muscle setting, Gua Sha-tissue scraping, An Mo-visceral manipulation, and Jing Point Therapy -channel point manipulation.
4. **Doctor of Medical Qigong Therapy (D.M.Q.):** Specializes in the five main modalities of Chinese Medical Qigong: distance Qi emission therapy, self-regulation prescription therapy, Qigong massage therapy, healing sound therapy, and invisible needle therapy.

MEDICAL QIGONG EXAMINATION AND CLINICAL QUALIFICATIONS IN CHINA

At one time, there existed numerous Medical Qigong colleges throughout China within various Traditional Chinese Medical Universities. Upon completing academic and clinical qualifications, Medical Qigong students had to pass five proficiency examinations before being allowed to graduate. After graduation, the students then entered specific Traditional Chinese Medical hospitals to complete their clinical internship for their doctorate.

The following five Medical Qigong proficiency examinations were used to determine the students' energetic potential. They were included in the final exams at the Hai Dian University in Beijing, China, and were also used throughout China by various Traditional Chinese Medical Universities.

The five proficiency examinations used to test the graduates energetic and alchemical skills (before allowing them to complete their internship at a resident hospital) include: decreasing the alcohol content in a cup of wine, neutralizing the acid in a glass of water to which a capsule of ascorbic acid has been added, imprinting an image of the palm on x-ray film, changing the alkaline component of red litmus paper, and changing the acidic component of blue litmus paper, described as follows:

1. **Decreasing the alcohol content in a cup of wine:** Wine is poured into two cups on a table in front of the student. The student must then purge and reduce the alcohol content in one cup. The student may also be asked to increase the alcohol content in the second cup (this is achieved through transferring the alcohol from the first cup into the second cup) (Figure 1.39).

2. **Neutralizing the acid in a glass of water to which a capsule of ascorbic acid has been added:** A glass of water containing a dissolved Vitamin C tablet is placed on a table in front of the student. The student must purge the Vitamin C water, neutralizing its acidic content (Figure 1.40).

3. **Imprinting an image of the palm on an x-ray film:** A piece of x-ray film is wrapped with a towel and placed on a table in front of the student. The student must place his or her hand over the towel and emit Qi into the x-ray film. Once the x-ray film has been developed, an image of the student's palm must be visible on the film (Figure 1.41).

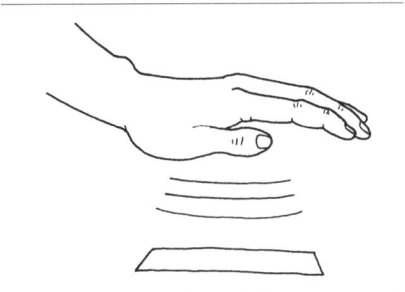

4. **Changing the acidic component of red litmus paper:** A strip of red litmus paper is placed inside a glass flask, and floats in an acidic solution. The student must place his or her hand over the strip of red litmus paper and emit Qi into the acidic solution, increasing or decreasing its acidic nature depending on the examining doctor's request (Figure 1.42).

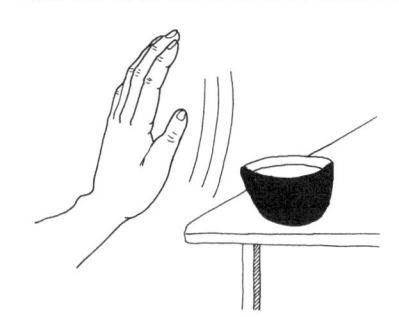

Figure 1.39. Decreasing the alcohol content in a cup of wine

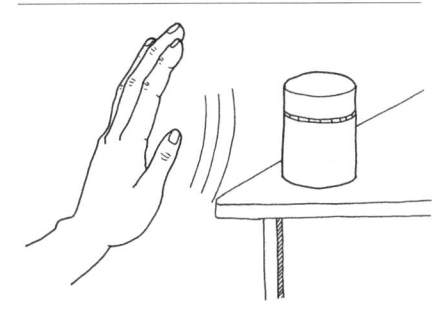

Figure 1.40. Neutralizing the acid in a glass of water to which a capsule of ascorbic acid has been added

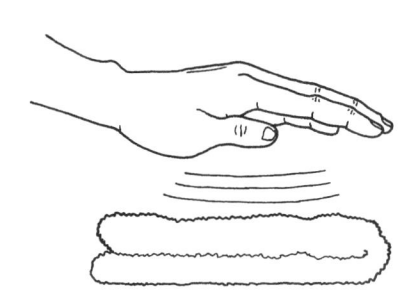

Figure 1.41. Imprinting an image of the palm on x-ray film

Figure 1.42. Changing the acidic component of red litmus paper

5. **Changing the alkaline component of blue litmus paper:** A strip of blue litmus paper is placed inside a glass flask, and floats in an alkaline solution. The student must place his or her hand over the strip of blue litmus paper and emit Qi into the alkaline solution, increasing or decreasing its alkaline nature depending on the examining doctor's request (Figure 1.43).

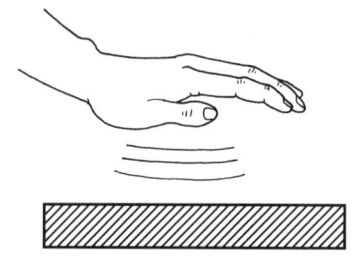

Figure 1.43. Changing the alkaline component of blue litmus paper

MEDICAL QIGONG TRAINING IN THE U. S.

Currently, the most clinically active and academically complete Medical Qigong schools operating within the United States stem from the International Institute of Medical Qigong (I.I.M.Q.), with several branches extending throughout North America, Belgium, Bermuda, Canada, England, France, Ireland, Israel and Sweden (see I.I.M.Q. Academic Directory).

Programs are comprised of three to four years of classes in Medical Qigong therapy, plus clinical internship. Also include are classes, labs, and seminars on Traditional Chinese Medical theory, and the foundations of Chinese medicine for internal diseases according to *the Yellow Emperor's Inner Canon: Magical Pivot and Essential Questions*, and *the Canon of Perplexities*.

Classes include energetic anatomy and physiology, diagnosis and symptomatology, energetic psychology, Qigong pathology and Medical Qigong therapy, Other related modalities include: a basic understanding of herbal medicine, acupuncture therapy, and Chinese massage. Classes in Western anatomy and physiology, Western internal diseases, and health and recovery are also required.

The International Institute of Medical Qigong was founded by Professor Jerry Alan Johnson, Ph.D., D.T.C.M. (China), in 1993. In 1996, the institute was established as a satellite school and an overseas branch of the Medical Qigong college at the Hai Dian University in Beijing China.

MEDICAL QIGONG TRAINING IN T.C.M. COLLEGES

In the Spring of 1999, Professor Johnson accepted the position of Dean of Medical Qigong Science from the Five Branches Institute, College and Clinic of Traditional Chinese Medicine, in Santa Cruz, California. At the Five Branches College, Professor Johnson incorporated two programs from the I.I.M.Q. into the Five Branches T.C.M. curriculum: A two year, 200 hour Medical Qigong Practitioner (M.Q.P.) certification program, and an ongoing Medical Qigong clinic open to the public.

In May of 2003, Professor Johnson accepted the position of Dean of Medical Qigong Science from The Academy For Five Element Acupuncture, in Hallandale, Florida. At the Florida acupuncture college, Professor Johnson incorporated three programs from the I.I.M.Q. into the Five Element T.C.M. curriculum: A 200 hour Medical Qigong Practitioner (M.Q.P.) certification program, A 500 hour Medical Qigong Therapist (M.Q.T.) certification program; and an ongoing Medical Qigong clinic (see Appendix 2 in the back of the book).

Additionally, in August of 2004, Professor Johnson implemented a 200 hour Medical Qigong Practitioner program within the Belgium College of Traditional Chinese Medicine.

In May of 2005, another 200 hour Medical Qigong Practitioner (M.Q.P.) certification program and ongoing Medical Qigong Clinic was started at the Acupuncture and Integrative Medicine College in Berkeley, California (see Appendix 2).

TRADITIONAL CHINESE MEDICINE AND MEDICAL QIGONG THERAPY

Medical Qigong therapy is the oldest of the four branches of Traditional Chinese Medicine and provides the energetic foundation from which the other branches of T.C.M. (acupuncture therapy, herbal therapy, and massage therapy) originated. It is through the energetic understanding inherent in Medical Qigong practice that the other

CHAPTER 1: INTRODUCTION TO MEDICAL QIGONG

Four Main Branches of Traditional Chinese Medicine

- Acupuncture Therapy
  1. Needling
  2. Cupping
  3. Bloodletting
  4. Moxa Burning
  5. Magnet Therapy

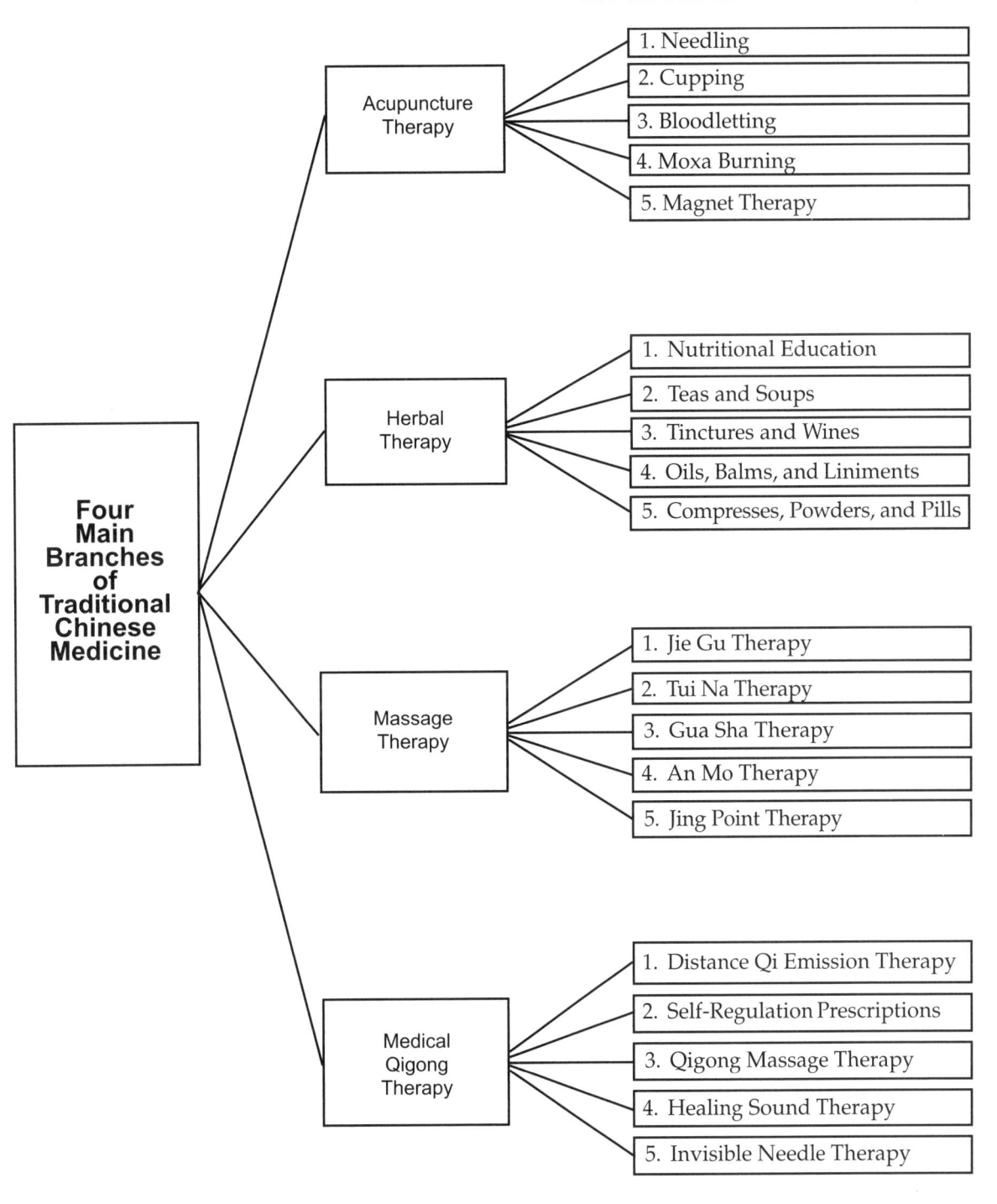

- Herbal Therapy
  1. Nutritional Education
  2. Teas and Soups
  3. Tinctures and Wines
  4. Oils, Balms, and Liniments
  5. Compresses, Powders, and Pills

- Massage Therapy
  1. Jie Gu Therapy
  2. Tui Na Therapy
  3. Gua Sha Therapy
  4. An Mo Therapy
  5. Jing Point Therapy

- Medical Qigong Therapy
  1. Distance Qi Emission Therapy
  2. Self-Regulation Prescriptions
  3. Qigong Massage Therapy
  4. Healing Sound Therapy
  5. Invisible Needle Therapy

Figure 1.44. The Four Main Branches of Traditional Chinese Medicine

branches of Traditional Chinese Medicine become elevated to a spiritual path of self-realization and internal transformation (Figure 1.44). Doctors of Traditional Chinese Medicine address the patients' physical, energetic, and spiritual needs simultaneously. According to the principles of Traditional Chinese Medicine, the root cause of all disease can be traced to a critical imbalance within the body's vital energies. Therefore, the best way to prevent or cure disease requires establishing a healthy energetic balance and harmony between the body's energy field and the forces of nature and the cosmos.

Traditional Chinese Medicine is divided into four branches of healing: Acupuncture, Herbology and Dietetics, Massage therapy, and Medical Qigong therapy. All of the four main branches are built on the same foundation of energetic diagnosis known as the "Five Main Roots of Traditional Chinese Medicine." The Five Main Roots are the theoretical framework used for internal organ diagnosis, and are described as follows: Six Stages Theory, Five Element Theory, Eight Principles Theory, Triple Burners Theory, and Four Levels Theory.

Acupuncture

According to historical records, the use of stone acupuncture needles and moxibustion in China dates as far back as the New Stone Age. Later, bone

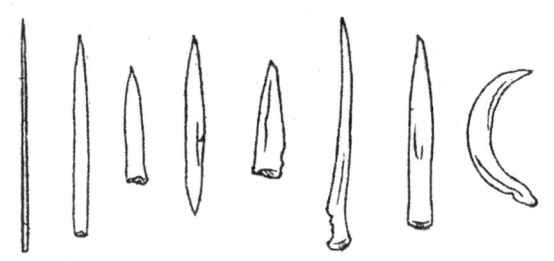

Figure 1.45. Ancient Bone Needles used in Acupuncture Treatments

and bamboo needles were commonly used as acupuncture instruments (Figure 1. 45). When the ancient Chinese began to use pottery, ceramic needles entered into the clinic, and were used to puncture certain shallow points on the skin.

The shapes, lengths and uses of "nine special needles" were written about during the Warring States Period (475-221 B.C.), and described in the *Huangdi Neijing*. These nine ancient needles are described as follows (Figure 1.46):

- **Di Needles:** These needles are used for pressing
- **Rounded Needles:** These needles are used to massage certain points
- **Round and Sharp Needles:** These needles are used for quick puncturing
- **Chun Needles:** These needles are used for piercing shallow points

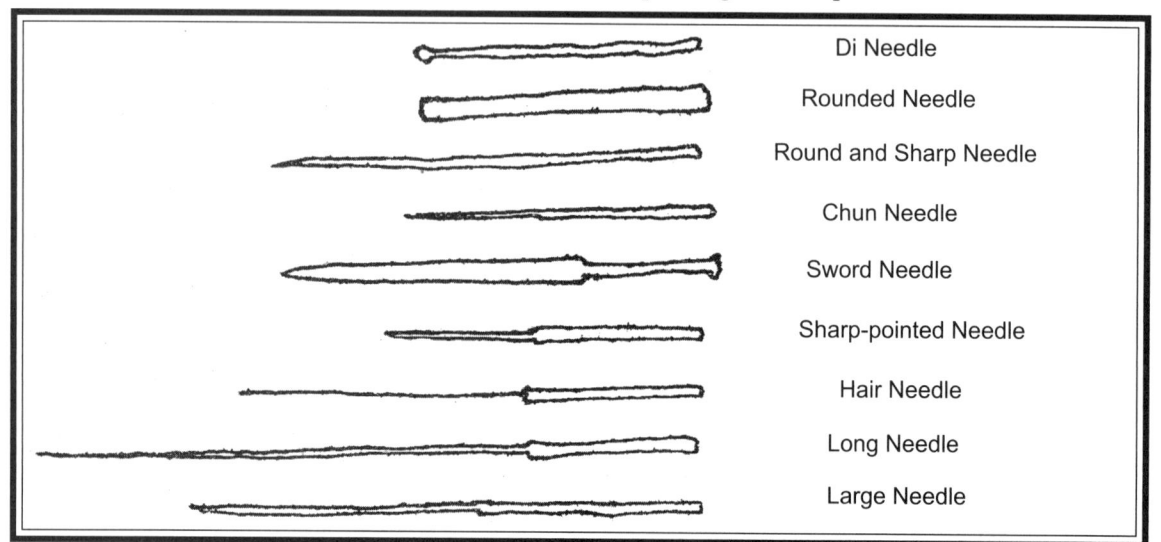

Figure 1.46. The Nine Ancient Bone Needles

- **Sword Needles:** These needles are used for cutting and discharging pus
- **Sharp-pointed Needles:** These needles are used for bloodletting
- **Hair Needles:** These needles are used for a variety of applications
- **Long Needles:** These needles are used for puncturing thick muscles
- **Large Needles:** These needles are used for puncturing joints

The specific application of these nine needles expanded the clinical practice and potential uses of acupuncture therapy. By inserting various types of needles into specific points, the acupuncturist would manipulate the patient's Qi in order to achieve an overall energetic and physical balance. In an acute or emergency situation, the life threatening symptoms were treated first, after which the focus was directed to disperse and remove stagnations, strengthen deficient conditions, and then return the patient's energetic fields and physical tissues back to a state of harmony.

The acupuncture points are specific areas within the body and on the body's surface where Qi emerges from deep energetic pools within the body's organs and tissues. The Qi moves along specific pathways known as channels and collaterals. Collaterals are the smaller streams of Qi that branch from the main energetic rivers (the meridians or channels). Each primary channel takes its name from one of the six Yin or six Yang organs to which it corresponds. Each organ has two channels, one on each side of the body.

Often in Chinese medical diagrams, one will see abbreviations referring to specific energetic points. The names of these points are based upon the specific channel on which the point lies and its location along the channel. The first points on each side of the Gall Bladder channels (GB), for example, are "GB-1." Some channels contain over 60 points, each numbered sequentially from beginning to end. These points are also given descriptive names according to their location and energetic affect upon the body when treated. The GB-1 points, for example, are located next to the eyes, on the outer canthus, level with the pupils, and are called Tongziliao, or "pupil's seam."

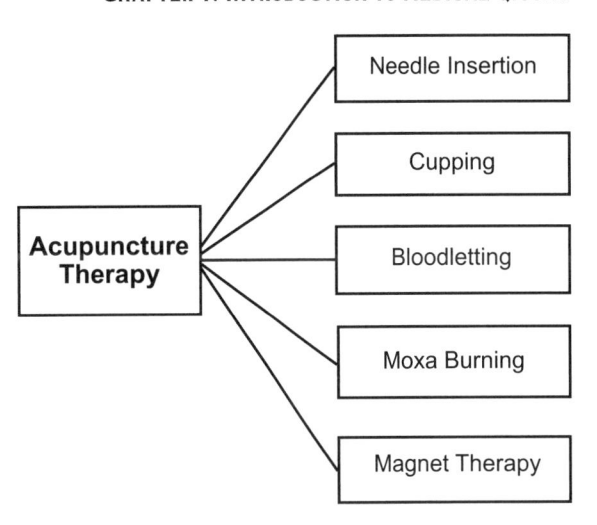

Figure 1.47. The Five Main Branches of Chinese Acupuncture Therapy

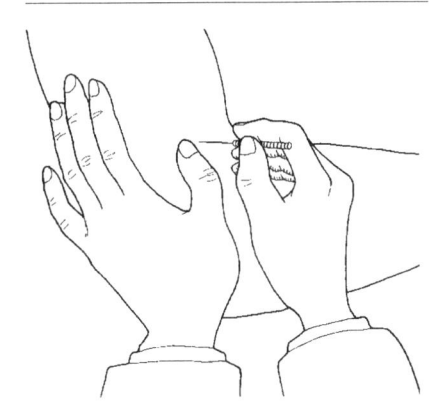

Figure 1.48. A doctor inserts an acupuncture needle into the patient's channel point. Acupuncture needles of various sizes are used to stimulate the energy flow for the tonification of Deficient Qi or the reduction of Excess Qi.

Acupuncture therapy includes five major treatment techniques: needling, cupping, bloodletting, moxa burning, and magnet healing, described as follows (Figure 1.47):

1. **Needle Insertion Therapy** utilizes acupuncture needles of various sizes that are inserted into channel points. These points are tiny areas where the Qi pools along the streams of an energy channel. The use of needles stimulates the nerves and energy flow to Tonify Deficient Qi or reduce Excess Qi (Figure 1.48).

2. **Cupping Therapy** utilizes wooden, clay, or glass cups that adhere to the patient's skin through suction. This suction drains and removes pathogenic Qi via the body's pores. This technique can also be used to tonify specific areas of the body. This modality of treatment has been successfully combined with bloodletting to treat acute sprains accompanied by Blood stagnation (Figure 1.49).

3. **Bloodletting Therapy** is induced with instruments such as Blood needles or seven- and five-star hammers to remove Toxic Qi, Blood stagnation, Heat, and other pathogenic factors. The hammer has five to seven sharp projections that pierce the skin. The doctor pricks the points and superficial channels to cause slight bleeding (sometimes called cutaneous needle puncturing). The acupuncturist diagnoses and then monitors the patient's condition by the different shades of the patient's Blood. Trapped or diseased Blood (usually dark red or black) is released until a healthy color is observed (ruby red). This therapy is considered useful for treating disorders of the nervous system, physical trauma, and extremely serious febrile diseases (Figure 1.50).

4. **Moxa Burning Therapy** consists of three types of ignited herbal therapy: moxa cones, rolled moxa sticks, and moxa that is inserted on top of acupuncture needles. The moxa herb (mugwort) is held over specific channel points to infuse heat and Qi into specific body areas for tonification and improving immune function. This technique is also used to expel Cold in order to disperse Blood stagnation (Figure 1.51).

5. **Magnetic Therapy** utilizes magnetic patches or strips that are attached to various points on the channels of the patient's body to stimulate a response in the electromagnetic field. The magnets are applied to specific points for a period of 3–5 days, removed for one day, then reapplied. Whether used for tonification or sedation, this therapy facilitates constant treatment of the channel point. Magnet therapy has been used since the Tang Dynasty (618–907 A.D.) (Figure 1.52).

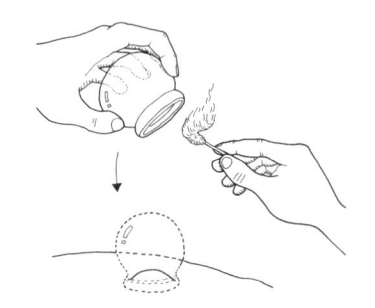

Figure 1.49. In cupping, heated air is directed into wooden, clay, or glass cups which are then placed on the patient's skin. The rapidly cooling air creates a suction force that drains and removes pathogenic Qi to the body's surface and out the pores.

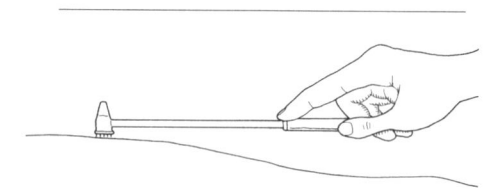

Figure 1.50. The doctor lightly taps with the Five-Star Hammer that has five sharp projections to pierce the skin and cause slight bleeding. The color of the patient's blood provides the doctor with information about the patient's condition.

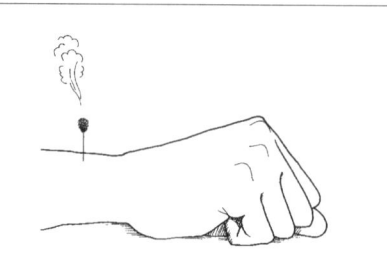

Figure 1.51. The doctor inserts a needle with burning moxa (herbal cones/sticks) on top of it. Burning moxa may also be held over specific channel points or placed directly on the skin.

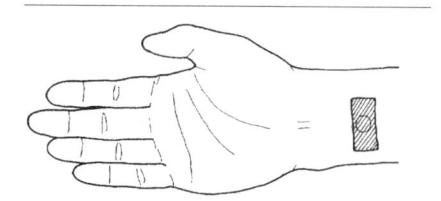

Figure 1.52. A magnetic patch is worn on the wrist. Magnets may be attached to various parts of the body or may be worn in shoes or wristbands.

HERBOLOGY

Herbal formulas have been used successfully to treat a variety of illnesses for over 5000 years. Much of the Chinese medical research on pharmacology organized during the Qin (221-206 B.C.) and Han (206 B.C.-220 A.D.) Dynasties was recorded in the *Canon of Materia Medica of Shen Nong* (also known as the Canon of Herbal Medicine). In this text, it contained 252 plants, 67 animals, and 46 minerals, and included a brief description of the places of each herb's origin, secondary names, the specific forms and properties of each herb, and the curative powers of each part of the plant, animal or mineral (Figure 1.53).

Historically, herbal medicine was the precursor of pharmaceutical medicines in most cultures. Today, herbs still provide the source and inspiration for the majority of the pharmaceuticals used in modern Western medicine, including those utilized for the treatment of viral and bacterial diseases, pain, tumors, chronic diseases, internal and external tissue regeneration, and many other infirmities.

Herbology is both a science and an art. An herbalist spends many years studying the herbs used to create herbal formulas. The herbalist must also understand the energetic effects of each individual herb, and their synergistic effects when combined.

Herbs can be used for tonifying, purging, dispersing, warming, cooling, nourishing the Yin, nourishing the Yang, and clearing heat, as well as moving Qi, Blood, Phlegm, and Fluids within the body. They cause the Qi in the body to either ascend or descend, affecting the upper or lower portions of the body. Thus, Chinese herbs are categorized according to the nature and effect that they produce on the Qi of the body.

Chinese medicine prescribes specific parts of plants (flowers, leaves, stems, seeds, roots, bark, etc.) for particular medicinal purposes. Parts of trees, shrubs, herbs, vines, and flowers are selected for their specific properties (hot, warm, neutral, cool, and cold) and taste (sour, bitter, sweet, pungent, and salty). These properties either tonify or disperse Qi and Blood.

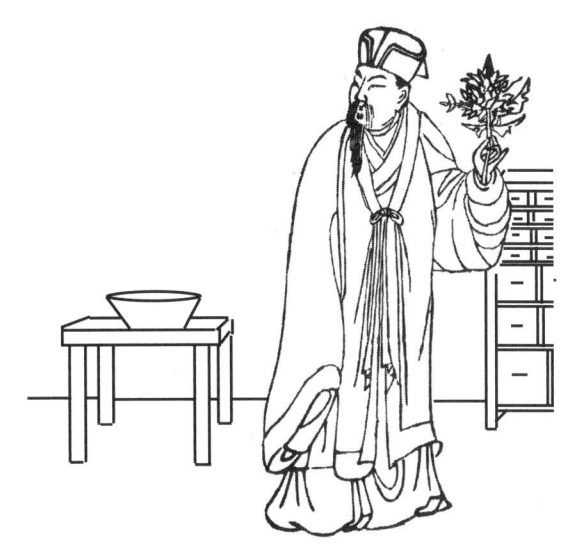

Figure 1.53. Herbology is both a science and an art

Chinese medical herbology includes the cultivation and gathering of seeds, grains, fruits, flowers, leaves, barks, stems, and roots. Non-herbal components such as minerals, fish, animals, or insect parts are sometimes added to enhance the herbs' healing effect.

Chinese herbs cure energetically by moving Qi in the channels. Each herb enters specific channels and affects different internal organs. Herbs are therefore an extremely powerful healing modality. The herbalist uses herbs to tonify (strengthen) and move Qi and Blood as well as eliminate heat from the patient's Blood. When tailored to an individual's constitution or combined into a formula for specific symptoms, herbs can be an invaluable aid in restoring and maintaining the health of the body. Taking an improper herb or herbal formula can have potentially deleterious effects.

Chinese herbal therapy includes five major clinical applications: nutritional education (food and diet); teas and soups (tang); tinctures and wines (jin); oils, balms, and liniments (you and gao); and compresses, powders (san), and pills (wan), which are described as follows (Figure 1.54):

1. **Nutritional Education** is stressed to assist patients in choosing foods for the body's nour-

ishment and optimum health, as well as for the treatment of disease. Foods have many healing properties similar to herbs and can be used as seasonal prescriptions. An old Chinese saying stresses the importance of diet by asking the question, "Are herbs food or food herbs?"

2. **Teas and Soups** are water-based herbal formulas traditionally prepared from raw or processed herbal ingredients. These are traditionally ingested for the treatment of internal and external disorders whether acute or chronic in nature.

3. **Tinctures and Wines** are both alcohol-based herbal formulas. Tinctures are concentrated alcohol-based formulas prepared from raw herbs that are used in small doses for treatment (similar to teas and soups). Wines are traditionally applied externally to alleviate pain or ingested as a tonic, depending on the specific formula and the disease being treated.

4. **Oils, Balms, and Liniments** are oil-based herbal formulas usually applied externally for the treatment of muscle, tendon, and ligament trauma, to alleviate pain, disperse Excess Qi, or to draw Qi into specific areas for tonification.

5. **Compresses, Powders, and Pills** consist of herbs that have been pulverized into a powder. Compresses are made into a paste or poultice and are then applied externally for the treatment of acute or chronic injuries. Powdered herbs can also be formed into teas, crackers, cakes, pastries and honey-based candies. They are ingested for internal organ tonification and rebalancing of the body's energy systems. Pills are herbs specifically prepared from traditional formulas, rolled into little balls, and orally ingested for the treatment of internal disorders.

SUPERIOR, MEDIUM AND INFERIOR HERBS

Up until the Song Dynasty (960-1279 A.D.), Chinese herbs (Materia Medica) were traditionally grouped into three classes: superior herbs, medium herbs and inferior herbs (see Volume 2, Chapter 13), described as follows (Figure 1.55):

• **Superior Herbs:** These herbs consisted of 120

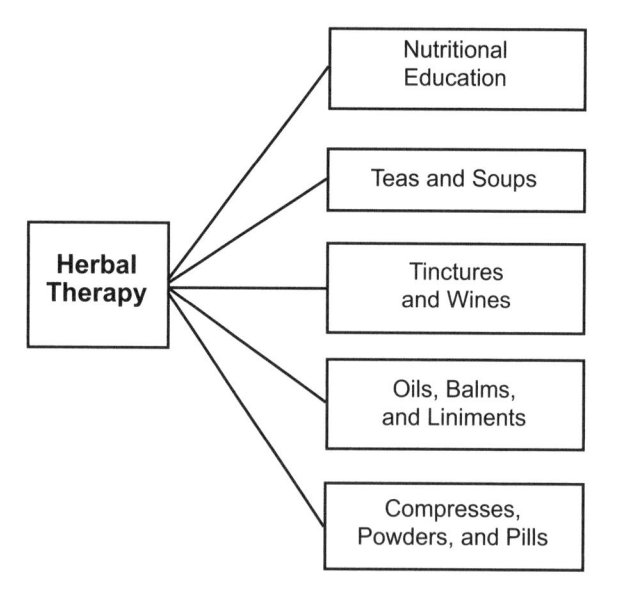

Figure 1.54. The Five Main Branches of Chinese Herbal Therapy

varieties of superior types of medical substances. Considered in ancient times as the "ruling medicines," these herbs were said to cause the individual to awaken his or her innate vital powers and help to fulfill the person's life purpose. Superior herbs were also said to have a beneficial effect on the body's Jing, Qi and Shen by making the body light, preventing old age, prolonging life, forestalling hunger and creating advanced spirit travel abilities. An example of a Superior herb is knotted fungus.

• **Medium Herbs:** These herbs consisted of 120 varieties of moderate types of medical substances. Considered in ancient times as "ministerial medicines," these herbs were said to enrich and nurture the individual's essential nature, replenish deficiencies and cure illnesses. These herbs, however, should not be taken over a long period of time. A few examples of Medium herbs are bitter ginseng, Chinese angelica, and scallions.

• **Inferior Herbs:** These herbs consisted of 120 varieties of inferior types of medical substances. Considered in ancient times as "assistant medicines," these herbs are mostly

CHAPTER 1: INTRODUCTION TO MEDICAL QIGONG

Superior Herbs "Ruling Medicines"	Awaken innate vital powers and help people fulfill their life purpose
Medium Herbs "Ministerial Medicines"	Enrich and nurtur the individual's essential nature, replenish deficiencies and cure illnesses
Inferior Herbs "Assistant Medicines"	Toxic herbs, used to treat Qi, Blood and Body Fluids

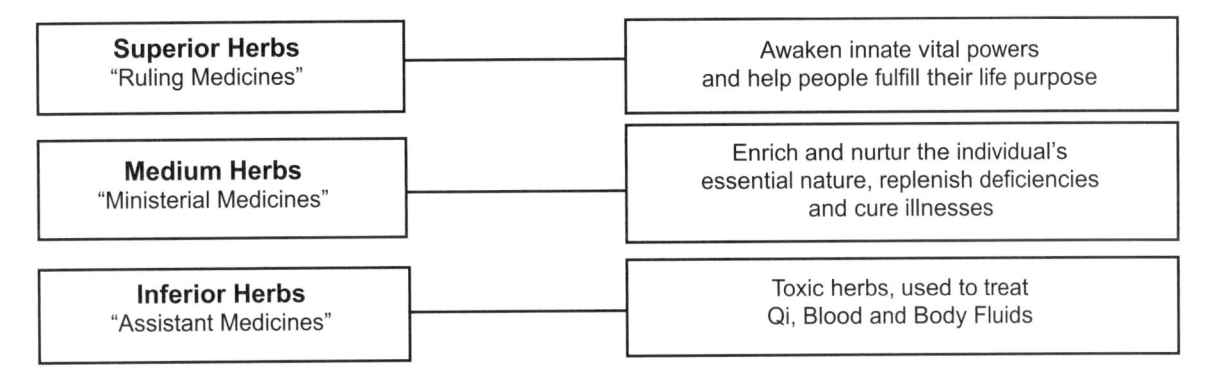

Figure 1.55. The Three Traditional Classes of Chinese Herbs (Materia Medica)

toxic and must be taken with precautions when used to treat an individual's disease. Inferior herbs were said to have an effect on the body's Qi, Blood and Fluids. A few examples of Inferior herbs are aconite, peach pit, and plum pit.

During China's Six Dynasties period (420-581 A.D.), the main concern of a doctor was maintaining a patient's health by means of diet, herbal prescriptions and physical exercise. As a result, two types of medical literature developed in China: books that focused on nourishing life and the classics of diet.

CHINESE MASSAGE THERAPY

Chinese Massage Therapy is a term used to describe all tissue manipulation techniques currently used in the People's Republic of China. In ancient China, during the Qin (221-206 B.C.) and Han (206 B.C.-220 A.D.) Dynasties, several books on the clinical use of massage were compiled. For example, according to historical records, a ten-volume treatise, known as *The Massage of Huang Di and Qi Bo* was written, revealing the effective clinical applications of specific massage techniques. In 1973 A.D., *Prescriptions for 52 Cases* was unearthed in a tomb from the Han Dynasty. This book included documentation of massage therapy used to treat and cure specific chronic diseased states and acute first aid. By the Northern Wei Dynasty (386-533 A.D.), Massage Therapy had become part of the four official medical departments within China's imperial medical colleges.

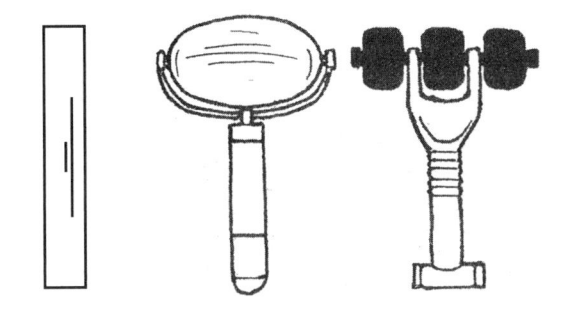

Figure 1.56. Ancient Chinese Massage Tools

Chinese Massage Therapy consists of five popular systems that include manipulation of the skin, muscles, tendons, joints, nerves, and inner fascia, in addition to the manipulation of the body's internal organs and organ systems.

Ancient Chinese Massage Therapy is the historical and inspirational source of modern Swedish massage, Shiatsu, myofascial trigger point therapy, reflexology, chiropractic therapy, osteopathy and neuromuscular therapy.

As a clinical modality, Chinese Massage Therapy can be used either as a preventative treatment or to heal acute and chronic injuries. Chinese Massage Therapy focuses on improving the structural alignment of the body and on healing soft-tissue injuries. By applying specific methods of tissue manipulation, obstructions in the channels' pathways can be removed, thus promoting and increasing the circulation of Qi and Blood (Figure 1.56). It also corrects deviant functions of the internal organs, nerves, and joints. These treat-

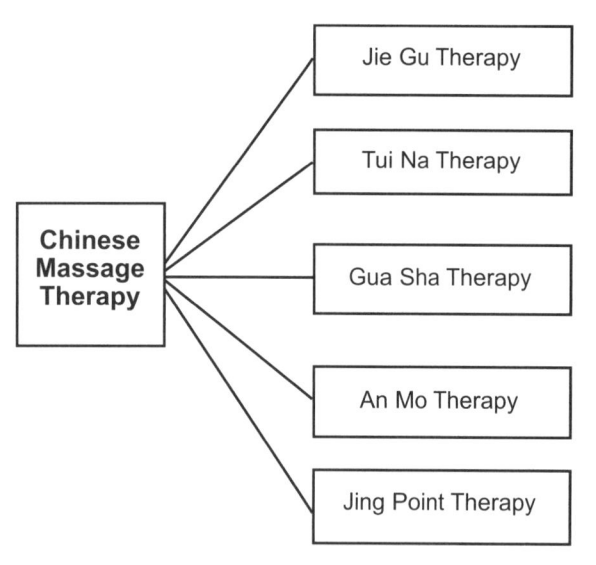

VOLUME 1, SECTION 1: FOUNDATIONS OF CHINESE ENERGETIC MEDICINE

Figure 1.57. The Five Main Branches of Chinese Massage

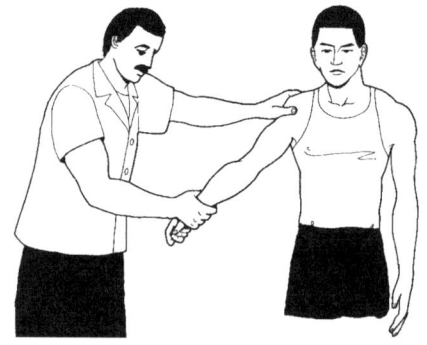

Figure 1.58. Jie Gu Therapy is used to set the bones and ligaments in order to unblock and release trapped junctions of Qi and Blood at the patient's joints.

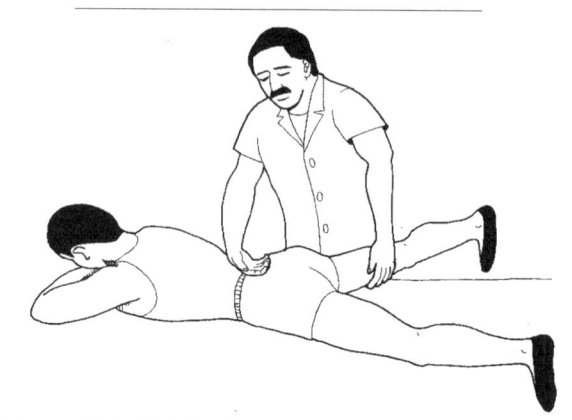

Figure 1.59. Tui Na Therapy is used to adjust the muscles and focuses on external tissue manipulation of the muscles and tendons in order to correct abnormal Qi circulation within the body's muscular system.

ment modalities utilized in Chinese Massage are similar to those used in chiropractic, osteopathy, Western physical therapy, and sports massage therapy.

Chinese Massage Therapy is divided into five different schools of instruction: Jie Gu, Tui Na, Gua Sha, An Mo, and Jing Point therapy. Jie Gu, Tui Na, and Gua Sha employ external tissue manipulations; these three external manipulations are used to treat the Bones, muscles, ligaments, and tendons, and also to treat fevers. An Mo and Jing Point therapy utilize soft-tissue manipulation and are used primarily to treat disorders of the internal organs and energy pathways (Figure 1.57).

1. **Jie Gu Therapy** is used for bone setting and to adjust the patient's body alignment. The literal translation for Jie Gu is "knotted bone," which describes the art of manipulating the Bones and ligaments to unblock and release the trapped junctions of Blood and Qi channels in the patient's joints (Figure 1.58).
2. **Tui Na Therapy** focuses on external tissue manipulation and the adjustment of the muscles and tendons to correct abnormal Qi circulation within the body's muscular system. Tui Na is translated as "push and grasp," and was developed primarily for correcting the misalignment of the body's Bones and muscles due to traumatic physical injuries. The popular practice of "reflexology" is historically rooted in the use of Tui Na therapy in Chinese pediatric care (Figure 1.59).
3. **Gua Sha Therapy** is used to regulate febrile conditions, such as flu, cholera and malaria, and to treat trauma and musculoskeletal conditions. Gua is translated as "to scrape or scratch" and Sha is defined as "cholera," or sand-like maculae (referring to the red discoloration that is raised on the skin by the application of scraping). This therapy focuses on external surface tissue scraping, usually on the

posterior aspect of the neck and thoracic areas (Figure 1.60).

Gua Sha Therapy is commonly used for promoting Qi and Blood circulation, removing toxins, clearing heat, cooling the Blood, removing stagnation, and dissolving masses. A jade scraper (a spoon or utensil with smooth edges will do) is used for purifying the Qi and transforming the Shen (Spirit). A water buffalo horn is commonly used for pulling heat and toxins from the patient's body (occasionally ceramic is used, but never glass or plastic).

4. **An Mo Therapy** is used for internal organ regulation. An Mo focuses primarily on Qi extension and soft-tissue and internal organ manipulation. Although the literal translation means to "press and rub," this therapy focuses primarily on internal visceral manipulation, concentrating directly on the treatment of specific internal diseases (Figure 1.61).

5. **Jing Point Therapy** is employed for channel and internal organ regulation. Jing point therapy uses pressing, pinching, clapping, and tapping techniques on specific energetic points and energetic channels. These techniques are used to promote Qi and Blood circulation, balance the body's Yin and Yang energy, tonify weak organs, dredge the channels, and expel pathogenic factors (Figure 1.62).

MEDICAL QIGONG THERAPY

Over the past two millennia, many doctors of Tradition Chinese Medicine, martial arts masters, monks and priests have contributed to the expansion of Chinese Medical Qigong. The objectives for healing disease in Medical Qigong training are as follows:

- First, eliminate internal pathogenic factors (the accumulation of excessive emotions such as anger, grief, worry, fear, etc.) as well as external pathogenic factors (the invasion of Cold, Hot, Damp, etc., from the environment).
- Second, increase or decrease the patient's relative Qi levels, as needed to counteract the deficient or excess condition within the internal organs and channels.

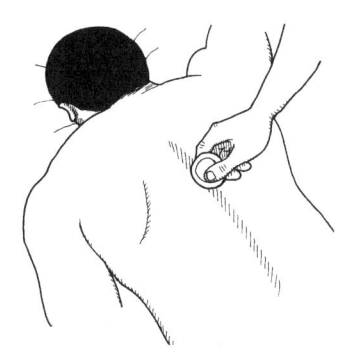

Figure 1.60. Gua Sha Therapy is commonly used for clearing heat, cooling the blood, removing stagnant Qi and Blood, and dissolving masses.

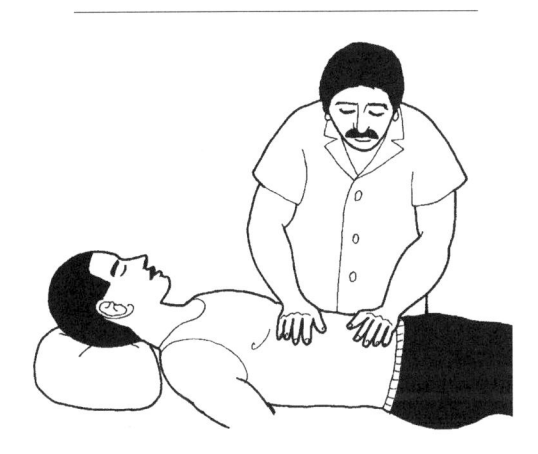

Figure 1.61. An Mo Therapy allows for internal visceral regulation and concentrates directly on treating specific Internal organ diseases.

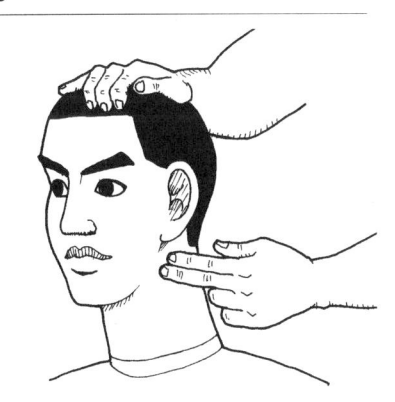

Figure 1.62. Jing Point Therapy is used to promote Qi and Blood circulation, balance the body's Yin and Yang energy, tonify weak organs, dredge the channels, and expel pathogenic factors.

- Third, regulate and balance the patient's Yin and Yang energy to bring the body into harmony.

Medical Qigong therapy consists of regulating the body's three external Wei Qi fields (physical, mental/emotional and spiritual), and the four internal fields of life-force energy (Wind of Nurturing Qi, Sea of Blood, Sea of Marrow, and the center core Taiji Pole). Some of the most common diseases treated in Medical Qigong clinics are: diabetes, arthritis, high blood pressure, breast and ovarian cysts and tumors, migraine headaches, fibromyalgia, insomnia, acute abdominal pain, prostatitis, irritable bowel syndrome, deep tissue obstruction, muscle atrophy, brain tumors, stroke, coma retrieval, and certain types of cancer. The Medical Qigong treatment focuses on relieving pain, detoxifying the body of toxic emotions (e.g., excessive anger, fear, worry, etc.), correcting internal organ dysfunctions, and balancing excess or deficient Qi and Blood conditions.

Ancient Chinese Medical Qigong therapy was divided into three levels of treatment, corresponding to Heaven, Earth and Man. Which clinical methods and internal powers were used depended on the healer's own personal internal cultivation and understanding of energetic and spiritual principles. Medical Qigong Therapy is where the medical skills of treating patients and the energetic and spiritual intuitive skills of shamanism united, creating a complete and balanced form of energetic medicine.

Medical Qigong therapy uses five major clinical modalities: Distance Qi Emission Therapy, Self-Regulation Prescriptions, Qigong Massage Therapy, Healing Sound Therapy, and Invisible Needle Therapy (Figure 1.63).

1. **Distance Qi Emission** requires the Qigong doctor to manipulate a patient's Qi by focusing on the energetic properties of the patient's channels, collaterals, and points, as well as internal organs, from a distance of several inches, several feet, or even many miles away (Figure 1.64).
2. **Self-Regulation Prescriptions** are Qigong exercises that include Dao Yin postures, movements, respiratory patterns, sound vibrations, and mental visualizations. Medical Qigong Prescription Exercises are given to patients to augment the benefits of a Medical Qigong treatment. Patients then use these Qigong techniques to regulate and maintain their own health between treatments, using various lying, sitting, standing and moving postures. The patients may also use their own spiritual belief system as a healing tool (Figure 1.65).
3. **Qigong Massage** is a soft-tissue regulation technique that differs from Tui Na or An Mo (Chinese external massage therapy), in that

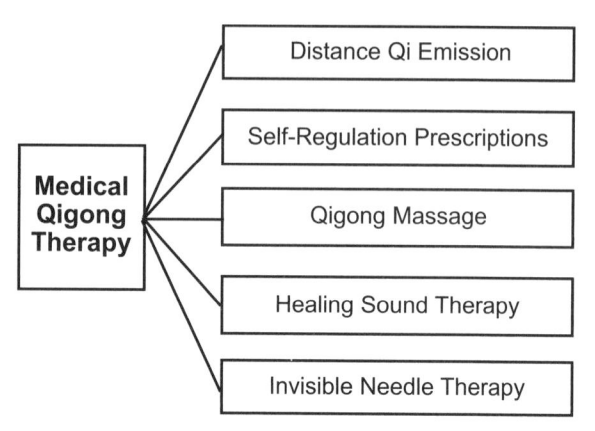

Figure 1.63. The Five Main Branches of Chinese Medical Qigong Therapy

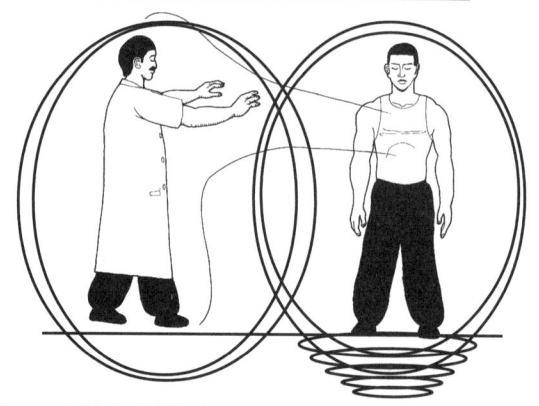

Figure 1.64. In Qi Emission Therapy, the Qigong doctor manipulates a patient's Qi by focusing on the energetic properties of the patient's channels, collaterals, and points from a distance of several inches, several feet, or even many miles.

CHAPTER 1: INTRODUCTION TO MEDICAL QIGONG

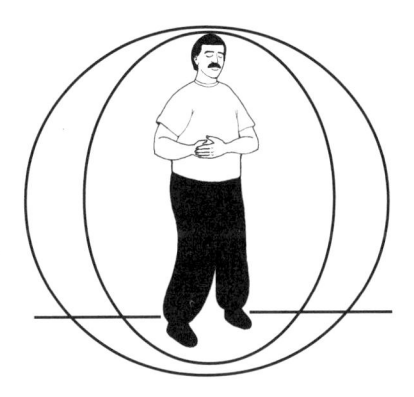

Figure 1.65. In Self-Regulation Prescriptions, the patients are required to self-regulate by performing Medical Qigong prescription exercises (postures, movements, breathing exercises, sounds, visualizations, etc.). Here the patient regulates his own Liver Qi.

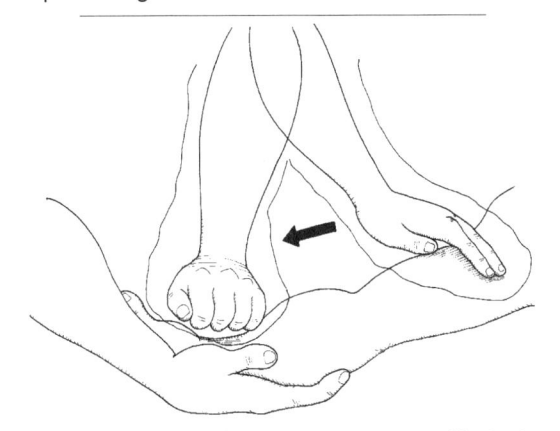

Figure 1.66. In Qigong Massage, the doctor softly dredges the patient's external channels in order to release stagnant energy from the internal channels, which serve as pathways for Qi transference.

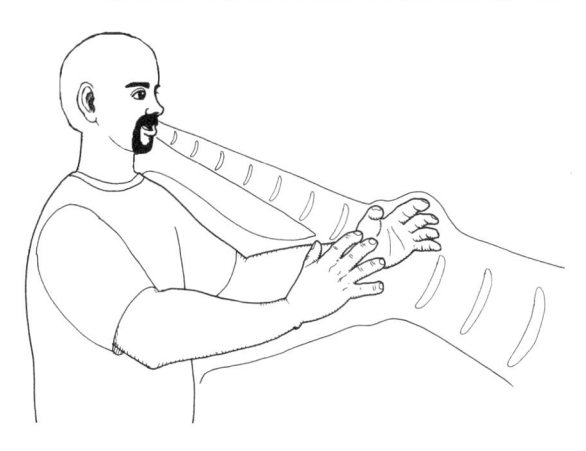

Figure 1.67. With Healing Sound Therapy, the doctor projects his or her voice deep into the patient's tissues, creating a vibrational resonance that purges the stagnant energy trapped deep within the viscera.

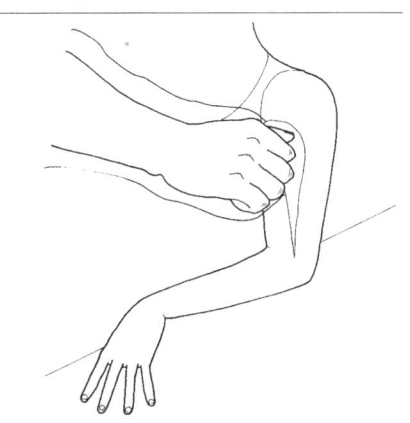

Figure 1.68. In Invisible Needle Therapy, the doctor visualizes inserting energetic acupuncture needles into the patient's channel points in order to stimulate the patient's Qi.

the doctor's hand skims the patient's body as lightly as a feather, never exceeding the pressure one would place on an eyeball. The light skimming action is used to dredge the patient's external channel Qi, causing energy to be released from the internal channels themselves which serve as pathways for Qi transference (Figure 1.66).
4. **Healing Sound Therapy** is one of the most powerful tools used in Medical Qigong for breaking up energetic stagnations. It requires the doctor to project sound vibration deep into the patient's tissues. When the sound resonation penetrates the patient's body it causes massive chaotic vibrational patterns that disrupt the body's accepted "normal" energetic flow. This energetic disruption softens and liquefies the patient's stagnant Qi, making it easier to purge and disperse (Figure 1.67).
5. **Invisible Needle Therapy** involves the visualization of energetic needles of light being inserted into specific points on the patient's body. The needles of light are used to stimulate and direct the patient's Qi (Figure 1.68).

Chapter 2
Understanding Ancient Chinese Metaphysics

Introduction

In 1993, when I began my internship at the Xi Yuan Hospital in Beijing, China. I became aware that most Chinese Medical Qigong doctors took a different approach to basic Western anatomy and physiology than that which is commonly encountered in the United States. When I asked why more attention was not paid to the subject I was told, "The perspective and priority we place on gross physical anatomy and physiology is quite different from yours -- Westerners only study the dead -- we study life, the living pools, rivers, and currents of life-force energy that can only be found in the living body."

Ancient Chinese medicine believed that when an individual dies, the substance or energy that gave the body life returns to its original source (back to Heaven and Earth), and all that remains of the individual is a mass of lifeless tissue. In this model, the tangible and the energetic exist in a binary, cohesive relationship.

When studying Chinese energetic medicine, a Qigong doctor must understand the concept of "life-force energy" in order to comprehend, diagnose, treat and prescribe the appropriate form of Medical Qigong therapy for the patient.

The concept of the energetic formation of the human body is new to Western thought, which has primarily focused on that which is physically tangible. The philosophical foundation of Traditional Chinese Medicine, on the other hand, includes the study of the whole human being with all of his or her aspects: physical, mental, emotional, energetic, and spiritual. This concept of energetic anatomy focuses not only on understanding the tangible physical form of human tissue, but also on comprehending the various contributing vitality and energetic fields that affect and govern the body (Figure 2.1). In China, Medical Qigong doctors continually study the effects of these energies, as well as their interrelationship with Heavenly and Earthly energetic influences.

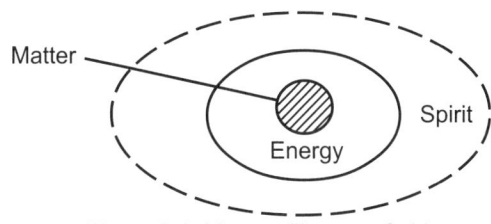

Figure 2.1. Matter - Energy - Spirit

In 1998, while visiting with friends at a local Medical Qigong Clinic in Beijing, I was fortunate to spend the entire day with a "founding father" of the World Academic Society of Medical Qigong. We spoke at great length about ancient Chinese Medicine, the energetic formation of existence, the descent of the Eternal Soul (Shen Xian) and the creation of the Human Soul (Yuan Shen). I would like to now present this great grandmaster's gift of insights into ancient Daoist forbidden knowledge regarding energetic and spiritual transformations.

The first part of this chapter will explore early Chinese understandings of the medical, energetic and spiritual aspects of the formation of the universe. This will include the original concepts of the Dao (Divine), Wuji (Infinite Space), Taiji (Yin and Yang), Bagua (Eight Trigrams), Wu Xing (Five Phases) and the three worlds of spirit, energy and matter.

The second part of this chapter will explore ancient Chinese understandings of the medical, energetic and spiritual aspects of the formation of the human body. This includes the ancient concepts of the Dao (Divine), Shen Ling (Supernatural Spirit), Zhi Yi Tian (the Will and Intent of Heaven), Shen Xian (Eternal Soul), Yuan Shen (Original Soul), Wu Jing Shen (Five Essence Spirits), Shen Zhi (Soul's acquired personality), energetic embryology (from conception to birth), and the three bodies of matter, energy and spirit.

The Energetic Formation of the Universe

Throughout the history of ancient China, there have been numerous theories as to creation of "Heaven, Earth and Man," as well as the creation and formation of the human soul.

The following ancient Daoist theory flourished during the Spring and Autumn Period (770-476 B.C.) in China. The theory begins with the concept of the Dao.

The Dao: Divine

The ancient Chinese believed that all life emerged from the Dao's eternal existence and would someday dissolve back into its infinite light. According to Guan Zi, the Prime Minister of the State of Qi, who lived during the Spring and Autumn Period (770-476 B.C.), "the Dao has neither root nor stem, no leaf nor flower, but all ten thousand things are born of and grow from it. It comes to rest in the compassionate Heart. In the tranquil Mind and harmonized Qi is where the Dao abides."

The Dao, or "Way," can be translated both as a spiritual approach to the Divine, or as the infinitely subtle realm and presence of the Divine underlying all things. According to ancient Chinese esoteric teachings, the energetic vibration and light pertaining to the Dao (Divine) is imprinted in every particle, and that whatever exists (i.e. all of creation) is simply an expression and manifestation of the Divine (Figure 2.2).

The Dao is also believed to be in every single particle of "Mind;" the Mind being the means through which the Divine manifests itself. The "Mind" exists as an infinite ocean of vibration within the Wuji (infinite space), ranging from the "highest" levels of vibration, down to the gross material plane.

The ancient Chinese believed that before conception, an individual existed as an integral part of the Dao. We were with the Divine, formless and undifferentiated, and not subject to the physical laws of birth, growth, death or decay. At conception, we became less conscious of this connection, and the "Way" therefore refers to making the journey back to conscious wholeness and integration with the cosmic order of creation and with the Divine after our birth.

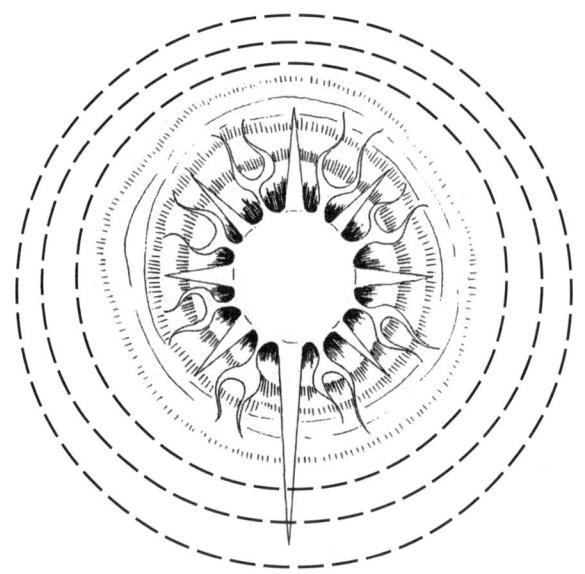

Figure 2.2. The Infinite Dao or Divine

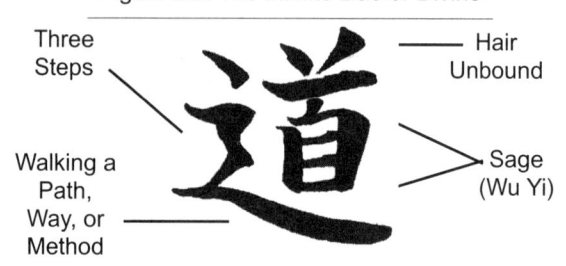

Figure 2.3. The Chinese character for "Dao," The Way of Harmony with Heaven, Earth and the Divine

- Three Steps
- Hair Unbound
- Walking a Path, Way, or Method
- Sage (Wu Yi)

The Concept of "Dao" Ideogram

The ancient Chinese character for Dao depicts a wise sage, with hair unbound (like that of the Wu Yi) walking a path, way, method, or principle (Figure 2.3). It was viewed by many ancient Daoist Qigong masters as an act of deliberately evoking something through magic rather than a symbolic gesture. The "path" is associated with the three footsteps, evoking a magical dance step (traditionally the left "Yang" foot begins the ritual, facing south and moves towards the eastern rising sun). Therefore, the ideograph suggests that the action is made by one who possesses privileged knowledge with directed purpose.

The ancient meaning conveyed by this ideograph can be translated as "the way that one comes to see and understand oneself in relationship with the universe or cosmos (Heaven), environment (Earth) and the Divine." The study of ancient Chinese Daoism was not a religion, but a way and means of maintaining the harmony between this world (the Physical Plane) and the worlds beyond (the Energetic and Spiritual Planes).

THREE ENERGETIC SUBDIVISIONS OF THE DAO

Within its vast energetic sea, the Dao gives birth to two energetic polarities, Heaven (Yang) and Earth (Yin). The Yang energy of Heaven arises from the sea of primordial chaos, radiating downward, with an active quality. The Yin energy of Earth, being passive, receives and interacts energetically with the influences of Heaven.

The concept of "Dao" in Medical Qigong can be better understood by observing its energetic influence as three subdivisions: the Dao of Heaven, the Dao of Earth, and the Dao of Man. Each of these energetic realities fits into the other's energetic form, creating a multidimensional unity (Figure 2.4). The energetic fields of Heaven (created from the energetic influences of the sun, moon and stars) envelop and affect the energetic fields of the Earth (causing energetic movement within the wind, water and soil); the energetic fields of the Earth in turn envelop and influence the energetic fields of Man (causing energetic movement within the body's Essence, Energy and Spirit).

THE DAO AS THE CHONG: CENTER

In ancient China, the Dao was considered energetically and spiritually as "Chong," the perfectly blended center. The Dao, therefore, exists as the center of all things, maintaining its existence throughout time and space.

The energy existing between Heaven (Yang) and Earth (Yin) is considered "Chong Qi" (or the "Energy of the Dao"). It exists within the infinite space of the Wuji as an energetic mist, blending within the infinite Void, between the energetic fields of Heaven and Earth (Figure 2.5).

The ancient Chinese believed that the qualities of these two universal poles (Yin and Yang)

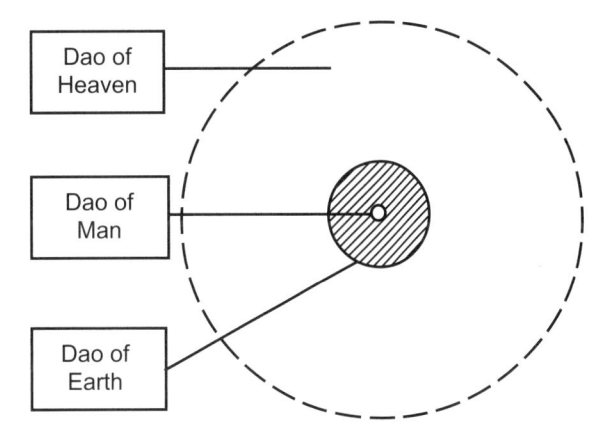

Figure 2.4. Each of the energetic realms fits into the other's energetic form creating a multidimensional unity.

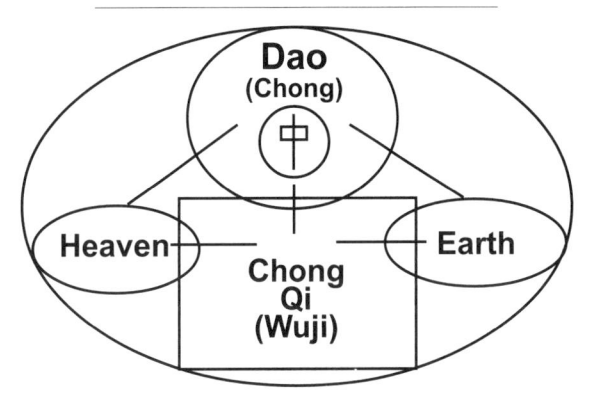

Figure 2.5. The Primordial Dao is composed of Heaven, Earth and Chong Qi.

are continually blended together through the whirling energetic vortex of the Chong Qi (Wuji). Therefore, Heaven, Earth and Wuji compose the fundamental unity of the energetic matrix known as the "Primordial Dao," existing before the evolution of material existence.

THE DAO WITHIN THE BODY

As a microcosm, the human body takes the place of the Wuji, mediating between the energies of Heaven and Earth. Just as the energy of the Wuji blends the energy of Heaven and Earth, so too does the energy of the Mingmen blend the energy of the body's Kidney Yin and Kidney Yang, producing the Essence (Jing), Energy (Qi) and Spirit (Shen) of life (Figure 2.6).

VOLUME 1, SECTION 1: FOUNDATIONS OF CHINESE ENERGETIC MEDICINE

As a science, Chinese medicine studies the functional relationship between the cells, tissues, organs and organ systems and their relationship with the energetic influences of Heaven, Earth and Man. This is considered the primary focus, rather than studying the physical material substance of the cells and tissues. The ancient Chinese believed that the energy of the Eternal Dao exists within the "infinite space" or Wuji, located within the body's tissues, cells, and molecules. Finding harmony between the energetic essence of the Dao and the body's Jing, Qi, and Shen brings health.

To the ancient Daoists, the Three Treasures of Man (Essence, Energy and Spirit) were believed to have two existing properties, one half (Yin) existing on Earth in tangible form, the other half (Yang) existing in Heaven in spiritual form. Possession and harmonization of the Earthly half enabled the individual to summon the Heavenly half. Through the union of Heaven (Yang) and Earth (Yin) the individual could transform him or herself and bring about a state of renewal. This was accomplished by consciously directing and controlling the energy (Qi) that acted as a medium between matter and spirit (Figure 2.7).

THE WUJI: INFINITE SPACE

In the ancient Chinese ideograms for Wuji (infinite space embodied in between matter, energy and spirit), the character "Wu" translates as "nothing or without," and the character "Ji" translates as "the ultimate or extreme." Together, the term "Wuji" translates as "ultimate emptiness," and describes the vast expansiveness of infinite space. In ancient China, this concept was symbolically represented by the formation of a never-ending circle (Figure 2.8).

The Wuji is the state of no boundaries, the state of pure and complete oneness. Its essence is that of emptiness (as depicted by the empty circle) which relates to the awareness aspect of our Shen Xian (Eternal Soul).

The ancient Chinese believed that the Wuji, extending from the Divine, is an infinite ocean of microscopic vibrations, from which all the realms of creation and all the different energetic worlds are constructed. Like an invisible web, it is through

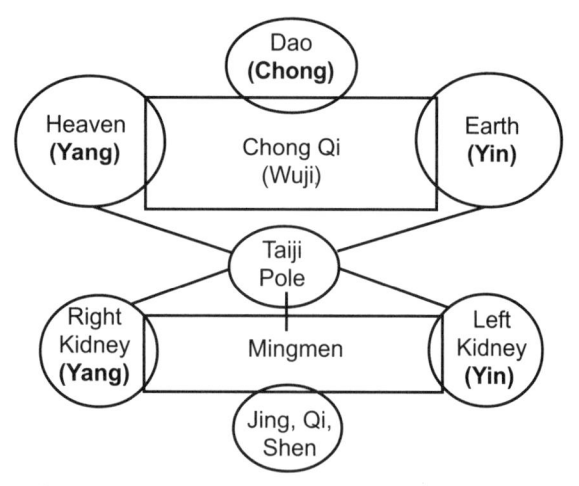

Figure 2.6. The Primordial Relationships with Human Energetic Correspondences

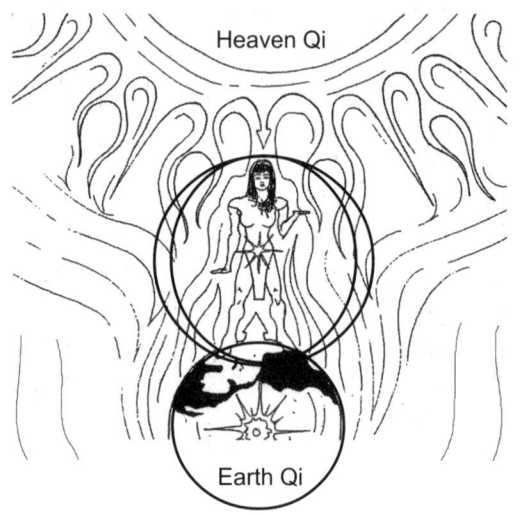

Figure 2.7. An individual's energetic field is suspended between the two energy fields of Heaven and Earth.

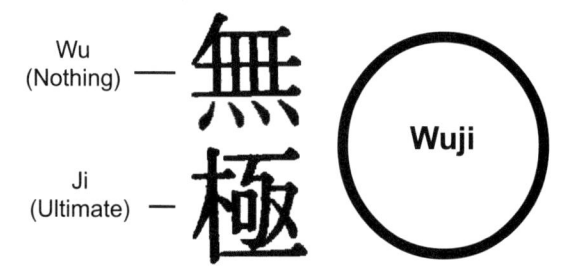

Figure 2.8. The Chinese characters for "Wuji," The Ultimate Emptiness of Infinite Space

CHAPTER 2: UNDERSTANDING ANCIENT CHINESE METAPHYSICS

The Body's Chemical and Electrical Messages Are Expressed Through Five Levels of Bio-Information Contained Within the Wuji

- Dao: Divine Energy
- Wuji: Infinite Space
- Shen: Spiritual Energy
- Qi: Intangible Energy
- Jing: Form or Tangible Matter

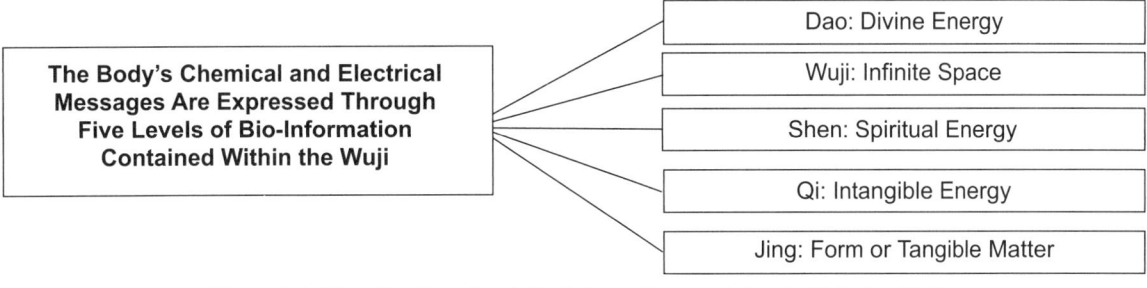

Figure 2.9. The Five Levels of Bio-information contained within the Wuji

the Wuji that the Divine manifests its infinite form.

The ancient Daoist cannon *Huainan Zi*, describes the existence of the Wuji and states, "In ancient times, before Heaven and Earth even existed, there were only images without forms; profound, opaque, vast, immobile, impalpable and still. There was a haziness, infinite, unfathomable and abysmal. A vast deep to which no one knew the door."

In the metaphysical realm, the Yang within Heaven corresponds to time, while the Yin within Earth corresponds to space. Through the quiescent states of prayer and meditation, the ancient Chinese Qigong masters were able to dissolve their energy into the infinite space of the Wuji and reconnect with the Dao, transcending both time (Yang) and space (Yin). Through stillness of Mind, one can realize the boundless ocean of vibrations connected to everything contained within the Wuji.

THE KNOWLEDGE STORED WITHIN THE WUJI

On the most fundamental level, all things are constructed of quantum energy, constantly exchanging information within the Wuji's inexhaustible energetic field. All matter in the universe is interconnected by energetic waves contained within the Wuji's sea of energy, which transcend the manifestations of time and space.

The stable state of matter depends on the dynamic interchange of subatomic particles flowing within the Wuji for its very existence. Similar to ripples on a pond, energetic waves are expressed by periodic oscillations, moving through the medium of the Wuji on a subatomic level. Each energetic wave is encoded with information. The Wuji field creates a medium enabling the molecules to communicate with each other in oscillating frequencies. As molecules slow down, they give off radiation and release encoded wave information about the history of matter.

THE MESSAGE: XIN XI

In ancient China, the body's encoded bio-information was known as Xin Xi, or "the message," which was not limited by the confines of space or time. This message referred to the energy fields that flow into, away from, and within the Wuji.

This bio-informational resonance was believed to contain information that could be subdivided into five levels of energetic expression, described as follows (Figure 2.9): Jing (form or tangible matter), Qi (intangible energy), Shen (spiritual energy), Wuji (infinite space) and the Dao (Divine energy).

The Wuji records the vibrational resonance of every action (including all thought and emotion), as well as light and sound. These energetic impressions are stored within the spiritual plane. These records exist as impressions in the spiritual dimension, providing a kind of accessible filing system for those who wish to access information about past history, past lives, or even for the examination of their own spiritual progress.

While deep in meditation, the energetic stimulation of the third ventricle of the Qigong doctor's Brain will stimulate the hypothalamic limbic system, allowing him or her admittance into this subtle energetic field of knowledge.

The body is composed of literally billions of energetic molecules. Each molecule is a hologram of ancestral particles, knowledge, and experiences existing throughout time and spanning our entire history as we know it. These molecules gather to form and create matter. They serve a specific purpose for life transitions and energetic interactions and then dissolve and transform back into Qi and Shen. Each molecule stores energetic experiences that can be later accessed through spiritual intention.

In energetic embryology, as the molecules gather to form a fetus, energy and ancestral history are stored within the tissues and cells of the child. This energy is gathered via the environmental, universal, maternal and paternal energetic fields.

By connecting to the energy field of a patient, the Qigong doctor is able to access specific information about the patient through an internal connection to the patterns and impressions contained within the patient's energetic space. This allows the doctor to study and learn about the patient's past history of disease patterns, as well as the information contained within the molecular structures of the patient's tissues.

SENDING MESSAGES

Qigong doctors access the knowledge needed to treat patients by remaining receptive to the messages stored within the patient's Jing, Qi, and Shen, and those resonating throughout the surrounding energetic space (Wuji). When the Qigong doctors emit healing energy to the patient, they are sending subatomic healing messages encoded within the Qi. When these messages are received by the patient's cells, the healing process is initiated.

Within the energy of the Wuji is the history of knowledge gathered and stored since the beginning of time. In Medical Qigong practices, accessing the knowledge of the Wuji is the Chinese equivalent of the Indian concept of accessing the knowledge of the Akashic Records. "Akasha" is a Sanskrit term roughly equivalent to "Wuji" that is used to describe the all-pervasive space of the universe. The infinite space of the Wuji is expressed either through internal or external dimensional perceptions, described as follows (Figure 2.10):

- The Internal Perceptional Dimension of Wuji: This Wuji is perceived through enveloping, penetrating, and descending deep into the

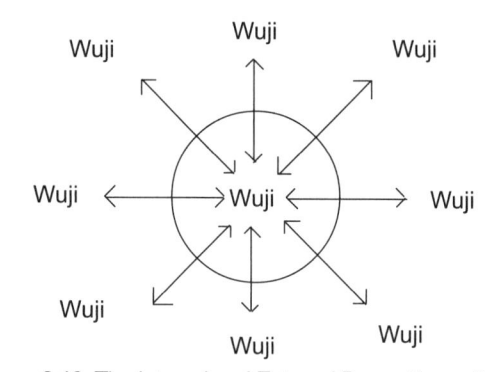

Figure 2.10. The Internal and External Perceptions of Wuji

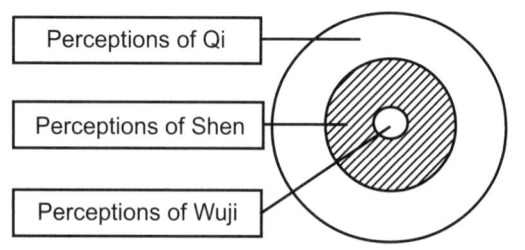

Figure 2.11. Wuji, Qi and Shen form a Trinity of Intuitive and Psychic Power.

internal aspect of an object. It is not limited by the object's material plane (or matter) and clinically can be associated with the enveloping and penetrating of the internal human form. Matter can be described as consisting of more space then actual physical form and its energetic properties can be infinitely divided. Contained within this energetic and spiritual Wuji field are the imprinted forms and foundations for structure or matter. Also contained within this energetic field is the body's personality by way of physical form, sensation, perception, mental formation, and consciousness.

- The External Perceptional Dimension of Wuji: The Wuji is external, unlimited, and beyond all description. It is unbound by the material, yet contains all material things. It is the vehicle for all life, resonating through sound and light, and permeating everything in the universe.

In the practice of Medical Qigong, the Wuji is one of three universal principles, along with Qi and Shen, which form a trinity of intuitive and

Tai
(Supreme)

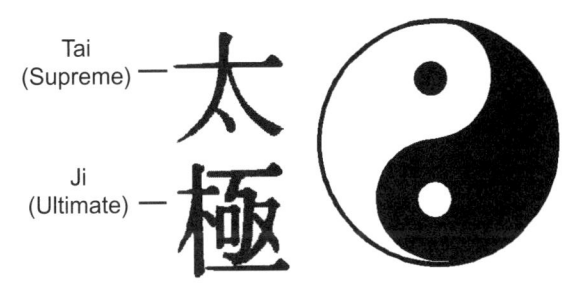

Ji
(Ultimate)

Figure 2.12. The Chinese Characters for "Taiji," The Supreme Ultimate

Yang Depicts the Bright Sunny Side of a Hill or River Bank	Yang	Yin	Yin Depicts the Dark Shady Side of a Hill or River Bank
	Active	Passive	
	Creative	Receptive	
	Masculine	Feminine	
	Back	Front	
	Left	Right	
	Fire	Water	
	Hot	Cold	
	Dry	Wet	
	Hard	Soft	
	Light	Heavy	
	Bright	Dark	
	Heaven	Earth	
	Sun	Moon	
	White	Black	

The Chinese Yang (Heaven) and Yin (Earth) Symbols: The Yang is represented by white, Yin is represented by black, and the center of the circle represents the Eternal Dao within the Wuji.

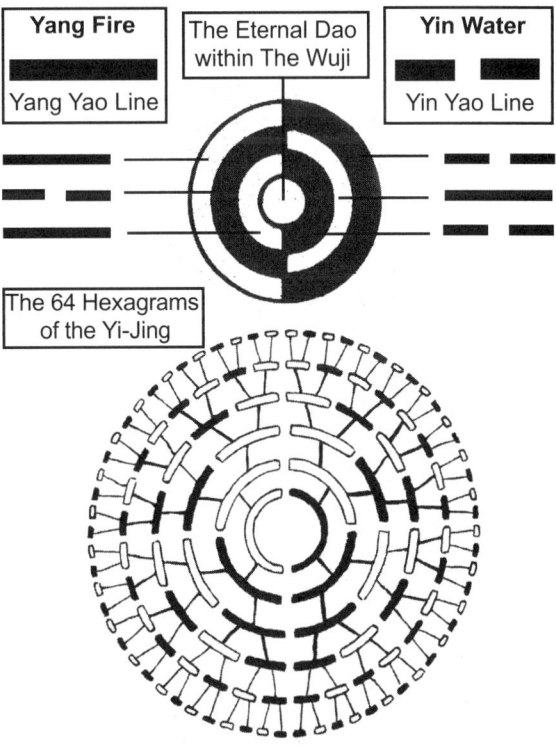

Figure 2.13. The ever-changing energy of the Yin and Yang form the 64 Hexagrams of the Yi-Jing

Chapter 2: Understanding Ancient Chinese Metaphysics

psychic power. These three universal principles also manifest in the human soul, allowing divine thought to infuse matter (Figure 2.11).

TAIJI: SUPREME ULTIMATE

The first record of the Taiji symbol was derived from the ancient book, *The Harmony in The Book of Changes*, written by Wei Boyang in the Eastern Han Dynasty (25 B.C.-225 A.D.). When deciphering the ancient Chinese characters for Taiji (the transformation of Yin and Yang energy), the character "Tai" translates as "great or supreme," and the character "Ji," as in Wuji, translates as "the ultimate or extreme." Together, the term "Taiji" can be translated as "the supreme ultimate," and represents the infinite, ultimate state of transformation (Yin transforming into Yang and Yang transforming into Yin). Both Yin and Yang represent opposite yet complementary energetic qualities.

There is an ancient Chinese saying, "the Dao governs the real, and Yin and Yang are transitory manifestations of it." The reunion of Yin and Yang are necessary for the unified existence of a human being. Therefore, energetically, Taiji is considered to be the origin of change or movement, which initiates "creation" (Figure 2.12).

The ancient Chinese ideogram of Yang depicts the bright, sunny side of a hill or river bank; Yin is depicted as the dark, shady side of a hill or river bank (Figure 2.13). Yin exists within Yang, and Yang within Yin. Yang energetically manifests as active, creative, masculine, hot, hard, light, Heaven, white and bright. Yin energetically manifests as passive, receptive, feminine, cold, soft, dark, Earth, black and shadow. The dynamic bal-

VOLUME 1, SECTION 1: FOUNDATIONS OF CHINESE ENERGETIC MEDICINE

Yin and Yang

Yang
―――
Immaterial
Produces Energy

- Tai Yang (Greater Yang)
- Shao Yang (Lesser Yang)

Energy ―――
Energy ―――
Yang within Yang

Energy ―――
Form ― ―
Yin within Yang

Yin
― ―
Material
Produces Form

- Tai Yin (Greater Yin)
- Shao Yin (Lesser Yin)

Form ― ―
Form ― ―
Yin within Yin

Form ― ―
Energy ―――
Yang within Yin

External Body Movement

Internal Energy Movement

The Prenatal Bagua Trigrams

Summer
(8) Heaven (Qian)
(7) Lake (Dui) — (1) Wind (Xun)
(6) Fire (Li) — (2) Water (Kan)
(5) Thunder (Zhen) — (3) Mountain (Gen)
(4) Earth (Kun)
Winter

Spring / Autumn

The Prenatal Bagua Trigrams
Eight Dimensions or Phases of Energy
Polar Opposites: Yin (1-4) across from Yang (5-8).
This Cycle of Harmony Relates to the
World of Thoughts and Ideas. The Opposite
Energetic Forces are Responsible for the
Creation of All Phenomena.

The Postnatal Bagua Trigrams

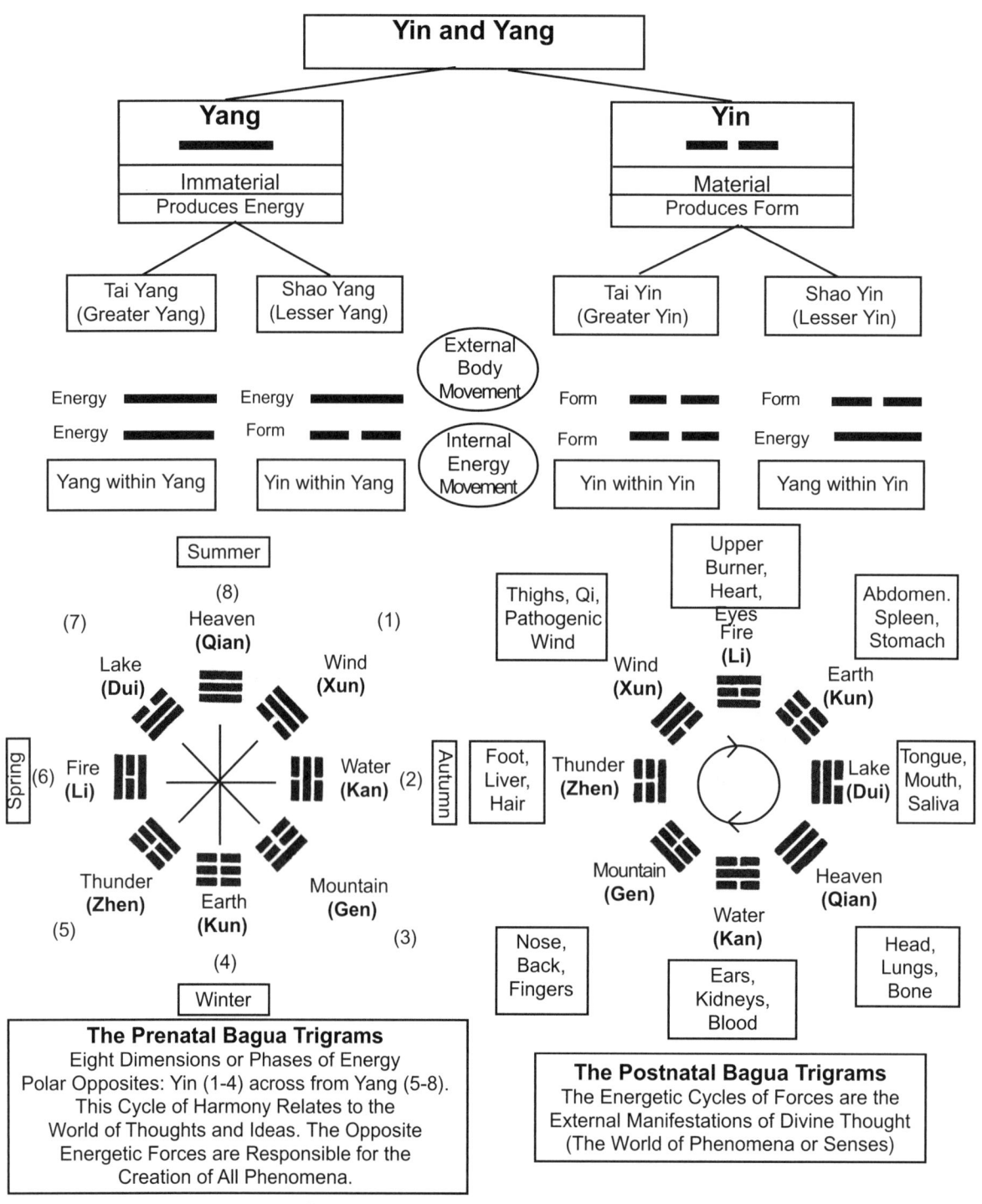

- Thighs, Qi, Pathogenic Wind — Wind (Xun)
- Upper Burner, Heart, Eyes — Fire (Li)
- Abdomen, Spleen, Stomach — Earth (Kun)
- Foot, Liver, Hair — Thunder (Zhen)
- Tongue, Mouth, Saliva — Lake (Dui)
- Nose, Back, Fingers — Mountain (Gen)
- Ears, Kidneys, Blood — Water (Kan)
- Head, Lungs, Bone — Heaven (Qian)

The Postnatal Bagua Trigrams
The Energetic Cycles of Forces are the
External Manifestations of Divine Thought
(The World of Phenomena or Senses)

Figure 2.14. The Ancient Daoist Concept of Yin and Yang Expressing the Four Phases of Universal Energy and Manifesting Through the Prenatal and Postnatal Bagua Trigrams (Pre-Five Element Theory).

Chapter 2: Understanding Ancient Chinese Metaphysics

ance of Yin and Yang constantly changes and transforms the body's life-force energy.

All matter is composed of different relative proportions of Yin and Yang energy. Within the infinite space of the Wuji, both Yin and Yang energy gather or disperse to balance the forces of nature.

Taiji Within the Human Body

In ancient Chinese medicine, the theory of Yin and Yang energy represents the duality of balance and harmony within the body, as well as within the universe. All comprehensions of Traditional Chinese Medical physiology, pathology and treatment can be expressed through the clinical understanding of Yin and Yang energetics (see Volume 3, Chapter 22).

In the Medical Qigong clinic, the body's tissues are believed to have an energetic influence and are typically classified in terms of Yin and Yang. Every person has both Yin and Yang elements within them but will tend to be predominantly one or the other in terms of personality, physique, life-style preferences, speech patterns and mannerisms. Within a general constitution, there will be more subtle fluctuations along the Yin and Yang continuum as the body reacts to external and internal energetic movements. For example, when designing the patient's exercise program, diet, or herbal remedies, it is necessary to first determine whether the patient is predominantly Yin or Yang in constitution.

The ancient Daoists understood that from the Wuji, the Dao creates Yin and Yang, which in turn gives birth to four phases of universal energy (Great Yang, Lesser Yang, Great Yin and Lesser Yin). The four phases of universal energy give birth to the eight natural forces of the Bagua (Heaven, Thunder, Water, Mountain, Earth, Wind, Fire and Lake). These four phases also form the energetic bases of the prenatal and postnatal transformations, manifested in the form of eight energetic actions (known as the Bagua Trigrams). These eight prenatal and postnatal energetic actions act as a template for all creation and can be further combined in order to form the ever-changing energetic patterns of the 64 Hexagrams of the Yi-Jing (Figure 2.14).

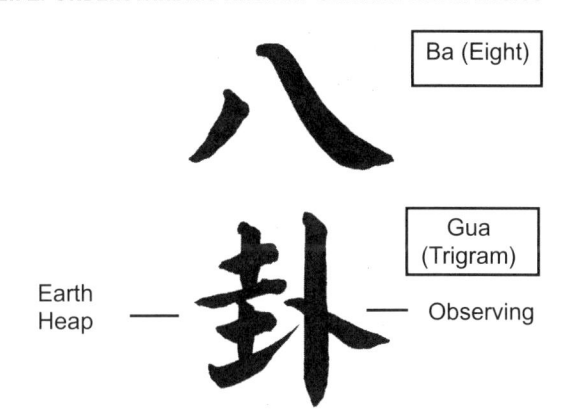

Figure 2.15. The Chinese Characters for "Bagua," The Eight Trigrams

Bagua: Eight Trigrams

In ancient times, the Bagua (Eight Trigrams) was the symbol originally used for observing the movements of the sun and moon. When observing the ancient Chinese characters for Bagua (the eight ancient Daoist energetic structures of life), the character "Ba" translates as "eight," and the character "Gua" translates as "trigram." Together, the term "Bagua" can be translated as "Eight Trigrams," and is considered a template for the basic laws of all energetic movements and transformations (Figure 2.15).

The character "Gua" is composed of two ideographs, on the right is the radical meaning "to observe," on the left is the radical "Gui" meaning "earth heap." The Gui (earth heap) was used in ancient times to measure the shadows in order to record ancient calendars (the ancient Chinese form of a sundial).

Each trigram is composed of three "yao" lines: a solid yao line (---) is considered Yang, a broken yao line (- -) is considered Yin. Each "yao" represents a basic unit of the Eight Trigrams, and has three meanings, sunlight, moonlight and the mutual projection of the sun and moon. The Yao Trigram itself is the symbol of the sun and moon's movement.

The Eight Trigram Inner Circle Yao lines of the Prenatal Bagua configuration begins and ends with Heaven (Qian) and Earth (Kun). From extreme Yin, located at the bottom Kun Trigram, to

53

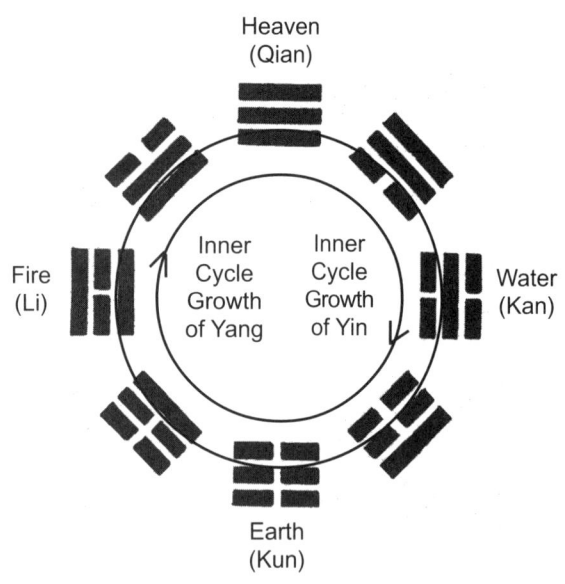

VOLUME 1, SECTION 1: FOUNDATIONS OF CHINESE ENERGETIC MEDICINE

Figure 2.16. The Inner Circle of the Prenatal Bagua Represents the Seasonal Yin and Yang Heavenly Cycles of the Sun.

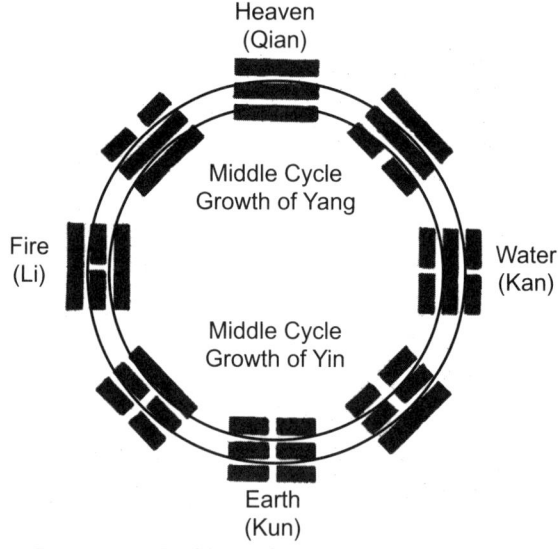

Figure 2.17. The Middle Circle of the Prenatal Bagua Represents the Yin and Yang Earthly Cycles of each day.

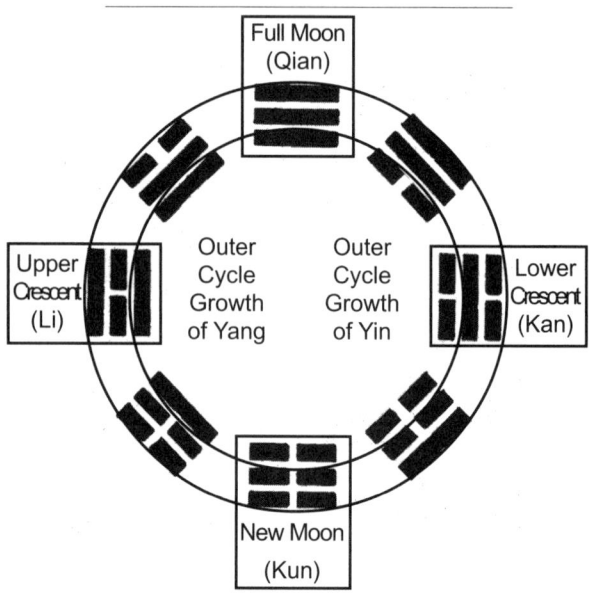

Figure 2.18. The Outer Circle of the Prenatal Bagua Represents the Yin and Yang Cycles of the Moon observed each Month.

extreme Yang, located at the top Qian Trigram, the transforming powers of Yin and Yang are expressed through the sun's movement during the seasonal year (Figure 2.16).

The Eight Trigram Middle Circle Yao lines of the Prenatal Bagua configuration begins and ends with Water (Kan) and Fire (Li), and represents the growth and decline of Yin and Yang during the Earth's revolution within each day and year (Figure 2.17).

The Eight Trigram Outer Circle Yao lines of the Prenatal Bagua configuration is composed of both the middle and outer Yaos. It represents the Yin and Yang energy of the moon's movement, observed and recorded each month (Figure 2.18).

The development of the Eight Trigrams is attributed to Fu Xi, the legendary emperor of ancient China during the Age of the Five Rulers (2852 B.C.). The Eight Trigrams were used in early forms of divination before the hexagrams were created. The movements of Heaven, Earth and all living things were depicted by two Eight Trigram images: Early Heaven (Prenatal) Bagua, which manifests the energetic "nature" of things, and Later Heaven (Postnatal) Bagua, which depicts the creation of all phenomena.

The Eight Trigrams are assigned to specific stages of cellular division within the forming zygote (explained later in this chapter). Additionally, each of the Eight Trigrams is assigned to one of the Eight Extraordinary Vessels responsible for fetal growth, causing specific areas of fetal tissue to develop. This Eight Trigram energetic pattern is evident in the structural formation of the Magic Square (Figure 2.19).

When viewing the Prenatal Bagua pattern, the energetic natures assigned to each specific trigram give the image of oppositely paired phases (Heaven-Earth, Lake-Mountain, Fire-Water, Thunder-Wind).

THE WU XING: FIVE ELEMENTS

When observing the ancient Chinese characters for Wuxing (the five energetic phenomena of life), the character "Wu" translates as "five," and the character "Xing" translates as "movement, process, manifestation, or phase." Together, the term "Wuxing" can be translated as "Five Elements," and is considered an energetic template based on the study of five phases or processes of Qi transformation (Figure 2.20). They classify all tangible and intangible substances into five specific categories, used for observation, study, diagnosis and treatment (five senses, five viscera, five emotions, five virtues, five flavors, five seasons and five phases of energetic transition) (see Volume 3, Chapter 24).

THE FIVE PURE LIGHTS

The "Gross" Five Elements (Wood, Fire, Earth, Metal and Water) are used to explain, classify, and characterize all natural phenomena. There are four primary laws of universal cycles in Five Element theory (creating, controlling, invading, and insulting). The original nature of the "True" Five Elements, however, exists as pure elemental light within the Wuji. According to ancient Daoist texts, "when Yin and Yang divided, the Five Pure Lights shot forth; spontaneously born from the infinite space of the Wuji, they appear as rays of light that came before the creation of the world."

The ancient Daoists believed that the energetic and spiritual components of the Five Elements existed as "Five Pure Lights," which emanated as a subtle expression of the "primordial luminosity" of the Dao. The "Five Pure Lights" were considered the energies from which all other energies (including visible light) arose. As they transform to become the various dimensions of existence (matter, energy and spirit) they form the different realms or worlds in which we exist.

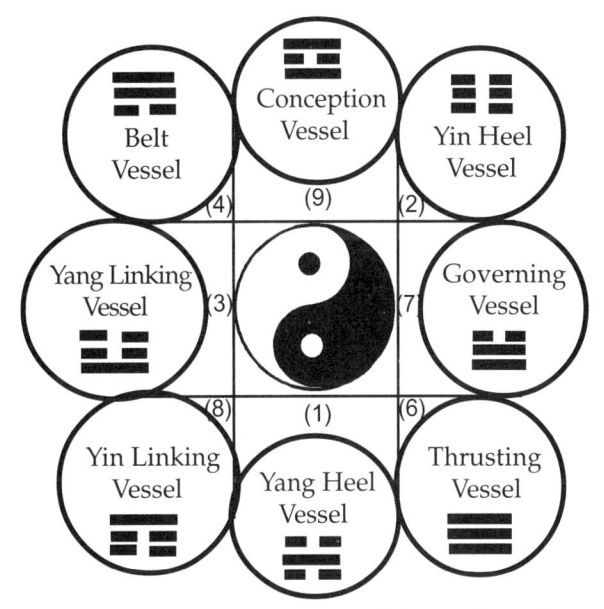

Figure 2.19. The Postnatal Eight Trigrams Form the Magic Square

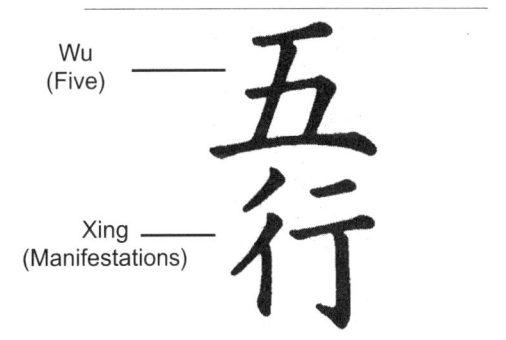

Figure 2.20. The Chinese Characters for "Wuxing," The Five Elements

According to energetic embryology, at the time of conception an individual will begin the energetic accumulation of the Five Elements in order to construct the physical body. As the Five Elements begin to form the physical body, the energetic and spiritual components of the True Five Elements (responsible for the creation and formation of prenatal tissues) establish their relationship with the forming tissues on a spiritual, energetic, and physical level. Internally, the Five Pure Lights begin to manifest into the Jing level of the organs and become the Prenatal Wu Jing Shen (Five Original Spirits). The Prenatal Wu Jing

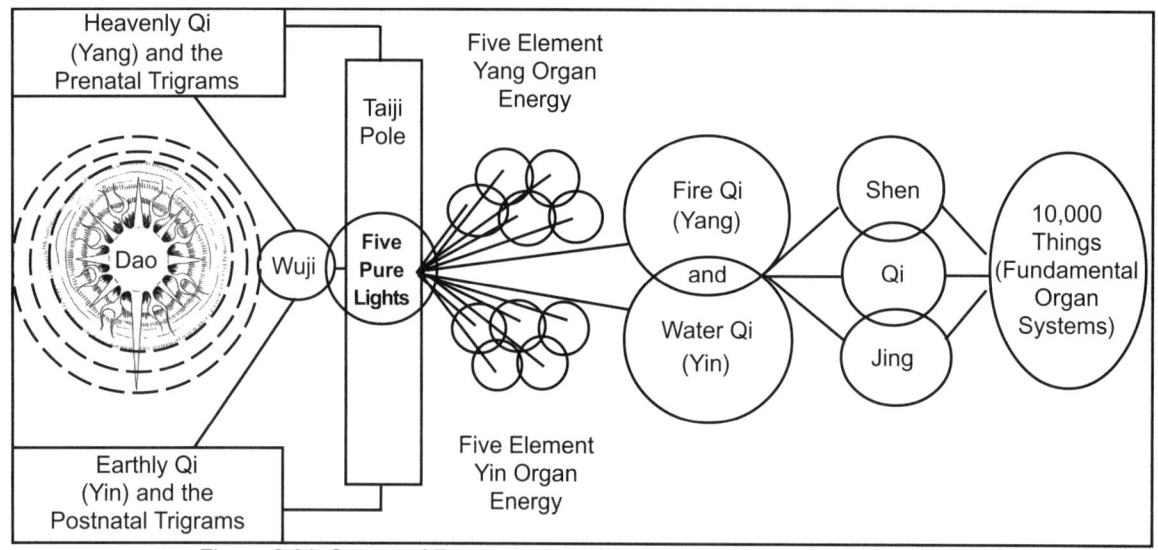

Figure 2.21. Stages of Energetic Transformation Forming the Human Body

Shen also inhabit the five branches of the body, the five fingers of each hand, the five toes of each foot, and the five internal senses.

Within the human body, the energetic qualities of the Five Elements are divided into Yin (solid) and Yang (hollow) organ energies. These elemental energies sustain the tissues and establish the foundation for the body's internal organ systems (e.g., digestive system, cardiovascular system, reproductive system, endocrine system, nervous system, etc.) (Figure 2.21).

THE PHYSICAL, ENERGETIC AND SPIRITUAL WORLDS

To review, from the Eternal Dao emerges the Wuji (Infinite Space). From the Wuji emerges the Taiji. The Wuji provides the energetic medium which joins both matter and spirit, as well as the energetic matrix through which all things exist. The energetic and spiritual fields of the Wuji are classified according to the specific characteristics and laws of universal cycles set forth by the energetic and spiritual natures of the Bagua (Eight Trigrams) and the Wuxing (Five Elements).

The energetic subdivisions of matter, energy and spirit create the foundation for the existence of worlds within worlds, separated by their different vibrational frequencies. As outlined in the ancient Chinese saying, "as above so below," just as the human body is made of a physical body, energetic body and spiritual body there is also a physical universe, energetic universe and spiritual universe (Figure 2.22).

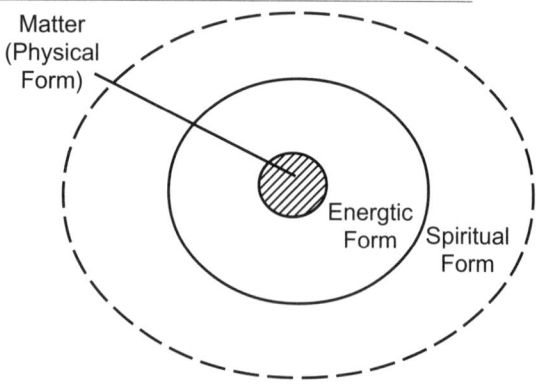

Figure 2.22. As the human body is made of a Physical Body, Energetic Body and Spiritual Body, there is also a Physical Universe, Energetic Universe and Spiritual Universe.

THE PHYSICAL WORLD

The physical or "material" body exists within the physical world (the third dimensional world of matter). This is the level of experience that has both form and substance, and that which is accessible through the ordinary senses. The physical world expresses itself through three realms: the

CHAPTER 2: UNDERSTANDING ANCIENT CHINESE METAPHYSICS

Wu Xing (Five Elements): Fire, Wood, Earth, Water, Metal

Wuji (The Infinite Space of the Dao)

Taiji (The Division of Yin and Yang)

Bagua (Postnatal Eight Trigrams): Wind (Xun), Fire (Li), Earth (Kun), Thunder (Zhen), Lake (Dui), Mountain (Gen), Water (Kan), Heaven (Qian)

The Spiritual World	The Energetic World	The Physical World
The Spiritual Body belongs to the fifth dimensional world, wherein time and space are transcended. It is a world of unexpressed forms, a world of "ideas."	The Energetic Body belongs to the fourth dimensional world which is considered a malleable material world existing within an accelerated energetic state.	The Physical Body belongs to the third dimensional world and appears to be solid because it vibrates on the same frequency as matter.

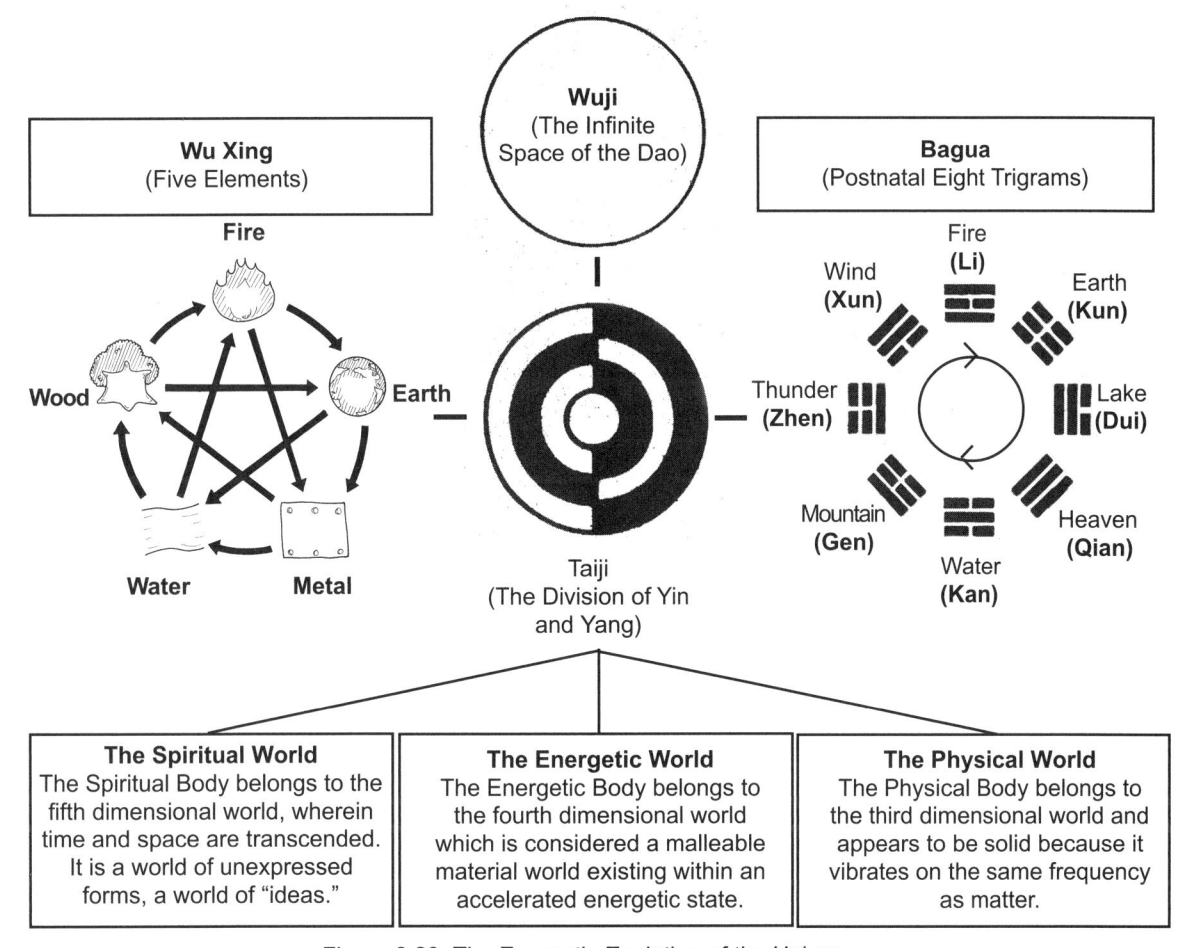

Figure 2.23. The Energetic Evolution of the Universe

physical realm of people, things, and events.

The physical world appears to be solid because it vibrates on the same frequency as matter. Everything which exists in the physical world has an energetic and spiritual counterpart.

THE ENERGETIC WORLD

The energetic body exists within the energetic world (the fourth dimensional world). This is the level of experience that has form but no substance (e.g., dreams, thoughts, desires) and substance but no form (e.g., energy). The energetic world exists and expresses itself through three realms: the energetic realm of Heaven, Earth, and Man (Figure 2.23).

The energetic world is also considered a type of physical world, existing within an accelerated energetic state. It is considered to be a world that exists at a higher level of vibration than the material world.

The energetic world cannot exist by itself, as its energetic field lives as an infinite malleable substance. This energetic dimension is constantly being programed and shaped by thought and intention. Everything that exists within the energetic world must have within itself a spiritual aspect because energetic matter or substance cannot obtain shape or color unless it acquires it from the spiritual world. The energetic world is like a mirror which can have no shape unless it is joined to the spirit world which shapes it. The energetic

VOLUME 1, SECTION 1: FOUNDATIONS OF CHINESE ENERGETIC MEDICINE

```
Spiritual ─┬─ Fifth Dimension          ┌─ (9) Realm of the Dao (Divine)
  Body     │  Higher Spiritual World   └─ (8) Realm of the Shen Ling
           │                           ┌─ (7) Realm of the Immortals
           │                           ├─ (6) Realm of the Shen Xian      Nine
           └─ Fifth Dimension          ├─ (5) Realm of the Zhi Yi Tian    Levels
              Lower Spiritual World    └─ (4) Realm of the Yuan Shen      of
                                                                          Heaven

Energetic ─── Fourth Dimension     ┌─ (3) Realm of the Spirit Entities
  Body         Energetic World     ├─ (2) Realm of the Nature Spirits
                                   ├─ (1) Realm of the Ghosts
                                   └─ (9) Realm of the Underworld

                                   ┌─ (8) Realm of Thoughts/Emotions
                                   ├─ (7) Realm of Form
                                   ├─ (6) Realm of Space                  Nine
Physical ─── Third Dimension       ├─ (5) Realm of Light                  Levels
  Body        Physical World       ├─ (4) Realm of Energy                 of
                                   ├─ (3) Realm of Cells                  Earth
                                   ├─ (2) Realm of Matter
                                   └─ (1) Realm of Particles
```

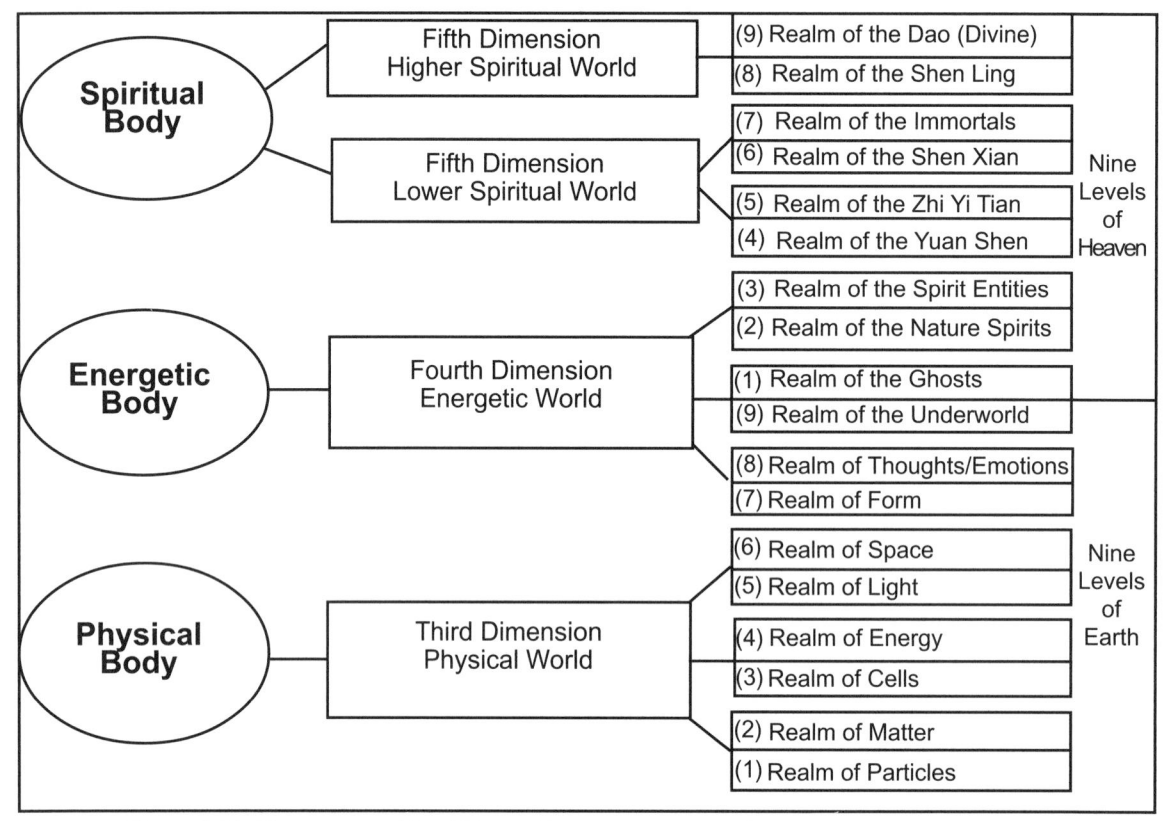

Figure 2.24. There are worlds within worlds, separated by different vibrational frequencies.

---

world can be conceived of as a blank sheet of paper upon which everything in the physical and spiritual worlds are reflected. Likewise, both the physical and energetic worlds are mirrors that reflect what is within the spiritual world. The physical Earth, for example, has behind it an energetic Earth (the Earth as it exists within the fourth dimension) and a spiritual Earth (the Earth as it exists within the fifth dimension).

In the energetic world, space does not exist. Within the energetic and spiritual worlds every cell and particle feels and perceives. One is therefore able to absorb the thoughts of others without the need for language. In other words, communication takes place directly from cell to cell and mind to mind. Within both the energetic and spiritual worlds, space is transcended and one can move instantly from one side of the Earth to the other. One can also be several places at once.

THE SPIRITUAL WORLD

The spiritual body exists within the spiritual world (the fifth dimensional world). This is the level of experience that has neither form nor substance. The spiritual world resonates at a more subtle and accelerated state than the energetic world. The spiritual world is the realm of the Dao, expressing itself through three realms: the spiritual realm of the universe, time and space.

In the spiritual world, time and space are transcended. When traveling within the energetic and spiritual dimensions everything manifests simply by focusing intention. Manifestation from the higher vibrational resonance of the lower spiritual worlds extending to the lowest vibrational resonance of the physical world is defined by form and shape (Figure 2.24). The higher spiritual worlds do have shape (to a lesser degree), but are not limited to the confines of shaped forms. This is a world of unexpressed forms, a world of "ideas."

Energetic Formation of the Human Body

Throughout China's history, there have been numerous theories as to the creation of "Heaven, Earth and Man," and the creation and formation of the human soul. The concept of the energetic formation of the human body, mind and soul, as well as its spiritual evolution has spawned numerous religions throughout the millennia. In Daoism, ancient symbols and metaphors are used to describe the various internal transformations of energy and spirit.

The following ancient Daoist theory regarding the creation and formation of the human body flourished in China during the Spring and Autumn Period (770-476 B.C.).

The Dao: Divine

The ancient Daoists believed that the energetic and spiritual form of the Divine was a vibrant luminous fire, composed of an infinite number of Shen Ling (supernatural spirits) surrounding its center core (Figure 2.25). The Shen Ling emanate from the Dao as a myriad of Divine fragments or rays, also called "Sparks of the Supreme Fire." The Shen Ling were considered the "Messengers of the Divine" and were in turn surrounded by an infinite number of Shen Xian (Eternal Souls).

The Light of the "Dao"

When the Eternal Dao begins to manifest itself within the relative universe of the Wuji (Infinite Space), its energetic nature appears as clear light which dispels darkness. When the Dao manifests its Divine nature as a pure and tangible physical form, it appears as a spiritually enlightened being (saint or immortal).

Shen Ling: Supernatural Spirit

In ancient China, the Wu Yi shamans believed that the Dao existed both within the individual and within the Heavens (as above so below). This "River of God," or "Heart of Dao," was located in the center core (Taiji Pole) of an individual. This is why the Wu Yi were often represented as being partially divided, becoming energetically and

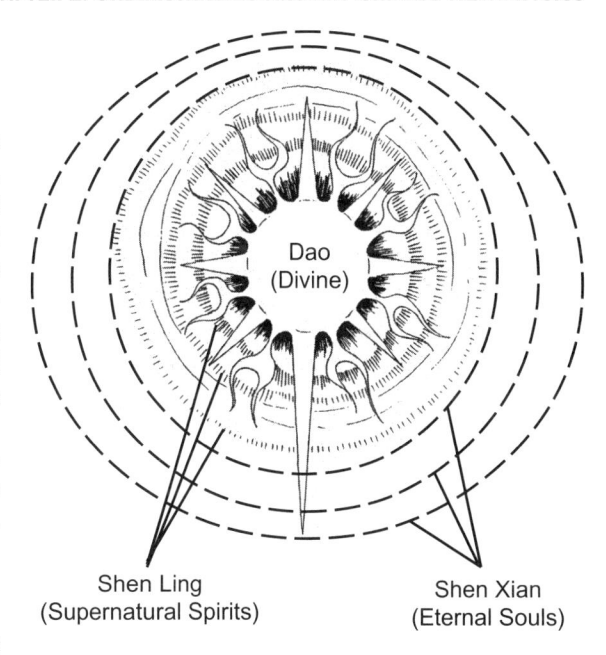

Figure 2.25. The Infinite Dao or Divine

spiritually whole only when possessed by the other half of their celestial spirit.

The word "Shen" means god, deity, spirit, and mind. In ancient China, it sometimes was used in order to depict the religious function of worshipping the ancestors by pulling down the heavenly influences of the sun, moon and stars. By incorporating these heavenly bodies into themselves, the ancient Chinese believed that they could establish an auspicious role in life. The Chinese ideogram for Shen is depicted by two characters: positioned on the right is a character representing the alternating expression of natural forces; positioned to the left is a character representing the unfolding of things under the authority and influence of Heaven. The ideograph depicts the heavenly influence that penetrates and instructs the core of the Heart, or "that which descends from the sky and passes through the body" (Figure 2.26).

The Chinese character "Ling" describes the spiritual quality of the Dao and is translated as "supernatural or magical." In contemporary religion it is equivalent to the "power of the Holy Spirit," and is responsible for healing and miracles.

The ideograph for "Ling" consists of three characters. The top radical "Yu" translates to mean rain. The three squares in the center of the character are three mouth radicals "Kou," which originally stood for "the calling of rain." The bottom character "Wu" translates as "magician or sorcerer" (Figure 2.27). Together, the three ideographs (Yu, Kou and Wu) depict the image of the Wu Yi doctors dancing, chanting and supplicating to the Heavenly Spirits (Shen Ling) for rain.

Together, the Chinese characters Shen Ling can be translated as "supernatural spirit," "gods" or "deities," and represents the living power of the Divine. The ancient Chinese believed that before creation, an individual's essence was energetically formed of Ling Zi (ultra-small heavenly particles that circulate throughout the universe). At conception, the individual's Ling lowers its vibrational essence in order to combine with the sperm and ovum to form the human soul and Original Spirit (Yuan Shen).

The *Ancient Book of Lu* states that "even a blade of grass or clump of dirt contains Ling Qi." Ling Qi is the spiritual energy that envelops and forms all things. In order to connect with and perceive the Ling Qi contained within the environment, an individual must first cultivate his or her own personal Ling Qi.

THE WU YI AND THE SHEN LING

The ancient Chinese believed that the supernatural spiritual quality of the Wu Yi doctor's own Ling (being spiritually Yin) would reconnect with the supernatural spiritual quality of the Dao (being spiritually Yang) and become energetically and spiritually whole. This energetic and spiritual union allowed the Wu Yi doctor access to supernatural powers, allowing him or her the ability to influence nature. One example of the Wu Yi doctor's ability to control nature was the skill of bringing rain, brought about in one of two ways: "direct influence" or "indirect influence," which are described as follows:

- **Direct Influence:** Brought about through the control and manipulation of Heavenly Qi (clouds), resulting in rain. This would occur if the Wu Yi doctor's energy and spiritual integrity were powerful and De (virtue) was pure.
- **Indirect Influence:** Brought about through the supplication for rain. Having found favor with the Dao, the Heavenly Spirits (Shen Ling) would be sanctioned to bring rain per the request of the Wu Yi.

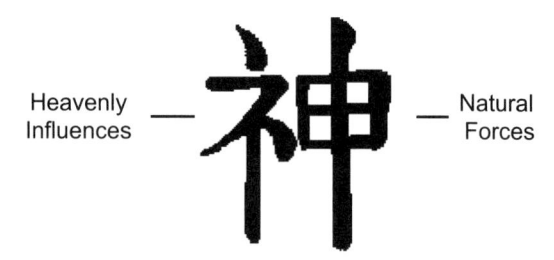

Figure 2.26. The Chinese Character for "Shen," Spirit

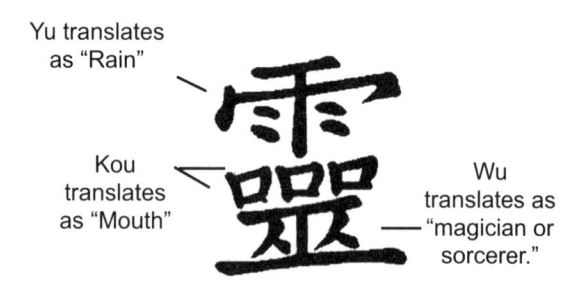

Figure 2.27. The Chinese Character for "Ling," Magical

SHEN XIAN: ETERNAL SOUL

The Eternal Soul (Shen Xian) has an infinite source of vitality derived from the high-frequency force of the Divine or Dao. The Eternal Soul's quest for knowledge and experience within the three planes of existence (physical, energetic and spiritual) as a human soul (Yuan Shen) has always been a topic of controversy and debate.

As previously mentioned, the Chinese ideogram for Shen can be translated as "god, deity, spirit or mind." The Chinese ideogram for Xian can be translated as "celestial being, immortal, or heavenly soul." It is depicted by two characters: positioned on the right is a character for "mountain"; positioned to the left is a character depicting "man". The ideograph depicts the "immortals" said to have lived in ancient times, high in the sacred mountains of China. Together, Shen

Xian can be translated as "Eternal Soul" (Figure 2.28).

The Shen Xian (Eternal Soul) is sometimes considered a component of the Shen Ling (Supernatural Spirit) that reincarnates. As the Shen Ling is rooted in the light of the Divine, so the Shen Xian is guided by the direction of the Shen Ling.

FROM ETERNAL SOUL TO HUMAN SOUL

After passing through the Zhi Yi Tian ("will and intent of heaven"), the Shen Xian (Eternal Soul) will be absorbed into the mother's egg at the time of conception in the form of a Yuan Shen (human soul). Although spiritual in nature, the Shen Xian is also connected to the Wuji, and is considered a separate entity, apart from the body.

During fetal development, the Shen Xian will be rooted in the area of the individual's Heart and Middle Dantian by a silver cord, which itself is rooted within the body's Taiji Pole. It is the Shen Xian that creates and roots the body's Taiji Pole within the forming tissue cells. The Taiji Pole is described as "emitting the spark of the Supreme Fire" (or Light of God) and is considered a divine fragment of God or the Dao (hence its internal connection to the Shen Ling). It is from this divine resonating light that the body's Taiji Pole becomes energized and all Three Dantians become interconnected. The rooting of the Shen Xian into the physical body as a human soul (Yuan Shen) is, therefore, considered the first manifestation of the divine source within the human body (Figure 2.29).

Whole-body consciousness is the main characteristic of the Shen Xian. The Shen Xian radiates through the physical, energetic, and psycho-emotional domains of human existence. Without the interactive process of the Shen Xian, energy would have no specific direction and would remain in meaningless activity. The Shen Xian radiates energy in all directions, and is responsible for growth, formation, vitality and health throughout the body.

ENERGETIC MANIFESTATION

The Shen Xian manifests its innate qualities as energetic movement, functioning through the physical form. The Shen Xian is expressed through the Yuan Shen and is connected to all parts of the body. The light of the Shen Xian is revealed through the sparkle, or Shen in the eyes. Through the influence of the Shen Xian, all of the body's energetic processes seek wholeness. The Shen Xian knows exactly what is needed for health preservation and survival in every situation.

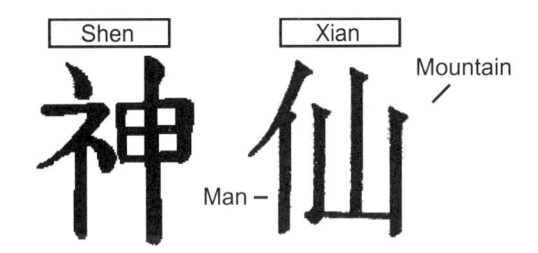

Figure 2.28. The Chinese Characters for "Shen Xian," Immortal Soul

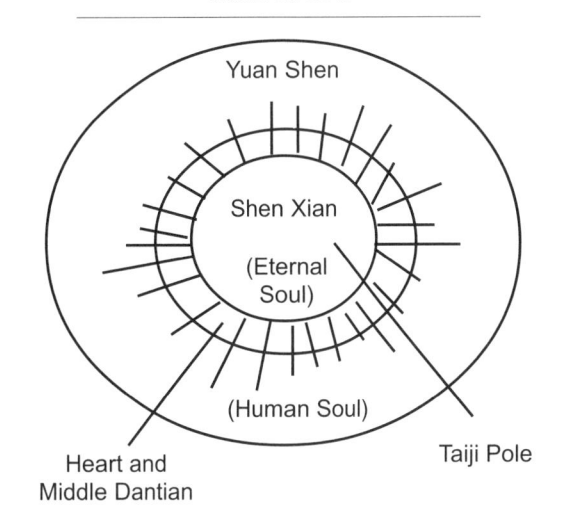

Figure 2.29. The Shen Xian is rooted in the area of the individual's Heart and Middle Dantian by a silver cord, which itself is rooted within the body's Taiji Pole.

When conserved and amplified through spiritual practice, the energy of the Shen Xian reveals a bright radiant quality which permeates and penetrates the cells, tissues, organs, and external energy fields. These energetic fields create a strong luminous shield of energy capable of guarding the Qigong doctor's body against an attack by hostile or pathogenic energy by enabling it to:

- ward off the invasion of external pathogens and harmful electromagnetic fields
- ward off the negative influences of malevolent spirits

- ward off ill intentions and spiritual malice projected unconsciously or deliberately by others
- ward off the parasitic influences of demonic forces

Soul Travel

To receive spiritual guidance and insight, the Shen Xian can leave the material body in the form of a "soul body," departing from the physical body while in deep meditation. The silver cord, which is connected to the soul body, is located at the fifth and sixth thoracic vertebrae. This physical area is the place on the spine where the silver cord lifts when an individual soul travels. This area also corresponds to the back of the Heart center, between Ling Tai GV-10 (Soul's Platform) and Shen Dao GV-11 (Spirit's Gate).

The journey of the Shen Xian is based on the spiritual evolution of the individual. The individual's ability to sojourn into other dimensions of existence depends on his or her capability to relax and increase the level of vibrational frequency.

When the Qigong doctor meditates, the Yuan Shen reconnects with its Shen Xian and consciously enters a spiritual realm wherein the doctor perceives the ideal of things (intention and thought) rather than the things themselves. The doctor no longer depends on the senses, but upon a clear inner-vision that perceives the whole picture. It is within this spiritual state that higher knowledge unfolds through divine intelligence, allowing all things to reveal their true nature.

Yin and Yang Aspects of the Shen Xian

On the spiritual plane, when referring to the energetic dynamics of the Shen Xian, there are two basic movements, described as follows:

1. **Yin:** The downward movement from the energy of the Dao releasing the Eternal Soul, traveling through the Wuji, transforming into a human soul, and finally to the energetic form of the body's Original Spirit.
2. **Yang:** The upward movement of the Original Spirit towards the reunion and fusion with the Dao.

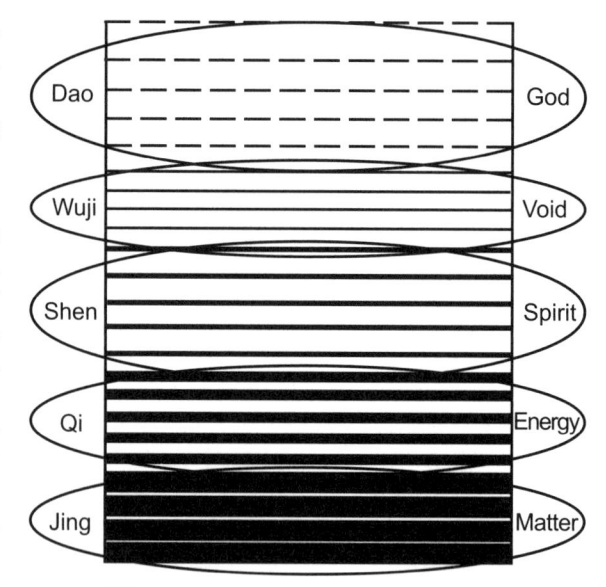

Figure 2.30. The Five Energetic Fields

The Yin Aspect of the Eternal Soul

The Yin aspect of the Eternal Soul spirals downward, resulting in the transformation of spiritual energy from the highest to the lowest divine energetic frequencies. Within this spiritual transformational process, there is a corresponding decrease in consciousness. The lowest frequency creates matter and is the basis for prenatal transformations.

At the higher energetic frequencies, the principles by which Qi operates are difficult to perceive if the individual's lower state of consciousness does not resonate in harmony with the information being presented. However, as energy slows down its resonance, it is more readily perceived by the five senses. This gives matter the quality of hardness, form, and smell, and also allows individuals to observe its energetic patterning (Figure 2.30).

The Yang Aspect of the Eternal Soul

The Yang aspects of the Eternal Soul spiral upward resulting in the transformation of spiritual energy from the lowest level of consciousness to the highest divine energetic frequencies. The highest frequency creates spiritual consciousness and is the primary goal of postnatal transformation.

Spiritual evolution involves a progressive opening of all the body's energy centers (Three Dantians and Twelve Chakra Gates) along the Taiji Pole, until a state of absolute unity of body, mind, emotion, energy, and spirit is achieved, and enlightenment is attained.

In the evolutionary process of the soul, stability and change become as one when there is a deep connection and internal commitment to integrated wholeness. The soul serves as a pivotal point for the body's Jing, Qi, Shen, Body Fluids, connective tissues, thoughts and emotions, all of which express the multidimensional aspects of the soul. Without a deep energetic and spiritual connection for transformation and change, the patient can experience a psychic splitting of his or her energies. The part of the patient that is open to change (Yuan Shen) will experience resistance from the part that demands stability and desires to maintain the denial system (Shen Zhi).

Zhi Yi Tian:
Will and Intent of Heaven

When a Shen Xian (Eternal Soul) descends into the "worlds of creation" for the purpose of acquiring experiences, it must first decrease its vibrational resonance in order to develop into a Yuan Shen (human soul). This is accomplished by passing through an energetic field commonly called the Zhi Yi Tian ("will and intent of heaven"). After passing through this energetic veil, the vibrational levels of the Shen Xian are lowered in order to transform the energetic nature of the Eternal Soul into a human soul.

The Chinese ideogram "Zhi" is composed of two characters: the character on the bottom is the Heart, while the character above it depicts a plant beginning to rise upward from the soil. Together, both characters depict the continuous and persistent intention of the Heart to develop towards a desired goal. The plant represents the process of life's development through the unity of both will and intention (Figure 2.31).

The Chinese ideogram "Yi" is composed of two characters: the character on the bottom is the Heart, and the one on the top represents a musical note or sound ("Yin"). Together, both characters describe the Heart's intention to think, speak or act (Figure 2.32).

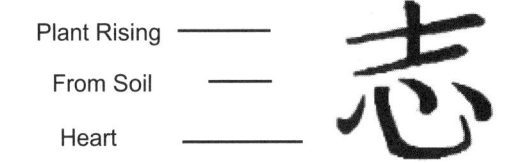

Figure 2.31. The Chinese Character for "Zhi," Will

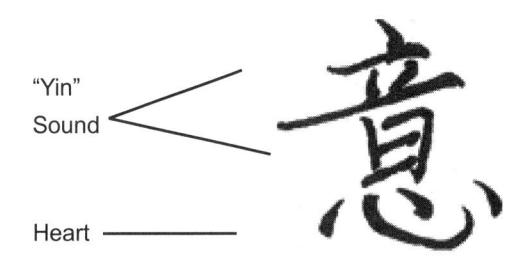

Figure 2.32. The Chinese Character for "Yi," Intent

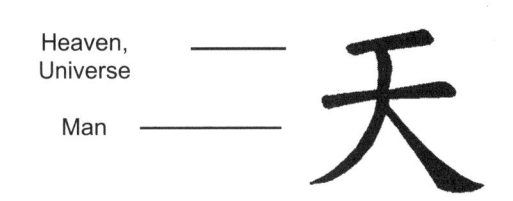

Figure 2.33. The Chinese Character for "Tian," Heaven

The Chinese ideogram "Tian" is composed of two characters: on the bottom is the character "Ren," meaning "man or humanity," which is expressed through the image of a person with both arms and legs outstretched. On the top is a single line representing the sky or Heaven above and the vastness of space. Together, both characters can be translated as god, divine, heaven, celestial, sky and weather governing (over) man; representing the spiritual and energetic firmament covering humanity (Figure 2.33).

Zhi Yi Tian can be translated as Heaven's will and intent, Heaven's design or Heaven's plan, and signifies the spiritual transformation occurring when individuals embrace Divine Will.

YUAN SHEN: HUMAN SOUL

The Chinese ideogram for "Yuan" can be translated as "primary" or "original." The Chinese ideogram for Shen can be translated as "god, deity, spirit or mind." Together, Yuan Shen can be translated as the "Original Spirit," and is considered the Yang aspect of the Human Soul (Figure 2.34).

As the Shen Xian descends into the material world, it fuses the energetic natures of the Dao, Wuji and Taiji, with the structural energetic natures of the Ba Gua and Wu Xing. These energetic components combine and fuse into the body's tissue cells via the formation of the individual's Taiji Pole, which is created when the sperm penetrates the egg (see Embryology Section, this Chapter).

The vibrational levels of the Shen Xian must slow down to resonate with the frequencies of the lower dimensions and maintain physical form. This allows the Shen Xian to acquire experiences within the world of time and space as a human soul. The ancient Daoists believed that we, as living organisms, are pure spirit, and that we have dressed ourselves with form via the Mind in order to manifest as a part of creation. As we live within the Wuji, we are suspended between Heaven and Earth on the material plane and are affected by universal and environmental energetic phenomena.

When the mother's and father's Jing, Qi and Shen combine during conception, the energy of the Dao is drawn into the mother's womb in order to orchestrate the forming of the embryo. While in the womb, the fetus continues to transform and develop the culminated Jing, Qi and Shen, while remaining in a state of quiescence.

THE YUAN SHEN AND SHEN XIAN

The ancient Chinese also believed that the Yuan Shen (the human soul's original personality) is expressed as the lower aspect of the Shen Xian (Eternal Soul) upon which incarnate experiences will be recorded once it has been absorbed into the mother's egg upon conception. Sometimes described as the "feet of the Eternal Soul," the Yuan Shen represents the expressions of the Shen Xian's personality, containing within itself the Divine consciousness. It supervises the life and experiences of the individual's temporary Shen Zhi (acquired personality, also known as Huode Shen).

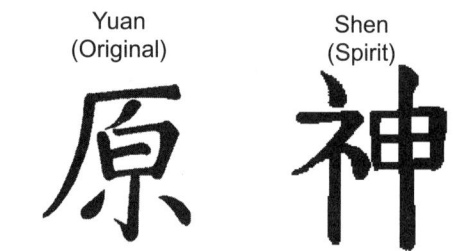

Figure 2.34. The Chinese Character for "Yuan Shen," Original Spirit

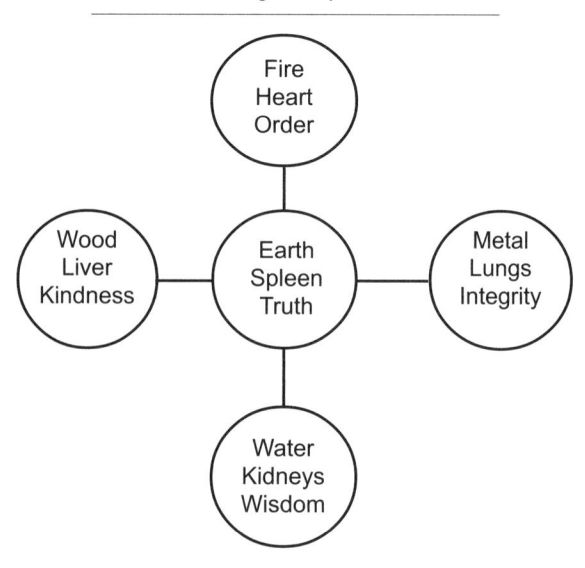

Figure 2.35. Once the energies of the fetus's Yin (Water) and Yang (Fire) divide and begin the work of internal tissue construction, the spiritual energy of the Five Lights take residence within the Five Yin Organs.

THE WUJING SHEN

Once the energies of the fetus' Yin (Water) and Yang (Fire) divide and begin the work of internal tissue construction, the spiritual energy of the Five Lights take residence within the Five Yin Organs (Liver, Heart, Spleen, Lungs, and Kidneys). Upon taking residence, the Five Lights begin absorbing and utilizing the various energies radiating from the heavenly and earthly Five Elements (Wood, Fire, Earth, Metal, and Water) in order to continue building the fetus' internal energetic fields (Figure 2.35).

The "congenital mind" (Yuan Shen) is integrated and sustained by the embryo's "five spiritual essences," or Prenatal Wu Jing Shen (see Volume 2, Chapter 14), which are in turn created from the energy of the five Yin organs. The Yuan Shen is then rooted in the combined Jing, Qi, and Shen that the mother and father provided upon conception. The combined Jing, Qi, and Shen also provides the basis for the formation of the "acquired mind" (Shen Zhi), which is integrated and sustained by the individual's Postnatal Wu Jing Shen.

The spiritual energies of the Five Elements differ in that they represent either the congenital mind of the Prenatal Wu Jing Shen (pertaining to the congenital five virtues of kindness, order, truth, integrity, and wisdom), or the temporal acquired mind of the Postnatal Wu Jing Shen (pertaining to the five acquired emotional states of anger, joy, worry, grief, and fear). The ancient Daoists believed that the cultivation of the Prenatal Wu Jing Shen produced sages, while the unbridled state of the Postnatal Wu Jing Shen produced ordinary people.

The acquired mental states of the Postnatal Five Elements attack and overcome one another, while the spiritual virtues of the Prenatal Wu Jing Shen nourish and support each other. When the spiritual virtues of the Prenatal Wu Jing Shen nourish and support each other they become integrated within the celestial design, causing the spiritual energies of the Five Elements to fuse as one energy.

In the ancient Daoist text *Understanding Reality*, the Chinese masters of esoteric magic wrote, "When the spiritual energies of the Five Elements are assembled, the great Dao may be attained." The work of assembling the spiritual energies of the Five Elements requires the individual to extract the spiritual virtues of the Prenatal Wu Jing Shen (benevolence, justice, courtesy, truthfulness, and wisdom) from the acquired mental states of the Postnatal Wu Jing Shen (anger, joy, worry, grief, and fear).

ENERGETIC MANIFESTATION

The Shen Xian (Eternal Soul) radiates from the interior of the Taiji Pole via the Yuan Shen. This spiritual light energetically crystallizes to form the individual's Spiritual Body, which gradually becomes conscious and awakens into action, affecting the body's Jing and Qi. The Spirit Body envelops the Physical and Energetic Bodies and communicates through the individual's innermost thoughts, feeling sensations and emotions.

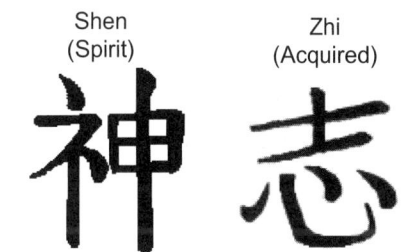

Figure 2.36. The Chinese Character for "Shen Zhi," Acquired Spirit

The body's Jing, Qi and Shen are temporal while being enveloped, fused and housed in the physical form. These Three Treasures (Jing, Qi and Shen) will eventually separate when the individual dies. The Jing and the Yin aspect of the Qi will dissolve back into the Earth, while the Yang aspect of the Qi and the Yuan Shen will ascend to Heaven along with the Shen Xian. The ancient Chinese believed that the Yuan Shen, being an expression of the Shen Xian, was a temporal part of the body.

SHEN ZHI: ACQUIRED SPIRIT

As previously mentioned, the Chinese ideogram for Shen can be translated as "god, deity, spirit, or mind." The Chinese ideogram for "Zhi" can be translated as "will and intention." Together, Shen Zhi can be translated as the "spirit's acquired will" or "acquired mind," and is considered the Yin aspect of the human soul. The Shen Zhi is reflected in the experiences of the individual's acquired knowledge and patterns (Figure 2.36).

As the human soul descends into the "world of physical matter" it is temporarily expressed through an acquired Shen Zhi, also known as the acquired personality. The Shen Zhi experiences a myriad of emotions and desires, forming a unique personality characteristic that learns to interpret and interact within its environment for the sake of survival (Figure 2.37).

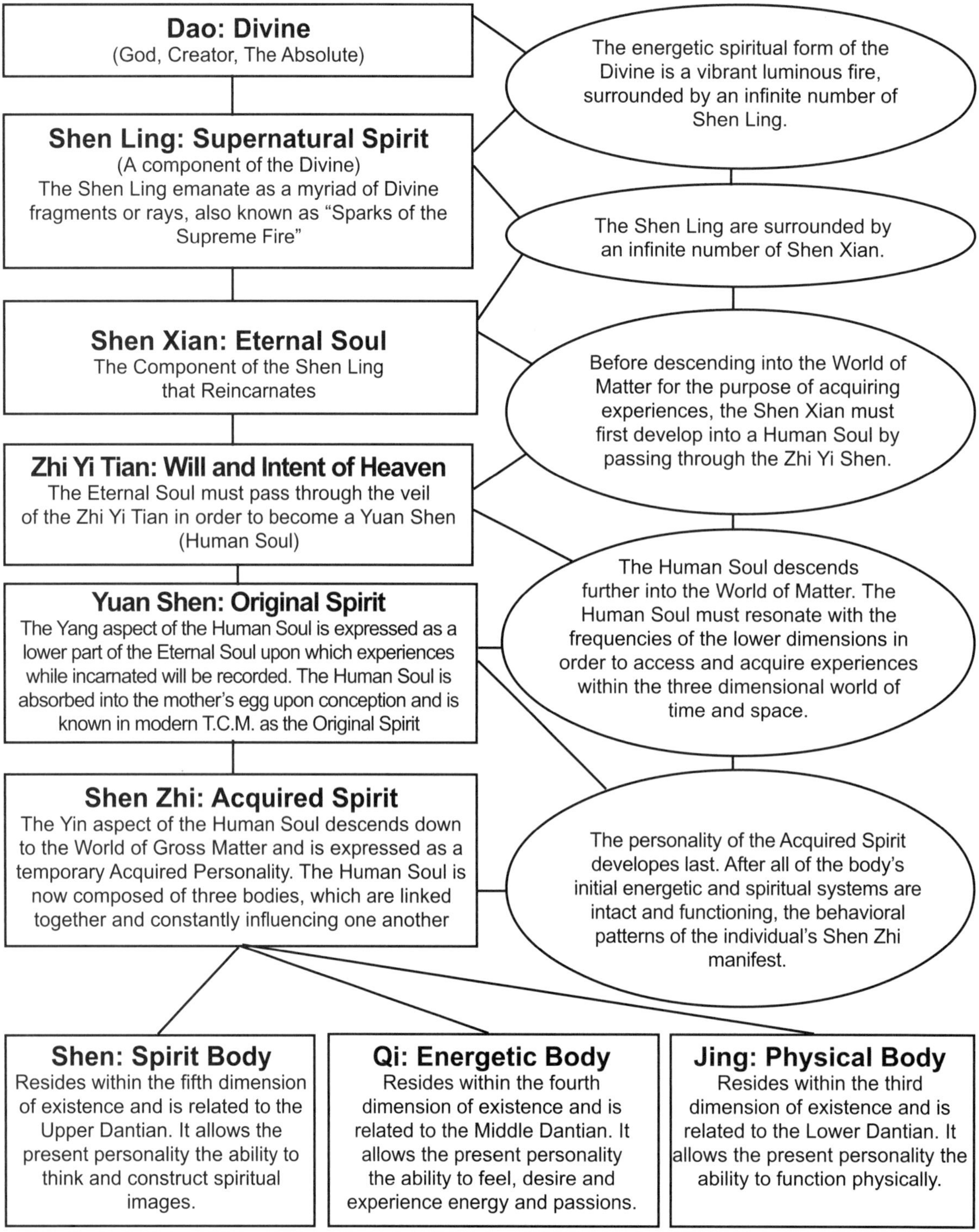

VOLUME 1, SECTION 1: FOUNDATIONS OF CHINESE ENERGETIC MEDICINE

Dao: Divine
(God, Creator, The Absolute)

The energetic spiritual form of the Divine is a vibrant luminous fire, surrounded by an infinite number of Shen Ling.

Shen Ling: Supernatural Spirit
(A component of the Divine)
The Shen Ling emanate as a myriad of Divine fragments or rays, also known as "Sparks of the Supreme Fire"

The Shen Ling are surrounded by an infinite number of Shen Xian.

Shen Xian: Eternal Soul
The Component of the Shen Ling that Reincarnates

Before descending into the World of Matter for the purpose of acquiring experiences, the Shen Xian must first develop into a Human Soul by passing through the Zhi Yi Shen.

Zhi Yi Tian: Will and Intent of Heaven
The Eternal Soul must pass through the veil of the Zhi Yi Tian in order to become a Yuan Shen (Human Soul)

Yuan Shen: Original Spirit
The Yang aspect of the Human Soul is expressed as a lower part of the Eternal Soul upon which experiences while incarnated will be recorded. The Human Soul is absorbed into the mother's egg upon conception and is known in modern T.C.M. as the Original Spirit

The Human Soul descends further into the World of Matter. The Human Soul must resonate with the frequencies of the lower dimensions in order to access and acquire experiences within the three dimensional world of time and space.

Shen Zhi: Acquired Spirit
The Yin aspect of the Human Soul descends down to the World of Gross Matter and is expressed as a temporary Acquired Personality. The Human Soul is now composed of three bodies, which are linked together and constantly influencing one another

The personality of the Acquired Spirit developes last. After all of the body's initial energetic and spiritual systems are intact and functioning, the behavioral patterns of the individual's Shen Zhi manifest.

Shen: Spirit Body
Resides within the fifth dimension of existence and is related to the Upper Dantian. It allows the present personality the ability to think and construct spiritual images.

Qi: Energetic Body
Resides within the fourth dimension of existence and is related to the Middle Dantian. It allows the present personality the ability to feel, desire and experience energy and passions.

Jing: Physical Body
Resides within the third dimension of existence and is related to the Lower Dantian. It allows the present personality the ability to function physically.

Figure 2.37. The Spiritual Evolution of the Soul

The Prenatal Wu Jing Shen helps to create and support the spiritual virtues of the Yuan Shen, and in a similar fashion, the Postnatal Wu Jing Shen helps to create and support the acquired thoughts and emotions of the Shen Zhi. At the moment of the infant's first cry, the ancient Daoists believed that the acquired conscious spirit (Shen Zhi) becomes activated as the Postnatal Qi enters into the opening of the mouth and nose and energetically merges with the baby's original spirit (Yuan Shen). The congenital Yuan Shen depends on the acquired Shen Zhi to exist, while the Shen Zhi depends on the Yuan Shen for effective awareness.

The ancient Daoists believed that the Shen Zhi's behavioral patterns are developed last, after all of the body's initial energetic and spiritual systems are intact and functioning. As the Shen Zhi is considered the lowest expression of the Divine within the individual, it is continually evolving, striving to become one with the human soul that resides within the Taiji Pole. It is believed that together the individual's Shen Zhi and Yuan Shen complete the Yin and Yang aspects of the human soul. Together, they gather the sum total of all thoughts, emotions, and experiences that the human soul accumulates from the moment of its descent into matter at conception.

The various personality characteristics of each of the individual's Shen are sometimes described as "soul extensions" because they manifest within the individual's energetic field and tend to influence his or her behavior and perception. The Yuan Shen is influenced primarily by the Hun (Ethereal Soul) while the Shen Zhi is influenced primarily by the Po (Corporeal Soul) (see end of Chapter).

The Three Bodies

The human soul is enveloped by and composed of three bodies. These three bodies are linked together, constantly influencing one another. While in the mother's Uterus, the human soul is initially enveloped in a spiritual body. Then an energetic body is formed within the spiritual body. Finally, the physical body is constructed within the energetic and spiritual bodies. This allows the individual to live within the lower levels of creation. All three bodies have substance,

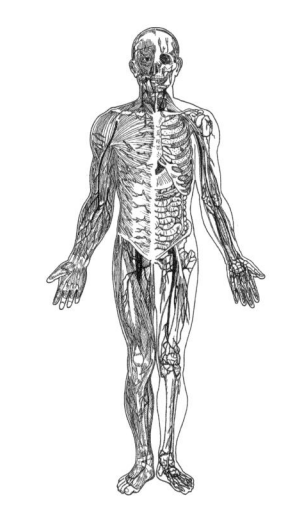

Figure 2.38. Jing: the "Material" Body

yet they exist at different levels of vibration.

It is important to remember that the human soul was not created at the time of birth. Being a part of the Divine, all souls have existed since the beginning of time. Every birth is a rebirth of the Eternal Soul which has already existed, and will continue to incarnate.

The body serves as a medium of transformation for the Shen Xian. The soul extends and expresses itself through consciousness and physical form. As we grow and change, the human soul maintains stability by providing the energetic blueprint for orderly development.

The Physical Body

The physical body exists within the physical or material world and is associated with Jing (Essence). This is the level of experience that has both form and substance, and which is accessible through the five ordinary senses. It is within the physical body that we express our energetic patterns through the vibrational resonance of the tissue cells. The physical body's Wei Qi field is rooted in the Lower Dantian and obeys the laws of three dimensionality, meaning that it can only occupy one position in space.

Every particle, atom and cell of the physical body has its energetic and spiritual counterpart. As mentioned earlier, the energetic body and spiritual bodies together serve as a womb within which the physical body is formed (Figure 2.38).

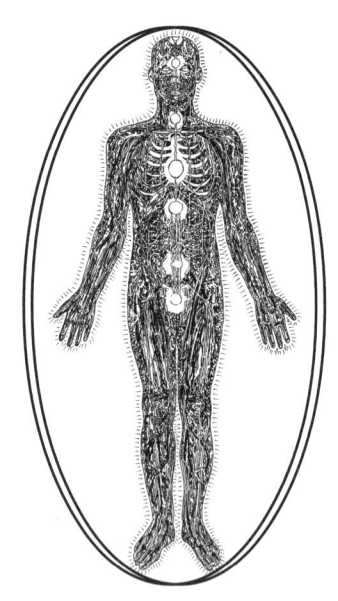

VOLUME 1, SECTION 1: FOUNDATIONS OF CHINESE ENERGETIC MEDICINE

Figure 2.39. Qi: the "Energetic" Body
(Inspired by the original artwork of Alex Grey)

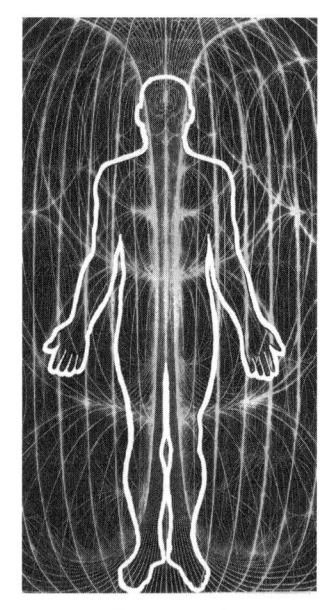

Figure 2.40. Shen: the "Spiritual" Body
(Inspired by the original artwork of Alex Grey)

THE ENERGETIC BODY

The energetic body exists within the fourth dimensional world and is associated with Qi (energy). This is the level of experience that has form but no substance (e.g., dreams) and substance but no form (e.g., energy). It is through the Energetic Body that we express our feelings, sentiments and desires. The energetic body's field is rooted in the Middle Dantian (Figure 2.39).

The energetic body is composed of energetic matter and is built cell by cell in the mould of the body's internal and external energetic fields. Even the smallest physical detail of the physical body is projected into the energetic body with the exception of any wounds or physical mutilations.

THE SPIRITUAL BODY

The spiritual body exists within the fifth dimensional world and is associated with Shen (spirit). This is the level of experience that has neither form nor substance. It resonates at a higher and more subtle level than the Energetic World. It is through the Spiritual Body that we express our thoughts and intentions. The spiritual body's energetic field is rooted in the Upper Dantian. There are two aspects to the spiritual body: The lower spiritual body and the higher spiritual body. The lower spiritual body has shape and form, while the higher spiritual body is shapeless (Figure 2.40).

OVERVIEW

The ancient Chinese understanding of the physical, energetic, and spiritual transformations occurring within the formations of the universe and the human body laid the foundation for modern Traditional Chinese Medicine. Although there is great variation in both the terminologies used and the spiritual practices associated with this knowledge, the practical clinical applications still contain the essence of the ancient Daoist theories behind them.

A Medical Qigong doctor, for example, will always diagnose from observing the patient's spiritual, mental, emotional, energetic, and physical interactions with cosmic (Heavenly) and environmental (Earthly) influences. This diagnosis will include the patient's interactions with all of the aforementioned aspects: the Dao (Divine), Wuji (Infinite Space), Taiji (Yin and Yang), Bagua (Eight Trigrams), Wu Xing (Five Phases) the Three Worlds (matter, energy and spirit), and the Three Bodies (physical, energetic, and spiritual) (Figure 2.41).

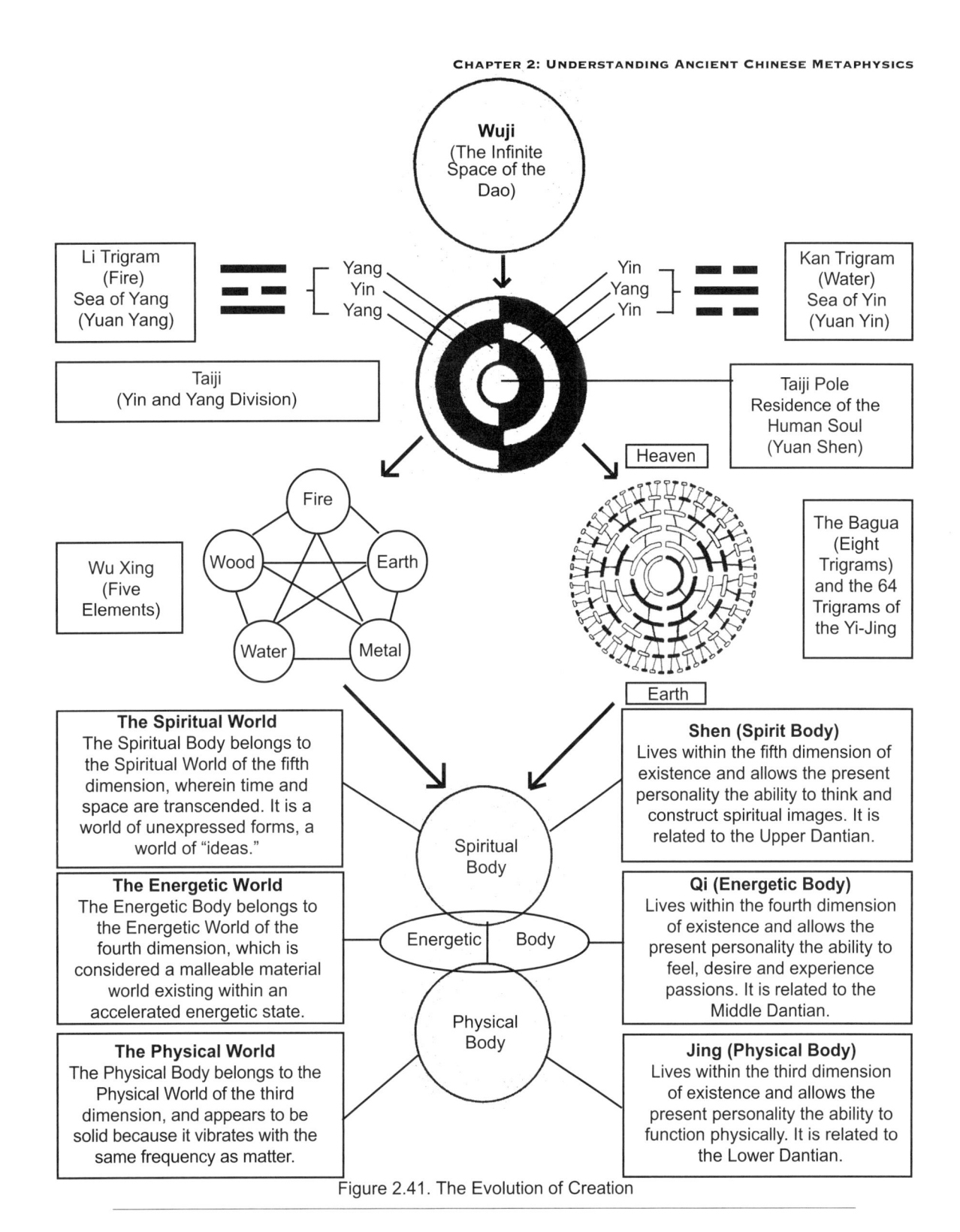

CHAPTER 2: UNDERSTANDING ANCIENT CHINESE METAPHYSICS

Wuji (The Infinite Space of the Dao)

Li Trigram (Fire) Sea of Yang (Yuan Yang) — Yang Yin Yang

Kan Trigram (Water) Sea of Yin (Yuan Yin) — Yin Yang Yin

Taiji (Yin and Yang Division)

Taiji Pole Residence of the Human Soul (Yuan Shen)

Heaven

Wu Xing (Five Elements): Fire, Wood, Earth, Water, Metal

The Bagua (Eight Trigrams) and the 64 Trigrams of the Yi-Jing

Earth

The Spiritual World
The Spiritual Body belongs to the Spiritual World of the fifth dimension, wherein time and space are transcended. It is a world of unexpressed forms, a world of "ideas."

Shen (Spirit Body)
Lives within the fifth dimension of existence and allows the present personality the ability to think and construct spiritual images. It is related to the Upper Dantian.

The Energetic World
The Energetic Body belongs to the Energetic World of the fourth dimension, which is considered a malleable material world existing within an accelerated energetic state.

Qi (Energetic Body)
Lives within the fourth dimension of existence and allows the present personality the ability to feel, desire and experience passions. It is related to the Middle Dantian.

The Physical World
The Physical Body belongs to the Physical World of the third dimension, and appears to be solid because it vibrates with the same frequency as matter.

Jing (Physical Body)
Lives within the third dimension of existence and allows the present personality the ability to function physically. It is related to the Lower Dantian.

Spiritual Body — Energetic Body — Physical Body

Figure 2.41. The Evolution of Creation

Energetic Embryological Development

The study of the embryological development of the body's inner fascia and organ tissues illuminates many of the ideas about energy, health, and disease contained within Traditional Chinese Medicine. The ancient Chinese doctors understood through energetic embryology that original patterns created during tissue formation remain operative throughout adulthood. Thus, the cells, tissues, and organs of the human body continue to interrelate according to the energetic patterning that begins at conception. As an embryo develops, it passes through several stages of formation causing it to recreate the patterning of remote ancestral energetic traits. This type of heredity is a form of unconscious organic memory.

Essentially, Heaven (the universal energy related to the sun, moon, and stars) and Earth (the environmental energy related to the earth, water and wind) both emit powerful energetic fields that influence the formation of life. If we consider Heaven Qi to be electropositive and Earth Qi to be electronegative, we can begin to understand the duality of these energetic fields and their pull on the human body. One can think of the body as being suspended between these two enormous fields of energy (Figure 2.42). As the energetic field of the sun cascades downward, the Earth's core extends its energetic field upwards through the Earth's crust. Man is therefore suspended between the electrically positive energy field of Heaven and the electrically negative energy field of Earth and is affected accordingly by both celestial and environmental phenomena.

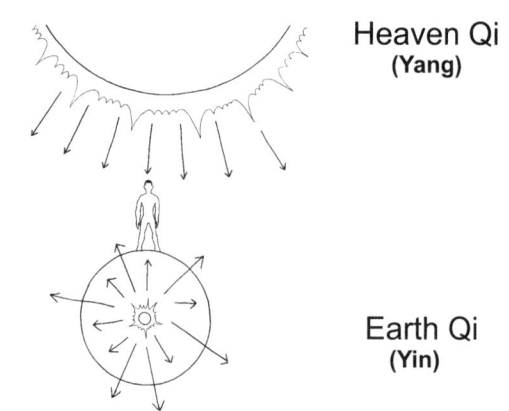

Figure 2.42. The human energetic field is suspended between the two energy fields of Heaven and Earth.

Interactions of Essence, Energy and Spirit

The *Yellow Emperor's Classic of Internal Medicine* states that woman's physiology is dominated by Blood, which serves as the foundation of her menstrual cycle, fertility, pregnancy, and childbirth. It further states that man's physiology is dominated by Qi, which serves as the basis of his strength, fertility, endurance, and virility.

A myriad of energetic interactions begin at the

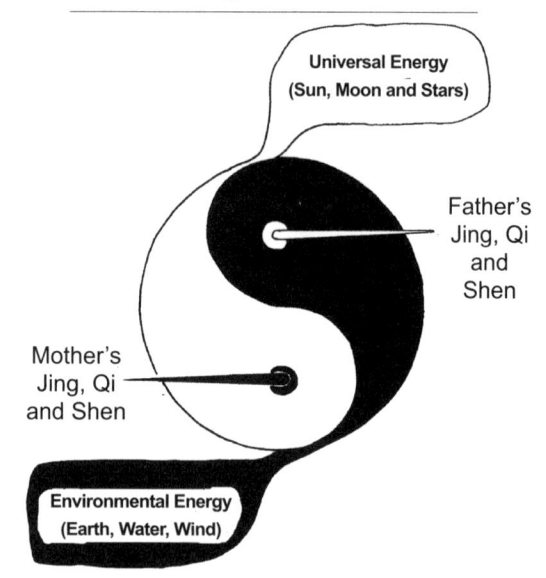

Figure 2.43. The blending of the energies of Heaven (Universal Qi) and Earth (Environmental Qi) with the energies of the father and mother creates a fusion of Yin and Yang energies within the body's tissues and cells during creation. These energies are responsible, on a psychophysical level, for transferring talents and traits from generation to generation.

moment of conception. At conception, the energies of Heaven and Earth, as well as the energies of the mother and father, exert a powerful influence on the state and patterning of the zygote. These four energies condense upon impact and form the nucleus of the cellular patterning of the new life (Figure 2.43). Every part of the resulting human body is affected by this energetic patterning.

In the *Yellow Emperor's Classic of Internal Medicine* it is also written that, "When the Jing (Essence) of Yin and Yang Qi merges (the blending of the sperm and the egg), before the fetus changes into its dominant sex, the two Kidney orbs grow first." Both Kidneys are formed like two halves of a bean, with the Original Qi (Yuan Qi) located between them. At one time, the left Kidney orb was called the "true" Kidney, while the right orb was considered the Mingmen (Gate of Life, Fate, or Destiny). The Mingmen is said to store the energy of the man's sperm essence, or the woman's egg essence (their Postnatal Jing). During the Ming dynasty, however, the theory of the Mingmen Fire occupying the space between the two Kidneys became more popular.

Around the age of fourteen, a girl's Conception Vessel grows to maturity and fully energizes her Xin (Heart), and her menses begins. Around the age of sixteen, a boy's Governing Vessel becomes mature and fully energizes his Kidneys, and his body produces mature semen.

The body's Yuan Qi (Prenatal Qi) is the representation of the energetic forces of Heaven and Earth as imprinted within the Jing at the moment of conception. As the Shen rises from the Jing, it creates the internal polarity of the body's Yuan Yin and Yuan Yang, associated with the Kidney's Original Qi. An old Chinese saying in Medical Qigong states that, "When people are born, Heaven gives them Jing and Shen (Spirit) -- which align to form the mind -- and Earth gives them Bones and shape, which unite to form the body. When joined together, these two sources of energy cause human beings to develop. When people die, their Essence and Spirit return to Heaven, and their Bones and shape go back to Earth."

During birth, pairs of channels from the mother's internal organs carry Qi that creates and nourishes the baby at each stage of development. Receiving its sustenance through the umbilical cord, the developing child's navel, Kidneys, and lower abdominal area become the collection points for Prenatal Qi (energy stored within the baby's body before it is born, also known as Yuan Qi).

Every life begins with inherent strengths and weaknesses. Energetically, it is believed that if the mother achieves orgasm during conception, the child's constitution will be stronger. This is due to a greater release of the combined energetic and spiritual forces of the mother and father's Jing, Qi and Shen as they enter into the physical tissues of the Uterus. As this released energy combines with the mother's Lower Dantian Qi, the forming zygote is allowed maximum energetic potential. Likewise, it is also believed that if the mother does not orgasm during conception, the child's energetic constitution will be relatively weaker.

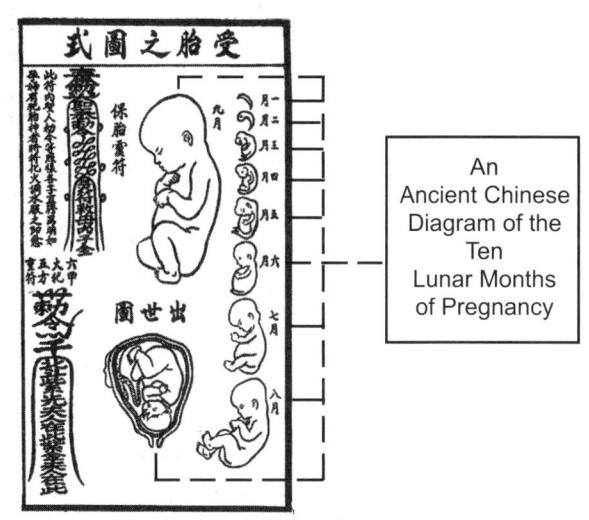

Figure 2.44. In ancient China, talismans were sometimes used to insure safe and healthy fetal development.

Prenatal care is mandatory for the healthy formation of the embryo. Before cell division, the DNA mass must be duplicated exactly in order to transfer normal genetic characteristics to the next generation. Although both parents contribute to the cellular DNA of the forming embryo, it is the mother who is solely responsible for contributing the mitochondrial DNA. Although heredity plays a large part in the transference of both parents' genetic history, a weakness in the mother's energy channels can result in congenital toxins, or other problems that the fetus may acquire during one of the corresponding stages of development.

In ancient China, talismans were sometimes given to pregnant women in order to ward off pathogenic influences, protect the womb against evil spirits, and to secure the health and safety of the developing child (Figure 2.44).

VOLUME 1, SECTION 1: FOUNDATIONS OF CHINESE ENERGETIC MEDICINE

DAOIST PERSPECTIVES ON EARLY EMBRYOLOGICAL DEVELOPMENT

The following is an ancient Chinese Daoist perspective of embryological development combined with modern Western anatomical understandings of fertilization and cell division (Figure 2.45).

- In essence, all life arises directly from the ocean of Qi that exists within the infinite space of the Wuji. Similarly, the woman's Bao (Uterus) is the ocean of Qi from which all humanity is created (Lower Dantian), and can also represent the infinite space of the Wuji, in terms of embryological development (see Uterus, Chapter 7).
- As the sperm breaks through the cell membrane of the ovum, it loses its tail and transforms into the male pronucleus (Yang). Once the male pronucleus (Yang) joins the female pronucleus (Yin), the first cellular division occurs. Both the female (Yin) and male (Yang) membranes of the two pronuclei fuse and then absorb into each other, and the zygote divides into "blastomeres." This energetic transformation causes the zygote to undergo its normal cellular division within 36 hours after fertilization.
- The blastomeres further divide into several distinct layers (later becoming the body's various energetic organs and systems). Within 48 hours, the next cellular division occurs, manifesting the development of the Four Phases of Universal Energy.
- Within 60 hours after conception, eight cells have developed and form what is known as a morula (a mass of blastomeres). According to Daoist belief, this energetic transformation relates to the eight energetic powers of the Prenatal Bagua Trigram configuration. By the end of the third day (72 hours), there are sixteen cells, a microcosm functioning under the macrocosmic influence of the energetic fields of Heaven and Earth. This corresponds to the interactions of the Prenatal and Postnatal Bagua Trigrams and the energetic cycles of the Magic Square.
- After five days, the dense cluster of cells has

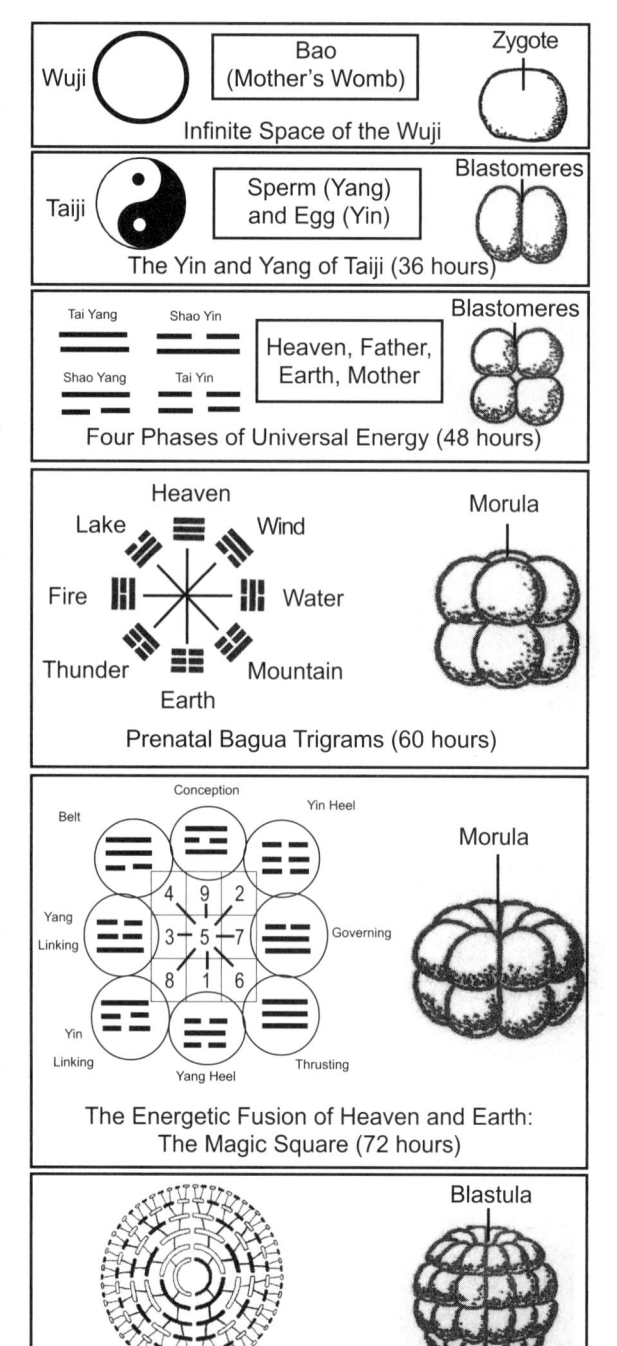

Figure 2.45. Embryological Development from an Ancient Daoist and Modern Medical Perspective

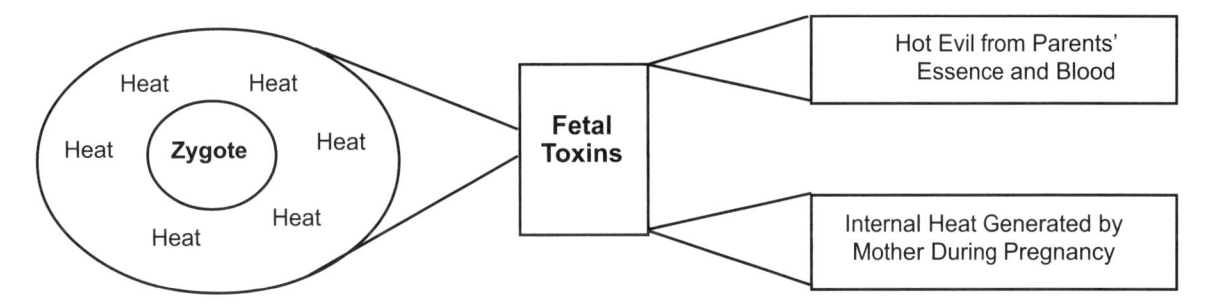

Figure 2.46. The External Invasion of Fetal Toxins

developed into a hollow ball of cells known as a blastula and enters the uterine cavity. This completes the 64 Prenatal and Postnatal Bagua Trigram energetic formation of the Yi-Jing.

Understanding Fetal Toxins

The external invasion of pathogenic toxins (known as fetal toxins in this context) can penetrate the zygote with latent heat that can cause diseases to appear during early fetal or childhood development. Fetal toxins can manifest as either emotional or physical pathogenic patterns. It is therefore important for both parents, but especially the mother, to strive towards strength and health at the time of conception and throughout the pregnancy. Toxins can be transferred to the embryo in-utero in one of two ways:

- Either the mother or father can transfer toxins at the moment of conception. Toxins transferred from the parents can create an inherited toxicity due to a retention of Hot Evil from either of the parents' Essence and Blood.
- Internal Heat generated by the mother during pregnancy can lead to fetal toxins. Toxins can be caused from either internal or external stresses placed on the mother due to repressed emotions, poor diet, unbalanced life-style, overwork, or negative environmental influences (Figure 2.46).

During pregnancy, the fetus is aware of both light and sound and also feels the mother's reaction to the surrounding environmental energy fields. The fetus is strongly influenced by its mother's physical activities, as well as her mental, emotional, and spiritual states.

It is necessary that the parents provide a harmonious and supportive environment for the mother and the unborn child in order to improve its physical, emotional, and mental health. This is called "fetal education" in Traditional Chinese Medicine. Doctors of T.C.M. believe that fetal education is important to ensure optimum development of the child's Prenatal Essence, Energy, and Spirit. This viewpoint is validated by the fact that the Heart and Uterus are directly connected via the mother's internal channels, allowing abundant Qi and Blood to flow into the Uterus. Anything that influences the mother's mind, emotions, and spirit affects her Heart, travels to the Uterus, and can then affect the fetus.

The Body's Developmental Sequence

The following description of the body's developmental sequence is only one of the many theories used in Chinese energetic embryology. The ancient Chinese did not have a comprehension of the body's cells and cellular division. However, energetic theories have postulated that the channels were formed at the earliest stages of cell division, creating an energy matrix for the developing fetus. The following theory was taught at the Hai Dian Medical Qigong College in Beijing, China as part of the Energetic Embryological course.

Creation of Yin and Yang

The ancient Daoist understanding of human creation is described as follows: Once the Absolute has divided (when the zygote experiences its first cellular division), clear Yang energy rises, creating the image of Heaven (Yang Qi begins to ascend and initiates the creation of the body's energetic and spiritual matrices). Opaque Yin energy descends, creating the energetic forms on Earth (Yin energy begins to sink and initiates the creation of the material matrix of the body's physical organs and tissues).

After the first cellular division, the fetus will begin the energetic accumulation of the Five Elements in order to construct the physical, energetic, and spiritual bodies. As the Five Elements begin to construct the physical body, the energetic and spiritual components of the Five Pure Lights begin to thicken the energetic mass (Jing), forming the internal organs and organ systems of which the Five Elements take residence.

PRENATAL YIN AND YANG FORMATIONS

Within the forming fetus, the energetic qualities of the Jing of the Five Elements are further divided into Major Yang and Major Yin components. The Jing of the Five Elemental energies are responsible for producing the foundation of the Major Yang and Major Yin formation.

The Jing of the Elemental energies of Wood and Fire produce Major Yang. The congenital Wood Jing (Hun) and congenital Fire Jing (Shen) influence the production and formation of the "River of Yang Qi" (Governing Vessel).

The Jing of the Elemental energies of Metal and Water produce Major Yin. The congenital Metal Jing (Po) and congenital Water Jing (Zhi) influence the production and formation of the "River of Yin Qi" (Conception Vessel) (Figure 2.47).

THE FIVE ELEMENTAL JING FORMATIONS

Beginning in the fourth lunar month and continuing until the ninth lunar month, each of the Five Element's energetic natures and their associated spiritual characteristics will be progressively activated and developed within the fetus' body. The Prenatal Wu Jing Shen represent the most subtle level of energetic expression manifesting within the spiritual matrix of the human body.

The Chinese characters for Jing Shen are described as follows. The first Chinese ideograph depicts the image for Jing (Essence), and consists of two characters. Positioned to the left is a picture of a bursting and decomposing grain of rice (or millet). Positioned to the right is the character

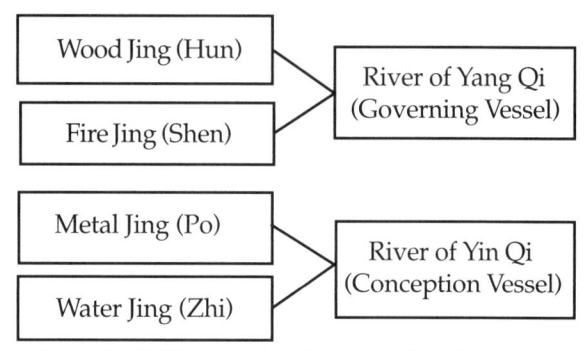

Figure 2.47. The Creative Process of the Body's Yin and Yang Formation

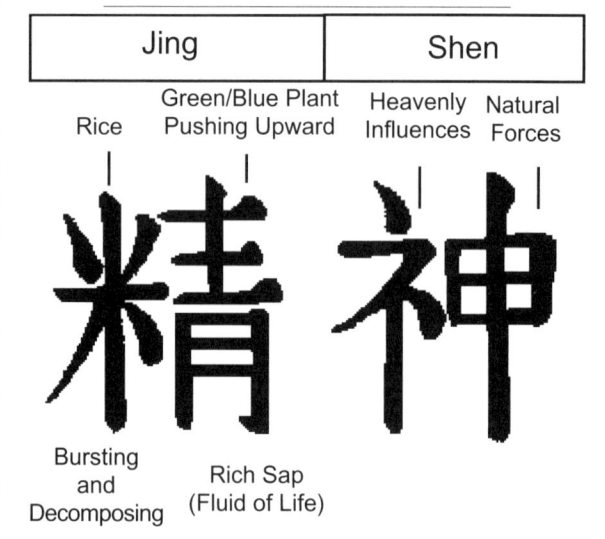

Figure 2.48. The Chinese Characters for "Jing Shen"

"Qing" (green/blue), depicting a young sapling being pushed upward and outward from the soil by its pure life-force Essence. This ideograph depicts decomposing food essence being absorbed into the soil and assimilated by the sapling's root system in order to produce and support life (Figure 2.48).

The second Chinese ideogram depicts the image for Shen (Spirit), and consists of two characters: positioned on the right is a character depicting the alternating expression of natural forces; positioned to the left is a character depicting the unfolding of things under the authority and influence of Heaven. This ideograph depicts the Heavenly influence that permeates and instructs

Jing	Formation	Energetic Property	Disorders
Water Jing Fourth Lunar Month	The Water Jing governs the genetic developmental aspect of the fetal growth, encompasses the fetus' unconscious reservoir of intuitive intelligence, will, and life-force energy, and relates to divine love, power, and spirit.	Harmonization of Kidney Yin and Yang Energy	Any faltering of Water Jing is associated with pervasive or subtle neurological disorders as well as a predisposition to severe psychological disorders (e.g., schizophrenia). Water (Kidney) Jing Deficiency can cause retardation or Congenital Qi Deficiency (i.e., Deficiency in the Sea of Marrow). This, in turn, can lead to Down Syndrome, Attention Deficit Disorder (ADD) and other learning disabilities.
Fire Jing Fifth Lunar Month	The Fire Jing promotes emotional and spiritual well-being by generating, controlling, protecting, integrating, dividing and harmonizing the internal energies of the fetus.	Harmonization of Fire and Water Energy	Any faltering of Fire Jing energy is associated with problems of right (Yin) and left (Yang) brain communication, such as internal imbalances between the rational male energy and intuitive female energy.
Metal Jing Sixth Lunar Month	The Metal Jing stabilizes the sinews and connective tissues and governs the ability to form and maintain emotional bonding with others.	Harmonization of Corporeal Soul and Ethereal Soul for Interaction and Survival	Any faltering of the Metal Jing energy is associated with problems of emotional attachment such as autism.
Wood Jing Seventh Lunar Month	The Wood Jing supervises the assertion and direction of the fetus' emotional and spiritual aspects.		Any faltering of the Wood Jing energy is associated with psychological problems such as passive-aggressive personality disorder.
Earth Jing Eighth Lunar Month	The Earth Jing energy supervises the quality and maturation of the fetus' emotional and spiritual bonding and boundaries.	Integration of Intention to Direct Spiritual Forces	Any faltering of the Earth Jing energy is associated with problems of severe psychological disturbances, such as schizophrenia.

Figure 2.49. The Creative Process of the Body's Prenatal Jing Formation

the core of the Heart, or "that which descends from the sky and passes through the body."

The body's Jing fastens the Shen into place by fusing each spiritual aspect with a particular Yin organ orb, thus creating a pathway for physical and energetic expression. For this reason, any deficiency in Prenatal Jing formation can create Postnatal problems (Figure 2.49). The first Jing to enter its orb and begin its energetic function is the Water Jing.

WATER JING FORMATION

During the fourth lunar month (16 weeks), the Water Jing energy governs the genetic developmental aspect of the fetal growth. This energy encompasses the fetus' unconscious reservoir of intuitive intelligence, will, and life-force energy. It also energetically relates to divine love, power, and spirit. Any faltering of the Water Jing energy (due to the influence of fetal toxins, stress, trauma or malnutrition) is associated with both pervasive and subtle neurological disorders, as well as a predisposition to severe psychological disorders, such as schizophrenia.

According to the *Magical Pivot*, "When the seminal essence is complete, it gives birth to the formation of the Brain and Marrow. Then the Bones solidify, the channels begin to nourish, the muscles begin to strengthen, the flesh begins to become a wall, the skin begins to firm and the hair begins to grow." Any deficiency in Water (Kidney) Jing can cause retardation or Congenital Qi Deficiency (i.e., Deficiency in the Sea of Marrow). This, in turn, can lead to Down Syndrome, Attention Deficit Disorder (ADD) and other learning disabilities. These psychological disturbances may be evident at birth or develop later in life.

FIRE JING FORMATION

During the fifth lunar month (20 weeks), the Fire Jing energy generates and controls, protects and integrates, as well as divides and harmonizes the fetus' internal energies. Because it promotes emotional and spiritual well-being, any faltering of the Fire Jing energy is associated with problems of right (Yin) and left (Yang) Brain communication, such as internal imbalances between the rational male energy and intuitive female energy. These psychological disturbances may be evident at birth or develop later in life.

METAL JING FORMATION

During the sixth lunar month (24 weeks), the Metal Jing is established in the fetus' body, stabilizing the sinews and connective tissues. The Metal Jing energy is also responsible for fetal tissue and structural formation, and the ability to form and maintain emotional bonds. Any faltering of the Metal Jing energy is associated with problems of emotional attachment, such as autism. These psychological disturbances may be evident at birth or develop later in life.

WOOD JING FORMATION

During the seventh lunar month (28 weeks), the Wood Jing is beginning to be incorporated into the fetus' body. The Wood Jing energy governs the assertion and direction of the fetus' emotional and spiritual aspects. Any faltering of the Wood

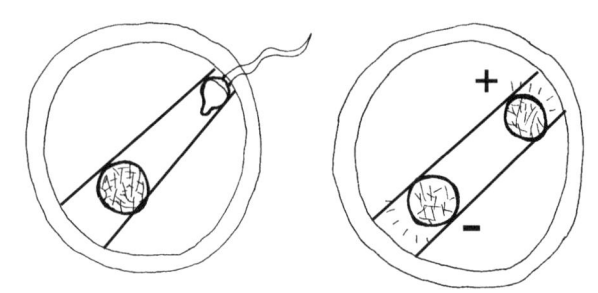

Figure 2.50. The human body is primarily composed of water. The Essence of man (sperm) and woman (egg) unite in the uterine sea to form the fetus. The egg is polarized at the entry point of the sperm, creating the original polar axis (the *Taiji Pole*) which determines the complex pattern of cellular division that occurs along this polar axis throughout development.

Jing energy is associated with psychological problems, such as passive-aggressive personality disorder. These psychological disturbances may be evident at birth or develop later in life.

EARTH JING FORMATION

During the eighth lunar month (32 weeks), the fetus receives the Zong (Essential) Qi from the mother's Spleen; This is the energy collected from Heaven and Earth that accumulates within the chest. At this stage, the Earth Jing begins to complete the formation of the skin.

The Earth Jing energy governs the quality and maturation of the fetus' emotional and spiritual bonding and boundaries. Any faltering of the Earth Jing energy is associated with problems of severe psychological disturbances, such as schizophrenia. These psychological disturbances may be evident at birth or develop later in life.

JING, QI AND SHEN FORMATION

Three important energies combine in the developing fetus: Jing (Essence), Qi (Energy), and Shen (Spirit). Jing is the body's foundational substance and is responsible for nourishing the tissues. Qi emerges from the circulation of the Jing moving through the tissues and supports the body's metabolism. Shen governs the body, energizes the Qi and forms a solid connection of internal light and vibrational energy (see Volume 2, Chapter 14).

Both parents contribute energetically to the baby's conception (Figure 2.50). Both the father's sperm and the mother's egg consist of Jing (Essence), Qi (Energy), and Shen (Spirit). This combination of Jing, Qi, and Shen from each parent is collectively referred to as father Qi, and mother Qi. The combination of father Qi and mother Qi is known as Yuan Qi, or Original Qi, and represents the energetic matrix from which all individuals are developed and maintained.

While studying synchronistic and coherent excitations in microtubules, Italian nanobiologist Ezio Insinna has proposed that centrioles (small tubular structures responsible for holding the cell structure in place) are virtually immortal oscillators or wave generators. Within the embryo, these energetic waves are set into motion by the father's Jing, Qi, and Shen when they fuse with the mother's Jing, Qi, and Shen. They will continue to pulse throughout the life of the individual. During the first stage of the embryo's development, the centrioles' vibrational pattern begins at a particular frequency, affecting both cell formation and metabolism. This frequency changes as the child matures, producing corresponding changes in metabolism and cell formation.

The quality and quantity of Original Qi that the baby receives at conception depends on three main factors:
- The purity and potency of the parents' genetic plasma (sperm and egg)
- The condition of both parents' health and vitality and the state of their physical, mental, emotional, and spiritual relationship at the time of conception
- The spiritual factors surrounding the conception (i.e., karma that is brought into this life by the incoming soul and the environment)

FERTILIZATION

As the sperm (containing the energetic patterns of the father's Jing, Qi and Shen) fertilizes the egg (containing the energetic patterns of the mother's Jing, Qi and Shen), Heaven Qi (containing the universal energetic patterns of the sun, moon and stars) and Earth Qi (containing the environmental energetic patterns of the soil, water and wind) all blend together within the zygote. The swirling and blending of these four energies

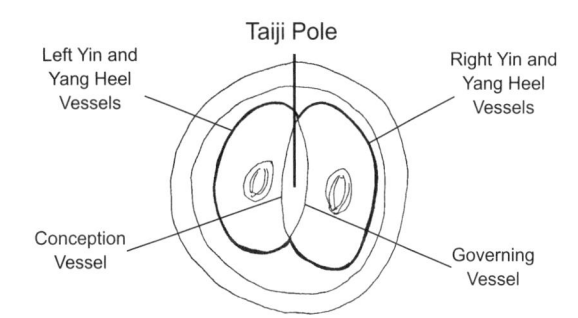

Figure 2.51. During the first cellular division, the field of energy in the polar axis is related to the Yuan Qi, from which the Conception and Governing Vessels form the seas of Yin and Yang energy. The Yin Heel and Yang Heel Vessels are also established during the first cellular division, forming the left and right sides. The development of the zygote's exterior is controlled by the Yang Linking Vessels. The development of the zygote's interior is controlled by the Yin Linking Vessels.

form energetic pools (which will later evolve into organs), rivers (which later evolve into channels), and streams (which later evolve into collaterals).

When the sperm unites with the egg, it produces a polar axis that creates an energetic vortex within and around the zygote (similar to the energetic vortex created by the axis of the Earth). This energetic vortex forms the central Taiji Pole by drawing Qi from Heaven and Earth into the zygote, allowing the human soul to enter into the fetus' body.

EIGHT EXTRAORDINARY VESSEL FORMATION

With the first cell division, the energetic polarization of the zygote determines a ventral and dorsal surface, which become the embryo's Conception and Governing Vessels, respectively (Figure 2.51). At this point, the Governing Vessel controls the cell divisions that eventually form the back of the body, while the Conception Vessel controls the cell divisions forming the front of the body. This first cell division also establishes a right and left side. Here, the Heel Vessels control the balance of Yin and Yang energy development in the two sides of the body.

The Belt Vessel and Thrusting Vessels form at the time of the second cell division. The four vessels formed at this point (Governing Vessel, Conception Vessel, Thrusting Vessels, and Belt Vessel) are interlinked for the production, circulation, and regulation of the body's Jing-Essence. With the formation of these four vessels, the body's entire energy system becomes established and is maintained (Figure 2.52).

During embryonic formation, the Yang Linking Vessels are responsible for the exterior development of the embryo, while the Yin Linking Vessels are responsible for the interior development. Each of the Eight Extraordinary Vessels has a specific role in the development of the embryo:

1. The Governing Vessel (Du Mai) controls development of the body's back.
2. The Conception Vessel (Ren Mai) controls development of the body's front.
3. The Thrusting Vessels (Chong Mai) carry energy through the center of the body, control the body's center core, and regulate Blood.
4. The Yang Heel Vessels (Yang Qiao Mai) control the development of the body's right and left Yang energy.
5. The Yin Heel Vessels (Yin Qiao Mai) control the development of the body's right and left Yin energy.
6. The Yang Linking Vessels (Yang Wei Mai) control the development of the Exterior of the body, and correlate to the energy of Heaven.
7. The Yin Linking Vessels (Yin Wei Mai) control the development of the Interior of the body, and correlate to the energy of Earth.
8. The Belt Vessel (Dai Mai) binds all the channels together.

These eight vessels—Governing, Conception, Thrusting, Yang Heel, Yin Heel, Yang Linking, Yin Linking, and Belt—are also known as the Eight Extraordinary Vessels or the Eight Prenatal Vessels.

The Eight Extraordinary Vessels form a vortex of energy at the center of the embryo's body centered in the area between what will become the left and right Kidneys (see Chapter 6). The Taiji Pole and Thrusting Vessels are at the center of this vortex and will form the Sea of Five Yin and Six Yang Organs, the Sea of Twelve Primary Channels, and the Sea of Blood. The body's Qi and Blood are energetically distributed through small channels or rivers of energy from the Taiji Pole and the Thrusting Vessels. This energetic vortex creates the energy for the growth of the embryo's physical form (Figure 2.53).

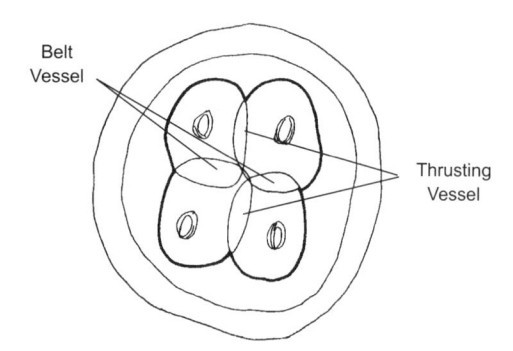

Figure 2.52. The second cellular division is associated with the development of the Belt Vessel and the Thrusting Vessel.

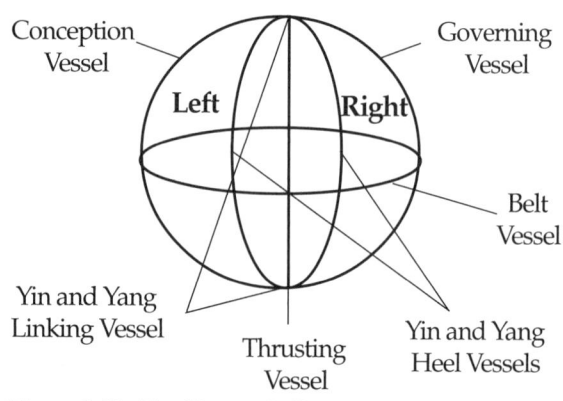

Figure 2.53. The Energetic Embryological Flow of the Eight Extraordinary Vessels

YIN AND YANG CHANNEL FORMATION

After the initial cell division is complete, the embryo's Yang channels and Yin channels begin the development and formation of the embryo's tissues and organs. These twenty channels are divided into two separate groups of energetic rivers known as the Eight Extraordinary Vessels and Twelve Primary Channels. As the embryo develops into a fetus and continues to grow, the twenty channels also continue to develop.

During the formation of the embryo, nine Yang channels begin to flow from the Governing Vessel (Sea of Yang Qi) and form the nine Yang rivers known as the Urinary Bladder Channel, Gall Bladder Channel, Stomach Channel, Small Intestine Channel, Triple Burner Channel, Large Intestine Channel, Yang Heel Vessel, Yang Link-

CHAPTER 2: UNDERSTANDING ANCIENT CHINESE METAPHYSICS

Lunar Month	Mother's Channels	Channel's Activity	Energetic Activity
Month 1	Liver Channels	Stops menses, begins embryonic growth	Energies combine at conception, channels nourish development of the embryo
Month 2	Gall Bladder Channels	Saturates embryo with Jing	Embryonic Qi transforms into amniotic fluid and the mesenteric membrane develops
Month 3	Pericardium Channels	Mother's Qi and Body Fluids purify and cleanse the fetal Shen	Yang Qi rises, the Hun and Po prepare the fetus' internal organs, heartbeat is now detected
Month 4	Triple Burner Channels	The Yin Organs develop	Water Jing is incorporated into fetus' body
Month 5	Spleen Channels	The Five Agents enter the Five Orbs (Yin Organs)	Fire Jing is incorporated into fetus' body
Month 6	Stomach Channels	The Six Pitches are established within the Six Storage Areas	Metal Jing is incorporated into fetus' body
Month 7	Lung Channels	Seven Essential Stars open orifices to the light from Heaven and Earth	Wood Jing is incorporated into fetus' body
Month 8	Large Intestine Channels	The Heart is harmonized and the breath is quieted	Earth Jing is incorporated into fetus' body
Month 9	Kidney Channels	The Kidney Channels control the energetic intake from the umbilicus	Energetic boundaries completed
Month 10	Urinary Bladder Channels	The spatial cavities surrounding major organs are completed	Heaven and Earth Qi settle into baby's Lower Dantian and birth begins

Figure 2.54. Prenatal Energy Development

ing Vessel, and Belt Vessel.

The nine Yin channels that flow from the Conception Vessel (Sea of Yin Qi) and form the nine Yin rivers are known as the Kidney Channel, Liver Channel, Spleen Channel, Heart Channel, Pericardium Channel, Lung Channel, Yin Heel Vessel, Yin Linking Vessel, and Thrusting Vessel (see Chapter 8).

THE TEN LUNAR MONTHS OF CREATION

The following description of the sequence of embryological development was presented by the Chinese Medical Qigong expert Dr. Chao Yuan Fang during the Sui Dynasty, around 610 A.D. In this model, pregnancy is measured in ten lunar months spanning the forty weeks of a normal pregnancy (Figure 2.54).

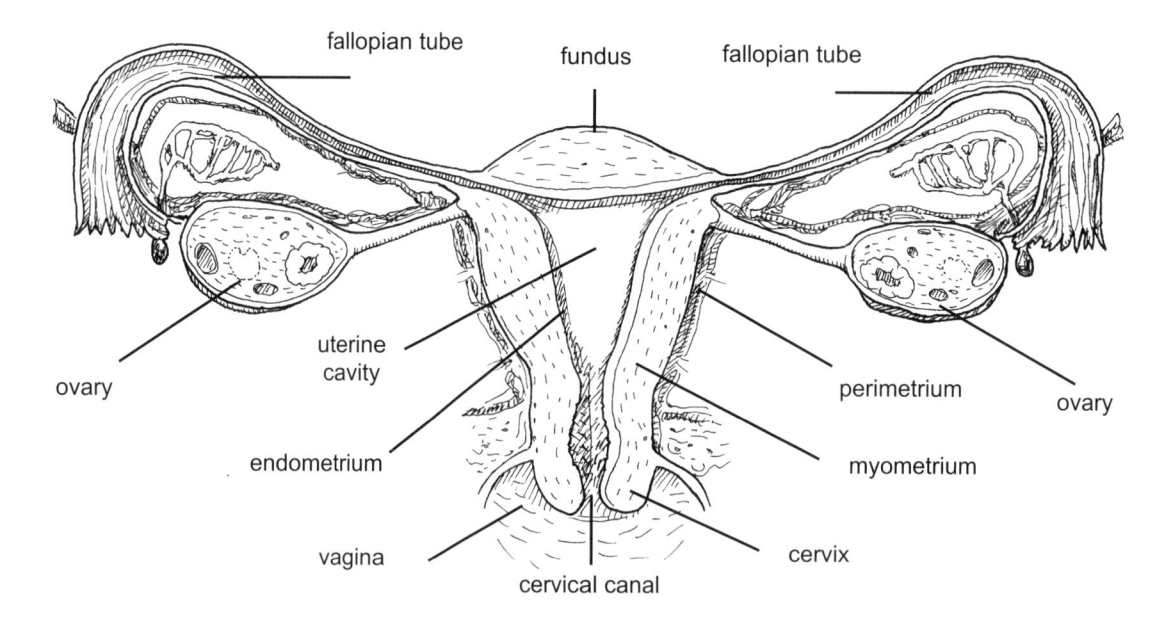

Figure 2.55. The Female Reproductive Organs, including the Uterus, Fallopian Tubes, and Ovaries (Inspired by the original artwork of Dr. Frank H. Netter).

MONTH ONE

Once a young woman's Uterus becomes fully developed she begins her menstrual cycle. When an egg is released from her ovary pregnancy can occur, and fetal growth will follow (Figure 2.55).

The first lunar month of pregnancy is traditionally called the "beginning of form" stage and refers to the formation of the Jing of the placenta. This stage also covers conception and early cell division and is described as the progression of "mingling, clotting, solidifying, and rounding."

The ancient Chinese believed that there is only primal generative energy (Prenatal Qi) in the mother's womb. This primal generative energy is responsible for the congealing and nurturing of the forming embryo, seeing it through to completion.

During conception, when the Yin and Yang energies of both parents interact within the womb, in the midst of the darkness there is a point of divine living potential which comes forth from the Dao, merging from out of the infinite space of the Wuji. This is what is known to the ancient Daoists as the "primordial, true, unified generative energy of creation." This energy of creation enters into the sperm and egg, fusing them as one. The ancient Daoist texts say, "formless, it produces form; immaterial, it produces substance. The internal organs, sense organs, and various parts of the body all naturally evolve because of this energy of creation, becoming complete."

In the mother's womb, it is the primordial, true, unified generative energy of creation (Yuan Qi) that causes the embryo to congeal and form, then nourishes the embryo, and eventually causes it to become complete. At this stage in development, although there is human form, there is no development of the acquired mind, only the true, congenital mind (Yuan Shen) exists.

THE UTERUS

In Traditional Chinese Medicine, the physiological functions of a woman's Uterus is connected to her Heart, Liver, Spleen, Kidneys, Conception and Thrusting Vessels. The Uterus connects to the Kidneys (which provide the Uterus with Jing), the Conception Vessel (which provides the Uterus with Qi and nourishes the fetus), and

CHAPTER 2: UNDERSTANDING ANCIENT CHINESE METAPHYSICS

the Thrusting Channel (which provides the Uterus with Blood). When the Jing of the Kidneys is sufficient, the menstrual period will occur regularly, making pregnancy and fetal growth possible. The Qi and Blood of the Twelve Primary Channels pass into the Uterus through the Thrusting and Conception Vessels, affecting the amount of menstrual flow and its cycle.

THE UTERUS AND THE LOWER DANTIAN

It is important to realize that each individual was conceived in the heart of the Uterus, which is considered the center of a woman's Lower Dantian (Sea of Qi). Given its Yin nature and close proximity to the Earth, the Lower Dantian itself is considered a center of consciousness, and is more kinesthetic or physical in nature (Figure 2.56).

From a Medical Qigong perspective (and Daoist inner alchemy), the Earth energy is gathered in the Uterus and Lower Dantian area. The Uterus is associated with the development of the fetus' forming tissues, allowing the Eternal Soul (Shen Xian) the ability to acquire a lower vibrational resonance in order to experience life on the gross material plane. The quiescent state from which the fetus develops translates to the Prenatal energetic state of prayer, meditation and sleep. These three energetic states form the foundation for the creation and formation of Prenatal Jing, Qi and Shen.

The Uterus and Lower Dantian are the major storage area for the various types of Kidney energies (i.e., Qi of the ovaries). It is the place where Qi is housed, the body's Mingmen Fire is aroused, the Kidney Yin and Yang Qi is gathered, and the Yuan Qi (also called Source Qi or Original Qi) is stored. The Yuan Qi is the foundation of all the other types of Qi in the body. The Yuan Qi is closely linked with the Prenatal Essence (Yuan Jing). Together, the Yuan Qi and Yuan Jing determine our overall health, vitality, stamina, and life span of the individual.

CHINESE CHARACTER FOR UTERUS

The ideograph depicting the Chinese characters for the Uterus, "Bao," is described as follows (Figure 2.57):

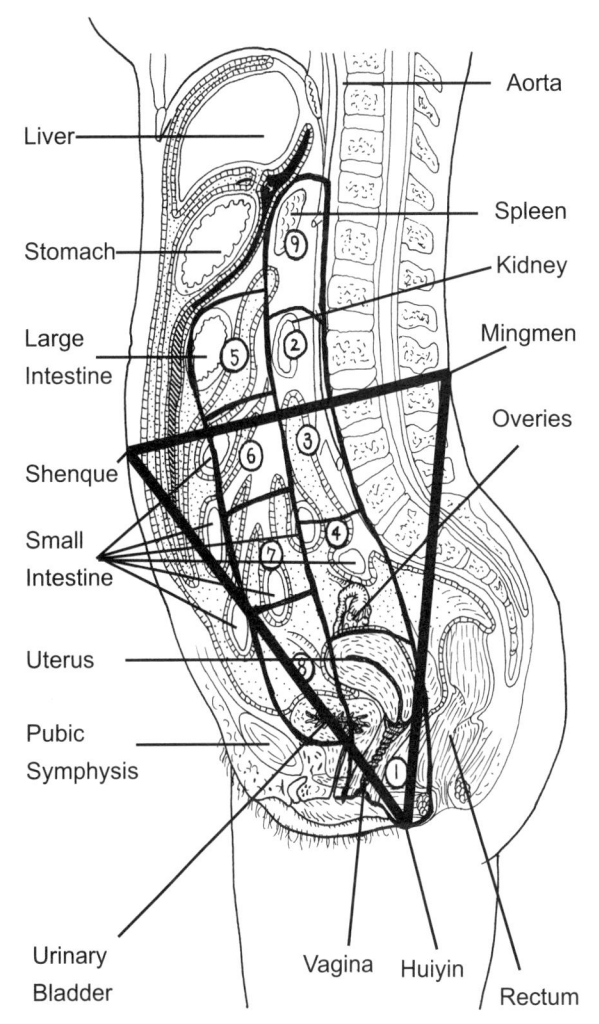

Figure 2.56. The Nine Chambers of the Lower Dantian are shown here in the female body. Each number encompasses the entire chamber. (Inspired by the original artwork of Dr. Frank H. Netter).

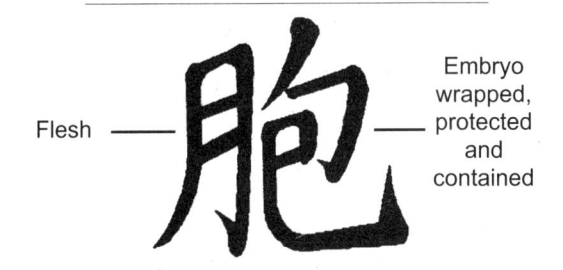

Figure 2.57. The Chinese Ideograph for "Bao," Uterus

- The Chinese character that depicts the ideogram for "Bao" is composed of two images: The character on the left can be translated as body tissue, muscle or flesh (depicting a form of connective tissue). The character on the right means to wrap, and refers to a bag or sack. Together, both characters are used to depict the Uterus and represent an embryo wrapped, protected and contained inside the mother's belly. In ancient China, the character for Bao was sometimes used to refer to the Urinary Bladder, placenta, or Uterus.

THE ROLE OF THE MOTHER'S LIVER CHANNELS

At conception, the mother's Liver Channels stop her menses and begin to nourish the growth of her embryo (Figure 2.58). During pregnancy, the mother's Blood is transformed into Jing (Essence) that nourishes the mother's as well as the embryo's body. The mother's Liver Channels cause Essence and Blood to coagulate in her womb. This Blood coagulation continues after the initial cellular division.

MOTHER'S SHEN

The mother's Shen (Spirit) becomes part of a threefold activity and is described as follows:

- First, the mother's Shen projects through the umbilical cord, sustaining and energizing the production of Jing, Qi, Shen, Blood and Body Fluids for the embryo (Figure 2.59).
- Second, the mother's Shen influences the embryo's Yuan Jing (Original Essence) and the embryo's Yuan Qi (Original Energy), forming the embryo's Yuan Shen (Original Spirit). This Yuan Shen appears as multicolored light and contains the inherited patterns and knowledge of the ancestors, including talents, skills, and natural abilities. This knowledge is stored deep within the embryo's cells, tissues, and consciousness.
- Third, the mother's Shen influences the embryo's Qi and Blood, and stimulates and awakens the embryo's Yuan Shen (Original Spirit). This energetic light manifests through the mother's skin and is associated with the "glow" shining through her eyes after conception.

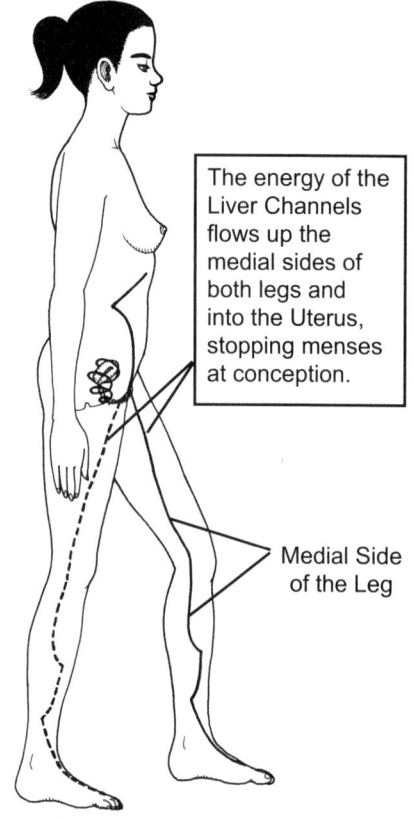

The energy of the Liver Channels flows up the medial sides of both legs and into the Uterus, stopping menses at conception.

Medial Side of the Leg

Figure 2.58. The mother's and father's Essence (Jing), Energy (Qi), and Spirit (Shen) blend with Heaven and Earth energies during the fusion of the sperm and egg. During the first lunar month, the mother's Liver Channels stop her menses and begin the embryonic growth cycle.

Yuan Jing (Original Essence)
Yuan Qi (Original Energy)
Taiji Pole
Yuan Shen (Original Spirit)
Three Dantians

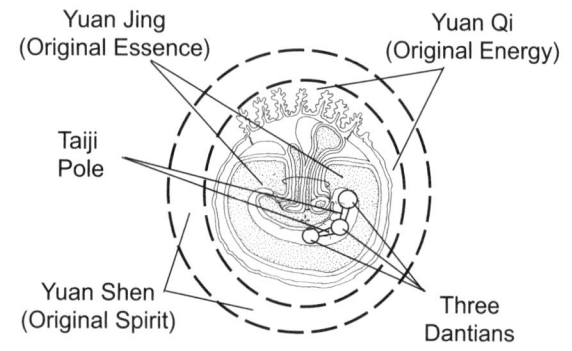

Figure 2.59. Sustained through the umbilical cord, the embryo absorbs the mother's Blood, Essence, Energy, and Spirit.

Month Two

The second lunar month of pregnancy is traditionally called the "beginning to gel" stage and refers to the completion of the formation of the "first shape" of the embryo.

The Role of the Mother's Gall Bladder Channels

The mother's Gall Bladder Channels are responsible for the development of the mesenteric membrane sac (Figure 2.60). The Gall Bladder Channels also saturate the embryo, Uterus, and placenta with Jing, causing the embryonic Qi to become denser until it transforms into a thick liquid (amniotic fluid).

This external (embryonic) fluid helps regulate the embryo's internal Body Fluids. The amniotic fluid that surrounds the embryo also acts as an energetic condenser, retaining and magnifying the Qi and Shen that is flowing into the mother's womb. At this stage, the embryo begins to take shape inside the uterine lining, developing basic structural features (Figure 2.61). The umbilical cord and placenta are now formed. Additionally, the Lungs, Liver, Kidneys, and major Blood Vessels are beginning to form.

Energetic Formation

With the formation of the major Blood Vessels, the Yin and Yang energies begin to occupy the embryo's channels. As the embryo's internal and external Yin and Yang energies actively balance themselves, the following occurs:

- The energy that will later coalesce into Lung Qi moves to the upper part of the body.
- The Original Qi (Yuan Qi) of the Kidneys begins to collect deep in the center of the body.
- The Earth Qi, absorbed by the embryo from the mother's exposure to the outside environment, begins to collect in the lower front and upper back areas of the embryo's body.

During embryonic formation, each distinct energy is naturally drawn to the appropriate area within the embryo's developing body, creating its own unique boundaries and pools of Qi. These pools and boundaries will later form the major internal organs and external tissues, in addition to the energetic spatial cavities that surround them.

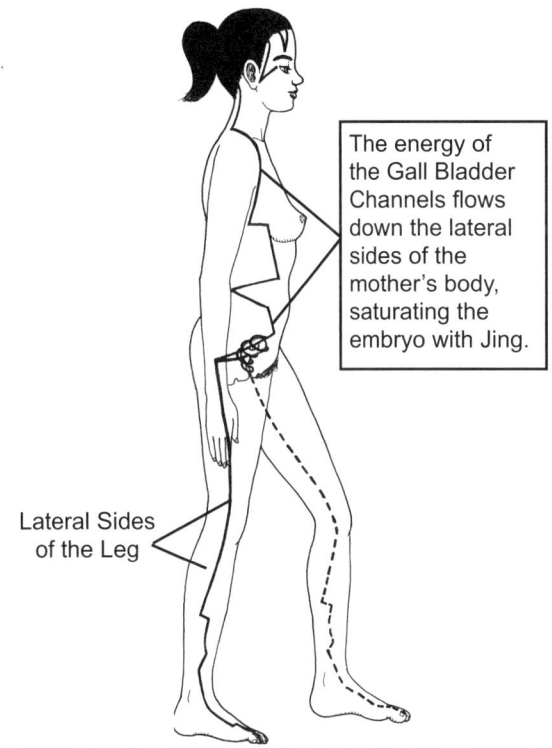

Figure 2.60. The mother's Gall Bladder Channels saturate the embryo with Jing during the second lunar month, causing the embryonic Qi to transform into amniotic fluid. The embryo begins to take shape as the energetic boundaries, pools, spatial cavities, channels and collaterals, internal and external spiritual, energetic and physical forms begin to manifest.

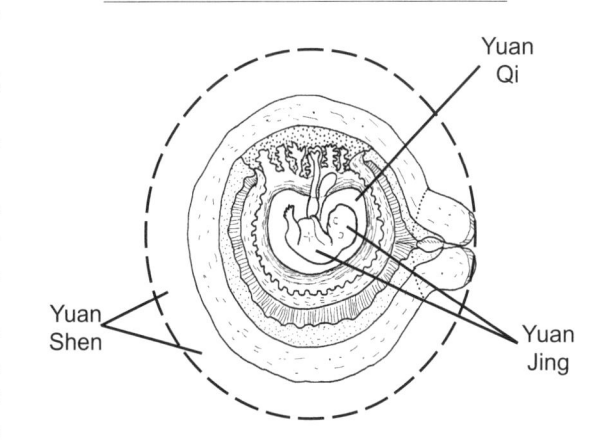

Figure 2.61. During the second month, the embryo begins to take shape as the energetic boundaries begin to form.

The areas where the energetic pools settle and begin to create a balance within themselves are the precursors to the body's internal organ systems. During this creative process, internal movement creates tiny energetic currents, eddies, and whirlpools that flow throughout the entire body. As the energy shifts, seeking balance, the larger pools of energy begin to condense, forming the internal organs, Brain, Bones, and skin.

Once the energetic pools and rivers have formed, all of the currents and eddies evolve to form the energetic channels and collaterals throughout the developing body. These energetic currents will move in accordance with the mother's respiratory patterns until the moment of birth. Upon the child's first breath, the energetic currents will follow the rhythmic patterns of the child's respiration. As these currents continue to spiral within the channels, energetic points are established according to the body's subtle energetic blueprint. Some of these areas spiral outward (positive polarity) to form energetic exit points, while others spiral inward (negative polarity) to form energetic entry points.

Month Three

The third lunar month of pregnancy is traditionally called the "beginning of the pregnant Uterus" stage. During this period, the embryo becomes a fetus and begins micro-movement. Its heartbeat can now be detected.

The Role of the Mother's Pericardium Channels

The mother's Pericardium Channels control the presence and amount of Jing and Shen in the vessels, channels, and collaterals of the fetus (Figure 2.62). The Jing and Shen that flow from the mother into the fetus are rooted in the Qi of her Blood. The combination of the mother's Qi and Body Fluids purifies and cleanses the Shen of the fetus. This purifying action transforms into Heat, causing the fetus' Yang Qi to arouse the Hun (the body's Ethereal Soul) into life. During the third lunar month, the Prenatal Five Agents (Wu Jing Shen) begin to energetically awaken.

Energetic Formation

As the Prenatal Jing and Blood combine, the

The energy of the Pericardium Channels flows from the Heart down the center of the mother's body into the Uterus, cleansing the Shen of the fetus.

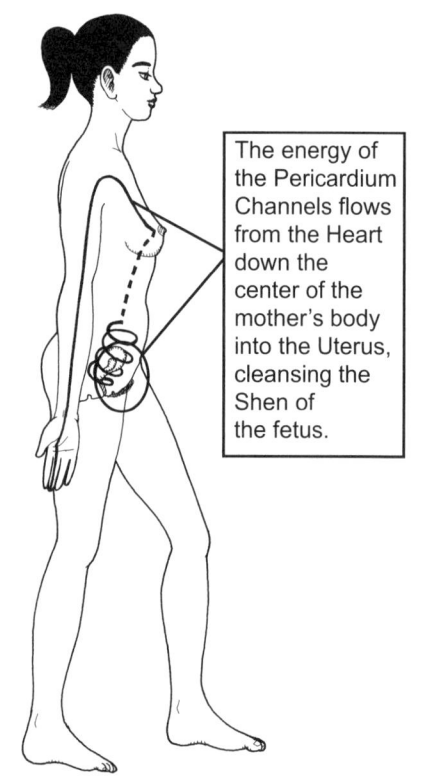

Figure 2.62. The mother's Pericardium Channels govern the third lunar month of creation. During this phase, the mother's Qi and body fluids purify and cleanse the fetus's Shen (Spirit). The Hun from Heaven and the Po from Earth are established within the fetus's internal organs.

fetus' Shen is further refined. The energy of the Hun (Three Ethereal Souls) was sometimes referred to by the ancient Daoists as an aspect of the Supernatural Shen, because they flow with the movement of the Blood. The energy of the Po (Seven Corporeal Souls) was sometimes referred to as a Moving Shen, because they follow the movement of the Jing. Combined, the energetic functions of the Hun, acting as a Supernatural Shen, were considered to be the "active impulse," while the energetic functions of the Po, acting as a Moving Shen, were considered to be the "enabling mover" of the body's Jing, Qi, and Shen.

Tissue Formation

At the end of the third month, the internal organs, limbs, and external sex organs of the fetus are fully formed, and the nails have developed.

MONTH FOUR

During the fourth lunar month, the mother's Triple Burner Channels, which are connected to the Yang organs, stabilize the Blood Vessels of the fetus (Figure 2.63). At this stage, the Water Jing is beginning to be accepted by the fetus' body, enabling the development of the Yin organs.

THE ROLE OF THE MOTHER'S TRIPLE BURNER CHANNELS

The mother's Triple Burner Channels direct the development of the fascia and connective tissues of the fetus. This process is referred to as "the development of Qi and Blood penetrating to the ears and eyes and circulating throughout the fetus' channels and connecting vessels."

WATER JING FORMATION

Beginning in the fourth month and continuing through the ninth month, the energetic nature and specific spiritual characteristics of each of the Prenatal Wu Jing Shen are progressively activated and developed within the fetus' body.

The Jing of the Water Element is the first of the Wu Jing Shen to energize the developing fetus and become active in tissue formation. As previously mentioned, during the fourth lunar month, the Water Jing energy governs the genetic development of the fetus. This energy encompasses the fetus' unconscious reservoir of intuitive intelligence, will, and life-force energy, and relates to divine love, power, and spirit. Any faltering of the Water Jing energy (due to the influence of fetal toxins, stress, trauma or malnutrition) is associated with both pervasive and subtle neurological disorders, as well as a predisposition to severe psychological disorders.

According to the *Magical Pivot*, "When the seminal essence is complete, it gives birth to the formation of the Brain and Marrow. Then the Bones solidify, the channels begin to nourish, the muscles begin to strengthen, the flesh begins to become a wall, the skin begins to firm and the hair begins to grow." Any deficiency in Water (Kidney) Jing can cause retardation or Congenital Qi Deficiency (i.e., Deficiency in the Sea of Marrow). This, in turn, can lead to Down Syndrome, Attention Deficit Disorder (ADD) and learning disabili-

The energy of the Triple Burner Channels flows up both arms into the Heart and down the center of the mother's body into the Uterus, directing the development and formation of the fascia and connective tissue of the fetus.

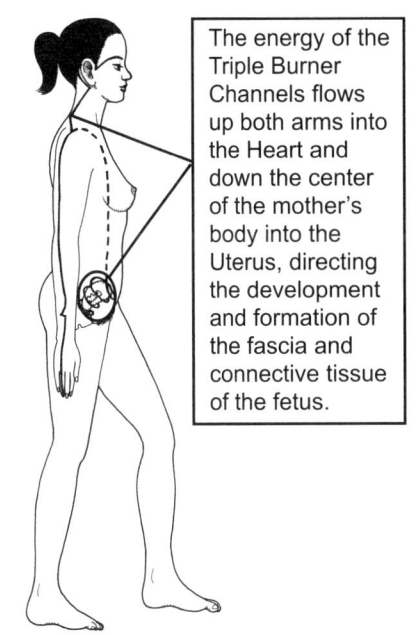

Figure 2.63. The mother's Triple Burner Channels govern the fourth lunar month of creation. The Water Jing (Essence) is accepted by the fetus' body.

ties. These psychological disturbances may be evident at birth or develop later in life.

TISSUE FORMATION

Through the later stages of fetal development, the embryo's relatively homogenous tissues transform into the more mature differentiated tissues of the fetus. The structures and boundaries of the maturing tissues (muscles, Bones, and organs, etc.) are defined and maintained by the fetus' connective tissue (fascia). Accordingly, a very large part of the body consists of connective tissue and membranes functioning to support and define the body's internal and external structures.

As the different structures of the body are defined by fascial boundaries (which border each other), these same tissues and structures are woven together through a vast network of interpenetrating connective tissue that pervades the entire body. This internal network facilitates the body's intercellular communication. These structures connect to every part of the fetus' body, forming a vast energetic and physical system capable of regulating and transforming the body's Jing, Qi, and Shen.

Month Five

During the fifth lunar month, the mother's Spleen Channels are responsible for completing the development of the four limbs (Figure 2.64). At this stage, the fetus begins to have its own respiratory movement. At this stage, the Fire Jing is accepted into the fetus, creating internal energy that stabilizes the Qi of the five Yin organs.

The Role of the Mother's Spleen Channels

The mother's Spleen Channels direct the development and completion of the four limbs.

Fire Jing Formation

During the fifth lunar month, the Fire Jing energy generates and controls, protects and integrates, as well as divides and harmonizes the fetus' internal energies. Because it promotes emotional and spiritual well-being, any faltering of the Fire Jing energy is associated with problems of right (Yin) and left (Yang) Brain communication, such as internal imbalances between the rational male energy and intuitive female energy. These psychological disturbances may be evident at birth or develop later in life.

Energetic Formation of the Five Orbs

At this stage of development, the Prenatal Five Agents (Five Virtues) are distributed to the Five Orbs through the influence on the Middle Hun, "Shang Ling" (see end of Chapter). The Five Orbs are both spatial cavities (i.e., internal organ tissue chambers) and extended spheres of energetic influence. These Orbs refer to pools of Essence, Qi and Blood, as well as to the channels and Body Fluids of each of the five Yin organs. Additionally, the energetic Orb of each Yin organ also includes the corresponding tissues, emotions and spiritual qualities that are extended throughout the entire body, and are not limited to the organ itself (see Chapter 8). The Prenatal Five Agents are distributed as follows (Figure 2.65):

- Kindness to the Liver
- Order to the Heart
- Trust to the Spleen
- Integrity to the Lungs
- Wisdom to the Kidneys

The even distribution and balance of the Prenatal Five Agents allows the energetic nature of

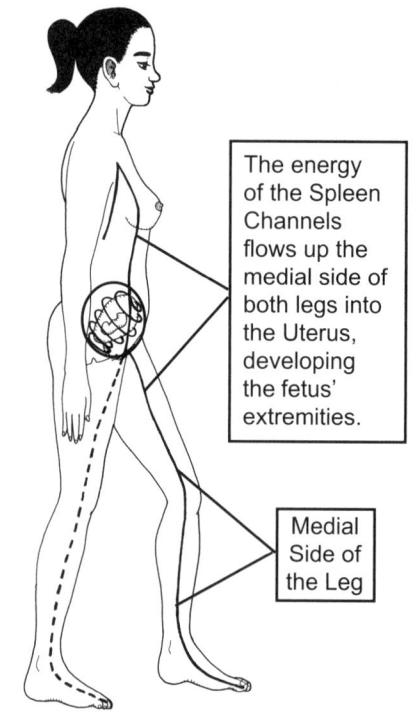

The energy of the Spleen Channels flows up the medial side of both legs into the Uterus, developing the fetus' extremities.

Medial Side of the Leg

Figure 2.64. The mother's Spleen Channels are responsible for the fifth lunar month of creation. The development of the fetus' four limbs is completed. The Five Agents are distributed within the fetus's Five Orbs (five Yin organs). The Fire Jing is accepted by the fetus' body.

Five Agents (Five Virtues):
- Kindness of the Liver
- Order of the Heart
- Trust of the Spleen
- Integrity of the Lungs
- Wisdom of the Kidneys

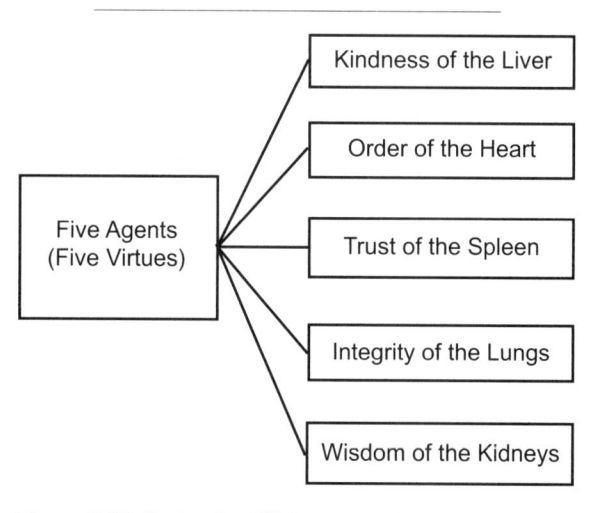

Figure 2.65. During the fifth lunar month, the Five Agents are distributed into the Five Orbs through the influence on the Middle Hun (Shang Ling).

the Hun to stabilize within the fetus' organs, creating peace and order within the fetus' Shen.

TISSUE FORMATION

At the end of the fifth month, the fetus' body systems develop rapidly. Its head is less disproportionate to the rest of the body, and the mother often feels the spontaneous muscular movements of the fetus.

MONTH SIX

During the sixth lunar month, the mother's Stomach Channels govern the development of the fetus and the Six Pitches are established within the body's storage areas. At this stage, the Metal Jing is beginning to be accepted by the fetus' body.

THE ROLE OF THE MOTHER'S STOMACH CHANNELS

In the sixth lunar month of creation, the mother's Stomach Channels begin to establish the fetus' muscles (Figure 2.66).

METAL JING FORMATION

As previously mentioned, during the sixth lunar month, the Metal Jing is established in the fetus' body, stabilizing the sinews and connective tissues. The Metal Jing energy is responsible for fetal tissue and structural formation, and the ability to form and maintain emotional bonds with others. Any faltering of the Metal Jing energy is associated with problems of emotional attachment, such as autism. These psychological disturbances may be evident at birth or develop later in life.

FORMATION OF THE SIX STORAGE AREAS

During the sixth month, the Yang organs begin to develop (i.e., the Stomach, Gall Bladder, Small Intestine, Large Intestine, Urinary Bladder, and Triple Burners). The Six Storage Areas of the body's Yang organs are constantly filling and emptying. Each of the Yang organs receive, move, transform, digest, or excrete substances, described as follows (Figure 2.67):

1. **The Stomach stores the food.** This Yang organ is responsible for receiving, storing, rotting, and ripening food.
2. **The Gall Bladder stores and excretes bile.** This Yang organ is responsible for storing and

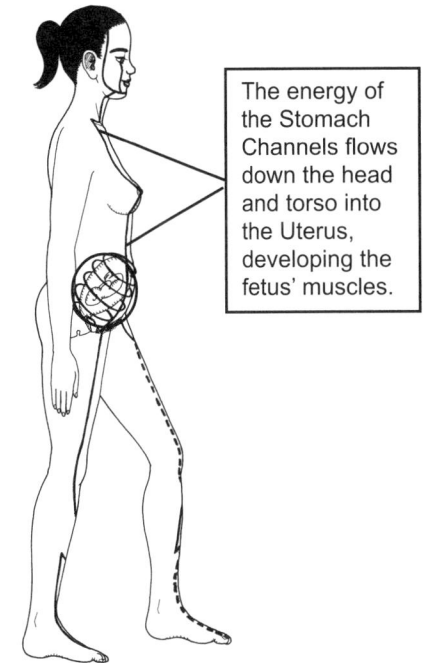

Figure 2.66. The mother's Stomach Channels govern the sixth lunar month of creation. The Six Pitches are established within the body's storage areas, and the Metal Jing is accepted by the fetus' body.

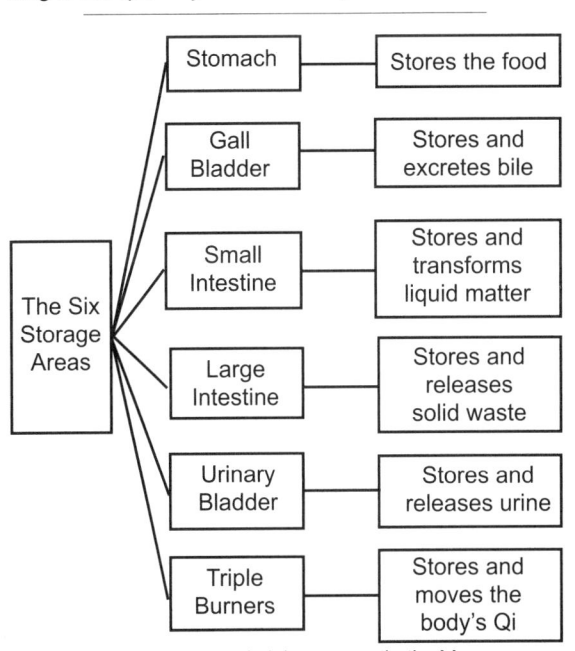

Figure 2.67. During the sixth lunar month, the Yang organs develop the Six Storage Areas.

releasing bile into the Small Intestine.

3. **The Small Intestine stores and transforms liquid matter.** This Yang organ receives, stores, transforms, and digests food and releases its waste products into the Large Intestine.
4. **The Large Intestine stores the solid waste.** This Yang organ receives, stores, and absorbs food and releases waste.
5. **The Urinary Bladder stores, and releases the urine.** This Yang organ is responsible for receiving, storing, and releasing urine.
6. **The Triple Burners store the body's Qi.** These three areas of the body receive, store, absorb, and move Qi.

Formation of the Six Energetic Pitches

The Six Pitches nourish the Qi and both support and stabilize the Lower Burners (see Triple Burners, Chapter 8). They are established within the Six Storage Areas, also known as the Six Yang Organs.

The Six Pitches are six specific tone resonances (notes) that vibrate within the body's internal organs, stimulating specific organ and tissue areas. These Six Pitches relate to the Five Prenatal (Heaven) Elemental Sounds of "Jue" (Wood), "Zhi" (Fire), "Gong" (Earth), "Shang" (Metal), and "Yu" (Water) (see Chapter 4). The sixth note, "Xi," relates to the Postnatal (Earth) Fire Element and corresponds to the Pericardium and Triple Burners. The ancient Chinese used these Six Pitches for specific clinical treatments. The sound "Yu" for example, spoken in a low tone, will vibrate and influence the lower abdominal area and is used for the treatment of Kidney and Urinary Bladder problems.

Tissue Formation

In the sixth lunar month of formation, the fetus' eyelids separate, the eyelashes form, and the skin becomes wrinkled.

Month Seven

The mother's Lung Channels govern the seventh lunar month of creation. The Seven Essential Stars open the fetus' orifices to let in the light from Heaven and Earth. At this stage, the Wood Jing is beginning to be accepted by the fetus' body.

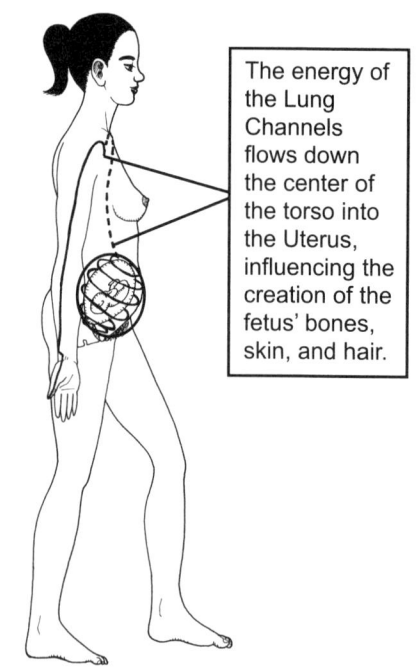

Figure 2.68. The mother's Lung Channels govern the seventh lunar month of creation. The Seven Essential Stars open the fetus' orifices to let in the light from Heaven and Earth. The Wood Jing is accepted by the fetus' body.

The Role of the Mother's Lung Channels

During the seventh lunar month, the mother's Lung Channels create the Bones, skin, and hair (Figure 2.68).

Wood Jing Formation

As previously mentioned, during the seventh lunar month, the Wood Jing is beginning to be incorporated into the fetus' body. The Wood Jing energy governs the assertion and direction of the fetus' emotional and spiritual aspects. Any faltering of the Wood Jing energy is associated with psychological problems, such as passive-aggressive personality disorder. These psychological disturbances may be evident at birth or develop later in life.

Seven Essential Stars

In the seventh lunar month, the fetus' Stomach and Intestines are stabilized, and the Seven Essential Stars open the body's upper orifices to absorb the light from Heaven and Earth. These

CHAPTER 2: UNDERSTANDING ANCIENT CHINESE METAPHYSICS

The Body's Six Openings			
1. Eyes	—	Absorb images into the Liver	—	Affects the Hun (Three Ethereal Souls)
2. Ears	—	Absorb sounds into the Kidneys	—	Affects the Zhi (Will Power)
3. Nose	—	Absorbs smells into the Lungs	—	Affects the Po (Seven Corporeal Souls)
4. Mouth	—	Absorbs tastes into the Spleen	—	Affects the Yi (Intent/Intellect)
5. Physical Body	—	Absorbs sensations into the Heart	—	Affects the Shen (Mind and Emotions)
6. Spirit	—	Absorbs sensations into the Heart	—	Affects the Shen (Mind and Emotions)

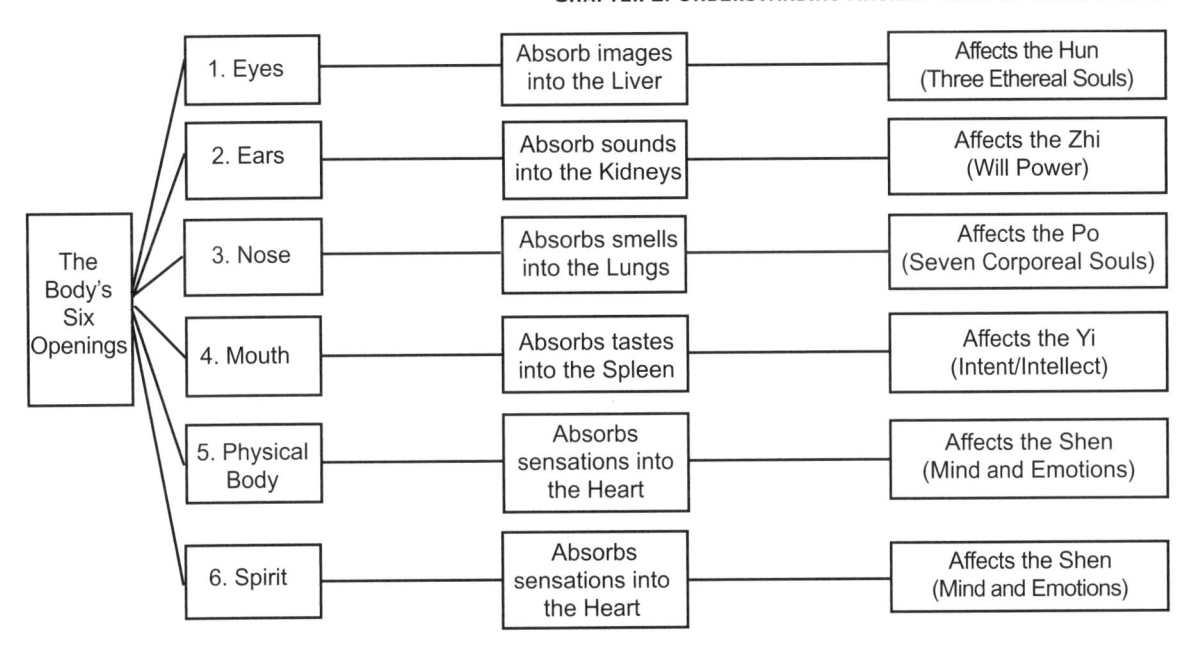

Figure 2.69. During the seventh lunar month, the body's Six Openings are stimulated into energetic awakening.

stars consist of the sun, the moon, and the five planets (Mars, Venus, Mercury, Saturn, and Jupiter). Each star is associated with one of the body's upper orifices:

- The Right Ear: Saturn
- The Left Ear: Jupiter
- The Right Nostril: Mars
- The Left Nostril: Venus
- The Right Eye: Moon
- The Left Eye: Sun
- The Mouth: Mercury

These orifices serve as receiving and projecting energetic portals for Jing, Qi, and Shen. They also serve as messengers of the body's Five Yin Organs. Thus, the Liver expresses "itself" through observation, the Heart through speech, the Spleen through taste, the Lungs through smell, and the Kidneys through hearing. These energetic messages are received by the body's Wu Jing Shen and emotionally, as well as energetically interact through the body's Six Openings.

THE BODY'S SIX OPENINGS

The energetic messages received through the body's Six Openings are described as follows (Figure 2.69:

1. The eyes absorb images into the Liver which affect the Hun (The Three Ethereal Souls).
2. The ears absorb sounds into the Kidneys which affect the Zhi (Will Power).
3. The nose absorbs smells into the Lungs which affect the Po (The Seven Corporeal Souls).
4. The mouth absorbs tastes into the Spleen which affect the Yi (Intent/Intellect).
5. The physical body absorbs sensations into the tissues which affect the Shen (Mind and Emotions).
6. The spirit (along with the physical body) absorbs sensations into the Heart which also affect the Shen (Mind and Emotions).

TISSUE FORMATION

During the seventh lunar month, there is a substantial increase in the weight of the fetus, and its head and body are even more proportionate. At this point, the fetus can survive if born prematurely (between 27 and 28 weeks); however, its temperature regulation (a function of the hypothalamus) and the lungs' production of surfactant (a phospholipid substance important in controlling the surface tension of the air-liquid emulsion present in the lungs) is still inadequate.

Month Eight

The mother's Large Intestine Channels govern the eighth lunar month of creation. During the eighth lunar month, the mother's Large Intestine Channels complete the formation of the fetus' skin, harmonizing the Heart (the Shen) and quieting the breath. At this stage, the Earth Jing is accepted by the fetus' body.

The Role of the Mother's Large Intestine Channels

The mother's Large Intestine Channels control the fetus' orifices. At this stage in development, the fetus' flesh is formed (Figure 2.70). The formation and consolidation of the fetus' Jing is now complete. The fetus' Zhen (True) Qi is now fully developed and circulates in the body's channels and collaterals, nourishing the Yin and Yang organs, and fighting disease.

Earth Jing Formation

As previously mentioned, during the eighth lunar month, the fetus receives the Zong (Essential) Qi from the mother's Spleen. Zong Qi is energy collected from Heaven and Earth which accumulates within the chest. At this stage, the Earth Jing is accepted by the fetus' body, completing the formation of the skin.

The Earth Jing energy governs the quality and maturation of the fetus' emotional and spiritual bonding and boundaries. Any faltering of the Earth Jing energy is associated with problems of severe psychological disturbances, such as schizophrenia. These psychological disturbances may be evident at birth or develop later in life.

Tissue Formation

At the end of the eighth month, the Bones of the fetus' head are soft, the skin is less wrinkled, and there is subcutaneous fat deposited throughout the body. If the fetus is a male, its testes will now descend into the scrotum.

At this stage, the fetus will normally assume an upside-down position in preparation for birth. If the fetus is born prematurely, its chances for survival are now much greater.

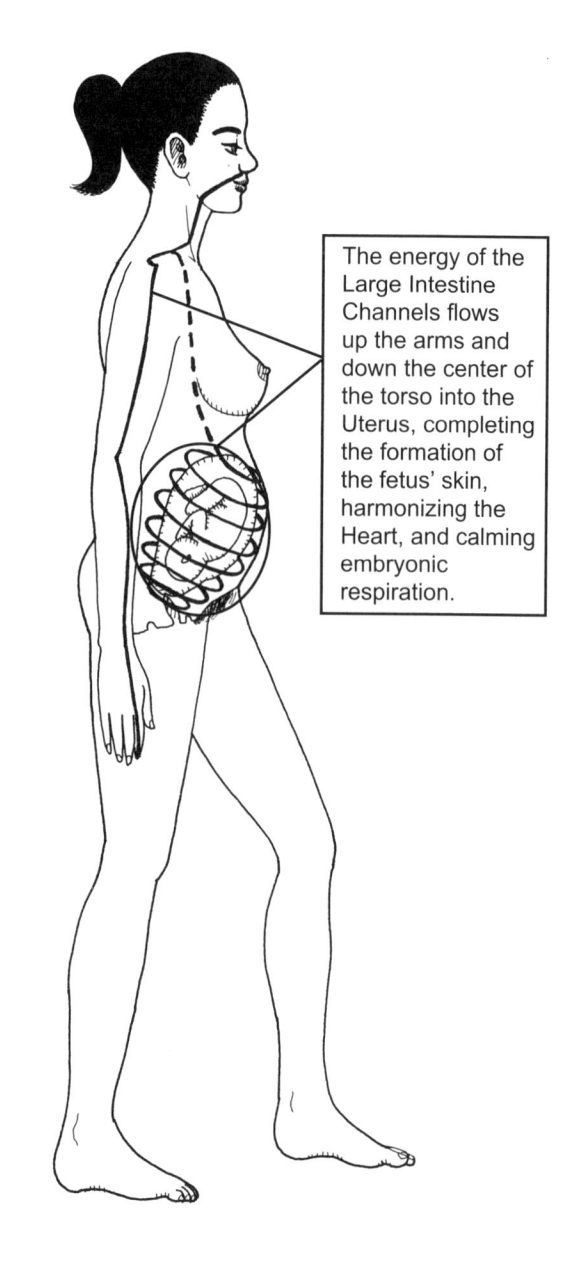

The energy of the Large Intestine Channels flows up the arms and down the center of the torso into the Uterus, completing the formation of the fetus' skin, harmonizing the Heart, and calming embryonic respiration.

Figure 2.70. The mother's Large Intestine Channels govern the eighth lunar month of creation. At this stage, the Earth Jing is accepted by the fetus's body.

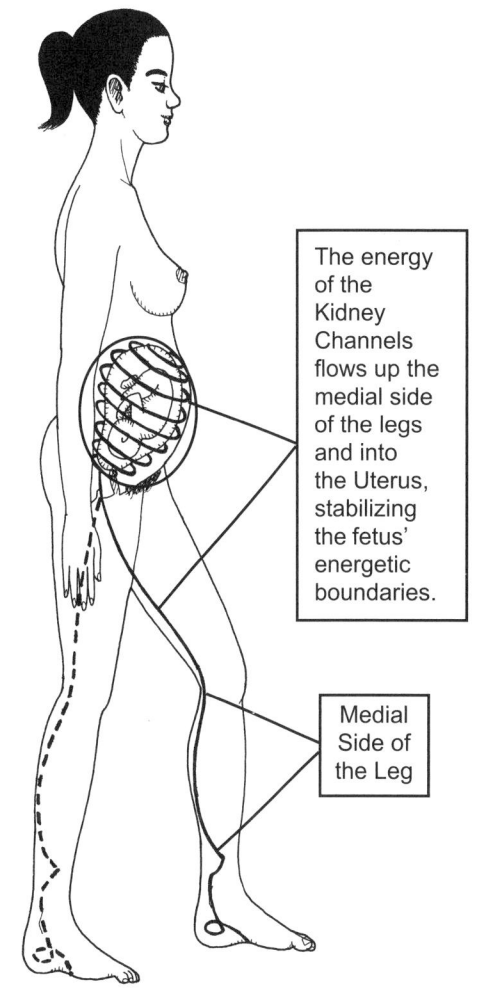

MONTH NINE

The mother's Kidney Channels govern the ninth lunar month of creation. At this stage, all of the fetus' spatial cavities and energetic boundaries are now firmly established.

KIDNEY CHANNEL'S RESPONSIBILITY

During the ninth lunar month, the mother's Kidney Channels control the amount of energy the fetus absorbs from the mother through the umbilicus (Figure 2.71).

FUNCTION OF THE UMBILICAL CORD

The fetus absorbs Qi and the nutrition derived from the mother's Blood by way of the umbilical vein which connects to the fetus' Liver. From the Liver, nutrients are processed and absorbed into the Blood to be distributed throughout the fetus.

The umbilical cord attaches to the placenta from the abdomen of the fetus. The placenta, which forms on the uterine wall after the first week of pregnancy, consists of tissues from both the mother and the embryo. Within the placenta, Qi and nutrients are transported from the mother's Blood to the Blood of the fetus. Although the circulation of the two come close, they never actually connect.

The function of the umbilical cord is to remove waste products and pass food, energy, and oxygen from the mother's bloodstream to the fetus. The mother's Kidney Channels regulate the flow of Qi and Shen into the fetus through the umbilical cord.

After the umbilical cord has been severed, the fetus' umbilical veins still remain. These umbilical veins eventually become the ligamentum teres that connect from the umbilicus, up along the interior surface of the abdominal wall, through the free margin of the falciform ligament to the right and left lobes of the Liver. This maintains the baby's connection between its Liver and its Lower Dantian (navel).

ENERGETIC FORMATION

In the ninth month, the Internal Palaces and the Nine Dantian Chambers (nine internal Dantian cavities) are created within each of the fetus' Three Dantians, and are established to keep the fetus'

The energy of the Kidney Channels flows up the medial side of the legs and into the Uterus, stabilizing the fetus' energetic boundaries.

Medial Side of the Leg

Figure 2.71. The mother's Kidney Channels govern the ninth lunar month of creation. At this stage, all of the fetus' spatial cavities and energetic boundaries are now firmly established.

Jing (Essence) safe.

At this stage of energetic formation, all of the fetus' energetic spatial cavities (internal organ tissue chambers) and energetic boundaries are arranged to prepare the fetus for its birth.

TISSUE FORMATION

In the ninth month, additional subcutaneous fat accumulates throughout the fetus' body. Externally, the fetus' fingernails will extend to the tips of the fingers and sometimes beyond.

MONTH TEN

The mother's Urinary Bladder Channels govern the tenth lunar month of creation. At this stage, the baby's Dantians and the spatial cavities that surround the major organs are completely developed to maintain the safety of the fetus' Jing. Heaven and Earth Qi settle into the fetus' Lower Dantian in preparation for birth.

THE ROLE OF THE MOTHER'S URINARY BLADDER CHANNELS

During the tenth lunar month, the mother's Urinary Bladder Channels harmonize all five Yin organs (Liver, Heart, Spleen, Lungs, and Kidneys) and five Yang organs (Gall Bladder, Small Intestine, Stomach, Large Intestine, and Urinary Bladder) (Figure 2.72).

ENERGETIC FORMATION

After ten lunar months in the womb, the fetus' Three Dantians are fully established. Also, the energy of the Wu Jing Shen are now active within the internal spatial cavities that surround the major organs. The internal spatial cavities are developed to maintain the safety of the fetus' Jing. The fetus is now ready to be released into the world.

The process of birth begins when Heaven Qi and Earth Qi settle into the fetus' Lower Dantian (Figure 2.73). The ancient Chinese described the birth transition as "a ripe melon falling off the stem," noting that the fetus breaks out of its amniotic sac and emerges head first towards the Earth and with its feet towards the Heavens.

With its first cry, the infant comes in contact with the environmental air. As the infant inhales, the air (considered Postnatal Qi), mixes with the infant's innate primordial original energy (Yuan Qi, also considered Prenatal Qi). The ancient Daoists believed that the innate Prenatal Qi supports the tissues of the body, while the acquired Postnatal Qi supports the tissue's function. The Postnatal Qi depends on the Prenatal Qi to support the respiratory system (breathing in and out), while the Prenatal Qi depends on the Postnatal Qi to nurture the vascular system.

At the moment of the infant's first cry, the ancient Daoists also believed that the acquired conscious spirit (Shen Zhi) enters into the opening and

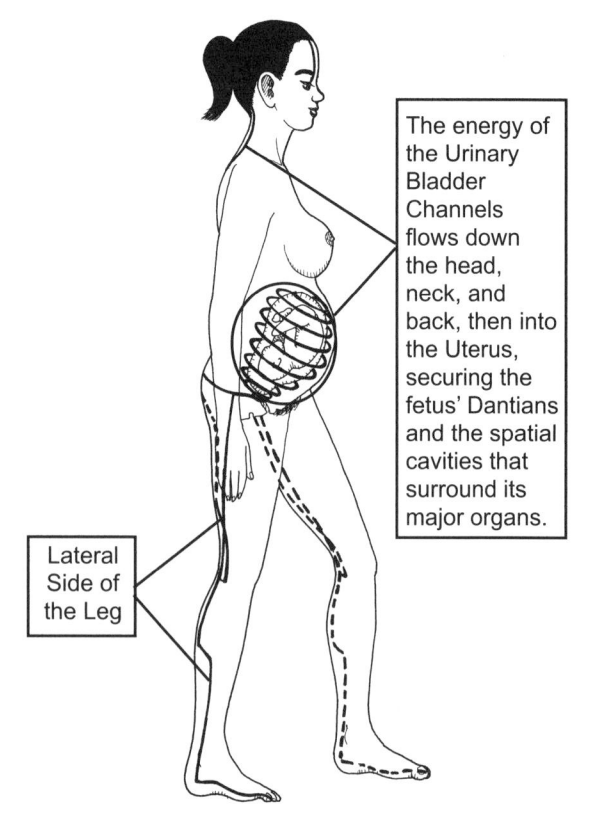

Figure 2.72. The mother's Urinary Bladder Channels govern the tenth lunar month of creation. At this stage, the fetus' Dantians and the spatial cavities that surround the major organs are completely developed to maintain the safety of the fetus' Jing.

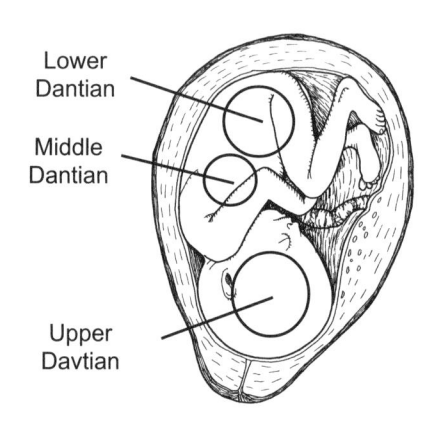

Figure 2.73. Heaven and Earth Qi settle into the fetus' Lower Dantian and the process of birth begins.

merges with the baby's primordial original spirit (Yuan Shen). The congenital Yuan Shen depends on the acquired Shen Zhi to exist, while the Shen Zhi depends on the Yuan Shen for awareness.

Postnatal Energy Development

According to ancient Daoists thought, the moment the baby cries, the "sealed enclosure" of Early Heaven is broken and the baby's Yuan Jing, Yuan Qi, and Yuan Shen divide into three separate entities. This division causes the energy of baby's Fire (Shen) to separate from its Water (Jing), and begins the Later Heaven patterns of energetic existence.

The ancient Daoists also believed that at the moment of birth, the conscious Acquired Spirit (Shen Zhi) merges with the child's Original Spirit (Yuan Shen). The Yuan Shen depends on the Shen Zhi to survive within its new environment, while the Shen Zhi depends on the Yuan Shen for effective awareness.

The energy of the Po are responsible for the first physiological processes after birth, allowing the child's eyes to see, ears to hear, and Heart to perceive. The Po also govern the movements of the hands and feet, as well as the baby's breathing patterns.

The Medical Qigong doctor studies the ten lunar month process of fetal developmental to create a foundation for understanding the formation of the patient's physical and energetic structure. This knowledge also aide in the comprehension of the initial formation of the Five Elemental Constitutions. The Five Elemental Constitutions are described in the next chapter of this volume.

Postnatal Channel Function

During prenatal development, the Eight Extraordinary Vessels (see Chapter 6) are responsible for transporting, transforming, and producing Qi and Blood for the fetus, while the Twelve Primary Channels (see Chapter 8) are still in the process of gradual development. While in utero, the energetic activity generated from the fetus' Lower Dantian and Eight Extraordinary Vessels resonates throughout its body, creating tissue development.

Once the umbilical cord is severed, the primary focus of energy shifts from the Lower Dantian to the Middle Dantian (located in the

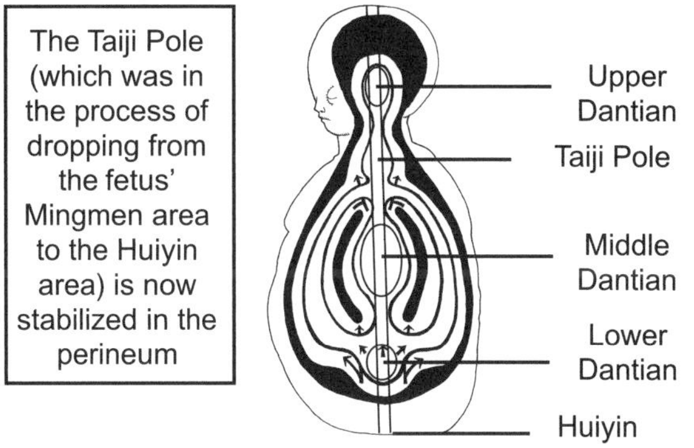

Figure 2.74. As the fetus develops, the Eight Extraordinary Vessels govern the development of the Twelve Primary Channels.

baby's chest area). In ancient China, it was believed that the energetic influence of Early Heaven begins to mix with the acquired influence of Later Heaven at the moment of the child's first breath. These energies combine within the chest and activate the "genetic" potential stored within the child's Original (Yuan) Qi.

After birth, Gu Qi (energy derived from air, food, and drink) is created within the baby's Stomach while it nurses. The baby is no longer receiving nourishment from the mother internally via the umbilical cord, but is now receiving external nourishment, transforming it into Gu Qi through the Stomach and Spleen. Gradual development of the baby's Spleen and Stomach is important, and the air, food, and drink that the mother consumes will directly affect the nursing baby if she breast-feeds.

As the Gu Qi establishes itself within the baby's Stomach and Spleen, it helps to form Qi and Blood. The Qi and Blood then become energized and flow within the Twelve Primary Channels, nourishing the organs and tissues. The Twelve Primary Channels will now assume the responsibility of circulating Qi and Blood throughout the baby's entire physical and energetic structure. The Eight Extraordinary Vessels shift their function from sustaining and directing tissue development to regulating the baby's Channel Qi. Additionally, the Taiji Pole which was in the process of dropping from the fetus' Mingmen area to the Huiyin area is now stabilized in the perineum (Figure 2.74).

ENERGETIC FUNCTIONS OF THE TAIJI POLE

The natural resonant vibration of the baby's Taiji Pole (energetic core) initiates an energetic expansion and contraction. This projection and reception simultaneously affects the baby at five distinct levels: physical, mental, emotional, energetic, and spiritual. Balanced physical growth will only occur when all five levels are in equilibrium. The physical body is generally the slowest realm to respond to growth and change. Matter does not move at the same rate as energy, mind, or spirit; thus, the energy, mind, and spirit must wait patiently for the physical body to evolve before progressing as a whole.

ENERGETIC FLOW OF THE MICROCOSMIC ORBIT

In ancient China, it was taught that at birth the individual's original nature (known as De, or virtue) is stored within the five Yin organs' Prenatal Wu Jing Shen, and was directed by the Yuan Shen (congenital mind) of the Heart (rooted in the Middle Dantian). Additionally, the individual's destiny (known as Ming) is stored within his or her Kidneys and rooted in the Lower Dantian. The Upper Dantian, acting as a spiritual axis, facilitates the subtle influences of energetic and spiritual awakenings, as well as divine insights needed to guide and direct the individual's spiritual path (life purpose).

The term "Microcosmic Orbit" generally refers to the flow of energy moving through the Governing Vessel (Sea of Yang) and the Conception Vessel (Sea of Yin). One of the functions of the Microcosmic Orbit is to connect the energetic and spiritual centers of the Three Dantians. Once an individual has been born, his or her Microcosmic Orbit will naturally flow in the direction of the Water cycle, with the energy moving up the front of the body (Conception Vessel) and down the back (Governing Vessel). This energetic movement naturally facilitates the child's spiritual, intuitive, and psychic perceptions. This energetic pattern generally continues until the child reaches puberty, at which time the energy reverses its direction and flows up the back (Governing Vessel) and down the front (Conception Vessel) which is the direction of the Fire cycle. This energetic switch in direction facilitates the child's cognitive development and the ability to control emotions and impulses. The time of the Microcosmic Orbit's energetic reversal varies depending on the child's physical constitution, state of health, and his or her environment.

Children have a natural tendency towards psychic and intuitive insights due to a number of factors, which are described as follows (Figure 2.75):

1. The flow of energy moving through the child's Water Cycle maintains the child's psychic and intuitive insights.
2. The overactive Hun going in and out the child's body allows him or her to see into the Spirit world.
3. The child's connection to the energetic resonances of the Taiji Pole and center core (Eternal Soul) is still open and subconsciously active. This allows the child to receive energy and information directly from his or her Eternal Soul.
4. The child's superior cranial sutures are still open, allowing his or her Taiji Pole to be more receptive to the vibrational resonance of the subtle energetic fields, hence facilitating the child's ability to spirit travel (Figure 2.76).

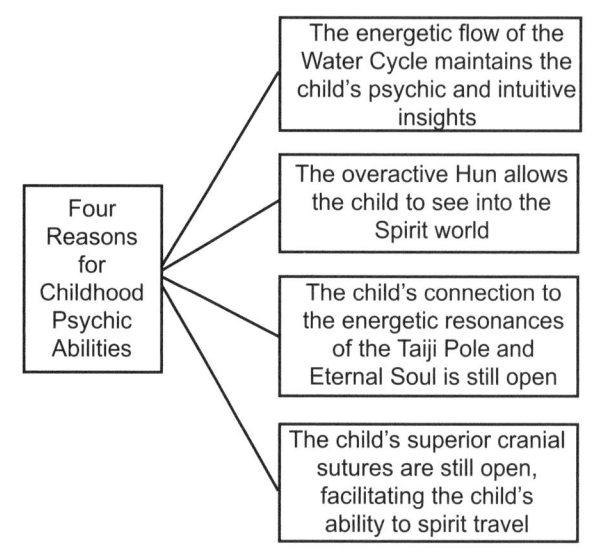

Figure 2.75. Children have a natural tendency towards psychic and intuitive insights.

Four Reasons for Childhood Psychic Abilities:
- The energetic flow of the Water Cycle maintains the child's psychic and intuitive insights
- The overactive Hun allows the child to see into the Spirit world
- The child's connection to the energetic resonances of the Taiji Pole and Eternal Soul is still open
- The child's superior cranial sutures are still open, facilitating the child's ability to spirit travel

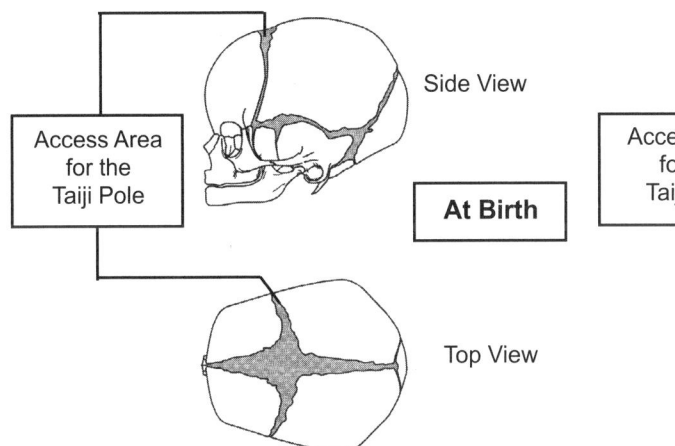

Chapter 2: Understanding Ancient Chinese Metaphysics

Figure 2.76. At birth, the baby's superior cranial sutures are completely open and susceptible to the vibrational resonance of the subtle energetic world.

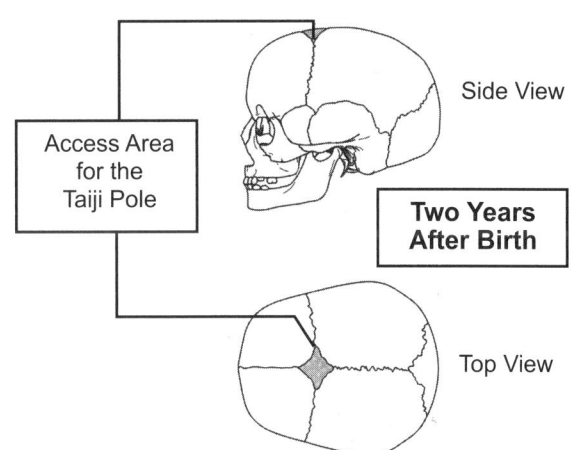

Figure 2.77. After two years, the baby's superior cranial sutures close, making the child less susceptible to the vibrational resonance of the subtle energetic world.

The soft apertures (fontanels) in the baby's skull slowly begin to close during the third month after birth. Several Qigong Masters believe that psychic and intuitive insights, as well as the ability to spirit travel, gradually wane as the baby's superior cranial sutures continue to close. In Tibetan Qigong practices (specifically in the teachings used to prepare an individual for death), the individual's superior cranial sutures are trained to become once again soft in order to facilitate the final exit of the Eternal Soul (Figure 2.77).

Congenital or Acquired Disorders

Understanding the energetic process of fetal development provides the Qigong doctor with an overview of the energetic components of tissues, organs, and channel function. This understanding is essential for diagnosing the causes of a disease, whether it is either congenital or acquired in origin. Unlike Western medicine, Chinese medicine treats the root of the illness and not just its manifested symptoms. Both congenital and acquired factors should be considered in every case. This is necessary because both the origin and development of a disease may result from either a congenital or acquired source, or a combination of both.

Congenital Disorders

In Medical Qigong channel therapy, cases of congenital Qi deficiency or congenital disorders of Qi flow are treated by Tonifying (strengthening) the Eight Extraordinary Vessels. In some cases, it is necessary to first Purge the pathogenic energy from the Eight Extraordinary Vessels before Tonifying to consolidate and regulate the patient's Prenatal Qi.

Acquired Diseases

The patient can generally be cured of acquired diseases when an effective selection of points and Qi emission methods are used for Purgation, Tonification, and Regulation according to the imbalances of Qi circulating within the Twelve Primary Channels.

Prenatal and Postnatal Energetic Patterns

In ancient China, an individual's physical, energetic, and spiritual strengths and weaknesses, as well as his or her destiny were believed to be influenced by both Yang and Yin energetic patterns. The Prenatal energetic patterns were believed to originate at the moment of conception and were considered Yang, while the Postnatal patterns were seen to originate at the moment of birth and were considered Yin.

The ancient Chinese calculated the strength or weakness of an individual's Prenatal (congeni-

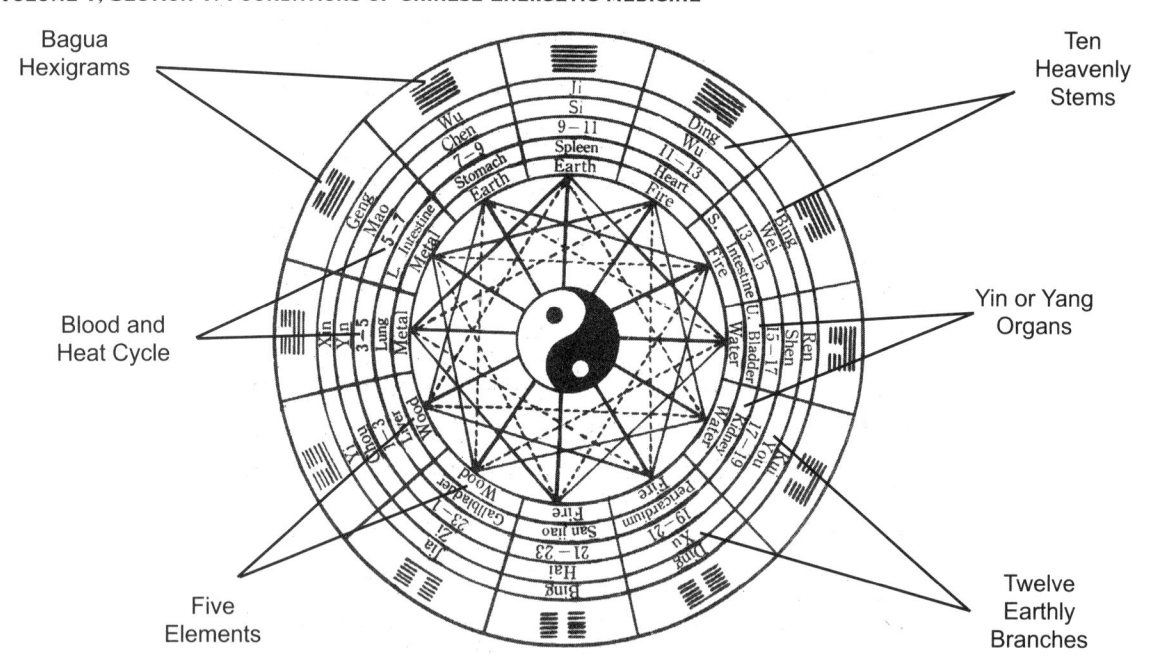

VOLUME 1, SECTION 1: FOUNDATIONS OF CHINESE ENERGETIC MEDICINE

Figure 2.78. After birth, the Daily Qi, Blood, and Heat Cycle is constantly being influenced by the interactions of the Celestial and environmental energetic fields.

tal) and Postnatal (acquired) energetic patterns according to interactions of the Heavenly and Earthly energetic fields. These energetic and spiritual interactions were manifested through the influences of the Ten Heavenly Stems and the Twelve Earthly Branches.

As the internal organs develop within the forming fetus, the Ten Heavenly Stems are responsible for the Prenatal regulation of all Jing formation, growth and internal power. The Twelve Earthly Branches are responsible for Postnatal interactions with the universal (Heaven) and environmental (Earth) energetic fields. The Ten Heavenly Stems and the Twelve Earthly Branches are described as follows:

- **The Ten Heavenly Stems** relate to the energies of Heaven and are represented in "Man" as the Yin and Yang aspects of the Five Element organs of Wood, Fire, Earth, Metal, and Water. The first and second stems correspond to the Wood Element, beginning with the Gall Bladder (Yang stem) and the Liver (Yin stem). The third and forth stems correspond to the Fire Element, beginning with the Small Intestine (Yang stem) and Heart (Yin stem). The fifth and sixth stems correspond to the Earth Element, beginning with the Stomach (Yang stem) and Spleen (Yin stem). The seventh and eighth stems correspond to the Metal Element, beginning with the Large Intestine (Yang stem) and Lungs (Yin stem). The ninth and tenth stems correspond to the Water Element, beginning with the Urinary Bladder (Yang stem) and Kidneys (Yin stem) (Figure 2.78).

- **The Twelve Earthly Branches** are Earth energies and are represented in "Man" as the Twelve Primary Channels. They also represent the ancient Chinese systems of time, space, and fate calculation (known as Ming Shu).

CONCEPTION AND THE PRENATAL ANCESTRAL TRAITS

According to ancient Chinese esoteric teachings, when the sperm joins with the ovum at conception, a polar axis is created that forms the embryo's Taiji Pole. The energetic vortex thus created draws universal and environmental energies, as well as the Eternal Soul (Shen Xian) into the em-

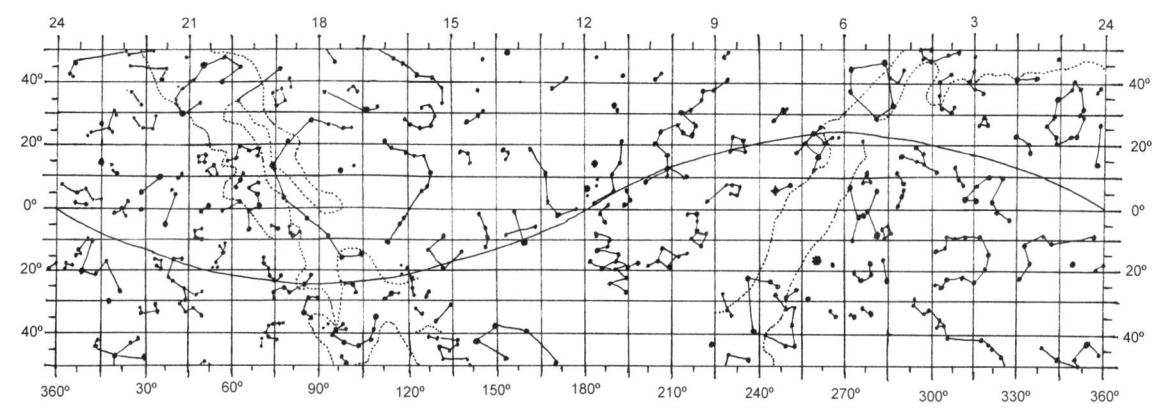

Figure 2.79. The Pathway of the Earth through the Twenty-Eight Constellations influences Prenatal Jing, Qi and Shen formation.

bryo. The Prenatal energetic patterns of the body are determined at the time and place of conception. As a general rule, to determine the time of conception, the ancient Wu Yi would count back forty weeks from the time of birth. The time and place of conception establishes the inherent strength or weakness of an individual's spiritual constitution, as well as his or her ancestral traits (food preferences, manner of dress, preferences of art, spiritual beliefs, affinity for certain cultures, and so on).

It is for this reason that the time and location of conception also determines the nature of the ancestral spiritual influence on the individual. As the Divine infuses the fetus' soul, the energy of the Eternal Soul (Shen Xian) combines with the environmental spiritual influences of the geographic location (the Orient, Europe, North America, etc.). This infusion of geographic spiritual energy creates within the individual a predisposition towards specific ancestral traits and cultural attractions.

At conception and throughout pregnancy, the mother absorbs the natural environmental energy through respiration (breathing Qi through the mouth, nose, and pores), digestion (absorbing nutrients from the food and soil), and visual/auditory absorption (observing and experiencing the surrounding environment). The entire history of each cultural environment is encoded within the natural energetic fields contained within that environment. Therefore, an individual conceived in the Orient may find him or herself unconsciously drawn to the social and cultural patterns and influences of that particular Asian population. This subconscious energetic attraction is considered a natural phenomenon due to the subtle influences of the location's spiritual and ancestral vibrations. The subconscious energetic attraction can indirectly affect an individual in several ways, described as follows:

1. The natural environment surrounding the location of an individual at conception exerts a strong influence on his or her environmental preferences. This often manifests as a general preference or attraction to environmental patterns and locations similar to those at conception. People conceived by the ocean, for example, may find within themselves an unconscious need to live by the ocean. Likewise, people conceived in the mountains, valleys, tropics, deserts, etc. may find feelings of peace or ease envelop them when visiting such places.

2. The time of an individual's conception also exerts a strong influence. The energetic formation, strength and weaknesses of the fetus' internal organs are also determined by the positions of the sun, moon, and stars at the moment of conception. These Heavenly energies affect on the fetus at the time of conception and continue influencing the fetus' formation throughout the entire pregnancy.

The Heavenly influences on Prenatal Jing, Qi and Shen formation can be understood by mapping the pathway of the Earth through the Twenty-Eight Constellations (Figure 2.79).

BIRTH AND THE POSTNATAL ENERGETIC PATTERNS

The ancient Chinese believed that after birth, the degree to which an individual can draw upon and absorb spiritual energy depends on his or her karma (the momentum of previous intentions, thoughts and actions which manifest as destiny).

The Postnatal energetic patterns of the body are determined by the time and place of birth. The time and place of birth also mark the beginning of the individual's energetic biorhythms (physical, emotional, and intellectual cycles).

These biorhythms are developed according to the energetic influence of the Heavens (position of the sun, moon, planets and stars), as well as the energetic influence of the Earth (i.e., geographic location: mountains, valleys, desert, ocean, etc.). This infusion of the Earth's geographic energy and Heaven's stellar energy creates within the individual a predisposition towards specific psychological traits, described as follows:

1. **The location of birth** strongly influences the individual's desire to seek or surround him or herself with a similar environment.
2. **The time of birth** may also have an unconscious influence on the individual's living patterns. For example, some individuals born at night often become "night people," while others born in the morning function better during the morning hours.

The body's biorhythms, which react to universal and environmental energetic vibrations, are divided into three distinct cycles and energy flows (Figure 2.80). Each rhythm follows a cyclical process of waxing and waning, creating times of physical, emotional, and intellectual peaks, as well as times of reflection and withdrawn behavior. These three cycles begin at the moment of birth and continue with regularity until death. The conditions of the cycle are divided into positive (the first, waxing half) and negative (the second, waning half) attributes. These rhythms influence the time during which many illnesses occur or worsen, as well as how fast a medication takes effect and how long the effect lasts. Therefore, Medical Qigong therapy, as well as herbal therapy are prescribed at specific times of the day in order to enhance the ef-

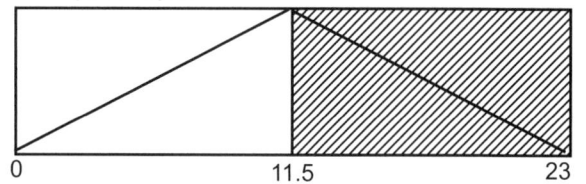

Physical Cycle

The Physical Cycle is 23 days long. The first 11.5 days are the positive side of the cycle, in which the individual experiences an increase physical strength and endurance. The second 11.5 days are the negative side of the cycle, marked by a gradual decrease in the level of endurance, and a tendency towards fatigue.

Emotional Cycle

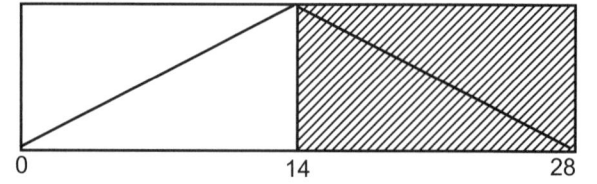

The Emotional Cycle is 28 days long. The first 14 days are the positive side of the cycle, in which the individual feels increasingly optimistic, cheerful, and cooperative. For the second 14 days, a negative stage of the cycle results in a tendency to be more moody, irritable, or pessimistic.

Intellectual Cycle

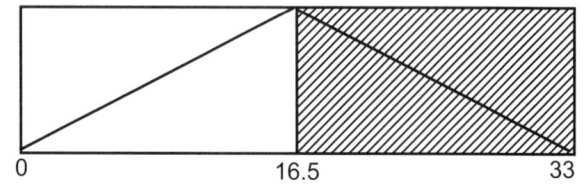

The Intellectual Cycle is 33 days long. The first 16.5 days are the positive side of the cycle, in which the individual experiences greater success in learning new material and pursuing creative, and intellectual activities. The next 16.5 days are the negative side of the cycle, in which the individual is encouraged to review old material rather than attempting to learn new concepts.

Figure 2.80. The physical, emotional, and intellectual cycles begin at birth.

fect on the patient's body.

The body's biorhythms are but one example of the influence of Heavenly energy on the physical, emotional, and intellectual cycles of mankind. By understanding the energetic potential of the cycles of the sun, moon, and stars, the Qigong doctor can direct the universal energy of Heaven to regulate and balance the patient's Qi.

Additionally, by understanding the energetic potential of local seasonal changes, the Qigong doctor can direct the environmental energy of Earth to regulate and balance the patient's Qi.

ANCIENT DAOIST ARCHETYPES OF THE HUMAN SOUL

Ancient Chinese medicine describes the Eternal Soul (Shen Xian) as consisting of three spiritual energies called the "Lords of the Three Dantians," which oversee the influences of the individual's human soul (Yuan Shen). This terminology is metaphoric, in that it is used to describe the various energetic aspects of the human soul.

Once the human soul has established its residence within the Taiji Pole, it separates its Yin and Yang spiritual energy into three distinct spiritual aspects. These three spiritual aspects oversee the differing internal energies and powers of the body's Three Dantians. They are referred to in esoteric Daoist traditions as the Lords of the Three Dantians: Tai Yi, Si Ming, and Xia Tao Kang. They are named according to their function: Tai Yi translates as Great Divinity, Si Ming translates as The Administrator of Destiny, and Xia Tao Kang translates as Below Healthy Peach (Life).

During conception, these three spiritual energies are given to each individual from the divine to maintain the spiritual residence of the Yuan Shen. These three energies reside in the innermost subtle aspects of the body and are described as follows:

1. **The Tai Yi (Great Divinity)** resides within the Upper Dantian in the region between the eyes, in the area known as the "Celestial Realm," and is considered the Lord of the Nei Wan (Innermost Palace). Tai Yi governs a multitude of the body's spirits (causing an individual's

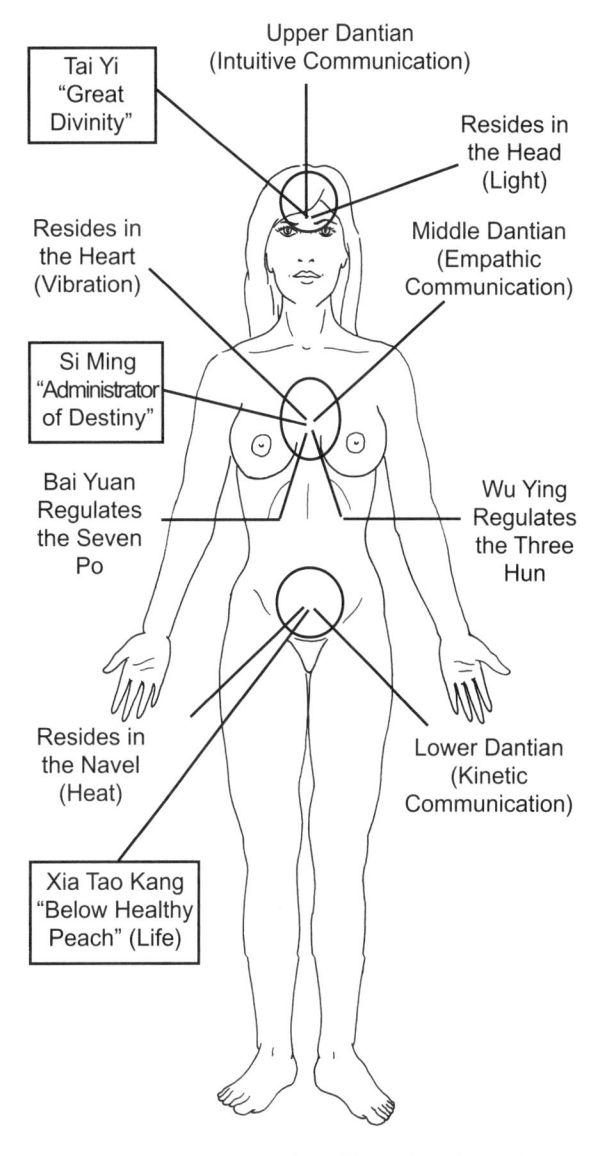

Figure 2.81. The Lords of the Three Dantians: Tai Yi, Si Ming, and Xia Tao Kang

Yuan Shen to shine externally), and rules all the activities of the mind (including the potential of the enlightened mind). Tai Yi facilitates awareness of the Three Ethereal Souls (Hun) and advocates personal spiritual enlightenment (Figure 2.81).

2. **The Si Ming (The Administrator of Destiny)** resides within the Middle Dantian in the region

of the Heart, in the area known as the "Terrestrial Realm." Si Ming regulates the body's Qi, and is the source of the mind and its emotional connections. Si Ming challenges our reactions to various internal and external obstacles. Although Si Ming controls and maintains the residence of the human soul, the body's Shen is free to make decisions that affect life and health based upon the individual's free-will (the interaction between the Yuan Shen and the Shen Zhi). Thus, the individual's free-will manifests through his or her thoughts and actions. Si Ming also controls the spiritual energies of Wu Ying and Bai Yuan which affect the body's Jing, Qi, and Shen via the breath.

- **The Spirit Wu Ying (Without Excess)** occupies the left side of the body and regulates the Three Ethereal Souls (Hun). In ancient China, the Three Hun were called Tai Guang (Eminent Light), Shang Ling (Pleasant Soul) and Yu Jing (Hidden Essence).
- **The Spirit Bai Yuan (Pure Origin)** occupies the right side of the body and regulates the Seven Corporeal Souls (Po). In ancient China, the Seven Po were known as Flying Poison, Unclean Evil, Stinking Lungs, Corpse Dog, Fallen Arrow, Yin Bird and Devouring Robber.

3. **The Xia Tao Kang (Below Healthy Peach/Life)** resides within the Lower Dantian in the region of the navel, in the area known as the "Water Realm." It is responsible for procreation and for the preservation of the body's Jing.

THE ETHEREAL SOUL AND CORPOREAL SOUL

In Western culture, an individual's internal dialogues are sometimes associated with the spiritual influences of good or evil. In Chinese medicine, internal dialogues influencing the patient's psyche are also divided into good and evil. These spiritual and emotional influences are considered to be the specific good and evil characteristics of the patient's Hun (Ethereal Soul) and Po (Corporeal Soul). The spiritual components and influences of the Hun and Po are considered to be separate entities, or archetypes, acting upon the patient's Shen and affecting the human soul.

These two archetypes are regarded as spirit souls that can exert a positive or negative influence on a person's life according to the nature of the individual's human soul. The positive or good internal influences are manifested through the Hun, while the negative or primal internal influences are generally manifested through the Po. The Hun or Po can either motivate or hinder personal growth, as well as cause illness and even the demise of the body.

The Hun (coming from Heaven) and the Po (coming from Earth) are both established within the fetus's internal organs at conception, yet they remain dormant until the third lunar month after conception. This is because at the third lunar month, the fetus' organs Orbs are sufficiently formed to house, support and maintain the spiritual energies of the Wu Jing Shen. One ancient belief is that the Hun and Po, although residing in the fetus, frequently leave and return together to gather and absorb universal and environmental Qi. The Hun will naturally connect with celestial spiritual beings, as well as with the Divine. The Po will naturally connect with nature spirits and environmental spirits.

The Three Ethereal Souls are collectively referred to as the Hun. Traditional Chinese Medicine therefore often refers to the Hun as a singular entity. The Seven Corporeal Souls are traditionally referred to as the Po, with the assumption that this term depicts all seven Po. Traditional Chinese Medicine, therefore often refers to the Po as a singular entity.

THE HUN: THREE ETHEREAL SOULS

The Liver stores the Hun, also called the Three Ethereal Souls. The Hun are rooted within the Liver, specifically the Liver Yin and the Liver Blood. The Hun represent spiritual consciousness, provide the energetic movement of the Mind, and are associated with the Qi of Heaven and the Five Agents.

The Chinese have maintained that there are three Hun since the Han Dynasty (206 B.C. - 220 A.D.). The Hun represent energetic and spiritual activities operating at three levels of influence, which directly inspire and are inspired by the Shen.

The Three Hun originate from Heaven, which the ancient Chinese considered a state of subtle and nonmaterial energies and beings (Figure 2.82). Therefore, the Hun are a part of the spiritual aspects of an individual that can spirit travel. Additionally, upon the death of the body, the energetic spiritual essence of the Hun ascends back to Heaven.

Although they reside in the Liver Orb, the Hun also resonate from the Three Dantians (like a vaporous mist extending from the Liver and filling the body's three Dantians). The Hun are energetically associated with the following: Yang, Heavenly soul, bright, light, Shen, constructive emotions and inspirations.

Chinese Ideogram for the Hun

The ideogram for the Hun has two parts. The character to the right represents the Earthly spirits, Gui (Ghost), depicted by a head suspended above a vaporous form of a body with an appendage (symbolizing the whirlwind that accompanies the movements of the Earthly spirits). The character to the left is the image for clouds, seen as vapor rising from the Earth and gathering in the Heavens (Figure 2.83). The Hun move within the body as freely as clouds, following the Yi (Will) of the "Heavenly breath, within the celestial vault" (following the will of the Eternal Soul stored within the Heart and originating in the Taiji Pole).

From this ideogram we also get a distinct picture of the spirit (Hun) rising to the Heavens. The Eternal Soul (Shen Xian) is considered energetically and spiritually different from the Hun in classical Chinese philosophy. In that context, the Eternal Soul is seen as the more personal of the two, while the term "spirit" (as in the Hun and Po) is seen as more universal temperaments or archetypes. The ancient medical classics state that there are Three Ethereal Souls (Hun) and Seven Corporeal Souls (Po) which symbolize different attributes of the human being. The Hun's spiritual

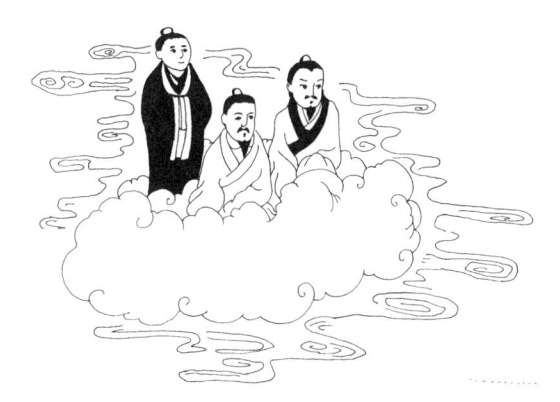

Figure 2.82. The Three Ethereal Souls of the Hun are named (1) Tai Kuang (2) Shang Ling (3) Yu Jing. The Hun represent spiritual consciousness, provide the energetic movement of the mind, and are associated with Qi of Heaven and the Five Agents. The Hun are the spiritual part of Man which ascends to Heaven after death.

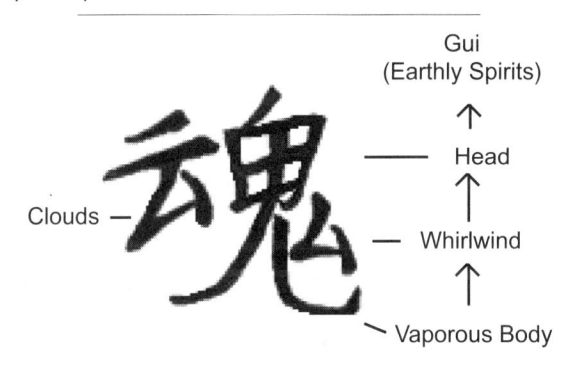

Figure 2.83. The Chinese character for "Hun," also known as the Ethereal Soul or Cloud Soul

energy is said to be able to leave the body and then return, thus indicating a relationship with out-of-body travel into the spirit world.

Tai Guan, Shang Ling, and Yu Jing

In ancient China, the Daoists described the Three Hun as having different personalities specific to the spiritual responsibilities of an individual's incarnated soul. The Three Ethereal Souls were called Tai Guang, Shang Ling, and Yu Jing; they are described as follows:

1. **Tai Guang:** The Hun known as Tai Guang resides within the Upper Dantian and is situated in the cranial cavity just below the Baihui GV-20 ("One Hundred Meetings") point. Tai Guang literally means "eminent light," and it

is considered to be the highest expression of Yin and Yang energy harmonized within the human form. It is connected energetically with the Upper Dantian and Heaven, and strives for physical, mental, emotional, and spiritual purity.

2. **Shang Ling:** The Hun known as Shang Ling resides within the Middle Dantian. It is situated in the Heart and the corresponding vessels, and is linked to the body's Five Agents. Shang Ling literally means "pleasant soul," and it is considered to be transformed Yin energy. It is connected with the Middle Dantian and is the expression of the Hun concerned with compassion towards others. It is through the influence of the Hun Shang Ling that the five virtues of each of the Five Agents manifest.

The Five Agents of Shang Ling

The Five Agents influence our desire to be involved in a variety of social interests and responsibilities. The Five Agents are energies that are linked to a person's moral qualities; they can be categorized as the five congenital virtues of the five Yin organs (Prenatal Wu Jing Shen). The Five Agents are similarly categorized into Five Elements. The psycho-emotional virtues of the Prenatal Wu Jing Shen and the acquired thoughts, beliefs and emotional states of the Postnatal Wu Jing Shen are both stored within the body's five Yin organs. Both influences are felt and expressed as the child grows into adulthood. When one of the internal organs is stimulated, a Yang (positive) or Yin (negative) psycho-emotional reaction is created. Psycho-emotional energetic interactions are feelings expressed through either the positive moral qualities of the congenital Prenatal Wu Jing Shen (the Five Agents of kindness, order, trust, integrity, and wisdom) or the negative emotional experiences of the acquired Postnatal Wu Jing Shen (the five emotional states of anger, excitement, worry, grief, and fear).

The Five Agents are commonly known as the Prenatal Wu Jing Shen (Congenital Five Essence Spirits: Hun, Shen, Yi, Po, and Zhi) and are stored within the energetic elemental natures of the

Yin Organ	Element	Congenital Agent	Acquired Emotion
Liver	Wood	Kindness	Anger
Heart	Fire	Order	Excitement
Spleen	Earth	Trust	Worry
Lungs	Metal	Integrity	Grief
Kidneys	Water	Wisdom	Fear

Figure 2.84. The Five Virtues of the Five Yin Organs

body's Jing. The Five Elemental energies (Wood, Fire, Earth, Metal, and Water) that internally support the Five Agents encompass not only the tissues of the physical body, but all of the phenomena of nature, combining and recombining in infinite ways to produce our manifested existence (Figure 2.84). The internal blending of the Five Elements along with the Prenatal Wu Jing Shen are described as follows:

- **The Wood Agent: The Virtue of Kindness.** This Agent represents the Prenatal virtues of love, benevolence, kindness, patience, unselfishness and compassion. This congenital agent is connected to the Hun and is stored in the Liver. The Wood Element also affects the Liver and Gall Bladder organs and the flow of energy in the Liver and Gall Bladder Channels. The Wood Agent governs the energy of the tendons, ligaments, small muscles, peripheral nerves, iris of the eyes, vision, tears, bile, nails, and external genitalia. After birth, through the influence of the Po, the Liver stores the acquired Postnatal emotions of frustration, irritability, stubbornness, anger, blame, rage, resentment, rudeness, impatience, jealousy and depression. When excess anger is eliminated, the congenital energies of benevolence, compassion, and love for others flourish and emanate from the Liver Orb, through the influence of the Hun.

- **The Fire Agent: The Virtue of Order.** This agent fosters social harmony and represents the Prenatal virtues of peace, pleasure, joy, contentment, tranquility and boundary setting. This congenital agent is connected to the

Shen-Spirit and is stored in the Heart. The Fire Element also affects the Heart, Small Intestine, Pericardium and Triple Burners, as well as the flow of energy in each of these channels. The Fire Agent governs the energy of the Blood Vessels, complexion, perspiration, and the tongue. After birth, through the influence of the Po, the Heart stores the acquired Postnatal emotions of nervousness, excitement, shock, anxiety, overexcitement, heartache and mania. Eliminating excess nervousness allows the congenital energies of order, forgiveness, and peace to be experienced. The environment is then conducive for contentment and orderliness, which allows self-esteem to grow, through the influence of the Hun.

- **The Earth Agent: The Virtue of Trust.** This agent represents the Prenatal virtues of faith, honesty, openness, acceptance, virtue and truthfulness. This congenital agent is connected to the Yi-Intention (thoughts and ideas) and stored within the Spleen. It affects the Spleen and Stomach organs and the flow of energy in the Spleen and Stomach Channels. The Earth Agent also governs the energy of the large muscles, lymph, saliva secretions, mouth, lips, and taste. After birth, through the influence of the Po, the Spleen stores the acquired Postnatal emotions of worry, remorse, regret, obsessiveness, self-doubt, self-centeredness and suspicion. Eliminating excess worry allows the congenital energies of trust and peace of mind to flourish, through the influence of the Hun.

- **The Metal Agent: The Virtue of Integrity.** This agent represents the Prenatal virtues of righteousness, dignity, generosity and social responsibility. This congenital agent is connected to the Po-Seven Corporeal Souls and is stored in the Lungs. It affects the Lung and Large Intestine organs and the flow of energy in the Lung and Large Intestine Channels. The Metal Agent also governs the energy of the skin and mucous membranes, body hair, nose, and the sense of smell. After birth, through the influence of the Po, the Lungs store the acquired Postnatal emotions of grief, sorrow, sadness, shame, disappointment, self-pity, guilt, and despair. Once excess sorrow is relieved, the congenital energies of justice, righteousness, integrity, dignity, and social responsibility flourish under the influence of the Hun.

- **The Water Agent: The Virtue of Wisdom.** This agent represents the Prenatal virtues of rationality, clear perception, self-understanding, self-confidence and wisdom. This congenital agent is connected to the Zhi-Will (mental drive and determination) and is stored in the Kidneys. It affects the Kidney and Urinary Bladder organs and the flow of energy in the Kidney and Urinary Bladder Channels. The Water Agent also governs the energy of the Brain, inner ear, hearing, spinal cord, cerebrospinal fluid, Bones, Bone Marrow, ovaries, testes, head and pubic hair, anus, urethra and sexual fluids. After birth, through the influence of the Po, the Kidneys store the acquired Postnatal emotions of fear, paranoia, terror, panic, horror, loneliness, and insecurity. Once excess fear is eliminated, the congenital energies of the mind become rational and wise under the influence of the Hun.

3. **Yu Jing:** The Hun known as Yu Jing resides in the Lower Dantian. Yu Jing literally means "hidden essence." This Hun is considered mixed (or combined) Yin energy. It is connected to the Lower Dantian and is associated with the Earth, producing our desire for enjoying life's pleasures and comforts, as well as the desire for the purity of life.

FUNCTIONS OF THE HUN

The Hun have eight primary functions: the Hun control sleep and dreaming; The Hun assist the Shen in mental activities; the Hun maintain balance in one's emotional life (under the leadership of the Shen); the Hun are responsible for the eyes; the Hun influence a person's courage; the Hun control planning and the sense of direction (with the aid of the Shen); the Hun control Spirit Travel; and upon death, the Hun document and report the actions, thoughts and deeds of the in-

```
                                    ┌─────────────────────────────────────────────────┐
                                    │ The Hun control sleep and dreaming              │
                                    ├─────────────────────────────────────────────────┤
                                    │ The Hun assist the Shen in mental activities    │
                                    ├─────────────────────────────────────────────────┤
    ┌──────────────┐                │ The Hun maintain balance in one's emotional life│
    │    The       │                │ (under the leadership of the Shen)              │
    │ Liver Stores │                ├─────────────────────────────────────────────────┤
    │   the Hun:   │───────────────▶│ The Hun are responsible for the eyes            │
    │    Three     │                ├─────────────────────────────────────────────────┤
    │   Ethereal   │                │ The Hun influence a person's courage            │
    │    Souls     │                ├─────────────────────────────────────────────────┤
    └──────────────┘                │ The Hun control planning and the sense of       │
                                    │ direction (with the aid of the Shen)            │
                                    ├─────────────────────────────────────────────────┤
                                    │ The Hun control Spirit Travel                   │
                                    ├─────────────────────────────────────────────────┤
                                    │ Upon death, the Hun document and report the     │
                                    │ actions, thoughts and deeds of an individual to │
                                    │ the spirits of destiny to determine the person's│
                                    │ degree of cultivated virtue                     │
                                    └─────────────────────────────────────────────────┘
```

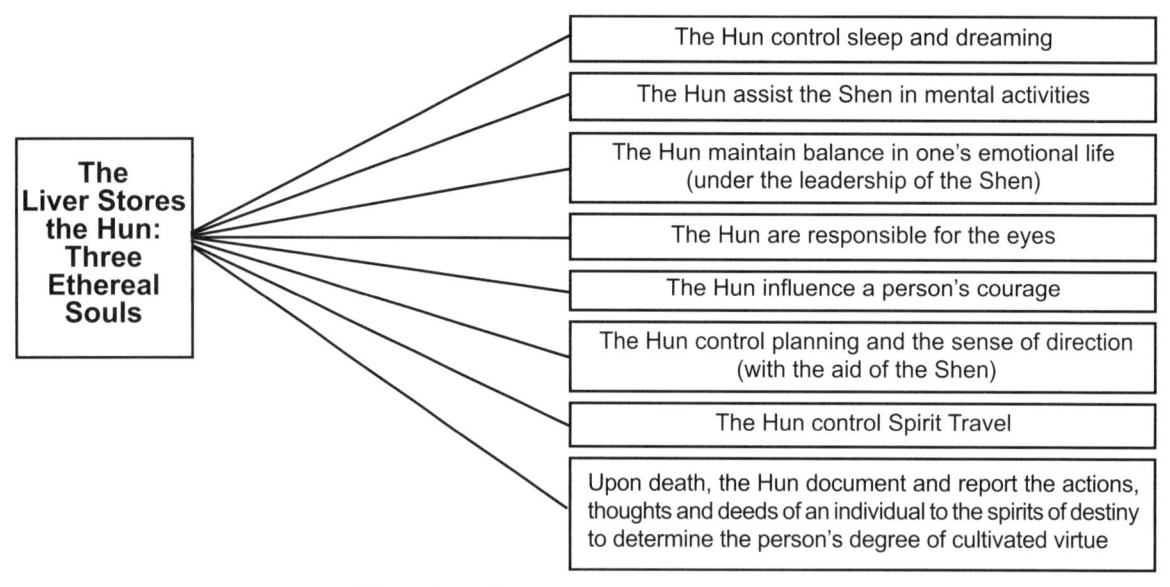

Figure 2.85. The Eight Functions of the Hun

dividual to the spirits of destiny to determine the person's degree of cultivated virtue (Figure 2.85). These eight functions of the Hun are described as follows:

1. **The Hun control sleep and dreaming:** They reside in the eyes during the day and lodge in the Liver at night. When residing in the eyes, they see; when lodging in the Liver, they dream. Dreams are the roaming of the body's Hun. It is the nature of the Hun to wander. At night the Hun must be anchored and rooted in the Liver; for this reason the Liver Blood and Liver Yin must be strong. If the Liver Blood and Liver Yin are not strong, the Hun wander, and the person dreams too much or has unpleasant dreams. Patients who suffer from severe Yin Deficiency may experience a floating sensation just before falling asleep. This symptom is due to the Hun not being adequately rooted in the patients' Yin.

Dreams are an example of the information gathered during the Hun's out of body travels. The ancient Chinese understood that the body's Hun can instantaneously traverse the Nine Levels of Heaven or Nine Levels of Earth.

The Hun store the sum total of past experiences. The expressions of the Hun are manifested through images, symbols, and ideas from the divine, as well as through the energetic state of the Wuji. These images, symbols, and ideas are stored in the individual's mind, affecting his or her spiritual life. Without this interaction, the patient's inner mental and spiritual life would become deficient in ideas, images, and dreams.

The Hun not only control dreams, but also daydreaming, as well as the ideals, aims, and the overall direction of an individual's life. The absence of these dreams, objectives and goals results in feelings of worthlessness and depression.

If the body's Liver Yin is depleted, the Hun are deprived of their residence, resulting in such conditions as fear, excessive daydreaming, insomnia, and a lack of sense of direction or purpose in life (one of the main features of depression).

Traditionally, sleepwalking is associated with the Hun. When sleepwalking, the body's Shen is not active and functioning; instead, the Hun are moving the individual. This is why a common treatment for a patient who suffers from sleepwalking involves the emission of Qi into the patient's Hunmen UB-47

(Door of the Hun). In modern research, however, some Qigong doctors have begun to theorize that the Po may also take an active role in sleep walking, especially when the sleep state involves violent actions (e.g., patients who thrash about, hurt people, or destroy things when sleeping).

If the patient does not sleep well because the Hun are wandering, the Qigong doctor can prescribe sour and astringing herbs (i.e., Bai Shao, Mu Li, Suan Zao Ren) which affect the Liver and encourage the Hun back into the body.

2. **The Hun assist the Shen in mental activities:** This relationship is very important, as the energy of the Shen and the Hun must continually be coordinated. The Shen is related to rational thinking and inspiration. The Hun give the Shen a sense of direction and project the Shen outwards. The Shen needs to direct the Hun to condense and "gather the Hun." The Hun give the Shen its movement and direction, encouraging the Shen to relate with people, to socialize and to bond. The Hun, in turn need to be gathered and restrained by the Shen. If the Shen is weak and does not control the Hun, the Hun will move about too much, resulting in the individual having many ideas but never accomplishing anything, leading to frustration.

It is essential that the Shen allow the Hun to move in and out of the body, though it is equally important for the Hun to give the Shen direction and purpose. The Hun inspire us and give us dreams. That is why the words "movement," "coming and going," and "swimming" are often used in connection with the Hun. In fact, many doctors say that the Hun are actually the coming and going of the body's Shen. When the spirit of one person enters another's body, as in a medium in trance, it is the individual's Hun that comes in, while the host's Shen is temporarily disabled.

Because knowledge is dependent on the awareness of the Three Ethereal Souls, the Hun are therefore considered the collectors of information. The Hun however, do not interpret, rationalize, or analyze the knowledge they collect; they pass on the information to the Shen, which is responsible for rational thinking, intuition, and inspiration. The Shen helps distinguish between useful and irrelevant information.

There is an interesting connection between the Hun controlling sleep and dreaming, and the Hun being rooted in the Liver Blood and Yin. The Hun's movement in and out of the Liver governs the free flow of Liver Qi, and the free flow of Liver Qi is a manifestation of the swimming energy of the Hun as it moves in and out of the tissues. Therefore, if the Liver Yin or Liver Blood are deficient, the Hun cannot move freely and the individual will experience restlessness (especially at night).

3. **The Hun maintain balance in the individual's emotional life under the leadership of the Shen:** It is normal for everyone to experience emotions in life. The Hun are responsible for maintaining a balance so that the emotions do not become excessive, which can cause disease. The Hun have a regulatory function closely related to the balance between Liver Blood (Yin) and Liver Qi (Yang).

The Postnatal Shen discriminates, while the Hun does not. The relationship between the Shen and the Hun is very similar to the concepts of the conscious-mind and unconscious-mind in Jungian terms. The Hun are a repository of images and archetypes connecting the (personal) subconscious mind with the collective unconscious. If the Hun are unsettled, then the Shen (consciousness) is cut off, confused, isolated, aimless, sterile, and without dreams.

The movement of ideas in the body has to be controlled or it can lead to madness. Madness can occur to the degree that the Shen doesn't control the Hun, resulting in an uncontrolled amount of emotional, mental, and spiritual input. All of the energies and symbols coming through the Hun have to be integrated and assimilated, otherwise there can be serious mental illness and possibly psychosis (except in the case of young children who are continually full of ideas, have active imaginations, and are also able to integrate and assimilate these energies and symbols at a phenomenal rate). In a child, the Hun are very active, and the Shen is not as restraining; so there is a continuous flow of energies streaming from the unconscious world of symbols into the child's consciousness without causing psychological problems.

4. **The Hun are responsible for the eyes:** When the Hun wander in through the eyes, the eyes can see. The Hun give us vision, both mentally and spiritually.

5. **The Hun influence a person's courage:** If the Hun are not strong, the person is timid and fearful. If the Hun are strong, the person is fearless, can face difficulties in life, and can take appropriate action. A patient with weak Hun will have difficulty gathering information, making decisions, and will lack courage. The patient may also become easily discouraged or apathetic.

6. **The Hun control planning and the sense of direction with the aid of the Shen:** The mental and spiritual confusion about one's role in life (what to do, what goals to set, etc.) can be compared to the aimless wandering of the Hun; this is a feature of depression. If the Liver is strong while the Hun are firmly rooted, the person has a clear sense of direction.

7. **The Hun control Spirit Travel:** By housing the Shen for "spirit travel" (the spirit journeying outside the physical body), it is possible for the Qigong doctor to consciously direct the Hun's travelling. This is different from soul travel, which is the human soul journeying outside the physical body while connected to the Middle Dantian by a silver "cord of life." The Hun, accompanied by the individual's consciousness, act as one unit which is sometimes referred to as the spirit-soul. The spirit-soul allows the doctor to know the exact location of the "spirit routes" travelled when it leaves the body. Otherwise, when the Hun wander, the individual "Shens out" and has no recollection of where he or she has been when in the spiritual realms.

The Hun and Po are expressions of the body's "true spirit." The ancient Chinese believe that, in the presence of a disorder (either physical, mental, emotional, or spiritual) the Hun sometimes fly away (like startled birds in a yard). This vacancy of the Hun causes the body's Corporeal Soul (Po) to either stir about thoughtlessly in the absence of effective control (clinically known as "disassociation" or commonly called "spacing out"), or to become animalistic in nature and attack or flee for the sake of survival.

8. **The Hun are spiritual souls and leave the body, ascending back to Heaven, at the time of death:** Upon death, the Hun exit the body through the Baihui at the top of the head and ascend to the Big Dipper. While at the Big Dipper, the Hun will report the individual's actions, thoughts and deeds from his or her lifetime to the celestial spirits that preside over the individual's destiny. The celestial spirits will then determine the degree to which the individual had cultivated virtue during that incarnation.

THE SPIRITUAL AWARENESS OF THE HUN

The Hun spiritually and energetically respond to the energetic grids of Heaven (universal energetic fields). The stars and planets within these Heavenly grids exert an influence on the Hun causing each individual's body to react to certain astrological configurations (full moon, new moon, equinox and solstice). An individual's positive or negative emotional reactions are sometimes based on the affinity of the vibrational rate of the Hun with the energies of a particular astrological alignment.

The Hun are classified as Yang spirits; they can be cultivated and refined. Imagination, visualization, and positive affirmation in the form of prayer and incantations (Mantras), meditation, and Hand Seals (Mudras) are traditionally used to awaken and establish an active relationship with the Three Ethereal Souls. Energetically, the Hun can be stimulated through the Hunmen UB-47 ("Gate to the Hun") points located on the back of the body below the shoulders. These points are used clinically to treat difficult or chronic disorders by regulating Liver Qi flow.

CHAPTER 2: UNDERSTANDING ANCIENT CHINESE METAPHYSICS

THE PO: THE SEVEN CORPOREAL SOULS

The Lungs store the Po, the Seven Corporeal Souls, which are physical in nature and are connected to the body's Jing and Qi. The word Po is defined as "the soul of vigor, animation, or life." The Po are closely linked to the body's Jing (Essence), and manifest through the body's Essence in the form of hearing, sight, and tactile sensations. The Po are considered to be the soul of the senses.

The Seven Corporeal Souls are energetically associated to the following: Yin, Earthly soul, shadow, heaviness, Jing, negative emotions and negative inspirations. They are the Earthly aspects of the human soul, and are considered the counterpart of the Hun. The energetic functions of the Po pertain to the individual's animal nature and his or her instincts and drives (Figure 2.86). The Po are passionate and advocate experiencing life in its fullest measure. Being attached to the physical body, they are, however, in a constant state of dying.

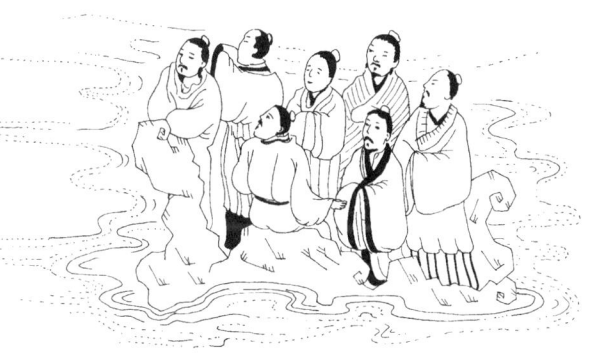

Figure 2.86. The Seven Corporeal Souls are composed of the Seven Po.

CHINESE IDEOGRAM OF THE PO

There are two parts to the Po ideogram. The character to the right represents the Earthly spirits-Gui (ghost), depicted by a head suspended above a vaporous form of a body with an appendage (symbolizing the whirlwind that accompanies the movements of the Earthly spirits). The character to the left is the image for the color white. The color white can be represented by the image of dried bones lying on the Earth (Figure 2.87). Thus, the Po are linked with a descending movement of energy and with the Jing. The Seven Corporeal Souls are also said "to come and go, enter and exit," in association with the body's essences.

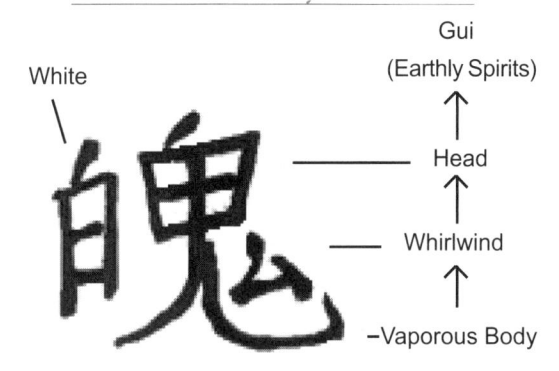

Figure 2.87. The Chinese character for "Po," also known as the Corporeal Soul, or White Soul

FUNCTIONS OF THE PO

The Po have six primary functions: the Po are the somatic expressions of the Eternal Soul related to the reflexive nervous system and limbic system (the "reptilian brain"); the Po are responsible for all physiological processes during childhood; the Po are related to weeping and crying; the Po are closely linked to breathing; the Po are connected to sexuality on the level of sensation; and the Po leave the body via the anus (considered to be the "door of the Po") upon death. Spiritually, the Seven Corporeal Souls are the counterpart of the Hun and can be described as follows (Figure 2.88):

1. **The Po are the somatic expressions of the Human Soul:** They are related to the reflexive nervous system and limbic system (the "reptilian brain"). They manifest through the body's sensations of feeling, hearing, and seeing. The Po have an impulsive tendency towards action and correspond to the deep animal instincts within the Mind (personal subconscious) and cells. Our reflexes are a Po reaction. They also provide us with the animal strength and resources necessary to mobilize the body and perform incredible feats of power. The "animal within" is driven by the Po. They are the manifestation of the body's Jing in the sphere of sensations and feelings. Just as the Three Hun provide the individual with the energetic movement for the Shen, the Po provide the individual with the energetic

```
                    ┌─────────────────────────────────────┐
                    │ The Po are the somatic expressions  │
                    │        of the Eternal Soul          │
                    ├─────────────────────────────────────┤
                    │ The Po are responsible for all      │
 ┌──────────────┐   │ physiological processes in childhood│
 │ The Lungs    │   ├─────────────────────────────────────┤
 │ store the    │   │ The Po are related to weeping and   │
 │ Po:          │──▶│             crying                  │
 │ Seven        │   ├─────────────────────────────────────┤
 │ Corporeal    │   │ The Po are closely linked to        │
 │ Souls        │   │             breathing               │
 └──────────────┘   ├─────────────────────────────────────┤
                    │ The Po are connected to sexuality   │
                    │       on the level of sensation     │
                    ├─────────────────────────────────────┤
                    │ The Po leave the body via the anus  │
                    │ (considered the "Door of the Po")   │
                    │           upon death                │
                    └─────────────────────────────────────┘
```

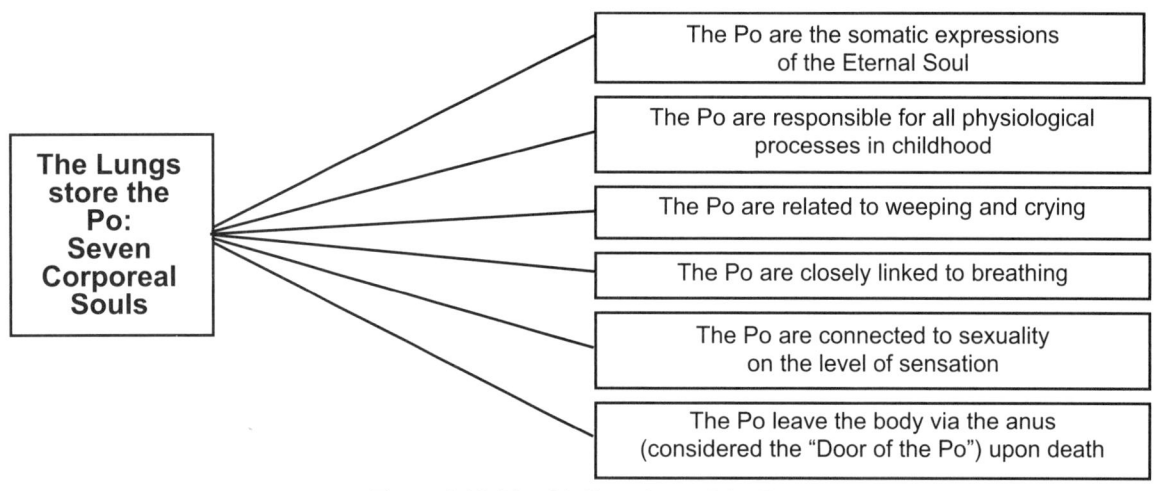

Figure 2.88. The Six Functions of the Po

movement of the body's Jing.

2. **The Po are responsible for all physiological processes during childhood:** In the beginning of life, the Po are responsible for the sensations of pain and itching (growing pains). The Po serve as the intermediary between the Jing and the body's other vital substances. At conception, the energetic interactions of the body's transforming Jing not only create the embryo but also establish the Po within the tissues. The Po are stored in the Lungs and they remain attached to the body until death, at which point their energy disintegrates and disperses into the Earth within a few days.

3. **The Po are related to weeping and crying:** The connection between the Po and Lungs is very important from an emotional point of view. When the Po's movement in the Lungs is constricted, grief and sadness are suppressed in the chest through shallow breathing. Additionally, if the patient feels dull and depressed upon waking, it is a sign that his or her Shen is clinging to the body. In other words, the patient's Shen is constricted by the excessive energy of the Po.

4. **The Po are closely linked to breathing:** The Po influence the sympathetic and parasympathetic nervous systems. Because the Po reside in the Lungs, all forms of breath control are methods used to regulate the Po, calm the Shen, and allow access to the higher Hun states. The movement of the breath is the pulsation of the Po. Each emotional change the body experiences correlates to a shift in the body's respiratory pattern. The quality of Qi and its circulation is dependent upon the method of breathing (depth, speed, duration and rhythm). To support the greatest longevity possible, it is important to utilize long, slow, and even breaths. The breath (air from Heaven) interacts with the Po in the Lungs, and plays a significant role in the Heaven-Man-Earth concept of balancing the emotions.

The virtues of the Lungs are righteousness and courage. These virtues give a person the drive and strength to do the "right thing" when the need arises. These virtues manifest and promote good health when a balanced energetic alignment with the Po is achieved (the alignment between the Lungs' breathing pattern and the Po).

5. **The Po are connected to sexuality on the level of sensation:** The Po are linked to the basic instincts and perceptions of the body. All instinctive sexual reactions and passions come under the authority of the Po. The Po provide the fundamental biological energy and are the source of biological needs and impulses. They are driven by basic instincts and urges, and their sole concern is the immediate satisfaction of

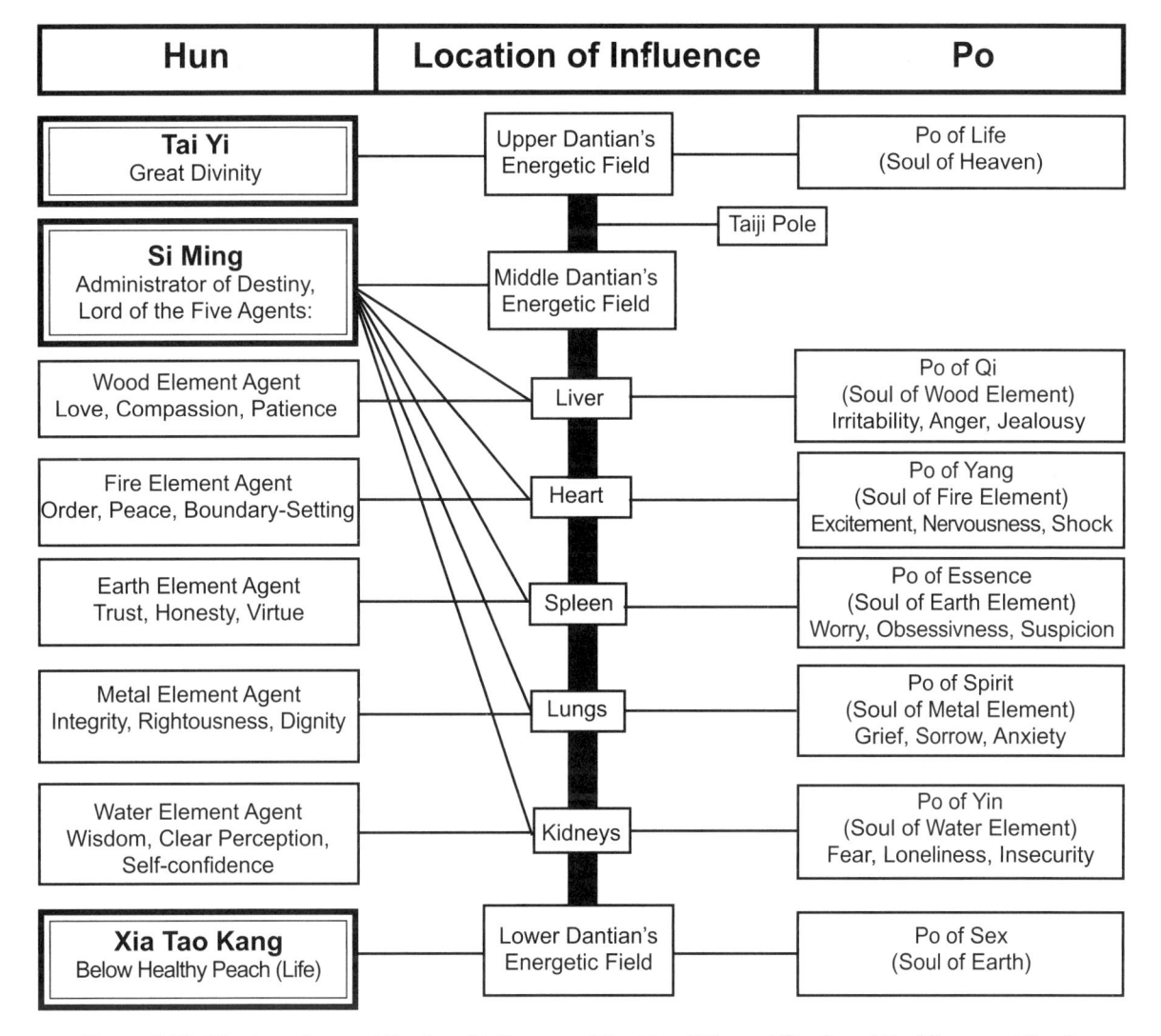

CHAPTER 2: UNDERSTANDING ANCIENT CHINESE METAPHYSICS

Hun	Location of Influence	Po
Tai Yi — Great Divinity	Upper Dantian's Energetic Field	Po of Life (Soul of Heaven)
	Taiji Pole	
Si Ming — Administrator of Destiny, Lord of the Five Agents:	Middle Dantian's Energetic Field	
Wood Element Agent — Love, Compassion, Patience	Liver	Po of Qi (Soul of Wood Element) Irritability, Anger, Jealousy
Fire Element Agent — Order, Peace, Boundary-Setting	Heart	Po of Yang (Soul of Fire Element) Excitement, Nervousness, Shock
Earth Element Agent — Trust, Honesty, Virtue	Spleen	Po of Essence (Soul of Earth Element) Worry, Obsessivness, Suspicion
Metal Element Agent — Integrity, Rightousness, Dignity	Lungs	Po of Spirit (Soul of Metal Element) Grief, Sorrow, Anxiety
Water Element Agent — Wisdom, Clear Perception, Self-confidence	Kidneys	Po of Yin (Soul of Water Element) Fear, Loneliness, Insecurity
Xia Tao Kang — Below Healthy Peach (Life)	Lower Dantian's Energetic Field	Po of Sex (Soul of Earth)

Figure 2.89. The Location and Realm of Influence of the Hun (Ethereal Soul) and Po (Corporeal Soul)

biological needs and impulses (emotional and physical survival, reproductive urges, etc.). Most self-destructive behavior, such as an attraction to unhealthy and dangerous life-styles, is due to imbalances of the Po.

6. **The Po leave the body via the anus upon death:** Since the Corporeal Souls have a relationship with the Lungs and Large Intestine, the anus is considered the Po Men or "the door of the Po." The anus acts as a doorway for the elimination of the waste products from the five Yin organs by draining off impure liquids and waste. Upon death, the Po return back to the Earth, descending out the body through the individual's anus.

ANATOMICAL LOCATION OF THE PO

The Po are a composite of Seven Corporeal Souls which originate from Earth, are housed within the Lungs, and reside in specific areas in the body. The Seven Po are located along the line between the Huiyin (CV-1) and the Baihui (GV-20) points, embracing the body's Taiji Pole (also called the "Center Thrusting Channel") at the following locations (Figure 2.89):

1. **The Po of Life (Soul of Heaven)** is considered the Po of the Upper Dantian. It is located below the Baihui (GV-20) point in the Ni Wan Palace (Hall of the Upper Dantian) area.
2. **The Po of Qi (Soul of the Five Element Wood)** is considered the Po of the Liver. It is located below the diaphragm. This Po is the counterpart to the Hun's Wood Agent (the virtue of kindness: love, benevolence and compassion). This Po manifests through the acquired emotions of anger, irritability, blame, rage, resentment, jealousy and depression.
3. **The Po of Yang (Soul of the Five Element Fire)** is considered the Po of the Heart. It is located anterior to the Mingmen (GV-4) point behind the Taiji Pole. This Po is the counterpart to the Hun's Fire Agent (the virtue of order: peace and boundary setting). This Po manifests through the acquired emotions of nervousness, shock, and excitement.
4. **The Po of Essence (Soul of the Five Element Earth)** is considered the Po of the Spleen. It is located at the midpoint of the Taiji Pole. This Po is the counterpart to the Hun's Earth Agent (the virtue of trust: faith, honesty openness, acceptance and truthfulness). This Po manifests through the acquired emotions of worry, regret, remorse, obsessiveness, and self-doubt.
5. **The Po of the Spirit (Soul of the Five Element Metal)** is considered the Po of the Lungs. It is located posterior to the Tanzhong (CV-17) point inside the mediastinum near the Middle Dantian. This Po is the counterpart to the Hun's Metal Agent (the virtue of integrity: righteousness, dignity, generosity and social responsibility). This Po manifests through the acquired emotions of grief, anxiety, sadness, shame, disappointment, guilt and despair.
6. **The Po of Yin (Soul of the Five Element Water)** is considered the Po of the Kidneys. It is located between the navel and the Taiji Pole. This Po is the counterpart to the Hun's Water Agent (the virtue of wisdom: rationality, clear perception and self-understanding). This Po manifests through the acquired emotions of fear, loneliness, and insecurity.
7. **The Po of Sex (Soul of Earth)** is considered the Po of the Lower Dantian. It is the only one not located within the Taiji Pole but is also located at the bottom of the feet in the Yongquan (Kd-1) points. It is considered a neighbor of the Po of Essence because of its relationship and energetic connection to Earth.

Negative Attributes of the Po

The Po's nature is one of survival, and their energies can be directed towards self-preservation or self-destruction (devouring and robbing the body of life-force energy). In ancient China, it was believed that the Po would sometimes desire to rejoin the damp, dark underground springs whose moist, heavy nature they share. Therefore, the Po would seek to undermine and rid themselves of the constraining human body that they were presently inhabiting. This was accomplished while their host was asleep and the Hun were spirit-traveling. The Po would beckon to passing ghosts and disease-demons, inviting them into the individual's body to take possession and work towards the destruction of the body.

Therefore, the Seven Corporeal Souls (Po) were sometimes called the "seven animals," the "seven sentient souls of the body," or the "seven turbid demons." When afflicted or not kept in check, the animal natures of the seven Po quickly become restless and hostile. In this context, the Po are given different names to express the different negative thoughts and emotions specific to each Corporeal Soul. Each Po has a characteristic mantra that it whispers to an individual's mind for influence and control. The Po's seven turbid demon natures are described as follows (Figure 2.90):

1. **Fei Du (Flying Poison):** The Fei Du Po manifests through feelings of anger and rage. The indignation and wrath that it helps to generate can produce hostile, destructive, and violently aggressive reactions. This Po can cause an individual to suddenly explode with venomous thoughts and evil intentions.
2. **Chu Hui (Sprouting Filth):** The Chu Hui Po manifests through haughty behavior and feelings of pride and arrogance.

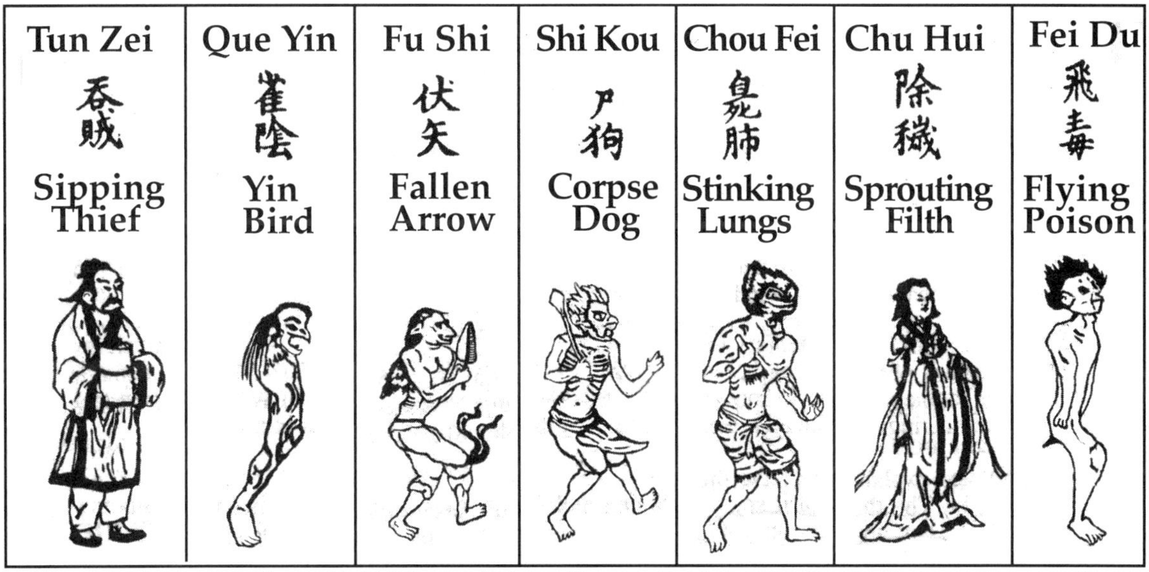

Tun Zei 吞賊 Sipping Thief	Que Yin 雀陰 Yin Bird	Fu Shi 伏矢 Fallen Arrow	Shi Kou 尸狗 Corpse Dog	Chou Fei 臭肺 Stinking Lungs	Chu Hui 除穢 Sprouting Filth	Fei Du 飛毒 Flying Poison

Figure 2.90. The Po's Seven Turbid Demon Natures (Source: *Taishang Chu Sanshi Jiuchong Baoshen Jing*, Highest Scripture of the Great One and the True One)

3. **Chou Fei (Stinking Lungs):** The Chou Fei Po manifests as hopelessness, and it smells of death. It destroys hope and faith, and feeds on ignorance, which can lead to a sense of despair, spiritual apathy or inactivity. It manifests through victimization and martyrdom.
4. **Shi Kou (Corpse Dog):** The Shi Kou Po manifests through feelings of greed. It is expressed through selfish desires and covetous actions.
5. **Fu Shi (Fallen Arrow):** The Fu Shi Po manifests through feelings of lust. It entices the individual by tempting or luring him or her into a desirable place or situation through unethical actions. It then creates distress in the form of guilt which generates shame. This spirit further creates anxiety and fear of being discredited, dishonored, or disgraced, and then immediately generates the feeling that attempting to correct the situation is fruitless. It also manifests in addictions and compulsions.
6. **Que Yin (Yin Bird):** The Que Yin Po torments the individual by causing him or her to experience extreme pain and severe anguish by dwelling on unresolved past emotional issues, present anxieties, and future fears. Also known as the "night tormentor," it is especially active at night, manifesting via nightmares, restless sleep, and insomnia.
7. **Tun Zei (Sipping Thief):** The Tun Zei Po manifests by stealing the individual's lifeforce energy and devouring it through negative judgements and bitter emotions such as jealousy, envy, and resentment.

THE SPIRITUAL AWARENESS OF THE PO

The Po are classified as Yin spirits and they can be controlled and refined through breathing exercises and quiescent meditations. When the fetus begins its movement, its Yin energy tranquilizes the Po which act as guardians of the fetus' body. The seven Po help to develop the growth of consciousness by providing obstacles to test the individual's faith and devotion. Many times the Seven Corporeal Souls will work in conjunction with hostile external energetic forces to test the individual's spiritual endurance.

Energetically, the Po can be accessed through the Pohu (Door to the Po) UB-42 point located on the back of the body and between the shoulders. This point is also used clinically to treat energetic imbalances of the Lungs. The energetic nature of the Po responds to the energetic grids of the Earth,

Figure 2.91

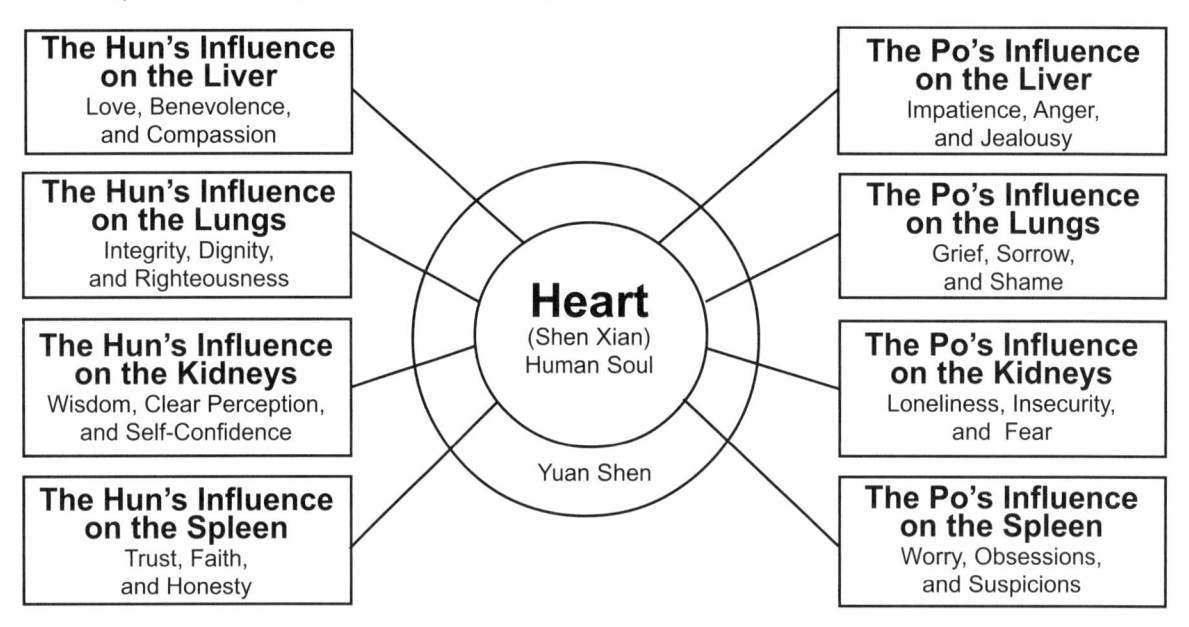

Hun's Influences (Left side):
- The Hun's Influence on the Liver: Love, Benevolence, and Compassion
- The Hun's Influence on the Lungs: Integrity, Dignity, and Righteousness
- The Hun's Influence on the Kidneys: Wisdom, Clear Perception, and Self-Confidence
- The Hun's Influence on the Spleen: Trust, Faith, and Honesty

Center: Heart (Shen Xian) Human Soul / Yuan Shen

Po's Influences (Right side):
- The Po's Influence on the Liver: Impatience, Anger, and Jealousy
- The Po's Influence on the Lungs: Grief, Sorrow, and Shame
- The Po's Influence on the Kidneys: Loneliness, Insecurity, and Fear
- The Po's Influence on the Spleen: Worry, Obsessions, and Suspicions

Figure 2.91. The Influence of the Hun and Po on the Yuan Shen

---

and can cause an individual to resonate in harmony or disharmony with certain ecological configurations (mountains, ocean, forest, valley, etc.). An individual's attraction to a particular environment, or a feeling of not belonging there, depend on the vibratory affinity (or lack thereof) between the individual's Po and the environmental energy of a particular area.

THE EFFECT OF THE HUN AND PO ON THE YUAN SHEN

In Medical Qigong therapy, the human soul (Shen Xian) is seen as being strongly influenced by two main divisions of internal spiritual energies, the Hun (Ethereal Soul) and the Po (Corporeal Soul).

The Yuan Shen is a manifestation and expression of the human soul, and is primarily affected by the energetic and spiritual influences of the Hun and Po. The combination of intuitive perceptions provided by the Hun (Yang Souls) and the Po (Yin Souls) create the foundational input for the body's Original Spirit (Yuan Shen). It is through this input that the Yuan Shen organizes and controls the psycho-emotional aspect of the body's five Yin organs (Figure 2.91).

The ancient Chinese viewed the Shen as the emperor; the Hun as a loyal minister; and the Po as a powerful general. If the general (Po) is left in control (being only concerned with the survival of self and the body), he or she will start to spiritually and energetically dominate the individual's thoughts, emotions and actions (a condition commonly referred to as "a rebellious general controlling a weak emperor").

When the general (Po) dominates the individual's thoughts, emotions and actions, the individual's acquired mind (Shen Zhi) takes over, and the individual becomes overly concerned with his or her own survival. Thus, the individual becomes absorbed in the protection and maintenance of his or her ego. In this context, the purpose of spiritual cultivation is to subdue and control the rebellious general and transform him into a servant. Once the inner government is orderly, the strong and violent nature of the Po becomes tame. Then, through the wise council of the loyal minister (Hun), the individual's Shen can walk a path of virtue.

Virtue is the enlightened path that leads the individual's Shen. Therefore, by cultivating virtue, the individual's consciousness becomes dominated by the council of the loyal minister (Hun) and produces healthy choices for the Yuan Shen.

When the Hun control the energy body and are nourished by the Five Virtues, the energy body then becomes a vehicle for the Heart's Shen. When the Heart's Shen is no longer dominated by the Yin and Yang souls (Hun and Po) and the destructive aspects of the acquired Five Element emotions, the individual returns to an awareness of his or her connection to the universe (Wuji) and the Divine. This state of balanced consciousness is sustained through prayer and meditation.

THE YUAN SHEN AND SPIRIT TRAVEL

The initial separation of the individual's energy body or "dream body" from the physical body generally leaves the patient's Shen in a weakened state (referred to as Yin Shen). The weakened Yin Shen must be protected. This Yin Shen is part of the Hun and leaves the body naturally whenever the patient is weak, sick, in shock, or asleep. It may also leave during the early stages of Qigong meditation or Taijiquan (Tai Chi Ch'uan) practice, as the practitioner encounters blocks and obstacles within the unconscious mind.

The spiritual travels of the Yin Shen are generally confined to the lower spiritual planes, and a scattered Yin Shen sometimes needs to be reclaimed through "soul retrieval." Once the Shen has been cultivated, refined, strengthened, fortified, and controlled through the proper development of the energy body, it is then referred to as a Yang Shen, sometimes referred to as a Shenming ("bright spirit" or "spirit of light"). When the energy body spirit travels, the developed Yang Shen can transverse the Nine Levels of Heaven or the Nine Levels of Earth in an instant (Figure 2.92).

The terms Ling Qi ("supernatural energy"), Ling Hun ("supernatural soul") and Ling Shen ("supernatural spirit") are ancient expressions used to describe the Yang Soul manifesting effective power and influence, either while residing in an individual, or being in a disembodied state.

Accordingly, the expression of the Ling is believed to be the very manifestation of the human soul. According to *The Book of Rites of the Senior Tai*, compiled by the Daoist Tai De during the Xia Dynasty (2205-1600 B.C.), historically the Shen and Ling are believed to be the origin of all living beings.

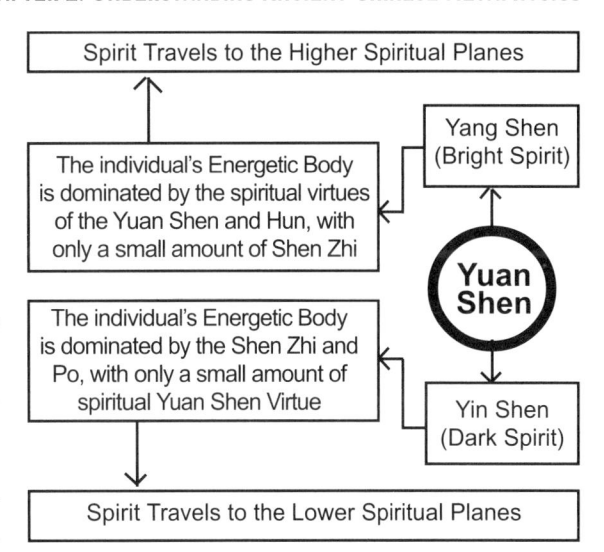

Figure 2.92. The Yuan Shen and Spirit Travel

The Nine Levels of Heaven and Earth

The Nine Levels of Heaven are nine spiritual planes which exist within Heaven's energetic grids. In the lower levels of the energetic grids there are enlightened beings coexisting with other spiritual entities. The Nine Levels of Earth are nine spiritual planes which exist within the Earth's energetic grids. In these levels of Earthly spiritual planes there exists various dimensions of animal, vegetable, and mineral powers, as well as Earthly spiritual beings.

THE CONCEPT OF SPIRITUAL VIRTUE

In ancient China, the concept of an individual's virtue (De) and his or her destiny (Ming) were closely connected. Destiny (associated with the Yuan Jing, Qi and Shen) was believed to originate from Heaven at the time of birth, after which it was stored in the individual's Mingmen (Gate of Destiny) area between the Kidneys (Figure 2.93). The individual's Ming becomes the spark of life and the dynamic potential underlying his or her thoughts and actions. Although the subtle impulses emanating from the individual's Ming are generally hidden from the conscious mind, through Shengong meditations a deeper realm of understanding can be intuitively discovered and accessed.

It is up to the individual to consistently act in accordance with his or her Ming throughout life. This action is based on the individual's conscious use of his or her intention (Yi). The intent to remain congruent with the "will and intent of heaven" (Zhi Yi Tian) is what gives the individual virtue (De). It is through the development of his or her virtue that the individual establishes a healthy relationship with the Dao, Heaven and the spirit world.

THE FIVE LIMITATIONS

The ancient Chinese believed that as the human soul journeys into the material world, it begins to lose its divine connection with the Dao. Once the individual is born, he or she begins to replace the subtle interconnections of the spiritual-self with those of the sensory survival instincts of the material self (Po).

As the Eternal Soul envelopes itself within its physical housing, the spiritual core becomes veiled by the illusionary existence of matter, space, and time. At this point in the individual's orientation and spiritual adjustment, the energetic fields of matter begin to dominate the individual's Yuan Shen (original spirit), giving rise to the birth and development of the individual's Shen Zhi (acquired personality). Along with the individual's disconnection from his or her spiritual core and the development of the Shen Zhi, are also included the development and formation of the belief in five specific limitations. These five specific limitations inhibit the individual's personal power and potential, and are described as follows:

- The belief in the limitation of the individual's power and potential to accomplish all things.
- The belief in the limitation of the individual's power and potential to know all things.
- The limitation of the ability to utilize the individual's power and potential by creating desire and attachment, thus giving rise to unceasing discontentment.
- The limitation of utilizing the individual's power and potential by creating the illusion

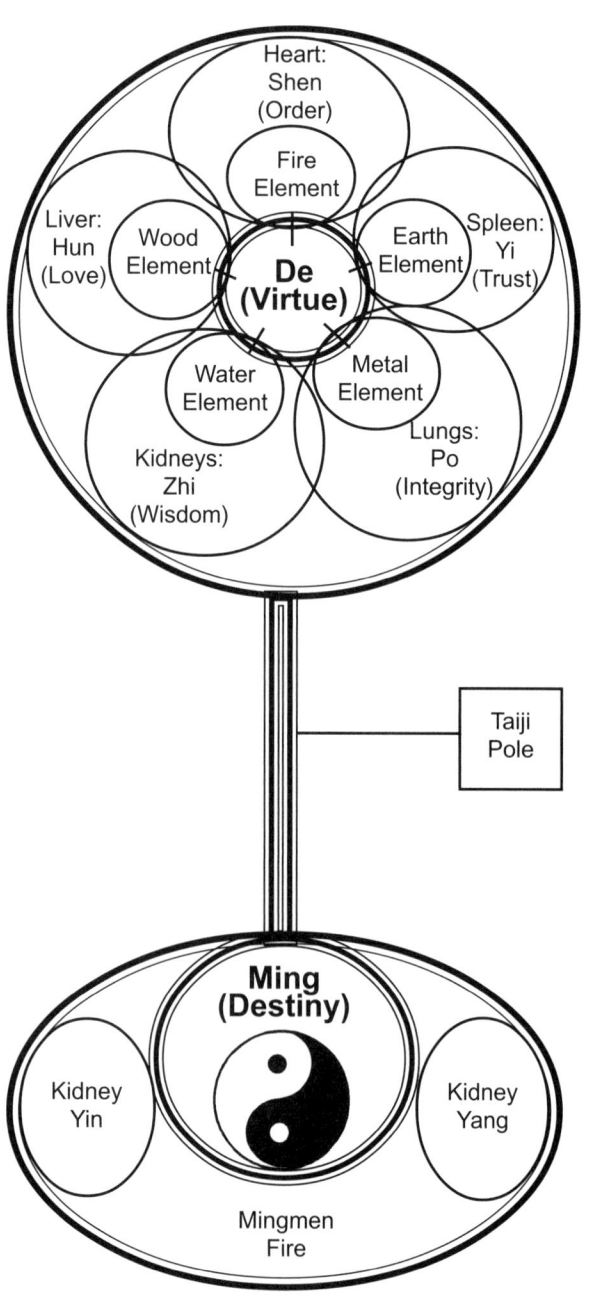

Figure 2.93. After the Five Lights escort the human soul into the world of matter, the Eternal Soul's De (virtue) rises upward, to later become the spiritual energy of the Five Agents, rooted within the five Yin organs. Simultaneously, the Eternal Soul's Ming (destiny) sinks downward to become stored between the Kidneys, rooted within the individual's Ministerial Fire.

of time related life changes (e.g., birth, growth, maturation, waning and death).
- The limitation of utilizing the individual's free will by creating fate, thus binding an individual to the endless cycles of birth and death.

The development of the belief in the five specific limitations causes the individual's subtle connection to the soul to "fall asleep," whereby allowing certain unique survival patterns to become initiated, facilitating the creation and development of the individual's ego. The Shen Zhi's investment in emotional and mental survival allows the individual's ego the ability to develop and acquire its unique personality.

The conscious state of the ego operates through the individual's physical body via the senses and analytical mind. The subconscious state of the ego operates through the individual's spiritual body via the dream state. When the individual is in a deep sleep or a meditative state, the ego retires into the energetic body in the form of inner awareness.

In order to reconnect with the divine, a spiritual "awakening" must occur, allowing the individual to remember and reexamine his or her lost spiritual state of existence. Once this "awakening" occurs, the individual must then come to the realization that he or she no longer needs to be attached to the acquired ego, acquired intellect, acquired memories, and acquired thought patterns. These four principles (acquired ego, intellect, memories, and thought patterns) constitute the medium through which the individual's consciousness and Shen Zhi act. It is the human consciousness that distinguishes the domain of man, separating him or her from the animal, plant and mineral kingdoms.

The individual's relationship with the ego is considered the paradox of creation. Although the ego binds an individual to the material plane of existence, it also allows for objective experiences. On the other hand, the ego must be completely eradicated in order to allow the individual the ability to reconnect with the true self (human soul), and to begin experiencing true liberation through increased spiritual intuition.

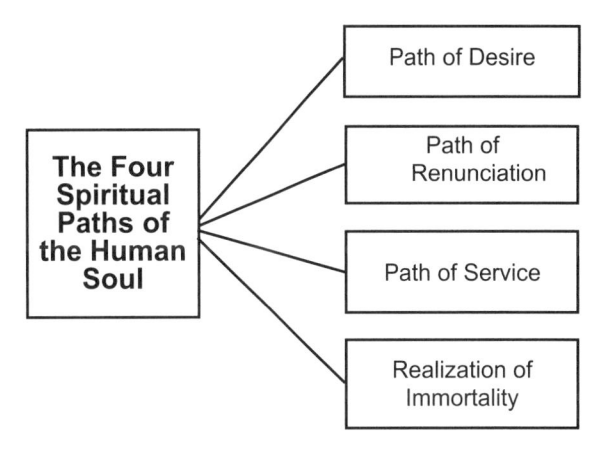

Figure 2.94. The Four Spiritual Paths of the Human Soul

FOUR SPIRITUAL PATHS OF THE HUMAN SOUL

The ancient Chinese believed that the initial Jodo ("will of heaven") or "true" purpose for the human soul's journey into the material world is to evolve through four stages of spiritual transformations: the Path of Desire, the Path of Renunciation, the Path of Service and the Realization of Immortality (Figure 2.94). These four spiritual paths allow the individual to uncover and control the acquired patterns of the ego, to deepen the energetic and spiritual connections with the Heavenly and Earthly realms, and augment a relationship with the divine. These four spiritual paths are described as follows:

1. **The Path of Desire:** The first challenge for the young human soul is to overcome the pursuit of the "four worms:" pleasure, wealth, fame and power. These four "worms" are said to eat away at the individual's spiritual growth. Each has its own inherited limitations and illusions and none of them can ever be fully satisfied. These illusions, however, are considered to be necessary obstacles for the experience and development of young souls. As the soul matures, it will eventually overcome the fascination of the Path of Desire and seek something more fulfilling.

2. **The Path of Renunciation:** The next stage that the human soul will experience is the Path of Renunciation. This entails avoiding any indulgences that interfere with the spiritual growth of the individual.

3. **The Path of Service:** At this stage, the individual has overcome the fascinations of pleasure and success, and genuinely devotes him or herself to the role of service. As the individual continues to mature spiritually, however, he or she will eventually recognize that society is finite and that even patriotism, and all forms of social as well as communal activities cannot fully satisfy the human soul.
4. **The Realization of Immortality:** At this final stage, the human soul understands "infinite beingness," experiencing and comprehending the infinite awareness and bliss present within his or her own core self. This realization allows the individual to feel and experience connectedness with the divine and to all creation.

THE DEATH ROOTS OF THE WOMB

In ancient China, Daoist mystics believed that Man was formed through the union of Yin and Yang, created from the interaction of contrary energetic movements originating from Heaven and Earth. The energy of Heaven is animated by Yang clockwise descending movements, while the energy of Earth is animated by Yin counterclockwise ascending movements.

According to the ancient Daoist text, *The Book of the Superior Transformations of the Cinnabar Nine into the Essence of the Embryo*, as the embryo develops, it receives (on a month to month basis) the "nine breaths" of the Nine Primordial Heavens. These nine breaths are responsible for the spiralling energetic transformations that occur during the process of Jing, Qi, and Shen embryonic development. Once the nine Heavenly breaths are all present, birth occurs in the tenth lunar month.

Progressive development of the fetus during pregnancy is attributed to the intervention of a divine influx of spiralling Yin and Yang energy, known as the "motion of the nine revolutions of cinnabar." Mankind is therefore believed to be the product of the energetic condensation of the spiritual breaths of the Nine Heavens, which are knotted and contained inside a person's Jing, transformed into spirit, and then formed into a human being.

During the time of pregnancy, these congenital knots (twelve in number) were considered by the ancient Daoists to be the "death roots of the womb." According to same ancient text, an individual's life also contains a "morbid" breath, and its energetic root is tightly formed into these twelve embryonic knots. Therefore, an individual also receives death at the same time that he or she receives life.

The ancient Daoists believed that these twelve embryonic knots have twelve nodules, and are divided into three groups of four, described as follows:

- **The Upper Four Nodules:** these knots are located in the Upper Dantian, eyes, cheeks, and mouth.
- **The Middle Four Nodules:** these knots are located in the viscera, Stomach, Large Intestine, and Small Intestine.
- **The Lower Four Nodules:** these knots are located in the Urinary Bladder, reproductive organs, anus, and feet.

The ancient Daoists believe that when an individual's fate was cut short, it was because the twelve embryonic knots became too tight, causing the morbid breath to be released.

THE FINAL EXIT OF THE HUMAN SOUL

From the most ancient times, the Chinese have considered death itself as a temporary state of transition which may be followed by the return of the Eternal Soul. At the time of death, the individual will begin to release his or her energetic accumulations of the Five Elements that constitute the energetic matrix of his or her physical, energetic and spiritual bodies. Each Element will disperse back into nature. As the Five Elements begin to decompose, the physical body, the energetic body, and the spiritual components of the true Five Elements (responsible for the energetic creation and formation of the Prenatal tissues) return back to their original nature as pure elemental light, dissolving into the Wuji. The individual's released human soul and original spirit are returned back into the energetic spiritual form of a Ling Zi, and are released back to the Wuji. Once released, the Ling Zi travels through the Six Realms to be reincarnated in a new form.

As the tissues of the physical body begin to die, the Yuan Shen prepares the human soul for its final journey home. This internal movement of the patient's spiritual energies is crucial. At the time of death, it is important that the human soul disconnects from the Heart and Middle Dantian area, and exits the dying patient through the Baihui area at the top of the head.

The ancient Chinese believed that the human soul can exit the body through one of nine orifices. According to Zhu Yunyang's *Commentary on the Can Dong Qi*, by Wei Boyang (142 A.D.), the nine orifices that connect an individual to the Later Heaven world of sensory experiences include the left eye, ear, and nostril, the right eye, ear, and nostril, the mouth and two excretory organs (anus and urethra).

It was believed that the area from which the patient's soul exits the body is determined by the state of his or her spiritual attachment or evolution (i.e., if the patient is attached to vision, he or she will be more inclined to leave through the eyes, etc.). This ancient Daoist belief preferred that the individual depart the body through the Baihui at the top of the head in order to avoid dissolving into the lower energetic realms of existence.

PREPARATION FOR DEATH

In China, when the Medical Qigong doctor is assisting a terminally ill patient, treatment focuses primarily on purging stagnant spiritual energy from the patient's body. Spiritual purging is required to purify and cleanse the patient's human soul. As the patient's soul is cleansed, and all material, emotional, and spiritual attachments to this life are released, the patient becomes peaceful. The patient attains a sense of completion and welcomes the final adventure of going home. The last rites performed by various clergy and ministers in Western culture serve a similar purpose.

The Qigong doctor then guides and encourages the patient's human soul to leave the body through the top of the head (Baihui). Souls that are more highly evolved exit the body through the top of the head, while souls of lesser evolution exit the body through lower portions of the physical structure.

The formation of a Gui or ghost is said to emerge from the untransformed energy of the human soul, manifested from the individual's Po (see Volume 2, Chapter 20). The ancient Chinese considered death to be a separation of Yin and Yang. As a individual ages, for example, the Yin increases at the expense of the Yang, and death marks the total separation of the two. Likewise, the human soul also contains both elements of Yin and Yang. The Yin aspect of the soul is called a Gui (ghost) the Yang aspect of the soul is called a Shen (spirit).

Emanating from the human soul is the individual's Yuan Shen. The Shen consists of Yang substance and is associated with the body's Qi and the Hun of Heaven; the individual's Gui consists of Yin substance and is associated with the Po and Earth. The union of the energetic and spiritual substances of the individual's Gui and Shen constitutes the matrix of his or her internal being, allowing for the connection and absorption of both universal and environmental Five Element energies. According to writings from Wei Liaoweng during the Yuan Dynasty (1279-1368 A.D.), "The Hun joins and gathers energy into a mass while the Po unites and consolidates it."

Upon the death of the physical body, the Hun ascend, becoming a Shen and return to Heaven, the Po descend becoming a Gui and return to Earth, while the energy of Tai Yi and Xia Tao Kang envelop the Eternal Soul (stored in Si Ming). These three spiritual energies (Tai Yi, Xia Tao Kang, and Si Ming) blend together, combining into one energy that completes the integration of the human soul (Figure 2.95).

The human soul leaves the body as a shining Shenming ("bright spirit" or "spirit of light") and returns to the source from which it came, through the tunnel of light, the energetic field of the Zhi Yi Tian (Will and Intent of Heaven) and back towards the divine light.

At this phase, the Eternal Soul experiences the judgement and subsequent consequences of the individual's actions and non-actions when it was in the form of a human soul. Otherwise, if it still possesses strong emotional attachments, the human soul cannot elevate its vibrational resonance and it becomes stuck in the lower vibrational plane, wandering the Earth in its Yin form as a Gui (ghost).

Spiritual Energy	Resides in	Associated Dantian	Purpose	
Tai Yi Great Divinity	the head as light	Upper Dantian (intuitive communication)	Governs the body's spirits, makes life shine forth, and encourages mankind to know the spirits of his or her Three Ethereal Souls	
Si Ming Administrator of Destiny	the Heart as vibration	Dantian Middle Dantian (empathic communication)	The Eternal Soul—regulates the primal energy of life (Qi) and is the source of emotions and the mind Controls the Wu Ying and Bai Yuan Spirits	Wu Ying (Without Essence), occupies the left side of the body and regulates the Three Hun (Ethereal Souls), associated with the Liver
				Bai Yuan (Pure Origin) occupies the right side of the body and regulates the Seven Po (Corporeal Souls), associated with the Lungs
Xia Tao Kang Below Healthy Peach (life)	the navel as heat	Lower Dantian (kinetic communication)	Preserves the root of the body's Essence (Jing)	

Figure 2.95. The patient's human soul resides in his or her Taiji Pole, and relates with Si Ming, the Administrator of Destiny. Upon the death of the physical body, the three Hun return to Heaven and the seven Po return to Earth, while the energy of Tai Yi and Xia Tao Kang envelop the Eternal Soul (stored in Si Ming) and combine into one energy. The human soul leaves the body through the particular gate (solar plexus, third eye, or top of the head) associated with the patient's degree of spiritual evolution, and returns through the tunnel of light to the divine.

In China, when an individual dies, there is a traditional ceremony performed called, "Zhao Hun" or "the calling of the Hun." This ceremony entails someone (a relative or loved one) going to the roof of the deceased individual's house and calling to the deceased person's Hun, begging it to return to its body. If the Hun do not return, then the Po will then begin their descent into the Earth and the body's tissues will start to decay. In order to insure that the Po stay in the body after it has been buried (and that they will not come out to annoy the living) the relatives seal all of the orifices (exits) of the body, in order to trap the Po inside. Generally, the orifices of the body are plugged with either jade or rice (depending on the deceased individual's financial status).

OVERVIEW

One of the unique aspects of ancient Chinese medicine is that it addresses all aspects of the individual's body, energy and spirit. It explores in great detail the spiritual transformations that take place during the body's Prenatal development, the relationship of fetal development to the formation of the adult body, and to the dying and after-death states. Ancient Chinese medicine further addresses the potential of spiritual involvement as a cause or cure of specific psychophysical diseases. It is through the complete study of an individual's physical, mental, emotional, energetic, and spiritual aspects that doctors of Medical Qigong therapy ascertain when and how to treat their patients.

Every human is a multidimensional being, existing within three energetic fields. The energetic forms of Jing, Qi and Shen compose our present personality yet exist within three different dimensions of vibrational frequencies. These energetic fields are linked together by their corresponding relationships to the alchemic transformations that maintain their vitality.

The metaphysical abilities of the individual's Shen are spiritual manifestations of the Eternal Soul. Once the Qigong doctor regulates his or her

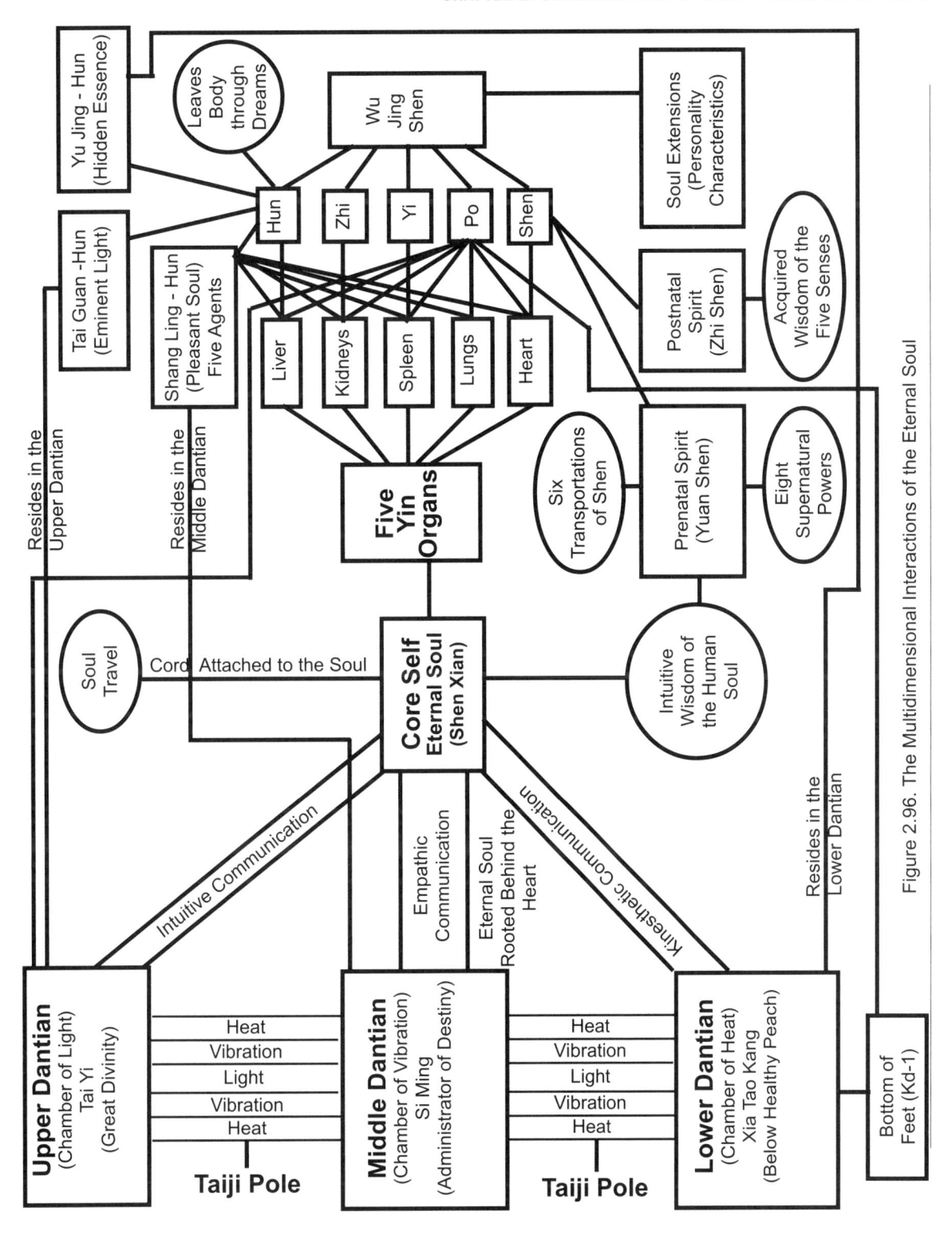

CHAPTER 2: UNDERSTANDING ANCIENT CHINESE METAPHYSICS

Figure 2.96. The Multidimensional Interactions of the Eternal Soul

own spiritual life, these abilities become natural and internalized, giving way to the development of advanced diagnostic abilities. A chart describing the interaction of the body's Eternal Soul with the energetic functions of the Three Dantians and Five Yin Organs' Wu Jing Shen (Five Essence Spirits) is located at Figure 2.96.

Chapter 3
Tissue Formation and Development

Fascial Development and Energy Flow

According to the *American Medical Association Encyclopedia of Medicine*, "fascia is the fibrous connective tissue that surrounds many structures in the body. One layer of the tissue, known as the superficial fascia, envelops the entire body just beneath the skin. Another layer, the deep fascia, encloses muscles, forming a sheath for individual muscles, and also separates them into groups. The deep fascia also holds in place the soft organs, such as the Kidneys. The thick fascia in the palm of the hand and sole of the foot have a cushioning, protective function."

In Traditional Chinese Medicine, the fascia is referred to as Huang, meaning any membranous tissue. Fascial development is divided into two stages: prenatal (congenital) and postnatal (acquired). The prenatal fascia is fixed and determined by the combination of the parents' Jing, Qi, and Shen. The postnatal fascia is formed through diet, exercise, and environmental stresses.

Qi is stored within the tissues and inner fascial layers, where it envelops and protects the body's internal organs. Energy that has been stored within the body's organs is available through the fascia to nourish the patient's body, mind, emotions, energy, and spirit. The body consists of three tissue layers, described as follows (Figure 3.1):
1. The first and innermost layer is made of the internal organs which produce and transform Qi.
2. The second layer consists of the body's fascia, tendons, ligaments, and Bones which assist in transporting Qi to the extremities.
3. The third and outermost layer of tissue consists of the muscles and skin, where Wei (Protective) Qi circulates to protect the organism from invasion of external pathogens (Cold, Heat, Wind, and Dampness, etc.).

Outermost Layer	Second Layer	Innermost Layer of Tissue
Muscles and Skin where Wei Qi circulates to protect the body from invasion of External Pathogens	Fascia, Tendons, Ligaments, and Bones which assist in Transporting Qi to the Extremities	Internal Organs which Produce and Transform Qi

Figure 3.1 The Three Tissue Layers of the Body

After being generated within the body's internal organs, Qi is distributed throughout the body's entire energetic network through the channels and collaterals, via the fascia. Each organ has its own layers of weblike fascia that cover, connect, protect, and nourish its tissues. Fascia also forms the energetic chambers of the body's organs and channel systems. Qi flows between the fascial sheaths and along the channel systems.

The fascia can form adhesions through trauma, infection, surgery, disease, or chronic muscular tension. These fascial adhesions restrict the flow of Qi and Blood to the tissues, thereby accelerating the aging process.

In its various forms, the fascia is the basic connective element that weaves together all other body tissues. It is the fascia that ultimately determines and maintains the body's structure. This structure is in part an adaptation and response of the body's fascial network to the stresses of the external environment. Therefore, our internal and external constitutions are formed, in part, by conditions from the environment that affect the innermost layers of fascial development. Traditional

```
                          ┌──────────────────────────────────────────────┐
                          │ Diagnosis according to the Prenatal and      │
                          │            Postnatal Influences              │
                          └──────────────────────────────────────────────┘
┌──────────────┐         
│    The       │          ┌──────────────────────────────────────────────┐
│ Three Types  │──────────│ Diagnosis according to the Five Element      │
│   of Body    │          │                Influences                    │
│Classifications│         └──────────────────────────────────────────────┘
└──────────────┘         
                          ┌──────────────────────────────────────────────┐
                          │ Diagnosis according to the Yin or Yang       │
                          │                Influences                    │
                          └──────────────────────────────────────────────┘
```

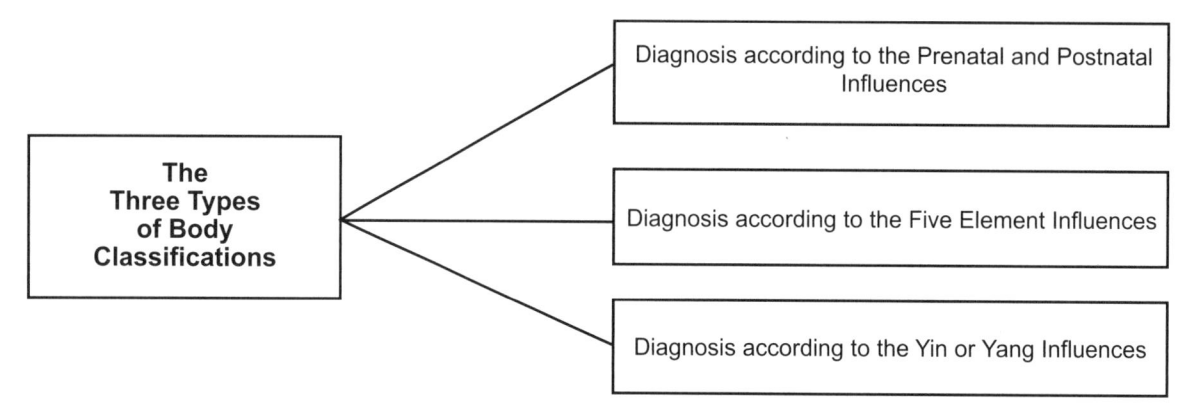

Figure 3.2 The ancient Chinese doctors taught three different ways of classifying and diagnosing the energetic patterns of an individual's body shape and tissue formation.

Chinese Medicine divides the observation and diagnosis of the physical characteristics and patterns of the body's inner fascia into Yin and Yang structures and Five Elemental constitutions.

THE THREE TYPES OF BODY CLASSIFICATIONS OF ANCIENT CHINA

The ancient Chinese doctors taught three different ways of classifying and diagnosing the energetic patterns of an individual's body shape and tissue formation: diagnosis according to the prenatal and postnatal influences, diagnosis according to the Five Element influences, and diagnosis according to the Yin or Yang influences. These three unique classifications are described as follows (Figure 3.2):

- **Diagnosis according to the Prenatal and Postnatal Influences:** In this type of diagnosis, the doctor observed the influence of the specific strengths or weaknesses initiated by both the patient's Prenatal and Postnatal constitutional formations. This type of diagnosis determined each patient's inclination towards specific congenital or acquired diseases.
- **Diagnosis according to the Five Element Influences:** In this type of diagnosis, the doctor observed the energetic formation and influence of the patient's Five Element constitution. This type of diagnosis determined each element's continual influence (balanced, excessive or deficient) on the patient's Jing, Qi and Shen.
- **Diagnosis according to the Yin or Yang Influences:** In this type of diagnosis, the doctor observed the dominant Yin and Yang formation of the patient's constitution. This type of diagnosis determined the overall dominant energetically induced patterns of the patient's tissues (introverted, extraverted or balanced state).

To better comprehend the ancient Chinese classification of the human body's physical development and structural formations, it is important to begin with an understanding of ancient Chinese alchemy.

YIN AND YANG STRUCTURAL FORMATION

Chinese philosophy teaches that the universe is composed of a duality of opposing forces or energies known as Yin and Yang. Everything in the natural world contains both Yin and Yang. Yin and Yang are interdependent; Yin cannot grow without Yang, and Yang cannot develop without Yin. The energetic transformation of Yin into Yang and Yang into Yin produces the various changes observed in matter and form (see Chapter 1, page 6).

Accordingly, Yin and Yang are also the principles governing all things within the human body. Life and death originate from the energies of Yin and Yang, and they are the forces that create all physiological change. In Medical Qigong therapy, the physical structure of the human body is divided into Yin and Yang organs, Yin and Yang

CHAPTER 3: TISSUE FORMATION AND DEVELOPMENT

	Yang	Yin
Attributes	Active, Creative, Masculine, Fire, Hot, Heaven, Light	Passive, Receptive, Feminine, Water, Cold, Earth, Dark
Organs	The Six Hollow Yang Organs: Gall Bladder, Small Intestine, Stomach, Large Intestine, Urinary Bladder, and Triple Burners	The Five Solid Yin Organs: Liver, Heart, Spleen, Lungs, and Kidneys
Respiration	Exhalation	Inhalation
Time of Day	The 12 Hour Yang Cycle: From 11 p.m. (Before Midnight) to 11 a.m. (Before High Noon)	The 12 Hour Yin Cycle: From 11 a.m. (Before Noon) to 11 p.m. (Before Midnight)
Seasons	Spring and Summer	Autumn and Winter
Pathological Movement	Turbid Yang Flows Upward like Fire	Turbid Yin Flows Downward like Water
Normal Movement	Heavenly Yang Flows Downward From the Sky	Earthly Yin Flows Upward from the Soil

Figure 3.3 Yin and Yang are the governing forces of the body.

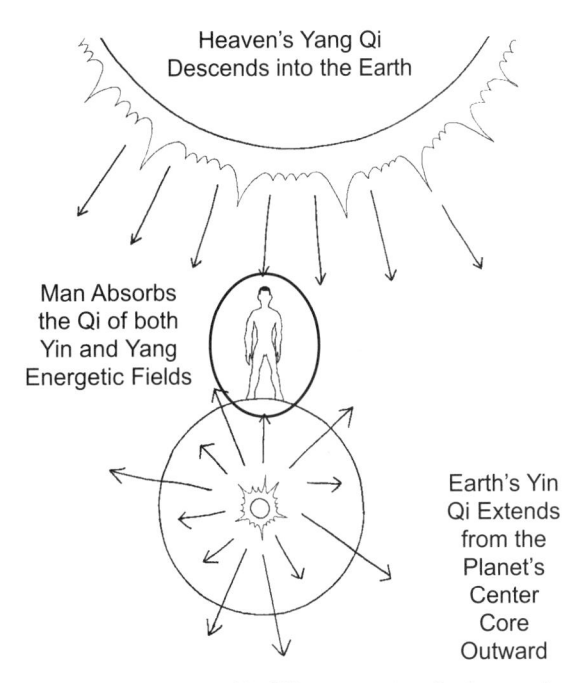

Figure 3.4 The Yang Qi of Heaven naturally descends, and the Yin Qi of the Earth naturally ascends.

substances, and Yin and Yang energetic functions (e.g., Qi that expands and flows outward is Yang, while Qi that contracts and flows inward is Yin).

Yin and Yang are in a constant state of waxing and waning (Figure 3.3). If this waxing and waning exceeds the body's natural energetic limitations and the body loses its dynamic equilibrium, deficiency or excess of either Yin or Yang will occur, leading to the development of abnormalities and illness.

The Yin Qi of the Earth naturally ascends. The Earth Qi enters into the Kidney, Liver and Spleen Channels of the legs and ascends into the body (Figure 3.4). When Yin Qi becomes pathological, weak or destructive, it becomes turbid and moves downward, descending like cascading water. Descending Spleen Qi due to deficiency, for example, can cause tiredness, incontinence, diarrhea, edema or prolapse of the viscera.

The Yang Qi of Heaven naturally descends. Heaven Qi enters the Stomach, Urinary Bladder and Gall Bladder Channels and flowing downward into the Earth. When Yang Qi becomes pathological, weak or destructive, it ascends like the flames of a fire moving upward. For example, Rebellious Stomach Qi ascends, causing nausea and vomiting. Another example of pathogenic Yang Qi ascending would be the temperature of a rising fever.

YIN AND YANG ANATOMICAL ASPECTS

The ancient Chinese doctors were among the first to develop a standardized system to describe the various anatomical features, locations and regions of the human body using Yin and Yang terminologies.

Similar to Western anatomy, Traditional Chinese Medicine also divides the body into aspects or planes. In T.C.M., these classifications are divided into Yin and Yang physical planes and anatomical directions. These divisions aid the Qigong doctor in defining and categorizing the patient's tissues and body structure, and also assist in determining the collection and movement of Qi (i.e., energy moving into and coalescing in the Yin or Yang areas of the patient's body). The structural aspects are categorized as follows:

- The cranial or superior aspect (top half) of the body's structure is considered Yang; the caudal or inferior portion of the body (bottom half)

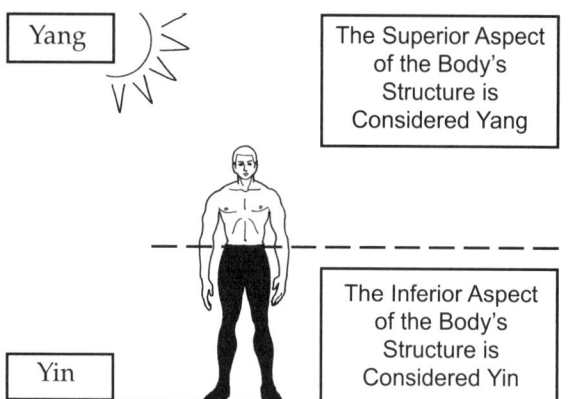

VOLUME 1, SECTION 1: FOUNDATIONS OF CHINESE ENERGETIC MEDICINE

Figure 3.5. The superior (upper) aspect of the body's structure is Yang; the inferior (lower) portion is Yin. Think of the sun shining on the upper torso, illuminating the body from the waist to the head, while the lower torso, from the hips downward, is in the shade.

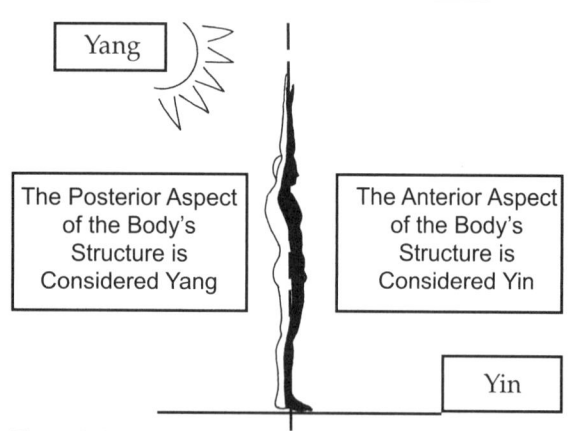

Figure 3.6. The posterior portion (back) of the body is Yang; the anterior portion (front) is Yin. Think of the sun shining on the back while the front of the body is in the shade.

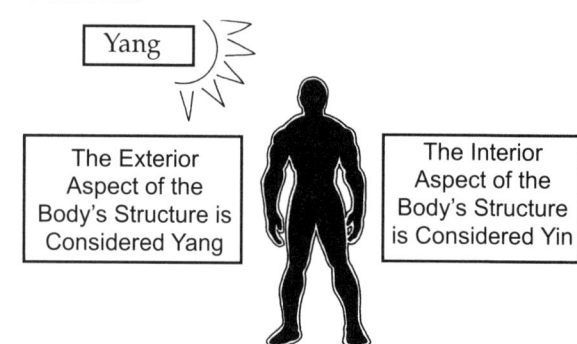

Figure 3.7. The superficial aspect (exterior) of the body is Yang; the deep portion (interior) of the body is Yin. Think of the sun shining on the external surfaces of the body while the internal organs remain in the dark.

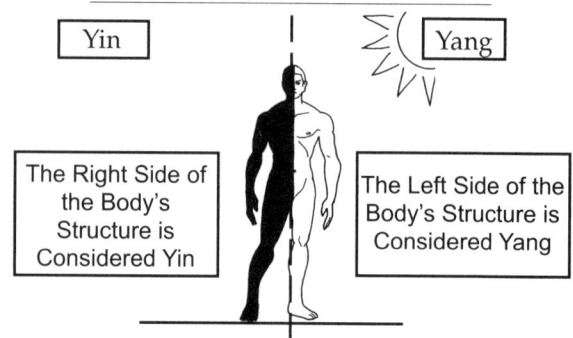

Figure 3.8. The left side of the body is Yang; the right side is Yin. Think of facing south in the morning while practicing Medical Qigong. The sun will rise in the east, illuminating the left side (Yang) while the right side remains shaded (Yin).

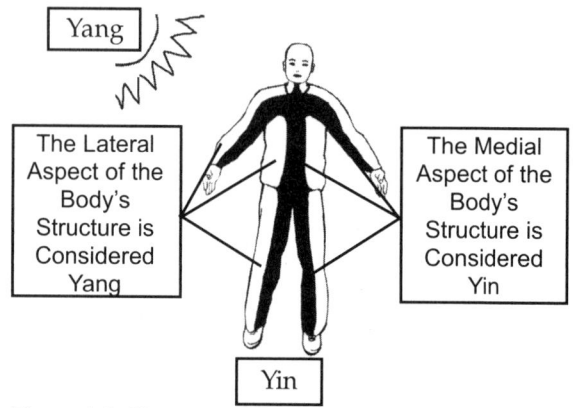

Figure 3.9. The lateral aspect (further from the center) of the body is Yang; the medial portion (middle) is Yin. Think of the sun shining on the furthest part of the external tissues, while the center is still in the shade.

is considered Yin (Figure 3.5)
- The posterior or dorsal portion (back side) of the body is Yang; the anterior or ventral portion (front side) is Yin (Figure 3.6)
- The superficial aspect (exterior) of the body is Yang; the deep portion (interior) of the body is Yin (Figure 3.7)
- The left side of the body is Yang; the right side is Yin (Figure 3.8)
- The lateral aspect (further from the center) of the body is Yang; the medial portion (middle) is Yin (Figure 3.9)

124

These structural Yin and Yang aspects are defined in relationship to each other (Figure 3.10). It is important to remember this relativity when considering the anatomical aspects of Yin and Yang. In clinical observation, for example, Yin and Yang are mostly used to describe the dominant nature or quality of something. The most common mistake is to view Yin and Yang as representing the fixed nature of people, places or things, rather than the quality or nature of these objects.

Yin and Yang are in a constant state of change, always waxing and waning. Two points of reference alone are not enough to sufficiently classify the many phases and stages of physical and energetic transformation. For example, day (Yang) can be further divided into dawn (waxing Yang), midday (peaking Yang), and late afternoon (waning Yang); while night (Yin) can be further divided into late afternoon (waxing Yin), midnight (peaking Yin), and dawn (waning Yin).

Yang	Yin
Superior (Upper)	Inferior (Lower)
Posterior (Back)	Anterior (Front)
Superficial (External)	Deep (Internal)
Left Side	Right Side
Lateral (Away from Center)	Medial (Middle)

Figure 3.10. The Yin and Yang Anatomical Aspects

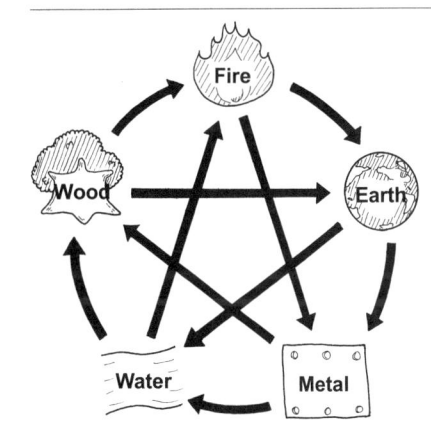

THE BODY'S FIVE ELEMENTS

The body energetically contains the attributes of Five Elements (Wu Xing), also translated as the Five Phases. The Five Elements are: Wood, Fire, Earth, Metal, and Water (Figure 3.11). The Five Elements are used in Chinese medicine to paint a clear and natural image of the changing cycles of Yin and Yang (see Volume 3, Chapter 24). Furthermore, each of the Five Elements can also be divided into Yin and Yang making a total of ten subdivisions. Wood, for example, can be subdivided into Yin Wood and Yang Wood.

The Chinese use the framework of the Five Elements to understand and categorize many different areas of knowledge and experience. This Five Element categorization includes the movements of the Heavens and the various land forms of the Earth, as well as the energetic workings of human anatomy, physiology, and psychology. As noted earlier, our organs and their associated energy channels are divided into Yin and Yang. In addition, each of the organs is also related to one of the Five Elements. The Liver and Gall Bladder relate to the Wood Element, the Heart and Small Intestine relate to the Fire Element, the Spleen and Stomach to the Earth Element, the Lungs and Large Intestine to the Metal Element, and the Kidneys and Urinary Bladder relate to the Water Element. These organs express the functional aspects of the Five Elements within the human body as they interact with each other to promote and maintain life.

Figure 3.11. The Five Elements (Wu Xing)

The Yin organs are said to store the Jing (Essence) of the Five Elements (see Chapter 2), though they share this essence with their elementally paired Yang organs. While the Yin organs serve as repositories that gather and store the Jing of the Five Elements, the Yang organs mobilize and utilize this Jing to perform various functions specific to each organ (transforming, transporting, etc.).

The Seven Emotions			
Chinese Word	English Translation	Associated Organ	Energetic Manifestations
Xi	Joy, Happiness, Delight, Excitement, Elation	Heart	Slows Down and Relaxes Qi
Nu	Irritation, Anger, Rage, Fury	Liver	Causes Qi to Rise
Si	Contemplation, Pensiveness, Worry, Mourning	Spleen	Causes Qi to Stagnate
You	Concern, Sorrow, Sadness, Anxiety, Depression	Lungs	Obstructs the Flow of Qi
Kong	Fear, Dread, Terror, Feeling Threatened or Intimidated	Kidneys	Causes Qi to Descend
Jing	Surprise, Fright, Alarm, Shock	Heart then Kidneys	Scatters and Deranges the Qi
Bei	Melancholy, Sadness, Sorrow, Grief	Lungs	Disperses and Consumes the Qi

Figure 3.12. The Seven Emotions

The Yin organs also store the Five Agents (the Five Virtues) and are more easily disrupted than the Yang organs by the seven emotions (anger, excitement, worry, grief, sadness, fear, and shock).

When in excess, the body's emotions can create an energetic imbalance, which in turn can cause a destructive physical pattern within the body (Figure 3.12). An example of this process is excessive anger leading to hypertension.

The emotions are said to be the motivational force behind energy transformation within each individual. People will have a different reaction to specific emotional changes based on their dominant Five Elemental pattern. There are five internal organ emotions associated with the energy of the Five Elements:
1. Anger: Liver - Wood
2. Excitement: Heart - Fire
3. Worry: Spleen - Earth
4. Grief and Sorrow: Lungs - Metal
5. Fear: Kidneys - Water

The energies of the Five Elements shape all aspects of a human being: physical, energetic, mental, emotional, and spiritual.

Congenital Constitutions

Most individuals are born with a dominant elemental pattern which will determine that individual's physical, energetic, and psycho-emotional constitution. When excess or deficient, the body's emotions can create an energetic imbalance, which in turn can lead to a destructive physical pattern within the body.

Pattern (Li) and Energy (Qi)

The ancient Chinese believed that the two fundamental properties of nature, "Li" (pattern) and "Qi" (energy) establish the foundation of all existence. Throughout the universe there can be no Qi without Li, nor Li without Qi. Li is the Dao that organizes all form (Xing) from above (Heavens) and from below (Earth). Li is the foundational roots from which all things are produced. Qi is the instrument that composes all form from below (Earth), and provides the tools and raw material from which all things are made. Therefore, all things must receive Li (cosmic and organic patterning) in their moment of coming into existence, and obtain their specific nature and form (Xing) through energy and matter.

It was believed that an individual's Li was molded through the assistance of the "Five Pure Lights," which were responsible for assisting the Eternal Soul in molding the Five Element Jings (Essences) into "Wu Cai" (five materials), manifesting on the gross material plane as five types of tissue formations (Wood, Fire, Earth, Metal, and Water).

The previous chapter on energetic embryology describes the different Five Elemental Jings (Essences) and how they enter the fetus via each of the mother's organs from the fourth to the eight lunar months of pregnancy. Depending on the relative strength or weakness of the mother's internal organ energies during her pregnancy, the fetus will inherit a greater or lesser amount of elemental Jing from the mother. If the mother's Liver energy is dominant, then the child will have a tendency to develop a Wood constitution; if her Kidney energy is dominant, then the child develops a Water constitution, and so forth.

Ancient Chinese astrology states that the various Heavenly influences present at the time of conception and birth influence the relative Five Element strengths and weaknesses inherent in a newborn's constitution. Thus, the astrological influences at conception and birth as well as the prenatal maternal transmission of Jing, Qi, and Shen determine each person's congenital constitution.

After birth, the Prenatal Jing is cultivated and sustained through prayer, meditation, physical exercise, and sleep, which are described as follows:
- In prayer, the Jing is given guidance, direction and purpose
- In meditation, the Jing is refined
- In physical exercise, the Jing is nourished, energized and cleansed through alternating Yin and Yang movements
- In sleep, the Jing is replenished

In Medical Qigong theory, the health of the Prenatal Jing determines the physical and energetic balance of the overall constitution, the level of vitality and resistance to disease, as well as the mental and emotional natures of the individual. The Prenatal Jing, with its unique balance of the Five Elements, becomes the foundation for an individual's Qi and Shen.

The congenital influence is, however, not absolute. Postnatal factors, such as diet, life-style, environmental influences, and internal belief structures all either support or undermine the health and balance of the individual's constitution. Thus, patients with congenital deficiencies can still improve their health by prayer, meditation, Medical Qigong, adequate sleep, proper diet and exercise, herbs, medicines, stress management, and other therapeutic modalities.

On the negative side, patients with strong inherited constitutions may still develop serious constitutional imbalances through intemperate life-styles such as chronic stress, overwork, excessive sexual activity, or poor eating habits. Therefore, the Qigong doctor must consider both prenatal (congenital) and postnatal (acquired) constitutional factors in order to understand and differentiate between the patient's innate constitution and his or her current condition.

CLASSIFICATION OF THE FIVE ELEMENT PHYSICAL CONSTITUTIONS

The Five Elements, which are associated with the five Yin organs, have numerous physical, energetic and spiritual aspects. Each element is expressed through different emotions, temperaments, colors, tastes, body types, illnesses and thought patterns.

Over the centuries, much has been written in Chinese medical literature about the Five Element Constitutions. The following interpretation was developed by Dr. Zhou Qianchuan, a Daoist master from Qi Cheng Shan, reputed by some to be the master of *The Yellow Emperor's Classic of Internal Medicine*.

Dr. Zhou perceived that each of the Five Element Constitutions has both a characteristic physical appearance and a corresponding psycho-emotional profile. Through observing these characteristics, the Qigong doctor determines a patient's Five Element Constitution. From this diagnosis, the doctor discovers much about the balance or imbalance of the patient's physical and mental health.

In Traditional Chinese Medicine, an individual's body type and his or her psyche are closely intertwined. Physical aspects such as coloring, proportion, dominant tissue (muscle, fat, sinew, etc.), tone, movement, postural patterns, as well as general vitality, all express the patient's internal energetic and psycho-emotional matrices. The body type reveals the patient's innate personality and acquired personality, as well as his or her emotional history.

Dr. Zhou subdivided each of the Five Element Constitutions into three categories: balanced nature, Yin nature, and Yang nature. The ideal is to have a balanced nature regardless of one's element type. A Medical Qigong treatment addresses the mental, emotional, and spiritual balance of the five constitutions. Since the Mind (Shen) is closely tied with the Jing and the Qi, it is not enough to simply tell patients how to change their personality to restore balance. The Qigong doctor must work with patients on all levels (physical, energetic, mental, emotional, and spiritual) to help them to restore balance. Specific healing methods are discussed at length in later chapters. The Qigong doctor normally selects treatment principles based on the Five Element Creative (Figure 3.13) and Controlling (Figure 3.14) Cycles to help restore balance (see Volume 3, Chapter 24).

For instance, a patient with a Yin Earth nature might tend to have weak or Deficient Spleen energy. Therapeutically, the Qigong doctor would choose one of the three following treatments:
1. Direct Tonification of the Earth Element
2. Tonification of the Fire Element in accordance with the principle, "To nourish the child, strengthen the mother"
3. Disperse or reduce the Wood Element (Wood, the "grandmother," may be overcontrolling Earth, the "grandson")

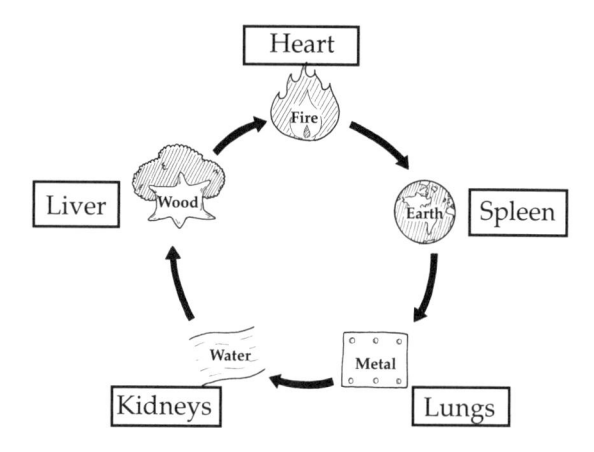

Figure 3.13. The Five Element Creative Cycle

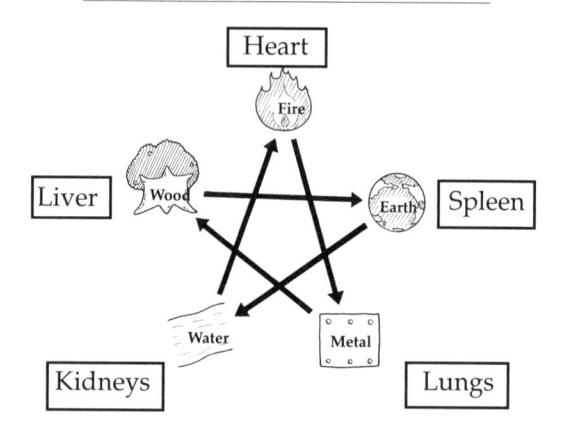

Figure 3.14. The Five Element Controlling Cycle

A patient with a Yang Earth nature might tend to have Excess Earth energy. In this case, the Qigong doctor would:
1. Use a Purging method to reduce the Earth Element
2. Strengthen the Wood Element, supporting the Wood in order to control the Earth (the weak "grandmother" may be unable to restrain an overly strong "grandson" without help).

THE WOOD CONSTITUTION

WOOD PERSONALITY

The Wood personality can be divided into three subdivisions, which are described as follows:

CHAPTER 3: TISSUE FORMATION AND DEVELOPMENT

1. **A Balanced Wood Nature:** Predisposes individuals to be confident, strong, independent, and intuitive, with a clear understanding of themselves and their goals. They are patient, able to allow things to develop naturally, and express their personality in a relaxed and harmonious way. They are kind when communicating with others, creative, free-flowing in self-expression, and display merciful and unselfish traits when dealing with the needs of others. They are able to establish and maintain healthy and proper boundaries (Figure 3.15).

2. **A Yin Wood Nature:** Predisposes individuals to feel externally insecure and to be overcautious. They have a tendency to worry and have a weak sense of their own abilities and potential. They are unassertive and are unsure of their identities and life purpose. They also have difficulty expressing their egos and have weak boundaries. They are timid, lack confidence, and display considerable doubt (Figure 3.16).

TREATMENT FOR YIN WOOD NATURE INDIVIDUALS:

Treatment involves establishing a sense of inner strength and security by teaching them self-trust and building self-esteem. These individuals need to strengthen their boundaries so that they no longer allow the intrusion or domination from others. They need to learn to trust in their intuition, develop a greater degree of confidence, enhance their personal power, and find a stronger sense of spiritual growth.

3. **A Yang Wood Nature:** Predisposes individuals to manifest their internal insecurities through irritability and impatience. Such individuals are intolerant, rude, stubborn, selfish, and tend to expand their egos without consideration for others. They are domineering, angry, aggressive, and generally known as overachievers; however, they are easily frustrated and depressed. Their self-esteem is elevated by acquiring higher social, political or otherwise influential positions, or by bullying others (Figure 3.17).

Balanced Wood Nature:
- confident, strong, independent, and intuitive
- patient, kind, and understanding of themselves and their goals
- relaxed and harmonious
- merciful and unselfish
- creative and free-flowing in self-expression
- maintains healthy and proper boundaries

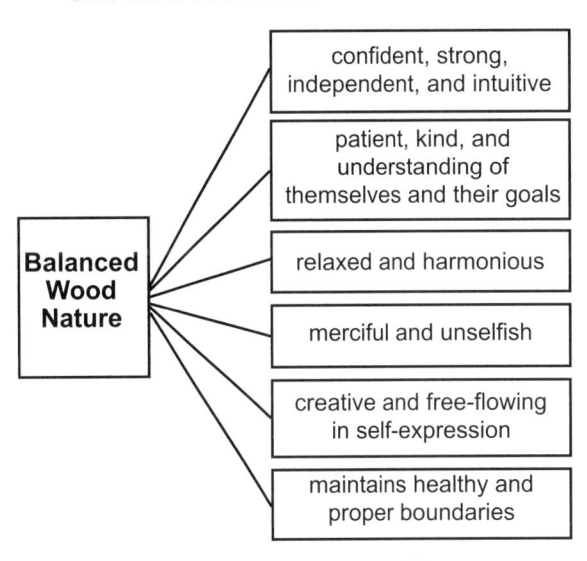

Figure 3.15. Balanced Wood Nature

Yin Wood Nature:
- externally insecure and overcautious
- worries and has a weak sense of own abilities and potential
- unassertive and unsure of own identity and life purpose
- has weak boundaries, timid, lack confidence, and displays considerable doubt

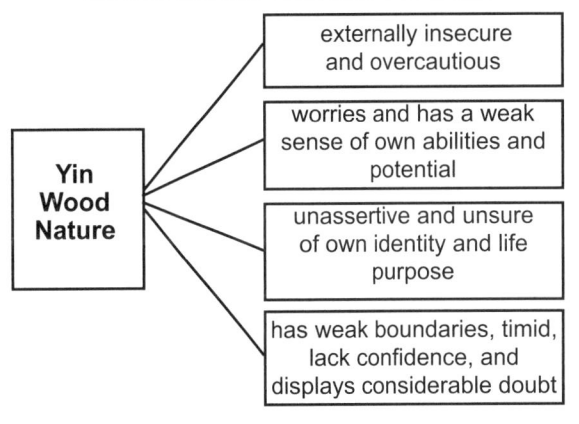

Figure 3.16. Yin Wood Nature

Yang Wood Nature:
- acts irritable and impatient, intolerant, rude, stubborn, and selfish
- domineering, angry, and aggressive
- overachievers, easily frustrated and depressed
- bullies others

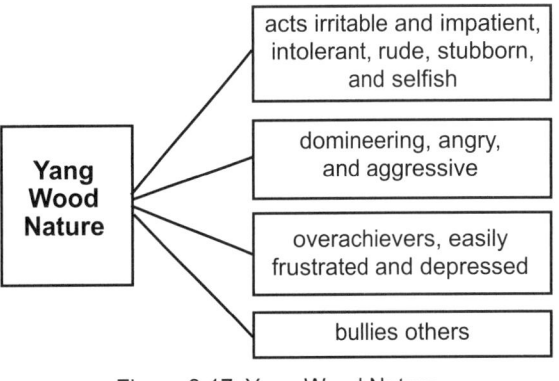

Figure 3.17. Yang Wood Nature

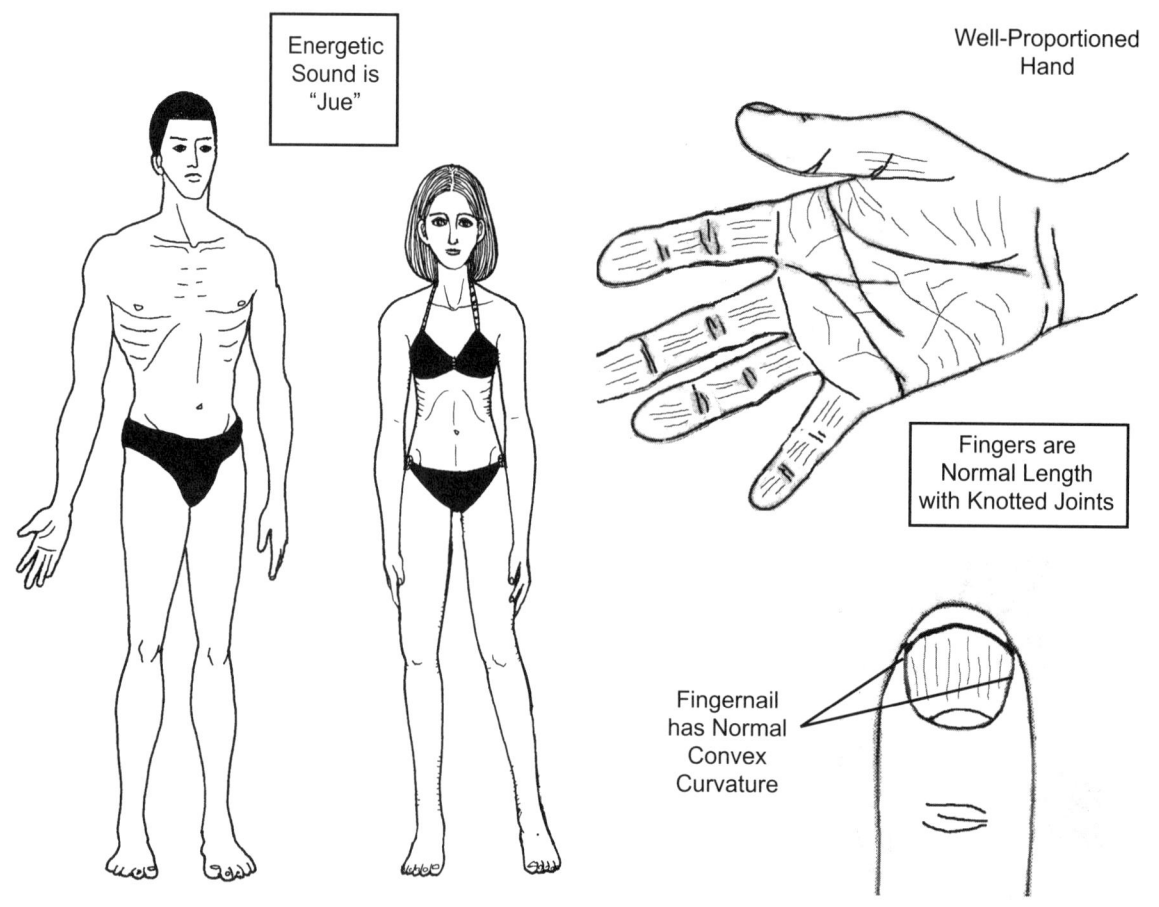

Figure 3.18. Wood Constitution in Males and Females

Figure 3.19. Wood Constitution Hand Features

Treatment for Yang Wood Nature Individuals:

Treatment should focus on cultivating humility, reverence, and inner peace, as well as consciously blending and harmonizing with life (following the Dao). In situations of conflict, they need to learn to relax, slow down, and act out of stillness. These individuals must learn to surrender to a higher will, and rely on their own spiritual intuition and inner direction. It is also important for them to learn to respect others.

Wood Outer Appearance

Wood constitution types usually have a subtle shade of green/blue in their complexion. They have a tall and sinewy body with a small head and a long face. They also have small, nicely formed hands and feet, broad shoulders, small torsos and a straight, flat back (Figure 3.18).

The hands of a Wood Constitution individual generally have a well-proportioned structure with average length fingers and knotted joints. The fingernails tend to have a normal convex curvature (Figure 3.19).

By nature, they enjoy spring and summer but generally dislike autumn and winter. This preference is due to the inherent vulnerabilities of the Wood constitution, making them especially susceptible to pathogenic invasion and disease during these seasons. Their dominant features include strong sinews and a green-blue facial color. Their energetic sound is "jue."

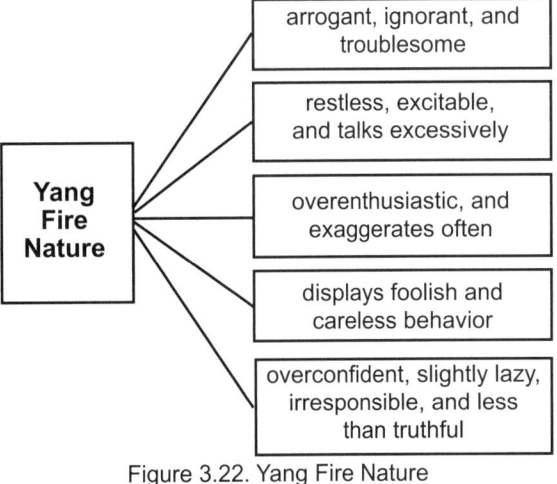

The Fire Constitution

Fire Personality

The Fire personality can be divided into three subdivisions, which are described as follows:

1. **A Balanced Fire Nature:** Predisposes individuals to be trusting, open-minded, complacent, social, unconcerned about wealth, and fond of beauty. They love themselves and others and are very expressive of their affection. They are calm, peaceful, happy, lively, spontaneous, funny, and fun to be with (Figure 3.20).

2. **A Yin Fire Nature:** Predisposes individuals to be solemn and depressed. They usually lack interest in life and have a tendency to become isolated, feeling unloved and unlovable (Figure 3.21).

Treatment for Yin Fire nature individuals:

Treatment requires teaching them how to store and conserve their energy, avoid extremes and apply the principle of moderation to all aspects of their life. They also need to engage in activities that create personal enjoyment, and find simple pleasures that awaken their affection. Individuals of a Yin Fire Nature can further benefit from learning how to express their feelings, wants, and needs.

3. **A Yang Fire Nature:** Predisposes individuals to be arrogant, ignorant, and troublesome. They are restless and excitable, and tend to talk excessively. Individuals of a Yang Fire Nature are overenthusiastic, exaggerate often, and generally display foolish and careless behavior. They are socially and sexually overactive and seek every opportunity to assert themselves. These individuals are often overconfident, slightly lazy, irresponsible, and less than truthful. They can easily go from mania to exhaustion, and then burnout and become suicidal (e.g., bipolar disorder) (Figure 3.22).

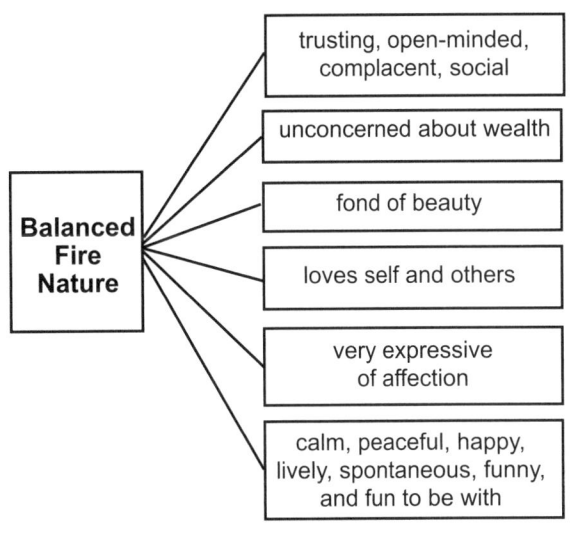

Figure 3.20. Balanced Fire Nature

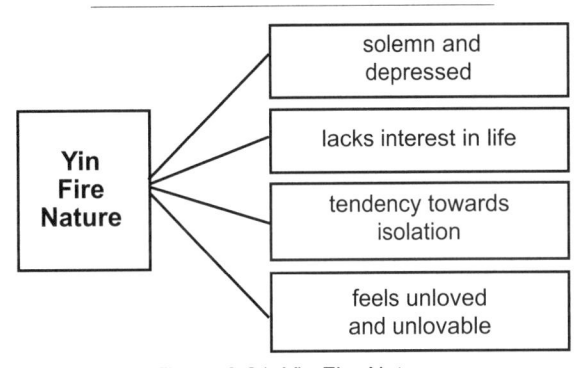

Figure 3.21. Yin Fire Nature

Figure 3.22. Yang Fire Nature

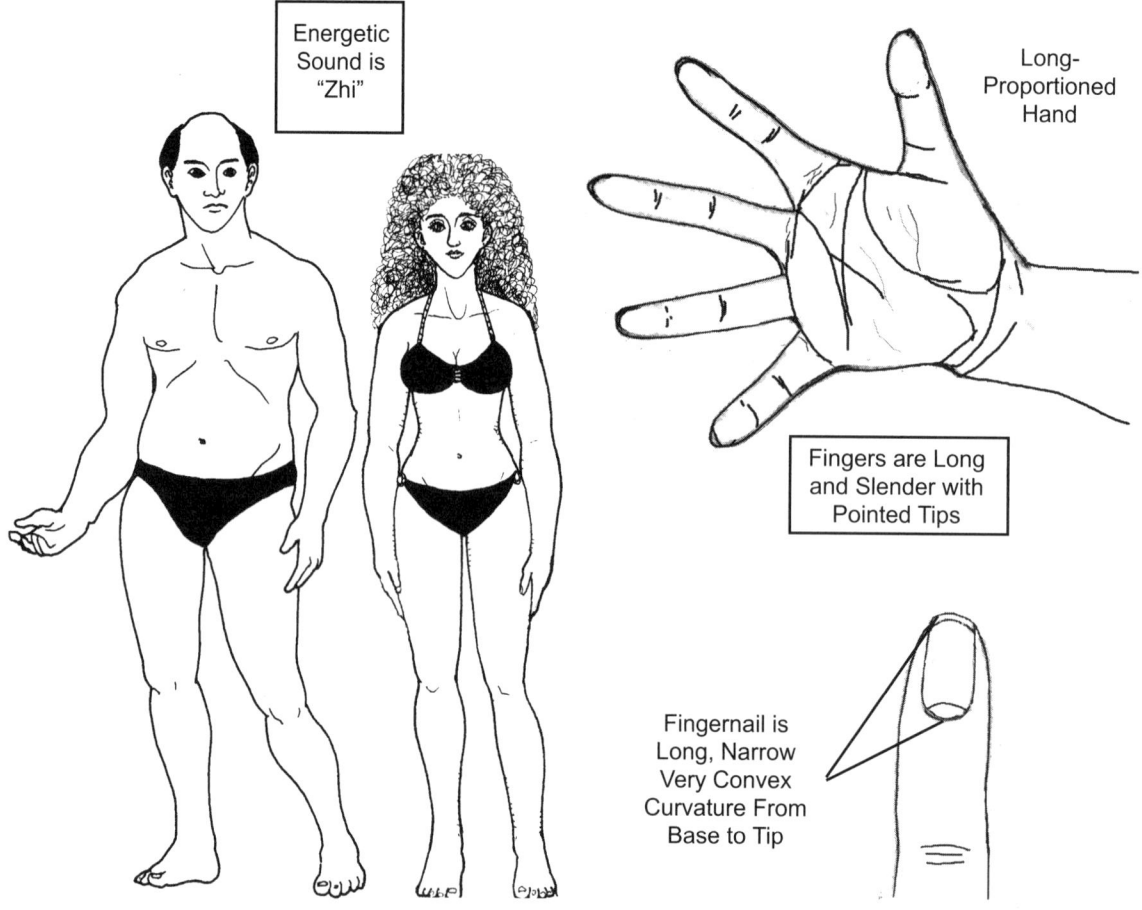

Figure 3.23. Fire Constitution in Males and Females

Figure 3.24. Fire Constitution Hand Features

TREATMENT FOR YANG FIRE NATURE INDIVIDUALS:

Treatment requires teaching them to learn how to stop, slow down, and look for their contentment from within. They should balance their feelings of love with contemplation and wisdom, avoid over-enthusiasm, and allow their inner spirit to radiate through in a more steady and sober manner.

FIRE OUTER APPEARANCE

Fire constitution types usually have a subtle shade of red in their complexion. They usually have broad paravertebral muscles and well-proportioned upper back, shoulders, buttocks, thighs and abdomen. They have small pointed heads, thin faces, pointed chins, small hands and feet, wide teeth, and curly or scanty hair, or no hair on top of their head (Figure 3.23).

The hands of a Fire Constitution individual generally have a long-proportioned structure with fingers that are long, slender and flexible. The finger tips are pointed. The fingernails tend to be long and narrow, with a very convex curvature from base to tip (Figure 3.24).

By nature, they enjoy spring and summer but dislike autumn and winter. This preference is due to the inherent vulnerabilities of the Fire constitution, making them especially susceptible to pathogenic invasion and disease during these seasons. Their dominant features include a strong circulatory system and a red facial color. Their energetic sound is "zhi."

THE EARTH CONSTITUTION

EARTH PERSONALITY

The Earth personality can be divided into three subdivisions, which are described as follows:

1. **A Balanced Earth Nature:** Predisposes individuals to lead quiet, stable, and peaceful lives, unconcerned about fame or wealth. They are easygoing, calm, generous, forgiving, sincere, and unambitious. They usually have open minds and rarely live in fear or make excessive demands. Individuals of a Balanced Earth Nature are analytical, logical and practical; and they use sound reasoning to communicate their opinions to others. They are adaptable to changing situations, and rarely use coercion to achieve power. They are kind and gentle with an earnest and well-mannered attitude. These individuals are pleasant, sweet, sympathetic, caring, and able to maintain healthy boundaries (Figure 3.25).

2. **A Yin Earth Nature:** Predisposes individuals to worry endlessly, becoming suspicious and self-centered. They think too much and rarely follow through with actions that manifest their decisions. Because they feel empty inside, they find it difficult to be nurturing to themselves and others (Figure 3.26).

TREATMENT FOR YIN EARTH NATURE INDIVIDUALS:

Treatment requires teaching them to learn how to let go of their inner feelings of worry and defensiveness. These individuals need to examine their assumptions, connect with their physical bodies, come out of their shells, and begin to live in the real world. They need to replace their negative thought patterns with positive affirmations, realistically look at their true potential and abilities, and learn how to take action and follow through.

3. **A Yang Earth Nature:** Predisposes individuals to cling to others. They are co-dependent, pushy, and possessive. Such individuals try to dominate in a passive-aggressive way while limiting the independence of others (Figure 3.27).

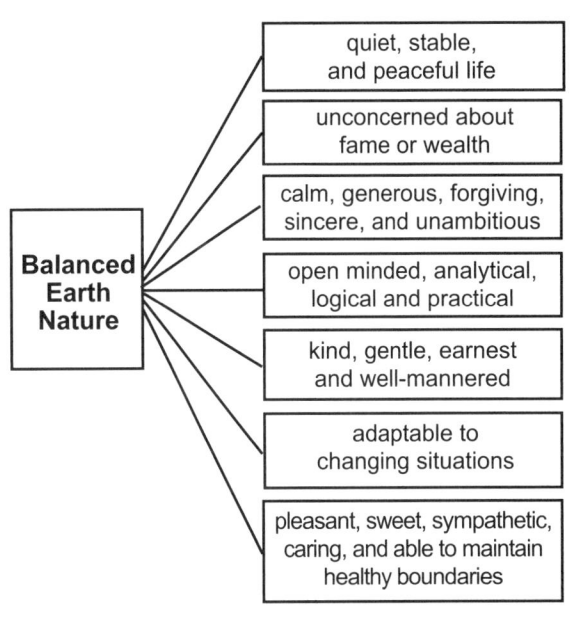

Figure 3.25. Balanced Earth Nature

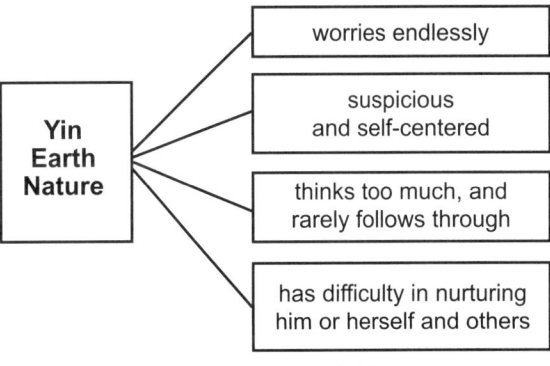

Figure 3.26. Yin Earth Nature

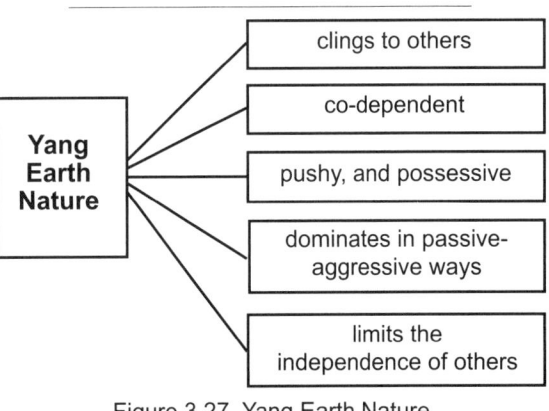

Figure 3.27. Yang Earth Nature

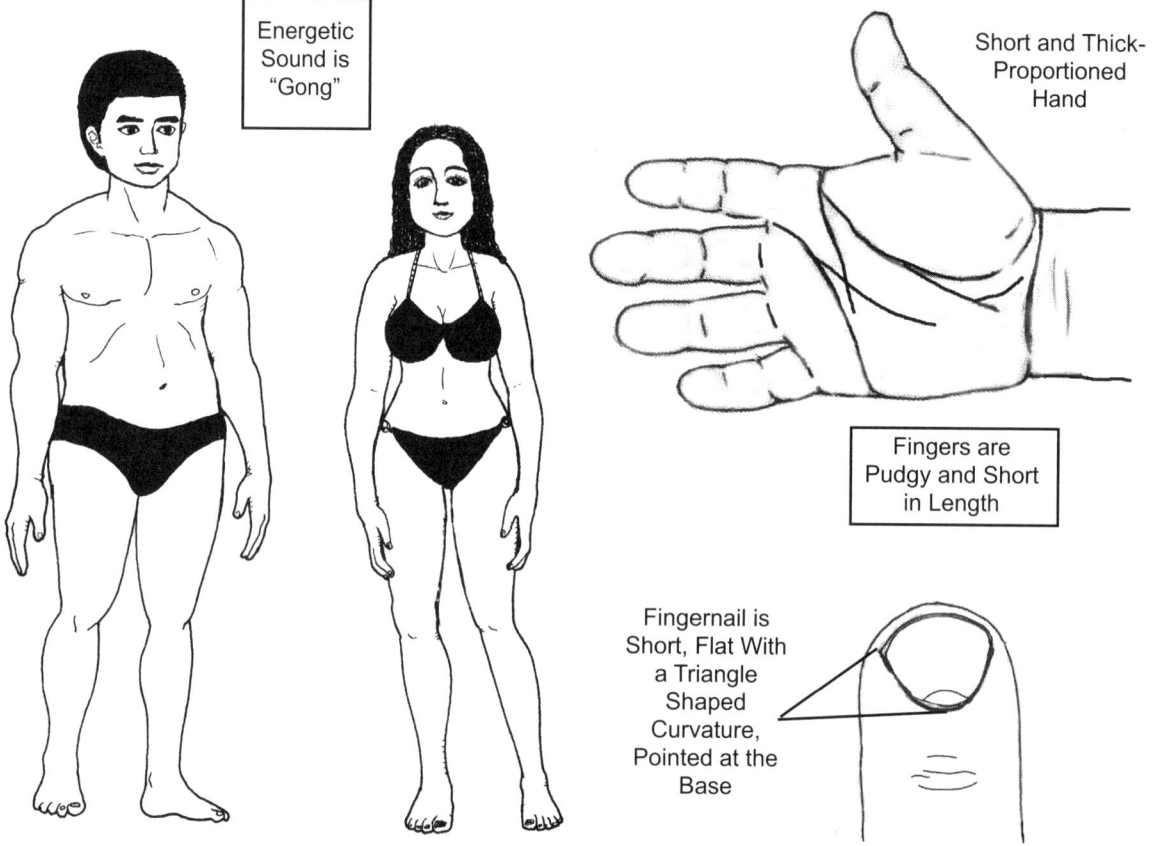

Figure 3.28. Earth Constitution in Males and Females

Figure 3.29. Earth Constitution Hand Features

TREATMENT FOR YANG EARTH NATURE INDIVIDUALS:

Treatment consists of teaching them to develop their inner strength in order to control the feelings of fear, insecurity, and inner emptiness that make them want to hold on to others. They need to create and establish love as a source of security from within themselves. They need to learn how to be themselves regardless of the praise of others. They must learn to become emotionally independent.

EARTH OUTER APPEARANCE

Earth constitution types usually have a subtle shade of yellow in their complexion. They usually have a somewhat large body, large head, round shaped face, wide jaw, well developed shoulders and back, large abdomen, strong thighs and calf muscles, and small hands and feet (Figure 3.28). They are categorized as having excessive flesh, with upper and lower limbs mutually well-proportioned.

The hands of an Earth Constitution individual generally have a short, thick proportioned structure with fingers that are thick, pudgy and short in length. The fingernails tend to be short and flat, with a slightly convex curvature and a triangular shape beginning at the nail base (Figure 3.29).

By nature, they enjoy autumn and winter but dislike spring and summer. This preference is due to the inherent vulnerabilities of the Earth constitution, making them especially susceptible to pathogenic invasion and disease during these seasons. Their dominant features include strong muscles and yellow or light brown facial color. Their energetic sound is "gong."

The Metal Constitution

Metal Personality

The Metal personality can be divided into three subdivisions, which are described as follows:

1. **A Balanced Metal Nature:** Predisposes individuals to process grief, enabling them to let go of past emotional baggage. They believe that they cannot be in the present without cleaning up and being released from their past. They are able to gain knowledge and wisdom by gathering and releasing their emotional bonds while learning and growing from each experience of intimacy and connection. They participate fully in life and form new bonds without fear of loss. They are also generous, just, and bright (Figure 3.30).

2. **A Yin Metal Nature:** Predisposes individuals to have a difficult time creating lasting bonds. They are fearful of establishing new relationships due to past losses and emotional trauma. They avoid joining with others and withdraw from active social participation. Living in remorse, they grieve over lost opportunities and relationships. They can be haughty and coldhearted. They are jealous, cunning, sneaky, and furtive. They become angry when they do not have things that others possess. Covetous and socially isolated, they try to obtain happiness by possessing people, places and things (Figure 3.31).

Treatment for Yin Metal nature individuals:

Treatment requires teaching them how to strengthen their physical body, as well as the energy of their Heart, Spleen, and Lower Dantian. They also need to strengthen their abilities to form close emotional bonds with people, reduce their fears of rejection and abandonment, and cultivate the strength, courage and ability to let go of their past hurts. They need to open themselves emotionally to experience the warmth and compassion of life.

3. **A Yang Metal Nature:** Predisposes individuals to suppress their emotions and hold on to grief. They are generally considered whiners and complainers, talking to others about their

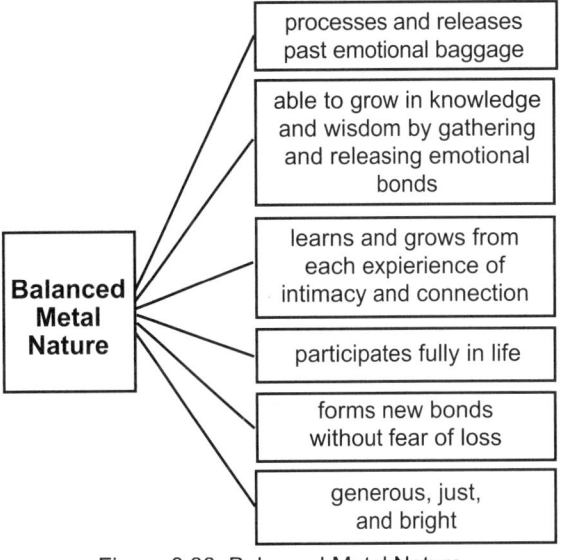

Figure 3.30. Balanced Metal Nature

Figure 3.31. Yin Metal Nature

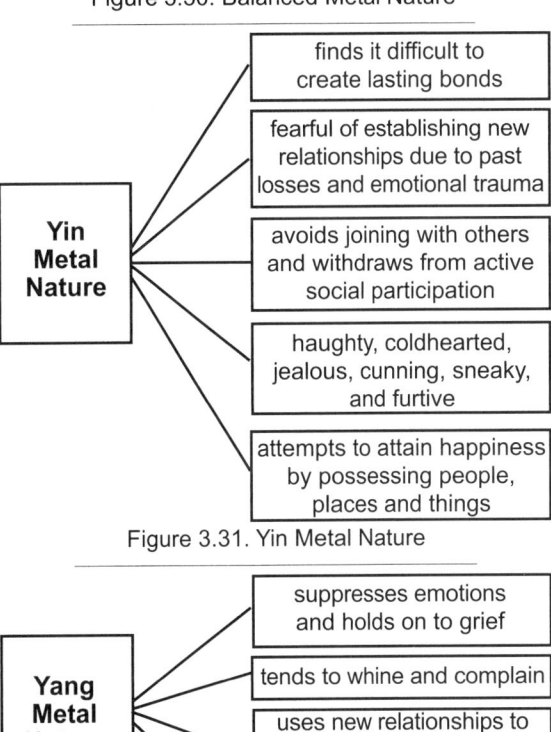

Figure 3.32. Yang Metal Nature

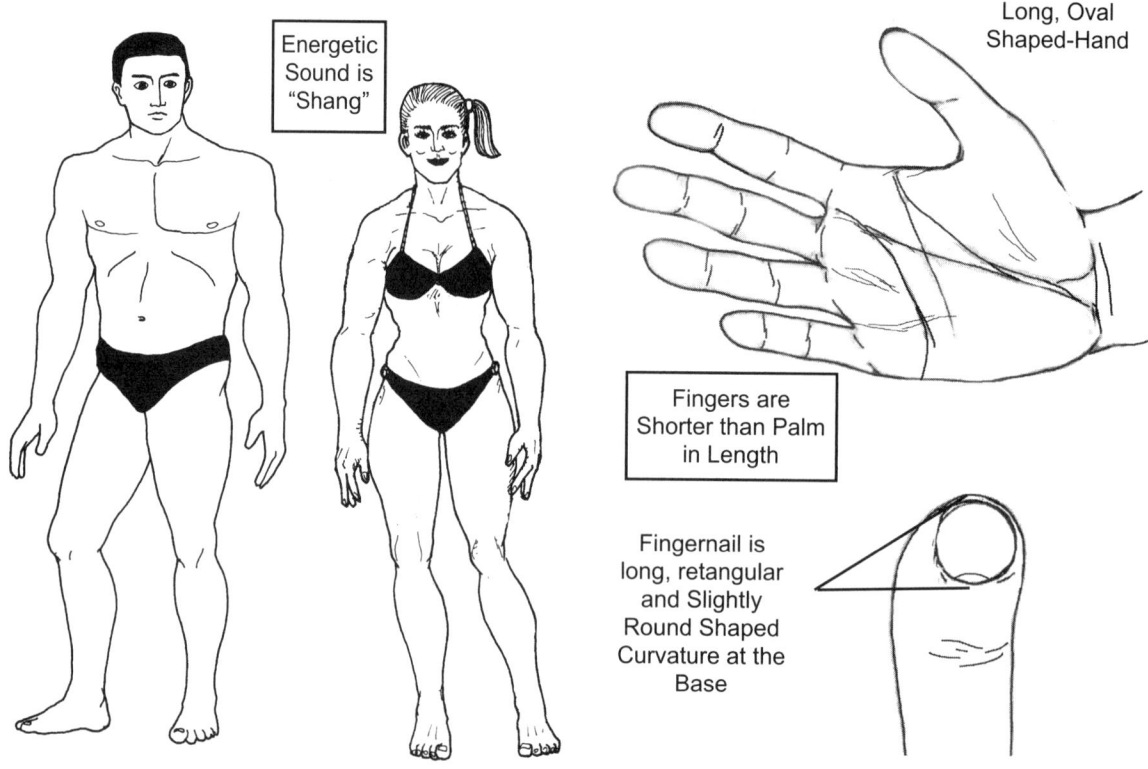

Figure 3.33. Metal Constitution in Males and Females

Figure 3.34. Metal Constitution Hand Features

problems in order to unload grief and control the situation. They use new relationships as an emotional bandage to avoid the unprocessed grief of their past relationships. They are also overly meticulous, independent, and strong-willed (Figure 3.32).

Treatment for Yang Metal nature individuals:

Treatment requires teaching them how to let go of the need to control and suppress their feelings, while allowing them to genuinely grieve over past wounds. They need to face the truth and be honest about their feelings, instead of selfishly using people and new relationships to cover up their grief. They also need to develop sympathy for the pain and sorrows of others and to put their own feelings of grief into a broader, healthier perspective.

Metal Outer Appearance

Metal constitution types usually have a subtle shade of white in their complexion. They usually have a relatively small head, square-shaped face with a triangular jaw, broad and square shoulders and upper back, flat abdomen, a strong voice, and a strong, muscular build (Figure 3.33).

The hands of a Metal Constitution individual generally have an oval shaped structure with a long palm, and fingers that are proportionally longer than the palm. The fingernails tend to be long with a rectangular curvature and sharp edges, and are slightly rounded at the nail base (Figure 3.34).

By nature, they enjoy autumn and winter but dislike spring and summer. This preference is due to the inherent vulnerabilities of the Metal constitution, making them especially susceptible to pathogenic invasion and disease during these seasons. Their dominant features include strong Lungs and white facial color. Their energetic sound is "shang."

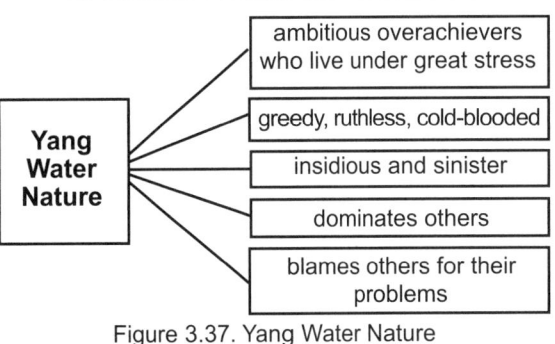

The Water Constitution

Water Personality

The Water personality can be divided into three subdivisions, which are described as follows:

1. **A Balanced Water Nature:** Predisposes individuals to be skilled negotiators who are not discouraged by difficulty and do not take foolish risks. They are sympathetic and loyal to their employers and their friends. They have a clear perspective and are sensitive and intuitive. They are powerful, tender, and soft. They have a firm will and know their boundaries and limitations. They are known for their inner strength and strong faith in themselves (Figure 3.35).

2. **A Yin Water Nature:** Predisposes individuals to lack spiritual, emotional, mental, and physical energy. They give up on life and surrender the control of their own destinies to inertia and external circumstances. They lack the determination to achieve their goals, doing everything halfheartedly, and becoming easily discouraged by difficult challenges (Figure 3.36).

Treatment for Yin Water nature individuals:

Treatment requires teaching them how to conserve and strengthen their energy by not reaching beyond their capacity. They need to learn to break down larger tasks into small sections that they can realistically complete. These individuals must learn how to follow their projects through to completion, and avoid procrastination. They also need to find the strength to overcome their fear of failure by learning to take action through the completion of their goals.

3. **A Yang Water Nature:** Predisposes individuals to be ambitious overachievers and to live under great stress. They lack consideration for others and can be reckless and foolhardy. They can also be greedy, ruthless, and cold-blooded. Seemingly modest, they can be insidious and sinister, concealing their true emotions by suppressing deeply rooted fears. Because they fear loss of control, they believe that their safety lies in their power and ability to dominate others. They habitually act in a self-serv-

Balanced Water Nature:
- skilled negotiators
- not discouraged by difficulty and do not take foolish risks
- sympathetic and loyal to employers and friends
- sensitive and intuitive
- powerful, tender, and soft
- firm will and know their boundaries and limitations
- strong inner strength and strong faith in themselves

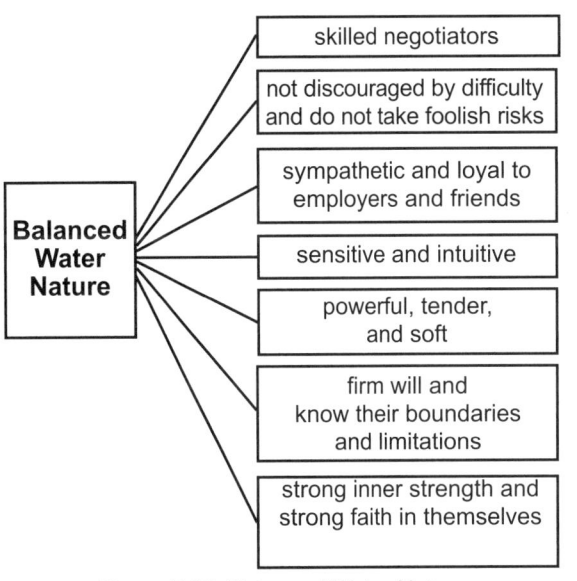

Figure 3.35. Balanced Water Nature

Yin Water Nature:
- lacks spiritual, emotional, mental, and physical energy
- gives up on life
- surrenders the control of own destinies to inertia and external circumstances
- lacks the determination to achieve their goals, doing everything halfheartedly
- becomes easily discouraged by difficult challenges

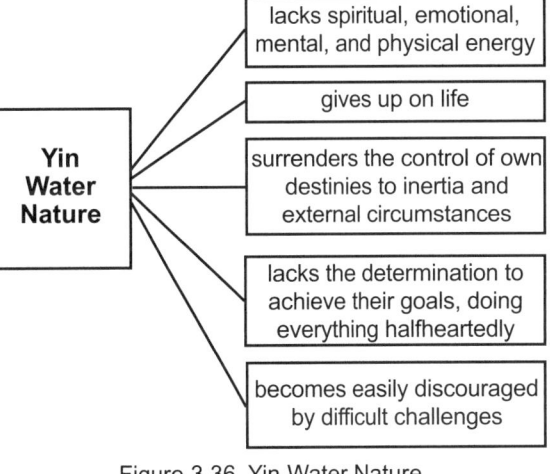

Figure 3.36. Yin Water Nature

Yang Water Nature:
- ambitious overachievers who live under great stress
- greedy, ruthless, cold-blooded
- insidious and sinister
- dominates others
- blames others for their problems

Figure 3.37. Yang Water Nature

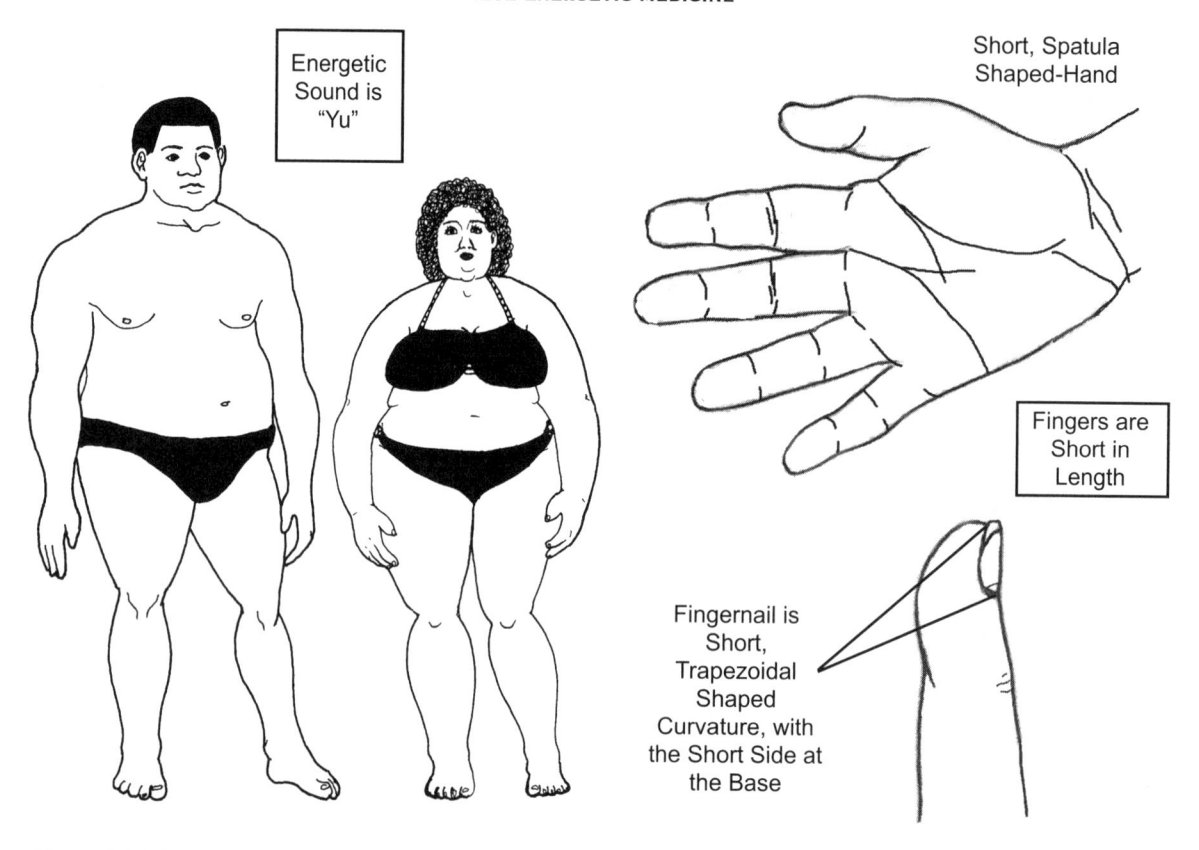

Figure 3.38. Water Constitution in Males and Females

Figure 3.39. Water Constitution Hand Features

ing manner and blame others for their problems (Figure 3.37).

TREATMENT FOR YANG WATER NATURE INDIVIDUALS:

Treatment consists of teaching them to learn how to act from inner stillness and gain strength and courage from their true selves. It is essential that they learn to surrender their ego and trust in the processes of the divine. They need to learn how to gain consideration for themselves and others, as well as how to open their hearts and begin to love. They also need to emotionally and physically slow down and to balance their activities with rest.

WATER OUTER APPEARANCE

Water constitution types usually have a relatively dark complexion. They usually have a big round face with a broad, angular chin and jaw, large head, long back, large abdomen and substantial body mass (Figure 3.38). They have a long upper back and unbalanced or uneven physical features.

The hands of a Water Constitution individual generally have a short proportioned structure with short fingers. The fingernails tend to have a short convex curvature, with a trapezoidal shape beginning with the short side at the nail base (Figure 3.39).

By nature, they enjoy autumn and winter but dislike spring and summer. This preference is due to the inherent vulnerabilities of the Water constitution, making them especially susceptible to pathogenic invasion and disease during these seasons. Their dominant features include their digestive system and black or dark facial color. Their energetic sound is "yu."

COMBINED CONSTITUTIONS

The Yellow Emperor's physician, Shao Shi, taught that the Five Element Constitutions consist of both internal and external energetic forms based on the strength and energetic development of the individual's Jing, Qi, and Blood. This system recognizes twenty five constitutional types. Thus, each the five basic Element Constitutions has an apparent external constitution, as well as a hidden internal aspect (Wood, Fire, Earth, Metal, or Water).

After determining the patient's physical constitution, the individual is then classified in terms of five different colors (green/blue, red, yellow, white or black), and further classified according to the five Prenatal (Heavenly) notes (Jue, Gong, Zhi, Shang or Yu).

The Five Element Constitutions are guidelines which aid the Qigong doctor in evaluating the patient. These guidelines are not fixed, and the doctor is likely to encounter combinations of two or more of these elements within one patient.

When several constitutions combine in an individual, the combination may be congenital or acquired in nature. The Qigong doctor must evaluate the patient, differentiating between his or her congenital and acquired tissue formations. For example, a woman who has large hips (Water), and a small chest and shoulders (Wood), probably inherited this structure from her parents. This woman's physical structure and personality would then be considered to be a combination of both Water and Wood (depending on which internal organ characteristic dominates).

A female patient who is a swimmer, on the other hand, may be congenitally Wood, but may have developed a dominant Metal upper physique through years of physical training. If, through intense physical activity, someone acquires a Metal physique, he or she may also acquire a Metal personality. This depends on the psychological predisposition rooted within his or her internal organs.

The external physical structure serves as a visual guide to congenital and acquired patterning, balance, and internal organ interactions.

PERSONALITY CONSTITUTIONS OF THE EIGHT EXTRAORDINARY VESSELS

Another system of identifying personality traits is in the observation the four personality constitutions of the Eight Extraordinary Vessels.

By observing the patient's personality and overall energetic and emotional demeanor, the Qigong doctor can determine which organ or organ system is deficient, and which is excess. Based on this information, the Qigong doctor can establish an appropriate treatment plan.

In this system, the Qigong doctor observes the patient's dominant Yin or Yang emotional characteristics to determine which of the Eight Extraordinary Vessels are governing his or her present emotional state. These personality traits can change or appear in different combinations based on the interaction of acquired and congenital organ energy patterns. Thus, organ patterns and personality traits may change with the patient's age (maturation) or situation (environment).

THE PATHOLOGICAL PERSONALITY TYPE OF THE GOVERNING AND YANG HEEL VESSELS

The Governing (Du) and Yang Heel (Yang Qiao) Extraordinary Vessels are located on the back and lateral sides of the body. They affect the Urinary Bladder, Stomach, and Gall Bladder Channels. To access the flow of energy within the Governing and Yang Heel Vessels, the Qigong doctor stimulates the patient's SI-3 and UB-62 points simultaneously (see Chapter 6).

The pathological personality types of the Governing and Yang Heel Vessels are divided into Yin (deficient) and Yang (excess) emotional profiles, described as follows:

1. **Patients with Deficient Qi in the Governing and Yang Heel Vessels** tend to be weak-willed and "spineless." They tend to be overly submissive and easily give up their personal power. They lack determination, courage, clarity, and inner strength, and have no control over their lives. They participate as little as possible in life for fear of failure (Figure 3.40).

2. **Patients with Excess Qi in the Governing and Yang Heel Vessels** tend to be tense, overpressured, stiff, rigid, inflexible, stubborn, and

awkward. They are narrow-minded and over-controlling. Fearful of letting go, they overcompensate by attempting to restrict reality (Figure 3.41).

THE PATHOLOGICAL PERSONALITY TYPE OF THE CONCEPTION AND YIN HEEL VESSELS

The Conception Vessel (Ren) and Yin Heel (Yin Qiao) Extraordinary Vessels are located on the front and inside of the body. They affect the Lung and Kidney Channels, which in turn affect the Kidneys, Lungs, and Heart organs. To access the energy within Conception and Yin Heel Vessels, the Qigong doctor stimulates the patient's Lu-7 and Kd-6 points simultaneously. The pathological personality types of the Conception and Yin Heel Vessels are divided into Yin (deficient) and Yang (excess) emotional profiles, described as follows:

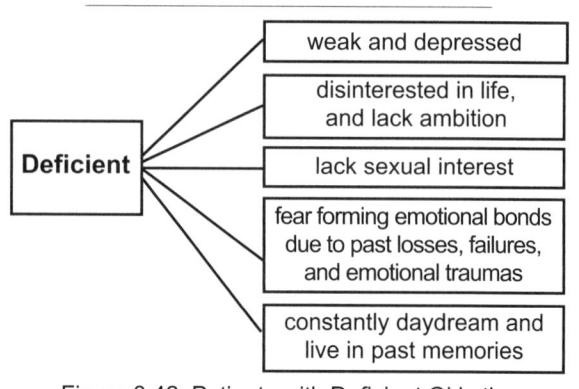

1. **Patients with Deficient Qi in the Conception and Yin Heel Vessels** tend to be weak and depressed. They live in the past, are disinterested in life, have no ambition, and also lack sexual interest. It is hard for them to form new relationships because they fear forming emotional bonds due to past losses, failures, and emotional traumas. They constantly daydream and live in their own world of past memories (Figure 3.42).

2. **Patients with Excess Qi in the Conception and Yin Heel Vessels** tend to participate in life but hold on to and suppress their grief. They fail to let go of emotional attachments and fear being alone. Female patients with this energetic pattern usually develop Qi stagnations resulting in breast cysts, tumors, and cancer, as well as uterine fibroids and uterine cancer (Figure 3.43).

THE PATHOLOGICAL PERSONALITY TYPE OF THE BELT AND YANG LINKING VESSELS

The Belt (Dai) and Yang Linking (Yang Wei) Extraordinary Vessels are located around the waist and on the outside of the body. They affect the Gall Bladder and Triple Burner Channels which in turn affect the Kidneys, Liver, and Gall Bladder organs. To access the energy within the Belt and Yang Linking Vessels, the Qigong doctor stimulates the patient's GB-41 and TB-5 points si-

Deficient
- weak-willed and "spineless"
- overly submissive and easily give up their personal power
- lack determination, courage, clarity, and inner strength
- lack control over their lives
- participate as little as possible in life for fear of failure

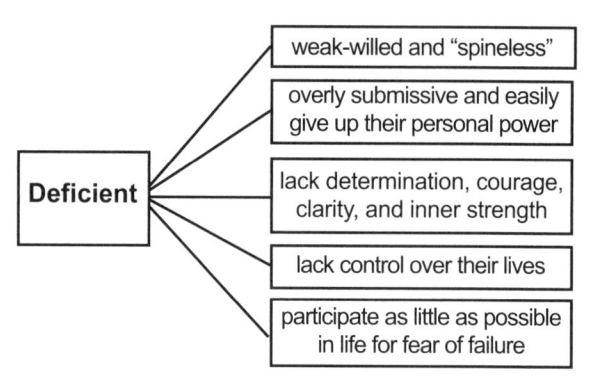

Figure 3.40. Patients with Deficient Qi in the Governing and Yang Heel Vessels

Excess
- tense, overpressured, stiff, rigid, inflexible, stubborn, and awkward
- narrow-minded and overcontrolling
- fearful of letting go

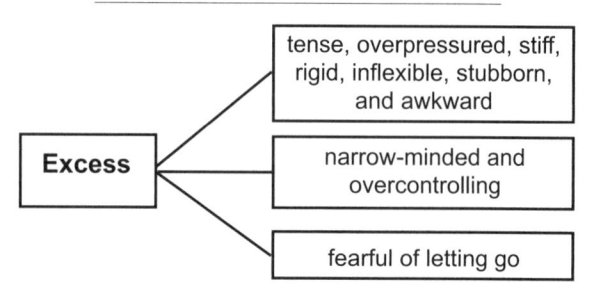

Figure 3.41. Patients with Excess Qi in the Governing and Yang Heel Vessels

Deficient
- weak and depressed
- disinterested in life, and lack ambition
- lack sexual interest
- fear forming emotional bonds due to past losses, failures, and emotional traumas
- constantly daydream and live in past memories

Figure 3.42. Patients with Deficient Qi in the Conception and Yin Heel Vessels

Excess
- retain and suppress grief
- fail to let go of emotional attachments and fear being alone

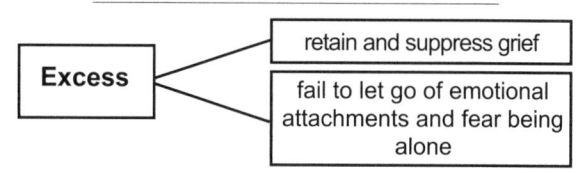

Figure 3.43. Patients with Excess Qi in the Conception and Yin Heel Vessels

multaneously. The pathological personality types of the Belt and Yang Linking Vessels are divided into Yin (deficient) and Yang (excess) emotional profiles, described as follows:

1. **Patients with Deficient Qi in the Belt and Yang Linking Vessels** are considered weak, indecisive, and unproductive. They fear criticism and are touchy, snappy, irritable, and hypersensitive. They also have low self-esteem and also lack sexual interest (Figure 3.44).
2. **Patients with Excess Qi in the in the Belt and Yang Linking Vessels** are aggressive, angry, resentful, bitter, and vindictive. They tend to be opinionated, inflexible, intolerant, domineering, selfish, and frustrated. Their sex life is based on anger or rage (Figure 3.45).

THE PATHOLOGICAL PERSONALITY TYPE OF THE THRUSTING AND YIN LINKING VESSELS

The Thrusting (Chong) and Yin Linking (Yin Wei) Extraordinary Vessels are located within the center of the body (internally) and on the medial and anterior aspects of the body (externally). They affect the Kidney and Stomach Channels which, in turn, affect the Kidneys, Spleen, and Heart organs. To access the energy within the Thrusting and Yin Linking Vessels, the Qigong doctor stimulates the patient's Sp-4 and Pc-6 points simultaneously. The pathological personality types of the Thrusting and Yin Linking Vessels are divided into Yin (deficient) and Yang (excess) emotional profiles, described as follows:

1. **Patients with Deficient Thrusting and Yin Linking Vessels** are physically and emotionally weak. They quickly become exhausted and depressed. It is easy for them to have their feelings hurt, and they take a long time to recover from emotional upsets. Their internal emotional world is constructed of fear, anxiety, worry, and tension. They do not connect well with the outside world or gain much pleasure from life or relationships (Figure 3.46).
2. **Patients with an Excess in the Thrusting and Yin Linking Vessels** tend to participate in life but have difficulty expressing their affection and communicating their needs in relationships. They are inclined to have stagnant Qi

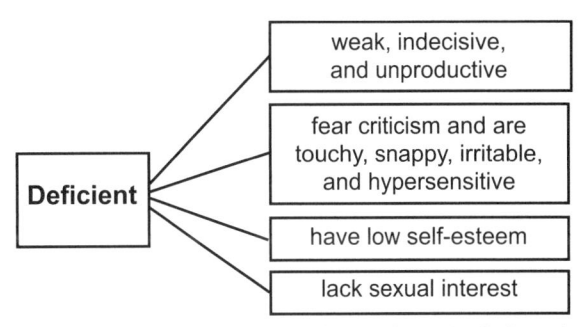

Figure 3.44. Patients with Deficient Qi in the Belt and Yang Linking Vessels

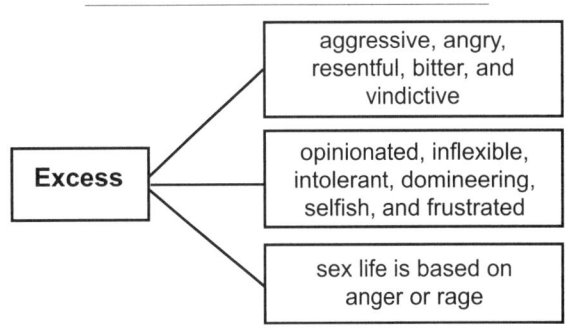

Figure 3.45. Patients with Excess Qi in the Belt and Yang Linking Vessels

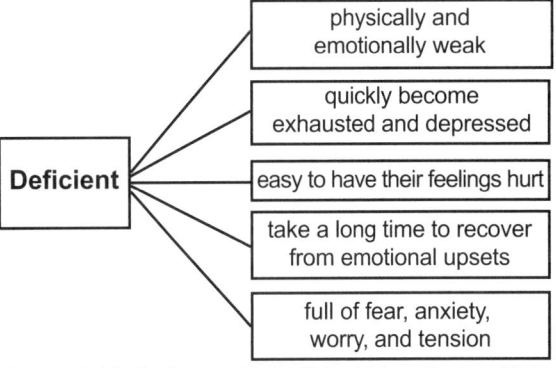

Figure 3.46. Patients with Deficient Thrusting and Yin Linking Vessels

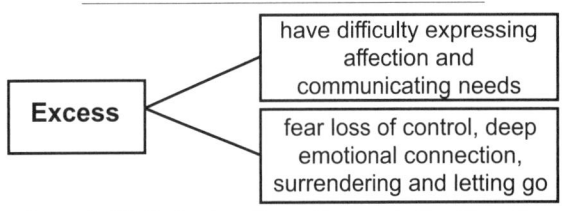

Figure 3.47. Patients with an Excess in the Thrusting and Yin Linking Vessels

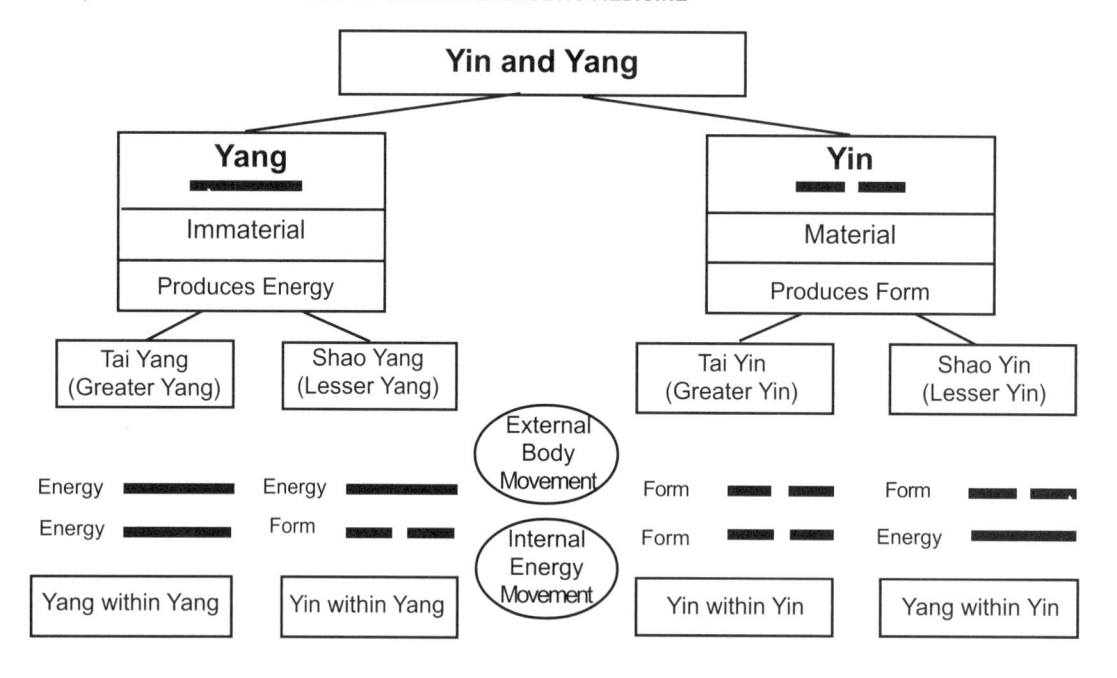

Figure 3.48. Yin and Yang Expressing the Four Phases of Universal Energy

and Blood in the chest, epigastrium, or Uterus due to fear, anxiety, worry, and sorrow. In their personal relationships, they fear loss of control and cannot make a commitment or a deep emotional connection with others. They also fear surrendering and letting go in their love and sexual relationships (Figure 3.47).

Yin and Yang and the Yao Image

In certain cases involving surgery, congenital deformity, or traumas, it is neither possible, nor advisable to directly treat certain areas of the patient's body. The Qigong doctor must then choose an indirect method of treatment to ensure better results. One such method available to the Qigong doctor involves an understanding of the Yao image and its correlation to a patient's physical and energetic anatomy. In order to better comprehend the complexity of this diagnostic and treatment modality, the Qigong doctor must first understand the energetic origin of the Yao images.

All matter is composed of different proportions of Yin and Yang energy (Figure 3.48). Within the infinite space of the Wuji, Yin and Yang energy continually gathers and disperses, giving rise to all forces and cycles of change in the universe. This interaction of Yin and Yang energy develops and transforms into four phases (or stages) of universal energy: Greater Yin, Lesser Yin, Greater Yang, and Lesser Yang. These four phases can be explained as follows (Figure 3.49):

1. **Greater Yin (Tai Yin)** is associated with midnight and the new moon phase. Modern physicists associate the Greater Yin with a weak nuclear force.
2. **Lesser Yin (Shao Yin)** is associated with sunset and the waning moon phase. Modern physicists associate the Lesser Yin with a heavy force and gravity.
3. **Greater Yang (Tai Yang)** is associated with high noon and the full moon phase. Modern physicists associate the Greater Yang with a strong nuclear force.
4. **Lesser Yang (Shao Yang)** is associated with sunrise and the waxing moon phase. Modern physicists associate the Lesser Yang with electromagnetism and a light force.

These four solar and lunar energetic phases

transform themselves into the energies of the eight foundational trigrams. These trigrams further combine to form sixty-four hexagrams and create the ancient binary system known as the Yi-Jing (I-Ching) or *Book of Changes*. The formation and patterning of these energetic powers (or stages) vary according to the composition of Yin and Yang expressed through the energetic symbols of the Yao.

A Yao is a line that represents either Yin or Yang energy. The lines fall into two categories:
- **The negative Yao** is symbolized by broken lines (- -) and relates to Yin energy
- **The positive Yao** is symbolized by solid lines (---) and relates to Yang energy

When these lines are stacked in combinations of three, they form trigrams (a group of three Yao lines). Hexagrams, or six lines, are formed when pairs of trigrams are joined. The lines are arranged from bottom to top, with the first Yao beginning on the bottom (Figure 3.50).

Ancient Daoist Prenatal and Postnatal Yao Formations

Ancient Daoist Qigong masters cultivated massive amounts of Qi and Shen by directing their attention towards the fusion of Kan (Kidney Water) and Li (Heart Fire). They believed that after an individual is born, his or her internal Qian (Heaven) Trigram changes from a pure Yang state (three solid Yao lines), to the Li (Heart Fire) Trigram, containing one Yin Yao between two Yang Yao lines. Additionally, the individual's internal Kun (Earth) Trigram also changes, transforming from a pure Yin state (three broken Yao lines) into the Kan (Kidney Water) Trigram, containing one Yang Yao between two Yin Yao lines (Figure 3.51)

The primary goal of the ancient Daoists was to fill the center of their Li (Heart Fire) Trigram with energy of the Yang gathered from the Kan (Kidney Water), and return the Li Trigram back into Qian (Heaven). Simultaneously, the Daoists would fill the center of the Kan (Kidney Water) Trigram with the energy of the Yin gathered from the Li (Heart Fire) and return the Kan Trigram back into Kun (Earth).

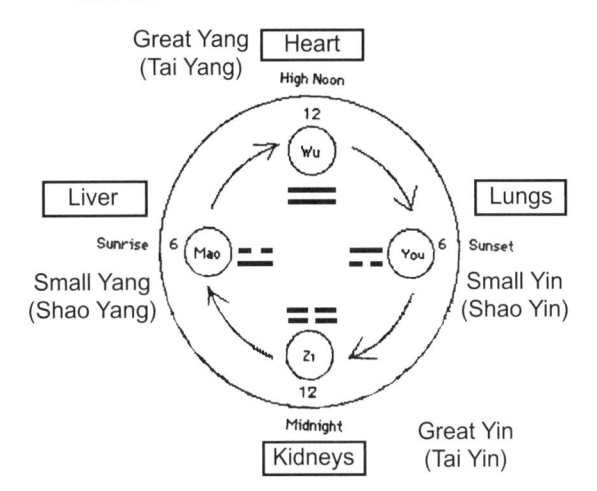

Figure 3.49. The Four Principal Time Periods

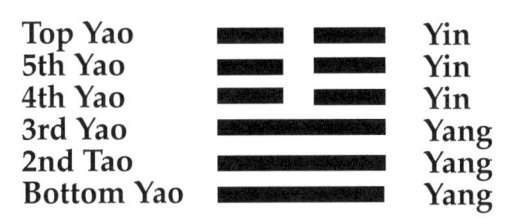

Figure 3.50. This diagram shows a hexagram composed of an upper and lower trigram. In this particular example, the upper trigram contains all Yin Yaos (symbolized by broken lines), while the lower trigram is composed of all Yang Yaos (symbolized by solid lines).

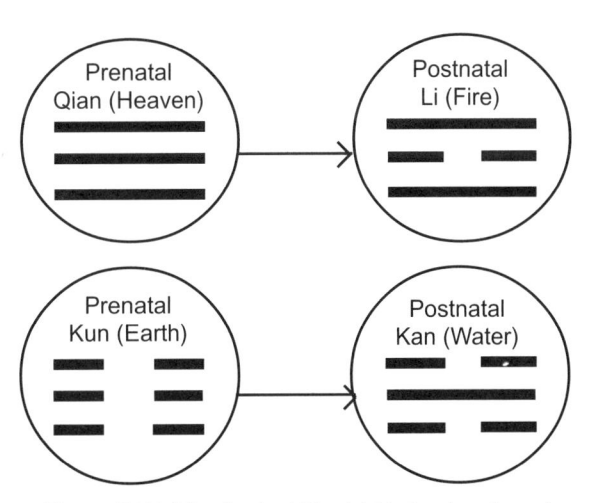

Figure 3.51. The Ancient Daoist Understanding of Prenatal and Postnatal Transformations.

Yao Image and Physical Anatomy

The Yao Trigrams and their relationship to the body's physical and energetic structure can be utilized by the Qigong doctor for both diagnosis and treatment. According to the ancient Daoists, the human body is subdivided into three regions: the lower region pertains to Earth; the middle region pertains to Man; and the upper region pertains to Heaven. Each region was further subdivided three more times. Each of the three subdivided levels contained the metaphysical aspect of the material, energetic and spiritual dimensions of Heaven (Shen: Spirit), Earth (Qi: Energy) and Man (Jing: Matter).

In one form of Medical Qigong Diagnosis, the doctor employs the Yao lines of the hexagram as a template and arranges Yin and Yang patterns alongside the patient's body. The arrangement of Yao images assists the doctor in recognizing the patient's physical and energetic imbalances. This type of Yao image diagnosis has been used in China for centuries.

Each Yao corresponds to a different region of the human body, as well as a different aspect of Qi. The system of energetic Yao correspondence with the physical body is described as follows:

1. **The two lowest Yaos** correspond physically to the feet and legs and energetically to the body's interaction with Earth Qi (soil, water and wind of the environment).
   - The 1st Yao extends from the feet to the knees.
   - The 2nd Yao extends from the knees to the upper thighs.
2. **The middle two Yaos** correspond physically to the lower and upper abdominal regions and energetically to the body's interaction with Human Qi (thoughts and emotional responses pertaining to Jing, Qi and Shen).
   - The 3rd Yao extends from the perineum to the navel.
   - The 4th Yao extends from the navel to the xiphoid process and the diaphragm.
3. **The upper two Yaos** correspond physically to the upper chest, neck, and head regions, and energetically to the body's interaction with Heaven Qi (sun, moon and stars of the universe).
   - The 5th Yao extends from the xiphoid process of the diaphragm to the top of the manubrium at the base of the throat.
   - The 6th Yao extends from the manubrium to the top of the head.

The ancient Qigong masters applied their knowledge of the hexagrams to explain the etiology, pathology, clinical manifestations and treatment principles of the patient's disease. Through observation and study, the Qigong doctor is able to determine the energetic and emotional associations the patient has with the surrounding environment. This diagnosis is achieved by observing the body's relationship to the three energetic Yao divisions of Heaven, Earth, and Man (Figure 3.52).

For example, if the patient's upper Yao is out of harmony with the patient's middle or lower Yaos, his or her energetic balance may be compromised. Such a patient is likely to experience a spiritual disconnection with his or her body. In this example, if the upper Yao is in a relatively excess condition, it will result in a Yang condition (restlessness) due to an excess spiritual "Heaven" state. If the patient's upper Yao is deficient, it will result in a Yin condition (tired) due to a deficient spiritual "Heaven" state.

Upper and Lower Hexagrams

In addition to applying the hexagrams to assess the body's relationship to Heaven, Earth, and Man, the ancient Chinese Qigong masters also studied two additional hexagrams for clinical evaluation. These hexagrams were known as the upper and lower hexagrams. In using the upper and lower hexagrams for diagnosis and treatment, the Qigong doctor further divided the patient's body into six upper Yaos and six lower Yaos. This division was used to determine the patient's dominant emotional and energetic patterns, and diagnosed where the patient's Qi was gathering, dispersing or stagnating.

In the Ming Dynasty (1368-1644), Tang Rongchuan stated in his book *Detailed Explanations of the Application of the Book of Changes to Medicine*, "In the clinical environment, the body may be divided into two different sets of hexagram constructions [the upper and the lower hexagram par-

Chapter 3: Tissue Formation and Development

- The top or 6th Yao is from the neck to the top of the head (Heaven)

- The 5th Yao is from the diaphragm to the neck (Heaven)

- The 4th Yao is from the navel to the diaphragm (Man)

- The 3rd Yao is the lower perineum to the navel (Man)

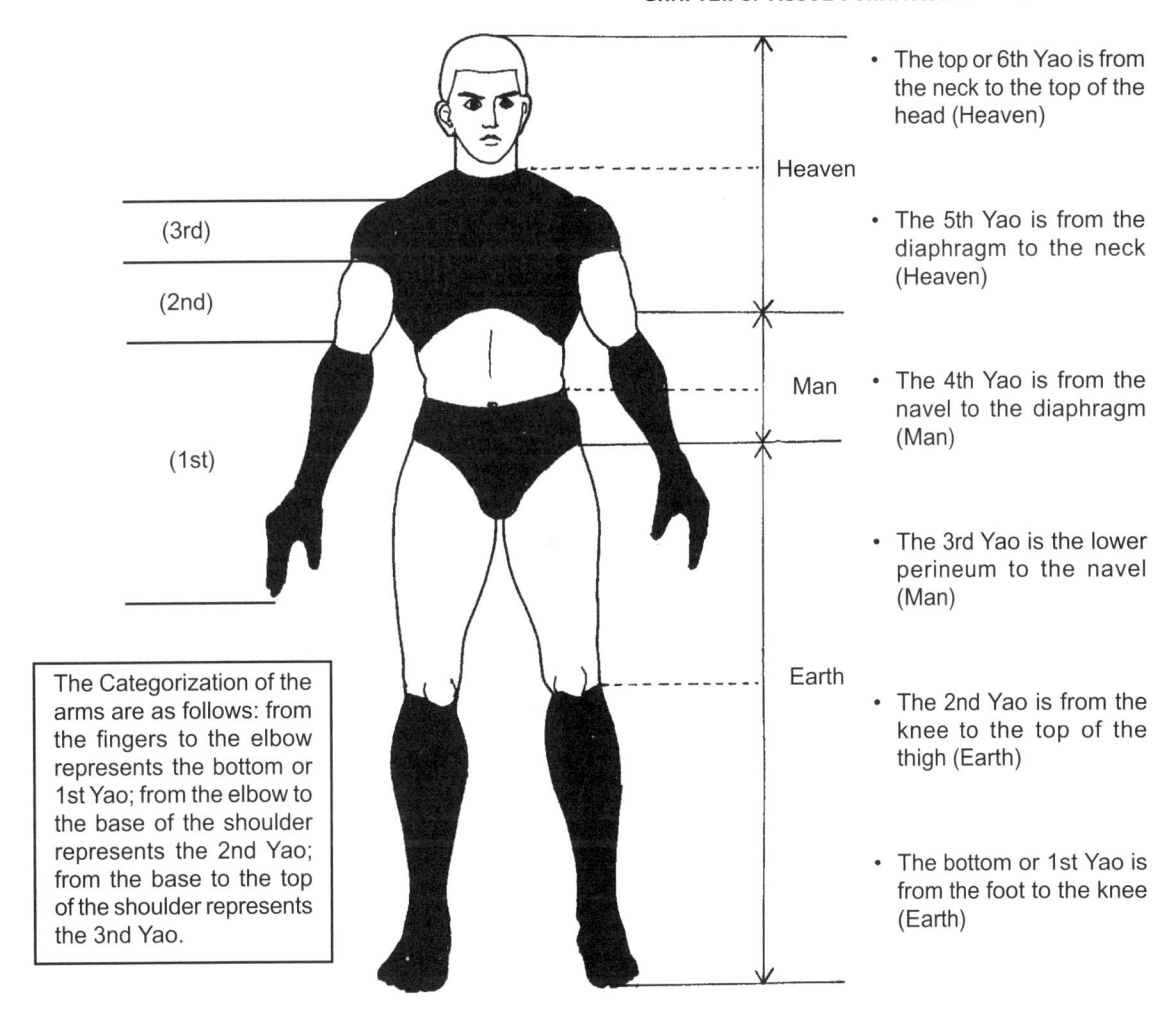

- The 2nd Yao is from the knee to the top of the thigh (Earth)

- The bottom or 1st Yao is from the foot to the knee (Earth)

The Categorization of the arms are as follows: from the fingers to the elbow represents the bottom or 1st Yao; from the elbow to the base of the shoulder represents the 2nd Yao; from the base to the top of the shoulder represents the 3nd Yao.

Figure 3.52. Yao Image and the Human Body

tition] for the purpose of making a diagnosis, detecting Qi, and for performing therapeutic Qigong treatments." This relationship of Yao positioning corresponds to both the channel system and the nervous system.

Physical disorders located within these hexagrams are generally expressed as symptoms manifesting in the extremities. If stagnant Qi or other abnormal conditions occur in any particular part of the body, an imbalance of both internal and external Qi may be detected in either its corresponding Yao area, or that specific Yao area of the body.

The body's upper torso, arms, neck, and head are divided into what is known as the upper hexagram partitions, while the body's lower limbs and torso are divided into the lower hexagram partitions. In this model, the six Yao of the upper hexagram interlock with the six Yao of the lower hexagram at the chest and abdomen. By applying these sets of hexagrams, the Qigong doctor has a template with which to understand the energetic patterning of patient's body.

The Upper Hexagram Construction

The upper hexagram extends from the base of the perineum to the top of the head. The six Yaos are organized as follows:

145

1. **The 1st or bottom Yao** encompasses the area from the pubic region to the navel. Reproductive, digestive, and urinary tract diseases are found in this area.
2. **The 2nd Yao** encompasses the area from the navel to the xiphoid process. Digestion, elimination, the distribution of nutrients, pancreatic diseases, problems with the Kidneys, adrenal glands, Liver, and Spleen are all found in this area.
3. **The 3rd Yao** encompasses the area from the xiphoid process to the clavicles at the base of the throat. Respiratory and circulatory diseases are found in this area.
4. **The 4th Yao** encompasses the area from the clavicles at the base of the throat to the tip of the nose. Teeth, jaw, and thyroid diseases are found in this area.
5. **The 5th Yao** encompasses the area from the tip of the nose to the eyebrow. Sinus problems, frontal headaches, and ear, nose, and eye diseases are found in this area.
6. **The 6th or top Yao** encompasses the area from the eyebrows to the top of the head. Headaches, brain tumors, and upper cranial dysfunctions are found in this area.

The Lower Hexagram Construction

The lower hexagram extends from the bottom of the patient's feet to the base of the patient's throat. The six Yaos are organized as follows:

1. **The 1st or bottom Yao** encompasses the area from the bottom of each foot to the ankle. Foot, toe, and ankle problems are found in this area.
2. **The 2nd Yao** encompasses the area from the ankles to the knees. Shin splints and calf and ankle problems are found in this area.
3. **The 3rd Yao** encompasses the area from the knees to the pubic symphysis. Thigh, knee, and quadriceps problems are found in this area.
4. **The 4th Yao** encompasses the area from the pubic region to the navel. Reproductive, digestive, and urinary tract diseases are found in this area.
5. **The 5th Yao** encompasses the area from the navel to the xiphoid process. Digestion, elimination, the distribution of nutrients, pancreatic diseases, problems with the Kidneys, adrenal glands, Liver, and Spleen are all found in this area.
6. **The 6th or top Yao** encompasses the area from the xiphoid process to the clavicles at the base of the throat. Respiratory and circulatory diseases are found in this area.

THERAPEUTIC USE OF THE YAOS

The entire body can be treated by focusing on one small area. When excess, deficient, or stagnant Qi occurs in one part of the body, the imbalance is detectable in that area or its corresponding region on the body's extremities. This ancient Chinese modality of treatment is the historical root of what is popularly called reflexology in the West.

When the Yao images are superimposed onto the patient's body, the patient can be diagnosed according to the Yin and Yang energetic symptoms expressed. This diagnosis can be either through the patient's extremities (hands, forearms, arms, feet, shins, and thighs), or through the six divisions located on the patient's torso and head. A Yao hexagram can additionally be visualized on specific locations of the patient's body such as the face, nose, ears, hand, or foot for diagnosis. The base of the palm, for example, corresponds to the lower abdominal area and reproductive organs, and relates to the 1st Yao in the hexagram applied to the hands. The six Yao areas of each hand provide a basis for diagnosis, treatment of diseases, and even for the perception and prediction of certain future diseases (Figure 3.53).

As an example of how the Qigong doctor can use the six Yaos of the body for Medical Qigong therapy, consider the following situation: an elderly patient with a problem in his prostate area visits the Qigong doctor. The prostate is located in the lower abdominal area, which is in the 1st Yao of the upper hexagram. Since the six Yao positions can be transferred to the hands and feet, the doctor knows that this particular Yao correlates with the 1st Yao of the foot. Therefore, the doctor may focus his or her attention on the foot as an energetic entry point into the patient's prostate area.

The diagram depicts the correspondence of the Yaos of the body to the Yaos of the hands and feet.

6. The third or last joint of the toes and fingers pertains to the top Yao and the energy of Heaven

5. The middle joint of the toes and fingers pertains to the 5th Yao and the energy of Heaven

4. The lower or first joint of the toes and fingers pertains to the 4th Yao and the energy of Man

3. The ball of the foot and the upper palm pertain to the 3rd Yao and the energy of Man

2. The instep of the foot and the mid-palm with the thumb pertain to the 2nd Yao and the energy of Earth

1. The heel and lower palm pertain to the bottom Yao and the energy of Earth

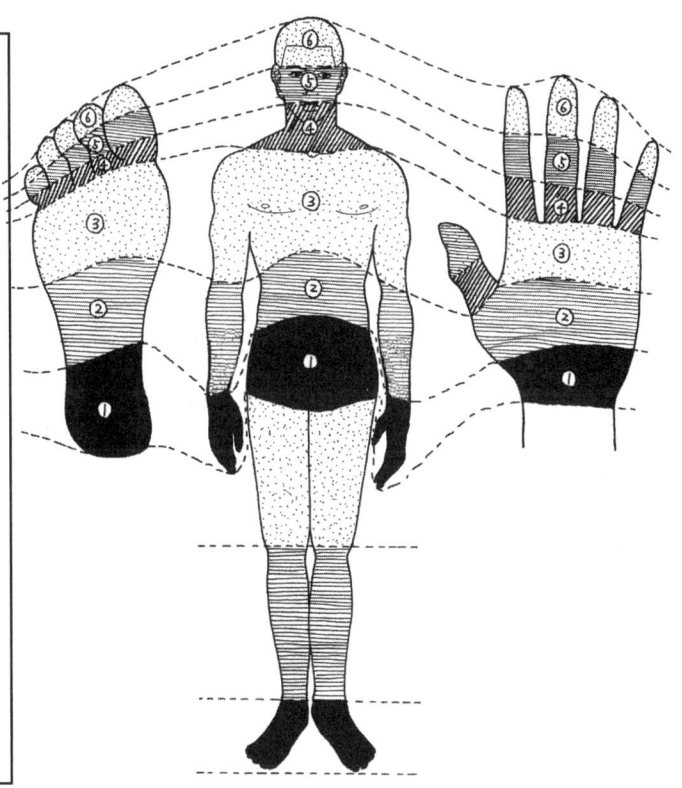

Figure 3.53. The Therapeutic Use of the Yaos

When dividing the foot into six Yaos, the Qigong doctor knows that the 1st Yao of the foot is the heel area. In order to treat the prostate gland, the doctor will focus his or her treatment on the patient's heel and ankle area. Alternatively, the doctor could have chosen the 1st Yao area of the hand, which is considered the 1st Yao position of the arm. Thus, the 1st Yao of the hand corresponds to the prostate and urogenital area.

Herbs and the Yaos

Herbs may also be classified and prescribed in accordance with the six Yao hexagram concept. With plants, the Yao correspondences are described as follows (Figure 3.54):
1. **The roots** correspond to the bottom or 1st Yao
2. **The stalk** corresponds to the 2nd Yao
3. **The upper stem** corresponds to the 3rd Yao
4. **The branches** correspond to the 4th Yao
5. **The leaves** correspond to the 5th Yao
6. **The flowers and fruit** correspond to the top or 6th Yao

When plants are used as medicine, the part of the plant corresponding to the number and position of the Yao manifests its healing properties through a particular energetic action, such as ascending, descending, floating, or sinking Qi. The achyranthes root (Niu Xi), for example, corresponds to the 1st Yao, and leads healing Qi downward; helping to heal the patient's lower back, knees and joints. The chrysanthemum flower (Ju Hua), on the other hand, corresponds to the top Yao, and leads healing Qi up into the patient's head and eyes.

Identifying Introverted and Extroverted Structures

Qi flows through the matrix of the connective tissue and adapts to the postural and structural demands of the body by changing the density and direction of the body's connective tissues and inner fasciae. Any postural habit creates an imprinted tissue memory in the supporting con-

VOLUME 1, SECTION 1: FOUNDATIONS OF CHINESE ENERGETIC MEDICINE

6. The fruit or flower of the herb pertains to the top Yao and the energy of Heaven

5. The leaf of the herb pertains to the 5th Yao and the energy of Heaven

4. The branch of the herb pertains to the 4th Yao and the energy of Man

3. The upper stem of the herb pertains to the 3rd Yao and the energy of Man

2. The stalk of the herb pertains to the 2nd Yao and the energy of Earth

1. The root of the herb pertains to the bottom Yao and the energy of Earth

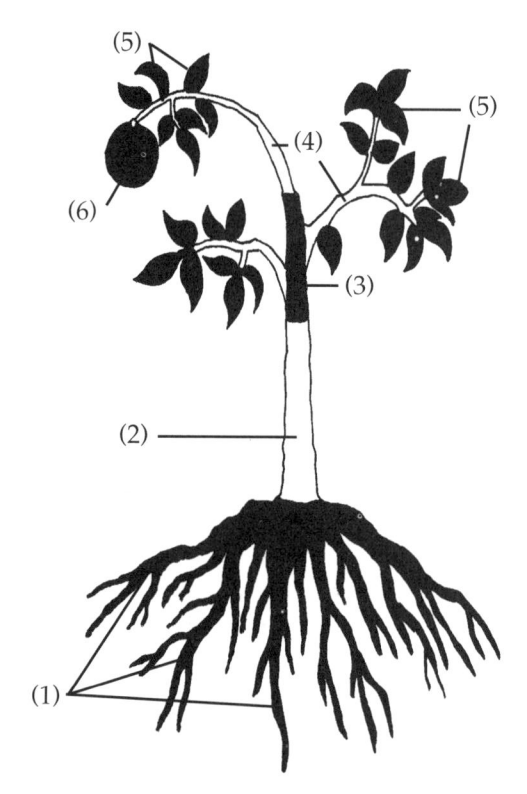

Figure 3.54. The Yao Image Applied to Plants

nective tissue, as well as an energetic memory in the supporting channels of Qi. These imprints can result in introverted or extroverted postural structures.

Each introverted (Yin) and extroverted (Yang) postural structure has a predictable impact on the myofascial webbing, as well as on the emotional disposition. Emotions create changes in posture, Qi flow, and breathing patterns and conversely, can be influenced by them. The patient's breathing pattern, emotional state and Qi flow affect his or her posture. Primary structural patterns are determined by the patient's habitual posture, which is in turn a composite of habitual breathing patterns, Qi flow and emotional states. All chronic stress creates postural imprinting or tissue memory and a corresponding energetic memory in the supporting Qi field.

INTROVERTED STRUCTURE

In a patient with an introverted structure, the back (Yang) area is rounded, and the his or her muscle structure is usually well-developed. The front of the body (Yin), especially around the chest and Heart area, is retracted, resulting in a narrow chest. The patient's head is generally held off-center, and his or her shoulders are sunken and slightly forward. Additionally, the patient's pelvis is tilted back with the genitals retracted (posterior tilt). This introverted condition is commonly referred to as "extended Yang and retracted Yin" of the upper torso (Figure 3.55).

EXTROVERTED STRUCTURE

In a patient with an extroverted structure, the back (Yang) area is retracted, while the front of the patient's body is expanded (Yin) and overly exposed. The head is usually held vertically, the

CHAPTER 3: TISSUE FORMATION AND DEVELOPMENT

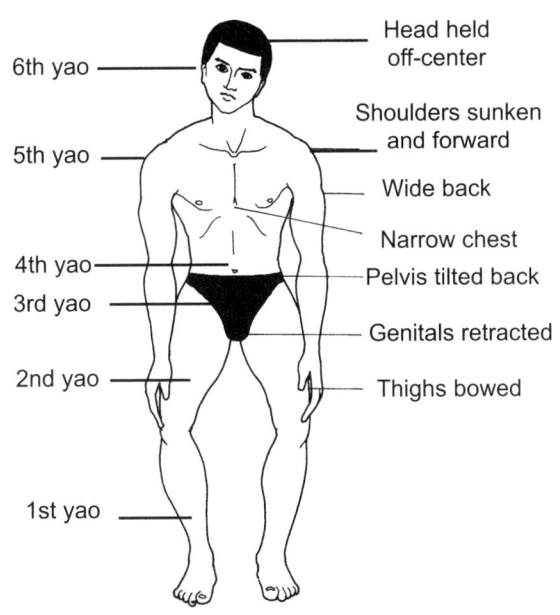

Figure 3.55. The Introverted Structure

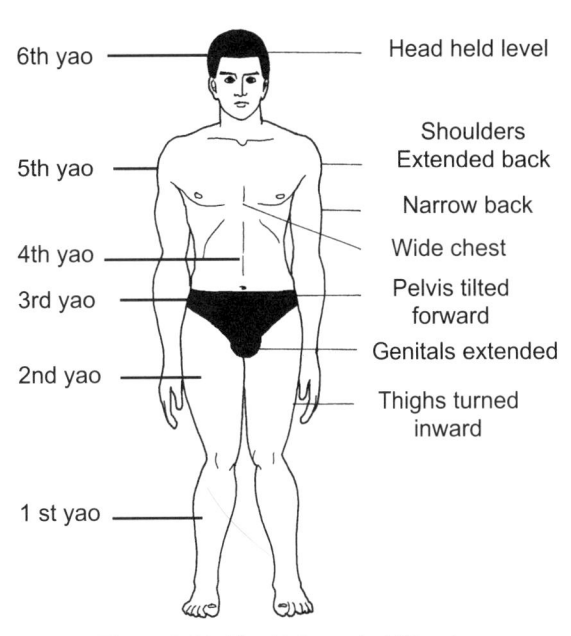

Figure 3.56. The Extroverted Structure

shoulders are slightly extended back and the chest is wide. Additionally, the patient's pelvis is tilted forward with genitals extended (anterior tilt). This extroverted condition is commonly referred to as "extended Yin and retracted Yang" of the upper back (Figure 3.56).

COMBINED STRUCTURAL FORMATIONS

As with the Five Element Constitutions, the introverted and extroverted structures provide guidelines for the Qigong doctor to evaluate the patient. These guidelines are not fixed, and the doctor is most likely to encounter combinations of introverted and extroverted structures in one patient. When two structures combine in an individual, the combination may be congenital or acquired in nature. The Qigong doctor must differentiate between a patient's congenital and acquired tissue formations.

CONGENITAL AND ACQUIRED CELLULAR PATTERNS

The Qigong doctor evaluates the patient's physical condition according to whether the patterns are congenital or acquired. The doctor may ask questions to determine whether the condition was acquired (through exposure to environmental pathogens, diet, trauma, occupation), or inherited (congenital or genetic in origin). This information aids the Qigong doctor in obtaining a deeper understanding of the patient's condition, and in helping the patient reprogram any dysfunctional congenital or acquired cellular patterns, described as follows:

1. **Congenital Cellular Patterns and Disease** predispositions are locked within the patient's congenital Jing, and can be released like a biological time-bomb. This is similar to the Western medical concept of genetic or inherited disease. The goal of Qigong treatment is to alter the toxic energetic pattern and to help the patient's body recognize that the formation of the disease is a "mistake." Then, the doctor will awaken and stimulate the creative healing potential of the patient's soul as it expresses itself through the tissues.

   In order to reprogram these patterns, the Qigong doctor prescribes guided meditations that involve vivid imagination, colorful visualizations, and positive affirmations. These images are used to identify diseased patterns and to release and return them to the divine light. While in the presence of the divine light, the Xie (toxic) Qi can either be energetically transformed and recycled back to the patient as healing energy, or be energetically disintegrated and scattered into the universe. That way when healing, the void left by the released pattern is filled from within by the resonant expression of the patient's soul. Patients with a family history of cancer, for example, can neutralize this tendency by correctly employing this type of Medical Qigong imagery.

2. **Acquired Cellular Patterns and Diseases** arise from either external exposure to pathogens or the chronic suppression of emotions. The initial goal of the Qigong doctor is to assist the patient in discovering the origin of his or her present disease. The next step is to teach the patient to alter the toxic patterns.

In order to reprogram these patterns, the Qigong doctor will have the patient attempt to identify and eliminate external pathogenic factors. Next, the Qigong doctor eliminates pathogens from the patient's body and energetic fields. Finally, the doctor will Tonify the patient's internal organ system, Wei Qi and Righteous Qi.

The patient must additionally address chronic patterns of emotional suppression. In order to reprogram these toxic patterns, the Qigong doctor will help the patient identify specific emotions related to the initial trauma from the patient's personal history. Then, the Qigong doctor will encourage the patient to release the suppressed energy through Medical Qigong exercises and prescription meditations. A patient who has been experiencing severe headaches due to a stressful work or family environment could benefit from this kind of treatment.

Summary

By observing the patient's physical and structural development, the Medical Qigong doctor will gain an understanding of the strengths and weaknesses of the patient's internal organs and immune system. The four patterns of physical development and structural formation described in this chapter (The Five Element Constitutions, the Yao Hexagram Formations, the Yin or Yang Structures, and the Congenital and Acquired Cellular Patterns) are summarized as follows.

1. First, the doctor begins to diagnose the patient's physical body according to the Five Element Constitutions and the dominant element. This helps the doctor to understand the condition of the patient's internal organs.
2. The doctor further divides the patient's body into six upper and lower Yaos to determine the dominant energetic and emotional patterns (where the patient's Qi is gathering, collecting, and stagnating).
3. The doctor evaluates the patient's external structure according to his or her body's Yin and Yang characteristics to understand whether the patient has a primarily introverted or extroverted physique.
4. The doctor determines whether the patient's condition is congenital, acquired, or a combination of both. This information helps the doctor understand the nature of the energetic and cellular patterns underlying the disease.

Chapter 4
The Five Energies of the Human Body

The study of various forms of Qi and energetic transformations has led to one of the greatest theories in physics - the Law of Conservation of Energy. The Law of Conservation of Energy states that "energy can neither be created or destroyed. It may be transformed from one form into another, but the total amount of energy in a given system never changes."

Physics defines four types of energy: mechanical, electromagnetic, chemical and thermal. All four types of energy interrelate and convert from one to another. Electricity, for example, can be converted into sound, light, mechanical energy, and heat. Conversely, sound, light, mechanical energy, and heat can all be reconverted into electricity.

Western science is philosophically rooted in the "enlightenment" obtained from the seventeenth century period of Western Europe. This knowledge is still, for the most part, founded on the scientific principles established by Sir Isaac Newton and Descartes, and relies heavily on logical and measurable scientific evidence and methods. This observation generally sees humanity as separate and relatively independent from the cycles and processes of nature and the environment, viewing energy as an impersonal and inanimate force. This current Western scientific view has led to a separation of the individual's spirit, mind and emotions from his or her body and physical experiences.

The ancient Chinese believed that all things were intimately connected in a vast unbroken harmony existing within the eternal matrix of the Dao. They perceived human beings as a microcosm of the universe that surrounded them, with the same essential forces that motivated the macrocosm. This ancient view of energy is much more akin to the theories of quantum physics. Both Chinese energetic theories and quantum physics hypothesize that energy cannot be studied without taking into account the mind's influence over it. Furthermore, as energy and matter are interchangeable, energetic behavior cannot be studied independently of matter.

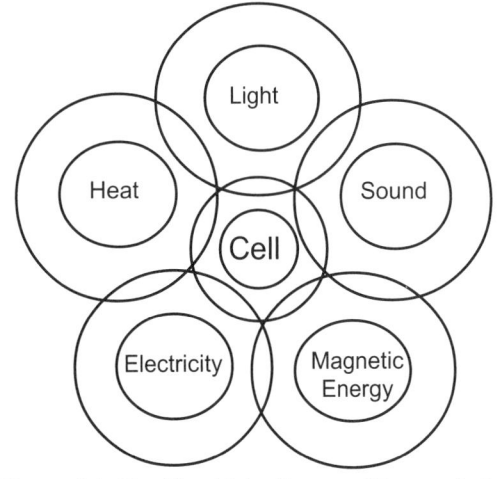

Figure 4.1. The Five Major Forms of Energy Active within the Human Body

From a Medical Qigong perspective, the entire human body is suffused with energy from the environment which is converted within the human organism. Light energy, for example, is absorbed, stored, and converted into various forms of energy within the body, similar to the way that plants absorb and convert light into chemical energy.

There are five major forms of energy active within the human body (Figure 4.1). Sound, light, magnetism, heat, and electricity envelop and sustain our internal experiences, as well as our interactions with the external world. These five energies sustain, govern and control our psychology and physiology, and also determine the subtle resonations of our energetic and spiritual fields. In Medical Qigong therapy, these energies are considered to be properties of the deeper spiritual real-

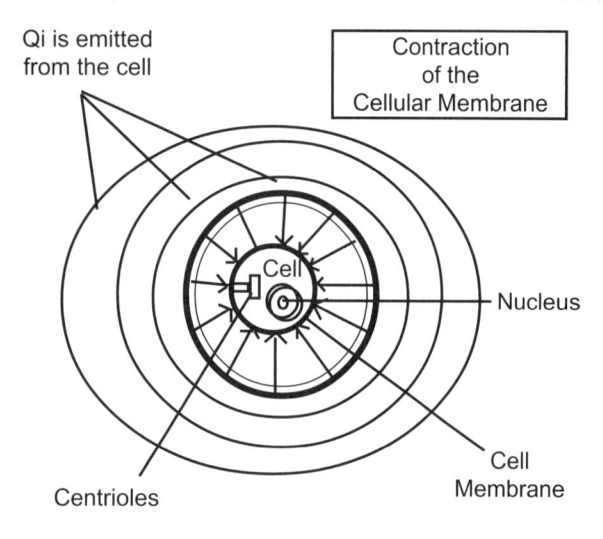

Figure 4.2. When a cell contracts, matter within the cell is released and transformed into energy.

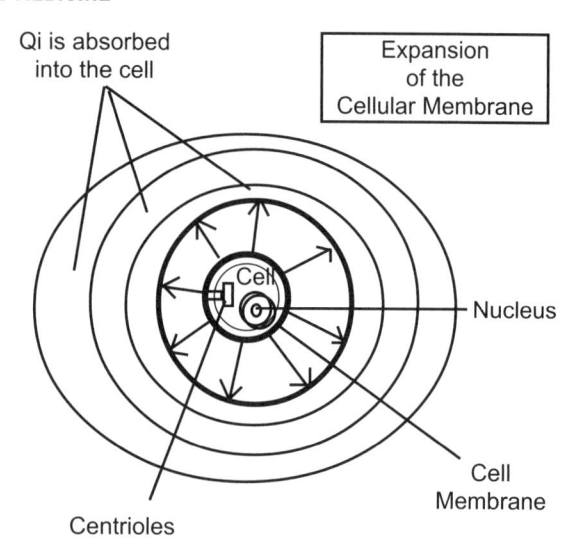

Figure 4.3. When a cell expands, energy is taken from outside the cell and transformed into matter within the cell.

ity that underlies and directs the physical reality. These energies are considered in both the diagnosis and treatment of illness. Extensive scientific research in China has concluded that the human body does indeed emit sound, light, magnetic energy, electricity, and heat.

CELLULAR VIBRATION AND THE FIVE ENERGIES OF THE HUMAN BODY

The condition and level of the body's overall health stems from the active patterns of cellular vibration within the tissues. The body's cells are constantly vibrating, expanding and contracting with the cycles and flow of the body's Qi. Throughout this process of cellular expansion and contraction, matter (in the form of Jing) is continually transforming into energy (in the form of Qi) and energy is continually transforming into matter.

When a cell contracts (cellular exhalation), matter within the cell is released and transformed into energy (Figure 4.2). When a cell expands (cellular inhalation), energy is taken from outside the cell and transformed into matter within the cell (Figure 4.3).

If a group of cells contracts too much (due to stress, overwork, caffeine or other stimulants, for example), an excessively large amount of energy is released from within the cells into the spaces surrounding the cells, resulting in a condition known clinically as "Qi Excess" (because more energy has been released than the body is able to utilize or process). Qi Excess can manifest through symptoms such as radiating heat. The accumulated Qi surrounding the cells can also obstruct the body's energetic flow, resulting in a condition clinically known as "Qi Stagnation." Qi Stagnation can manifest through symptoms such as pain, inflammation and swelling.

Conversely, if a group of cells expands too much (due to obesity, sleeping, lethargy, or depression), a great amount of energy is absorbed from the spaces surrounding the cells and is converted into matter within the cell. When too much matter is absorbed into the cell, an insufficiency of energy is created outside of the cells resulting in a condition known clinically as "Qi Deficiency." Qi Deficiency can manifest through symptoms such coldness, weakness, fatigue, and degenerative conditions.

Matter and energy rhythmically transform into each other within and around the cells. Constantly transforming back and forth, this cellular activity energetically influences the nearby cells, creating a sympathetic resonance that is unique to each type of tissue. The Chinese association of tissues, energies and emotions to the Orb of each Yin organ is based on this concept of sympathetic resonance, and not on the Western classification of tissues and tissue functions.

Traditional Chinese Medicine approaches disease with the understanding that the energy and cellular function of the tissues must both be harmonized in order to initiate healing. Every cell of the body responds to and produces sound, light, magnetic, electrical and heat. Thus, all tissues and functions of the body can be either positively or negatively influenced by the amount and quality of any one of the above five energies. The majority of celestial and environmental influences on the body (excluding more subtle aspects of the Shen) can be explained in terms of these energies. The effect of each type of energy on the body is described as follows (Figure 4.4):

- **Sound:** When the body is exposed to any type of sound resonance, the tissues and cell structures are influenced by that particular frequency or combination of frequencies. Therefore, tone frequency can be used clinically to Purge energetic excess or stagnation conditions, and calm the nervous system.
- **Light:** All living cells emit units of light called "bio-photons." Emitted light affects cellular membranes, and can be used clinically to Tonify energetic deficiencies.
- **Magnetic Energy:** The body's cells carry electromagnetic fields containing positive and negative polarities that both attract and repel each other. This results in a magnetic pull between the body's various types of Qi, tissues, organs, and extremities. Specific magnetic fields can be created to either attract (Tonify), repel (Purge), unify (Regulate) and direct the Qi created from within the cells.
- **Heat:** The heat within the body causes increased electron movement, resulting in the generation of more heat at the cellular level. Heat is also created as a by-product of cellular metabolism and can be used to increase the activity of Qi and Tonify an energetic deficiency.
- **Electricity:** The electromagnetic energy in the cells is continuously generated through the bio-chemical transformations of food and air, and is circulated by the electromagnetic fields generated by the tissues. Examples of the electrical energy in the body are found in the bioelectrical impulses of the nervous system and heart (measured by EEG and ECG respectively).

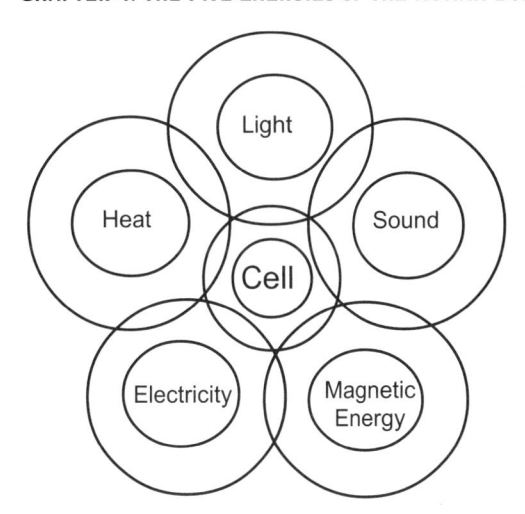

Figure 4.4. Each of the body's cells produces and responds to the vibrational resonance of sound, light, heat, magnetic and electric sensations.

SOUND ENERGY RESONANCES

Audible sound has three main energetic characteristics: pulse, wave and form. Every phenomenon, from molecular to cosmic, is the result of the combination and interaction of these three forces, described as follows:

- **Pulse:** The term "pulse" is used to describe the generating aspect of sound, arising from the energetic force of expansion and contraction. In musical terms, the pulse is expressed as the beat. The pulse is the fundamental field which simultaneously creates wave and form.
- **Wave:** A sound "wave" is represented in the rising (expanding) and falling (contracting) rhythms of an energetic pulse. The original pulse is always contained within the wave. Sound waves are measured in cycles per second (cps).

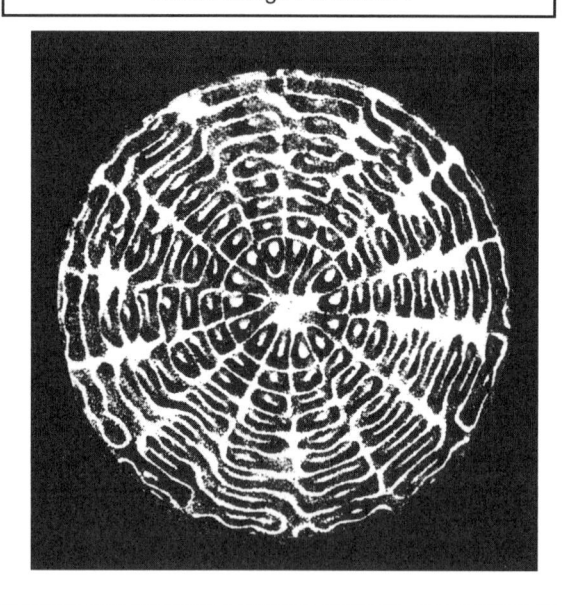

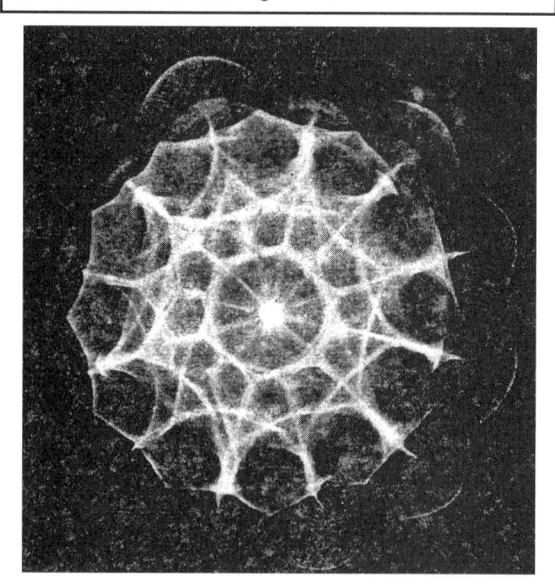

Sound Image From Sand	Sound Image From Water
Sound Image From Sand	Sound Image From Water

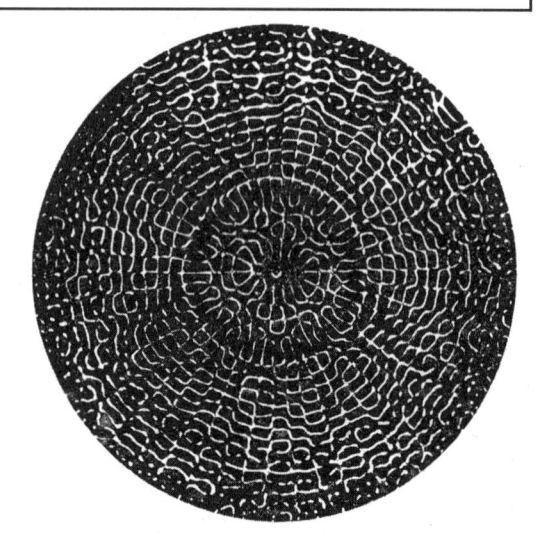

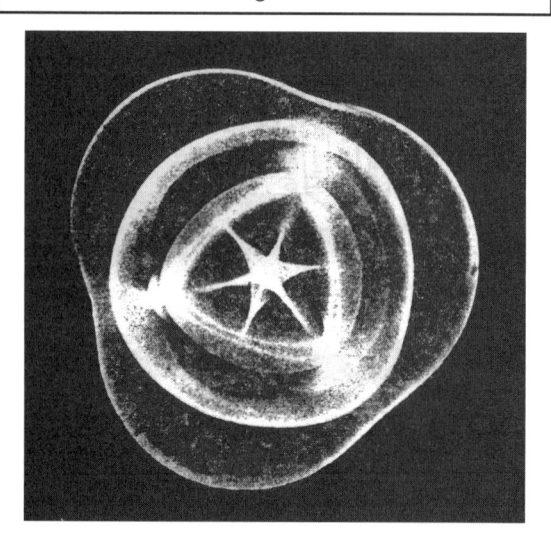

Figure 4.5. Dr. Hans Jenny's Sound Form Images (created from sand and water)

- **Form:** Sound "form" can be observed by subjecting matter to a continuous sound vibrational pattern. Research scientist, Dr. Hans Jenny, created sound form images by placing sand or water on a steel plate with a crystal sound oscillator attached to the bottom. The sound vibrates the steel plate and organizes the matter placed on it into various forms and patterns (Figure 4.5). Other research physicists have discovered similar phenomena using water, light and subatomic particles in conjunction with sound vibration.

SOUND ENERGY AND THE HUMAN BODY

Although the human body appears to be solid, it is roughly 75% liquid. All of matter is a manifestation of vibration and wave function. Both the solid and liquid aspects of the body are organized and defined by underlying vibrational patterns, which thus maintain the body's structural form. We are constructed of pulse (energetic fields), waves (energetic vibrations) and form (energetic particles).

Sound has a profound influence as an energetic code on the subtle body. Sound is capable of accessing consciousness and creating a link between matter and spirit. When the body is exposed to any type of sound resonance, the tissues and cell structures are affected by that particular frequency or combination of frequencies, which results in either a positive or negative automatic response.

The human body both receives and generates sound energy. These subtle sounds resonate from four distinct physical and energetic actions. The following subtle sounds are natural tones that resonate as a result of four physical energetic actions: breath, muscle movements, Qi movements and the pulsating sounds of the Taiji Pole, which are described as follows (Figure 4.6):

1. **Breathing** creates respiratory sound resonances that follow the inhaled and exhaled air through the lungs, mouth, and nose. The condition of the five Yin organs is reflected by the body's respiratory patterns, described as follows:
   - **Liver:** grunting, screaming, sighing
   - **Heart:** laughing, cooing
   - **Spleen:** singing, whistling, humming, gurgling, belching, hiccuping
   - **Lungs:** yawning, sneezing, sniffing, panting, sighing, sobbing, crying
   - **Kidneys:** groaning, whining, moaning, yelping, gasping, shivering
2. **Muscle Movements** create somatic and visceral sound resonances. These include the clicking of the joints, the beating of the heart, the movement of the Blood flowing through the veins and vessels, and the gurgling of the stomach and intestines.

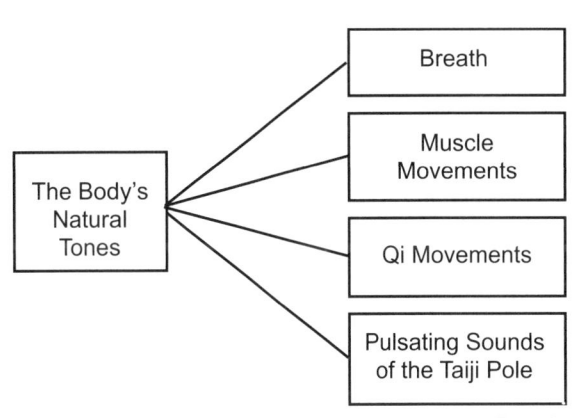

Figure 4.6. Natural Tones That Resonate as a Result of Four Physical Energetic Actions

3. **Qi Movements** can produce a more subtle type of energetic sound resonance. For example, when Liver Yang, Liver Fire, or Liver Wind rise, a high-pitched tone is heard in the ears. When the Kidney Yin is deficient, this sound is dull, like rushing wind.
4. **Energy Pulsating** within the Taiji Pole creates the most subtle sound vibrations within the human body. The vibrations resonating from within the body's Taiji Pole manifest as three distinct pulsating sounds, produced when the current of energy pulsating in the Taiji Pole interacts with the body's Upper, Middle and Lower Dantians. These sounds can be heard when an individual is in deep meditation.

THE ANATOMY OF LISTENING

Although the human body is capable of hearing, the ability to listen energetically is quite different. Sounds must be both perceived by the ear, as well as analyzed and decoded by the Brain.

Balance, Listening and Stimulation

According to French physician and otolaryngologist, Alfred Tomatis, there are three main functions of the ear: balance, listening and stimulation, described as follows (Figure 4.7):
- **Balance:** This involves the ear's function of maintaining equilibrium, tissue symmetry, and the integration of motor and sensory information.
- **Listening:** This involves the ear's function of analyzing and decoding vibrations from both

outside the body (cochlea) and inside the body (vestibular). This allows an individual to audibly perceive external sounds (such as language) and recreate them using the vocal cords.

The ear consists of three main structures: the outer ear, which is responsible for collecting and channeling sound; the middle ear, which is responsible for converting sound energy into mechanical energy, amplifying it and transferring it to the next inner chamber; and inner ear, which is responsible for both auditory and vestibular stimulation (Figure 4.8).

- **Stimulation:** This involves the ear's function of stimulating the central nervous system and the cortex of the Brain. The ear is connected with the 10th cranial nerve (vagus nerve) which affects the heart, larynx, bronchi and intestinal tract.

Turbid Sound and Clean Sound

In Medical Qigong therapy, there are two types of sound: turbid sound and clean sound, described as follows:

- **Turbid (Yin) Sound:** This type of sound is toxic to the body, resulting in fatigue to the listener.
- **Clean (Yang) Sound:** This type of sound is beneficial to the body, resulting in stimulating and charging the listener's central nervous system and the cortex of the Brain.

THE ANATOMY OF THE SPOKEN SOUND

Energetically, spoken sound is the result of a powerful spiritual interaction and energetic fusion involving the Brain (Kidney Water) and Heart (Heart Fire). It is therefore important for the Shen to guide and direct the spoken sound, as the projected voice is a direct manifestation of the individual's spirit and life-force energy.

In human physiology, the body creates sound vibration by controlling the flow of air as it passes through the larynx in the throat. The larynx, which is located the upper part of the trachea, contains the vocal cords, which consist of two strong bands of elastic tissue (another form of fascia) that are stretched across the larynx. The stream of exhaled air is transformed into controlled sound vibration

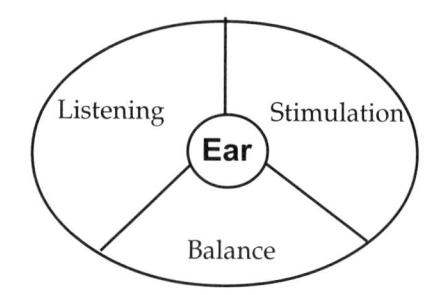

Figure 4.7. The Three Main Functions of the Ear

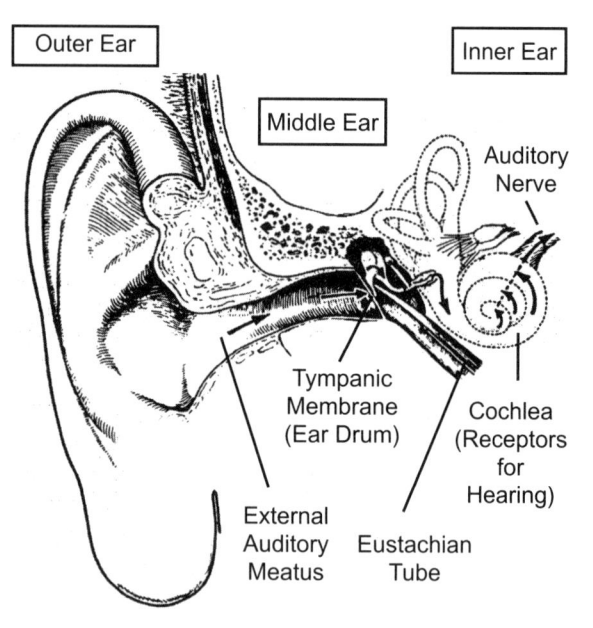

Figure 4.8. The ear consists of three main structures: the outer ear, which is responsible for collecting and channeling sound; the middle ear, which is responsible for converting sound energy into mechanical energy, amplifying it and transferring it to the next inner chamber; and inner ear, which is responsible for both auditory and vestibular stimulation
(Inspired by the original artwork of Wynn Kapit)

by regulating the amount of tension placed on the elastic membranes of the vocal cords. With the exhalation, Qi is released from the diaphragm, lungs, trachea and bronchi, and is modified and refined by the action of the larynx.

As the air is forced through the membranous folds of the larynx, a small amount of pressure builds up behind the closed membranes of the vocal cords and causes them to vibrate. This vibration creates controlled waves of sound that resonate within and around the body (Figure 4.9). These sound waves are further amplified through the primary "resonators" (consisting of the nasal, oral and throat cavities), and the secondary "resonators" (consisting of the chest cavities and chest Bones). The emitted sound is further shaped and augmented through primary "articulators" (consisting of the lips, teeth, gum ridges, hard palate, soft palate, tongue and uvula).

The resonating surfaces of the body's tissues act as initial vibrators of sound. Bone, cartilage, membrane and muscle have the potential of serving as living amplifiers and conductors. Thus, the structure and density of the body's tissues modify and enhance the quality of emitted sound. The harder the surface of the tissue, the stronger the energetic resonance. It is for this reason that the sounds made by a patient (language or otherwise) create an accurate and detailed map of the individual's internal physical structure. In addition to using sound as a diagnostic modality, the Qigong doctor is also able to use emitted sound for a variety of therapeutic purposes.

Sound Therapy Through Emitted Qi

As sound waves vibrate through the body, the liquid crystalline structures of the tissues transform the vibration into pulsed currents. These currents are then conducted throughout the body to various structures, organs and glands, according to the frequency and amplitude of the incoming wave signal. As the tissues change and transform due to the influence of sound wave vibrations, it automatically creates a corresponding change in the function and flow of energy in the body. Thus, sound vibrations have a profound effect on psychology, physiology, and the flow of the body's internal energy. Sound and tone resonation have been used for centuries as effective healing tools and are currently used as an integral part of modern Qigong Medicine.

Recent research on molecular water patterns has confirmed what the ancient Chinese sages have known for millennia, that the vibrational patterns of sound can disrupt the tissues' energetic patterns and can initiate a new energetic pattern. Depending on the type of projected sound vibration, the new pattern can either be healthy or destructive.

During extensive experimentations, a drop of water was subjected to the vibrational patterns of specific sounds. At a certain pitch, the drop of water's entire structure dissolved and immediately created (and maintained) an entirely different energetic pattern. Each time the sound pattern was altered, it initiated a chaotic energetic resonance into the water-drop form, causing the water-drop to disperse and reshape itself in accordance with the new projected sound pattern.

Five Ancient Chinese Pitches

For centuries in China, patients have used sound therapy to heal certain parts of the body. Used in this way, sound therapy stimulates the flow of Qi and Blood to move into and/or away from specific internal organs and tissues. This new move-

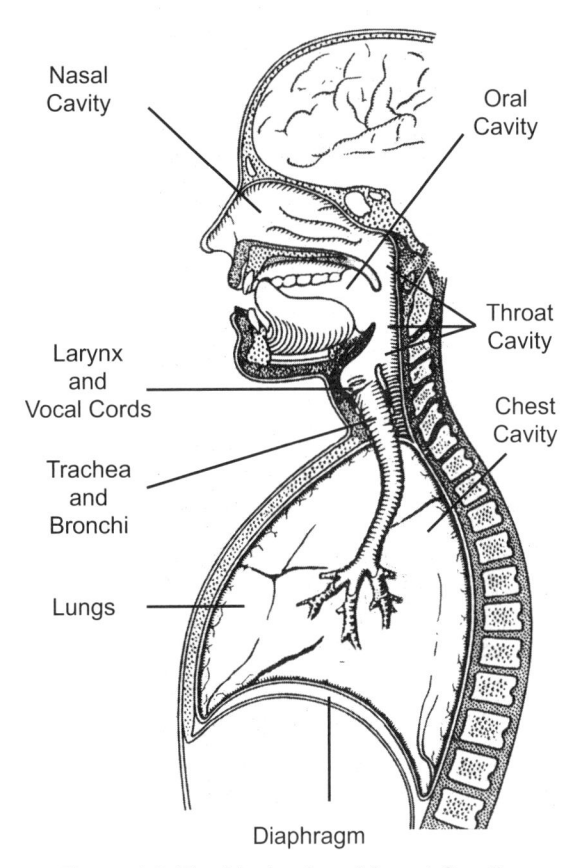

Figure 4.9. The Mechanics of Sound Creation

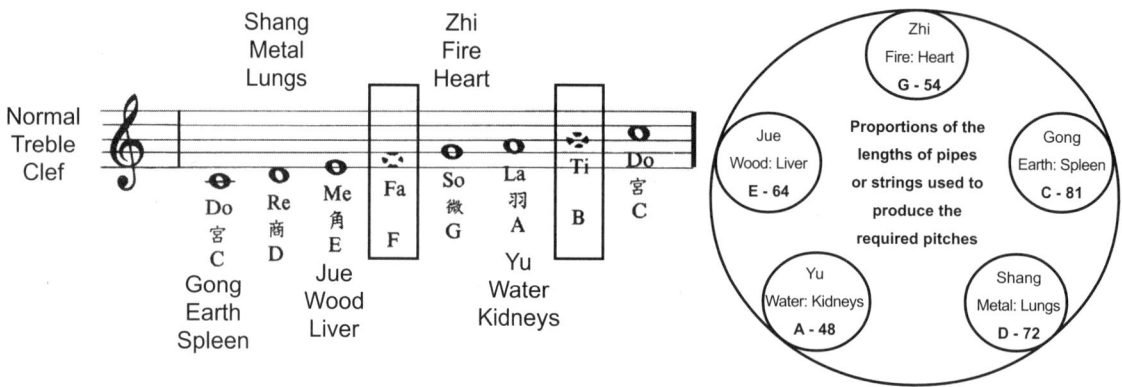

Figure 4.10. The Five Energetic Pitches and Their Corresponding Elements

ment of Qi and Blood is used to increase health and energetic balance within the patient. The primary healing sounds relate to the Five Agents and to the Five Element aspects of the patient's internal organs (Chapter 2). Each of the Five Elements has a note and is described as follows (Figure 4.10):
- Gong - C = Earth: Spleen
- Shang - D = Metal: Lungs
- Jue -   E = Wood: Liver
- Zhi -   G = Fire: Heart
- Yu -   A = Water: Kidneys

PROJECTED SOUND

The Qigong doctor can project powerful sound vibrations by focusing on the middle of all three Dantians, at the center of his or her Taiji Pole. With intention and focused concentration, the doctor can vibrate specific internal organs and combine these energies with the Qi of the Dantians to project powerful sound vibrations to treat the patient. The Qigong doctor practices vibrating sound therapy by:

1. **Audible Toning:** By audibly toning the healing sounds, the Qigong doctor can fill his or her energetic field with healing sound vibration. This energetic field of sound is then projected into his or her patient. Audible sound resonation is considered a Jing level energy projection and is generally used when the patient is armored or not energetically sensitive.

2. **Slightly Audible Toning:** By using slightly audibly healing tones (also known as "whispering sound therapy"), the Qigong doctor can project and release an emotional type of vibration into the patient. In this case, the Qigong doctor will begin by internally focusing his or her mind on the healing sound. As this internal sound fills the Qigong doctor's energetic field, it is then emitted into the patient's body. To increase the energetic intensity of the sound projection, the doctor needs only to increase the mind's intention and the pressure of his or her exhalation. Slightly audible sound resonation is considered a Qi level energy projection, and is generally used when the patient is energetically sensitive.

3. **Inaudible Toning:** By projecting the healing sounds with breath, in conjunction with focused mental intention (also known as "breath incantation"), the Qigong doctor can initiate deep yet subtle vibrations inside the patient's body. In this case, the Qigong doctor will begin by internally focusing his or her mind on the healing sound. As this internal sound fills the Qigong doctor's energetic field, it is then emitted into the patient's body through soft exhalation. To increase the intensity of the energetic sound projection, the doctor needs only to increase his or her mind's intention, and focus the vibration deeper into the patient's tissues. Inaudible sound resonation is considered a Shen level energy projection, and is generally used when the patient is energetically sensitive.

4. **Combined Toning:** Both the doctor and patient can simultaneously resonate the sound to enhance the synchronization of both their energy fields. As the Qigong doctor resonates

```
Sound Therapy ─┬─ Characteristic Sound Therapy ─── Sound Emitted From Musical Instruments
               ├─ Extraordinary Sound Therapy ──── Sound Emitted From Vocal Resonances
               └─ Infrasonic Sound Therapy ─────── Low Frequency Sound Waves Emitted From the Hands of Qigong Doctors
```

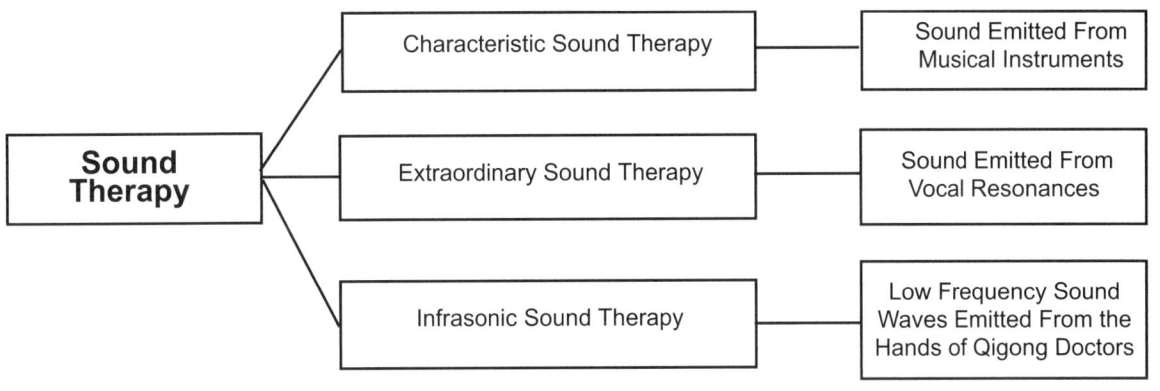

Figure 4.11. Three Sound Therapy Modalities

his or her own internal organs along with the patient, both the doctor and patient can modulate the sound and energy patterns as needed. Sometimes the Qigong doctor will combine color with the emitted sound in order to increase the sound's effect on the patient's tissues. This joint sound resonation is used in cases of extreme armoring in which the patient first needs to be brought to a state where he or she can feel the tissues vibrating.

THREE MODALITIES OF SOUND THERAPY

The healing sounds used by Qigong doctors are effective because they are based on an understanding of the multidimensional influence of sound on the human structure. The modulated nature of sound pulsation affects the energetic structures which shape and maintain the patient's physical structure. Once the patient's energetic structures have been disturbed, the body must immediately begin a reconstructive process, creating new energetic patterns to restructure and heal the tissues.

There are three modalities used for sound therapy, described as follows (Figure 4.11):

1. **Characteristic Sound Therapy:** This refers to the sound produced by musical instruments (flute, guitar, piano, drum, etc.) and their effects on the subconscious mind. This type of instrumental musical energy creates specific physical, emotional, and spiritual states in both the listener and within the energetic fields of the surrounding environment.
2. **Extraordinary Sound Therapy:** This refers to the vocal resonances used in chanting, prayer, and singing. Such techniques include the Daoist six-word healing sound method, Zhuang Zi's breath listening method, and Lao Zi's sound-voice method. This type of therapy uses the individual's energy to produce sound with directed intention and enhanced visualization. It is also practiced in conjunction with breathing techniques that are guided by the Yuan Shen (the intuitive consciousness of the spirit). All of these techniques are combined to achieve physiological and psychological transformation.
3. **Infrasonic Sound Therapy:** This refers to the low frequency sound waves emitted from the hands of Qigong doctors. These chaotic low frequency sound waves are inaudible to the human ear and are a vibrational by-product of the intense amount of Qi focused in a Qigong doctor's hands. This infrasonic sound resonance affects the central nervous system and alters the body's neurophysiological functions. Extensive research performed by Richard H. Lee of China Healthways Institute in Los Angeles, California, as well as research performed by the Beijing College of Traditional Chinese Medicine and the Department of Natural Science in Beijing, China, confirm that all humans have a very high degree of acoustic activity in the subsonic range below 20 Hertz (infrasonic). This subsonic level of sound vibration is the "hum" of human energy, similar to the alpha rhythm of an EEG. Qigong doctors may combine characteristic,

extraordinary, and infrasonic sound therapies into one treatment in order to facilitate a deep and thorough transformation within their patient's tissues. The choice of sound prescriptions varies according to each patient's cultural upbringing, religious beliefs, emotional temperament, and appreciation of energetic healing modalities.

Music and Sound Therapy

Since ancient times, masters of energetic medicine have known that musical patterns can affect an individual's health, character, morality and consciousness. An ancient Daoist text states that "each sound has something that it disturbs, calls, and causes to come." Because of this principle, the ancient Chinese used the power of music to tame wild animals, change the natural order of the world, provoke drought, or alter the course of the seasons.

When notes are arranged into rhythmical and melodic patterns, they can produce a positive or negative effect on the body's physical, mental, emotional and spiritual energetic fields. One of the books written in the Daoist Treaties on Ceremonial Usages, entitled *The Book of Music*, states that an individual's passions should be restrained by means of music.

The powerful effects of music are largely due to what is known as "entrainment." Entrainment is a principle in physics in which the stronger vibrations of one object (in this case, the musical instrument or voice) will cause the weaker vibrations of another object (the tissue cells) to change and begin oscillating at the same rate as the stronger object. Thus, the melody and rhythm of music can positively or negatively entrain an individual's body, mind, emotions and spirit by affecting the rhythms of his or her subtle energetic fields.

Another effect of music on the body's tissues is that of destabilizing pre-existing physical and energetic patterns by temporarily introducing a new and more powerful sound vibration. Any exposure to powerful sound resonation disturbs the body's energetic field and disrupts the individual's established patterns. This disruption is known in Medical Qigong therapy as "chaotic resonance." The principle of chaotic resonance can be applied therapeutically to disperse harmful physical and energetic patterns before the introduction of beneficial healing patterns. Similarly, unconscious exposure to fields of chaotic resonance can disrupt the body's natural pattern and rhythms.

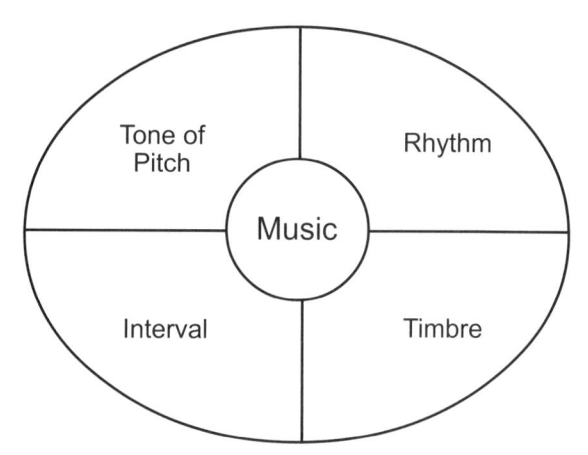

Figure 4.12. The Four Elements of Music that Induce a Physiological and Psychological Effect on the Body

Research has shown that the elements of music that induce a physiological and psychological effect on the body are: rhythm, tone or pitch, interval, and timbre, described as follows (Figure 4.12):

- **Rhythm:** This is the energetic beat and pulse. It has the most immediate and intense effect on the body, especially affecting the individual's pulse rate, skin temperature, blood pressure, muscle tension, emotions and brain-wave activity.
- **Tone or Pitch:** This is the specific rate of vibration that determines different notes.
- **Interval:** This is the distance between the notes, and creates the melody, as well as harmony.
- **Timbre:** This is the specific quality and nature of the sound that is produced from an instrument or a voice. In ancient China, the voice was divided into five basic timbres, each related to the energetic natures of the Five Elements.

Therapeutic Effects of Sound

Music and vocal harmonics have always been acknowledged as a powerful medium for emotional enhancement. Scientific studies have shown

CHAPTER 4: THE FIVE ENERGIES OF THE HUMAN BODY

```
                                    ┌─ Healing ──────────── Aids Digestion, Induces Sleep and
                                    │                        Treats Mental Disturbances
                Therapeutic         │
                Uses of ────────────┼─ Meditation ────────── Initiates Specific Altered
                Entrainment         │                        States of Consciousness
                                    │
The                                 └─ Religious ─────────── Initiates Positive Effects on the
Therapeutic                            Experience            Individual's Spirit (Yuan Shen)
Effects of ─┤                                                and Soul (Shen Xian)
Music
                                    ┌─ Physical ──────────── Disperses Physical Stagnations:
                                    │  Transformation        Cancer, Tumors, Cysts, Scar
                Therapeutic         │                        Tissue and Adhesions, etc.
                Uses of ────────────┤
                Chaotic             │  Energetic             Disperses Harmful Emotional
                Resonance           └─ (Thoughts and ─────── Patterns: Depression, Anger and
                                       Emotions)             Rage, Grief, Despair, Fear, Worry,
                                       Transformation        Shock, etc.
```

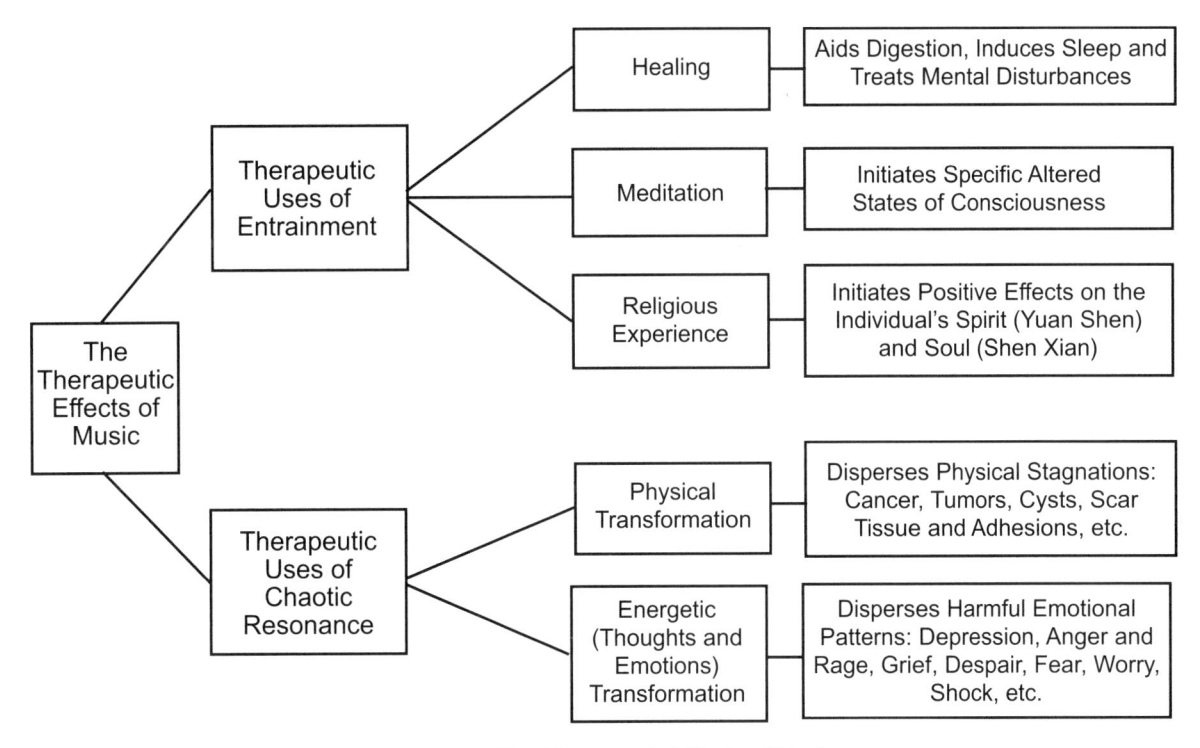

Figure 4.13. The Therapeutic Effects of Music

that plants grow faster, trees produce sweeter fruit, cows produce more milk and patients recover quicker when they are exposed to soft, mellow music. The therapeutic application of music and sound can be divided into two main categories: the therapeutic uses of entrainment, and the therapeutic uses of chaotic resonance (Figure 4.13):

The Therapeutic Uses of Entrainment

The principle of entrainment can be applied therapeutically to induce healing, meditation and religious experience, described as follows:

- **Healing:** Vocal harmonics have been shown to physiologically create changes in heartbeat, respiration and brain-wave patterns. Sounds and tones stimulate the cerebral centers creating a wide range of results including enhanced memory retention, facilitating certain emotions, stimulating creative inspirations, treating mental disturbances, aiding digestion, and inducing sleep.
- **Meditation:** Music and sound can initiate specific altered states of consciousness by influencing and directing the body's biorhythms and frequencies. When used as a healing modality, music and sound can cause subtle shifts and frequency coherence within the individual's Brain, Heart and internal organ systems. Examples range from shamanic trance to various other altered states.
- **Religious Experience:** For centuries, music and sound have been used to help people transcend the physical and social planes of awareness and enter into the archetypal realm of the spirit. The ancient Chinese Wu Yi doctors would use music and sound to initiate positive effects on the individual's Spirit (Yuan Shen) and Soul (Shen Xian).

The Therapeutic Uses of Chaotic Resonance

The principle of chaotic resonance can be applied therapeutically to induce physical transformation, and energetic (thoughts and emotions) transformation, described as follows:

- **Physical Transformation:** Sound therapy is often applied to disperse a wide variety of

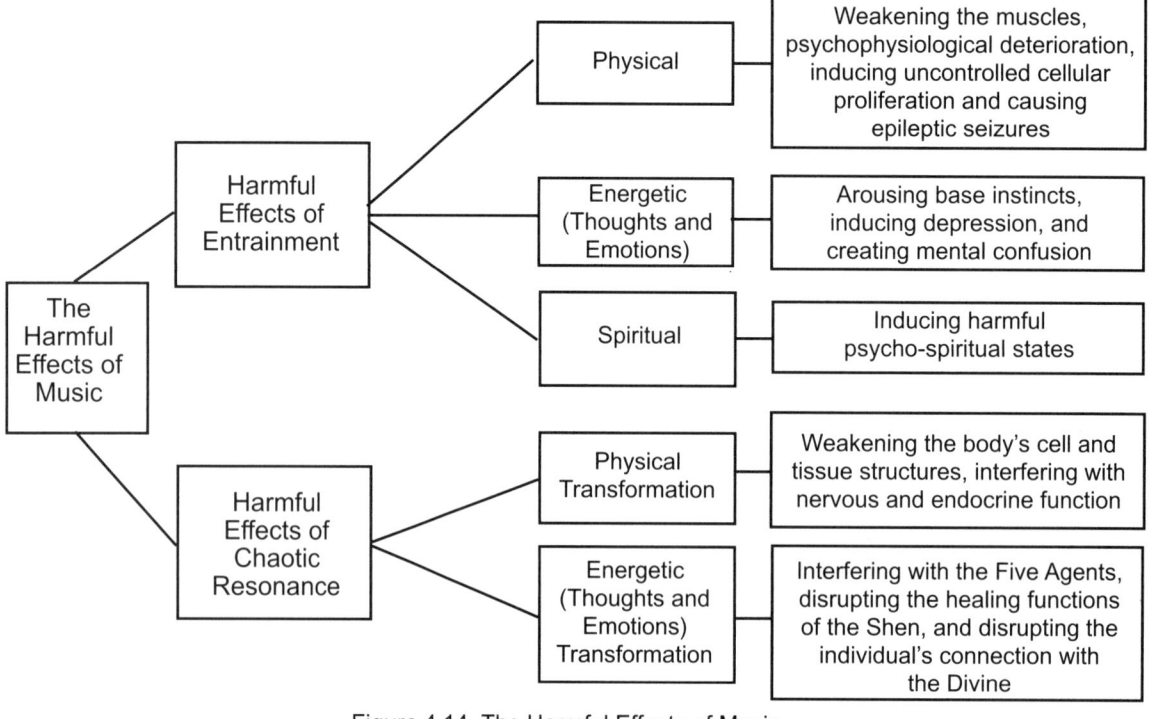

Figure 4.14. The Harmful Effects of Music

The Harmful Effects of Music

- **Harmful Effects of Entrainment**
  - Physical: Weakening the muscles, psychophysiological deterioration, inducing uncontrolled cellular proliferation and causing epileptic seizures
  - Energetic (Thoughts and Emotions): Arousing base instincts, inducing depression, and creating mental confusion
  - Spiritual: Inducing harmful psycho-spiritual states
- **Harmful Effects of Chaotic Resonance**
  - Physical Transformation: Weakening the body's cell and tissue structures, interfering with nervous and endocrine function
  - Energetic (Thoughts and Emotions) Transformation: Interfering with the Five Agents, disrupting the healing functions of the Shen, and disrupting the individual's connection with the Divine

---

physical stagnations. This is because of the susceptibility of the body's tissues to vibrational resonance. In Medical Qigong therapy, chaotic resonance is generally used in cases of stagnation to break up the cellular and energetic accumulations held within the liquid matrix of the body (see Volume 3, Chapter 39). Physical stagnations that have been proven to be especially responsive to Medical Qigong Sound Therapy include: cancer, tumors, cysts, scar tissue and fascial adhesions. Modern sound therapy treatment protocols include the use of sound to break up kidney stones and gallstones (shock-wave lithotripsy), and the use of ultrasound to relieve sore muscles.

- **Energetic (Thoughts and Emotions) Transformation:** The principle of chaotic resonance can be applied to disperse harmful energetic and emotional patterns. Examples include using chaotic resonance in the treatment of depression, anger, rage, grief, despair, fear, worry and shock.

HARMFUL EFFECTS

The improper or unconscious exposure to music and sound can damage or imbalance the individual's physical, energetic or spiritual well being. The harmful effects of music and sound can be divided into two main categories: the harmful effects of entrainment, and the harmful effects of chaotic resonance (Figure 4.14):

The Harmful Effects of Entrainment

The harmful effects of entrainment can be observed when exposure to music or sound creates an unhealthy or unnatural pattern of resonance within the body's tissues and energetic fields. Modern research has shown diseases and emotions to posses specific vibrational frequency patterns which can be accidently triggered by chronic exposure to any strong detrimental vibrational field.

The deleterious effects of entrainment are generally due to exposure to music or sound that is extreme in nature (too loud, too fast, too slow, etc.), or out of harmony with the body's natural frequencies. Examples include jackhammers, sirens, car horns, heavy machinery, heavy metal music, fast aerobic or trance dance music, and depressing musical compositions such as funeral marches. Such exposure can negatively affect the individual's physical, energetic, and spiritual health.

- **Physical:** Entrainment can have a negative effect on the body's physiology when the dominant vibration to which the individual is exposed creates patterns detrimental to proper cell and tissue structure. Examples of the harmful physical effects of entrainment include:
    1. A physical weakening of the muscles.
    2. Psychophysiological deterioration (syncopated rhythms).
    3. Uncontrollable cellular proliferation.
    4. Epileptic seizures in energetically hypersensitive individuals (certain rhythms).
- **Energetic (Thoughts and Emotions):** Entrainment can have a negative effect on the energetic field of the body by inciting toxic thoughts and emotions. This effect can be created with either harmful musical tones and patterns, or through disturbing lyrics that affect the individual's subconscious mind. Some examples of the harmful energetic effects of entrainment include:
    1. Arousing base instincts (aggression, and destructive behavior).
    2. Inducing states of depression or melancholy.
    3. Creating mental confusion.
- **Spiritual:** The physical and energetic effects of entrainment, in combination with the more subtle vibrations of will and intent, can negatively influence the individual's spiritual field by inducing harmful psycho-spiritual states.

The Harmful Effects of Chaotic Resonance

The harmful effects of chaotic resonance are observed when exposure to music or sound interferes with the body's physical structures or energetic patterns.

- **Physical:** Chaotic resonance can have a negative effect on the body's physiology when it interferes with the individual's normal internal rhythms. When these rhythms are disrupted, the ability of the body's systems to properly interact is compromised, resulting in general weakness, or specific tissue malfunction. Examples of the harmful physiological effects of chaotic resonance include:
    1. Weakening the body's cell and tissue structures.
    2. Interfering with the proper functioning of the body's electrical (nervous system) and chemical (endocrine system) communication systems.
- **Energetic and Spiritual:** The energetic and spiritual field patterns exist on a more subtle level, and are therefore more sensitive and susceptible to the effects of chaotic resonance. Examples of the harmful effects of chaotic resonance on the individual's energetic and spiritual fields include:
    1. Interfering with the proper functioning of the Five Agents.
    2. Disrupting the natural healing functions of the individual's Shen.
    3. Disrupting the individual's connection to the Divine.

Music in Ancient China

The ancient Daoists believed that music was the basis of everything; that all things, including the human body, were molded according to the music performed within its substance. According to this theory, a primordial sound emitted from a central spiritual source created the entire physical universe.

Masters of energetic medicine have known for centuries that musical patterns can affect an individual's health, character, morality and consciousness. "Sacred sounds" have been used for healing and spiritual endeavors (in combination with postures, rhythmic movements and chants) throughout the ages.

Music was also believed to have a powerful social and political influence. Confucius once stated that if the music of a kingdom changed, then its society would alter itself accordingly.

In ancient China, music therapy was focused on harmonizing the Five Elements within the body's Yin and Yang organs, and was also used in Feng Shui training to regulate mind and body imbalances stemming from seasonal changes. During autumn, for example, when dryness is prevalent and there is a transition from warm to cool, music was used to help stabilize the body in relation to the changing external conditions.

SECONDARY ACOUSTIC BIOLOGICAL RESPONSE

The following information was presented in Beijing, China by Professor Lu Yan Fang, a Medical Qigong doctor.

The frequency of sound is measured by the number of oscillations a sound wave makes in one second, called a hertz (Hz). Most individuals can consciously hear frequencies vibrating between the ranges of 30 Hz. to 20,000 Hz. Secondary sounds, however, are those sound vibrations that resonate outside of the hearing range of the human ear. One fascinating observation about secondary sounds is that they can travel long distances with little attenuation or distortion.

Secondary sounds were first discovered and scientifically measured during the 1930's. However, it was not until the 1960's that secondary sound started generating attention.

Initial studies regarding the biological effects of secondary sound on human tissue revealed that exposure to certain ranges of secondary sounds consistently caused damage to the structure and function of the human body. After laboratory studies showed that strong secondary sounds (beyond 150 dB) were harmful to biological tissues, the American Environmental Protection Agency (E.P.A.) began to set strict standards for secondary sounds released within the environment. These studies also concluded that secondary sounds vibrating below 130 dB were not harmful to the body.

To date, there have been few studies that have examined how secondary sounds affect the biological processes of the human tissues; nor has there been much investigation into the production of secondary sounds by the human body. The small amount of the scientific information that is available comes from the Peoples Republic of China, or is classified U.S. military research.

In 1983, a study began in the Peoples Republic of China, which included the investigation of more than 70 famous Medical Qigong masters. In this study, it was discovered that the human body actually emits a secondary sound signal. The average frequency emitted by the Qigong Masters measured in the secondary sound region of about 10 Hz.

In 1984, more than 100 repeated lab experiments revealed identical results of frequency distribution. Based on an analysis of these results, the first infrasonic Medical Qigong machines were constructed. These machines used electroacoustic technology to simulate the low frequency signal emitted by the Medical Qigong masters, and further increased the intensity of the signal. In the two years that followed, many clinical trials were performed incorporating the use of the "Infratonic Qigong Machine." Several hospitals (1,134 patients), and several animal studies were included. All tests revealed that weak secondary sounds can be beneficial to the human body. It was also discovered that infrasonic sound could be used as a basic substitute for Medical Qigong Qi emission therapy, which opened an exciting new door for medical science.

The Infratonic Qigong Machine can also have significant treatment value by promoting circulation, regulating Qi and Blood, opening the body's channel systems, and relieving pain.

A Qigong master is not alone in his or her ability to emit secondary acoustical signals, as most individuals can be taught to generate a similar energetic pattern. The human body is a receptor of secondary acoustical signals. It produces, delivers, emits, receives and controls various forms of low frequency energy. Very early in the development of Traditional Chinese Medicine, the effects of secondary acoustic signals had been demonstrated. Medical Qigong therapy, acupuncture, and Chinese therapeutic massage therapy all use aspects of this type of low frequency stimulation to influence the human body.

WESTERN SOUND THERAPY

Sound therapy is also being used in contemporary Western medicine, and we have hardly

begun to tap into its full healing potential. The following are some examples of current clinical modalities:
- music therapy for postoperative healing
- ultrasound therapy for sore muscles and back injuries
- shock-wave lithotripsy therapy for kidney stones and calcified gallstones

LIGHT ENERGY

Quantum theory arose from the concept that atoms absorb and emit light in quanta (portions or units of energy). A quantum is the smallest known indivisible unit in which waves of information and energy are either absorbed or emitted. A quantum of light is known as a photon, while a quantum of electricity is known as an electron.

Matter and the transformation of matter can be viewed as a result of light (photons) interacting with atoms and molecules. All matter absorbs, stores, produces, and transmits light. Matter and light are fundamentally inseparable. Matter is simply a denser form of energy and consciousness. All life on Earth, whether plant, animal, or human, is dependent upon light and its miraculous qualities for existence.

BIOPHOTONS

All living cells emit units of light called "biophotons." Biophoton emissions radiate from the internal organs, as well as from the body's surface tissues, to create the body's auric field. Over 50 years ago, Soviet scientists discovered that light carries biological information. In a 1995 documentary shown on Swiss/Italian television, Dr. Fritz-Albert Popp showed cells talking to each other in short and long bursts of light, similar to Morse code.

This interaction of light on the body's tissues and within the body's internal organs has a profound healing effect, especially when activated by the Qi emission from a Qigong doctor. When muscles or nerves are activated by Medical Qigong therapy or exercises, the intensity of the biophoton emission increases. Studies performed on the healing potential of light and color therapies have repeatedly demonstrated their clinical efficacy. Like sound resonance, light therapy is also being researched further as an addition to modern clinical medicine.

LIGHT AND ENERGETIC FIELDS

Research has shown that all living things emit a permanent current of photons, extending beyond the organism. The number of photons emitted are determined by the organism's position on the evolutionary scale, the more complex the organism, the fewer the photons being emitted. For example:
- Plants and animals generally emit 100 photons per square centimeter per second, at a wavelength of 200 to 800 nanometers. This corresponds to a very high frequency of electromagnetic wave.
- Humans normally emit only 10 photons per square centimeter per second, at a wavelength of 200 to 800 nanometers. This corresponds to a lower frequency of electromagnetic wave.

LIGHT AND FOOD

While studying photosynthesis, in which plants use light as their primary source of energy, Dr. Popp observed that as humans consume plant foods, they absorb and store the photons present within the plant structure. As the food is digested, it is metabolized into nutrients, carbon dioxide, water, and light that had been stored from the sun and was present during the plant's photosynthesis. The human body naturally absorbs and utilizes the nutrients and water, stores the light's electromagnetic waves, and removes the carbon dioxide. Once the energy of these photons is absorbed into the cells and tissues, it is distributed over the entire spectrum of the body's electromagnetic frequencies, adding to the energy present in all the molecules of the body. The most essential storehouse of light, and the major source of biophoton emission, is the body's DNA.

LIGHT AND DNA

Dr. Popp discovered that DNA is capable of sending out a large range of light frequencies, and that these frequencies produce various energetic effects within the body. The DNA acts as a master tuning fork, releasing specific frequencies that cause certain molecules within the tissues to resonate. This active resonation acts as a feedback system of communication through energetic waves which encode and transfer information. Dr. Popp reasoned that if the DNA is responsible for storing light, it would naturally be responsible for emitting more light once it was unwound.

LIGHT AND CANCER

Research conducted by Dr. Popp in 1970 revealed that compounds that are carcinogenic absorbed UV light, which then changed their DNA energetic frequency. Dr. Popp's research also confirmed that carcinogens reacted only to the light at a specific 380 nanometer wavelength. Further biological laboratory experiments showed that if you can blast a cell with UV light so that 99% of the cell is destroyed (including the DNA), you can almost entirely repair the damage in a single day by illuminating the cell with the same wavelength at a very weak intensity. This type of "photo-repair" works most efficiently at 380 nanometers, the very same wavelength to which the cancer causing compounds react.

Dr. Popp realized that the body must have some type of light that is responsible for photo-repair, and that a cancerous compound therefore causes cancer because it permanently blocks this light and scrambles its signal preventing photo-repair from happening.

THE BODY'S INTERNAL LIGHT

The body both absorbs and projects light energy. The divine light that enters at the time of conception continues to reside in the Taiji Pole throughout life. This light responds and reacts to the doctor's emitted therapeutic light energy. Emitted light and color are absorbed into the patient's body, causing the energies of Heaven and Earth to fuse inside the tissues. This facilitates the healing process.

In 1989, Russian research scientist Professor Kaznacheev proved that channels of light exists within the human body. These channels of light correspond to the ancient Chinese channel (meridian) system. He showed that these lines of light energy operate like mighty rivers of information, flowing in and around the body's tissues to create an energetic grid along which light quanta move.

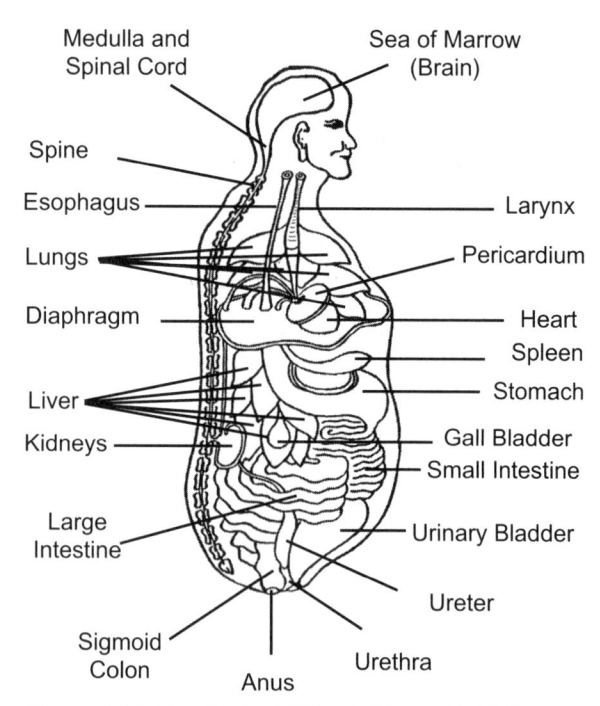

Figure 4.15. The Ancient "Chart of Inner Lights"

In Traditional Chinese Medicine, one of the most ancient illustrations used to depict the internal organs, routes of body fluids, and arteries is called the "Chart of Inner Lights" or "the chart for visualizing the true ones" (Figure 4.15). Charts such as these would depict the internal organs along with their energetic presence, (sometimes referred to as the "radiant one" residing within the organ). The internal organs and organ systems were sometimes referred to as "orbs of light" or "spheres of influence."

The ancient illustrations that depicted the body's energetic channels were traditionally called "Charts of the Halls of Light," and they showed the external pathways along which the body's Qi moved (Figure 4.16).

These detailed maps of Qi and Blood flow illustrated the energetic organs, as well as the body's Jing and Shen (which are rooted in the Blood). The Shen flows inside of the body, transforming into light and radiating from inside of the tissues outward. The light radiating out from the physical body spontaneously interacts with the mental, emotional, and spiritual light energy released from other beings.

THE INTERNAL LIGHT OF THE DANTIANS

Light energy can also be accumulated in the storage chambers of the Three Dantians, described as follows:

- **The Upper Dantian** is called the "peak of Yang energy" and is considered to be electropositive. It is the doorway to the chamber of Heavenly or Divine light. White light is stored and released from the Upper Dantian where the spiritual energy is stored. Once white light energy manifests, it should be drawn down the Taiji Pole and rooted into the center of the Lower Dantian. By using inner vision to focus the eyes on the center core of the body, the Qigong doctor can concentrate on the white light energy vibration and fuse this energy into one column of light stemming from the Upper Dantian to the Lower Dantian (Figure 4.17).
- **The Middle Dantian** is called the "blending of Yin and Yang energy" and is considered to be the transforming location of electronegative and electropositive energy. It contains the light of the Shen (Mind, thoughts and emotions) which forms the basis of human interaction and relationships.
- **The Lower Dantian** is called the "peak of Yin energy" and is considered to be electronegative. It is the body's most direct connection to the Earth. Accumulated Qi is generally stored as a golden glowing ball in the Lower Dantian.

With proper Qigong training and time, the Postnatal heat circulating up the Governing (Yang) Vessel and down the Conception (Yin) Vessel can awaken the Prenatal Qi stored in the Brain, causing it to unite with the body's nervous system. This is considered a full integration of Yin and Yang energy and manifests as a shimmering white light glowing in the center of the Upper Dantian. This glow is universally depicted in pictures of saints, prophets and celestial beings.

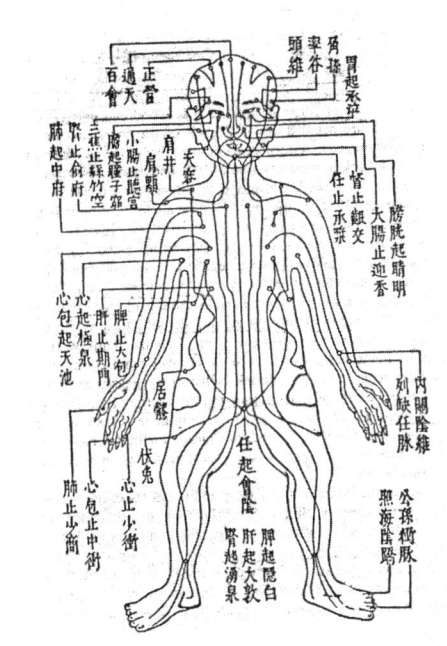

Figure 4.16. The Ancient "Chart of the Halls of Light"

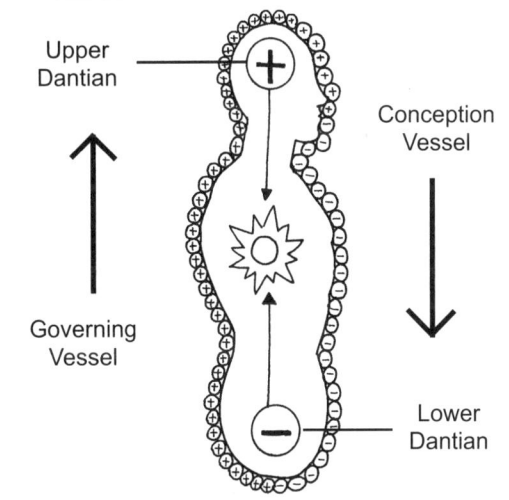

Figure 4.17. Light resonates within the body's Taiji Pole. From the body's Yang Governing Vessel flows a sea of electropositive energy. From the body's Yin Conception Vessel flows a sea of electronegative energy.

When the Microcosmic Orbit is completed (i.e., when the Governing and Conception Vessels are energetically fused), the first center column of light can be accessed via the body's five center Thrusting Channels into the Taiji pole. This col-

Level of Spiritual Light	Dimension of Existence	Source of Light	Manifestation of Light
(4th) Highest Level	Light Existing Within the Higher Spiritual World	Higher Spiritual Light Develops From the Fusion of the Individual's Heart and Mind with the Divine	Higher Spiritual Light is Not Associated with the Concept of "Seeing," but with "Illumination"
(3rd) Higher Level	Light Existing Within the Lower Spiritual World	Lower Spiritual Light Exists as a Continuation of Light Stemming from the Energetic World and the Energetic Frequencies of the Spiritual World	Lower Spiritual Light Manifests Through the Individual's Spiritual Consciousness
(2nd) Middle Level	Light Existing Within the Energetic World	The Light of the Energetic World Extends from the Vibration of Each Atom, Molecule and Cell	Nothing is Lit By Reflection Each Individual's Mind (Thought and Emotion) Creates Light
(1st) Lowest Level	Light of the Gross Material World	The Light of the Gross Material World is Governed by the Energy of the Sun	Light Vibrations Collide with Various Surfaces and Reflect Shapes, Colors, Sizes, Etc.

Figure 4.18. The Energetic Dimensions of Light

umn of light runs through the center of the body connecting all Three Dantians together, and contains several layers similar to that of an onion.

PHYSICAL LIGHT

The light of the material world (see Chapter 2) is governed by the energy of the sun. This type of light manifests as electromagnetic waves and particles, with energetic vibrations that ripple throughout space in all directions. These energetic vibrations are observed with our sense of physical sight. These vibrations of light collide with various surfaces and bounce back to reflect their shape, color, size, etc. The eyes, acting as light receptors, observe these various details and the Brain records the data.

Light of the material world manifests as both heat and color, and is projected through visible and invisible color spectrums. At one end of the spectrum is infrared light, capable of thermodynamic manifestation (giving off heat). At the other end of the spectrum is ultraviolet light, which gives off no heat, but enables photosynthesis (the absorption of light) in plants and is the mechanism for suntans in humans.

ENERGETIC LIGHT

The light existing within the energetic world is different from the light existing within the physical world. All of the planes and sub-planes of the energetic world are internally illuminated from within instead of reflecting what has been projected onto them. This light has two main aspects, described as follows (Figure 4.18):

1. In the energetic world, nothing is lit by reflection. Here the source of light is the very high frequency vibration of each atom, molecule and cell. This is a living light that is connected to, and essentially linked with shapes, sounds and consciousness.

2. The energetic world is a world of conscious thought and emotional energy. The brighter an individual's energetic light, the greater the feeling of satisfaction he or she experiences. This clear and unobstructed vibrational resonance produces a feeling of euphoria.

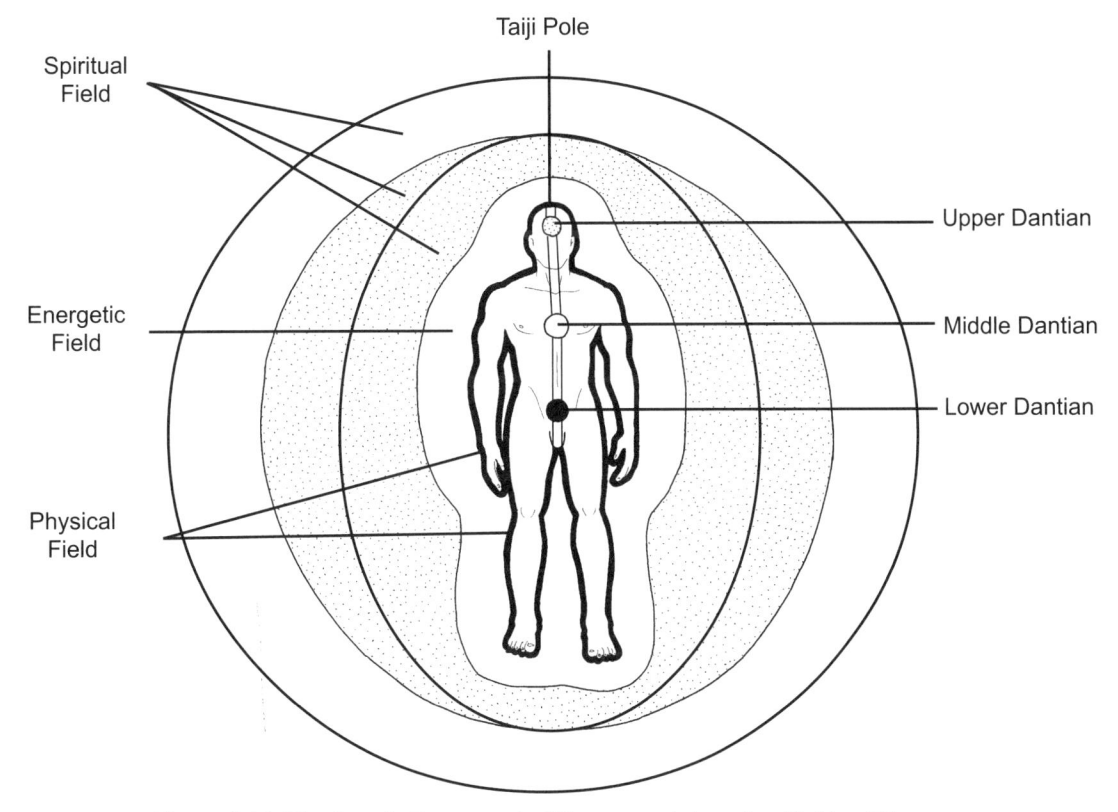

Figure 4.19. The Aura is Composed of Numerous Interacting Fields of Energy

SPIRITUAL LIGHT

Beyond the light of the energetic world (energetic light) exists the lower spiritual light and the higher spiritual light, described as follows:

1. The lower spiritual light forms a continuum with the energetic light, and corresponds to the lower frequencies of the spiritual world. The lower spiritual light manifests through the individual's spiritual consciousness.
2. The higher spiritual light is not associated with the ability of "seeing," but rather with the presence of "illumination." It is considered the true perception of "oneness," which comes from the fusion of an individual's Heart and Mind with the Divine. It manifests within a superluminal (faster than light) state of existence.

AURA COLORS

An "aura" is a field of luminous energy that surrounds all living things (people, animals and plants), and, to a lesser degree, all inanimate objects. Aura colors sometimes appear in the form of waves or patterns of energy (for example: evenly layered, blotchy, or mixed together). Aura colors are in a constant state of energetic flux, changing their colors and patterns with each shift in the patient's thoughts and emotions. These energetic colors merge and blend as they fluctuate, weaving in and around the patient's second field of Wei Qi (Figure 4.19).

A patient's auric field may be observed in the form of a transparent or opaque flow of Qi or as masses of different densities and colors. This may be used as a basis for determining the location and features of specific diseases. Each Yin and Yang organ has its own signature color vibration.

When the energy of an organ is healthy, the Qi color is clean, clear, and lucid. When an organ is diseased, its Qi becomes dark gray and turbid. These colors reveal whether an organ is in an abnormal condition and to what extent it has been affected.

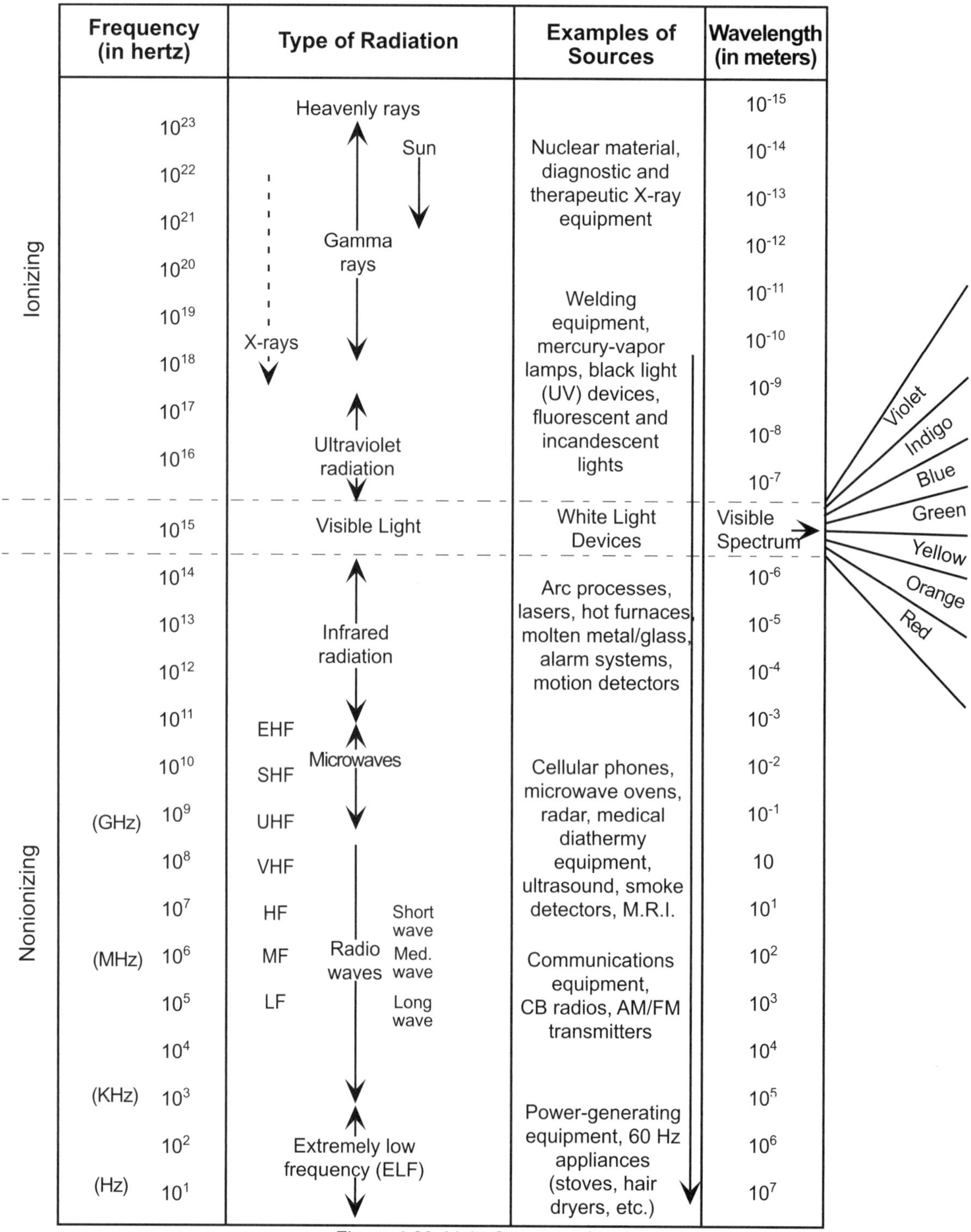

VOLUME 1, SECTION 1: FOUNDATIONS OF CHINESE ENERGETIC MEDICINE

Frequency (in hertz)	Type of Radiation	Examples of Sources	Wavelength (in meters)
Ionizing			
10^{23}	Heavenly rays ↑	Nuclear material, diagnostic and therapeutic X-ray equipment	10^{-15}
10^{22}	Sun ↓		10^{-14}
10^{21}			10^{-13}
10^{20}	Gamma rays		10^{-12}
10^{19}		Welding equipment, mercury-vapor lamps, black light (UV) devices, fluorescent and incandescent lights	10^{-11}
10^{18}	X-rays ↓		10^{-10}
10^{17}	↑		10^{-9}
10^{16}	Ultraviolet radiation ↓		10^{-8}
			10^{-7}
10^{15}	Visible Light	White Light Devices	Visible Spectrum
Nonionizing			
10^{14}	↑	Arc processes, lasers, hot furnaces, molten metal/glass, alarm systems, motion detectors	10^{-6}
10^{13}	Infrared radiation		10^{-5}
10^{12}	↓		10^{-4}
10^{11}	EHF		10^{-3}
(GHz) 10^{10}	SHF — Microwaves ↓	Cellular phones, microwave ovens, radar, medical diathermy equipment, ultrasound, smoke detectors, M.R.I.	10^{-2}
10^{9}	UHF		10^{-1}
10^{8}	VHF		10
10^{7}	HF — Short wave		10^{1}
(MHz) 10^{6}	MF — Radio waves — Med. wave	Communications equipment, CB radios, AM/FM transmitters	10^{2}
10^{5}	LF — Long wave		10^{3}
10^{4}	↓		10^{4}
(KHz) 10^{3}	↑	Power-generating equipment, 60 Hz appliances (stoves, hair dryers, etc.)	10^{5}
10^{2}	Extremely low frequency (ELF)		10^{6}
(Hz) 10^{1}	↓		10^{7}

Visible Spectrum: Violet, Indigo, Blue, Green, Yellow, Orange, Red

Figure 4.20. Light Spectrum Chart

Color Vibrational Classifications

The visible light spectrum is measured in nanometers (nm). A nanometer is one billionth of a meter. Colors are divided into approximately 700 bandwidths (or wavelengths) ranging from 290 to 990 nm. The variety of shifting colors can be interpreted according to their density and tone. The preceding chart displays the color frequency correlation in nanometers (Figure 4.20). All living organisms vibrate at a frequency with a wavelength between 300-2,000 nanometers. Specific colors emanate consistent frequencies and wave forms. The slower frequencies register in the infrared light spectrum, while the highest vibrational frequencies register in the ultraviolet light spectrum.

The Physiology of Visual Perception

The surrounding aperture of the eye, known as the "iris," expands and contracts around the pupil according to various energetic stimulations (Figure 4.21). As light enters the pupils, it converges on the retina at the back of the eye, creating a reversed image in two dimensions. These images are converted into electrical impulses that travel through the optic chiasm to various parts of the visual centers at the back of the Brain where they are then reversed and interpreted (Figure 4.22).

There are two types of nerve cell receptors located within the retina. These nerve cell receptors are known as rods and cones, described as follows:

- **Rods:** There are, on average, 10 million nerve cell receptors located on the periphery of the retina, with only one light sensitive pigment. The rods are responsible for nighttime vision; they discern the shadows between light and darkness, shape and movement.
- **Cones:** There are, on average, 3 million nerve cell receptors located at the center of the retina. On average, there receptors have three light sensitive pigments which respond to the red, green and blue wavelengths. The cones are responsible for daytime vision and can distinguish 7,500,000 different hues. However, if even a single set of these color receptive cones is missing from the retina, the patient will be unable to distinguish most colors and can be classified as color blind.

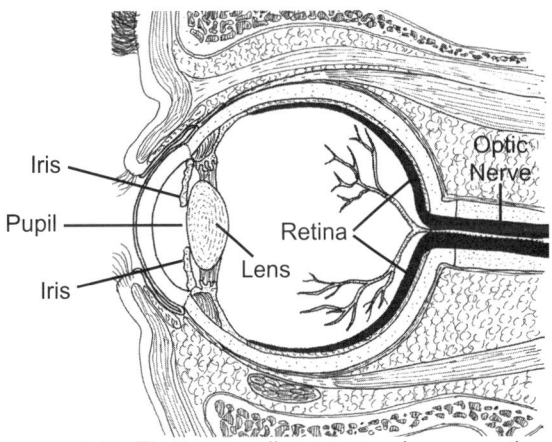

Figure 4.21. The surrounding aperture known as the "iris" expands and contracts around the pupil according to various types of stimulation (Inspired by the original artwork of Wynn Kapit).

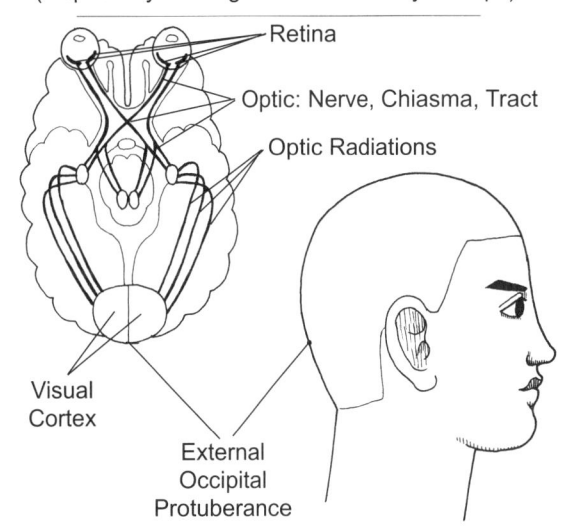

Figure 4.22. As light enters the pupils, it converges on the retina at the back of the eye, creating a reversed image in two dimensions (Inspired by the original artwork of Wynn Kapit).

Seeing Auras and Emotional Energy

Seeing auras is a visual phenomenon which can occur after many hours of regular Qigong training. This ability to see the external energy field is not limited to Medical Qigong training, as many people are born with this ability. The word "aura" literally means "breeze" manifesting as shimmering layers of luminous colored energy that circulate around and penetrate into the physical body. These colors are part of the body's biophoton emissions, which is radiant light energy that emanates from all living systems. These colors are constantly in motion, reflecting thoughts, feelings, emotional patterns, and environmental influences.

Through the stimulation and physical dilation of the occipital lobe of the Brain, the doctor begins to develop this unique visual ability. In the beginning stages, the doctor may see energy coming off the patient's body like steam. Later, brilliant, luminous colors become visible. The doctor is beginning to observe the infrared and ultraviolet radiation color patterns emitted by the patient's body. The infrared spectrum is just below the average person's visual spectrum, while the ultraviolet is just above the average visual spectrum. By stimulating and dilating the occipital lobe, the visual spectrum expands to include the infrared and ultraviolet frequencies, allowing the doctor to observe a much greater range of color.

It has been my personal observation that students who possess a large bump on the back of the cranium, specifically between the channel points GV-16 and GV-17, begin to see auras at a very early stage. These points are below and just above the external occipital protuberance and surround the internal branches of the occipital arteries, veins, and nerves. When energy fills this area, it stimulates and vibrates these nerves and arteries which causes the visual receptors of the Brain to perceive phenomena at a faster rate. This has the subjective effect of slowing down time.

These subtle perceptions are all possible due to the dilation of the occipital membranes. To maintain this dilation, the doctor must remain calm and relaxed. Any tension brought about by stress only diminishes this ability. Auras are generally seen through the peripheral field of vision, using the rods rather than the cones of the eyes. The rods are more sensitive to the low light levels than are the cones, which are more sensitive to color.

If the doctor begins to stare at any particular object, focused concentration will contract the occipital membranes, causing tension and pressure which can inhibit the dilation process. The secret in maintaining this altered state of observation is to anchor the mind deep into the ground. By focusing the mind on a specific point, the attention can be shifted to receiving and observing auras, or to extending energy without distraction.

Projecting Colored Light

When Qigong doctors connect with divine healing white light energy, they absorb massive quantities of this energy into their Taiji Pole. This white light energy prisms into eight colors of light and energy vibration. As the divine white light energy transforms into multicolored beams of light, the colors can be either absorbed to strengthen the internal organs or projected for Qi emission.

Qigong doctors project light of different colors by first drawing and gathering the divine light energy into their body via the Taiji Pole. They then focus on the divine light energy and either project it outward through the arms and the hands, or release it by visualizing the divine light traveling from out of the doctor's Yin Tang (Third Eye) area and into the patient's tissues.

The Qigong doctors use inner vision techniques to connect with the correct color for energy projection. One such technique allows the color to naturally develop by mentally focusing both eyes to the back of the head. The color that is observed in the back of the mind is then projected into the patient's body. This visualization technique is only performed after connecting with the patient's energetic field.

Light Therapy Through Emitted Qi

The human body produces light which is visible to both clairvoyants and Qigong doctors. In China, doctors of Traditional Chinese Medicine have discovered that light therapy is effective in treating certain diseases due to the fact that projected light is able to penetrate the tissues and interact with the patients' energetic fields.

Extending the image of the color is an important part of the Qigong doctor's ability to treat and heal patients. The colored light acts as a catalyst to bring specific aspects of the patient's unconscious thoughts and feelings to the surface.

To treat patients with emitted light therapy, the Qigong doctor first focuses his or her intention on visualizing and cultivating a certain color. By visualizing this specific color, the Qigong doctor is activating a particular aspect of the light energy within his or her own body. The doctor then focuses on projecting this healthy colored light into the patient's organs, channels, and organ systems.

Energetic color therapy utilizes eight healing colors, ranging from low frequency (red) to high frequency (violet) and white. These energetic projections are associated with the colors emanating from the body's Taiji Pole and range from dark to lighter color bands.

When projecting color vibrations, it is important to note that there are four levels, or intensities, of color gradations within each color (Figure 4.23). In the soft color range there are two levels: a light and a medium-light color, both of which are used for gentle, less potent projections (usually for healing and cleansing wounds). Medium-light color projections are especially effective for treating young children and the elderly. In the intense range, there are also two levels of intensity: a bright and a very bright color range, both of which are used for full-force projection (for destroying cells and pathogenic factors, or for stabilizing a deficient organ or organ area). The bright color is initially used to begin with; later, the very bright color is used as the patient's strength increases.

Research has demonstrated that the use of color in Qigong treatments can effectively change a patient's pulse rate, body rhythms, and depth of breathing. Advanced Qigong doctors modulate and switch energetic color projections during treatment. To avoid overstimulating the patient's tissues, the doctor starts with a lighter shade of color projection then increases the color's intensity until the desired affect is obtained.

Medical Qigong uses the following eight colors for energetic projection: red, orange, yellow, green, blue, indigo (dark blue), violet, and white. Based on the modern understanding of the prismatic division of light, color projection is categorized and described as follows (Figure 4.24):

1. **The Ruby Red Color:** This color has the longest wavelength of the visible colors and is associated with physical and material forces. It simultaneously heats and activates the body. The color red improves Blood circulation and can be used to stimulate the Small Intestine, Heart, Triple Burners and Pericardium organs and channels, as well as energize the body's Fire Element Qi. Red can be used to repair the body's tissues, Tonify Blood Deficiency, increase cellular growth, increase blood pressure, and increase the body's metabolic rate. Additionally, the color red can be used to vitalize the body's tissues, Blood, and the skeletal system. It can also be used for treating paralysis, broken Bones, and both internal and external wounds. The color red engenders strength, courage, passion and sensuality, and it counteracts depression, worry, and fear. It can have a positive influence in cases of debility and Blood disorders.

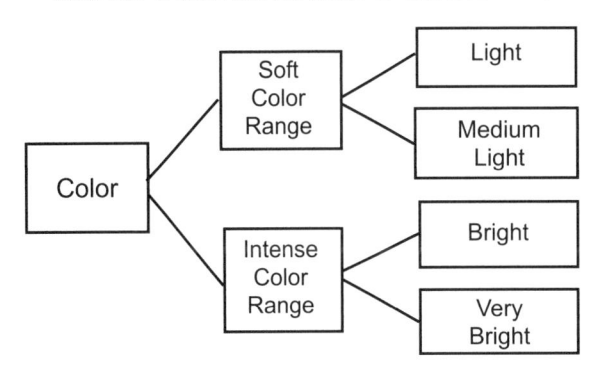

Figure 4.23. The Four Levels of Energetic Projection of Colored Light

Contraindications: The doctor must avoid using red colored Qi when treating patients who have hypertension, external bleeding, or when women are menstruating. The use of the color red is strictly prohibited in cases of Excess Heart Fire.

Generally, the color pink is used to tonify the Heart in cases where the color red is too strong. Pink can be used in small doses to relax and neutralize aggressive behavior, however, prolonged exposure will cause irritability, aggression and emotional distress.

2. **The Orange Color:** This color expels pathogenic factors and is often used for treating cysts and for disintegrating blood clots. The color orange can also be used to stimulate the Spleen and Stomach organs and channels. It

The Eight Colors of Light Projection

- White Color — Energizes, Purges and Strengthens Wei Qi
- Violet Color — Facilitates Rapid Healing of Difficult Infections
- Indigo Color — Knitting Bones and Creating Energetic Casts
- Blue Color — Cools the Body
- Green Color — Detoxifies and Disperses Pathogenic Qi
- Yellow Color — Stimulates Nerves, Reconstructs Cells, and Heals Wounds
- Orange Color — Expels Pathogenic Factors and Disintegrates Blood Clots
- Red Color — Heats and Activates the Body

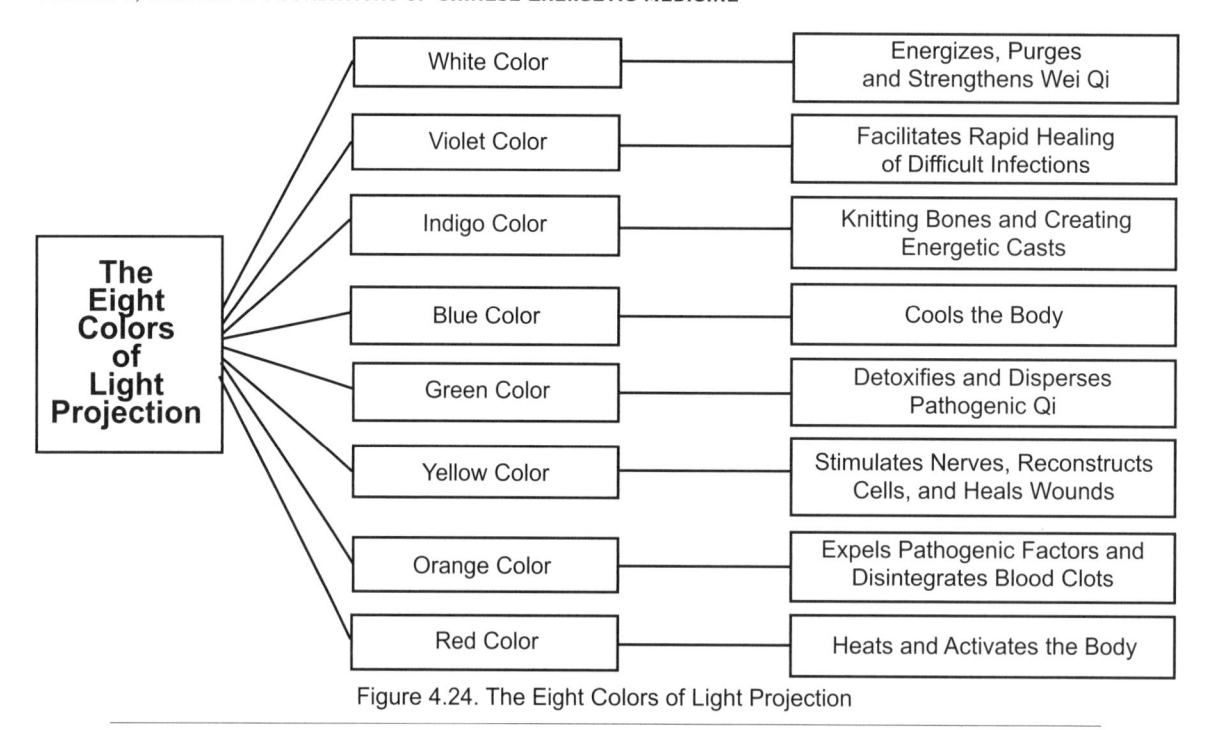

Figure 4.24. The Eight Colors of Light Projection

is associated with both Qi (energy) and Zhi (wisdom), and is considered to be a powerful tonic. The color orange engenders self-confidence, determination and optimism, and stimulates the visual expression of ideas.

Contraindications: The doctor must avoid projecting orange colored Qi into the Brain, eyes, or Heart of the patient. The color orange is extremely potent and may cause tissue damage when used improperly or in excess.

3. **The Lemon Yellow Color:** This color stimulates the nerves, reconstructs cells, and heals wounds. Yellow or orange yellow can be used to stimulate the Stomach and Spleen organs and channels, as well as the body's pancreas, digestive system and nervous system. The yellow color can be used to energize the body's Earth Element Qi. Yellow is also used in the treatment of skin rashes. The color yellow revitalizes and stimulates the Shen (spirit) and assists the mind in creating thoughts and visualizations. It engenders optimism, happiness, and a balanced outlook on life.

4. **The Emerald Green Color:** This color is soothing to the nerves and can be used as a tonic for the Heart. It can also be used to detoxify and disperse pathogenic Qi. Green can stimulate the Liver and Gall Bladder organs and channels, and energize the body's Wood Element Qi. The color green is associated with harmony and compassion, and engenders peace, sympathy, and kindness.

Green is also used in combination with other colors. For example, shades of green are combined with shades of orange for treating tumors. Green color vibration is generally not as powerful as orange and may be used on elderly patients, young children, or for a more gentle healing session.

5. **The Flame Blue Color:** This light color cools the body and is beneficial in soothing and calming anxiety. The light blue color can be used to stimulate the Urinary Bladder and Kidney organs and channels, as well as the body's reproductive system, skeletal system, throat, and thyroid gland. Light blue can also be used to energize the body's Water Element Qi. The light blue color can be used as a mild anesthetic, and

is also excellent for relieving inflammation, insomnia, headache, and fever. Additionally, the light blue color is used for slowing the metabolism, lowering blood pressure, perspiration, respiration and brain-wave activity. It is a spiritual color that engenders truth, devotion, serenity, peace, and religious aspirations.

6. **The Indigo Color:** This dark blue color has a deep penetrating property. It is generally used for knitting Bones, treating eye diseases, insomnia, mental disorders, nervous disorders, and for creating "energetic casts" (enveloping wounds and encapsulating specific internal organs). The dark blue indigo color can also be used to stimulate the Urinary Bladder and Kidney organs and channels, as well as the body's skeletal system, reproductive system, and pineal gland. The dark blue color can also be used to energize the body's Water Element Qi. The color indigo is a spiritual color that engenders inspiration and artistic creativity.

7. **The Violet (Reddish-Blue) Color:** This color has the shortest wavelength of all visible colors and is associated with spirituality, mysticism, intuition, psychic abilities, and enlightenment. It is known for its purifying force, which facilitates the rapid healing of difficult infections, such as pneumonia. It is also excellent for treating nervous disorders, mental diseases, neurosis, neuralgia, and epilepsy. Because of its ability to energetically dissolve into the Wuji, the color violet can sometimes be used to dissolve brain tumors (when used in short durations during treatment and then immediately removed).

8. **The White Color:** This color is a fusion of all other colors, and thus the most neutral. White is associated with purity, and is the most common color of light used by the Qigong doctor. It is useful for calming the mind, or for placing a protective field around the body or around a specific internal organ. White can be used to stimulate the Large Intestine and Lung organs and channels, as well as the body's respiratory system. The white color can also be used to energize the body's Metal Element Qi.

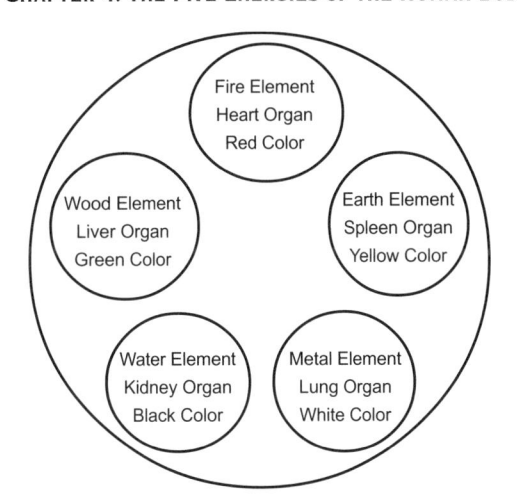

Figure 4.25. The Five Colors of the Five Yin Organs

USING HEALING COLOR IMAGERY

Meditations emphasizing specific colors (Wood: Liver-Green/Blue; Fire: Heart-Red; Earth: Spleen-Yellow or Light Brown; Metal: Lungs-White; and Water: Kidneys-Black or Dark Blue) can be prescribed to assist patients in their healing (Figure 4.25). The patients are instructed to visualize specific organ colors while the Qigong doctor projects that same color into their body and energetic fields. The patient may later be asked to repeat the visualization as a Medical Qigong homework prescription exercise. This treatment technique is successfully used for Tonifying, Regulating, or Purging all the body's major organs, and is often combined with healing sounds.

When using colors in therapeutic imagery, the patients are encouraged to first visualize the diseased organ as being dull, dark, and impure in color. In cases of Liver Heat, for example, patients might imagine a dull, turbid brownish-green tinged with red. For a Heart imbalance, the red color may be first imagined as a dull, weak or darkish red, tinged with brownish-red or purplish-red (like the color of stagnant Blood). Patients begin the meditation by concentrating on exhaling the impure, toxic colors. As the patients inhale, they imagine a pure, vibrant color flowing into their body from either the Heavens or the Earth, energizing and cleansing their body, internal organ and organ system (replacing the toxic energetic color of the diseased area).

EXPOSURE TO EXTERNAL COLOR FIELDS

In certain Five Element schools of color therapy, patients are required to sit and meditate in rooms painted in the color that relates to their specific condition. A healthy color is chosen in accordance with either the Five Element Creative Cycle or the Controlling Cycle, depending upon the nature of the patient's disease and which particular Yin organ (or organs) is involved. One example is using the Five Element Creative Cycle to tonify a patient's deficient organ. According to the theory of the Creative Cycle, one can stimulate and energize the "mother" Element in order to strengthen the "child" Element that follows it. A patient with a Liver imbalance, for example, can be placed in a dark blue room for tonifying the Kidneys (the Liver's "mother" organ). The Kidney (mother organ) color indigo (dark blue), is used to nourish the Liver (child organ). For a Liver Excess, the Qigong doctor would use the Five Element Controlling Cycle and place the patient in a white room, allowing the Lungs' (the grandmother) white Metal color to control the Liver Wood (the child) organ (Figure 4.26).

Additionally, the patient can wear or surround him or herself with certain Five Element colors to initiate healing (e.g., emerald green for Liver conditions).

FOOD AND COLOR

Another treatment method requires the presentation of food (diet) as a form of color and light therapy. In this treatment the doctor makes sure that the Five Element colors are present within the patient's food. Each color (i.e., Green/Blue for Liver, Red for Heart, Yellow or Light Brown for Spleen, White for Lungs, and Black or Dark Blue for Kidneys) will target and tonify the patient's organs.

Modern nutritional research demonstrates that the presence of specific vitamins and minerals in food is often associated with the color of the food itself. When eating the food, the patient focuses his or her intention on ingesting the color, light, and energy of the food being eaten.

USING DISTANCE AND RANGE

When using color projection, an important factor is the doctor's ability to maintain focused

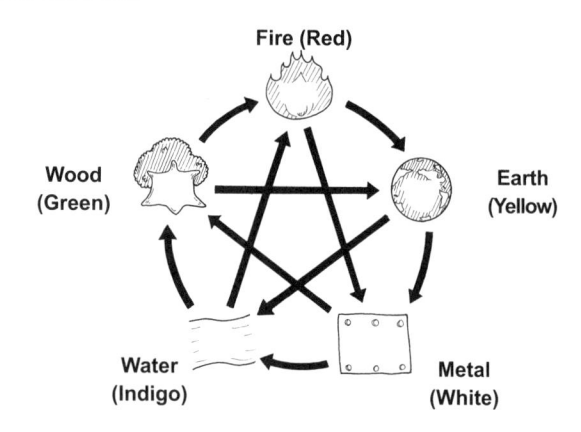

Figure 4.26. The Five Elements (Wu Xing)

attention. If the doctor becomes distracted or looses visual concentration, the color resonance being emitted becomes weakened, and the projected color transforms back into non-differentiated white-light energy.

WESTERN LIGHT THERAPY

In 1941, Harry Riley Spitler, M.D., O.D., performed extensive research on the way in which light influences the autonomic nervous system. Some of his findings are described as follows:
- Light has a regenerative effect on the body, increasing the growth rate of cells.
- Light affects the functioning of the pituitary gland.
- Environmental light can have an effect on the reproductive cycle.
- Light affects the tension between the sympathetic and the parasympathetic nervous system.
- Light influences hormone secretion and neurotransmitters.
- Light affects muscle responses (i.e., slowing or speeding up the heartbeat).
- There is a relationship between the frequency of light that enters into the eyes and the perception of pain.
- There is a relationship between the frequency of light that enters into the eyes, the vitamin A content, and the adaptation of the eyes to low degrees of light.
- There is a relationship between environmental light and the affects of the patient's hereditary potential.

Due to Dr. Spitler's research and the research of his colleagues, light therapy is currently being used in numerous forms by Western medicine. Some examples of light therapy are described as follows:
- Laser-light therapy surgery
- Full-spectrum light therapy for SAD (seasonal affective disorder)
- Color-light therapy for eye problems and various other illnesses
- UV-light therapy for "blue babies" with hyperbilirubinemia

MAGNETIC ENERGY

Magnetic energy is the energy contained within a magnetic field. A magnetic field is generated by the movement of electrical currents. An electromagnetic "field" is a matrix or medium which connects two or more points in space, and is usually represented by ripples or waves of energy. The concept of an electromagnetic field is represented by lines of "force" used to indicate direction, shape and influence.

The Earth, like the body, has both a Yin (magnetic) field and a Yang (electrical) charge. These energetic fields are interdependent. The magnetic field is caused by the movement of charged particles, and it spans the circumference of the Earth creating a strong electrical field (Figure 4.27). It is difficult to separate the energetic properties of magnetism and electricity, as they are practically two aspects of the same energetic field. However, by establishing different magnetic polarities (Yin and Yang), the Qigong doctor can influence the flow of electromagnetic energy in the body.

The Earth can be viewed as a giant geomagnetic energy field that contains both strong and weak areas. Generally, the energetic fields within specific areas are fixed and do not move (Figure 4.28). However, if an energetic field becomes weak (due to plate tectonic shifts, volcanic eruptions, military experimentation, etc.) nearby stronger fields expand, altering the area's overall energetic pattern.

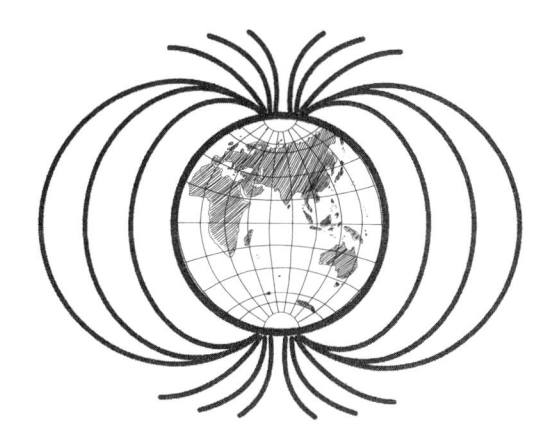

Figure 4.27. The Earth is enveloped with electromagnetic currents, affecting gravitational fields, weather, and vegetation.

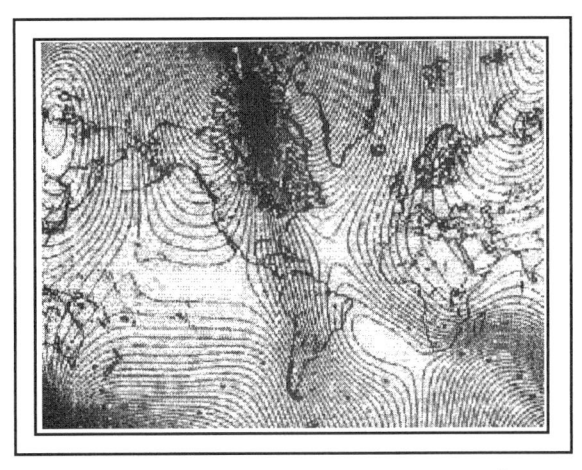

Figure 4.28. The Earth's magnetic field, according to US geologists in 1995.

MAGNETIC FIELDS AND THE BODY

Magnetism is produced by the body's energetic patterns, and can also influence the flows of energy currents in the body. As previously mentioned, the body's cells carry electromagnetic fields containing both positive and negative polarities that both attract and repel each other. This results in a magnetic pull between the body's various types of Qi, tissues, organs, and extremities. These tiny electromagnetic fields, when viewed as a whole, govern the body's electromagnetic interaction with the Earth. Clinical research in China demonstrates that the iron in the hemoglobin of the Blood is attracted to the magnetic pull of the body's tissues, as well as to the magnetic pull of the Earth.

Additionally, the body's emotional field is connected to the Earth's electromagnetic fields, and any shift in the Earth's field influences the individual's emotional temperament. This explains the change in moods and behavior historically associated with the phases of the moon. During the full moon, for example, there is a slight expansion and change in the Earth's magnetic field causing a corresponding change and expansion in human emotional fields.

The ancient Chinese believed that the Earth's energetic fields contained a type of "memory" imprinted within them. Thus, each geographical area contains its own resonant field of ancestral and environmental knowledge. The entire energetic history of any given area is encoded in the subtleties of its present energetic field, and can be accessed through Shengong (Spirit Skill) training.

Modern Research

Some modern researchers believe that the physical body's channel system (Chapters 6 and 8) charges its magnetic field through movement (the alternation of positive and negative pressure). It is further believed that the channel system creates an electrical field that attracts electrons into the body's Taiji Pole.

Richard Lee of the China Healthways Institute found that the magnetic substances (Yin) stored within the body's water molecules naturally align themselves with the flow of electrical energy (Yang) in the body's channels. When the body's magnetic energy field is low, these channels become weakened and the conductivity is lowered. This magnetic energy can be replenished either by ingesting and transforming energy from food, air, and water, or gathered directly from the Earth's magnetic field. The body's magnetic field is affected by the Earth's magnetic field through the energetic exchange occurring within both electromagnetic fields (Figure 4.29).

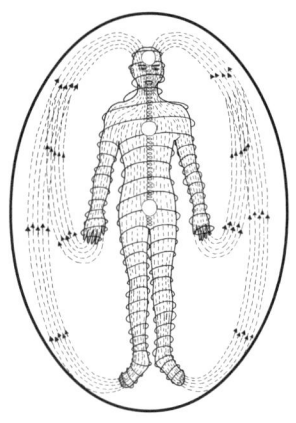

Figure 4.29. The body is enveloped with electromagnetic currents that influence both internal and external organ functions.

The Electromagnetic Effects of the Body's Taiji Pole

The body maintains its electromagnetic connection with the Earth through the energetic resonance of the Taiji Pole. Within the energetic structure of the body's Taiji Pole are located two major poles of energy. Each pole is located at opposite ends of the Taiji Pole (one is positioned at the top of the head and the other is positioned at the base of the perineum). The purpose of these energetic poles is to absorb Qi from the various universal and environmental fields, and connect and integrate that energy into the body's Three Dantians (see Chapter 5).

The two magnetic poles of the Upper Dantian and Lower Dantian have a different energy influx. The electromagnetic lines in the body's biofield begin at the top of the head where the Heaven Qi flows into the body and descends the Taiji Pole, ending at the base of the perineum (Figure 4.30). Consequently, the Earth energy is drawn upwards from the legs and perineum and flows into the Lower Dantian, eventually ending at the top of the head in the Upper Dantian. The bottom pole, located in the Lower Dantian, converts Jing (Essence) into Qi (Energy) and increases the body's overall life-force energy. The upper pole, located in the Upper Dantian, converts Shen (Spirit) into perceptual insight and spiritual light contained within the infinite space of the Wuji.

There are several ways in which the Qigong doctor can manipulate the electromagnetic field that surrounds the body. The doctor can directly absorb Heaven and Earth energy from the bottom of his or her feet, through the top of the head, and through both palms (called "absorbing Qi from the Five Gates").

The doctor can also gather and wrap different types of environmental energy around his or her body through creative visualization, which can increase the thickness and power of his or her electromagnetic field. This looping action is similar to wrapping a magnet with wire to increase its magnetic field potential (Figure 4.31). Stronger lines of magnetic force will be produced around the body, thus, creating a stronger "energy bubble" (Figure 4.32).

The direction of electromagnetic wrapping should be done in accordance with the natural flow of energy in the surrounding environmental fields. Each individual should be sensitive as to which method works best, as there are many techniques available depending on the doctor's intention and belief.

Magnetic Therapy Through Emitted Qi

Qigong doctors are trained to manipulate their patient's electromagnetic field by extending emitted energy into the patient's tissues. This stimulation of the body's magnetic field is extremely effective for regulating the flow of channel energy, and for stimulating the activity of the nervous system.

Magnetic therapy is also used in combination with acupuncture therapy. Acupuncturists use magnetic patches by placing them on various channel points on the patient's body, inducing energy flow and stimulating the patient's tissues.

The negative north pole of the magnet is placed in contact with the patient's skin when treating conditions of Excess Heat and stagnation. The negative north pole is found to have a cooling and calming effect on tissues. Herbal teas used for Purgation, dispersing, anti-inflammatory, or sedative properties can be enhanced by placing the tea on the negative north pole of a magnetized surface for a minimum of one hour before drinking.

The positive south pole of the magnet is placed

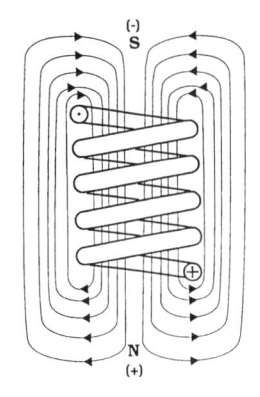

Figure 4.30. Magnetic field around an electrified spiral coil

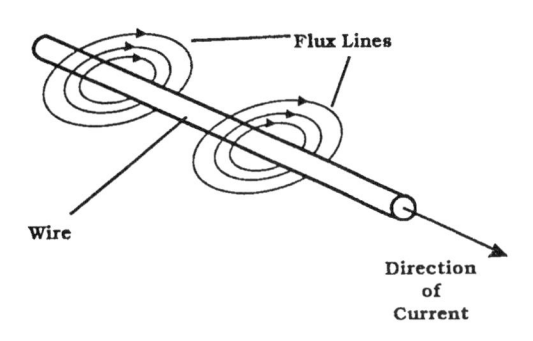

Figure 4.31. Flux lines around a current-carrying conductor

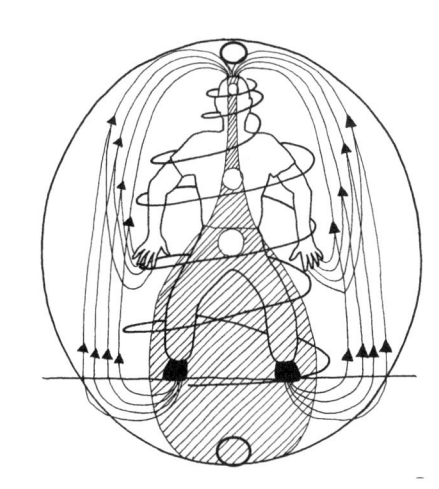

Figure 4.32. Qigong doctors can create a stronger energetic field by extending Qi into the Earth (like an anchor), increasing and expanding the Wei Qi field.

in contact with the patient's skin when treating deficiencies, Cold, and blockages. The positive south pole is said to have a stimulating and warming effect on tissues. Herbal teas used for warming and Tonification can be enhanced by placing the tea on the positive south pole of a magnetized surface for a minimum of one hour before drinking.

WESTERN MAGNETIC THERAPY

In 1990, Dr. Arthur Trappier submitted a paper entitled "Evaluating Perspectives on the Exposure Risks from Magnetic Fields" to the *Journal of the National Medical Association*. In his article, Dr. Trappier explained that exposing cancer cells to a negative magnetic field discourages the growth of the cancer, while exposing cancer cells to a positive magnetic field encourages their growth. Magnetic therapy is currently being used in Western medicine in a variety of clinical modalities, described as follows:

- Permanent magnet therapy for localized pain and inflammation relief
- Super-magnet therapy for stimulation of the thymus, and for immune system enhancement in cancer patients
- Pulsed magnetic therapy for the treatment of arthritic joints

HEAT

When electricity passes through any substance it produces heat. The amount of heat that is generated depends upon the resistance of the substance and the density of the current's flow. Heat is generated at the electron level by the friction created through molecular motion. By increasing the motion of the molecules, more heat is generated.

The molecules in living organisms are in constant motion, increasing or decreasing their rate of acceleration according to the external environmental temperature. In order for heat to have any effect on the body's temperature, enough Qi has to be transferred to increase the movement of the molecules within the tissue's cells.

The heat within the body causes increased electron movement, resulting in more heat being generated on a cellular level. Heat is also created as a by-product of cellular metabolism. The body's metabolism produces 75% of the energy created in the form of heat. Cellular activity is increased through electrical, magnetic, heat, sound, and light stimulation.

INTRODUCTION TO THE THREE FIRES

From a Medical Qigong perspective, heat in the body is generated from the accumulation of "Three Fires" which radiate from specific locations within the body. The Heart Fire is located within the body's chest cavity, the Kidney Fire is located within the abdominal cavity, and the Urinary Bladder Fire is located in the lower perineum. When the Heart Fire first awakens, the Kidney Fire responds to it and when the Kidney Fire moves, the Urinary Bladder Fire follows (Figure 4.33).

When these Three Fires follow their normal course of energetic movement, they direct and lead the body's life-force energy creating what the ancient Daoists called the "True Fire." Functionally, the Three Fires are responsible for regulating the Yin and Yang energy of the body by fusing the Five Element energies (stored within the body's five Yin organs) with the energy of the Three Dantians. As the Shen from the Heart Fire is drawn into the Lower Dantian, the Urinary Bladder Fire fuses with the Kidney Fire creating the body's True Fire. The True Fire causes the body's Jing to transform Qi within the Lower Dantian, and the Qi to transform into Shen within the Middle Dantian. Once the fusion of the Three Fires is complete, the mind, breath and body connections all become regulated.

REGIONS OF THE THREE FIRES

The Three Fires also represent the regions of vital heat responsible for the circulation of energy that sustains the human soul. The energy of the Three Fires is used for cultivation and spiritual liberation and is accessed through Medical Qigong Shengong practice, prayer, and meditation. The Three Fires are described as follows:

1. **The Heart Fire:** The Heart Fire is also called the Commanding Fire or the Emperor's Fire, and is located in the center of the chest. The Heart Fire is responsible for transforming Qi

CHAPTER 4: THE FIVE ENERGIES OF THE HUMAN BODY

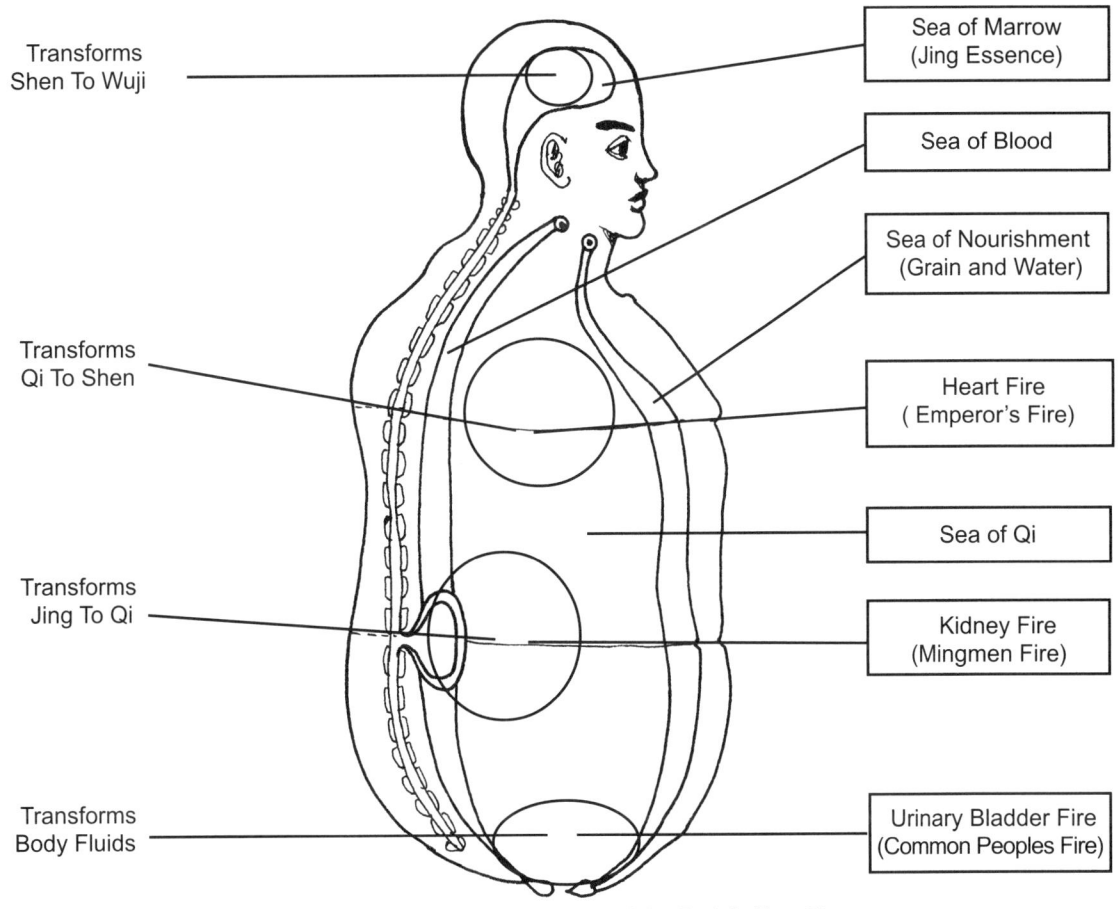

- Transforms Shen To Wuji
- Transforms Qi To Shen
- Transforms Jing To Qi
- Transforms Body Fluids

- Sea of Marrow (Jing Essence)
- Sea of Blood
- Sea of Nourishment (Grain and Water)
- Heart Fire (Emperor's Fire)
- Sea of Qi
- Kidney Fire (Mingmen Fire)
- Urinary Bladder Fire (Common Peoples Fire)

Figure 4.33. The Internal Formation of the Body's True Fire

into Shen, heating the internal organs in the Upper Burner, and energizing thought and emotion.

A deficiency of Heart Fire can lead to Shen Disturbances. Conversely, if the Heart Fire is in excess, Shen Disturbances will also occur.

2. **The Kidney Fire:** The Kidney Fire is also called the Ministerial Fire or the Mingmen Fire, and is located in the back of the body, just below the last floating rib and between the two Kidneys. The Kidney Fire is responsible for transforming Jing into Qi, heating the internal organs in the Middle and Lower Burners and is the "root" of the body's Yuan (Prenatal) Qi.

Qigong masters in ancient times regarded the Mingmen Fire as the motivating force of the body and paid special attention to its training during Qigong exercises.

A deficiency of the Mingmen Fire may lead to decreased sex-drive, hypogonadism, and impotency. Conversely, if the Mingmen Fire is in excess, increased sex-drive, sexual obsession, or hypergonadism can occur.

Dr. Zhao Xianke, an expert on medicine during the Ming dynasty period (1368-1644 A.D.), states that "the Mingmen Fire dominates all Twelve Primary Channels. Without it the Kidneys would be weak, the Spleen and Stomach could not digest food, the Liver and Gall Bladder would not provide any energy for thinking or planning, the urine and feces would not be moved, and the Heart would malfunction causing dizziness and endangering life."

3. **The Urinary Bladder Fire:** The Urinary Bladder Fire is also called the Common People's Fire, and is located in the lower abdominal area by the perineum. The Urinary Bladder Fire is responsible for heating the internal organs in the Lower Burners, evaporating water and transforming body fluids.

The purpose of the Three Fires is to transform and transport Jing, Qi and Shen throughout the body, transform and transport the energy of the Four Seas, provide heat to the internal organs within the Triple Burner, and assist in evaporating water and transforming Body Fluids. The physical locations of the Three Fires, coincide with the anatomical locations of the Triple Burners.

THE THREE FIRES AND THE TRIPLE BURNERS

The Three Fires are not the Triple Burners, which are a completely different energetic system. The purpose of the Triple Burners is to regulate the major internal organs, and differs from the purpose of the Three Fires as outlined above. The physical locations of the Three Fires, however, coincide with the locations of the Triple Burners (see Chapter 8).

HEAT THERAPY THROUGH EMITTED QI

Stimulating the body's tissues through heat therapy is extremely effective for treating deficient and Cold syndromes. In China, Qigong doctors use the extension of heat emitted through their field of electromagnetic energy, to stimulate their patients' tissues. This therapy helps to regulate the flow of the patients' channel energy and also tonifies the patient's Qi and Blood. Heat therapy is also used in the form of moxibustion as an adjunct to acupuncture therapy. Acupuncturists will use moxa sticks and/or cones, lighting and placing them over various channel points on the patient's body. This therapy induces Qi flow and stimulates the patient's tissues and channel points.

WESTERN HEAT THERAPY

Western medicine currently uses radiant and conductive heat therapy for vasodilation and pain relief. These heat therapies can further divided and categorized into dry-heat therapy and moist heat therapy.

Dry-heat therapies are described as follows:
• Dry packs
• Hot water bottles
• Heliotherapy-sun therapy
• Ultraviolet-heat therapy
• Infrared-heat therapy
• Diathermy therapy

Moist-heat therapies (hydrocolators) are described as follows:
• Hot bath packs
• Hot wet packs
• Hot foot baths
• Fomentations
• Poultices
• Vapor and paraffin baths

ELECTRICITY

The flow of electrons is called a current. A current produces a magnetic field, and likewise a magnetic field induces an electrical current when it moves in relation to a conductor. In Medical Qigong therapy, the body's channels are considered to be electrical circuits, and the points existing along each channel can be seen as booster amplifiers (or step-up transformers) that maintain the current's strength. According to Robert O. Becker, M.D., research scientist and author of the book *Cross Currents*, acupuncture needles have the capacity to act as antennae, drawing charged particles (ions) from the atmosphere and sending them into the body. The acupuncture needle delivers a low-level electrical stimulation to the channel points and can be used to charge up or decrease the energetic potential of these step-up transformers, thus affecting the energetic current flowing along the channel.

While researching the electromagnetic currents within the human body, Dr. Becker found that the human body is an excellent conductor of electricity, containing both alternating electrical currents (AC) and direct electrical currents (DC). The alternating current is responsible for the transformation of the body's magnetic field into the body's electrical field. The direct current is responsible for the body's positive (Yang) and negative (Yin) flow of electrical charges (Figure 4. 34).

The friction produced by rubbing the feet on

a carpet creates an electrical charge that is stored within the body until it touches another conductor (metal, another body, etc.) which releases the charge. This everyday occurrence demonstrates the storage, conduction, and discharging of electrons from the body. Any time electrons travel, heat or thermal radiation is produced.

According to Swedish physician and medical research scientist, Dr. Bjorn Nordenstrom, the biological circuits of the body are driven by accumulated charges, which, unlike a battery, oscillate between positive and negative. The body's system of channels and Blood Vessels act as insulated cables, while the blood plasma acts as a conductor.

The intercellular fluid in the body's permeable tissue conducts ions. The ion pumps and channels located in the plasma membrane of the cells are a key component of the body's electrical circuits. Every human thought and action is accompanied by the conduction of electrical signals along the fibers of the nervous system. In fact, life would not exist without this constant flow of ions across the membranes of cells.

The electromagnetic energy in the body's cells is continuously being generated from the biochemical transformation of food and air. It is circulated throughout the body by the electromagnetic fields generated from within the tissues. Perineural cells, or nerve sheaths, carry the direct current of the body's electricity. These cells are responsible for motivating the body to heal, regenerate, and repair itself. Healing is always affected by a change within the body's electromagnetic field. The rate and efficiency of healing is based on the strength and polarity of the body's energetic field. This electricity is one of the primary types of energy responsible for maintaining life itself.

THE BODY'S PIEZOELECTRIC QUALITIES

Vibratory wave energy is transformed in the human body by the piezoelectric properties (the ability to produce electricity or electrical polarity from the application of mechanical force) of tissues such as Bones and connective tissue containing crystalline structures. The helical molecules

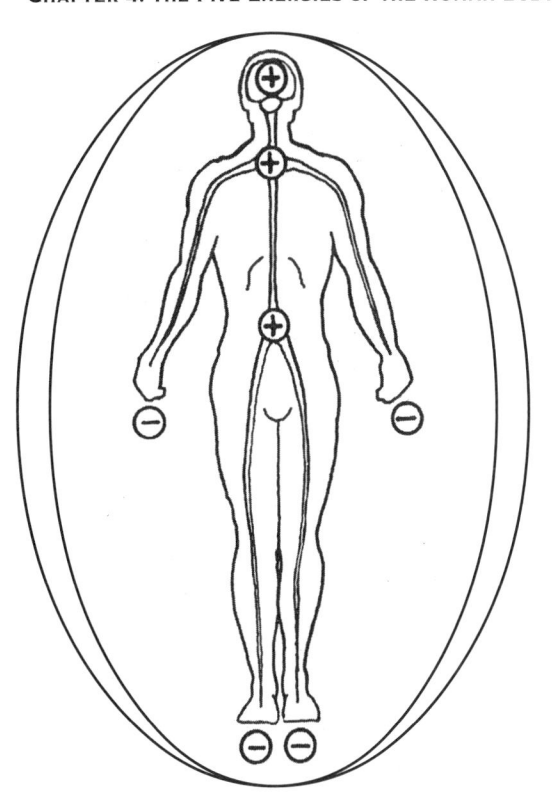

Figure 4.34. The Direct Current is responsible for the body's positive (Yang) and negative (Yin) flow of electrical charges.

such as DNA, keratin, collagen, actin and myosin all have piezoelectric qualities. Dr. Becker's research demonstrates that Bones are "piezoelectric," and that when Bones are stressed, mechanical energy is converted into electrical energy. He discovered that running a minute electrical current through a fractured Bone will stimulate the reproduction of the cells, creating a healing current similar to the body's natural healing mechanism.

According to Richard Lee of China Healthways Institute, electrostatic waves are observed in the body with both EEGs (electro-encephalograms) and EMGs (electromyograms). Therapies that affect the EEGs include sound therapy, meditation therapy, self-regulation Qigong therapy, and light therapy. By controlling their thoughts, Qigong doctors can affect the energy currents in their body and thus affect the EEG measurements. Experiments show that EEG measurements in test subjects receiving energy from healers tend to synchronize. Qigong doctors, when treating patients, can produce voltages as high as 190 volts, which is 100,000 times greater than regular EEG voltages.

The body's natural ability to gather, store, and move Qi increases the body's abilities to gather, store, and move electrical charges. The gathering of these electrical charges can cause a gradual buildup of electricity within the tissues and internal organs, and can develop into an excess Qi condition if not properly grounded or rooted.

Excess Qi conditions often manifest in mood swings and are responsible for the energetic circuit overloads that occur spontaneously within the body. Excess Qi may manifest as a sudden "explosion" or "release" of emotions such as rage, fear, grief, worry, fright, anxiety, and excitement.

If the treating doctor is not properly grounded or rooted, an excess electromagnetic charge can be released from the patient's internal tissues and become absorbed by the doctor's internal organs. This energetic reaction can cause an already overcharged internal organ to spontaneously release emotions. Sometimes the release can be physiological, (e.g., sudden sweating, blushing, twitching, jerking, yawning, sighing, burping, etc.). These are all examples of an internal organ seeking to regain homeostasis by discharging energy.

Research conducted on electromagnetic fields has revealed that electric blankets diminish the pineal gland's ability to produce melatonin. Since the body uses melatonin to combat cancer, this explains the relationship between the use of electric blankets and increased incidences of leukemia and Alzheimer's disease.

ELECTRICAL THERAPY THROUGH EMITTED QI

The idea that an electric current can stimulate bodily repair, alert defense mechanisms, and control the growth and function of cells is not a new concept in Western medicine. In fact, the use of bio-electromagnetism dates back at least 200 years. Electrotherapy has been found to be useful for relieving pain by signaling the Brain to activate and alter the body's neurochemicals. The insertion of electrically stimulating needles into a patient's body, for example, causes a release of endorphins and is used for pain management.

Medical Qigong, acupuncture, and Chinese massage likewise stimulate the peripheral and cutaneous nerves that carry sensory information through the spinal cord to the Brain. This stimulation of the cutaneous nerves activates the Brain's opiates (endorphins) and facilitates the closure of the body's pain-relay gates, stopping pain, and providing the neurological basis for anesthesia. Because Medical Qigong therapy also has an analgesic effect on the body's cutaneous tissues, it is increasingly being used in hospitals for preoperative and postoperative procedures.

WESTERN ELECTROTHERAPY

Western medicine is currently using electrotherapy in a variety of modalities, some of which are described as follows:

- Giga-TENS therapy for stimulation of healing
- TENS therapy for pain relief
- CES-cranial electro-stimulation therapy, for depression and substance abuse, etc.
- Micro-stimulation therapy for micro-current stimulation below the threshold of awareness, to stimulate nonspecific healing, the reduction of inflammation, and the harmonization of tissue polarity

Chapter 5
The Taiji Pole and Three Dantians

The Taiji Pole

The Taiji Pole flows from the Baihui point at the top of the head through the center core of the body to the Huiyin point at the base of the perineum. It is seen as a vertical column (or pole) of brilliant white light, full of vibration and energetic pulsation. The Taiji Pole roots the energy of the divine within the human body, envelops the spine, connects the Three Dantians, and links together the seven primary chakras (Figure 5.1).

In Chinese energetic embryology, as the father's sperm enters the mother's egg, it creates the upper or Heavenly vortex point of the Taiji Pole. At this early stage of development the Heavenly vortex begins drawing energy into the embryo's forming cells in order to create and link together the energetic structures of the Three Dantians. The Taiji Pole roots its column of white light energy into the Kidneys and the Mingmen area. In the embryo, this area is energetically stimulated by the Heavenly vortex allowing for the growth and development of the Kidney Orb. In ancient times, the Kidney Orb was also known as the "lotus bulb" or "seed of life," and was seen as the fundamental seed for all of the body's Yin and Yang energy. From the lotus seed, the spinal column develops and extends upwards to form the Brain. Hence the spinal column was known as the "lotus stem" or "stem of life," and the Brain was known as the "lotus flower."

As the fetus continues to grow and develop around the Taiji Pole, the body's tissues and energetic needs slowly begin to change. This causes the energetic root of the Taiji Pole to shift from its position located at the Mingmen area to the base of the perineum. After birth, the Taiji Pole is observed as a vertical column of brilliant white light surrounded by a spiraling veil of golden light.

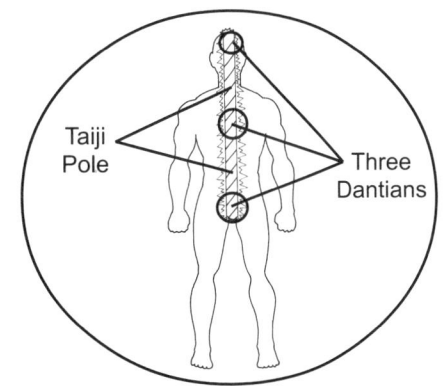

Figure 5.1. The Taiji Pole, located in the center core of the body, and extends from the base of the perineum to the top of the head.

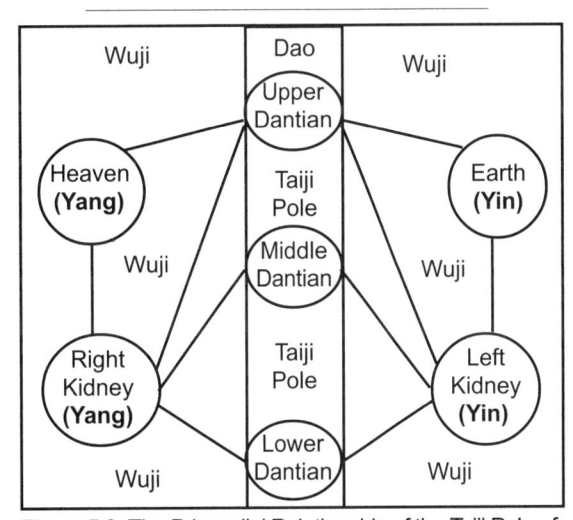

Figure 5.2. The Primordial Relationship of the Taiji Pole of Heaven and Its Human Energetic Correspondence to the Taiji Pole of Man

In ancient times, the Dao was considered the Chong (center) of all existence. As the Dao divided itself into the two polarities of Yin and Yang, Chong Qi (Wuji) - the energy existing between Yin and Yang was created (Figure 5.2). The Taiji Pole

185

is symbolic of the personalized energy of the living Dao. The left and right Kidneys represent the energetic nature of Yin and Yang, respectively. The Chong Qi, or Wuji, is seen as the energetic void that exists between the cells, tissues and organs.

THE TAIJI POLE OF HEAVEN, EARTH, AND MAN

The Taiji Pole of the body is comparable to the Taiji Pole (central axis) of the Earth. At the extremities of the Earth's Taiji Pole are the North and South Poles, which can be compared to the Baihui and Huiyin areas of the human body. The Earth's Taiji Pole (or central axis) aligns to the North Star.

The North Star is seen as the Taiji Pole of Heaven and is sometimes called the Pole Star, or the Taiji of Heaven. As previously mentioned, the original Chinese character for Taiji means "the supreme ultimate," and represents the ultimate state of transformation (Yin transforming into Yang and vice versa). While the original meaning of the Chinese character for Yin is the shady side of the mountain and Yang depicts the sunny side of the mountain, the center of the mountain's peak is considered a Taiji (the center of Yin and Yang) where both Yin and Yang meet (see Chapter 2).

The center core or midline of the Taiji is also called the "still-point," because although all of the changes of Yin and Yang occur in the Heavens within the course of a day, and all of the stars seem to make a 360 degree rotation (as the Earth rotates), the Pole Star remains stationary as Heaven's still-point. In a similar manner, the body's Taiji Pole is viewed as the still-point of Man, around which a person experiences all of the changes, transformations and developments of his or her life. Consequently, great stillness can be experienced when a Qigong practitioner gathers Qi and focuses attention into the Taiji Pole.

INTERNAL ENERGY INTERACTIONS

The Taiji Pole is responsible for absorbing the energy from Heaven and Earth and distributing the collected Qi into the body's major internal organs. Similar to the Earth's central axis, the Taiji Pole is divided into two main energetic polarities: The Five Portals of the Heavenly Yang Gate (the Baihui and Sishencong points), located at the top of the head, and the Five Portals of the Earthly

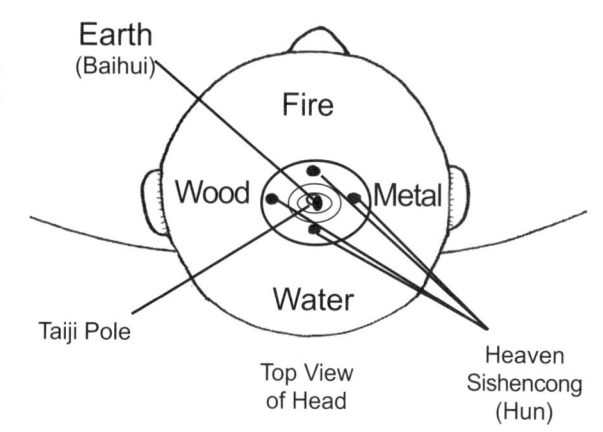

Figure 5.3. The Five Portals of the Heavenly Yang Gate are considered the gate of the Hun. Universal energy is absorbed into the Taiji Pole through the Five Portals of the Heavenly Yang Gate, located at the center of the Baihui ("One Hundred Meetings") and Sishencong ("Four Spirits Hearing") areas at the top of the head.

Gate (Changqiang GV-1, Huiyin CV-1, etc.) located at the perineum.

The Five Portals of the Heavenly Yang Gate are considered the gate of the Hun. Universal energy is absorbed into the Taiji Pole through the Five Portals of the Heavenly Yang Gate, located at the center of the Baihui ("One Hundred Meetings") and Sishencong ("Four Spirits Hearing") areas at the top of the head (Figure 5.3).

The Five Portals of the Earthly Yin Gate are considered the Gate of the Po. The environmental energy of the Earth is absorbed into the Taiji Pole through the Five Portals of the Earthly Yin Gate, located at the center of the anal sphincter, between the Huiyin ("Meeting of Yin") and the Changqiang ("Long Strength") areas, at the base of the perineum (Figure 5.4).

The Three Dantians, Five Jing-Shen, and the Eight Extraordinary Vessels all extend directly from the body's Taiji Pole. These vital energetic systems supply energy to all of the major organs and to the body's Twelve Primary Channels. As the Three Dantians absorb energy from the body's Taiji Pole, they also feed the body's Yin and Yang organs, Twelve Primary Channels, and Eight Extraordinary Vessels. Each individual Dantian is connected to the body's Taiji Pole and each is responsible for an alchemical transition in the process of converting Jing into Qi, Qi into Shen, Shen into Wuji, and converting Wuji back into the Dao (see Volume 2, Chapter 14).

The closer the Qigong doctor works to the patient's Taiji Pole, the more powerful the energies become. Accessing the patient's Taiji Pole, Three Dantians, and Eight Extraordinary Vessels promotes faster and more efficient treatment results than does emitting Qi directly into the patient's Twelve Primary Channels. This is because the Taiji Pole, Three Dantians, and Eight Extraordinary Vessels are the deepest energetic structures of the body.

THE FIVE THRUSTING CHANNELS

There are five internal Thrusting Channels that connect and traverse the body's center Taiji Pole. These five channels begin at the perineum and spiral upwards through the center of the body, flowing into the crown of the head. They connect the Baihui area at the top of the head to the Huiyin area at the bottom of the perineum, and though they lie in the very center of the body, they are more superficial than the Taiji Pole. These five internal channels absorb the Five Element energies from the universe and the environment (Wood, Fire, Earth, Metal and Water) into the body.

The four points that surround the Baihui, where the Thrusting Channels connect to the top of the head are known as the "Four Spirits Hearing," or the "Four Great Spirits of the Gate" (Sishencong). This name signifies the importance of these points as guardians of the human soul, as they control access to the body's Taiji Pole. In ancient times, the Taiji Pole was also known as the "Gate of Heaven," and only through deep meditation or death could the human soul leave its corporeal residence and travel into the physical, energetic or spiritual worlds. Throughout life, the Four Great Spirits of the Gate protect the human soul from spirit possession, and receive Heavenly energy as well as intuitive insights to guide and direct the human soul through the various challenges of life.

SPIRITUAL MANIFESTATIONS

In China, Qigong doctors describe the Taiji Pole as a holy place that practically defies descrip-

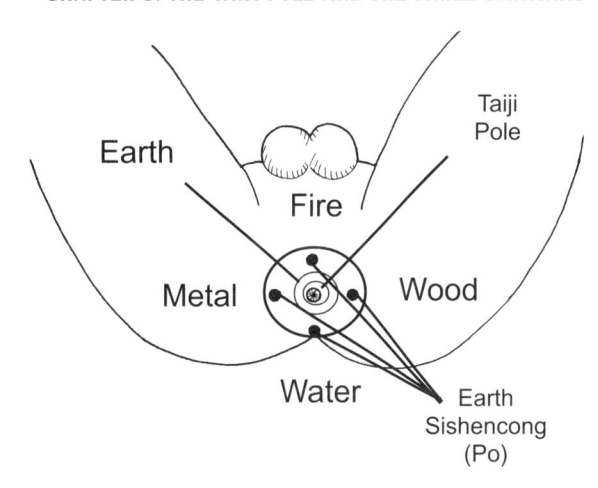

Figure 5.4. The Five Portals of the Earthly Yin Gate are considered the Gate of the Po. The environmental energy of the Earth is absorbed into the Taiji Pole through the Five Portals of the Earthly Yin Gate, located at the center of the anal sphincter, between the Huiyin ("Meeting of Yin") and the Changqiang ("Long Strength") areas, at the base of the perineum.

tion. Similar to an aquarium which is built to house and contain fish from the deep sea, it is the spiritual container of Divine light that houses the individual's Eternal Soul.

The Taiji Pole is a revered and sacred place, as it contains the essence of the patient's Eternal Soul (the patient's true self), devoid of all ego, masks, or defense mechanisms. When the body's internal and external energetic wave patterns become synchronized through prayer or meditation, a rhythmic pulsation occurs within the Taiji Pole. This pulse begins deep within the center core of the body and vibrates outward into infinite space connecting the individual with the Wuji and eventually with the Dao.

When a Qigong doctor penetrates the veil surrounding the center of a patient's Taiji Pole and extends intention into the light's core, he or she will often experience the sensation of falling into space or dissolving into the Wuji (infinite space). This sensation is followed by seeing flashing colored lights and moving shapes, as the surrounding core seems to dissolves into infinite space itself. Time and space dissolve and a feeling of being stretched into eternity occurs. This experience is considered a true connection in which the Wuji returns back to the Dao. The potential for this experience exists within everyone and can be accessed through deep prayer and meditation. It is quite a normal phenomenon within deep spiritual practices and is sometimes known as accessing the "River of God." The Qigong doctors may also feel a powerful stream of energy issuing from the top of the head, connecting the Taiji Pole with the energy of the divine.

MASKS AND DEFENSE MECHANISMS SURROUNDING THE CENTER CORE

When we are born, we are connected to a divine source of spiritual wisdom and power via our center core. As we age and seek to establish security in external social relationships, we gradually forget this internal connection. During this process, we create various masks and defense mechanisms that seek to shield us from our pain and self-hatred (shame). Throughout our lives, any time we repress the flow of feelings connected to an event (especially those that are painful or difficult), we instantly freeze the energy of that particular event and lock it within our cells and tissues. Because the external Wei Qi is composed of energy consciousness, a block of frozen psychic energy is formed within both the Wei Qi field and the internal tissues at the moment we inhibit feelings of pain. By walling off our wounds, we also wall off our connection to our deeper core self. We pretend not to feel the pain anymore and we block the memory of the event through denial. Thus, we prevent a natural resolution to the pain and the trauma of the event.

The amount of energy and life-force that we are able to feel and experience is directly related to the degree of connection to our center core. When we deny our true feelings, we disconnect from our core self and begin to identify with our created social masks (Figure 5.5). We may smile when we really feel angry, for example, or pretend to be indifferent to our hurts. We lose our creative ability when we deny this deeper connection because creative inspiration comes from our core. When we attempt to prevent the negative feelings of anger, pain, or fear, we also prevent ourselves from being able to experience a wide spectrum of the positive emotions, and negate the possibility of healing the physical, mental, and emotional aspects of an experience.

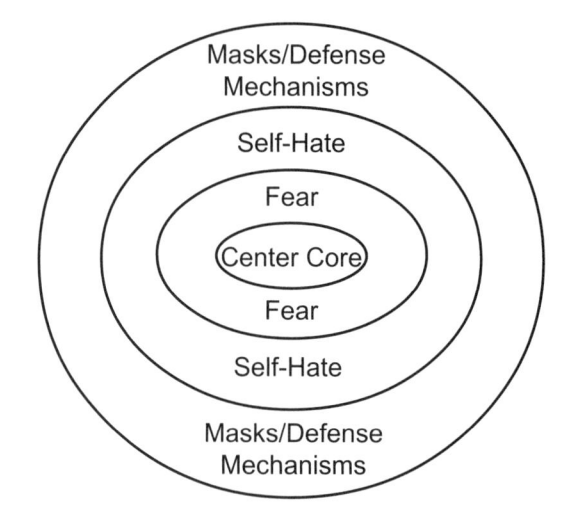

Figure 5.5. The center core self is surrounded by walls of fear, self-hatred and social masks, which act as trigger mechanisms for the wounded soul.

During Medical Qigong treatments, patients regress layer by layer through the pain and fear embedded in patterns of blocked energy that give rise to symptoms of disease. Even though the patient's emotional release may cause frightening memories, the pain decreases with the dispersal of the original trauma.

In clinical practice, most of the patients' pain comes not from the original trauma but from the unconscious belief system that was established to protect them from the original trauma. In other words, more pain and illness is created by the avoidance of working through the original trauma (denial) than was present in the original event itself. It requires enormous amounts of energy to suppress our true feelings, and each time we do so we simultaneously exhaust and injure ourselves. Any attempt at healing that does not address the deeper release of these emotional and energetic patterns from the tissues and psyche will ultimately be less effective.

Spiritual Awakening

When patients become aware of their internal connection to the divine, it is called a spiritual "awakening." As we become aware of our deeper self (energetically manifested through the Taiji Pole), we also awaken to a more objective awareness of the energetic and emotional patterns contained within the Three Dantians, and to the harmonies and imbalances existing between them. Our internal awareness has moved from the external social masks and defense mechanisms, through layers of self-hatred and fear, and is beginning to penetrate into our center core self. Our Shen Xian (Eternal Soul) begins to shine brighter and stronger from within us as we gradually reorganize various aspects of our internal being to align with our life purpose. Numerous physical, emotional, and energetic adjustments take place throughout this process.

Understanding the Energy Within the Taiji Pole

The role and content of the Taiji Pole can be understood metaphysically and mythologically, described as follows:

1. **Metaphysically:** The energy existing within the Taiji Pole contains the following metaphysical aspects:
   - the primordial energetic state before creation
   - the primordial energy of creation
   - the energetic principle of creation itself
   - the underlying energetic characteristic common to all created things

   Connecting with the energy of the Taiji Pole allows the individual the ability to access and experience the spiritual state of primordial oneness.

2. **Mythologically:** The energy contained within the Taiji Pole can be understood both as a part of the divine energy of Heaven, and as an aspect of the divine consciousness contained within each individual, or a combination of the two. According to ancient texts, the energy contained within the Taiji Pole is the divine energetic matrix of the universal Dao. Within the human body, the Taiji Pole is primarily identified as the energetic source of the Three Dantians. It is the personification of the central power of life and the universe expressed as the energetic combination of both spiritual and physical divinity, and exists simultaneously on the microcosmic and macrocosmic levels.

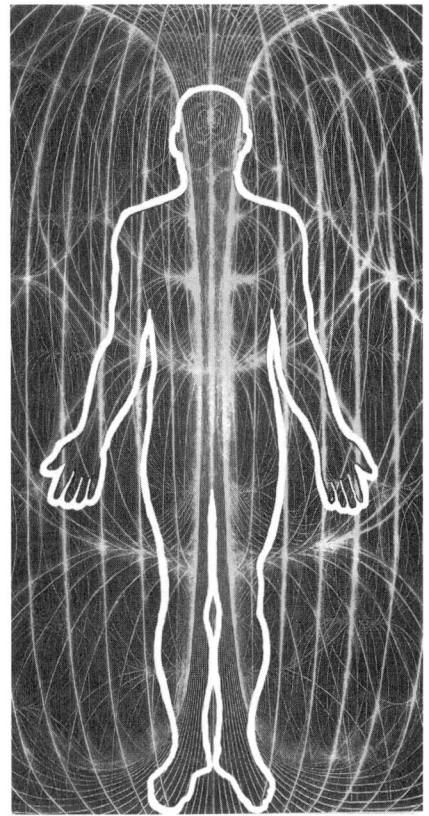

Figure 5.6. The Energy From Within the Taiji Pole Radiates Through the Physical, Energetic and Spiritual Bodies (Inspired by the original artwork of Alex Grey).

Ancient Daoist Qigong masters taught that focused concentration on the Taiji Pole was paramount, as within its very center lay the Supreme Ultimate (Taiji), hence omnipresent awareness. This was considered to be the individual's gateway to the entire universe and allowed simultaneous perception and control of all the subtle mechanisms of creation (Figure 5.6).

The following are seven methods of ancient Daoists esoteric Shengong practice, used to awaken the energetic and spiritual consciousness within the Taiji Pole. This progressive method of "Spiritual Awakening" is described as follows (Figure 5.7):

1. **The Dao and the Taiji Pole:** The individual visualizes the divine energy of the eternal Dao resonating within the center core of his or her body. When mastered, this meditation leads to the awakening of magical powers within oneself and over one's environment (e.g., multi-location, invulnerability, spirit travel, and extending one's life at will).

2. **Divine Light and the Taiji Pole:** The individual "awakens" and strengthens the energy in his or her Taiji Pole by visualizing the radiant light of the eternal Dao absorbed deep into the Taiji Pole's center core. When mastered, this meditation restores an individual's physical health and ultimately transforms his or her energy into spirit, fusing a mystical union with the eternal light of the Wuji (infinite space) that exists throughout the universe.

3. **Dao, the Taiji Pole, and the Postnatal Transformations:** The individual concentrates on feeling the rhythmic Postnatal Transformations (Jing to Qi, Qi to Shen, Shen to Wuji, and Wuji to Dao) of the Three Inner Treasures of Man. Consciously awakening to these rhythmic transformations occurring along the Taiji Pole brings about a state of internal and external harmony. When mastered, this awareness will allow the individual to further refine pure energy and spirit, eventually establishing a deep mystical union with the eternal Dao.

4. **The Dao, the Yuan Shen, and the Taiji Pole:** The individual controls his or her thoughts by surrendering the acquired mind (Shen Zhi) to the Dao, thus establishing a perfect unity of original mind (Yuan Shen) and Dao. When mastered, this meditation stabilizes one's thoughts, and the individual can obtain limitless energy within the body. This enables the transcendence of physical discomforts (hunger, thirst, pain, etc.) and mental turmoil (anger, worry, fear, etc.).

5. **The Dao, the Five Virtues of the Hun, and the Taiji Pole:** The individual controls his or her emotions in order to house the five spiritual components of the Wu Jing Shen, thereby attaining single-pointedness of mind and connecting with the eternal Dao. When mastered,

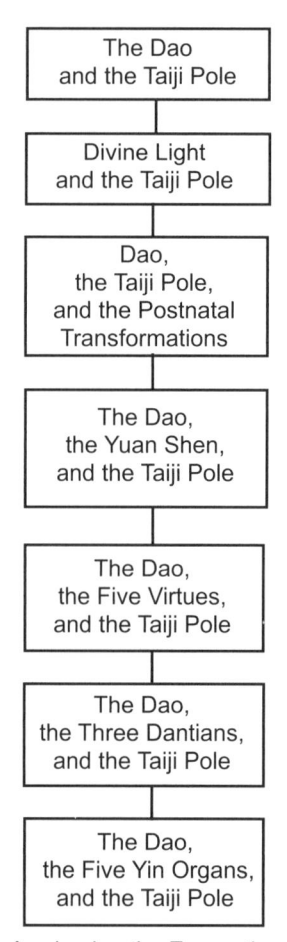

Figure 5.7. Awakening the Energetic and Spiritual Consciousness within the Taiji Pole

this meditation enhances the dominant spiritual presence of the individual's Hun. When the Hun are firmly rooted within the individual's being, he or she manifests a state of harmony and compassion during all activities, even in times of difficulty and misfortune.

6. **The Dao, the Three Dantians, and the Taiji Pole:** The individual visualizes the divine energy of the eternal Dao resonating within his or her center core and Three Dantians. When mastered, this meditation leads to the eternal survival of the individual's soul. Even though he or she experiences the death of the physical body on this earth, the memories of the individual's present personality will be preserved.

7. **The Dao, the Five Yin Organs, and the Taiji Pole:** The individual may visualize the divine energy of the eternal Dao resonating within the center core of his or her body and extending its energy outward into the five Yin organs. When mastered, this meditation leads to enhanced physical strength and increases the vitality of the internal organs.

THE TAIJI POLE AND THE CHAKRA SYSTEM

The body's major internal energy centers are rooted within the Taiji Pole which acts as the main channel of the body's energetic network. The Three Dantians are the energetic reservoirs that pool and contain the body's transforming energies. Located within the Taiji Pole and surrounded externally by the Three Dantians are the seven internal chakras.

Also located within the energetic field of the Taiji Pole, but existing outside the human body, are six spiritually oriented Transpersonal Chakras (three located above the head, and three located underneath the feet). Traditionally, the enlightenment and training of these external chakras was considered privileged information, taught only to senior adepts of esoteric Daoist magic. This knowledge is still generally kept hidden from the public. However, the inclusion of two of these external chakras allows for a more complete understanding of the body's internal and external energetic connections. Therefore, this chapter introduces the public to information that is even more carefully guarded; the location and function of the external Eighth and Ninth Chakras (see Volume 3, Chapter 37).

The energetic field of the external Eighth Chakra (also known as the first or lower "Heavenly Transpersonal Chakra"), is located above the top of the head, about a foot superior to the Crown Chakra. The energetic field of the external Ninth Chakra (also known as the first or lower "Earthly Transpersonal Chakra"), is located below the bottom of the feet, about a foot underneath the ground (Figure 5.8).

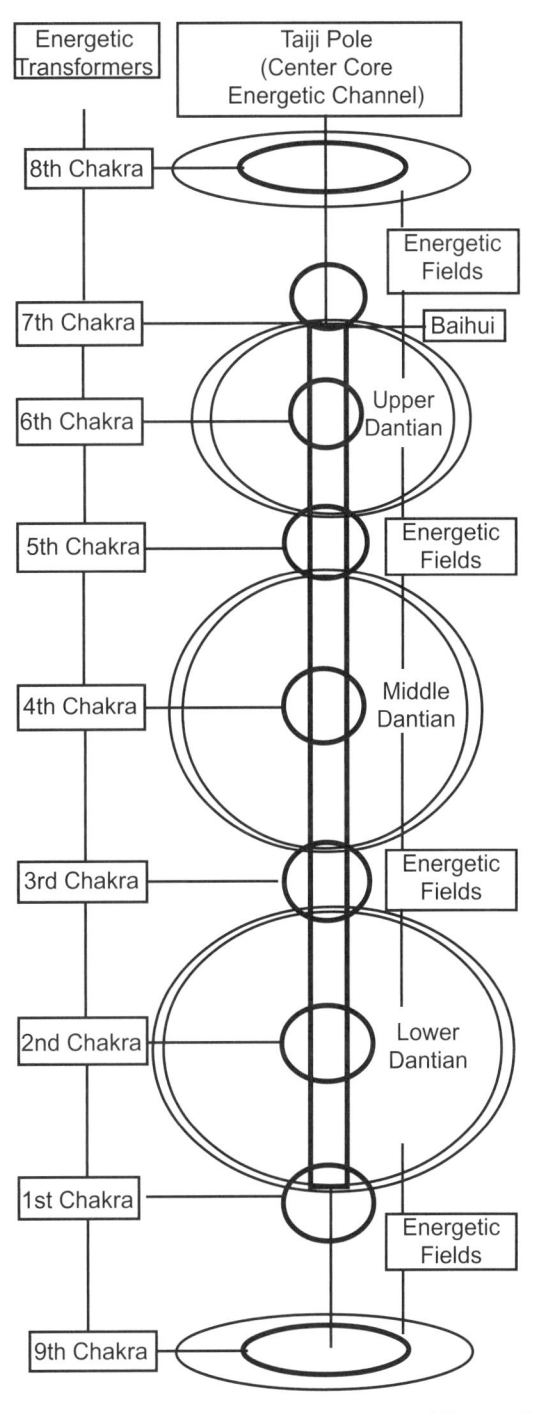

Figure 5.8. The Body's Interconnected Energetic System: The Taiji Pole, Seven Internal Chakras, The Three Dantians, and Two External Chakras

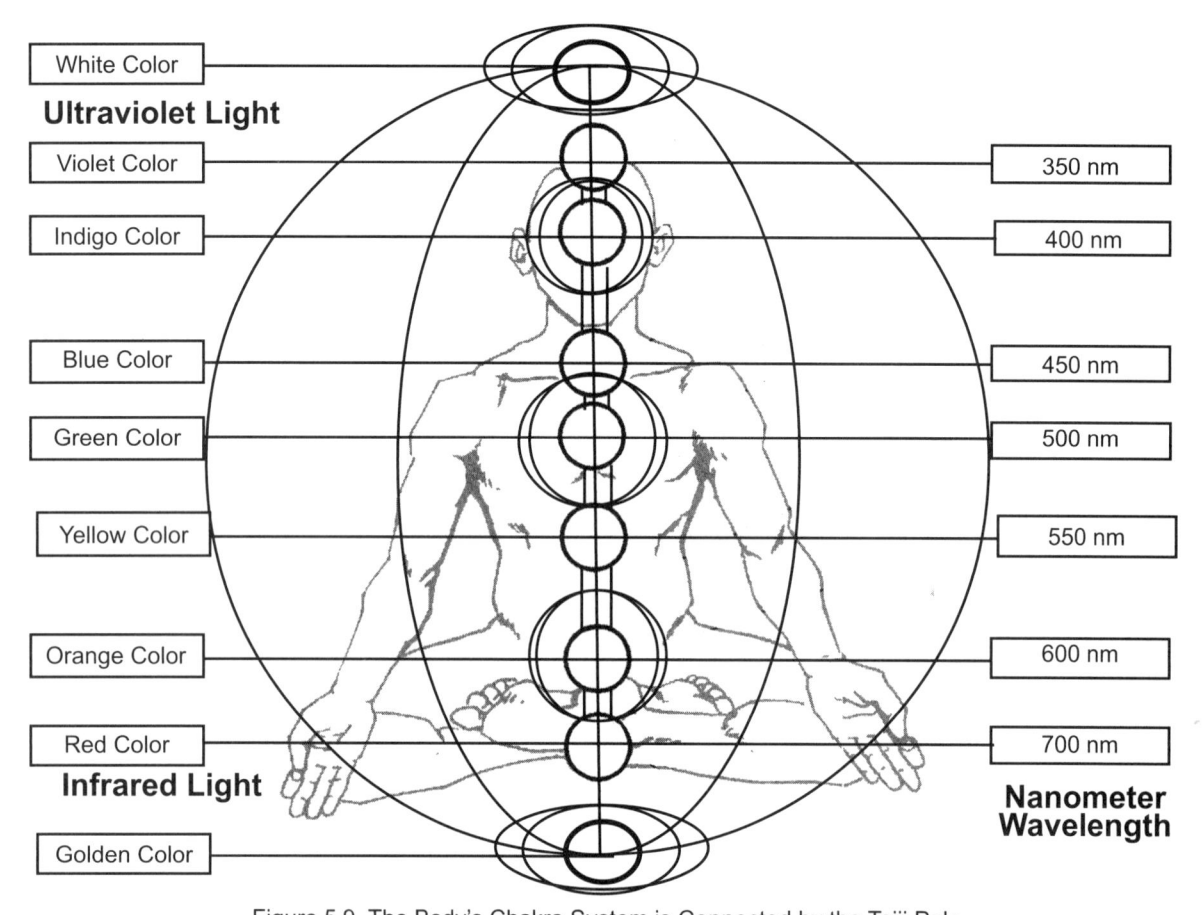

White Color	
Ultraviolet Light	
Violet Color	350 nm
Indigo Color	400 nm
Blue Color	450 nm
Green Color	500 nm
Yellow Color	550 nm
Orange Color	600 nm
Red Color	700 nm
Infrared Light	**Nanometer Wavelength**
Golden Color	

Figure 5.9. The Body's Chakra System is Connected by the Taiji Pole

The seven internal chakras act as energetic step-down transformers that draw charged energy from the Taiji Pole and differentiate it into various multidimensional fields specific to the role and function of each chakra.

Each of the seven internal chakras is positioned along the Taiji Pole, and manifests externally through twelve major energy gates located along the body's Governing and Conception Vessels. The front and back gates of chakras 2 through 6, and the gates of the root and crown chakras open to the energetic fields of the Heaven and Earth respectively.

The Taiji Pole is often compared to the body's main electrical channel and is considered the source of all prenatal life-force energy, as well as the residence of the human soul. The seven internal chakras are the energetic transformers that step-down the pure energy from the Taiji Pole into various forms of psychophysical energy, allowing the soul to express itself and interact at the various levels of human experience. The role of the chakras and the Taiji Pole can be understood by comparing the Taiji Pole to a prism. The Divine radiates the infinite pure white light of being into every individual's Taiji Pole via the external Eighth Chakra, which then refracts this light into seven internal fields of energy (Figure 5.9). This occurs in the same way that a prism splits a beam of white light into the seven colors of the rainbow.

The word chakra is Sanskrit for "wheel." The chakras are often described as small colored disks, usually about the size of a silver dollar, resonating from the Taiji Pole at the center of the body.

There are differing opinions as to the color correspondences for each chakra. In the mid-seventies, while conducting research at U.C.L.A. on the body's neuromuscular system and its relationship to emotions and energy fields, Dr. Valerie Hunt presented empirical data regarding the energetic frequencies and functioning of the body's chakra system. Specifically, Dr. Hunt's research covered how the chakras affect the body's aura field, state of health and disease, pain, and emotional states.

INTRODUCTION TO THE CHAKRAS

As outlined earlier, the Taiji Pole is the primary energetic channel through which the individual connects with the energy of the divine. It is for this reason that the Taiji Pole is considered to be the residence of the human soul, and the personalized expression of the divine. The energy of the human soul radiates outward from the Taiji Pole to interact with the world on many different levels or dimensions. In the chakra system, twelve primary dimensions are considered. Each of the chakras projects energy and information from the Taiji Pole (the Yang, active principle of creation) into the external world, and also receives energy and information (the Yin, receptive principle of assimilation) from the external world into the Taiji Pole. This enables the human soul the potential to engage and experience twelve distinct, though profoundly interrelated, dimensions of life.

Viewed as a compete system, the twelve chakras together act like an immensely complex hologram. A hologram is created by taking a single coherent beam of light (analogous to the Taiji Pole), and splitting it into two equal beams of light using a beam splitter. Both beams of light are then directed to reach an object at the exact same moment, and the resulting interference patterns of light are recorded on a photographic plate. When a beam of light is later passed through this photographic plate, the result is the appearance of a three dimensional image, a hologram of the object originally photographed.

In the chakra system, the divine light of the human soul is concentrated as a single beam in the individual's Taiji Pole, and this beam is simultaneously split into not two, but twelve distinct beams of energy. All of these beams interact to create a complex interference pattern that manifests as the individual's subtotal of experiences. As the individual's residual energetic patterns (karma) are stored within each of the seven internal chakras, he or she then experiences the effects of past karma as they resonate outward into life experiences. In the process of purifying the chakras, it is necessary for the individual to allow these patterns to arise naturally without attempting to repress or control them. Through consistent practice, the seven internal chakras existing within the center core of an individual's tissues will gradually release their dysfunctional patterns and attachments, thus allowing the light of the soul to resonate unobstructed into every aspect of the individual's life. This internal light is then manifested externally through the individual's twelve chakras.

Most people tend to be consciously aware of only the more tangible energetic experiences associated with the lower internal chakras, while remaining unconscious of the subtle energies of the upper internal chakras. This often occurs to such an extent that some people believe these more subtle levels of reality do not even exist. Nevertheless, all individuals are continually affected by the energetic patterns resonating from each of the twelve chakras, whether they are conscious of them or not.

YIN AND YANG AND THE SEVEN INTERNAL CHAKRAS

The Yin and Yang polarity of the seven internal chakras are generally opposite in men and women. The energetic progression of a woman starts and ends with a Yin (electronegative) charge. Therefore, a woman is considered to have a Yin energetic nature. The energetic pathway of a woman's Taiji Pole is generally described as follows (Figure 5.10):
- First Chakra: Yin (-) Reproductive Area
- Second Chakra: Yang (+) Navel Area
- Third Chakra: Yin (-) Yellow Court Area
- Fourth Chakra: Yang (+) Heart and Chest Area
- Fifth Chakra: Yin (-) Throat Area
- Sixth Chakra: Yang (+) Yin Tang Area (Third Eye)
- Seventh Chakra: Yin (-) Bai Hui Area (Top of the Head)

Taiji Pole	Polarity		Chakra Color
Chakra	Men	Women	Color
7th	+ Yang	− Yin	Violet
6th	− Yin	+ Yang	Indigo
5th	+ Yang	− Yin	Blue
4th	− Yin	+ Yang	Green
3rd	+ Yang	− Yin	Yellow
2nd	− Yin	+ Yang	Orange
1st	+ Yang	− Yin	Red

Figure 5.10. The energetic Yin and Yang polarity of the Seven Internal Chakras are opposite in men and women

The energetic progression of a man starts and ends with a Yang (electropositive) charge. Therefore, a man is considered to have a Yang energetic nature. The energetic pathway of a man's Taiji Pole is generally described as follows:
- First Chakra: Yang (+) Reproductive Area
- Second Chakra: Yin (-) Navel Area
- Third Chakra: Yang (+) Yellow Court Area
- Fourth Chakra: Yin (-) Heart and Chest Area
- Fifth Chakra: Yang (+) Throat Area
- Sixth Chakra: Yin (-) Yin Tang Area (Third Eye)
- Seventh Chakra: Yang (+) Bai Hui Area (Top of the Head)

COLOR AND SOUND

In certain Tibetan Buddhist Medical Qigong systems, emphasis is placed on combining specific colors and sounds with focused concentration on the energy centers existing along the Taiji Pole. The notes of the octaves are said to correspond to the color spectrums of the seven internal chakras. The seven notes, seven colors, and seven chakras are described as follows (Figure 5.11):

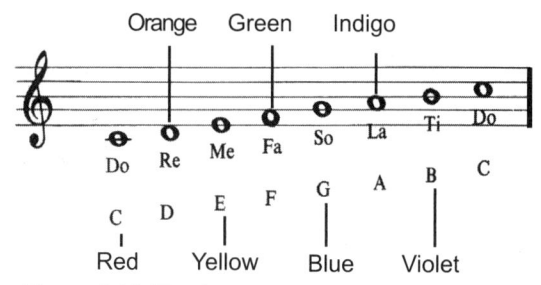

Figure 5.11. The Seven Colors Correlation to the Energetic Pitches

- **Do (C):** Red, the 1st Chakra
- **Re (D):** Orange, the 2nd Chakra
- **Me (E):** Yellow, the 3rd Chakra
- **Fa (F):** Green, the 4th Chakra
- **So (G):** Blue, the 5th Chakra
- **La (A):** Indigo, the 6th Chakra
- **Ti (B):** Violet, the 7th Chakra

The Qigong doctors are taught to play stringed or wind instruments while focusing on projecting specific colors (with the appropriate sounds) into a patient's body. The variations in the scale can produce combinations of colors and various hues, depending on whether the chord or scale is a major or minor. The three primary colors (red, yellow, and blue) correspond to the three fundamental notes of the scale (the first, third and fifth), which construct the matrix for the major cord.

AWAKENING THE SEVEN CHAKRAS

In general, all seven internal chakras are continually operating within every individual, though often in an impaired or dysfunctional manner. Full energetic awakening of the spiritual potential of any given chakra begins with the purgation of the dysfunctional aspects and imbalances of that particular chakra. This cleansing and releasing allows for the dormant potential inherent within each chakra to gradually manifest and integrate into the life and consciousness of the individual.

As each chakra is awakened, the individual will release the associated negative emotions and energetic patterns of that chakra in his or her journey to fully manifest the positive patterns and archetypes.

Each chakra contains an energetic storehouse of both positive and negative karma (patterns) which surface during the awakening process and

CHAPTER 5: THE TAIJI POLE AND THE THREE DANTIANS

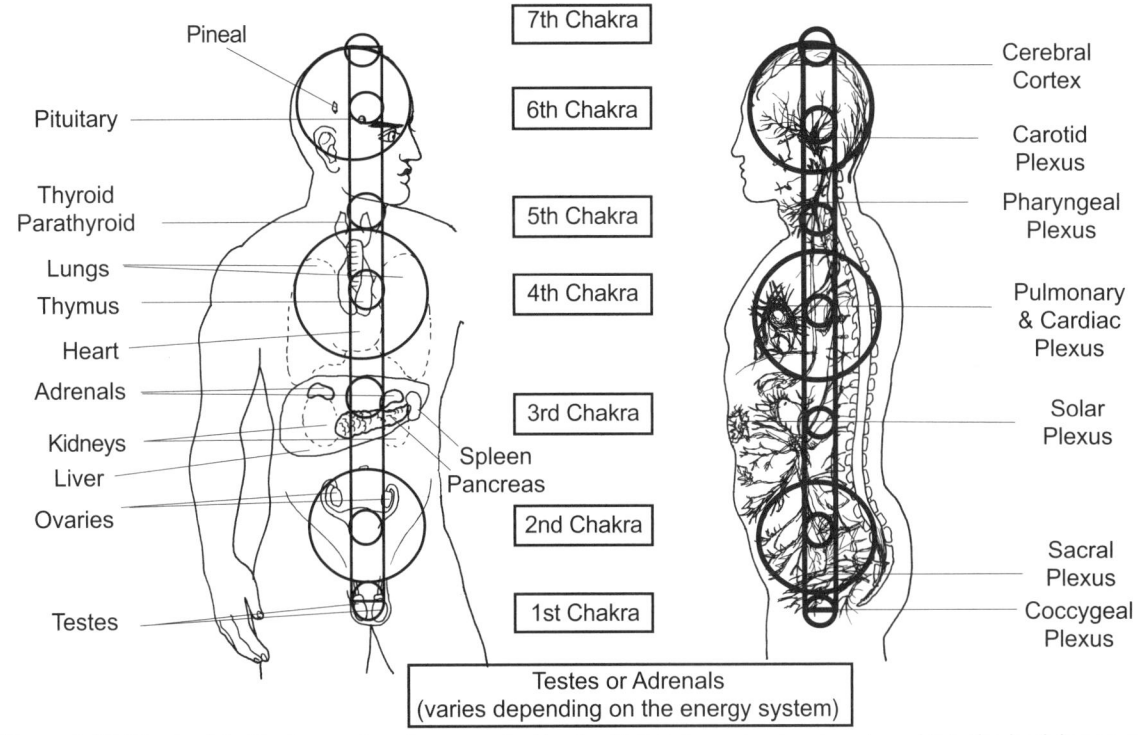

Figure 5.12. The body's Chakra system is connected by the Taiji Pole and extends outward into the body's nerve plexus, affecting the glandular system and both anterior and posterior external energetic fields.

must be released in order to allow the divine light of the individual to fully manifest. Though any or all of the chakras may be accumulating or releasing karma simultaneously, spiritual growth and evolution can be measured by the process of ascending the ladder of the chakras; cleansing, balancing and integrating the potential of each chakra before the one above it.

If an awakening happens too quickly (such as through recreational drug use, bizarre impact traumas to the head or tailbone areas, or the improper practice of psychophysical energetic exercises like Qigong and yoga), it can cause an explosion of suppressed emotional experiences and latent spiritual and energetic abilities that is too intense for the individual to handle. For this reason, in some systems the individual's 6th Chakra is considered, studied and awakened first. This enables the individual to be better prepared for the energetic and emotional experiences that he or she undergoes during the cleansing and awakening process, maintaining an overall sense of clarity and equanimity.

THE NERVE PLEXUSES OF THE SEVEN INTERNAL CHAKRAS

Each internal chakra has a physiological correlation, both with the major nerve plexuses within the spine, and with particular endocrine glands (Figure 5.12).

The three lower chakras are the centers of instinctual energies within the body and are broadly associated with the energy of the Earth and with physical survival. The three uppermost chakras are centers for higher spiritual development and are associated with spiritual evolution and the subtle energies of Heaven. The Heart Chakra rests in between the two Heaven and Earth poles, where the two energies meet and harmonize. The Heart Chakra mediates between the individual's physical and spiritual habits, needs and intentions.

FIRST CHAKRA

The First Chakra is located within the energetic field of the Lower Dantian. It relates to the Element Earth and the solid state of matter. This

195

chakra is associated with the sense of smell, and the color red. It connects to the Taiji Pole at the base of the perineum and exits at the top, or Crown Chakra. It is also associated with the control and development of the physical body sheath. It governs access to the physical (first) plane of reality.

The First Chakra is associated with the kinesthetic, tactile, and proprioceptive senses. This chakra is also energetically connected to both the Conception and Governing Vessels. The First Chakra relates to fear, security, and survival instincts (i.e., the "fight or flight" response). It also relates to tribal power, group acceptance, and the "grounding" or "rooting" of the body. It governs the downward and outward movement of energy from the body, especially excretion, orgasm and exhalation.

PHYSIOLOGICAL ASSOCIATIONS

The First Chakra is associated with the lower limbs and excretory organs. Though the First Chakra governs much of the energy of the reproductive organs (more so for men than for women), it is not usually linked with the emotionally charged energy of sexuality which is the realm of the Second Chakra. The First Chakra also supplies energy to the spinal column, adrenal glands (in some systems), testicles, ovaries, and Kidneys.

THE FIRST PSYCHIC KNOT

The first of three major psychic knots existing within the human energy system is located in the First Chakra, and corresponds to the energy of the Lower Dantian. These knots are more substantial than the chakras, and thus require more insight and discipline to work through. This first knot binds the human soul with attachment to physical survival, the desire for procreation and the fear of death. In order to release the deeply creative energy that is locked in this area, these attachments must be gradually overcome through discipline, spiritual insight and surrender.

BALANCED MANIFESTATION

When functioning properly, this chakra ensures the individual's ability to take care of himself or herself while respecting the needs of others and the needs of the Earth. This chakra will immediately open and release stored information and energy to ensure survival in the presence of danger or in any emergency situation.

PATHOLOGICAL MANIFESTATION

In its unbalanced state, the First Chakra often creates patterns of chronic fear and victimization, wherein the individual continually feels at the mercy of surrounding influences and is unable to stand on his or her own.

Energetic malfunctions and stored emotional trauma in this chakra can cause any of the following symptoms: lower back pain, sciatica, constipation, hemorrhoids, rectal tumors and cancer, testicular cancer, knee problems, and varicose veins.

ENERGETIC AWAKENING

This chakra is the seat, or storehouse, of what is known in the Yogic tradition as the "kundalini" energy. The word kundalini is derived from the term "kunda," which means "a pit or cavity." Kundalini is the internal manifestation of the energetic potential of the human soul sleeping within the un-awakened Taiji Pole. It is symbolically represented as a serpent coiled three and a half times at the base of the spine. The ancients believed that the entire cosmic experience, from creation to dissolution, is embedded within the folds of the coiled serpent. When the full potential of this energy is released, it travels up through the individual's central nervous system (in the physical body) and the Taiji Pole (in the energetic body).

When the kundalini energy is initially aroused, the individual is often subject to extreme swings of energy, perception, and emotion. Additionally, some people often report spiritual experiences and sensations of floating or levitation, as the body is beginning to run energy at higher frequencies which in turn causes the spirit to leave the physical body.

As the First Chakra awakens, the sense of smell may become extremely acute and strong odors may become unbearable. Other common experiences are feelings of warmth in the coccyx and sacral area, or a creeping sensation, as if something water-like were moving internally up the spine. In working through this chakra, the practitioner descends into the most primitive levels of consciousness, and must fully experience, understand, and integrate them.

SPIRITUAL POWERS

When the First Chakra is fully awakened, the ability of telekinesis begins to manifest, and one feels a strong connection with the energy of the Earth. The control over the First Chakra will manifest certain psychic experiences and spiritual powers, such as the ability to make the body as light as air for levitation and spirit travel.

SECOND CHAKRA

The Second Chakra area is considered the gateway of the Lower Dantian. It relates to the Water Element and the liquid state of matter. This chakra is associated with the color orange. It is also associated with the sense of taste, the tongue, and the hands (hence palmistry's strength in relating with the unconscious). It is associated with the intermediate plane of spiritual awareness.

The Second Chakra relates to the emotions, sexuality and the unconscious. It is associated with the True Qi and the energy that pervades the entire body. Energetically, the Second Chakra relates to the Lower Burner and corresponds to the first Wei Qi field.

The Second Chakra is the dominant energy center for sexuality and sensuality. It supplies the sexual organs (ovaries and testicles) and the immune system with energy. It is one of the energy centers for empathic perception, through which the individual is able to sense or feel the emotions of others. However, this chakra often manifests in unbalanced patterns characterized by neediness or co-dependency, which limits empathic perception. Instinctual sexual perception, as well as the ability to sense dangerous situations are examples of this level of empathy.

The Second Chakra governs the unconscious mind and the subterranean movement of karma. It is considered the main storehouse of the body's karma and mental impressions, including those accumulated from past lives.

PHYSIOLOGICAL ASSOCIATIONS

The Second Chakra is associated with the prostatic and uterovaginal nerve plexuses, as well as the reproductive organs. It also governs the Kidneys and the area of the lower back.

BALANCED MANIFESTATION

When functioning properly, the Second Chakra allows the ability to fully accept and experience one's feelings. A balanced Second Chakra allows the formation of relationships and communications that are free of emotional neediness or sexual enmeshment. When in balance, this center radiates a full and healthy sense of sexuality.

PATHOLOGICAL MANIFESTATION

In an unbalanced state, energy in the Second Chakra manifests as uncontrolled empathy, or the inability to differentiate one's own feelings from those of others. Unconscious repression of sexuality may give rise to overwhelming or disturbing sexual dreams, desires or fantasies. Feelings of a lack of self-worth and inner emptiness may drive a person into unhealthy or co-dependent relationships or situations. The martyr complex, for example, is rooted in an imbalance of energy in the Second Chakra.

Energetic malfunctions and stored emotional trauma in this chakra can cause lower back problems, frigidity, or impotence. Second Chakra dysfunction can also cause Kidney, ovarian, uterine, and Urinary Bladder, problems

ENERGETIC AWAKENING

In awakening the Second Chakra, individuals often experience extreme sleepiness, or may undergo a crisis when facing the roots of sexual desire. Women may also experience an extremely heightened emotional need to have a child. Relationships are revealed in a new light, and may become temporarily chaotic. When the Second Chakra opens, the individual may feel the release of sexual desires and fantasies, or experience waves of orgasm flowing through the entire body. Additionally, one may go through a period of experiencing an insatiable appetite for food and the process of eating.

SPIRITUAL POWERS

When the Second Chakra is fully awakened, the individual manifests the ability of clairsentience and the associated ability of psychometry (the ability to touch an object and know its history). The control over the Second Chakra will manifest certain psychic experiences and spiritual powers such as the ability to live for long periods of time without food or water.

THIRD CHAKRA

The Third Chakra area is associated with the Middle Dantian and is commonly referred to as the "Yellow Court" in Medical Qigong therapy. It relates to the Fire Element and the transformational qualities of Qi. This chakra relates to the sense of sight, and its energetic color is yellow. The Third Chakra is the body's main distribution point for psychic energies, and the primary center for personal power and self-image.

This chakra holds the energetic patterns and blueprints for storing issues of responsibility, self-esteem, personal honor and the fear of rejection. It is also a storage chamber for neglected emotional pain and anger. It is associated with the Heavenly plane of existence. It is also associated with the Middle Burner and those aspects of Ying Qi which are responsible for digestion and the fire of metabolic assimilation. It is also the area where the body's Qi transforms into Shen.

The Third Chakra is the place where the energy of inhalation (Yin) meets with the energy of exhalation (Yang). If the practitioner is able to unify these two energies, an alchemical explosion takes place that is simultaneously the full awakening of the Third Chakra and the initial rousing of the kundalini. This is why some texts say that the awakening of kundalini actually takes place in the Third Chakra, and that once it is awakened, this supercharged energy then gathers and drops down to the First Chakra to enter the spinal channel.

PHYSIOLOGICAL ASSOCIATIONS

The Third Chakra is associated with all the organs of the digestive system. It supplies energy to the Liver, Gall Bladder, Stomach, Spleen, pancreas, adrenal glands, and nervous system. Proper diet and fasting helps to purify this chakra, because when the digestive fire is not engaged in assimilating food, it is able to complete its other functions. Thus, when fasting or eating lightly, the digestive fire turns inward and begins cleaning and burning all the stagnant undigested foods, thoughts, and emotions trapped within the individual's digestive system. This accounts for feelings of heat, and hot purification when fasting.

BALANCED MANIFESTATION

When in balance, the Third Chakra has the appearance of a radiant sun. The individual experiences abundant physical energy, emotional stability, a strong metabolism and constitution, as well as the ability to work efficiently and complete desired tasks. Dynamism, energy, perseverance, achievement, metabolism, and strong digestion (including the digestion of thoughts and emotions) are all positive attributes of this chakra. In the same way that the sun shines its light onto all of the planets, the Third Chakra radiates energy throughout the entire cellular structure of the physical body, and supplies power to the vast network of energy channels within the energetic body.

PATHOLOGICAL MANIFESTATION

When out of balance, the Third Chakra looks like a dying fire or a pile of smoldering embers. This may manifest in symptoms such as poor health, depression, lack of motivation in life and an inability to work or follow through. In its unawakened state, the Third Chakra slowly burns and destroys the essence of the body over time, causing decay, disease, and death.

When the Third Chakra's energy gates open, feelings of power and waves of anger, rage, fear, greed, jealousy, judgment, or criticism can be released. Because this area is also associated with the desire for power and the ability to manifest one's ideas, sometimes the desire to destroy is also experienced. Energetic malfunctions and stored emotional trauma in this chakra can cause metabolic disorders, indigestion, ulcers, hypoglycemia, diabetes, disorders of the Liver and Gall Bladder, or adrenal problems.

ENERGETIC AWAKENING

Because the Third Chakra is the major distribution center for the physical energy of the body, when this center is energetically awakened, the practitioner is able to greatly (or indefinitely) extend his or her life-span. When this center is purified, the individual's body becomes disease free and luminous, and the consciousness does not easily fall back into lower states. During the awakening process of the lower three chakras, it is often difficult to maintain the quality of energetic focus required and the practitioner's energy often drops back to the base of the spine. Once the awakening of the Third Chakra is complete, however, it is naturally easier to harness the attention and the energy will either remain in one place or continue its upward journey towards the crown. There is also a corresponding shift in consciousness from being deeply enmeshed in one's own mental and emotional problems, to releasing them more easily and being able to comprehend, envision, and manifest one's greater spiritual potential.

Spiritual Powers

It is said that meditation on the Third Chakra leads to an understanding of the entire human physical framework and energetic system. The psychic powers that come with the awakening of this chakra are naturally lighter than those associated with the lower two chakras, which are still tinged by the darker aspects of the lower mind. The powers gained by the awakening of the Third Chakra include the ability to create and destroy, the acquisition of hidden treasures, control over the Fire Element, knowledge of one's own body, freedom from disease, and the ability to withdraw one's energy into the central channel at will.

Control over the Third Chakra will manifest certain psychic experiences and spiritual powers, allowing the individual to endure strong heat, and to consume large amounts of food without gaining weight.

Fourth Chakra

The Fourth Chakra area is associated with the Middle Dantian, the Air Element, and the gaseous state of matter. This chakra relates to the sense of touch, and the color green.

Energetically, this chakra relates to the Upper Burner and Zong Qi (Gathering Qi). It governs the field of mind and emotions, which corresponds to the second Wei Qi field, and to the human aura. It is associated with the first of the immortal planes of spiritual awareness.

This energy center is associated with love, compassion, empathy, clairsentience, and intuition. It is also responsible for the creative sciences and fine arts such as painting, dance, music, poetry, etc.

Physiological Associations

The Fourth Chakra is connected with the cardiac nerve plexus and it supplies energy to the Heart, Lungs, circulatory system, thymus gland, vagus nerve, diaphragm, and upper back.

Balanced Manifestation

A healthy Fourth Chakra manifests balance and harmony in relationships, and expresses itself in such qualities as affinity, compassion and selfless action. In the Fourth Chakra, the individual is effortlessly defining the external world in his or her own personal terms, whereas in the Third Chakra the individual is struggling to define his or her self in the terms of the external world.

In its positive form, the energy of the Fourth Chakra manifests as creativity, spiritual love, spiritual charity, and spiritual compassion (which is given effortlessly without attachment).

Pathological Manifestation

When out of balance, the energy in the Fourth Chakra can manifest as the inability to feel love for oneself, which then leads to insincerity, co-dependence, insecurity, and isolation. When unbalanced, this chakra is also associated with conditional love and insincere human charity, both of which reflect selfishness and personal attachment.

Energetic malfunctions and stored emotional trauma in this chakra can cause Heart and Lung diseases.

The Second Psychic Knot

The second psychic knot is located in the Fourth Chakra, and corresponds to the energy of the Middle Dantian. This knot holds the individual separate from, and therefore dependent on, the social surroundings. It represents the bondage of emotional attachment, co-dependence, and the need to be externally validated as a result of inherent lack of self love and acceptance. Until this knot is released, the individual's thoughts are generally enmeshed with patterns of emotional dependency, such as the fear of being negatively judged by others.

Energetic Awakening

The Fourth Chakra awakens when the individual's ego surrenders into boundless love. During this awakening, the individual's mental and emotional fields are purified and blended as they become aligned with the higher intention of the Eternal Soul.

In the process of awakening the Fourth Chakra, it is important to be in a supportive social environment and to avoid toxic relationships. At this stage of energetic opening, it is very easy to absorb the surrounding environmental Qi into one's body.

When this energy center opens, and the individual becomes aware of being attached to the personal ego, and the resulting catharsis can be both physically and emotionally painful. The individual may experience chest pain, feelings of a heavy weight on the chest, irregular heartbeat, or the spontaneous release of tears.

As the Fourth Chakra awakens there is a profound sense of peace and emotional ease. The individual's voice becomes subtle, enchanting, and imbued with emotion. Due to the emotional charge developed in both the voice and aura, he or she becomes very attractive and beautiful to others. He or she becomes creatively inspired and often inspires others. The ability to heal is greatly increased, and the practitioner develops a very sensitive touch. The internal and external acceptance of both good and bad, and a clearer understanding of each also develops.

Spiritual Powers

With the awakening of this chakra, the individual is able to control his or her thoughts and focus with deep mental and emotional concentration, thus effortlessly entering into higher states of meditation. Due to this potential of transcendent focus, the ability to escape preordained fate and to determine one's own destiny now becomes a reality. Voices and sounds originating from other realms are heard. Together with the Fifth Chakra, the Fourth Chakra rules clairaudience. The Fourth Chakra is also said to contain the "wish fulfilling tree", and upon awakening it, the individual is able to acquire whatever he or she thinks or desires.

Control over the Fourth Chakra will manifest certain psychic experiences and spiritual powers, such as energetically becoming light, soul projecting and understanding the language of birds.

Fifth Chakra

The Fifth Chakra area is associated with the Middle Dantian. It relates to infinite space (Wuji), and the space in which all the other Elements and their transitions take place. This chakra relates to the sense of hearing and its energetic color is blue. This energy center is associated with sound vibration, personal will, divine will, and divine communication. It is the center for clairaudience, and is also the source of the individual's inner voice.

This energy center governs the upward movement of Qi associated with movements of the head and with facial expressions. The Fifth Chakra, together with the Sixth Chakra, rules and regulates the intuitive mind. This can be conceptualized as being the perfect harmony between the conditioned (acquired) perceptions and the unconditioned (inherent or intuitive) perceptions of the mind. It is this form of mind that initiates and evolves psychic development. The Fifth Chakra is associated with the fifth or "immortal" plane of consciousness.

Physiological Associations

The Fifth Chakra supplies energy to the throat, thyroid and parathyroid glands, neck vertebrae, mouth, Lungs, and alimentary canal (the digestive tube from the mouth to the anus). It also relates to the ears and the vocal chords.

Balanced Manifestation

The Fifth Chakra together with the Sixth Chakra, governs the development of intellectual discrimination. Truth and untruth relate to the Fifth Chakra. In its positive form, the energy of the Fifth Chakra manifests as self-expression and the ability to communicate one's own truth to others clearly, honestly and directly. This chakra is the main center for creativity, and when it is balanced one will feel enthusiasm and a genuine interest in life.

Pathological Manifestation

When out of balance, the Fifth Chakra can interfere with the ability of the internal organs to release energy through the throat (voice) and arms, thus upsetting the harmony of Yin and Yang within the upper body.

Heat from Liver Fire sometimes gathers at the Fifth Chakra area, becoming entangled with Phlegm originating from the Lungs. Together, this combination of Phlegm and Fire forms an energetic knot within the throat, often referred to in Traditional Chinese Medicine as "Plum Pit Qi."

Emotionally, an individual may sometimes refuse to communicate or use silence for control and attention. Difficult feelings such as pain, depression, anger, or violence may be suppressed. The individual may feel a lack of creativity, or a mysterious creative weight or block that prevents the feeling of being fully alive. The mind may become cloudy and dull due to a lack of communication, leading to depression and despair.

Energetic malfunctions caused from stored emotional trauma in this chakra area can cause stiff neck, sore throat, thyroid problems, and swollen glands. The individual can sometimes experience coughing, or laryngitis.

ENERGETIC AWAKENING

When the Fifth Chakra opens, a compulsive urge to sing or chant may arise. When awakened, this chakra is said to be the center at which the "nectar of immortality" (which drips from one of the minor chakras in the head and flows down through the back of the roof of the mouth) is split into its pure and impure forms. The impure form is discarded as poison, while the pure form nourishes the body. As long as this center remains unawakened, the nectar remains undifferentiated and flows downward into the Third Chakra to be consumed by the digestive fire.

It is said that awakening the Fifth Chakra enables one to digest poisons and to overcome the need for food and drink; and by extension, to overcome the aging process. This center relates to the legendary fountain of youth, in that once one is able to go beyond food and drink (and to assimilate the "nectar of immortality"), one is in essence immortal. Thus, when the kundalini is within the Fifth Chakra, a spontaneous physical rejuvenation takes place. The sense of hearing becomes very sharp, mainly through the mind, as well as through the ears.

Additionally, it is said that with the awakening of this chakra, the individual obtains full knowledge of the past, present, and future. At this stage, the individual may have spontaneous experiences of feelings of the vastness of the Wuji.

SPIRITUAL POWERS

By meditating on the Fifth Chakra, the mind is said to become pure like infinite space (Wuji). The ability to communicate telepathically initially begins here, and is then refined within the Sixth Chakra.

Control over the Fifth Chakra will manifest certain psychic experiences and spiritual powers, such as the ability to hypnotize, the ability to look into (beyond and before) time, and the ability to dissolve into space. In some systems, the awakening of the Fifth Chakra leads to the ability to manifest the Eight Supernatural Powers (see Volume 2, Chapter 14).

SIXTH CHAKRA

The Sixth Chakra area is associated with the Upper Dantian. Its energetic elemental nature relates to light. This chakra relates to "mental seeing" (clairvoyance), and its energetic color is indigo. This energy center is responsible for enabling the individual to see auras, chakras, and other energetic images. This center is also responsible for mental telepathy, allowing the individual to sometimes know the patient's thoughts and feelings. The Sixth Chakra area is the center for psychic intuition (or "knowing without knowing"), clairvoyant seeing (inner vision), and energy projection.

The Sixth Chakra is considered to be the main chakra of the mind. Intellectual and intuitive, the Sixth Chakra is the root of the plane of duality within human experience. Defining and maintaining boundaries and opposites, this is the center at which the duality of egocentric self-contraction is transcended, and the merger of individual self with the divine self takes place. Along with the Fifth Chakra, the Sixth Chakra rules and regulates the intuition. The Sixth Chakra is associated with the plane of austerity, in which impurities are purified and burned away by means of non-attachment to perceptions of duality.

Physiological Associations

The Sixth Chakra is considered the energetic control center for all the rest of the body. This area of the body supplies energy to the lower Brain, ears, nose, eyes, and nervous system. Physically, this energy center also relates to the pituitary gland and the hypothalamus (which controls the body's endocrine system and the interaction between the body's endocrine system and nervous system).

The Third Psychic Knot

The Sixth Chakra is the home of the uppermost of three major energetic knots within the human energy system, and corresponds to the energy of the Upper Dantian. This knot holds the individual self separate from the divine identity. It is said to effectively block the practitioner's spiritual evolution until attachment to the duality of phenomena (pleasure and pain, desire and aversion, life and death etc.) is transcended.

Balanced Manifestation

A balanced Sixth Chakra manifests through the integration of the masculine qualities of discernment, intellectual analysis and clear knowledge, and the feminine qualities of intuition and imagination. This functional integration and its application allows the individual to recognize and ascertain deeper realms of wisdom.

Pathological Manifestation

An imbalance Sixth Chakra may manifest as over-intellectualization, or even psychic arrogance. One may have very firm views and opinions that he or she is unable to release, or see beyond. There is a tendency to rationalize and theorize one's way through life rather than directly engage in experience.

Blockages in the Sixth Chakra are reflected by very deep and hardened belief structures about the nature of creation itself, these being the root of nearly all other energetic patterns developed and embodied by the individual. Static and inaccurate interpretations of events, projections of personal fears (and other emotions or motivations) onto others may also occur. Recurring nightmares and delusional fantasies may further disconnect the individual from the real world.

Energetic Awakening

The process of awakening the Sixth Chakra involves the burning and purification of the fog of ignorance that clouds the mind. During this awakening, energetic releases can manifest through such symptoms as headaches, eye strain, pain around the eyes, distorted or blurred vision, and temporary blindness.

Each of the lower five chakras is associated with a physical sense, whereas the Sixth Chakra is associated with the intuitive sense of the mind itself. In an un-awakened individual, the mind gathers and organizes information based only on the five senses; however, when the Sixth Chakra is developed and awakened, the individual will have access to knowledge beyond sensory input. Such knowledge is non-local, being independent of time and space. One aspect of awakening the Sixth Chakra is the true perception, and subsequent interception, of karma.

Spiritual Powers

Once awakened, the Sixth Chakra is said to yield clairvoyance, refined telepathy, and a myriad of other minor powers. Here, the ability to visualize becomes so acute as to involve all five senses (those having been already mastered). One is able to see beyond duality and thus affect reality directly from the substratum of creation. With these faculties in place, one is able to visit other energetic and spiritual realms and to navigate through a very wide spectrum of consciousness.

Seventh Chakra

The Seventh Chakra area is associated with the Upper Dantian. Its energetic elemental nature relates to infinite space (Wuji), and its color is violet. This energy center is associated with spiritual knowledge, understanding, pure intuition, and ecstasy.

The Seventh Chakra is the primary gateway of the Taiji Pole to the divine, or "the door to kingdom of God." While the other Chakras are considered to be energetic transformers that modify and direct the energy contained within the Taiji Pole, the Seventh Chakra affects the energy of the Taiji Pole by controlling the flow of divine energy into the body.

The Seventh Chakra is associated with totality. It relates to bliss and complete enlightenment, beyond the uppermost reaches of the human realm. It is considered to be the lowest of the divine levels of consciousness.

Physiological Associations

The Seventh Chakra is located at the highest point of the Taiji Pole and supplies energy to the pineal gland and upper Brain.

Balanced Manifestation

When the Seventh Chakra is in balance, the individual experiences a strong and continuous connection with the divine, manifesting as a state of spiritual sanctuary, faith and inner peace.

Pathological Manifestation

When this chakra area is blocked or closed, the individual may feel useless or have no meaningful sense of purpose or direction in life. This is often associated with symptoms such as confusion, apathy, alienation, boredom, depression, or varying states of incomprehension.

Energetic Awakening

In ancient China, it was believed that when the Seventh Chakra's energetic center opened, it was like a golden flower opening, accompanied by a dazzling bright light and a strong, powerful feeling of connection with the divine.

It is often said that when the kundalini reaches the level of the Seventh Chakra, the individual transcends all human experiences and enters into the lower divine realms. Once this has taken place, it is essential to bring this energy down the front of the body and reconnect it with the First Chakra in order to function in the world as a fully awakened being.

Spiritual Powers

When the Seventh Chakra is awakened, one has access to the infinite knowledge of the Wuji, and is said to be beyond time and space.

Awakening The External Chakras

To review, the Divine radiates down the infinite pure white light of being into the Taiji Pole via the external chakras, which then refract this light into seven internal fields of energy. The following is a description of the various energetic properties and functions of two of the six external chakras that exist within the external energetic field of the body's Taiji Pole.

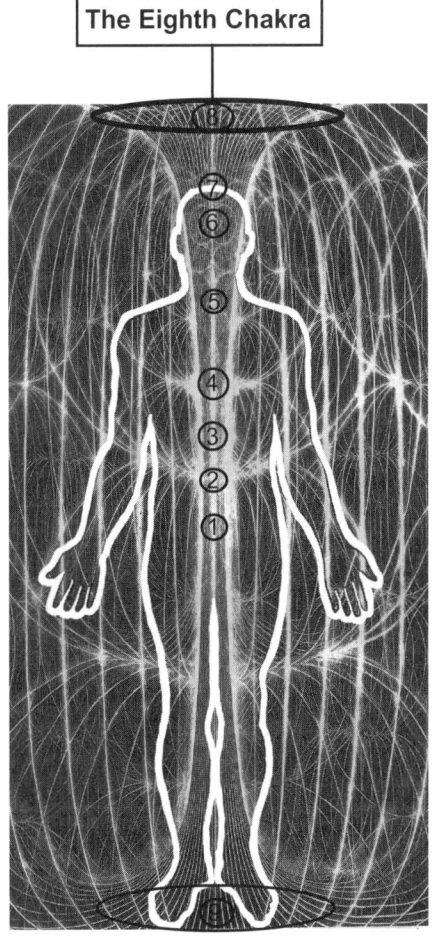

Figure 5.13. The Divine energy is received through the Eighth Chakra, which transforms and transfers this most subtle information to the individual's Taiji Pole. The Taiji Pole then radiates this information throughout the individual's physical, energetic and spiritual bodies (Inspired by the original artwork of Alex Grey).

The Eighth Chakra

In ancient China, the Eighth Chakra was traditionally known as one of the three Heavenly Transpersonal Points that exist above each individual's head (Figure 5.13). In general, the external Eighth Chakra spiritually operates within every individual, bringing deep spiritual insights and esoteric perceptions to light. It is considered to exist at a higher level of the divine consciousness, communicating with the individual's Yuan Shen.

The Eighth Chakra nourishes the Yang aspect of the individuals soul, and is responsible for transformations occurring during the Prenatal spiritual and energetic transitions of Dao to Wuji, Wuji to Shen, Shen to Qi and Qi to Jing.

The Divine radiates the infinite pure white light of being into every individual's Taiji Pole via the External Eighth Chakra, which then refracts this light into several internal fields of energy.

It is through the Eighth Chakra that the individual receives and absorbs the spiritual interactions of the Heavenly Five Elements that contribute to form the developing matrices of the individual's physical, energetic and spiritual bodies.

The energetic light of the Eighth Chakra is white, and represents the fusion of all the chakra colors. It relates to the spiritual body of bliss and complete enlightenment, beyond the uppermost reaches of the human realm.

ENERGETIC AWAKENING

The full energetic awakening of the Eighth Chakra's spiritual potential begins with the purgation of the dysfunctional aspects and imbalances of this particular chakra. This cleansing and releasing allows for the dormant potential inherent within the Eighth Chakra to gradually manifest, and integrates the individual's latent spiritual insights and powers into consciousness.

Additionally, it is from within the external energetic and spiritual field of the Eighth Chakra that the Medical Qigong doctor will create his or her Invisible Needles, used in advanced Medical Qigong Therapy. For example, when using the single Invisible Needle image, the Qigong doctor will imagine energetic needles of light existing within the celestial halo of his or her Eighth Chakra (see Volume 3, Chapter 37). This celestial halo is positioned above the doctor's head, located within the Heavenly Transpersonal Point of the Eighth Chakra. To use the energetic needle technique, the Qigong doctor reaches above his or her head and imagines plucking a splinter of light

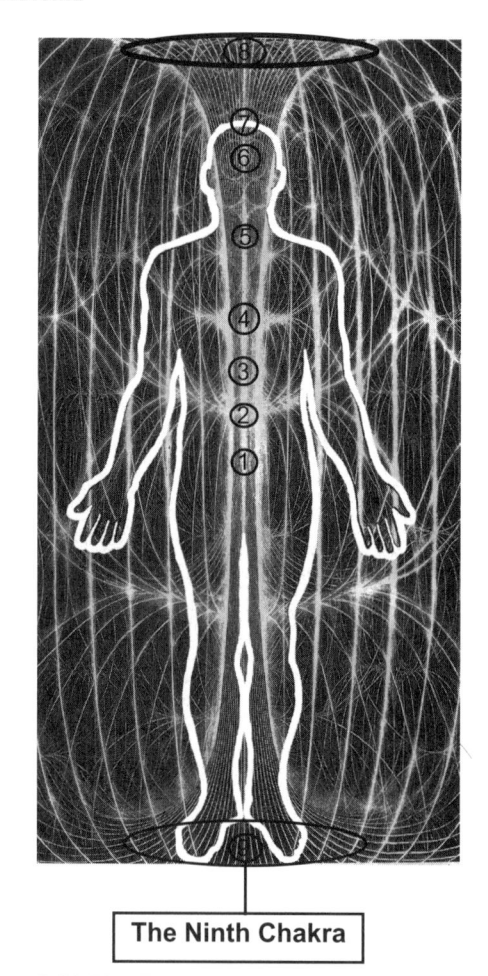

Figure 5.14. The Earthly energy is received through the Ninth Chakra, which transforms and transfers this most subtle information to the individual's Taiji Pole. The Taiji Pole then radiates this information throughout the physical, energetic and spiritual bodies. (Inspired by the original artwork of Alex Grey).

from the celestial halo. The splinter of light is transformed into a needle and then inserted into the patient's body.

SPIRITUAL POWERS

The Eighth Chakra is the primary spiritual gateway of the Taiji Pole to the Heavens, or "the immortal's door to the planet and star kingdoms." Once awakened, the Eighth Chakra is said to yield a direct connection to the infinite knowledge of the Dao, contained within the Heavenly realms.

THE NINTH CHAKRA

In ancient China, the Ninth Chakra was traditionally known as one of the three Earthly Transpersonal Points that exist beneath each individual's feet (Figure 5.14). In general, the external Ninth Chakra spiritually operates within every individual, bringing deep spiritual insights and esoteric perceptions to light. It is considered to exist at a higher level of the divine consciousness, communicating with the individual's Yuan Shen.

The Ninth Chakra nourishes the Yin aspect of the individuals soul, and is responsible for transformations occurring during the Postnatal spiritual and energetic transitions of Jing to Qi, Qi to Shen, Shen to Wuji, and Wuji to Dao.

It is through the Ninth Chakra that the individual receives and absorbs the spiritual interactions of the Earthly Five Elements that contribute to form the developing matrices of the individual's physical, energetic, and spiritual bodies.

The energetic color of the Ninth Chakra is golden yellow, and relates to the energetic body.

Energetic Awakening

Full energetic awakening of the Ninth Chakra's spiritual potential begins with the purgation of the dysfunctional aspects and imbalances of this particular chakra (such as Earthly karma dragged about like a dead weight). This cleansing and releasing allows for the dormant potential inherent within the Ninth Chakra to gradually manifest, and integrates the individual's latent spiritual insights and powers into consciousness.

Additionally, it is from within the external energetic and spiritual field of the Ninth Chakra that the Medical Qigong doctor creates his or her energetic connection and root into the specific energies of the Earth. For example, as the Qigong doctor sinks his Zhi (Will) and Yi (Intention) deep into the Earth, a corresponding energetic field expands outward from below his or her feet, encircling the doctor's entire physical body. This energetic bubble acts as a protective field, allowing the doctor to move about the clinic in a safe environment (Figure 5.15).

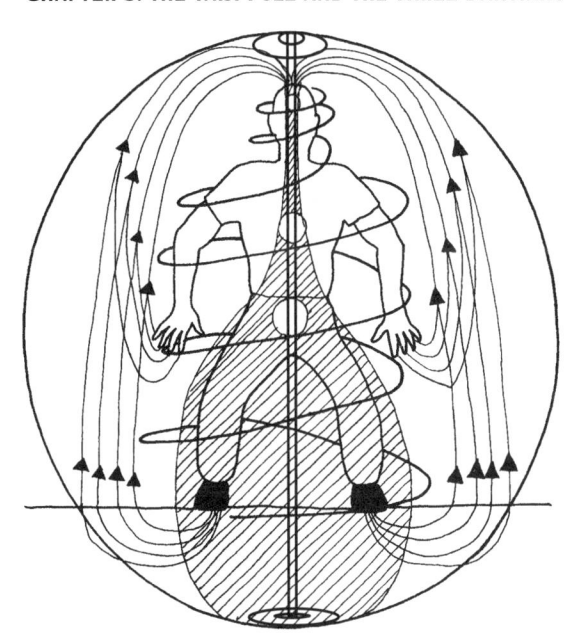

Figure 5.15. This energetic bubble acts as a protective energetic field, allowing the doctor to move about the clinic in a safe environment

Spiritual Powers

The Ninth Chakra is the primary spiritual gateway of the Taiji Pole to the Earth, or "the immortal's door to the plant and mineral kingdoms." Once awakened, the Ninth Chakra is said to yield a direct connection to the infinite knowledge of the Dao, contained within the Earthly realms.

There is a direct correlation between the nine chambers of the body's Three Dantians and the energetic fields of the nine chakras. When all nine chakras are completely open, each of the Dantian's nine chambers are said to be functioning a maximum potential. This allows the individual the unique ability to access the hidden esoteric knowledge and power stored within all of his or her three bodies (physical body, energetic body and spiritual body), as well as power and control over all three realms (the realm of matter, the realm of energy, and the realm of spiritual power).

THE TWELVE CHAKRA GATES AND THE THREE DANTIANS

Energetically, the chakra gates look like funnels or vortices of Qi extending outward from the body's Taiji Pole. Qigong doctors, sages, and healers have for centuries described these gates as resembling energetic wheels or vortexes within the subtle energy body. Each funnel extends and expands its energetic vortex outward into the body's Wei Qi field. As energy travels up and down the Taiji Pole, it creates an energetic pulse. This energetic pulse resonates from the body's seven chakras through the twelve chakra gates and can be felt several feet from the body. While the center of each chakra is actually located within the middle of the Taiji Pole, its field resonates outside the body through energetic gates embedded along the surface of the tissues, positioned along the pathways of the Conception and Governing Vessels.

The First Chakra is located at the perineum and has only one gate, as does the Seventh Chakra located at the top of the head. The Second, Third, Fourth, Fifth, and Sixth Chakras have two gates each, one on the front of the body and the other on the back of the body. These chakra Gates serve different energetic functions, and are described as follows:

1. **The Crown or Seventh Chakra Gate** is responsible for absorbing Heavenly Qi and light into the body, as well as energizing the body's Taiji Pole.
2. **The Front Chakra Gates** are responsible for the individual's feelings and emotions. They are related to the individual's Shen and the Heart Fire energy. They are connected to points along the Conception Vessel.
3. **The Back Chakra Gates** are responsible for the individual's willpower and determination. They are related to the individual's Zhi and the Kidney Water energy. They are connected to points along the Governing Vessel.
4. **The Base or First Chakra Gate** is responsible for absorbing Earthly Qi and heat into the body, as well as energizing the Taiji Pole.

Generally, when treating a patient, the Qigong doctor extends energy into the patient's back

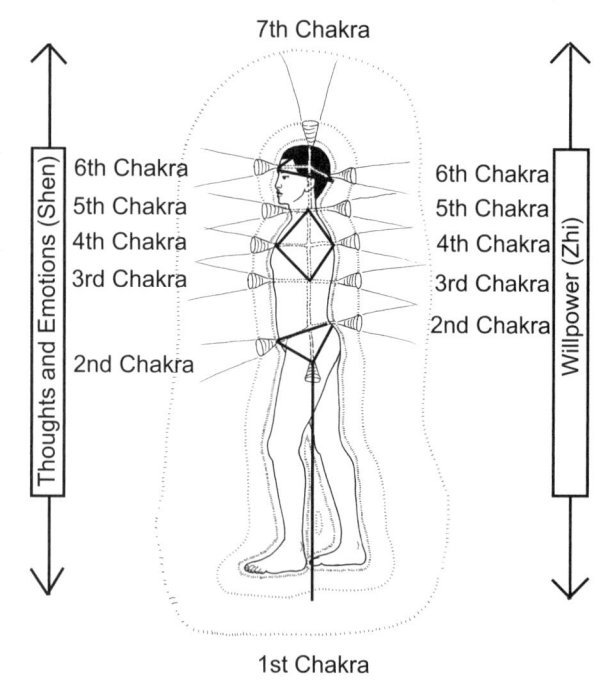

Figure 5.16. The body's Twelve Chakras Gates extend from the Taiji Pole and expand outward into the three external Wei Qi fields

chakra gates to stabilize the emotions and to regulate the patient's will and determination (Figure 5.16). The doctor can, for example, connect with the Heart Chakra back gate, located on the patient's Shendao, GV-11 point, to access the emotions stored within the Heart. The Front Chakra Gates are used to remove excess emotions from the patient's tissues. The Three Dantians system and the Seven Chakra system mutually compliment each other, both in their location of the energy centers and in their associated physical and energetic manifestations.

ENERGETIC FUNCTION

The twelve chakra gates serve as subtle energy distributors that help absorb and distribute environmental Qi to the patient's organs, tissues, and major nerve plexus areas closest to each gate. Each chakra gate connects to its own potential of psychic perception, interfaces with the body's nervous system, and is associated with a specific endocrine gland. Any energy extended by the

Qigong doctor towards a patient's chakra gate will affect the patient's physical body. As the doctor begins to energetically open the patient's chakra gates, the external chakra wheels begin to open and close in half-circle rotations, rhythmically moving with the Taiji Pole's energetic pulse. The action is similar to the centripetal (closing) and centrifugal (opening) action of the body's energetic channels.

A chakra gate can become stuck open, stuck closed, or tilt out of alignment from the Taiji Pole. Any of these conditions can cause Qi Deviations that may result in a distorted or obstructed flow of energy. This obstruction may cause physical, as well as psychological, stress or trauma.

Each opening of a chakra gate may result in a spontaneous emotional release. Some of these releases can involve painful memories that have been dislodged from the energetic filter (or veil) that envelops each gate. This energetic filter prevents external emotional traumas from entering into the body's center core.

The release of these emotional traumas can be overwhelming if the patient does not understand the nature of these healing transitions. Releases usually occur after the patient's system has been adequately balanced and energized by the Qigong doctor. The patient's system then functions with more energy and will effectively seek to release any and all trapped physical, emotional and energetic toxins. Qigong doctors should be aware of these energetic releases and assist their patients in working through the fears and pain as the Qi Deviations along the Taiji Pole are corrected. Sometimes these experiences unwind at a rapid rate, stimulating the patient's central and anterior nervous system; this can release a flood of mental images, emotions, and sensations accompanied by shaking, thrashing, and other unusual movements of the body.

THE BOTTOM CHAKRA GATE

The bottom or first chakra gate is located at the "Meeting of Yin" Huiyin CV-1 point (referring to the Earth Qi) and is rooted at the perineum in front of the anal sphincter. This energy center controls the reproductive system and the urogenital organs (Figure 5.17).

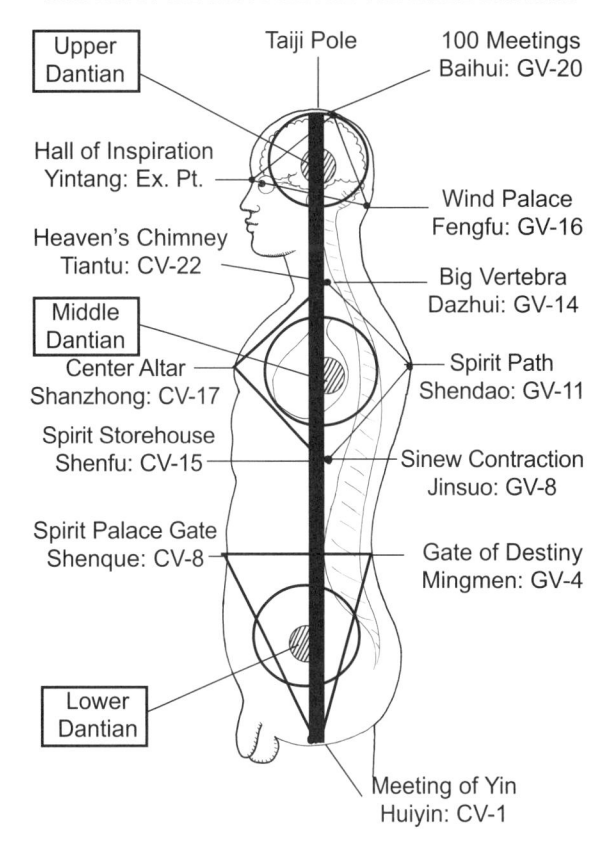

Figure 5.17. The Anatomical Locations of the Twelve Chakra Gates and the Taiji Pole

The first chakra gate accesses the Lower Dantian and is the bottom gate of the Taiji Pole. It is also connected to the Governing Vessel, Conception Vessel and Thrusting Vessel, and intersects with the Urinary Bladder Channel and Kidney Channel.

THE SECOND CHAKRA AND GATES

The second chakra core can be accessed through two energetic gates. The front gate is located at the "Spirit's Palace Gate" Shenque (CV-8) point and is rooted at the navel. The back gate is located at the "Gate of Destiny" Mingmen (GV-4) point and is rooted on the lower back.

THE THIRD CHAKRA AND GATES

The third chakra core can be accessed through two energetic gates. The front gate is located at the Yellow Court; in this system of chakra diagnosis, it is located at the solar plexus area at the "Spirit Storehouse" Shenfu (CV-15) point. The back gate is located at the "Sinew Contraction" Jinsuo GV-8 point and is rooted at the middle of the back.

THE FOURTH CHAKRA AND GATES

The fourth chakra core can be accessed through two energetic gates. The front gate is located at the "Center Altar" Shangzhong (CV-17) point (Heart Center) and is rooted at the center of the breastbone. The back gate is located at the "Spirit Path" Shendao (GV-11) point and is rooted on the back between the scapulae.

THE FIFTH CHAKRA AND GATES

The fifth chakra core can be accessed through two energetic gates. The front gate is located at the "Heaven's Chimney" Tiantu (CV-22) point (Throat Center) and is rooted just above the hollow of the throat. The back gate is located at the "Big Vertebra" and is rooted at the back at the base of the neck on the Dazhui (GV-14) point.

THE SIXTH CHAKRA AND GATES

The sixth chakra core can be accessed through two energetic gates. The front gate is located at the "Hall of Impression" Yintang point (Third-Eye Center) and is rooted at the middle of the forehead. The back gate is located on the back of the head between "Wind Palace" (GV-16) and "Brain's Door" (GV-17) at the external occipital protuberance.

THE UPPER CHAKRA GATE

The upper or top chakra gate is located at the "One Hundred Meetings" Baihui (GV-20) point (Crown Center) and is rooted at top of the head .

PRECAUTIONS

It is important for the student or patient to realize that when energetic reactions to opening the chakra gates happen, these are normal phenomena that occur temporarily during energetic and spiritual transformations. The student or patient should take certain precautions, however, such as finding a qualified Qigong doctor before beginning any type of energy training.

It is also important not to allow patients to experience these emotional transitions alone. Because these energy transitions, malfunctions, and deviations are new to the Western mode of thinking, they can easily be misdiagnosed by doctors unfamiliar with energetic medicine. Patients should be encouraged to find or establish a support group consisting of advanced energy workers familiar with the chakra system. Having a support group of experienced practitioners allows these emotional and spiritual transitions to occur in a safe environment where other experienced practitioners can monitor the patient's feelings and energy, if and when unfamiliar emotions start to emerge.

THE TWELVE EARTHLY BRANCHES AND THE TWELVE CHAKRA GATES

The body is viewed as a small and complete universe unto itself. The internal organs are influenced by the celestial movements of the sun, moon, planets, and stars. The Governing and Conception Vessels, where the twelve chakra gates are located, are also affected by the Heavenly cycles.

In ancient China, the day was divided into twelve separate time divisions. Each time division encompassed two hours of the day and was named after one of the Twelve Earthly Branches. These twelve time divisions were further organized into months and seasons (see Volume 2, Chapter 12). The ancient Qigong doctors discovered that the body's Qi and Blood mirror the Earth's seasonal ebb and flow, rising and falling like the lunar tides.

Each time period in the Twelve Earthly Branches system is regarded as having a specific influence on each of the Twelve Gates of the body's chakra system (Figure 5.18). The rhythmic variations of the waxing and waning of Qi and Blood are associated with the waxing and waning of Yin and Yang energy, as well as the circulation of Qi along the Microcosmic Orbit (Fire) cycle.

Each of the Twelve Chakra Gates relates to one of the Twelve Earthly Branches following the Fire Cycle of the Microcosmic Orbit (see Volume 4, Chapter 43). These twelve chakras gates extend their energy outward through the anterior and

Chapter 5: The Taiji Pole and The Three Dantians

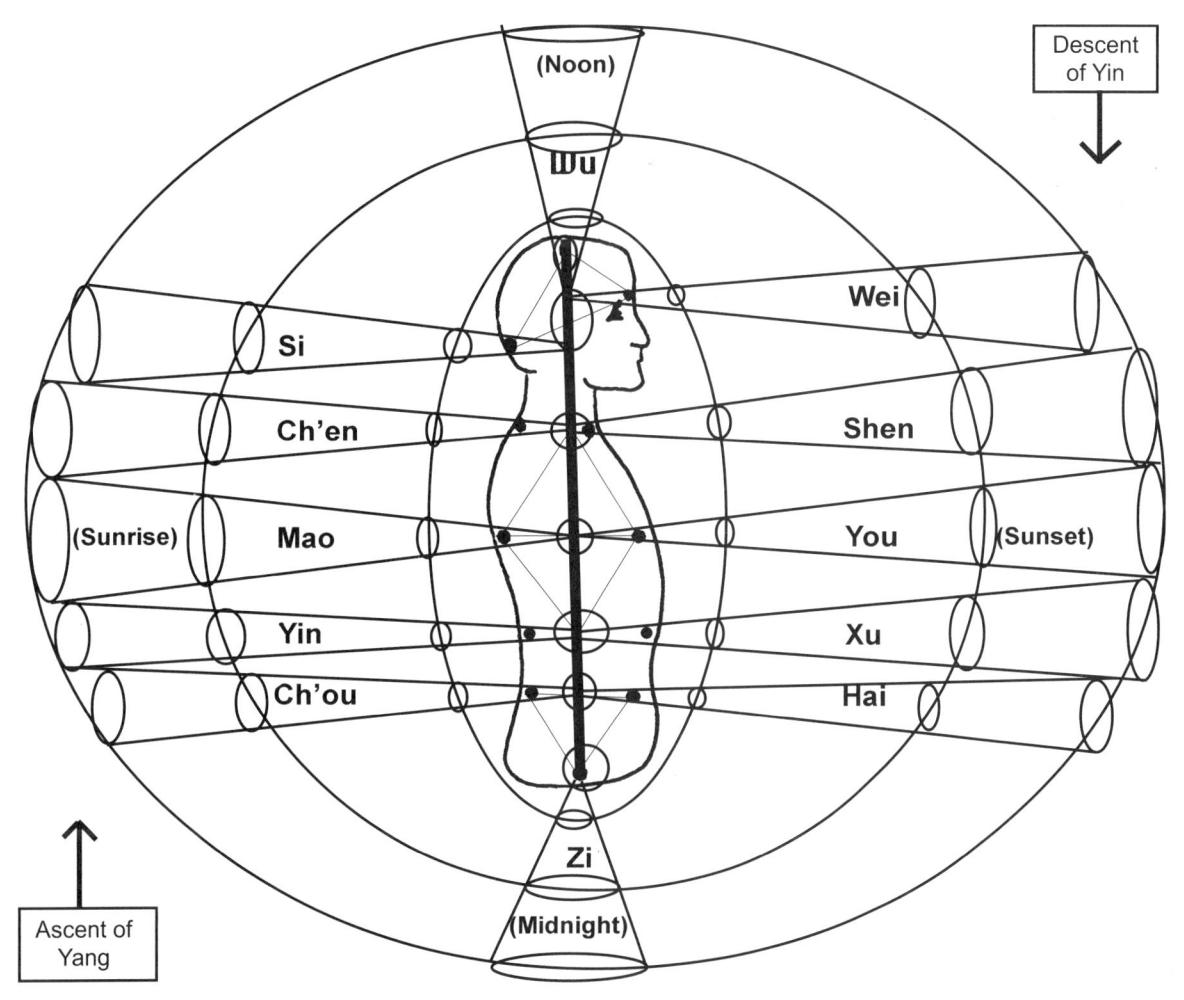

Figure 5.18. This figure shows the correspondence between the Twelve Earthly Branches and the Twelve Chakra Gates. The Governing Vessel and the Conception Vessel (flowing up the midline of the back and down the front of the body) correspond to the elliptic path of the sun along the Twelve Chakra Gates. The twelve time divisions of each day are related to one of the Twelve Earthly Branches and have a specific energetic influence on the corresponding chakra gate.

posterior fields of Qi, from the patient's Taiji Pole in the center of the body. Beginning at the bottom chakra gate (the "Zi" Branch, representing midnight), the energy follows the Fire Cycle of the Microcosmic Orbit, traveling up the Governing Vessel, following the ascent of Yang. After the Yang Qi reaches its peak, the Yin begins to grow. Starting at the upper chakra gate (the Wu Branch, representing noon time), the energy travels down the Conception Vessel following the descent of Yin.

Reconstructing The Chakra Gates

The protective energetic grid of a patient's chakra gate can sometimes be disfigured, torn, or even completely ripped away from the chakra gate itself (Figure 5.19). When the chakra gate's protective grid becomes damaged, the patient's energetic field is no longer able to repel the invasion of external pathogens from the body. Neither is the patient able to clearly direct energy out from the chakra, preventing the creative process of expression.

VOLUME 1, SECTION 1: FOUNDATIONS OF CHINESE ENERGETIC MEDICINE

In order to repair the damaged energetic grid, the Qigong doctor must first remove the chakra gate from the patient's body. This is accomplished by following the chakra gate reconstruction clinical procedure, described as follows:

- With the doctor's left palm, use the Qi Compression technique (Volume 3, Chapter 38) and stimulate the tissues several inches above the area of the damaged chakra's gate. The doctor will simultaneously use the Bellows Palm techniques (Volume 3, Chapter 35), with his or her right palm over the damaged chakra gate in a counterclockwise circular direction, to unwind and remove the chakra's gate.
- If the chakra gate is stuck or frozen within the patient's tissues and becomes difficult to remove from the body, the doctor can remove it by first wobbling it from side to side while applying pressure to the tissue area above the chakra Gate using the Bellows Palm technique.
- Next, the doctor will pulse white light energy into the chakra to lift and remove the chakra from its chamber. This energetic pulse should resemble the flashing of a strobe light.
- Once the chakra is free, it will reveal a complex root system that is embedded within the patient's energetic body. This energetic root system has subtle extensions into the spiritual body, as well as energy channels connecting with the patient's internal organs. The actual size of the chakra gate is about the diameter of a silver dollar, therefore it is important for the doctor to energetically expand its size in order to more effectively clean the filter.
- To clean the chakra filter, the doctor will hold the energetic body of the chakra gate with his or her left palm (like holding an ice cream cone) and begin to clean the chakra gate by manually dredging and purging the chakra filter. The chakra Gate can then be energized and reconstructed by connecting its energetic field to a column of divine healing white light energy.
- After the chakra gate has been cleansed, it is important to reduce its expanded size back

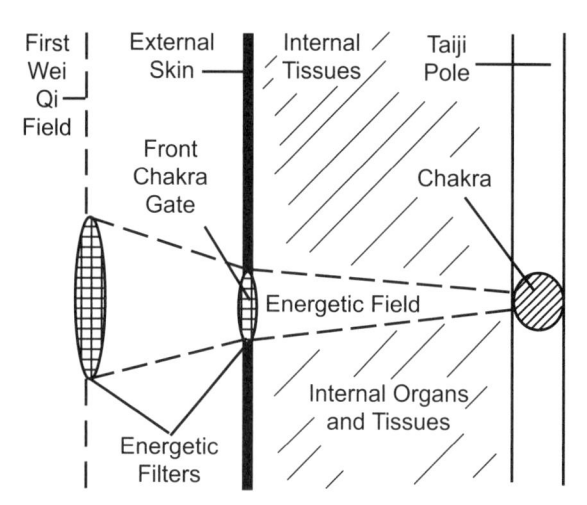

Figure 5.19. The Protective Energetic Grid of a Chakra Gate

to normal and reconnect it into the patient's body while simultaneously energizing the patient's Taiji Pole. This re-establishes the energetic function of the chakra gate by rooting it back into its energetic core. This is accomplished by holding the chakra gate with the right Bellows Palm (in order to secure it), mentally commanding it to shrink in size and gently placing it back into its proper residence. Simultaneously, the doctor's left hand should be placed on the patient's crown point (Baihui) in order to engage and integrate the chakra's energetic rhythm with the natural rhythm of the Taiji Pole.

- End the treatment by connecting with the divine and enveloping the patient with white light energy. Allow the Qi to flow into the Microcosmic Orbit (Fire Cycle) for several rotations. Then reconnect with the divine and allow the Qi to flow in the Microcosmic Orbit (Water Cycle) for several rotations. This concludes the treatment.

ENERGIZING THE CHAKRAS THROUGH THE TWELVE GATES

Vibration, color and sound are all interrelated and are a means of determining or monitoring the frequency of energy within the patient's chakra gates. By projecting the appropriate colors into the

210

CHAPTER 5: THE TAIJI POLE AND THE THREE DANTIANS

The Three Energetic Fields Taught Within the Ancient Daoist Traditions

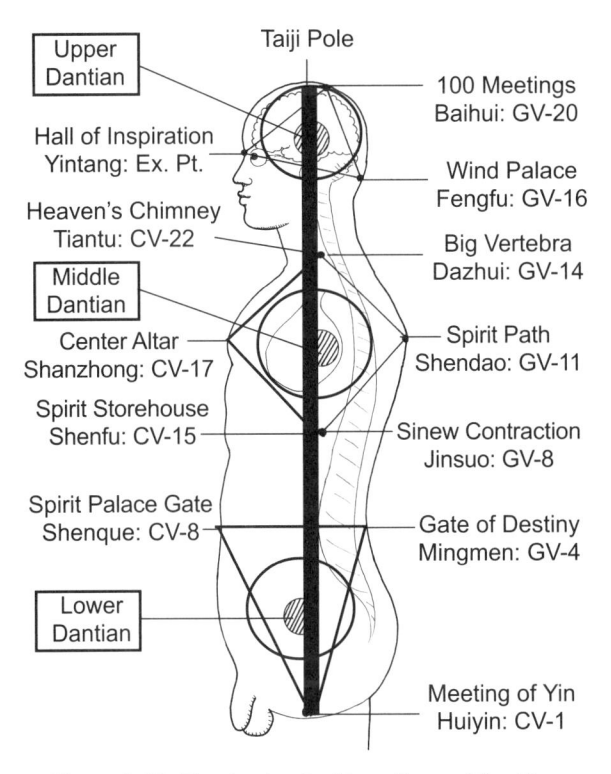

- Upper Dantian
- Taiji Pole
- Hall of Inspiration Yintang: Ex. Pt.
- Heaven's Chimney Tiantu: CV-22
- Middle Dantian
- Center Altar Shanzhong: CV-17
- Spirit Storehouse Shenfu: CV-15
- Spirit Palace Gate Shenque: CV-8
- Lower Dantian
- 100 Meetings Baihui: GV-20
- Wind Palace Fengfu: GV-16
- Big Vertebra Dazhui: GV-14
- Spirit Path Shendao: GV-11
- Sinew Contraction Jinsuo: GV-8
- Gate of Destiny Mingmen: GV-4
- Meeting of Yin Huiyin: CV-1

Figure 5.20. The Anatomical Locations of the Three Dantians and Taiji Pole According to Ancient Daoist Teachings

The Three Energetic Fields Taught Within the Ancient Buddhist and Yogic Traditions

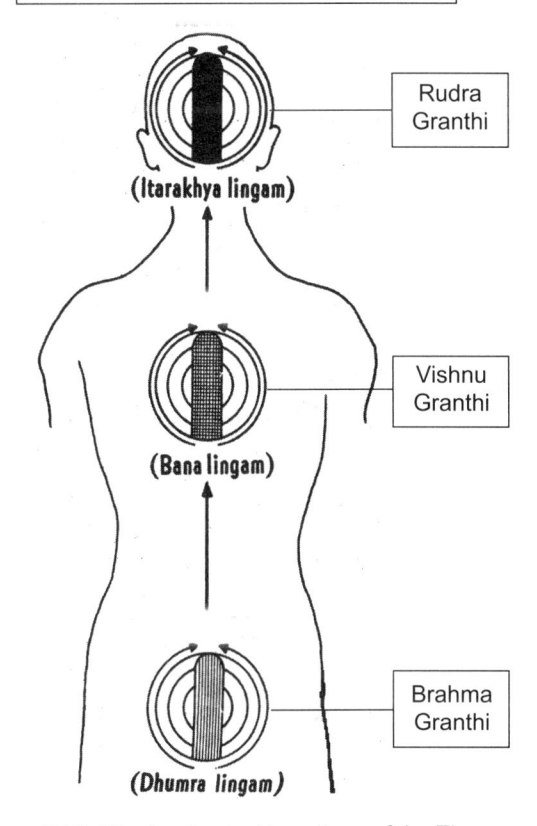

- (Itarakhya lingam) — Rudra Granthi
- (Bana lingam) — Vishnu Granthi
- (Dhumra lingam) — Brahma Granthi

Figure 5.21. The Anatomical Locations of the Three Dantians According to Ancient Buddhist Teachings

chakra gates, the Qigong doctor is able to re-energize the chakras, as well as Tonify their internal organ functions and stimulate the emotional components associated with the specific chakra areas.

THE THREE DANTIANS

According to ancient Daoist energetic anatomy and physiology, humans have three important energy centers that store and emit energy similar to the same way a battery stores and emits energy. These three centers are called the Three Dantians (Figure 5.20). The Three Dantians are strategically positioned along the Taiji Pole in order to facilitate maximum energy transference.

Although the chakra systems are more significant in the Buddhist and Yogic traditions, both of these spiritual disciplines commonly refer to the Three Dantian areas in their energetic practice. According to ancient Buddhist and Yogic traditions, these three areas contain the three psychic knots or "Granthi" where an individual's energy and spiritual consciousness interact and manifest in particular ways (Figure 5.21).

THE CHINESE CHARACTER FOR DANTIAN

The ideograph depicting the Chinese characters for "Dantian" is described as follows (Figure 5.22):

- The first character is the Chinese ideograph "Dan," which is generally translated as "red," "vermillion" or "cinnabar." Cinnabar, a bright red or vermillion mineral, is chemically known as mercury sulfide, and is the principal ore of mercury. Cinnabar was an important mineral in ancient China, as it was the source material for vermillion ink, manufactured exclusively for the use of the emperors. Cinnabar was, and still is, also used in Chinese medicine to sedate the Heart and calm the Shen, but always in small doses and for short periods due to its toxic nature. Cinnabar was also a vital elixir in Daoist alchemy, as it was discovered to contain an ideal balance of Yin and Yang properties.

- The second character is the Chinese ideograph "Tian," which is generally translated as "field," but can also be translated as "farmland." In Medical Qigong terms, Tian is referred to as a field of energy. Together, the characters for Dantian literally translates as "cinnabar field" or "field of elixir."

OUTER AND INNER ALCHEMY

Daoist alchemy, like Western alchemy, was practiced in two ways: outer alchemy (Wai Dan) and inner alchemy (Nei Dan). Outer alchemy was the ancestor of modern chemistry. Outer alchemists set up laboratories and experimented with many substances from mineral, animal, and plant sources with the goal of discovering how to turn base metals into gold. Secretly, they were also seeking to discover an elixir that would confer immortality or, at least greater longevity. In the process of this outer alchemical experimentation, the ancient Chinese discovered many exceptionally potent herbal medicines, in addition to other chemical formulas such as the formula for gunpowder.

Inner alchemy was concerned with purifying human nature and transforming the spirit into its most pure and radiant potential without the use of external agents. Qigong exercises and meditations were developed in order to circulate and gather the "inner elixirs" of Jing (sexual energy), Qi, and Shen (consciousness) at various locations within the body.

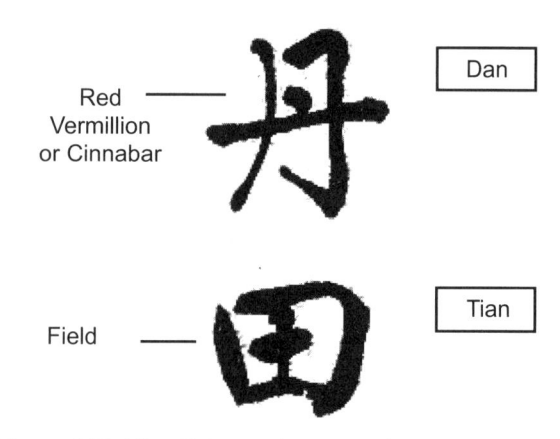

Figure 5.22. The Chinese characters for "Dantian."

These internal alchemists viewed the Three Dantians as inner crucibles or cauldrons, and employed them in the role of gathering and transforming vital substances, energies, and various aspects of awareness. All of the internal alchemy methods and formulas involve specific combinations of the body's Jing, Qi, and Shen (Figure 5.23). The inner alchemists kept their work hidden by using secret mineral code words such as "gold," "lead," and "cinnabar" to describe the movements and transformations of energetic and spiritual substances within the body.

The ultimate goal of internal alchemy is immortality, a complete transformation of the body's Jing, Qi, and Shen. Jing, Qi, and Shen are the three fundamental energies necessary for human life, and are collectively referred to as the "Three Treasures of Man." To accomplish this transformation, alchemists first gather and transform Jing into Qi in the Lower Dantian. They then gather and transform Qi into Shen in the Middle Dantian. Next, they transform Shen into Wuji (the absolute openness of infinite space) in the Upper Dantian. Finally, they merge Wuji into Dao (divine energy).

These transformations can be compared to the changes of water consistencies, which when heated, can change from solid ice, to liquid, to vapor. These progressive transformations are one example of the use of the Three Dantians as inner crucibles in the process of internal alchemy. Through extensive experimentation in the internal laboratory of the physical, energetic, and spiritual body, Daoist alchemists were able to become powerful sorcerers, augurs, and healers.

The Three Treasures of Man (Jing, Qi, and Shen) are also connected with the Three Outer Forces or Powers known as Heaven, Earth, and Man. Jing (reproductive essence) is the most substantial and therefore the most Yin of the three, and it is closely linked with Earth Qi. In Medical Qigong practice and Daoist inner alchemy, the Earth energy is gathered in the Lower Dantian and is associated with heat. Qi is closely connected with the atmospheric energy (a blend of Heaven and Earth energy), is gathered into the Middle Dantian and is associated with vibration. Shen (Spirit) is the most insubstantial, and therefore, the most Yang of the three. It corresponds with Heaven Qi, is gathered in the Upper Dantian, and is associated with light.

The Three Dantians are connected to each other through the Taiji Pole. The Taiji Pole acts as a passageway for communication between the Three Dantians and as a highway for the movement of the various life-force energies. The Eternal Soul is drawn into the body at the moment of conception through the Taiji Pole and departs through the Taiji Pole at death. The Taiji Pole also serves as a portal for the body's Hun.

Medical Qigong views the Three Dantians as vital centers for the cultivation of energy. They are important areas for diagnosis and self-healing, as well as for the therapeutic projection of Qi into patients. The Three Dantians have specific relationships to the Three Treasures of Jing, Qi, and Shen.

THE LOWER FIELD OF CINNABAR: XIA DANTIAN

The Lower Dantian is the Dantian most familiar to martial artists and meditators, as it is the first place on which they are trained to focus their concentration. It is regarded as the center of physical strength and the source of stamina. Called the "hara" in Japanese, it is located in the lower abdomen, in the center of the triangle formed by drawing a line between the navel, Mingmen (lower back), and perineum. These three points form a pyramid facing downward. This configuration allows the Lower Dantian to gather the energy from the Earth.

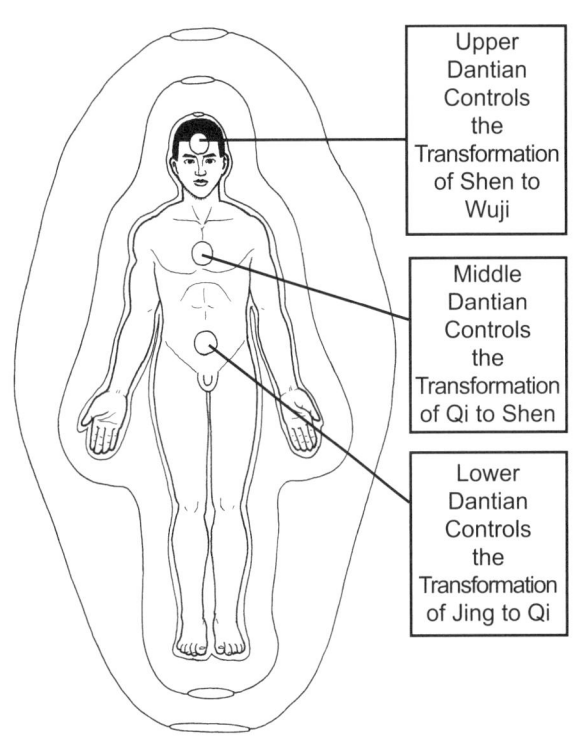

Figure 5.23. The Three Dantians and their relationship to the transformation of Jing, Qi, and Shen

The Lower Dantian is the major storage area for the various types of Kidney energies (i.e., Qi of the ovaries and testicles). The Kidney energies, in turn, are closely linked with the prenatal energies and provide the foundation for all other types of energy (Jing, Qi, Yin, and Yang, etc.) in the body.

The Lower Dantian is connected to the first level of Wei Qi. This level of Protective Qi circulates outside the body, extending roughly one inch beyond the body's tissues. As the Lower Dantian fills with Qi, the Wei Qi field naturally becomes thicker.

THE LOWER DANTIAN AND JING

The Lower Dantian collects Earth energy and is associated with Jing and the energy of the physical body. The Earth energy that is transformed in the Lower Dantian is a dense, full, thick energy. In the above analogy of the transformations of water, the energy in the Lower Dantian relates to ice, the densest state of water.

The Lower Dantian is closely linked to the Jing Gong (Essence Palace), which is located in the perineum, and serves as a reservoir of Jing. Our Prenatal Essence (Yuan Jing) determines our constitutional strengths and vitality and is stored in the Lower Dantian. It interacts with the Kidney energies to form Kidney Jing.

The Lower Dantian acts as a reservoir for heat and energy and is associated with the Kidneys. The Kidneys control the Water element in the body, and in alchemical terms, Jing is said to be analogous to the water in the cauldron. Through focused concentration and meditation, the Jing (essence) in the Lower Dantian is refined and transformed to produce Qi (energy). When sufficient heat is generated in the Lower Dantian as a result of the Heart and Mingmen Fire mixing with the Kidney Water, the alchemical transformation of Jing in the Lower Dantian area causes the water of the Jing to turn into the steam of Qi. This is one reason why the modern character for Qi is composed of the image of steam rising from rice that is bursting and decomposing (Volume 2, Chapter 14). This alchemical transformation is known as "changing Jing (essence) into Qi (energy)," and takes place within the Lower Dantian.

The Kidney energies are all closely intertwined: Kidney Jing, Kidney Qi, Kidney Yin, Kidney Yang, and Kidney Mingmen Fire. The Mingmen Fire, also called Kidney Yang, helps transform the Jing into steam (Kidney Qi).

Kidney Jing circulates throughout the body via the Eight Extraordinary Vessels, in particular the Governing Vessel, Conception Vessel, and Thrusting Vessels, all of which originate in the Lower Dantian.

Kidney Jing controls the reproductive energies and life cycles of the body. Some of the ancient alchemical texts describe the Lower Dantian in women as being located in the "Bao" or Uterus, illustrating the important role of the Uterus in relationship to the function of Jing in a woman's body. In men, the reproductive essence is located in the prostate and seminal vesicles, also known as the Jing Gong (Essence Palace) in Daoist alchemy. In some Daoist, Qigong, and Chinese medical literature, the term Kidneys is occasionally used as a synonym for the testes and ovaries.

The exact location of the Jing Gong differs in men and women due to the anatomical locations of the male and female reproductive organs. In men, this area is located in the center of the body at the level of the superior border of the pubic bone, posterior to the Qugu CV-2 (Crooked Bone) point. The Jing Gong area in women is located higher, centered in the Uterus, about an inch above the superior border of the pubic bone, posterior to the Zhongji CV-3 (Utmost Center) point.

This difference in location affects the production and storage of Jing. The testicles in the male cause the transformation of energy to occur lower in the body than it does in females. In females this transformation takes place in a slightly higher position due to the location of the woman's ovaries.

Jing is the most physical and material form of energy within the body and thus corresponds to Yin and to Earth energy. The Lower Dantian is the place where the Qi of the Earth is drawn into the body and transformed by heat.

THE LOWER DANTIAN AND QI

The Lower Dantian is often called "the Sea of Qi." It is the place where Qi is housed, the Mingmen Fire is aroused, the Kidney Yin and Yang Qi are gathered, and the Yuan Qi is stored. Also called Source Qi or Original Qi, the Yuan Qi is the foundation of all the other types of Qi in the body. The Yuan Qi is closely linked with the Prenatal Essence (Yuan Jing). Together, the Yuan Qi and Yuan Jing determine our overall health, vitality, stamina, and life span.

The Yuan Qi is the force behind the activity of all the organs and energies in the body. It is closely related to the Mingmen and works to provide body heat. The body's Yuan Qi is the catalytic agent for transforming the food we eat and the air we breath into Postnatal Qi. It also facilitates the production of Blood.

Yuan Qi is housed in the Lower Dantian, and flows to all the internal organs and channels via the Triple Burners. Yuan Qi is said to enter the

Twelve Primary Channels (the body's twelve major energy pathways) through the Yuan points (sometimes called Source points) in acupuncture theory.

Of the Three Dantians, the Lower Dantian is the closest to the Earth and is the most Yin; it is therefore the natural center for gathering and storing Earth Qi within the body. In Medical Qigong, once students have learned to conserve and circulate their own Qi, they can increase it by connecting to the unlimited reservoirs of Qi existing within the natural environment. Being the densest and easiest to feel, Earth energy is the first form of external Qi with which the Qigong practitioner connects. This energetic connection with the Earth is important for two main reasons, described as follows:

1. Qigong practitioners need the Yin grounding power of Earth Qi to counterbalance the more active Yang energy cultivated during Qigong exercises. Without grounding in Earth Qi, many Qigong practitioners develop Qi deviations in the form of excess heat.
2. Each person's supply of Qi is limited. When Qigong doctors extend their Qi to heal others, they deplete their personal store of Qi unless they are able to simultaneously replenish their supply from outside sources.

Even people who do not practice Medical Qigong naturally draw Earth Qi into their Lower Dantians as an unconscious action of survival and environmental adjustment. By practicing Qigong and directing conscious intent, the amount of Earth Qi drawn into the body can be vastly increased.

THE LOWER DANTIAN AND SHEN

Given its Yin nature and close proximity to the Earth, the Lower Dantian itself is considered a center of consciousness. This consciousness is more physical and kinesthetic than the consciousness of the Middle or Upper Dantian. As the Lower Dantian is the energetic home for both the lower Po and lower Hun, it is subject to specific patterns of influence, described as follows:

- **Influence of the Corporeal Soul (Po):** The body's Jing is connected with the Seven Corporeal Souls, which are collectively known as the Po. The Po control our survival instinct and the subconscious physical reflexes associated with survival. For this reason, martial artists spend many hours cultivating their Lower Dantians to create the integration of Jing, Qi, and Shen needed for the split-second clarity of focus required in life-and-death struggles.
- **Influence of the Ethereal Soul (Hun):** The Lower Dantian is the residence of the Lower Hun, called Yu Jing, or Hidden Essence. This Hun is associated with the Earth, producing our desire for enjoying life and comforts, as well as our ability to fully experience the pure passions of life.

THE LOWER DANTIAN AND KINESTHETIC AWARENESS

In addition to being the center of physical strength and the source of stamina, the Lower Dantian is also considered the "house" of physical (kinesthetic) feeling, communication and awareness. Kinesthetic communication is the level of awareness referred to as "the intuition of the physical body," and is stimulated by particular aspects of the subconscious. The subconscious mind picks up many signals from the environment that are not processed by the logical mind. The subconscious mind may react to these signals with spontaneous body movements, or with subtle but powerful emotional responses sometimes referred to as "gut feelings."

Kinesthesia is defined as "the sensory experiences mediated by nervous elements within the muscles, tendons and joints, and stimulated by bodily movements and tensions characterized by movement." It is this kinetic state of awareness that allows the Qigong doctor to naturally feel the patient's internal resonant vibrations. When the doctors' body suddenly feels hot or cold, starts shaking or trembling, this may indicate that the subconscious mind is trying to communicate, and is resonating with the location and condition of the diseased areas within the patient's tissues.

Often, the feelings experienced in the Lower Dantian are very subtle. For this reason, Qigong doctors are trained to establish a heightened degree of awareness of their own body, and are thus able to pick up subtle variations and energetic shifts within themselves and others. When doctors collect energy in the Lower Dantian, an increased awareness and sensitivity naturally occurs. Cultivating this ability requires the practice of paying attention to the physical body (training kinesthetic awareness). A high level of awareness of the physical body, the surrounding environment, and the relationship between the two, is required in order to maximize kinesthetic communication. When physical awareness is increased, feeling and kinesthetic body movements happen naturally. These subtle senses allow Qigong doctors to feel, smell, or hear energetic phenomena as they are released from the patient's diseased tissues.

THE LOWER DANTIAN AND SCIENCE

The Lower Dantian's "Brain," is known in Western terms as the enteric (intestinal) nervous system. According to research conducted by Dr. Michael Gershon, a professor of anatomy and cellular biology at Columbia Presbyterian Medical Center in New York, the Lower Dantian sends and receives impulses, records experiences, and responds to emotions. Its nerve cells are bathed in and influenced by the same type of neurotransmitters that exist in the Brain.

The entire nervous system mirrors the body's central nervous system and is a network of 100 million neurons (more neurons than the spinal cord), neurotransmitters, and proteins that can act independently of the body's Brain and can send messages, learn, remember, and produce feelings.

Dr. Gershon explains that major neurotransmitters like serotonin, dopamine, glutamine, norepinephrine, nitric oxide, enkephalins (one type of natural opiate), and benzodiazepines (psychoactive chemicals that relieve anxiety) are active within the neural system of the lower abdominal area. The lower abdomen also has two dozen small Brain proteins called neuropeptides. Dr. Gershon's research provides modern scientific verification of what Eastern wisdom has taught for millennia; that centers of consciousness exist at places in the body apart from the organ of the

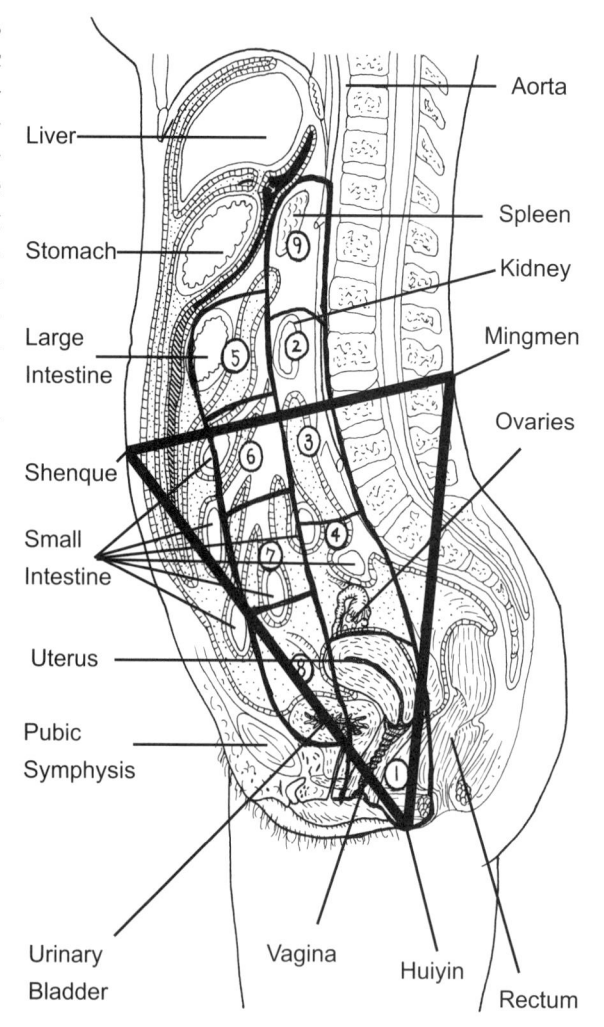

Figure 5.24. The Nine Chambers of the Lower Dantian are shown here in the female body.
(Inspired by the original artwork of Dr. Frank H. Netter).

Brain. The abdomen or Lower Dantian, is one of the these major centers of awareness.

ANATOMICAL LOCATION OF THE LOWER DANTIAN

The Lower Dantian is centered below the umbilicus, and inside the lower abdomen, forming a downward pointing triangle. Its boundaries are defined by the three lower chakra gates, described as follows (Figure 5.24 and Figure 5.25):

1. **Huiyin (Meeting of the Yin):** The lowest point of the Lower Dantian extends to the Huiyin CV-1 point at the perineum. This point is lo-

cated midway between the genitals (anterior Yin or Qianyin) and anus (posterior Yin or Houyin), traditionally known as the "Huiyin." The name "Huiyin" refers to the area on the body responsible for gathering and absorbing the Earth energy. This area is responsible for gathering the Yin energy into the body and Lower Dantian area via the three Yin leg channels (Liver, Spleen, and Kidney), and is the intersecting point for the Governing Vessel, Conception Vessel and Thrusting Vessels. This area is sometimes known as the lower gate of the Taiji Pole, or the bottom gate of the Lower Chakra.

2. **Shen Que (Spirit's Watch Tower):** The front area of the Lower Dantian is located posterior to the Shenque CV-8 point at the navel. The name refers to the place where the mother's Qi and Shen enter the embryo during fetal development. After the umbilical cord is cut, the cord extending out of the navel resembles a tower over the abdomen of the newborn, hence its name "Spiritual Tower." This area is sometimes known as the Front Dantian, or the front gate of the Second Chakra.

In ancient China, it was believed that the twisting of the umbilical cord and the internal coiling of the intestines around it followed the patterns of the energetic vortex known as the "Taizhong" (Supreme Center), which spiralled between Heaven (the fetus' head) and Earth (the fetus' lower abdomen). It was through the energetic movement of the Taizhong that all things polarized (becoming either Yin or Yang) and received their form. It was also believed that the Heavenly center of this energetic vortex (within the center of the umbilicus) was equal to the Pole Star in the sky, around which the constellations continually spin. Therefore, the area of the umbilicus was sometimes called "Tianshu," the "Pivot of Heaven," or the "Capital of the Spirit."

In Chinese cosmology, Yin and Yang and the three worlds of spirit, energy and matter polarize from the undifferentiated energetic center of the Wuji. As this energetic center begins to polarize, a spinning vortex is created,

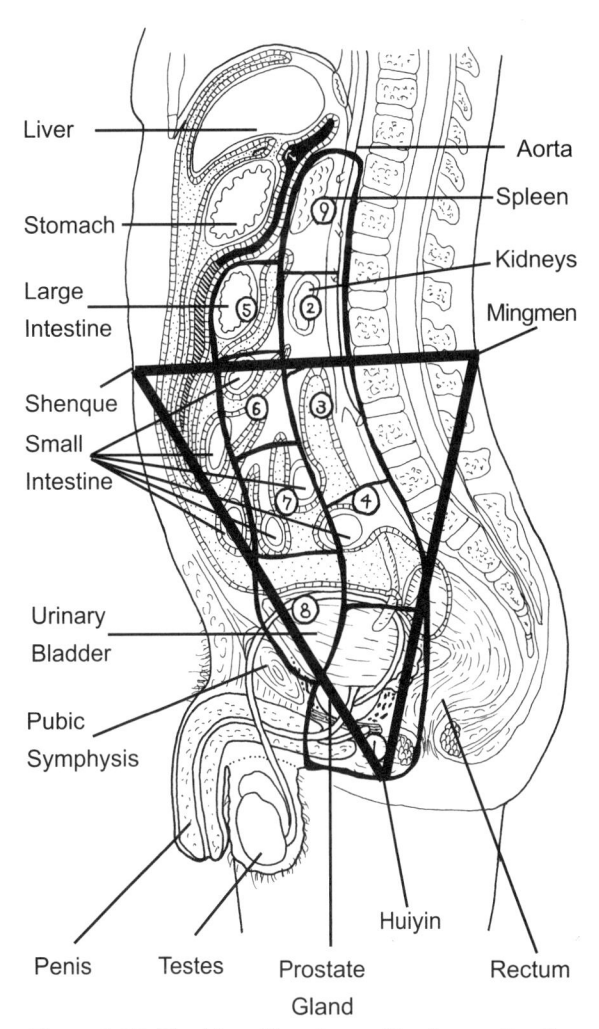

Figure 5.25. The Nine Chambers of the Lower Dantian are shown here in the male body.
(Inspired by the original artwork of Dr. Frank H. Netter).

setting the pattern that forms the energetic template for all things. In ancient Daoism, this energetic interaction set the foundation for the creation of the Prenatal and Postnatal Bagua, the original Eight Trigram formations of the Yi-Jing.

Due to this internal connection, the area of the navel is considered to be the lair of Qi and Shen, as energetically both Qi and Shen continually spin and manifest from the umbilical area the same way that the stars and constellations spin around the Pole Star. The ancient

Daoists considered the umbilical area the "root of preserving life," because the energetic treasure of its Qi and Shen flowed outwards to connect with all of the internal organs. An ancient Chinese saying states, "When the umbilicus opens, the body's internal organs can interact with the womb of Heaven and Earth."

According to ancient Daoist philosophy, once the umbilical cord is cut, Heaven and Earth separate; and the fetus' Yin (Earth: Water Qi) and Yang (Heaven: Fire Qi) polarities divide. The Yang Shen rises upward into the chest and Middle Dantian area and becomes the Fire of the Heart; the Yin Jing descends into the lower abdomen and Lower Dantian area and becomes the Water of the Kidneys (Figure 5.26).

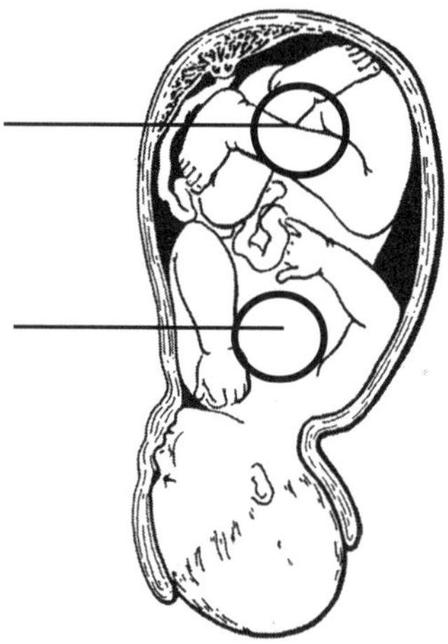

3. **Mingmen (Gate of Destiny):** The back area of the Lower Dantian is located at the Mingmen GV-4 point on the lower back, inferior to the second lumbar vertebra. The Mingmen (Gate of Life, Fate, or Destiny) is located between the Kidneys, and in ancient times it was also called the "Gate of Destiny," the "Door of Fate," the "Golden Portal," the "Mysterious Pass," and the "Door of all Hidden Mysteries." It was believed that all of creation passed through this gate as it emerged from the eternal Dao to form the individual's Taiji Pole upon conception. Physiologically, the ancient Daoists also believed that the spiritual function of the Mingmen empowers the individual with the ability of energetic interpenetration. This ability allows the individual to move within the energetic forms of Yin and Yang, Jing and Shen, as well as the energetic forms of the inner aspects of the early and later Heaven.

In ancient China, the concept of an individual's Virtue (De) and his or her Destiny (Ming) were closely connected. Destiny (associated with the Yuan Jing, Qi and Shen) was given by Heaven at birth and stored away in the individual's Mingmen area between the Kidneys. The individual's Ming becomes the spark of life and the dynamic potential existing behind his or her thoughts

Lower Dantian
Yin Jing Descends to Become the Kidney Water

Middle Dantian
Yang Shen Rises to Become the Heart Fire

Figure 5.26. Once the umbilical cord is cut, Heaven and Earth will separate, and the fetus' Yin (Earth: Water Qi) and Yang (Heaven: Fire Qi) polarities will divide. The Yang Shen rises upward into the chest and Middle Dantian area to become the Fire of the Heart; the Yin Jing descends into the lower abdomen and Lower Dantian area to become the Water of the Kidneys.

and actions. Although the subtle impulses emanating from the individual's Ming are generally hidden from the conscious mind, through Shengong Meditations a deeper realm of understanding can be intuitively discovered and accessed.

It is up to the individual to consistently act in accordance with his or her Ming throughout life. This action is based on the individual's conscious use of his or her Intention (Yi). The intention to remain congruent with the "Will and Intent of Heaven" (Zhi Yi Tian) is what gives the individual Virtue (De). It is through the development of his or her Virtue that the individual establishes a healthy relationship with the Dao, Heaven and the spiritual world.

The Mingmen is the root of Yuan Qi, and therefore determines life and death. The Mingmen provides one third of the body's "True Fire," supplies the heat for the Triple Burners, and is responsible for stabilizing the Kidneys and Lower Dantian. This anatomical area is sometimes known as the Back Dantian, or the back gate of the Second Chakra.

4. **Lower Dantian Center:** The center or middle

of the Dantian refers to its position located between the navel and Mingmen areas. Medical Qigong schools in China differ in their opinions as to where the center of the Lower Dantian is located. Some schools teach that the center of the Lower Dantian is affected by the different anatomical locations of the male and female reproductive organs. In these particular schools, students are taught that in men, the center of the Lower Dantian is located posterior to the Guanyuan CV-4 (Gate of Original Qi) point. The center of the Dantian area in a women is said to be located higher, posterior to the Qihai CV-6 (Sea of Qi) point, located within the center of the Bao or Uterus (see Chapter 7).

THE NINE CHAMBERS OF THE LOWER DANTIAN

The human body is viewed as a microcosmic replica of Heaven. Just as Heaven is said to be divided into nine different levels, each containing various palaces, our bodies are also said to contain palaces and chambers. The eight stars of the Big Dipper constellation and Polaris (North Star) are said to correspond to the nine chambers of each of the Three Dantians.

The functional aspects of the body's psyche were described by ancient Qigong masters as "spirits" that lived within the nine chambers of the Lower Dantian. These "spirits" linked the body's energetic channels and vital internal organs into an organic harmony of life-force energy. Qigong masters believed that as each Dantian became energized, it would initiate specific reactions within the body's energetic system, manifesting certain energetic and spiritual experiences within the practitioner's psyche.

Each of the nine chambers is several inches in diameter and is numbered in accordance with its energetic stimulation (see Figure 5.23 and Figure 5.24). The vertical abdominal set of Lower Dantian chambers relates to many cavities of the body's internal viscera. The nine chambers of the Lower Dantian are named as follows:
1. The Palace of Jade (Jade Stem or Jade Cave)
2. The Official Health Monitor (Kidneys)
3. The Minister of the Orchard Terrace
4. The Chamber of Moving Pearls
5. The Minister of House Cleaning (Large Intestine)
6. The Palace of Mystical Spirits (Small Intestine)
7. The Chamber of Mysterious Elixir
8. The Spirit of the Jade Court (Urinary Bladder)
9. The Spirit of the Yellow Court (Spleen)

TRAINING OF THE LOWER DANTIAN

All Qigong training begins with a focus on the Lower Dantian. In the beginning stages of Medical Qigong training, the doctor will encourage students to focus their mind and breath into the Lower Dantian. The purpose of this training is to gather the body's Yuan Qi into the Lower Dantian (called "returning to the source") to strengthen the foundational root of the body's energy.

Medical Qigong practitioners strive to gather and balance the Yin and Yang energy within the Lower Dantian. In ancient China, the union of Yin and Yang energy within the Lower Dantian was called "Dragon and Tiger swirling in the winding river." The ancient Daoist shamans believed that the "vital essence spirit" always appears in a bright white light energy within the Lower Dantian.

It is dangerous for Medical Qigong students to bypass the discipline of Lower Dantian cultivation training in an attempt to move quickly into the more advanced intuitive and psychic training of the Upper Dantian. Such an approach to training may lead to Qi deviations (see Volume 2, Chapters 19 and 20) and cause emotional instability.

THE MIDDLE FIELD OF CINNABAR: ZHONG DANTIAN

The Heart is the primary organ related to the Middle Dantian. The secondary organ of the Middle Dantian is the Lungs. In Medical Qigong, the thymus gland is also important to the Middle Dantian.

In children, the thymus gland is quite large. As the child matures into adulthood, the thymus gland shrinks in size. Until recently, Western biologists thought that the thymus gland became vestigial and inactive in adults. Beginning in the 1980's, however, with the onset of the AIDS epidemic and the increase in cancer cases, intensive new research was launched into the immune system. As a result, scientists discovered that the thymus gland plays a major role in maturing the white blood cells to become immunocompetent; thus thymus function continues throughout one's life.

The Middle Dantian collects Qi and represents the body's reservoir for mental and emotional vibrations and energy. The energy of Man that is transformed in the Middle Dantian has a fluid quality, like water.

A refining process also takes place in the Middle Dantian, transforming the fluid energy into more steam-like energy which is then transferred to the Upper Dantian. The Middle Dantian transforms Qi into Shen by bringing the transformed Qi into the Heart Fire. This alchemical process is commonly called "changing Qi into Shen" and refers to kinesthetic energy transforming into spiritual consciousness.

The Middle Dantian is connected to the second level of Wei Qi, circulating from one inch around the body to roughly one-and-a-half feet outside the body. As the Middle Dantian fills with Qi, the colors of the student's middle field of Wei Qi change, becoming even more pronounced. The reason for this change is that the Middle Dantian is connected to the Five Agents, which in turn govern the five Yin organs and organ emotions. As the students begin to experience various stresses and emotional releases, their aura (resonating from the internal organ, into the second energetic field) changes its colors.

THE MIDDLE DANTIAN AND JING

The Heart is related to the Fire element. The Heart derives its Yang Fire from Kidney Yang. Modern research in Chinese medicine equates the function of the adrenal glands to the traditional function of Kidney Yang. A parallel can be observed in Western physiology, in which the adrenal glands help to regulate the pace of the heart.

To keep the Heart Fire in balance, the Heart also needs Yin. Heart Yin is derived from Kidney Yin (Jing is one aspect of Kidney Yin).

In traditional Chinese physiology, the Heart is said to govern the Blood. Gu Qi (energy distilled from the consumption and transformation of food and drink) is a form of postnatal Jing, transformed by the Spleen and Stomach. Blood is composed of Ying (Nutritive) Qi (energy derived from food), Jing, and Fluids (see Volume 3, Chapter 23). The Kidneys also send prenatal Kidney Jing to the Heart to make Blood. Therefore, Jing – particularly postnatal Jing – is vital to the Heart's function of governing Blood.

THE MIDDLE DANTIAN AND QI

Similar to the Lower Dantian, the Middle Dantian is also considered to be a Sea of Qi. The Qi of the Middle Dantian is called Zong Qi. Zong Qi is translated as Ancestral Qi, Gathering Qi or Essential Qi. In English translation, it is sometimes confused with and mistranslated as the Original Qi (Yuan Qi), yet they are not the same. The Zong Qi is a form of Postnatal Qi, whereas the Yuan Qi is housed in the Lower Dantian and is a form of Prenatal Qi. Zong Qi and the Yuan Qi assist each other to maintain the healthy function of the Heart and Lungs.

The Zong Qi nourishes both the Heart and Lungs, controls the speech and the strength of the voice, and interacts with the Kidneys to aid in respiration. According to Traditional Chinese Medicine, the Kidneys assist the Lungs in grasping, holding, and stabilizing the breath during inhalation.

Qi and Blood are closely related. In Chinese medicine, it is often said, "Qi is the commander of Blood; Blood is the mother of Qi." Qi gives the Heart and Blood Vessels the strength to circulate Blood, and Qi gives life to the Blood itself. Blood, on the other hand, houses the Qi and carries it to all the cells in the body. When one loses Blood, one also loses Qi. Therefore, Qi and Blood are considered to be inseparable.

Qi is also inseparable from the mind and spirit. According to the teachings of ancient Tibetan Qigong masters, the channels are (metaphorically speaking) the roads, the Qi is the horse, and the mind is the rider. Through the process of refining the Qi, the mind and spirit are refined and purified. The Middle Dantian is the main focal point for the refinement of Qi into spirit.

In ancient China, the Middle Dantian was considered the primary location for women to focus on during meditation (the men were to focus on their Lower Dantian). The ancient Daoists believed that it was harmful for a woman to focus on her Lower Dantian for extended periods of time, especially during menses. In *The Treatise of Spiritual Alchemy for Women*, the Lower Dantian was considered to be an area for the woman to focus on only in the beginning stages of her practice. After completing the fusion of the Microcosmic and Macrocosmic Orbit meditations, a woman would then focus her attention on the Middle Dantian, located at center of her sternum. As the collected energy in her Middle Dantian overflows, it moves into her breasts, causing her nipples to become erect, and opening "one hundred energy channels within her body."

THE MIDDLE DANTIAN AND SHEN

Classically, the Chinese locate the mind in the Heart. In Chinese, the word for "mind" (Xin) is also the Chinese word for Heart. In Medical Qigong, a distinction is made between the acquired mind (Ren Xin) and the original mind (Yuan Xin).

The Middle Dantian is said to house the Shen, and to control all of the functions of Shen that are attributed to the Yin organs. Thus, the Heart is often referred to as the "Heavenly Emperor."

Throughout the world, people relate the Heart to emotions and feelings. Emotions and feelings are an important aspect of the spirit. All emotions have an effect on the Shen.

The human mind easily falls under the influence of the Po (the Seven Corporeal Souls) that are concerned with survival. When the Po dominate the Heart, their overexaggerated self-concern gives rise to a chronic state of fear, sadness, worry, anger, and defensive arrogance. These negative emotions are sometimes called "the five thieves" because even though negative emotions are necessary aspects of life, chronic states of negative emotions drain the Qi.

The Middle Dantian is the residence of the Middle Hun named Shang Ling or "Pleasant Soul." Shang Ling is situated in the Heart and is considered a soul that is concerned with the wellbeing of others. It is associated with the Five Agents and produces our desire to be involved in social activities and responsibilities.

The redeeming virtue of the Heart is a sense of propriety and discriminating awareness. The Hun (the Three Ethereal Souls) control the smooth flow of Qi throughout the body and are nourished by the Five Virtues of kindness, order, trust, integrity, and wisdom. These Five Virtues give peace and clarity to the Heart and allow the higher qualities of the Yuan Shen to overrule the Po.

An important relationship between the Middle Dantian and Shen is found in the Heart's role of governing the Blood. The ancient classics state that the Shen also resides in the Blood and pervades the body through Blood circulation. This relationship between Blood and Shen is one reason why anemic patients are often restless and suffer from insomnia. Many forms of spiritual unrest can be treated through nourishing the Heart Blood.

According to Dr. Candace Pert's information on neurotransmitters (stated in *Psychoneuro Immunology*), the brain and white blood cells both contain the same neurotransmitters and biochemical constituents that are prerequisites for the existence of consciousness awareness. The same neurotransmitters and biochemical constituents that are linked to consciousness are synthesized and created by the white blood cells. This correspondence indicates that not only do the brain and abdomen have their own consciousness and nervous systems, but the Blood does as well. This further implies that consciousness is possible anywhere in the body, substantiating the ancient Chinese understanding that consciousness is pervasive throughout the body via the Shen, which resides in the Blood.

THE MIDDLE DANTIAN AND EMPATHIC AWARENESS

The Middle Dantian is also considered the "house" of emotional (empathic) feeling, communication, and awareness. Emotional communication is experienced as empathy within the Heart. This empathy is the means by which the Qigong doctor will most frequently become aware of the emotional components of the patient's energetic blocks and imbalances.

Empathic communication is felt as an emotion and originates in the Heart and Middle Dantian area. When Qigong doctors focus on the Middle Dantian area, a line of communication is created with their higher self. We are all born with this ability, but as we grow older we tend to override this type of emotional communication with an exaggerated dependence on the logical mind. Through shock, disappointment, denial, and lack of use, impressions slowly diminish, eventually causing us to lose this natural empathic ability of communication. We generally disconnect from this higher perception as a response to the negative and mixed messages received from our parents and from society. The way to reconnect with the intuitive self is to look inward and become one with the true self that is connected to the divine.

THE MIDDLE DANTIAN AND SCIENCE

According to research conducted by Dr. Paul Pearsall, the history and impressions of the Heart (Middle Dantian) are recorded and stored in every cell of the human body as a sort of informational template of the soul. The Heart can literally perceive and react to the external world on its own.

According to bioscientific measurements, the Heart has five thousand times more electromagnetic power than the brain. It is considered to be the body's primary generator and transmitter of life-force energy, constantly sending out patterns of energetically "encoded" information that regulates the organs, tissues and cells. It beats approximately one hundred thousand times a day and forty million times a year. It propels more than two gallons of Blood per minute and transports about one hundred gallons of Blood per hour throughout the vascular system.

Recent discoveries from research conducted in the new field of neurocardiology (the study of the heart as a neurological, endocrine and immune organ) include the following:

- Neurotransmitters found in the brain have also been identified within the heart.
- Through hormones, neurotransmitters and "quantum energies" (Qi), the heart exerts as

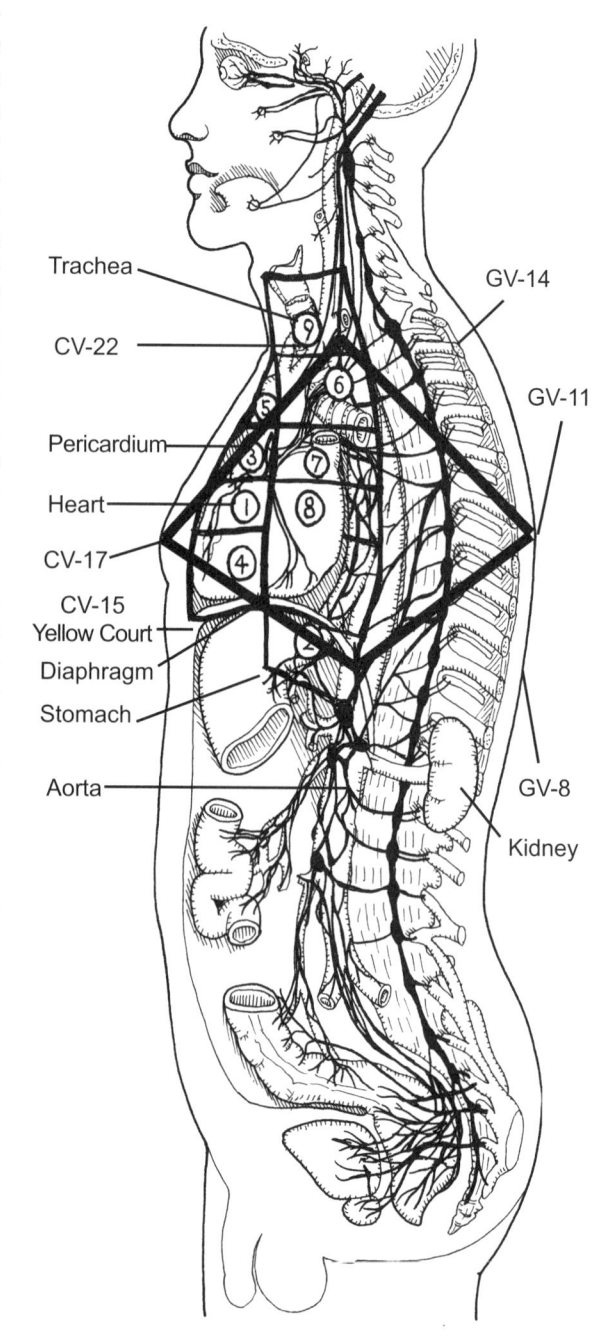

Figure 5.27. The Nine Chambers of the Middle Dantian are identical for men and women.
(Inspired by the original artwork of Dr. Frank H. Netter).

much control over the brain as the brain exerts over the heart.
- The heart requires constant environmental updates from the brain in order to organize the body's bioenergetic fields.
- The heart produces a neurohormone that communicates with the brain and immune system, influencing the thalamus, hypothalamus, pineal, and pituitary glands.

ANATOMICAL LOCATION OF THE MIDDLE DANTIAN

The Middle Dantian, having four points, is shaped like a tetrahedron: the top points toward the Upper Dantian and the Heavens, the bottom points toward the Lower Dantian and the Earth, and the sides point toward the front and back. These areas are described as follows (Figure 5.27):

1. **The Yellow Court (Huangting):** The front lower point of the Middle Dantian is located at the Spirit Storehouse (Shenfu) CV-15 point on the midline of the abdomen, just below the xiphoid bone on the sternum. This point is now commonly called the Turtledove Tail in modern Chinese acupuncture texts. This area is where the Postnatal Qi flows downwards through the Stomach Channels, and the Prenatal Qi flows upwards through the Kidney Channels. They converge with the Thrusting Vessel in order to balance the Fire and Water polarities of the Heart and Kidneys.

   According to the *Ling Shu* (Magical Pivot), this area is the Yuan (source or original) point of all the Yin organs, affecting the Yuan Qi of all five Yin organs. The Yellow Court nourishes the Yin organs, regulates the Heart and calms the spirit (especially in cases of Yin Deficiency). The Yellow Court is the connecting point for the Conception Vessel; it is the Mu point of the sexual organs and is sometimes known as the front gate of the Third Chakra.

   In ancient Daoist alchemy, this point was known as Shenfu, the Spirit Storehouse, and is the place where Qi transforms into Shen. Today this point is commonly called the "Yellow Court" (Huangting) because it reflects the emotions stored from the Heart. In ancient

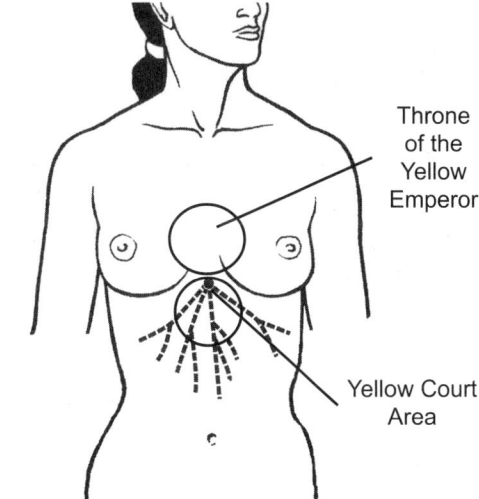

Figure 5.28. The Throne of the Yellow Emperor and Yellow Court Area

Chinese medicine, the Heart was often referred to as the "Yellow Emperor" or "Suspended Gold."

The responsibility of the Pericardium (known as the "Minister of Council", and the "Heart's Protector") was to store emotional experiences that the Heart was not yet ready to process into the emperor's courtyard. These emotions would stay outside the realm of the Heart within the courtyard (known as the "Yellow Court") until the Heart was ready to receive or face the information and experience (Figure 5.28).

Historically, there has been much confusion and disagreement as to the actual location of the Yellow Court. This confusion stems from the understanding that the Yellow Court is also a generalized term referring to the energetic centers of Qi transformation (the Three Dantians). Some Daoist traditions maintain that the Yellow Court and Middle Dantian are located in the same area, being both associated with the Heart. Other traditions assign the Yellow Court to the energetic functions of the Spleen.

In ancient China, the transformation of Qi into Shen occurring in the Yellow Court was considered the pivotal stage in energetic alchemy. The Yellow Court was the location where the emergence of the spiritual embryo (Taixi) takes place. Therefore, the exact location of the Yellow Court was historically kept secret. Because of the overlap of energies existing between the Heart and Spleen, only a true Daoist initiate would be able to clearly differentiate the exact location of the Yellow Court.

Energetically, the Yellow Court is believed to be a microcosmic replica of the Dao of the universe, as Yin and Yang polarities continually emerge from and return to it. According to Chinese alchemy, reuniting the Kan (Yang: Fire) and Li (Yin: Water) of the five Yin organs at the Yellow Court reconnected the individual with the energies of the former (Prenatal) and later (Postnatal) Heavenly Realms. This energetic reversal enabled the individual's Shen to "come and go between the physical and spiritual realms" (Figure 5.29).

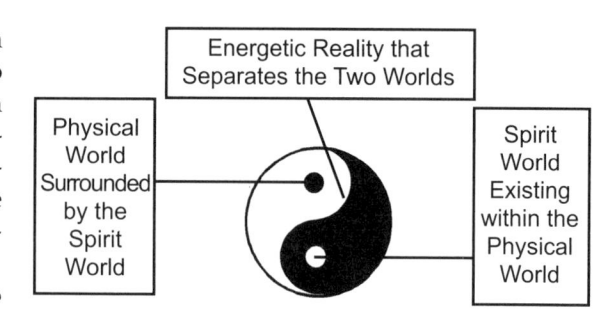

Figure 5.29. In ancient Chinese alchemy, the two circles within the Yin and Yang symbol represented the mysterious existence to the spirit world existing within the physical world, as well as the physical world surrounded by the spirit world. The center dividing line represented the energetic world, considered the bridge that separated the two worlds.

2. **Jinsuo (Sinew Contraction):** The back lower point of the Middle Dantian is located at the Jinsuo GV-8 point. The name of this point, Jinsuo (Sinew Contraction), refers to its relationship to the Liver, and is commonly used to treat Liver Wind and calm the spirit. This area is sometimes known as the back gate of the Third Chakra.

   Crossing the center of the torso, the horizontal axis between the front and back gates of the Yellow Court also intersects with the vertical axis of the great vortex of the Taiji Pole, connecting the energy of Heaven and Earth as it flows through the body.

3. **Shanzhong (Central Altar):** The front center point of the Middle Dantian is located at the Shanzhong CV-17 point on the middle of the sternum at the level of the fourth intercostal space. The name refers to the "place of worship" where the Shen resides. This area is sometimes known as the front gate of the Fourth Chakra.

4. **Shendao (Spirit Path):** The back center point of the Middle Dantian is located two inches up from the shoulder blades at the Shendao GV-11 point located at the hollow between the fifth and sixth thoracic vertebrae. This point's name refers to its use for direct access into the patient's Shen (within the Heart), and is especially used when the front of the Heart is armored. It is also the access point to the individual's moral virtues (associated with the Eternal Soul existing within the Heart) and his or her connection to the Dao (Divine) and De (Virtue). This area is sometimes known as the back gate of the Fourth Chakra.

5. **Tiantu (Heaven's Chimney):** The upper front point of the Middle Dantian is located at the Tiantu CV-22 point, at the base of the throat. The name refers to the cavity at the base of the throat that "pools" escaped Heaven Qi from the Lungs. It is the intersection point of the body's six Yin channels (Liver, Heart, Spleen, Lungs, Pericardium and Kidneys) and Conception Vessel. For this reason, it is considered an influential point in accessing the body's Yin Sea of Qi. This area is sometimes known as the front gate of the Fifth Chakra.

6. **Dazhui (Big Vertebra):** The upper back point is located on the Dazhui GV-14 (Big Vertebra) point on the back. The point's name refers to its location above the relatively large first thoracic vertebra and below the much smaller seventh cervical vertebra. It is the intersection point of the body's six Yang channels (Gall Bladder, Small Intestine, Stomach, Large Intestine, Triple Burners and Urinary Bladder)

and Governing Vessel. Therefore, it is considered an influential point of the body's Yang Sea of Qi. This area is sometimes known as the back gate of the Fifth Chakra.

7. **Middle Dantian Center:** The center of the Middle Dantian is located in the right atrium of the heart, centered between the sinoatrial node (SA node) and the atrioventricular node (AV node). The center of the heart is considered the seat of all emotions.

THE NINE CHAMBERS OF THE MIDDLE DANTIAN

The nine chambers (refer to Figure 5.26) of the Middle Dantian originate around the atria and ventricles of the heart, particularly the pericardial and pleural cavities. The Middle Dantian regulates the body's Heart-Mind connection. The Heart-Mind connection includes both the Shen and the all pervasive consciousness of the entire body. This connection determines the flow of Yuan Qi into the Yin and Yang aspects of both the structure and function of the body, mind and emotions. These functions within the psyche are controlled by the interaction of the body's Prenatal Wu Jing-Shen or Original Five Essence Spirits (Hun, Po, Zhi, Yi, and Shen). The energy of the Middle Dantian is also associated with the transforming and transporting energies of the Spleen and Stomach. The nine chambers of the Middle Dantian are named as follows:
1. The Chamber of Mysterious Elixir
2. The Lower Court of the Heart
3. The Chamber of the Ultimate
4. The Chamber of Splendor
5. The Cover of Heaven
6. The Chamber of Twelve Stories
7. The Chamber of Government
8. The Purple Chamber
9. Heaven's Chimney

TRAINING OF THE MIDDLE DANTIAN

In Medical Qigong training, students are encouraged to focus their mind and breath on the Middle Dantian to regulate the Heart. Techniques are used for treating deficient conditions by drawing Qi into the Heart and Middle Dantian area, and then regulating the body's energetic fields. For treating excess conditions, the students are instructed to lead and purge the Excess Qi from the Heart and Middle Dantian area and release it outward through the body's extremities. The purpose of this training is to release the toxic Excess Qi gathered in the patient's Heart and Yellow Court areas.

Students of Medical Qigong also focus on the Middle Dantian in order to train themselves to release their own psycho-emotional patterns. Only after sufficient development of the Middle Dantian does the Medical Qigong student have the maturity and sensitivity to correctly diagnose the patient's psycho-emotional patterns.

Medical Qigong practitioners strive to gather and balance both the Yin and Yang energy within the Middle Dantian. In ancient China, this union of Yin and Yang energy within the Middle Dantian was called, "The Sun and Moon reflecting on each other in the Yellow Palace." The ancient Chinese Daoist shamans believed that the "spirit of man," who stands as a liaison spirit between Heaven and Earth, always appears in a golden yellow light energy, and resides within the Middle Dantian.

THE UPPER FIELD OF CINNABAR: SHANG DANTIAN

The Upper Dantian collects the Qi of Heaven and represents the spiritual aspect of man and his connection to the divine. The Heaven energy that is transformed in the Upper Dantian has a thin, ethereal, vapor-like quality.

The Upper Dantian is connected to the third field of Wei Qi, circulating several feet outside the body. As the Upper Dantian fills with Qi, spiritual intuition and psychic perception increase.

In Chinese medical physiology, the Brain controls memory, concentration, sight, hearing, touch, and smell. These senses stay in close communication with the Heart and Shen. The Upper Dantian is also considered the house of spiritual (intuitive) communication, awareness, and feelings.

THE UPPER DANTIAN AND JING

The Jing and Qi form the material foundation for the Shen. In Chinese, the term Jing-Shen means mind or consciousness. Jing-Shen may also mean vigor, vitality, or drive. In China, doctors of both Western and Traditional Chinese Medicine use the term Jing-Shen Bing to refer to all types of mental illness. The term Shen is nearly always used with the understanding of the close relationship between the mind and spirit, even in the modern medical context.

The term Prenatal Wu Jing Shen is used in Medical Qigong to describe the body's Original Five Essence Spirits (Hun, Po, Zhi, Yi, and Shen). These five spirits combine the energetic essence of the five Yin organs in order to create the body's innate spiritual consciousness.

The Jing itself is considered the basis for, and ruler of, Marrow, which is defined in Chinese medicine as a substance derived from the Kidneys which nourishes the Brain and spinal cord and also forms the Bone Marrow. The Brain is one of the Six Extraordinary Organs and is called the "Sea of Marrow," as it is considered to be a form of Marrow. The Six Extraordinary Organs are hollow Yang organs that store Yin Jing. Deficiency of Jing may lead to poor concentration, poor memory, dizziness, and absentmindedness. Deficiency of Prenatal Jing is related to mental retardation and attention deficit disorder (ADD) in children.

In some styles of Qigong, the Jing is intentionally conserved and its energy is drawn upwards from the Lower Dantian through the spine to nourish the Brain. Such nourishment benefits the mind and enhances spiritual consciousness.

THE UPPER DANTIAN AND QI

The head is the most Yang aspect of the body since it is the part of the body closest to Heaven. The Qi that operates in the Upper Dantian is, therefore, Yang in nature. The Spleen and Kidneys send the Clear Yang Qi (pure, light, and insubstantial) upwards to the Brain to facilitate mental clarity and activity.

The Upper Dantian is also the place where the individual connects with the Yang Qi of Heaven. Qigong practitioners consciously absorb Heavenly Qi through the upper doorway, Baihui GV-20. Heaven Qi is composed of the Qi from the celestial bodies: the sun, moon, planets, and stars.

The Upper Dantian is located in the center of the Brain, in an area that encompasses the pineal, pituitary, thalamus, and hypothalamus glands.

The pineal gland and hypothalamus have been shown to be extremely sensitive to the influence of light. In his book, *The Body Electric*, Dr. Robert Becker cites experiments with bees and several species of birds that navigate by the light of the sun. In birds, this ability may be due to the fact that they have disproportionately large pineal glands. He also discovered that birds seem to have a backup system of navigation based upon a sensitivity to the electromagnetic fields of the Earth.

Light, electricity, and magnetism are three forms of energy that the Brain is naturally conditioned to automatically recognize, receive, and respond to. Additionally, the Brain also interacts with and generates the energy of light, electricity, and magnetism. These particular forms of energy stimulate the pineal, pituitary, thalamus, and hypothalamus glands, influencing the individual's mental and emotional state. The function and patterning of the Brain is dependent on the interactions of countless energetic structures within fields of light, electricity, and magnetism. Although the Brain is also influenced by heat and sound, it does not use or generate them to the degree that it generates light, electricity, and magnetism.

THE UPPER DANTIAN AND SHEN

We have already discussed the relationship of the Jing and the Shen with the Upper Dantian. Of particular interest to Daoist alchemists is the opening of the center of the Upper Dantian, called the "Crystal Room," as this is where psychic perceptions and intuitive awareness take place. Higher communications, experiences of intense bliss, and perceptions that transcend time and space are associated with the Upper Dantian. These experiences are particularly valuable to Qigong doctors, who are trained to use these heightened perceptions to diagnose illness. The efficacy of intuitive cognition is well documented in the works of C. Norman Shealy and Caroline Myss, who use the term "medical intuitive" to describe this paranormal ability.

The Upper Dantian is also the place where the Eternal Soul connects with the Wuji and with the Dao. The awareness associated with this union is beyond description, as this level of unity surpasses

CHAPTER 5: THE TAIJI POLE AND THE THREE DANTIANS

```
Center Core        →  Purity of Intention
True Self          →  No Hidden Agendas
Eternal Soul       →  Surrender to the Divine Will
                   →  Complete Trust and Faith (Believes and Expects)
                   →  Quiet and Receptive Stillness of Mind
```

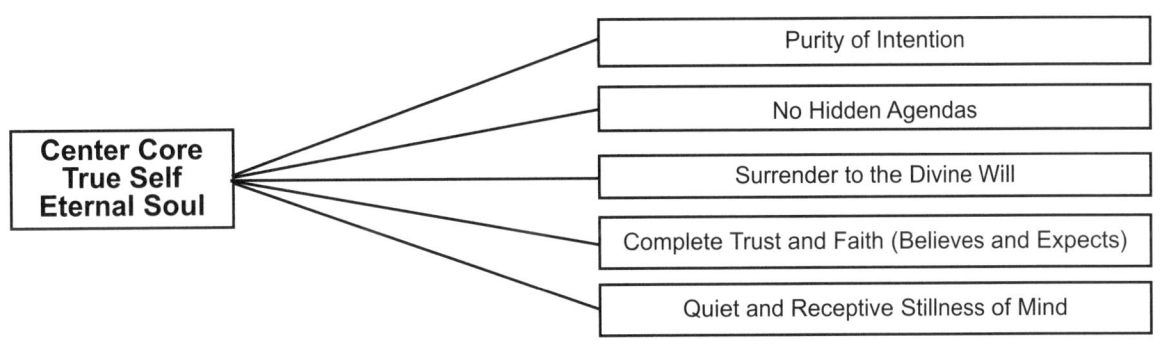

Figure 5.30. The Five Spiritual Principles Required for Open Communication With The Higher Self

conceptual thought and words.

Although the Upper Dantian is responsible for the fruition of intuitive and psychic perceptions, it is necessary to balance the combined energetic properties of all three Dantians in order to establish a reliable foundation for genuine psychic perception. The steam-like quality of the energy within the Upper Dantian fuses with the light that naturally resides within this center. As this combined energy disperses, it travels outward into the Wuji, returning back to the divine. This interaction (of the refined "steam" and the indwelling light) is also responsible for what the Chinese call "receiving the message," which describes the ability of connecting with a patient's subtle energy field to acquire hidden knowledge stored within the tissues.

While in a state of tranquility and inner peace, the Qigong doctor's Upper Dantian intuitively processes information from the environment and universe. This intuitive knowledge provides the Qigong doctor with a greater ability to explore his or her own consciousness, as well as the subtle subconscious patterns of the patient. The ancients called this ability "knowing without knowing."

The Upper Dantian is the residence of the upper Hun named Tai Guang or Eminent Light. This Hun naturally connects with Heaven and strives for physical, mental, emotional, and spiritual purity.

THE UPPER DANTIAN AND INTUITIVE AWARENESS

As the Shen is developed and the Upper Dantian is opened, spiritual communications may reveal themselves in a flash of an image or as a vision in the mind's eye. These images and visions are sometimes very brief and abstract. Correctly interpreting these images takes practice, as the images streaming from the Yuan Shen must be distinguished from the dreamlike wanderings of the subconscious and cannot be interpreted easily by the logical mind.

Qigong doctors must be able to distinguish between true and false messages reflected through their visions. True visions are received from the doctor's divine connection to the Dao or Wuji, while false visions reflect messages from the subconscious. The ability to accurately separate these visions is another example of "knowing without knowing."

Although intuitive communication from within is usually felt as a strong impulse, the Qigong doctor must learn to keep the logical mind from interfering by practicing spiritual meditations. These meditations involve techniques of establishing and strengthening clear links of communication with the higher self. They should be practiced repeatedly until this connection becomes a natural, recurring phenomenon, replacing the otherwise endless drone of the ego and the logical mind. The more one practices stilling the logical mind and circumventing the ego, the easier it becomes to receive a clear communication from the higher self. When the higher self initiates a communication, it does not demand or impose itself.

If an individual consistently ignores these subtle internal communications from the higher self, they often begin to manifest externally in various messages conveyed through people, places and things. These external messages often supercede the individual's own realm of internal intuition.

Five Spiritual Principles

Five spiritual principles must be in place before communication lines between the individual and the higher self become fully open and operational. These five spiritual principles are described as follows (Figure 5.30):

1. The individual must have purity of intention
2. The individual must have no hidden agendas
3. The individual must surrender to the Divine Will
4. The individual must have complete trust and faith in success (believes and expects)
5. The individual must have a quiet and receptive stillness of mind

The lines of communication with the higher self are severed by the logical mind through doubt, fear, and disbelief. Strong faith is required to open this line of communication. Faith requires no logical proof; if proof is needed, then doubts interfere and lead to failure. The logical mind cannot know absolute faith, as genuine faith must come from much deeper within one's true self. Any form of cynicism will lead to the stagnation of spiritual growth, for it strikes at the root of faith itself.

Faith is not something that can be forced. Even after practicing Medical Qigong for many years, Qigong doctors may still have to struggle with their own questions and doubts. Through dedicated practice, however, the seed of faith is firmly established, allowing it to grow and blossom. The opposite of faith is a combination of doubt and fear. Suppression and denial of fear builds and armors the ego, leading to further pain through isolation and confusion. When an individual acknowledges and accepts fear, he or she can overcome any obstacle through faith.

THE UPPER DANTIAN AND SCIENCE

The Upper Dantian, in particular the Brain, may contain more cellular connections than there are stars in the Milky Way constellation. The Brain never truly falls completely asleep, and it is sustained by different levels of subconscious awareness. Energetically, the Brain is constantly active.

It is in a state of perpetual readiness, designed to react, defend, or attack when it senses danger.

ANATOMICAL LOCATION OF THE UPPER DANTIAN

The Upper Dantian is centered in the head, approximately three inches posterior to the Yintang point between the eyebrows. It is shaped like an upright pyramid, facilitating the gathering of energy from Heaven. This pyramidal reservoir houses light. The anatomical locations of the Upper Dantian are described as follows:

1. **Yintang (Hall of Impression):** The front point of the Upper Dantian is the Yintang point. This name refers to the ancient Buddhist tradition of placing a red mark or "seal" over the Bright Hall, or Entrance of the Spirit. The ancient Buddhist tradition maintains that the Third Eye is roughly the size and shape of a large almond. Its left and right lids draw apart simultaneously to illuminate its chamber with spiritual light. The ancient Daoist text, *Huang Ting Jing* (The Yellow Court Classics), written during the Jin Dynasty (265-420 A.D.), refers to this point as "the square inch field of the square foot house." The square foot house refers to the human face, the square inch field refers to the chamber of the Bright Hall. The Yintang point represents wisdom and enlightenment, and is sometimes known as the front gate of the Sixth Chakra, or the Third Eye point.

2. **Fengfu (Wind Palace):** The back point of the Upper Dantian is located below the external occipital protuberance, on the Fengfu GV-16 (Wind Palace) point. This area is also connected with the UB-10 (Heavenly Pillar) points, positioned on either side slightly below the GV-16 point. The energy field connected to this point may be likened to an antenna receiving messages. It allows the Qigong doctor to regulate his or her state of consciousness and thereby tune-in to the various frequencies of consciousness existing within the universe.

The ancient Daoists taught that the two Celestial Pillar points (UB-10) were trance-medium channel points. In certain esoteric schools, these points are considered the main points through which spiritual entities could extend their Qi and Shen into the physical body. This area was therefore commonly used for spirit communication via language (i.e. "channeling").

The GV-16 point is a Sea of Marrow point used to affect the flow of Qi and Blood to the Brain. It is also a "Window of Heaven" point (one of eleven points used for treating Shen disturbances), as well as one of the "Thirteen Ghost Points" (used for treating spirit possession) identified by the famous Daoist physician Sun Simiao. Medical Qigong doctors have observed that individuals with a more prominent occipital protuberance tend to see auras more easily and develop psychic intuition faster. This area is sometimes known as the back gate of the Sixth Chakra.

3. **Baihui (One Hundred Meetings):** The highest point of the Upper Dantian is located on the vertex of the crown, on the Baihui GV-20 point. The name, "Baihui" refers to the ancient understanding that an individual can access and receive divine messages and spiritual intuitions through this point. The esoteric Daoists understand that the Baihui is one of the areas that directs the Heavenly Qi into the Chamber of Mysterious Elixir, located within the third ventricle of the Brain. The Baihui area is sometimes known as the upper gate of the Taiji Pole, or the upper gate of the Seventh Chakra.

It is also said that all of the body's major channels maintain a connecting vessel to the Baihui so that at death the Shen can leave the body through this upper doorway and ascend to the Heavenly realms.

According to legend, Huang Di (the Yellow Emperor), was credited as being the true originator of ancient Shamanistic or Magical Daoism. It is said that the Yellow Emperor would gather and meet with one hundred spirits and ten thousand souls at the "Mingtang" (The Hall of Light), located the ninth chamber of the Upper Dantian, in front of the Celestial Court. In energetic cosmology, the Yellow Emperor is believed to represent the human soul located within the inner chambers of the Heart, within the Middle Dantian.

Four times a year (during the equinoxes and solstices), the one hundred spirits and ten thousand souls would gather together at the meeting place of the Baihui and Sishencong (refer to Figure 5.3), allowing the human soul the ability to communicate with the spirit world at the Mingtang or Hall of Light. This interaction could be initiated in meditation by rolling the eyes upwards and focusing on the Mingtang or Hall of Light Chamber. The joining and crossing of the eyes at the Mingtang area allowed for the convergence of the individual's Hun (Ethereal Soul), Po (Corporeal Soul), and Yuan Shen (Original or Prenatal Spirit) to unite with the spiritual energy of the Dao.

In ancient Daoist alchemy, the energetic influence of the Mingtang was sometimes grouped together with the nose, occiput, throat, Heart, spinal column, and coccyx. These seven areas were known as the "Seven Gates" (Qimen), and were important gateways of energetic and spiritual interaction.

4. **Upper Dantian Center:** The center of the Upper Dantian is located in the pineal gland, which is a small, reddish-gray colored gland attached to the base of the third ventricle of the Brain, in front of the cerebellum. The pineal gland is a mass of nerve matter, containing corpuscles resembling nerve cells and small hard masses of calcareous particles. It is larger in children than in adults and more developed in women than in men. The pineal gland is the organ of telepathic communication, and receives its impressions through the medium of vibrations caused by thoughts projected from other individuals. When an individual thinks, he or she initiates a series of vibrations within the surrounding energy field which is radiated out from his or her body as energetic waves and pulses. Therefore, this area is considered the space where

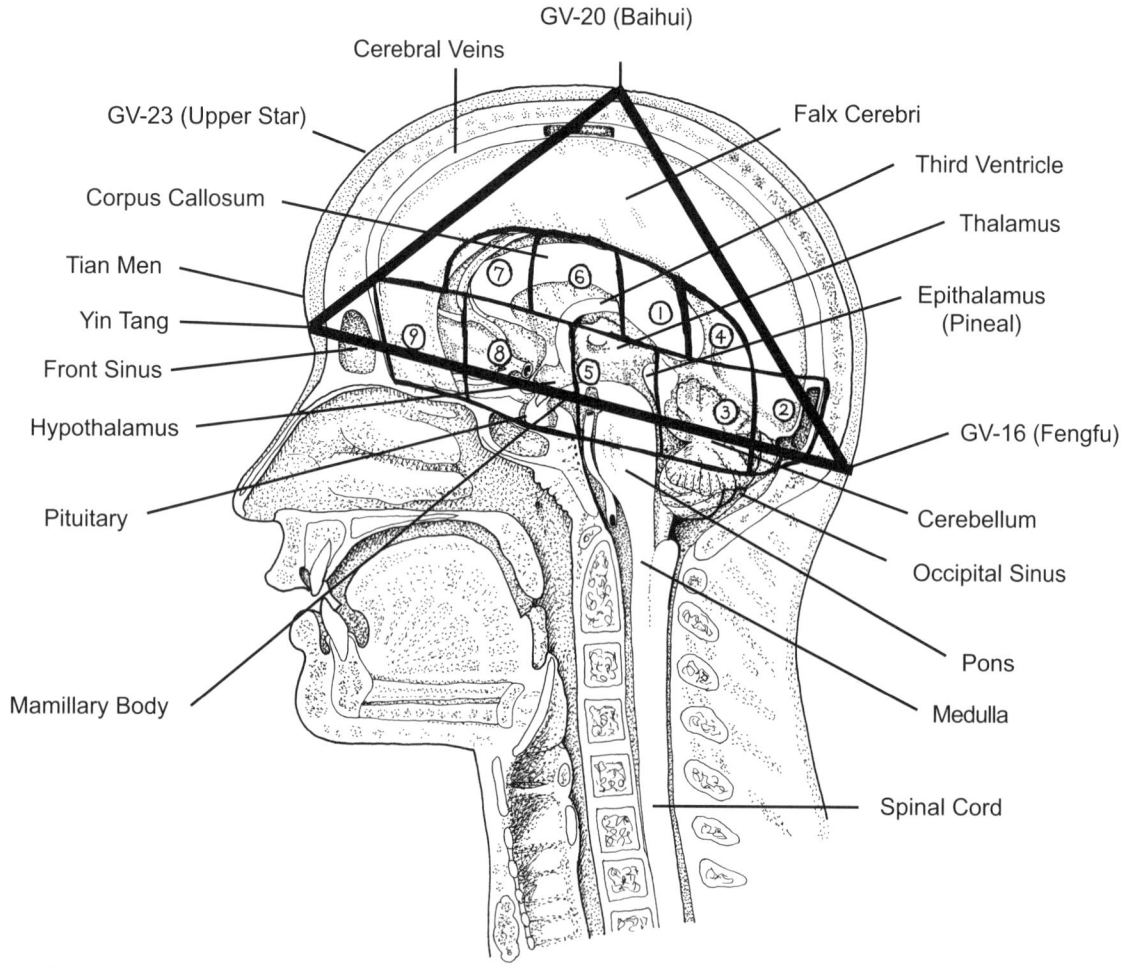

Figure 5.31. The Nine Chambers of the Upper Dantian are portrayed in this drawing. Each number encompasses the entire chamber.

the Shen transcends the limitations of form and merges with the infinite space of the Wuji. From the Wuji, the Shen then progresses towards reuniting with the Dao.

THE NINE CHAMBERS OF THE UPPER DANTIAN

The horizontal cephalic set of nine chambers located within the Upper Dantian corresponds with the structures and location of the different ventricles of the Brain (Figure 5.31). The nine chambers of the Upper Dantian are described as follows:

1. **The Palace of Mysterious Cinnabar (*Xuandan*):** also known as the Chamber of Mysterious Elixir and the Chamber of Mystical Medicine
2. **The Palace of the Jade Emperor (*Yuhuanggong*):** also known as the Original Cavity of the Spirit (*Yuan Shenshi*) and the Ancestral Cavity (*Zuqiao*)
3. **The Palace of Flowing Pearls (*Liuzhugong*):** also known as the Flowing Pearl Deity
4. **The Palace of the Supreme August (*Taihuang*):** also known as the Chamber of Splendor
5. **The Cinnabar Field (*Dantian*):** also known as the Hall of the Upper Dantian, the Upper Medicine Field, and the *Ni Wan* Palace

6. **The Palace of the Ultimate Truth (*Zhizhengong*):** also known as the Palace of the Limitless
7. **The Palace of the Celestial Court (*Tiantinggong*):** also known as the Cover of Heaven and the Heavenly Court Palace
8. **The Palace of the Grotto Chamber (*Dongfang*):** also known as the Profound Chamber and Chamber of Government
9. **The Hall of Light (*Mingtang*):** also known as the Entrance of the Spirit and the Bright Hall

TRAINING OF THE UPPER DANTIAN

In Medical Qigong, the training of the Upper Dantian is used for cultivating spiritual intuition and light. Upper Dantian training exercises are commonly known as Shengong meditations, and are the primary methods used for advancing the doctor's psychic ability (see Volume 2, Chapter 14).

The Qigong doctor may absorb universal and environmental Qi into the Upper Dantian through the Baihui, Yin Tang (Third Eye region), and the Tian Men (located in the center of the forehead) points. The energy is gathered and then directed as healing energy to the patient through either the Yin Tang or Tian Men points. The Shen can both exit and enter the body from the Upper Dantian by way of the Baihui, Yin Tang, or Tian Men (Heavenly Gate) areas.

Medical Qigong practitioners strive to gather and balance Yin and Yang energy within the Upper Dantian. In ancient China, the union of Yin and Yang energy within the Upper Dantian was called "The union of husband and wife in the bedchamber." The ancient Daoist shamans believed that the "primordial breath" (the basic life-giving substance within the body) always appeared as a blue-green light energy, residing as a luminous mist within the Ni-Wan Palace of the Upper Dantian.

In some Daoist traditions, it is said that when an individual's internal cultivation has reached an advanced stage, the inner apertures of the Upper Dantian's nine chambers naturally open. This energetic opening reveals nine small circular spheres revolving around the circumference of a large ball of light. This large ball of light corresponds to the sun and the nine smaller balls of light correspond to the nine planets, like a miniature version of the solar system.

ANCIENT DAOIST MEDITATIONS FOR ENERGIZING THE NINE UPPER DANTIAN CHAMBERS

Throughout all Daoist traditions, meditations that focus on each of the nine chambers of the Upper Dantian are extensively used for bringing about enlightenment. The internal principles attributed to the nine chambers of the Upper Dantian first appeared in the ancient Daoist text, *Sulingjing*, which states that the upper nine chambers (or palaces) can only be inhabited by divine deities (immortals) if the disciple practices internal visualization meditations. These internal visualization meditations actualize the presence of the divine deities, otherwise the nine chambers will remain vacant of divine spiritual power. Each of the divine deities not only inhabits a heavenly palace, but also governs the physical body in relationship to the specific palace that it occupies within the Brain. These nine divine deities are associated with the origin of the world, and are also responsible for the celestial Yin functions of specific internal organs, as well as the stages of development at the time of an individual's birth.

These nine cranial chambers measure one square inch in diameter, and are arranged within the Brain in two levels. Each of the nine chambers intercommunicate with each other, however, the Upper Cinnabar Field (or Ni Wan Chamber) also connects with the throat. The first level extends from the middle of the head between the eyebrows, and terminates at the back of the head, by the external occipital protuberance.

- **The Outer Gate, or *Yin Tang* (Hall of Impression):** The first level includes an outer passage or gate existing between the external world and the Hall of Light (the first inner chamber). The passage outside the Hall of Light is located three-tenths of an inch inside the head, and has a gateway on each side. To the right is the Yellow Portico, which contains a Purple Gate; to the left is the Scarlet Terrace, which contains a Green Chamber. There are two gate guards positioned at the entrance to the Brain cavities. The ancient Daoists believed that each gate contains an immortal that holds a small bell of liquid fire in their hand, which they shake to announce the arrival and departure of spirits (Figure 5.32).

- **Lower Level, First Chamber:** *Ming Tang* **(Hall of Light).** The first chamber is located behind the Outer Gate, and is known as the Hall of Light (Figure 5.33). The ancient Daoists believed that the Hall of Light chamber contains three male immortals that hold a red jade mirror in their mouths, and carry a small bell of red jade on their waist. They exhale red fire which quenches all those who are thirsty, and they illuminate the way when the disciple is spirit travelling during the night. The tinkling of their small bells is heard as far away as the celestial North Star. The sounds of these bells frightens enemies and causes demons and evil spirits to disappear. In order to achieve longevity, the Daoist adept must internally exhale the three immortals' red breath, which then travels throughout the disciple's body, enveloping and transforming his or her tissues into fire. As this internal fire sweeps through the adept's body, it becomes transformed into light, allowing the adept to spiritually and energetically die, and then become reborn again. In ancient China, this meditation was called "The Sun and Moon Purify the Body."
- **Lower Level, Second Chamber:** *Dongfang* **(Grotto Chamber).** The second chamber is located behind the Hall of Light Chamber, and is known as the Grotto Chamber. The ancient Daoists believed that the Grotto Chamber also contains three male immortals, two of which correspond to the Liver (Hun, Ethereal Soul) and Lungs (Po, Corporeal Soul).
- **Lower Level, Third Chamber:** *Dantian* **(Cinnabar Field).** The third chamber is located behind the Grotto Chamber, and is known as the Upper Dantian (or Nei Wan Chamber). The ancient Daoists believed that the Upper Dantian is one of the primary focal points of concentration to meditate on while practicing

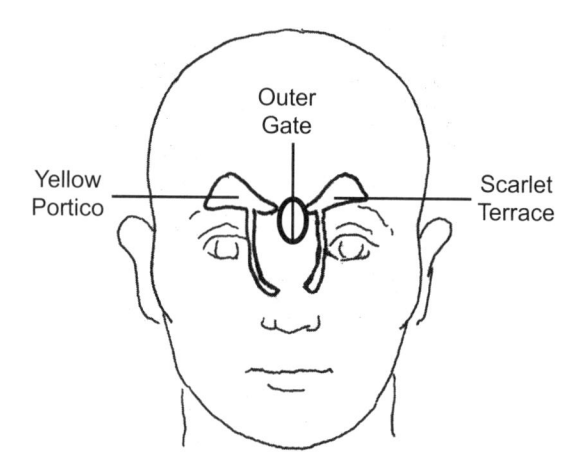

Figure 5.32. The Two Gates to the Inner Passage of the Hall of Lights
(Inspired by the original artwork of Wynn Kapit).

incantations. This is because the Upper Cinnabar Field is also energetically connected to the throat.

- **Lower Level, Fourth Chamber:** *Liuzhugong* **(Palace of Flowing Pearls).** The third chamber is located behind the Upper Dantian Chamber, and is known as the Palace of Flowing Pearls. The ancient Daoists believed that the Palace of Flowing Pearls contains male immortals.

After completing the various meditations on the first four chambers of the Upper Dantian, which are inhabited by masculine (Yang) deities, the Daoist adept then proceeds to practice specific meditations that stimulate the next four chambers of the Upper Dantian, which are inhabited by feminine (Yin) deities.

- **Lower Level, Fifth Chamber:** *Yuhuanggong* **(Palace of the Jade Emperor).** The fifth chamber is located behind the Palace of Flowing Pearls, and is known as the Palace of the Jade Emperor. It is the last chamber on the first level of the nine chambers of the Upper Dantian. The ancient Daoists believed that the Palace of the Jade Emperor is inhabited by the Holy Mother of the Jade Purity of Heaven.
- **Upper Level, First Chamber:** *Tiantinggong* **(Palace of the Celestial Court).** Located above

the Hall of Light, one inch above the eyebrows and two inches deep into the Brain, is the Palace of the Celestial Court. The ancient Daoists believed that the Palace of the Celestial Court is inhabited by the True Mother of the Great Purity of Heaven.

- **Upper Level, Second Chamber:** *Zhizhengong* **(Palace of Ultimate Truth).** Located behind the Palace of the Celestial Court, on the upper level, is the Palace of Ultimate Truth. The ancient Daoists believe that the Palace of Ultimate Truth is inhabited by the Imperial Concubine of the celestial North Star (Taiji Pole).
- **Upper Level, Fourth Chamber:** *Taihuang* **(Palace of Supreme August One).** Located behind the Palace of Mysterious Cinnabar, on the upper level, is the Palace of Supreme August. The ancient Daoists believe that the Palace of Supreme August is inhabited by the Imperial Empress on High.

Only after the meditation on the first four masculine deities (attributed to the Yang Trigrams of the Yi-Jing) should the Daoist adept attempt the meditate on the four feminine deities (attributed to the Yin Trigrams of the Yi-Jing). The combination of four masculine and four feminine deities spiritually establishes the energetic formation of the Prenatal Bagua, responsible for creation.

After meditation on the four feminine deities has been completed, only then should the adept attempt to meditate on the final chamber, the Palace of Mysterious Cinnabar, which contains the True Lord of the Supreme One.

- **Upper Level, Third Chamber:** *Xuandan* **(Palace of Mysterious Cinnabar).** Located behind the Palace of Ultimate Truth, on the upper level, is the Palace of Ultimate Truth. The ancient Daoists believed that the Palace of Mysterious Cinnabar is inhabited by the True Lord of the Supreme One.

THE ENERGETIC FUNCTIONS OF THE THREE DANTIANS

The primary functions of the Three Dantians is to gather, store, and transform life-force energy. The energy reservoirs of the Three Dantians are linked externally through the Governing and Conception Vessels and internally through the Thrusting Vessels and the Taiji Pole.

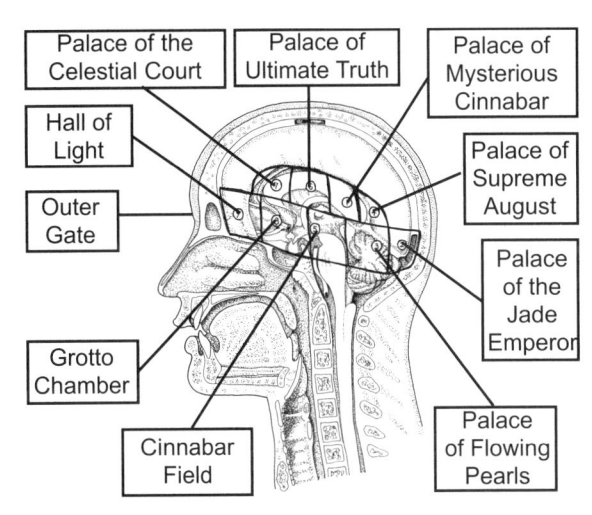

Figure 5.33. The Nine Chambers of the Upper Dantian

The center of each Dantian is penetrated by and attached to the Taiji Pole, which extends from the Baihui point at the top of the head to the Huiyin point at the perineum. The anatomical location of each of the Dantians corresponds to a physiological center for heat, light, magnetic and electrical vibration. The intensity and charge of this vibration is dependent on the individual's mental intention, posture, and respiration.

Qi moves into the body's Dantians through the body's Taiji Pole. The energy is then absorbed into the body's major organs and surrounding tissues as it flows through the Dantians and into the body's internal and external channels and collaterals. Energy is also absorbed from the external environment through the channels, tissues and organs, flowing into the Three Dantians and ultimately into the Taiji Pole.

Each Dantian acts like a reservoir, collecting energy and redistributing it into all of the internal organs. This energy projects through the surface of the body into the Wei Qi field. The same energy is also projected throughout the physical body, flowing through the energy channels, the nervous system and the endocrine glands, and

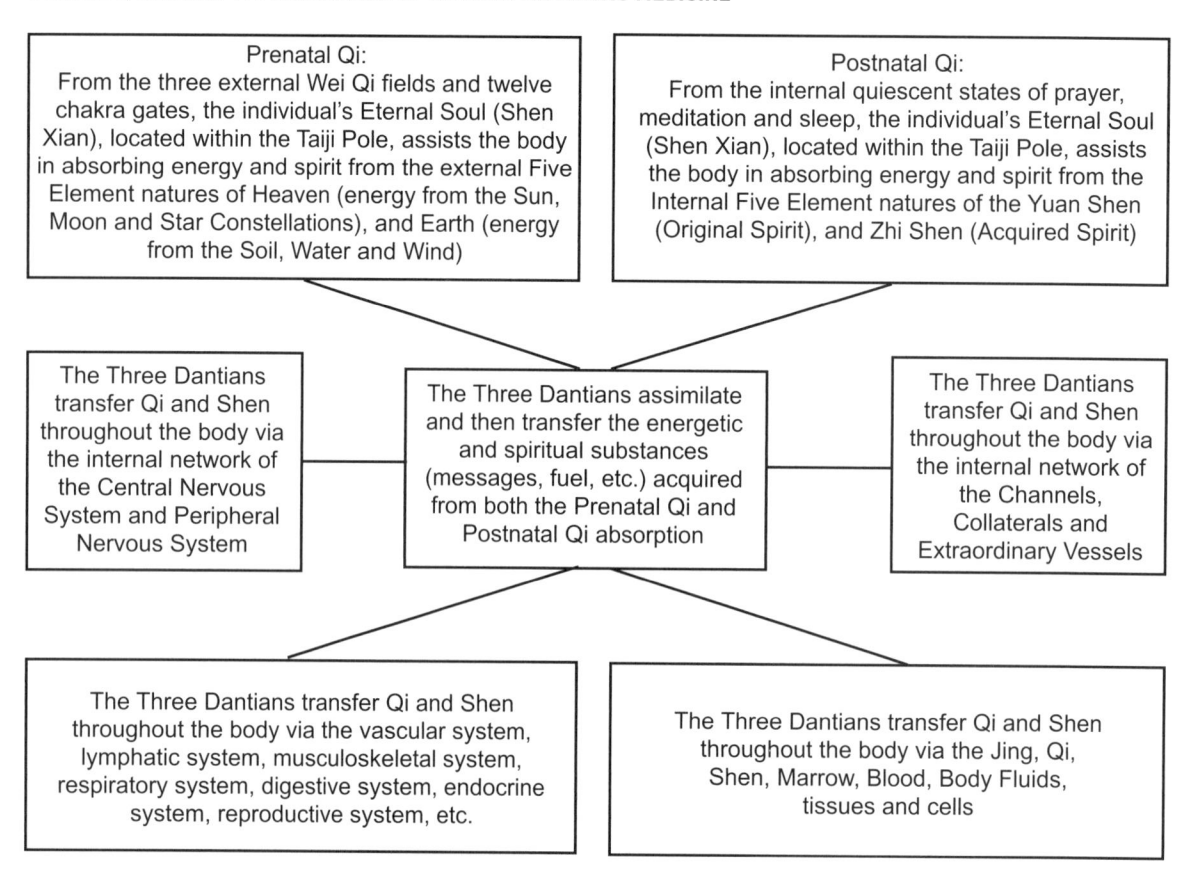

Figure 5.34. Qi Dispersion From the Center Taiji Pole Through the Dantians and into the Body

Prenatal Qi:
From the three external Wei Qi fields and twelve chakra gates, the individual's Eternal Soul (Shen Xian), located within the Taiji Pole, assists the body in absorbing energy and spirit from the external Five Element natures of Heaven (energy from the Sun, Moon and Star Constellations), and Earth (energy from the Soil, Water and Wind)

Postnatal Qi:
From the internal quiescent states of prayer, meditation and sleep, the individual's Eternal Soul (Shen Xian), located within the Taiji Pole, assists the body in absorbing energy and spirit from the Internal Five Element natures of the Yuan Shen (Original Spirit), and Zhi Shen (Acquired Spirit)

The Three Dantians assimilate and then transfer the energetic and spiritual substances (messages, fuel, etc.) acquired from both the Prenatal Qi and Postnatal Qi absorption

The Three Dantians transfer Qi and Shen throughout the body via the internal network of the Central Nervous System and Peripheral Nervous System

The Three Dantians transfer Qi and Shen throughout the body via the internal network of the Channels, Collaterals and Extraordinary Vessels

The Three Dantians transfer Qi and Shen throughout the body via the vascular system, lymphatic system, musculoskeletal system, respiratory system, digestive system, endocrine system, reproductive system, etc.

The Three Dantians transfer Qi and Shen throughout the body via the Jing, Qi, Shen, Marrow, Blood, Body Fluids, tissues and cells

---

then saturating the Blood to nourish the whole body (Figure 5.34).

This energy transformation can be visualized as follows: Qi flows into the body like rainwater flowing into a pond (the body absorbing and collecting Qi into the Dantians). The rainwater is then absorbed into the surrounding soil, foliage, and root systems (skin, tissues, and cells) before it gathers, collects, and pools into deep artesian wells (the Dantians). Pressure begins to build up as these artesian wells fill with the rainwater and eventually overflow, pouring into smaller pools (the organs) before combining with the rushing flow of underground streams (the channels).

Another popular analogy is to consider the Dantians as batteries, the body's Taiji Pole as a magnetic bar connecting the batteries together, the channels as the wires, and the Wei Qi fields as the electromagnetic fields manifesting from the energy contained within the structure.

Mental and emotional awareness of a specific tissue area can be heightened through increasing the flow of energy to that location. When energy fills the tissues, a cellular reaction causes the tissues to either store or release emotions, depending on the body's excess or deficient Qi.

If, by focused intention, Qi is increased in the Lower Dantian, the result is a heightened feeling of power and stability. If, by focused intention, Qi is increased in the Middle Dantian, the result is a heightened feeling of emotional awareness. If, by focused intention, Qi is increased in the Upper Dantian, a heightened spiritual awareness and sense of connection to the divine occurs. The health of the individual, and the strength of his or her energetic fields depends on the amount of energy present in the Three Dantians (Figure 5.35).

THE DANTIAN'S YIN AND YANG ENERGETIC CHAMBERS

Each of the Three Dantians can be divided into Yin and Yang energetic chambers. The Yang chambers relate to each Dantian's upper chambers and the spiritual aspects of the Hun. The Yin chambers relate to each Dantian's lower chambers and the carnal aspects of the Po. The chambers and their energetic potential are described as follows:

THE LOWER DANTIAN

1. **The Yang Energetic Chamber of the Lower Dantian** corresponds anatomically to the upper quadrant of the abdomen, located within the area of the small intestine in men and the Uterus in women. When influenced by the Hun, quiescence and serenity are enhanced.
2. **The Yin Energetic Chamber of the Lower Dantian** corresponds anatomically to the lower quadrant of the abdomen, which includes the reproductive organs, the urinary bladder, urethra, and anus. This chamber is responsible for reproduction and sexuality. When influenced by the body's Po, raw physical power and sexual vitality is aroused.

THE MIDDLE DANTIAN

1. **The Yang Energetic Chamber of the Middle Dantian** corresponds anatomically to the upper quadrant of the heart, which includes the left and right atrium, the upper portions of the left and right ventricles, and the atrioventricular node. This chamber is responsible for the spiritual attitudes and virtues associated with the Hun. The Hun are responsible for:
   - gathering and transmitting divine inspirations and spiritual insights
   - giving and receiving unconditional love
   - motivating spiritual growth through prayer, devotion, and commitment
2. **The Yin Energetic Chamber of the Middle Dantian** corresponds anatomically to the lower quadrant of the heart, which includes the left and right ventricles. This chamber is

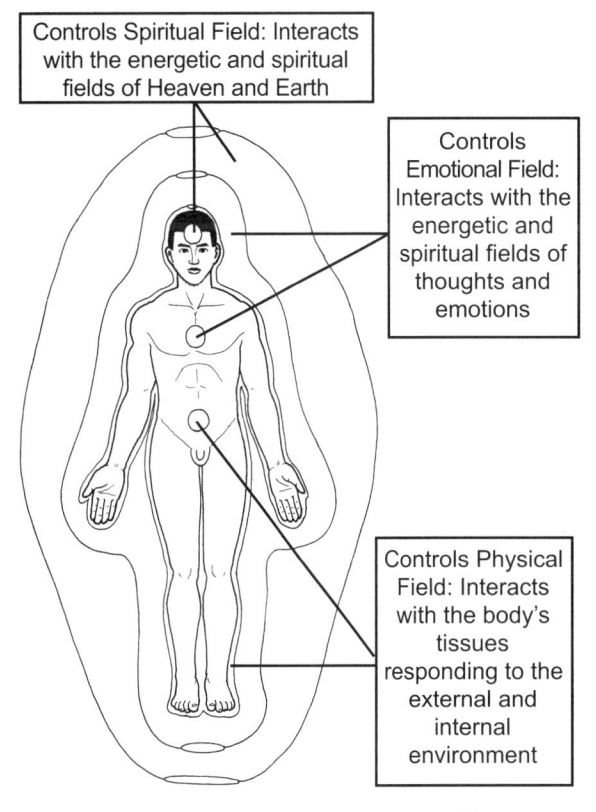

Figure 5.35. The Three Dantians and Their Relationship to the Three External Wei Qi Fields

responsible for sensual passions, conquests, and conditional love. It is associated with actions that are based on hidden agendas. These emotions are related to the Po's influence. The influence of both the Po and the Yin energetic chamber of the Upper Dantian activates, energizes, and enhances:
- biological drives (for food and self preservation)
- sexuality, lust, and desire
- sensuality

THE UPPER DANTIAN

1. **The Yang Energetic Chamber of the Upper Dantian** corresponds anatomically to the upper quadrant of the Brain, often referred to as the third ventricle or the higher Brain centers. When stimulated, the higher Brain centers manifest spiritual intuition and divine insight related to the influence of the Hun. Such insight

is responsible for spiritual growth and maturation. Activation of these higher Brain centers eventually leads to the emergence of extrasensory perceptions (ESP), such as clairvoyance, clairaudience, telepathy, psychokinesis, and eventually to spiritual enlightenment.

2. **The Yin Energetic Chamber of the Upper Dantian** corresponds anatomically to the lower quadrant of the Brain, often referred to as the "reptilian" brain. When stimulated, the reptilian brain activates the thalamus, hypothalamus, cerebellum, and cortex, which awakens the body's intuition, as well as our animalistic and primitive survival instincts. When the Yin energetic chamber dominates, the sensory, animalistic nature of the Po emerges in full force. This phenomenon sometimes occurs when coma patients begin to recover. As energy begins to fill the lower chambers of the Three Dantians, their initial reactions are basic and carnal in nature, i.e., to either engage in sexual activity or strike out in violence. As the Qi begins to fill the upper chambers of the Three Dantians, the energy balances in the patient's Taiji Pole, and the patients' impulses return back to normal.

THE DOCTOR'S PROJECTED AURA FIELDS AND THE THREE DANTIANS

In China, Qigong doctors are tested and categorized according to the predominant color of their Qi emissions. The healing color will depend upon which of the three Dantians is dominant (corresponding to either the Lower Dantian, Middle Dantian, or Upper Dantian), as well as the energetic strength and potential of the doctor being tested. The emitted color is observed in the visible-light spectrum projected from the Qigong doctor's hands (Figure 5.36).

RED EMITTED COLOR

Qigong doctors who have adequately trained their body and mind will emit a red radiant glow around their external energy field. The Qi will overflow from the Lower Dantian area, and the color red will dominate the aura. This is actually a normal aura color observed in most beginning

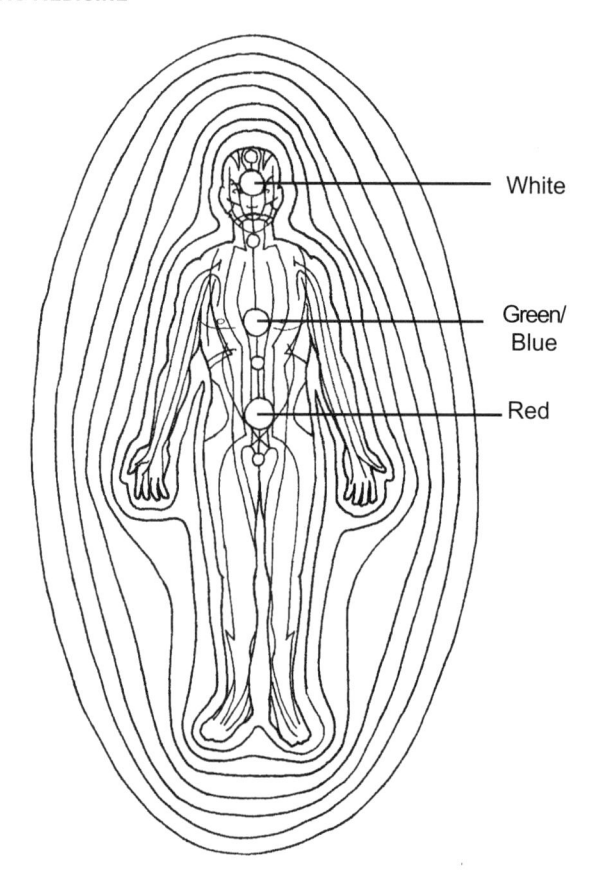

Figure 5.36. The Three Dantians and Their Relationship to the Three External Wei Qi Fields

Qigong doctors, indicating that the energy field is still too weak to treat serious diseases.

GREEN/BLUE EMITTED COLOR

Qigong doctors who have further refined their energy will emit a blue radiant glow around their energy field. These doctors' Qi will also overflow from the Middle Dantian area, and the color blue will dominate the aura. This aura color is observed in advanced Qigong doctors.

WHITE EMITTED COLOR

Energy emitted directly from the divine is generally white. This Qi emission is different from the indigo radiant glow and is a sign of divine intervention in the healing process. The color of this aura is considered the strongest and most powerful.

CHAPTER 5: THE TAIJI POLE AND THE THREE DANTIANS

The small cranial sutures ebb and flow within the rhythms of the energetic pulsation of the Upper Dantian

The bones of the sternum compress and release in conjunction with the rhythmic actions of the ribs, costal cartilage, and the intervertebral discs located between the thoracic vertebrae

The mobile symphysis pubis compresses and releases in conjunction with the rhythmic action of the sacrum and coccygeal bones

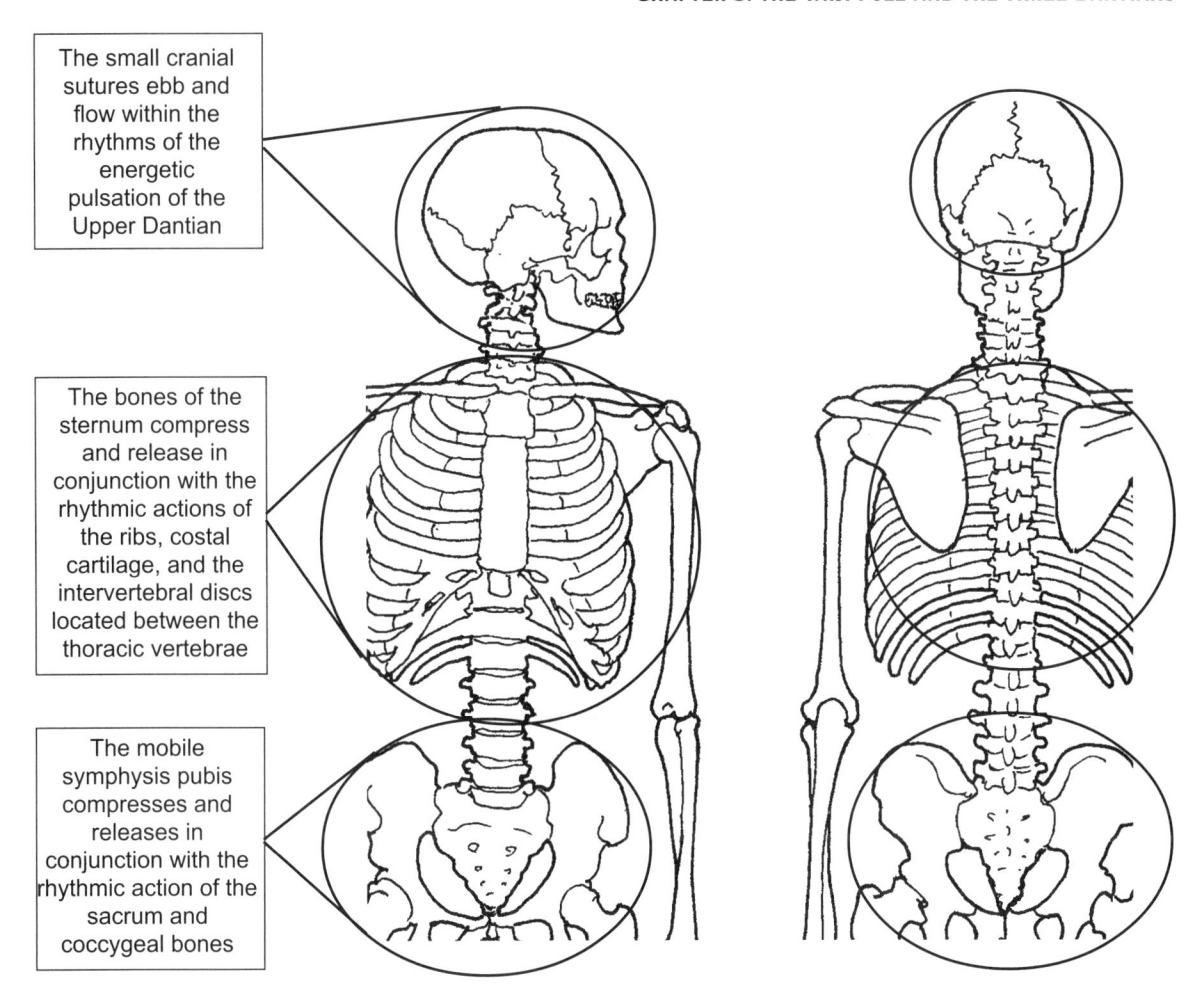

Figure 5.37. The Three Dantians and Their Relationship to the Movable Structure of the Bones

Instances of divine intervention can occur in any stage of the doctor's energetic development and are a testimony to the healing power and love of the divine.

Although every Qigong doctor uses a combination of all Three Dantians when projecting Qi into patients, the color of the aura surrounding the doctor's body reflects which Dantian's reservoir is predominantly used. Through time, patience, and much practice, the Qigong doctor will be able to transform from a red to a yellow, purple, blue, and eventually to a white-light healer.

THE MOVEABLE BONES OF THE THREE DANTIANS

When studying the specific anatomical locations of the Three Dantians, one can observe the structural interactions of the moveable Bones in relationship to the Dantian's energetic fields. As each Dantian energetically pulses, the surrounding tissues expand and contract with the rising (Yang) and the falling (Yin) rhythm of life. This ebb and flow of the human tissues moves in response to the energetic rhythm radiating from the body's center core. All life is sustained by this rhythmic function (Figure 5.37).

THE LOWER DANTIAN AND SACRAL RHYTHM

As the energy of Lower Dantian energetically pulses, the mobile joint of the symphysis pubis (interpubic joint) compresses and releases in conjunction with the rhythmic action of the sacrum and coccygeal Bones. This sacral rhythm initiates an energetic pulse that ripples up the spine, also stimulating the vibrational resonances within the Middle Dantian and Upper Dantians.

THE MIDDLE DANTIAN AND THORACIC RHYTHM

As the energy of Middle Dantian energetically pulses, the manubrium, the sternum body, and the xiphoid bone compress and release in conjunction with the rhythmic action initiated by the ribs and costal cartilage, and the intervertebral discs located between the thoracic vertebrae. This thoracic rhythm initiates an energetic pulse that ripples through the spine, also stimulating the vibrational resonances within the Lower Dantian and Upper Dantians.

THE UPPER DANTIAN AND CRANIAL RHYTHM

As the energy of Upper Dantian energetically pulses, the small sutures of the frontal, sphenoid, parietal, temporal, and occipital bones compress and release in conjunction with the rhythmic action initiated by the cerebral spinal fluid, and the dynamic action of the falx cerebri and tentorium cerebelli. This cranial rhythm initiates an energetic pulse that ripples through the spine, also stimulating the vibrational resonance within the Middle Dantian and Lower Dantians.

Chapter 6
The Eight Extraordinary Vessels

The Eight Extraordinary Vessels

In the Traditional Chinese Medicine colleges in China, when students of Medical Qigong are introduced to energetic anatomy and physiology, they focus their studies on the energy extending from the body's Taiji Pole, the Three Dantians, Eight Extraordinary Vessels, and Six Extraordinary Organs. These energy systems feed all of the vital organs, as well as the body's Twelve Primary Channels.

The Eight Extraordinary Vessels (Qi Jing Ba Mai) are the first vessels to form in the developing fetus and are also called the Eight Ancestral Channels, Eight Prenatal Channels, Eight Preheaven Channels, or Eight Psychic Channels. The ideograph depicting the Chinese characters for "Qi Jin Ba Mai" are described as follows (Figure 6.1):

- The first character is the Chinese ideograph "Qi," which is generally translated as "extraordinary," but can also be translated as surprising, strange, or marvellous. It is composed of three characters. Positioned on the top is a character "Da," meaning big or great; positioned on the bottom-right is a character "Ren" depicting a person; and positioned on the bottom-left is a character "Kuo," meaning mouth. As a whole, the ideograph depicts the actions of a startled person, having discovered something strange yet wonderful, falling backwards with their mouth open, with the expression of surprise

- The second character is the Chinese ideograph "Jing," which is generally translated as "channel," but can also be translated as meridian, to pass through, and the wrapping of a silk fiber or net. The word Jing carries a multitude of meanings, all of which are reflected within the many components of the character. Positioned to the left is the radical "Mi," used for silk, net or string-like objects. It depict threads that have

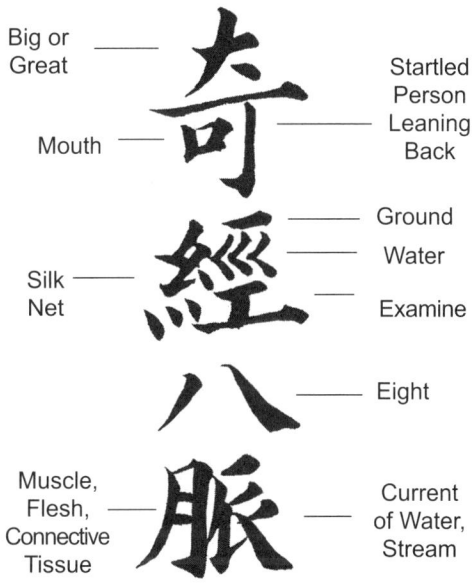

Figure 6.1. The Chinese Ideograph for "Qi Jing Ba Mai," the Eight Extraordinary Vessels

been twisted together to form a net, and refers to a silk rope that is tied around something, pulling and securing it, or the wrapping and enveloping of a silk net. Positioned on the top right portion of the character is the phonetic "Jing," which is sometimes used to denote the flow of underground water (the horizontal line on top represents the ground, while the three curved lines beneath it represent the flow of water). Positioned to the bottom-right is a modification of the ancient radical "Ting," meaning to examine the underground veins. As a whole, this ideograph describes the deep aquatic passageways or subterranean rivers (channels) which energetically knit together the internal fabric of the human body.

- The third character is the Chinese ideograph "Ba," which is generally translated as the

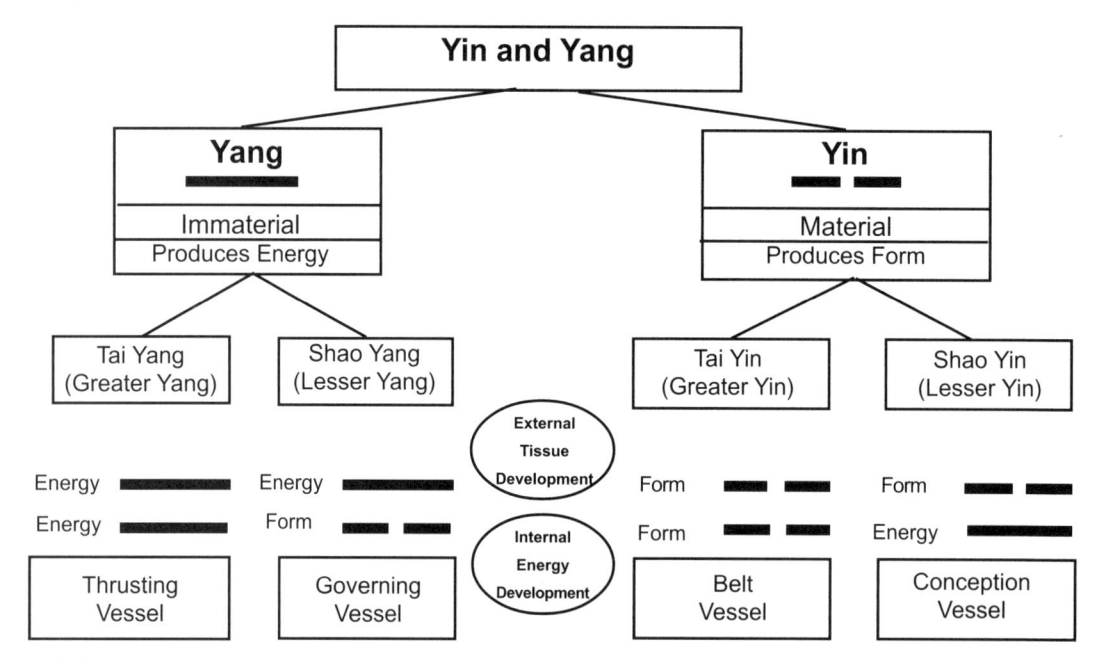

```
                        Yin and Yang
                       /            \
                   Yang              Yin
                   ▬▬▬               ▬ ▬
               Immaterial          Material
             Produces Energy    Produces Form
              /        \          /        \
        Tai Yang    Shao Yang   Tai Yin    Shao Yin
      (Greater Yang)(Lesser Yang)(Greater Yin)(Lesser Yin)
                       External
                        Tissue
  Energy ▬▬  Energy ▬▬ Development  Form ▬ ▬   Form ▬ ▬
  Energy ▬▬  Form   ▬ ▬ Internal    Form ▬ ▬   Energy ▬▬
                        Energy
                      Development
   Thrusting    Governing          Belt       Conception
    Vessel       Vessel           Vessel        Vessel
```

Figure 6.2. The Ancient Daoist Concept of Yin and Yang Expressing the Four Phases of Universal Energy and Manifesting Through the Four Foundational Vessels.

number "eight." The number eight is significant in many areas of ancient Chinese thought, such as the Eight Directions of the Prenatal (Heavenly) Trigrams, the Eight Directions of the Postnatal (Earthly) Trigrams, the Eight Directions of the Wind, Heaven and Earth (N, NE, E, SE, S, SW, W, NW), the Eight Directions of Perception (front, back, left, right, above, below, inside and outside the body), and the Eight Extraordinary Vessels.

- The fourth character is the Chinese ideograph "Mai," which is generally translated as "vessel." It is composed of two characters: the character to the left, "Ji" depicts the Chinese ideogram for body tissue, muscle or flesh (all of which are forms of connective tissue); the character on the right "Mai" depicts a current of water, stream, or branch of a river. As a whole, the character can be translated as arteries, veins or pulse, depicting a form of energetic circulation.

The Eight Extraordinary Vessels are given their names because they differ in energetic function from the Twelve Primary Channels. These eight vessels have an extraordinary ability to regulate the deeper energetic reservoirs of the body. These vessels represent the merging of the mother's and father's energy and the linking of the body's prenatal and postnatal energies. They interconnect all of the Twelve Primary Channels and circulate the Jing Qi (essence energy) throughout the body.

ENERGETIC EMBRYOLOGY

The energetic expansion and contraction of the Eight Extraordinary Vessels affects the creation and development of the baby's tissues up until the time of birth. In energetic embryology (see Chapter 2), the Eight Extraordinary Vessels can be subdivided into two groups: The Four Foundational Vessels and the Eight Secondary Formational Vessels, are described as follows:

- **The Four Foundational Vessels:** Comprised of the Thrusting Vessel, Governing Vessel, Conception Vessel and Belt Vessel, these four vessels are believed to be responsible for the first cellular divisions. The Thrusting Vessel is the oldest of these channels, having originated with the formation of the Taiji Pole when the father's sperm entered the mother's egg. The ancient Chinese believed that the Thrusting Vessel was

CHAPTER 6: THE EIGHT EXTRAORDINARY VESSELS

```
Thrusting Vessel ──── Left Yin Linking Vessels
                  ──── Right Yin Linking Vessels

Governing Vessel ──── Left Yang Heel Vessels
                  ──── Right Yang Heel Vessels

Belt Vessel      ──── Left Yang Linking Vessels
                  ──── Right Yang Linking Vessels

Conception Vessel ──── Left Yin Heel Vessels
                   ──── Right Yin Heel Vessels
```

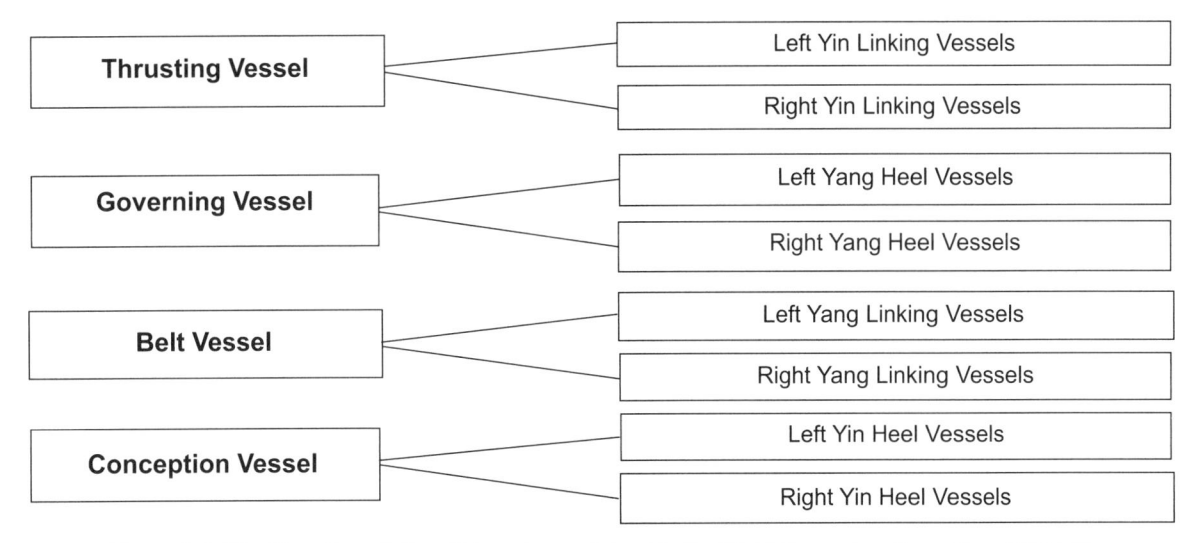

Figure 6.3. The Four Foundational Vessels are Joined to the Eight Secondary Formational Vessels

the original "root," allowing the other "branches" to spring forth (Figure 6.2).

- **The Eight Secondary Formational Vessels:** Comprised of the left and right Yin Linking Vessels, the left and right Yang Linking Vessels, the left and right Yin Heel Vessels and the left and right Yang Heel Vessels, these eight vessels are believed to be responsible for completing the energetic and physical structure of the fetus.

In Traditional Chinese Medicine, it is taught that the eight secondary formational vessels are joined to the four foundational vessels in the following manner (Figure 6.3):

- The Left and Right Yin Linking Vessels are coupled with the Thrusting Vessel
- The Left and Right Yang Linking Vessels are coupled with the Belt Vessel
- The Left and Right Yin Heel Vessels are coupled with the Conception Vessel
- The Left and Right Yang Heel Vessels are coupled with the Governing Vessel

The Thrusting Vessel, Belt Vessel, Yin Linking Vessels and Yang Linking Vessels are responsible for the organization of the internal embryonic tissues; whereas the Conception Vessel, Governing Vessel, Yin Heel Vessels and Yang Heel Vessels are responsible for both the internal embryonic tissues and the external energy formations.

THE THREE-DIMENSIONAL SPACE OF THE IMPREGNATED EGG

In energetic embryology, the three-dimensional space of the impregnated egg is viewed as an object with eight different surfaces along four axes. Each of the Eight Extraordinary Vessels corresponds with one of the following directions, described as follows: (Figure 6.4):

- Anterior/Posterior: Governing and Conception Vessels
- Superior/Inferior: Yin and Yang Linking Vessels
- Right/Left: Yin and Yang Heel Vessels
- Interior/Exterior: Thrusting and Belt Vessels

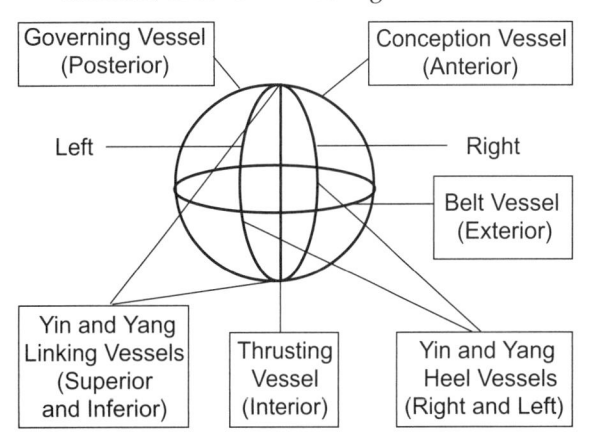

```
Governing Vessel (Posterior)     Conception Vessel (Anterior)
                      \         /
          Left ────────( sphere )──────── Right
                      /         \
                                  Belt Vessel (Exterior)

Yin and Yang            Thrusting        Yin and Yang
Linking Vessels         Vessel           Heel Vessels
(Superior               (Interior)       (Right and Left)
and Inferior)
```

Figure 6.4. A Model of the Flow of the Eight Extraordinary Vessels in Energetic Embryology

241

THE FUNCTION OF THE EIGHT EXTRAORDINARY VESSELS

The Eight Extraordinary Vessels have neither a direct connection nor a clear internal and external relationship with the internal organs. Similar to the Three Dantians' function of distributing the body's energy, these Eight Extraordinary Vessels are reservoirs that regulate the distribution and circulation of Jing and Qi inside the body. When these reservoirs become full, the energy overflows into the center channel or Taiji Pole. This stimulation of the Taiji Pole expands consciousness and increases perception and intuition. These vessels are the foundation of the body's energy, bridging the Yuan Qi (Original Prenatal Energy) with the body's postnatal energy.

The Eight Extraordinary Vessels have six main functions: They serve as reservoirs of Qi, store and circulate Jing Qi, circulate the Wei Qi, regulate the body's life cycles, integrate the six primary Yang organs with the six Extraordinary Organs and the Kidneys, and integrate the Four Seas with the body's internal energy flow. These functions are described as follows (Figure 6.5):

1. **Serve as Reservoirs of Qi:** The Eight Extraordinary Vessels criss-cross the body and weave together the Twelve Primary Channels, strengthening the energetic structure of the Twelve Primary Channels and regulating the flow of Qi and Blood within them. If the Qi and Blood of the Twelve Primary Channels becomes excessive, the overflow is absorbed into the Eight Extraordinary Vessels. The Eight Extraordinary Vessels act as Qi reservoirs receiving, storing and distributing the Excess Qi, thus regulating the body's overall energy flow. If the Qi flow of the Twelve Primary Channels becomes deficient, energy can be drawn from the reservoirs of energy stored within the Eight Extraordinary Vessels. In this way, the Eight Extraordinary Vessels maintain internal and external harmony by continually regulating and balancing the body's energy flow.

2. **Store and Circulate Jing Qi:** The Eight Extraordinary Vessels draw their energy from the Kidneys and are responsible for storing and circulating the body's Jing Qi throughout the tissues, particularly to the skin, hair, and the Six Extraordinary (Curious) Organs. The Six Extraordinary Organs are the Brain, Bone, Marrow, Blood Vessels, Gall Bladder and Uterus, also known as the Six Ancestral Organs.

3. **Circulate the Wei Qi:** The Eight Extraordinary Vessels aid in circulating the Wei (Protective) Qi, helping to protect the body against the invasion of external pathogens. The Governing, Conception, and Thrusting Vessels are primarily responsible for circulating the body's Wei Qi over the thorax, abdomen, and back.

    The Eight Extraordinary Vessels provide the link between the Kidney Jing and the Wei Qi. Although the Wei Qi is circulated by the Lungs, it has its root in the Kidneys. Thus the Kidneys play an important role in supporting the Lungs' function of circulating the body's Wei Qi. Due to the Kidneys function in supporting the Wei Qi field, the immune system can also become vulnerable to pathogenic factors, as well as allergies, and asthma. This energetic reaction demonstrates why the Kidneys are always at the root of latent Heat syndromes (chronic fatigue) caused by Kidney Deficiency.

4. **Regulate the Body's Life Cycles:** In the first chapter of *the Yellow Emperor's Classic of Internal Medicine*, it is stated that the life changes of women (every seven years) and men (every eight years) are governed by the Conception and Thrusting Vessels. The rhythms and cycles of life are related to the body's Jing and are thus greatly influenced by the Eight Extraordinary Vessels' role in moving and circulating the body's Jing (see Volume 2, Chapter 13).

5. **Integrate the Six Extraordinary Organs with the Six Primary Yang Organs:** The Eight Extraordinary Vessels provide the link between the body's Six Extraordinary (Curious) Organs (Brain, Bone, Marrow, Blood Vessels, Gall Bladder and Uterus), and the internal energy flow of the body's six primary Yang organs (Gall Bladder, Small Intestine, Stomach, Large

```
Eight Extraordinary Vessels
  ├── Serve as Reservoirs of Qi
  ├── Store and Circulate Jing Qi
  ├── Circulate the Wei Qi (Protective Energy)
  ├── Regulate the Body's Life Cycles
  ├── Integrate the Six Extraordinary Organs with the Six Primary Yang Organs and the Kidneys
  └── Integrate the Four Seas with the Body's Internal Energy Flow
```

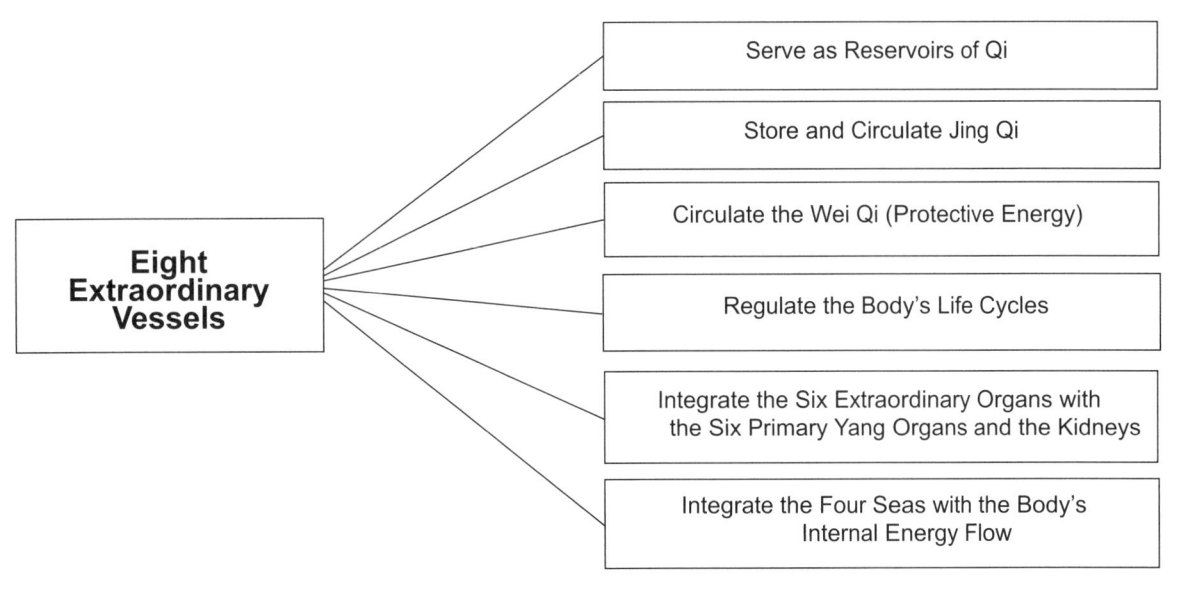

Figure 6.5. The Energetic Functions of the Eight Extraordinary Vessels

Intestine, Urinary Bladder and Triple Burners), in addition to the Kidneys. The integration of this internal connection is described as follows:

- The Brain is regulated by the Governing Vessel and the Yin and Yang Heel Vessels.
- The Uterus is regulated by the Thrusting and Conception Vessels.
- The Blood Vessels are regulated by the Thrusting Vessels.
- The Gall Bladder is regulated by the Belt Vessel.
- The Marrow is regulated by the Thrusting Vessels.
- The Bones are regulated by the Thrusting and Conception Vessels.

6. **Integrate the Four Seas with the Body's Internal Energy Flow:** The *Magical Pivot (Ling Shu)* states, "People have Four Seas: the Sea of Marrow, the Sea of Blood, the Sea of Qi, and the Sea of Grain and Water." The Eight Extraordinary Vessels provide the link between the body's Four Seas and the body's internal energy flow, described as follows:

- **The Sea of Marrow** consists of the Brain and spinal cord, and it is related to the Governing Vessel and the Yin and Yang Heel Vessels. The Sea of Marrow access points (GV-16 and GV-20) are located on the Governing Vessel. When the Sea of Marrow is excess, the patient will show signs of strength and increased power. When the Sea of Marrow is deficient, the patient may experience headaches, tinnitus, blurred vision, dizziness, weak legs, fatigue, or possible physical collapse.

- **The Sea of Qi** is located in the center of the chest and is regulated by the Conception Vessel. The Sea of Qi access point (CV-17) is located on the Conception Vessel. Some Medical Qigong schools maintain that there are two main reservoirs of Qi in the body: the Middle Dantian, being the Sea of Postnatal Qi; and the Lower Dantian (which is regulated by the Qihai CV-6 point) being the Sea of Prenatal Qi. When the Sea of Qi is in excess, the patient may experience a feeling of fullness in the chest, dyspnea (urgent breathing), and a red complexion. When the Sea of Qi is deficient, the patient may experience weakness, energy depletion and insufficient speech.

- **The Sea of Nourishment** (also known as the Sea of Grain and Water) is the Stomach, and is regulated by the Thrusting Vessels. The Sea of Nourishment access points (St-30) are located on the Stomach Channels. When the Sea of Water and Grain is in excess, the patient may experience a feeling of fullness or bloating in the abdomen. When the Sea of Water and Grain is deficient, the patient may experience a feeling of hunger with a corresponding inability to eat.

- **The Sea of Blood** (also known as the Sea of the Twelve Primary Channels) is related to the Thrusting Vessels, and the Liver organ. The Sea of Blood access points (Sp-10, St-37, St-39, and UB-11) are located on the Spleen, Stomach and Urinary Bladder Channels. When the Sea of Blood is in excess, the patient's mind is constantly thinking and his or her physical body may feel big and bulky. When the Sea of Blood is deficient, the patient's mind is constantly thinking and his or her physical body feels small.

THE EIGHT EXTRAORDINARY VESSELS AND MEDICAL QIGONG THERAPY

The energetic pathways, functions, and use of the Eight Extraordinary Vessels and their associated points are often quite different in Medical Qigong than those taught in acupuncture colleges, even though they may sometimes bear the same names.

Most acupuncturists, with the exception of some Japanese practitioners, often pay little attention to the Eight Extraordinary Vessels in diagnosis and treatment. One Medical Qigong doctor from China has claimed that a Chinese study showed that treatments based on the utilization of the Eight Extraordinary Vessels were far more effective than treatments utilizing standard Traditional Chinese Medical protocols. The results of this study, however, were not released because officials did not want to disturb the credibility of China's established T.C.M. institutions. The reason that Medical Qigong makes use of the Eight Extraordinary Vessels is that they are relatively easy to access through Qi Emission Therapy and Medical Qigong Self-Regulation prescription exercises.

The Eight Extraordinary Vessels have been of special importance to Medical Qigong practitioners for thousands of years. They are viewed as the foundation of the body's energy, and they bridge the body's Prenatal and Postnatal Qi. These Eight Extraordinary Vessels affect the body on the deepest levels of our basic constitutional energy. In Medical Qigong regulation exercises, opening the flow of energy through the Eight Extraordinary Vessels is a prerequisite for opening the energy flow in the Twelve Primary Channels. The major purpose of opening the Eight Extraordinary Vessels is to provide a container for storing the Three Forces of Heaven (universal energy), Earth (environmental energy), and Man (Jing: Essence, Qi: Energy, and Shen: Spirit).

It is essential for the Qigong doctors to open their Eight Extraordinary Vessels to attain mastery of their energetic body. The Microcosmic Orbit is introduced to use for purgation, fusion, tonification, and regulation of the Governing and Conception Vessels in the first stages of Qigong training. This exercise restores a healthy flow of energy throughout all of the channels and vessels creating a healthy and balanced body.

Qigong doctors receive more Qi, and the quality of their Blood changes, (in that its energetic potential contains more Qi) through the refinement of energy achieved by focusing on the development of the Eight Extraordinary Vessels. At this advanced stage of transformation, Qigong doctors then re-channel the flow of energy through their body's Three Dantians, including the "mystical pass," located within the Upper Dantian chambers of the Brain. When the flow of energy is directed to stimulate the Mystical Pass, the Qigong doctors acquire greater awareness and control over all of their bodies (physical, energetic, and spiritual). The doctors are then able to enhance their perception and communication with all the other energetic planes of existence (mineral, plant, animal, and human) and with the Dao (or divine).

CLINICAL MANIFESTATION AND USE

The Eight Extraordinary Vessels form and establish the energetic patterns for the tissues of the developing fetus, and for the entire body of the adult. The clinical use of the Eight Extraordinary Vessels can be divided into several different approaches of energy manipulation, all of which are aimed at changing the energetic patterns within the patient's tissues.

One approach divides the Eight Extraordinary Vessels into four pairs of Yin and Yang vessels. In this particular approach, the Eight Extraordinary Vessels are grouped according to the same polarity, with two pairs of Yin Vessels and two pairs of Yang Vessels. When paired this way, each set of the Yin and Yang Extraordinary Vessels has a common range of energetic actions in terms of the patient's body areas. These energetic actions and the pairing of the Eight Extraordinary Vessels are described as follows:

1. **The Conception and Yin Heel Vessels** affect the flow of energy to the patient's abdomen, chest, Lungs, throat, and face.
2. **The Governing and Yang Heel Vessels** affect the flow of energy to the back of the patient's legs, as well as to his or her back, spine, neck, head, eyes, and Brain.
3. **The Thrusting and Yin Linking Vessels** affect the flow of energy to the inner aspect of the patient's legs, as well as to his or her abdomen, Stomach, chest, and Heart.
4. **The Belt and Yang Linking Vessels** affect the flow of energy to the outer aspect of the patient's legs, as well as the sides of his or her body, the shoulders, and sides of the neck.

ENERGETIC FUNCTIONS

The Eight Extraordinary Vessels can also be categorized according to their energetic functions, which are described as follows:

1. **The Conception, Governing, and Thrusting Vessels** are considered the source of all the other Extraordinary Vessels. These three vessels affect the patient's energy at a deep constitutional level. They originate directly from the Kidneys and are connected to the body's Jing.
2. **The Yin and Yang Heel Vessels** are mutually complementary in that they both flow from the legs (controlling the condition of the muscles of the legs) into the eyes (controlling the muscles that open and close the eyes). Therefore, the Qigong doctor can treat energetic excess or deficient conditions in either the legs or eyes by simultaneously treating and regulating the Qi of the Yin and Yang Heel Vessels.
3. **The Yin and Yang Linking Vessels** complement each other by linking the body's Yin and Yang Channels.
4. **The Belt Vessel** is the only horizontal vessel in the body, encircling and connecting the main channels. For this reason, the Belt Vessel affects the circulation of energy throughout the entire body, especially within the legs and waist.

THE EIGHT EXTRAORDINARY VESSELS AND THE EIGHT CONFLUENT POINTS

The Eight Confluent points communicate with the Eight Extraordinary Vessels. In ancient China, there were two primary ways of accessing and utilizing the Eight Extraordinary Vessel Confluent Points: The Master - Coupled Point Combination and the Magic Square.

THE MASTER - COUPLED POINT COMBINATION

The Confluent points are divided into Master points and Coupled points. The Master point is the primary point chosen for treatment, while its Coupled point is the connecting or secondary point used to open the specific Vessel. Each of the Eight Extraordinary Vessels has both a Master and a Coupled Confluent point on either the upper or lower limbs.

All of the Eight Extraordinary Vessels can be treated in various combinations according to their specific Master and Coupled point locations (Figure 6.6). If, for example, the Qigong doctor causes Qi to flow from the patient's Master point on the hand (SI-3) to its Coupled point (UB-62) on the

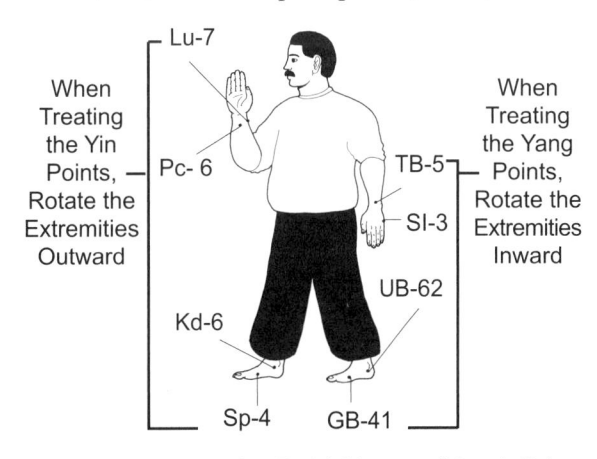

Figure 6.6. Locations of the Body's Master and Couple Points

foot, the Governing Vessel will open. After making the connection, the doctor will apply a slight traction to the arm and leg to further stimulate the opening of the channel and increase Qi and Blood flow. When stimulating the Yang Vessels, rotate the patient's arms and legs inward, towards the medial aspect of the body; when stimulating Yin Vessels rotate the patient's arms and legs outward, towards the lateral aspect of the body. It is important for the doctor to also focus his or her mind on opening the energetic flow of the Vessel that is being activated. To complete the treatment, the doctor must first remove stimulation from the Coupled point then disconnect from the Master point (Figure 6.7). There are two patterns used when applying the Master and Coupled Point combination: same side treatment and crossover treatment; described as follows:

1. **Same Side Treatment:** When treating the same side (same side arm and leg), the energetic stimulation will affect the specific side that is being treated. When using the same side treatment, the deficient or stagnant side is chosen first. This is immediately followed with the crossover treatment. The same side treatment is used to address energetic or physical asymmetries, and initiate a chaotic rhythm used in order to disrupt the established imbalance pattern of the patient's disease. Once the chaotic rhythm has been initiated, the Qigong doctor will then reprogram the patient's energetic body in order to facilitate a healthy re-patterning of the patient's physical body. Same side treatments are used in conditions such as stroke, multiple sclerosis, Bells palsy and Parkinson's disease.
2. **Crossover Treatment:** When treating with the crossover pattern (same arm and opposite leg) the doctor will focus on balancing the Qi and Blood within the stimulated Vessel. The crossover pattern is generally used in order to end a treatment, instilling balance and harmony within the patients body.

THE MAGIC SQUARE

Each of the Eight Extraordinary Vessels is also connected to one of the Eight Trigrams (or Eight

Channel	Open with Master Point	Complete with Couple Point
Governing	Hand (SI-3)	Foot (UB-62)
Conception	Hand (Lu-7)	Foot (Kd-6)
Thrusting	Foot (Sp-4)	Hand (Pc-6)
Belt	Foot (GB-41)	Hand (TB-5)
Yin Linking	Hand (Pc-6)	Foot (Sp-4)
Yang Linking	Hand (TB-5)	Foot (GB-41)
Yin Heel	Foot (Kd-6)	Hand (Lu-7)
Yang Heel	Foot (UB-62)	Hand (SI-3)

Figure 6.7. The Vessels with their Associated Master Points and Couple Points

Natural Manifestations) and can be energetically regulated through the use of the "Magic Square." In ancient Chinese medicine, the Lo Writings and their correspondences form a model or "Magic Square," which is the basis for the Ling Gui Ba Fa (The Eight Techniques of the Mysterious Turtle) system of acupuncture. In this system of energetic medicine, the Eight Confluent Points are associated with the Eight Trigrams.

The Eight Confluent Points are also where the Eight Extraordinary Vessels and Twelve Primary Channels intersect each other. The Ling Gui Ba Fa method describes the theory that all of the primary channel points on the body are dominated by the Shu Points, which are in turn dominated by the Eight Confluent Points. The Eight Confluent Points and their trigram correspondences are described as follows (Figure 6.8):

- **The Trigram Kan,** located at number 1, is associated with the Yang Heel Vessel, and the UB-62 point

- **The Trigram Kun,** located at number 2, is associated with the Yin Heel Vessel, and the Kd-6 point
- **The Trigram Zhen,** located at number 3, is associated with the Yang Linking Vessel, and the TB-5 point
- **The Trigram Xun,** located at number 4, is associated with the Belt Vessel, and the GB-41 point
- **The Bright Hall (Ming Tang),** located at number 5 on the center of the square, is associated with the Taiji Pole
- **The Trigram Qian,** located at number 6, is associated with the Thrusting Vessels, and the Sp-4 point
- **The Trigram Dui,** located at number 7, is associated with the Governing Vessel, and the SI-3 point
- **The Trigram Gen,** located at number 8, is associated with the Yin Linking Vessel, and the Pc-6 point
- **The Trigram Li,** located at number 9, is associated with the Conception Vessel, and the Lu-7 point

Eight Confluent Points

The Eight Confluent points are consistent with the Master Points of the Eight Extraordinary Vessels, and are described as follows:

- **Governing Vessel:** The Confluent point for the Governing Vessel is the SI-3 point. This point is used to treat mania-depression, epilepsy, occipital headache, and stiffness or pain of the spinal column. This point is also used to dispel febrile diseases and dispel External Wind Cold or Wind Heat.
- **Conception Vessel:** The Confluent point for the Conception Vessel is the Lu-7 point. This point is used to treat uterine, reproductive and urinary organ diseases.
- **Belt Vessel:** The Confluent point for the Belt Vessel is the GB-41 point. This point is used to treat breast abscesses, pain and distention of the breast, and menstrual disorders.
- **Thrusting Vessel:** The Confluent point for the Thrusting Vessel is the Sp-4 point. This point is used to treat acute abdominal pain (with cramping), vomiting and edema (especially

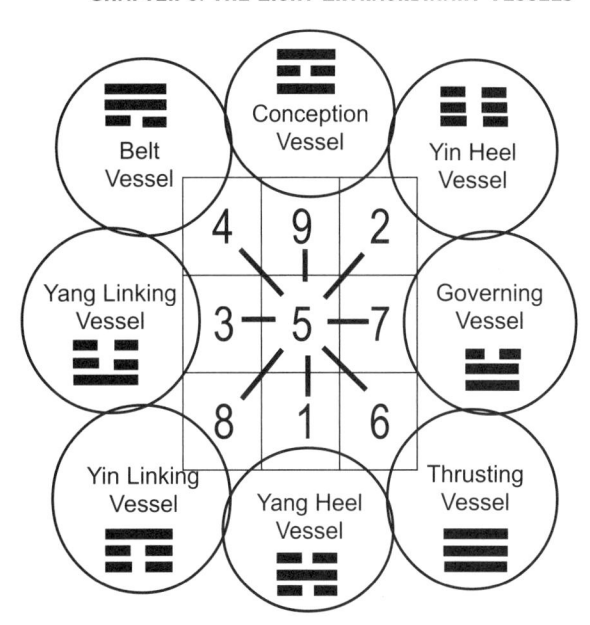

Figure 6.8. The Magic Square

of the face).
- **Yang Heel Vessel:** The Confluent point for the Yang Heel Vessel is the UB-62 point. This point is used to treat both External Wind Invasion and Internal Wind Invasion. External Wind invasion usually manifests in symptoms such as headaches and a stiff neck, while Internal Wind Invasion symptoms include insomnia, lockjaw, opisthotonos, Windstroke, epilepsy, upward staring eyes, deviations of the mouth and eyes, or hemiplegia.
- **Yin Heel Vessel:** The Confluent point for the Yin Heel Vessel is the Kd-6 point. This point is used to treat tightness and contraction of the inner aspect of the leg, chronic throat disorders (swelling, pain, difficulty swallowing), eye disorders and daytime epilepsy.
- **Yang Linking Vessel:** The Confluent point for the Yang Linking Vessel is the TB-5 point. This point is used to treat temporal, frontal, occipital and vertex headaches, as well as to dispel pathogenic factors located on the Exterior (Yang) portion of the body.
- **Yin Linking Vessel:** The Confluent point for the Yin Linking Vessel is the Pc-6 point. This point is used to treat pain in the Heart and chest, as well as pain in the lateral coastal region.

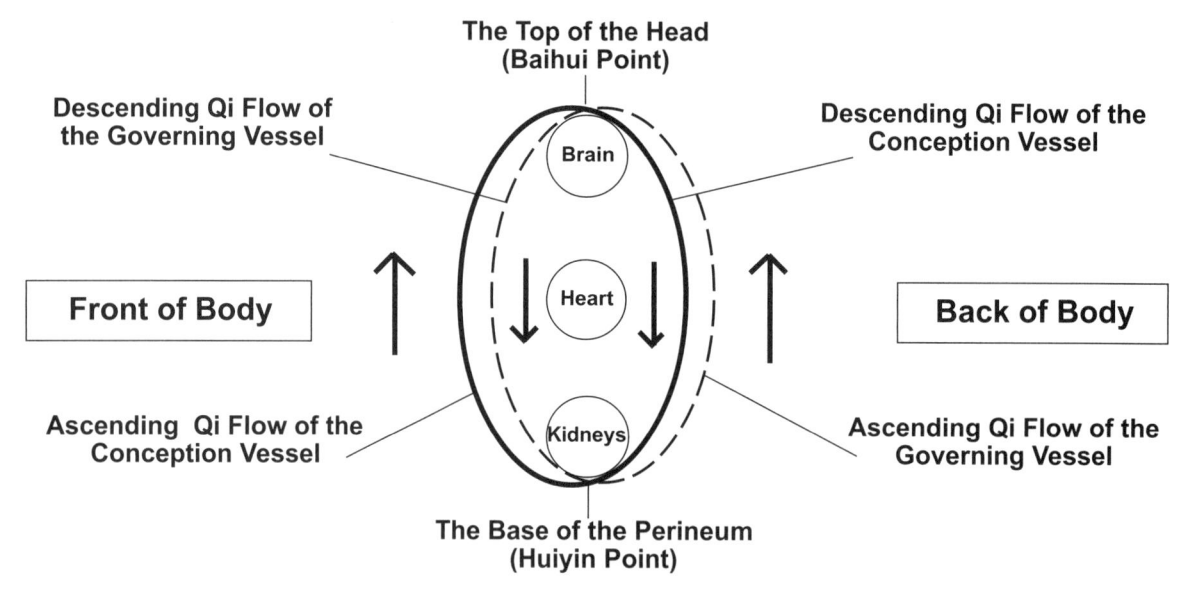

Figure 6.9. The Energetic Flow of the Conception and Governing Vessels

Governing and Conception Vessels: Du and Ren Mai

The Governing and Conception Vessels are the main rivers of the body's Yang and Yin energies, respectively. They are the polar aspects of the body, perfectly complementary, like midday and midnight. They are responsible for the formation of the holoblastic cleavage and the first cellular division of the fertilized ovum in embryological development (see Chapter 2).

In China, Dr. Li Shi Zhen was the first to believe that the Governing and Conception Vessels are two branches of the same source, an inseparable Yin-and-Yang, front-and-back duality. These vessels connect the Uterus with the Kidneys, Heart, and Brain.

They originate externally at the Huiyin CV-1 point, ascend the front and back of the torso, and form a small circle when the tip of the tongue touches the upper palate in the mouth and the anal sphincter is closed. Not only does this action complete the balance of Fire (Heart) and Water (Kidney) energy, it also increases the body's protective Wei Qi.

Regulating the Conception and Governing Vessels is a priority in Medical Qigong practice. The Qigong practitioner draws the Yang Fire and Yin Essence up and down his or her body, along these vessels, fusing the Water and Fire energies together. This fusion facilitates a Yin and Yang balance throughout the body.

The Governing and Conception Vessels each have energy pathways on both the anterior and posterior vertical midline of the body. Each vessel's pathway is a complete circle, being composed of an ascending and descending energetic flow. These two medial lines join at the extremes of the torso (the head and perineum), forming one complete circle of energetic current (Figure 6.9).

Both vessels are superimposed on each other. The energy of the Governing Vessel is predominant up the back and inferior down the front (interior to the Conception Vessel); the energy of the Conception Vessel is predominant up the front and inferior down the back of the body, where it flows interior to the Governing Vessel.

The energetic flow of the Conception Vessel corresponds to Yin, negative polarity, the female aspect, and responds to bass tones. The energetic flow of the Governing Vessel corresponds to Yang, positive polarity, the male aspect, and responds to treble tones.

The direction of the energetic movement of

these two vessels explains why there are two opposite methods of directing the flow of energy along the torso in various meditation systems of energy cultivation. One direction follows the Fire Cycle of the Microcosmic Orbit, moving Qi along the Governing Vessel, flowing up the spine and down the chest to energize and regulate the emotions and of the acquired mind (Shen Zhi). The other direction follows the Water Cycle of the Microcosmic Orbit, moving Qi along the Conception Vessel, flowing up the chest and down the spine to stimulate spiritual intuition and activate the perceptions of the congenital mind (Yuan Shen).

THE GOVERNING VESSEL: DU MAI

The word Du translates as "governing" and it refers to a general, or to someone who controls and is in charge. The Chinese character Du can also be translated as: to oversee, inspect, superintend or reprove; a viceroy or governor general; and the center or the middle seam on the back of a coat. The ideographs for Du Mai are described as follows (Figure 6.10):

- The first character is the Chinese ideograph "Du," which is composed of two parts. Positioned on the top are three separate characters depicting "upper" or "Yang," "small" and "again." This combination has been translated by some scholars as indicating one's father's younger brother or uncle. Positioned to the bottom is a character depicting a watchful eye. The authority of the Governing Vessel is not equal to the higher level of the Heart (emperor), but is that of a smaller governor or prime minister that answers to the emperor. This ideograph depicts the keen eyes of an inspector who watches and monitors on behalf of someone else, denoting that the Governing Vessel is responsible for overseeing or monitoring the Yang of the body, but is nevertheless subordinate to the Heart, or emperor.
- The second character is the Chinese ideograph "Mai," is generally translated as "vessel." It is composed of two characters: The character to the left, "Ji" depicts the Chinese ideograph for body tissue, muscle or flesh (all

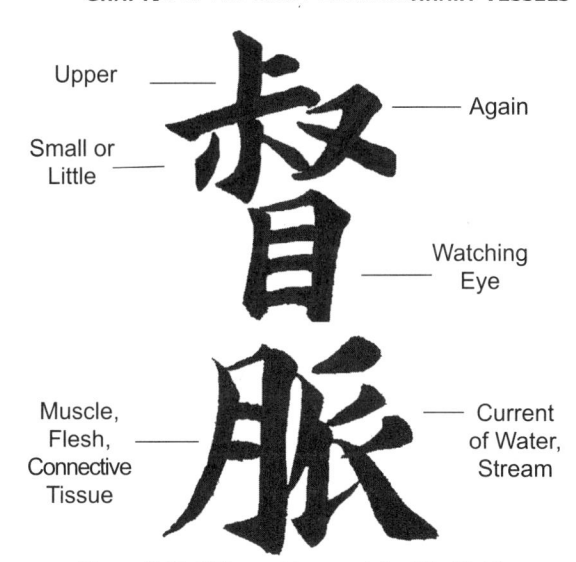

Figure 6.10. Chinese Ideograph for "Du Mai," the Governing Vessel

of which are forms of connective tissue). The character to the right, "Mai" depicts a current of water, stream, or branch of a river. As a whole, the character can be translated as arteries, veins or pulse, indicating a form of energetic circulation.

DEVELOPMENT

During the development of the embryo, the Governing Vessel is responsible for the formation of the medulla oblongata and cerebrum. It is also responsible for nourishing the Brain and the spinal cord, and for consolidating the Yuan Qi in the Kidneys.

The Governing Vessel controls all of the Yang channels in the body and therefore, is known as the Sea of Yang. Along its course, it intersects the three Yang channels of the hands and feet, as well as the Yang Linking (Wei) Vessels several times.

ENERGETIC PATHWAY

The Governing Vessel originates in the Lower Dantian in both men and women. It is composed of many energetic branches, described as follows:

- The primary channel of the Governing Vessel originates in the Lower Dantian (the center of the Uterus in women), emerges at the perineum (bottom gate of the Lower Dantian) and runs posteriorly along the midline of the sacrum. It travels along the interior of the spinal column to the lower back and the Mingmen GV-4 point (back gate of the Lower Dantian). From there it continues to the mid-back and at the Shendao GV-11 point (Back Gate of the Middle Dantian). From the Shendao point it continues to ascend the spinal column to the nape of the neck, where it enters the Brain at the Fengfu GV-16 point (back gate of the Upper Dantian). It further ascends over the head to the vertex at the Baihui GV-20 point (upper gate of the Upper Dantian), from which a branch of the Governing Vessel descends directly into the Brain to reconnect with the GV-16 point at the base of the skull. From the Baihui point the Governing Vessel progresses along the midline of the forehead, past the Yin Tang point (front gate of the Upper Dantian) to the bridge of the nose where it terminates at the junction of the upper lip at the gum.

- The first branch of the Governing Vessel originates in the Lower Dantian (the center of the Uterus in women), descends to the genitals and perineum (bottom gate of the Lower Dantian), encircles the anus and ascends the spinal column slightly internal to the primary channel of the Governing Vessel, entering the Kidneys and Mingmen area (back gate of the Lower Dantian).
- The second branch of the Governing Vessel originates in the Lower Dantian (the center of the Uterus in women), descends to the genitals and perineum (bottom gate of the Lower Dantian), envelops the external genitalia and ascends to the middle of the umbilicus (front gate of the Lower Dantian). From the umbilicus it further ascends up the chest, passing through the Heart and Middle Dantian, ascending through the throat to circle the mouth. After circling the mouth, it further ascends to the eyes, terminating just below the middle of the eyes at the Chengqi St-1 point.
- The third branch of the Governing Vessel originates from the inside of the eyes at the Jingming UB-1 point. From the UB-1 points, this vessel follows both of the Urinary Bladder Channels along the forehead, converges

Governs All the Yang Channels of the Body

Nourishes the Brain and Marrow

Consolidates the Yuan Qi in the Kidneys

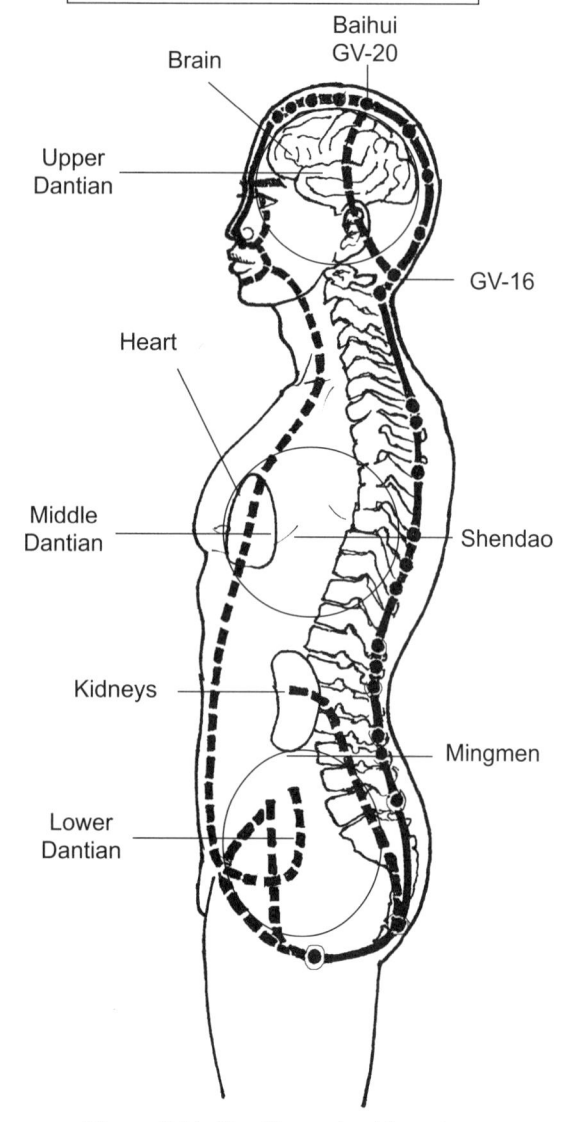

Figure 6.11. The Governing Vessel: Sea of All Yang Vessels (Side View)

CHAPTER 6: THE EIGHT EXTRAORDINARY VESSELS

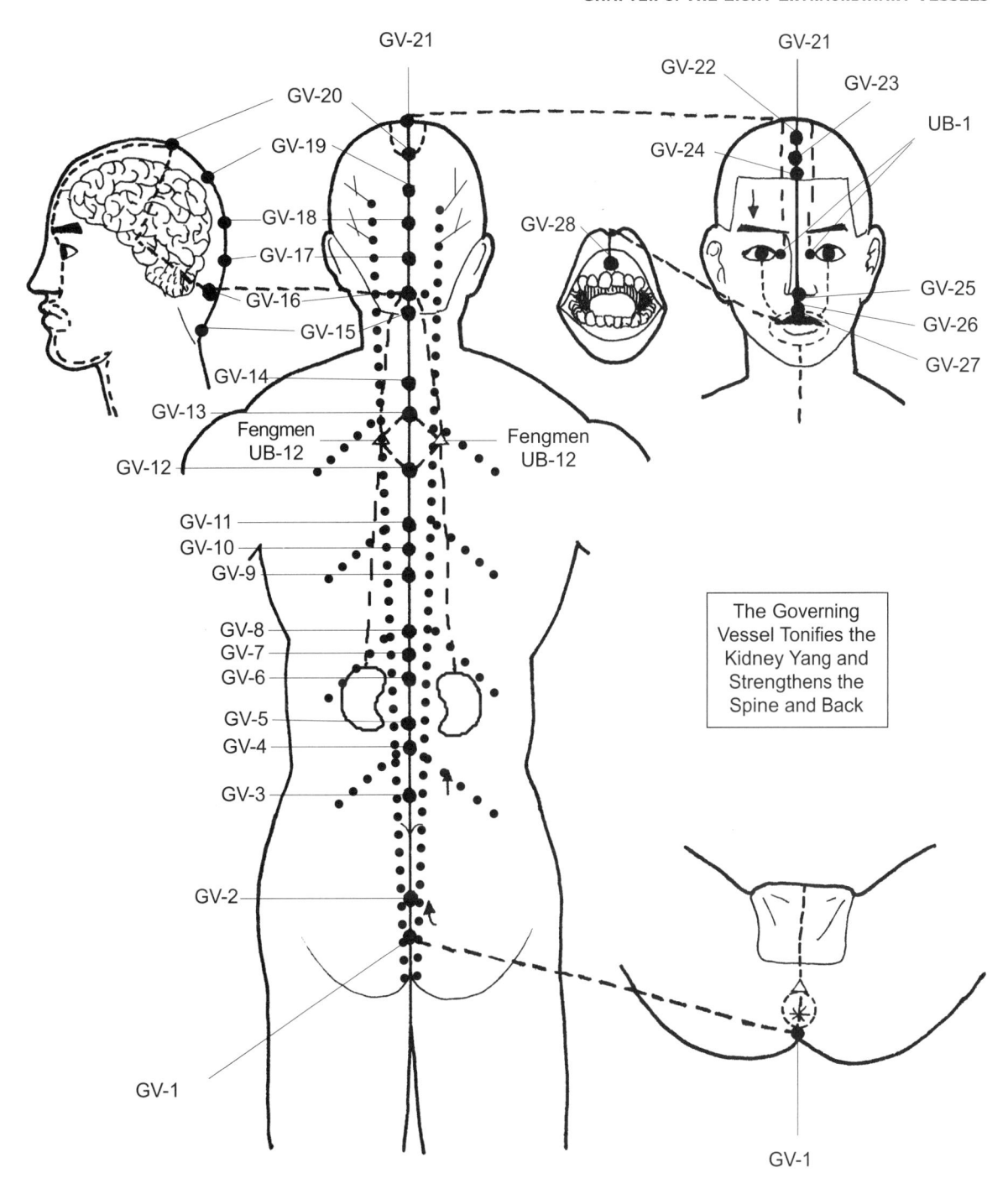

Figure 6.12. The Governing Vessel (GV)

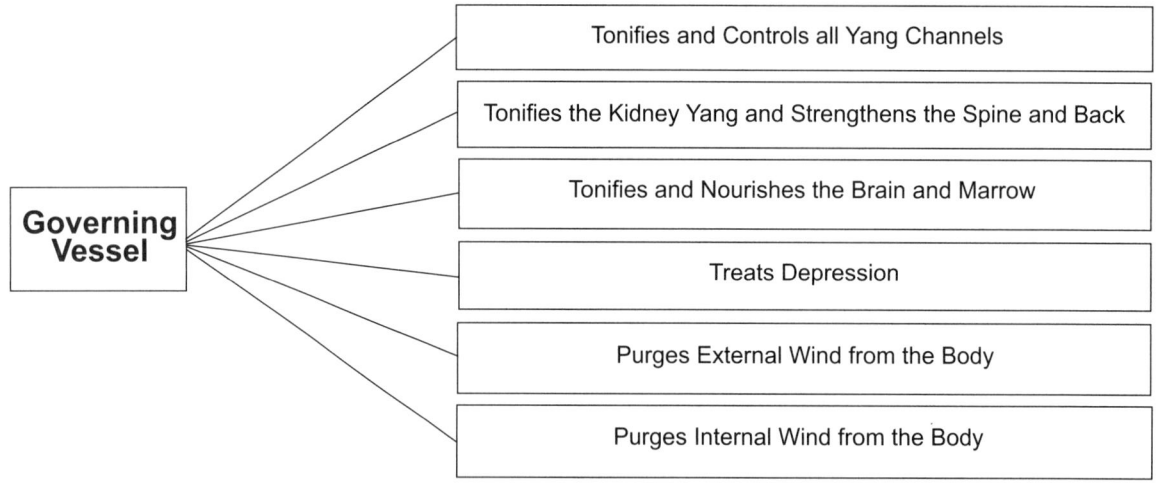

VOLUME 1, SECTION 1: FOUNDATIONS OF CHINESE ENERGETIC MEDICINE

Figure 6.13. The Functions and Clinical Uses of the Governing Vessel (GV)

Governing Vessel:
- Tonifies and Controls all Yang Channels
- Tonifies the Kidney Yang and Strengthens the Spine and Back
- Tonifies and Nourishes the Brain and Marrow
- Treats Depression
- Purges External Wind from the Body
- Purges Internal Wind from the Body

at the vertex of the Baihui GV-20 point (upper gate of the Upper Dantian), and descends to enter the Brain. From the Brain, the vessel emerges at the Fengfu GV-16 point (back gate of the Upper Dantian) and divides into two additional branches which descend the back. These branches pass through the Fengmen UB-12 points along the sides of the spine before entering into the Kidneys and Mingmen area (Figure 6.11 and 6.12).

- The Luo-Connecting Vessel of the Governing Vessel originates from the Changqiang GV-1 point at the perineum (bottom gate of the Lower Dantian) and ascends bilaterally along the sides of the spine to the Fengfu GV-16 point (back gate of the Upper Dantian) where it disperses over the occipital region.

CLINICAL MANIFESTATIONS

The Governing Vessel tonifies the Kidney Yang and strengthens the spine and back. When the Governing Vessel is in excess, the back becomes stiff; when it is depleted, the head becomes heavy, unstable, and shaky.

The functions and clinical uses of the patient's Governing Vessel are described as follows (Figure 6.13):

1. Tonifies and controls all the Yang Channels of the patient's body (particularly in relation to the Kidney Yang and the Brain).

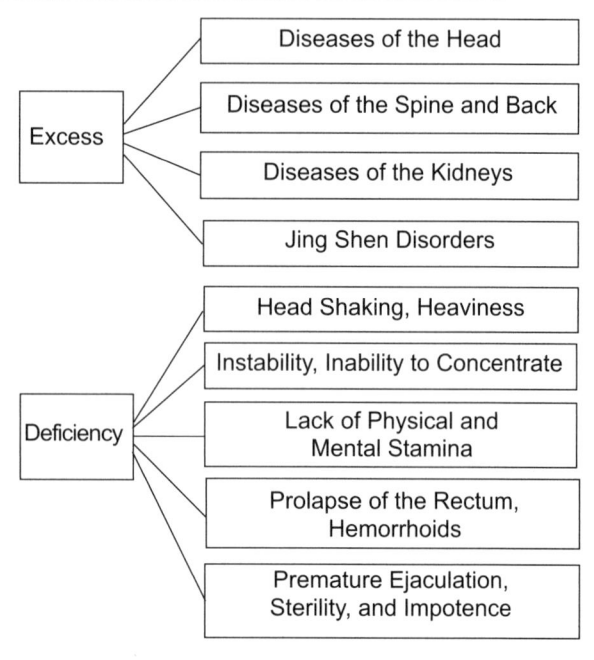

Figure 6.14. Pathological Manifestations of the Governing Vessel (GV)

Excess:
- Diseases of the Head
- Diseases of the Spine and Back
- Diseases of the Kidneys
- Jing Shen Disorders

Deficiency:
- Head Shaking, Heaviness
- Instability, Inability to Concentrate
- Lack of Physical and Mental Stamina
- Prolapse of the Rectum, Hemorrhoids
- Premature Ejaculation, Sterility, and Impotence

2. Tonifies the Kidney Yang and strengthens the patient's spine and back, especially in cases of chronic lower back pain due to Kidney Deficiency.
3. Tonifies and nourishes the patient's Brain and Marrow and treats such symptoms as poor memory, dizziness, and tinnitus.

252

4. Treats depression, due to the Governing Vessel's connection to the body's Jing (Kidneys and willpower), Qi (Heart awareness), and Shen (Spirit).
5. Purges External Wind from the patient's body when symptoms such as runny nose, headache, fever, and stiff neck are present.
6. Purges Internal Wind from the patient's body when symptoms such as dizziness, tremors, convulsions, epilepsy, or the condition of Wind Stroke are present.

In men, the Governing Vessel is generally treated by itself, and in women it is combined with the treatment of the Conception Vessel.

Pathological Manifestations

The main diseases associated with energetic malfunctions in the Governing Vessel are describes as follows (Figure 6.14):

1. **Symptoms of Excess** energy in the Governing Vessel include diseases of the head (apoplexy, aphasia, epilepsy, headaches, tetany), back, neck, and Kidneys (pain and stiffness in the spinal column), opisthotonos (spastic muscle movement), night sweating, and Jing Shen disorders (such as hyperexcitability, hallucinations).
2. **Symptoms of Deficient** energy in the Governing Vessel include the shaking of the head, feelings of general heaviness, instability, and an inability to concentrate. The patient may lack physical and mental stamina, display weakness of character, and may also experience prolapse of the rectum, hemorrhoids, premature ejaculation, sterility, or impotence.

The Conception Vessel: Ren Mai

The word Ren translates as "Conception," and refers to pregnancy, responsibility, or obligation. It can also mean "to accept or take charge." The ideographs for Ren Mai are described as follows (Figure 6.15):

- The first ideograph is the Chinese character "Ren," which is composed of two parts. Positioned on the left is the radical "Ren" for "person" or "human." Positioned on the right is the radical for "Ren" that is, etymologically speaking, a "working person." It depicts the image of a bamboo pole suspended on the shoulders of one who is walking on the road with a load hanging at each end. This suggests the meaning of enduring, bearing, or taking the burden of something. When combined with the previous radical for person, the overall meaning is that of bearing the burden of being human.
- The second character is the Chinese ideograph "Mai," which is generally translated as "vessel." It is composed of two characters: The character to the left, "Ji" depicts the Chinese ideogram for body tissue, muscle or flesh (all of which are forms of connective tissue). The character on the right "Mai" depicts a current of water, stream, or branch of a river. As a whole, the character can be translated as arteries, veins or pulse, indicating a form of energetic circulation.

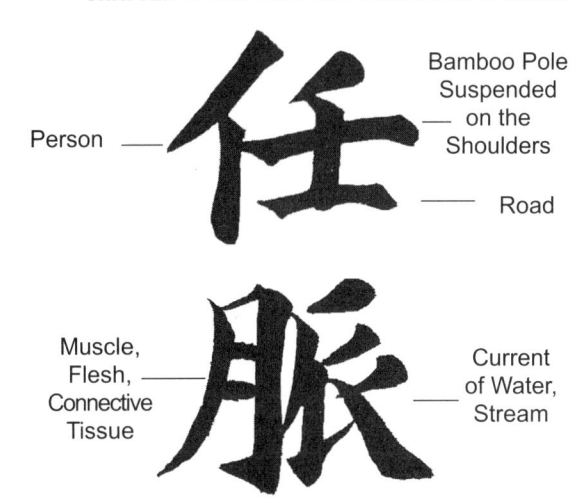

Figure 6.15. The Chinese Ideograph for "Ren Mai," the Conception Vessel

Development

The Conception Vessel originates from the Lower Dantian, and specifically in the Uterus for females. It nourishes the Yuan Qi of all five Yin organs. The Conception Vessel governs all the Yin channels of the body and for this reason it is called the Sea of Yin. It intersects the three Yin channels of the hands and feet, as well as the Yin Linking (Wei) Vessels several times.

Functionally, the Conception Vessel can be divided into three quadrants, described as follows:
- The upper third of the Conception Vessel on

Volume 1, Section 1: Foundations of Chinese Energetic Medicine

- Governs All the Yin Channels of the Body
- Nourishes the Yuan Qi of all Five Yin Organs
- Controls Respiratory Functions
- Controls Digestive Functions
- Controls Urogenital Functions

The internal branch of the Conception Vessel originates from the Lower Dantian. It descends into the pelvic cavity and then ascends the body along the spine, ending at the mouth.

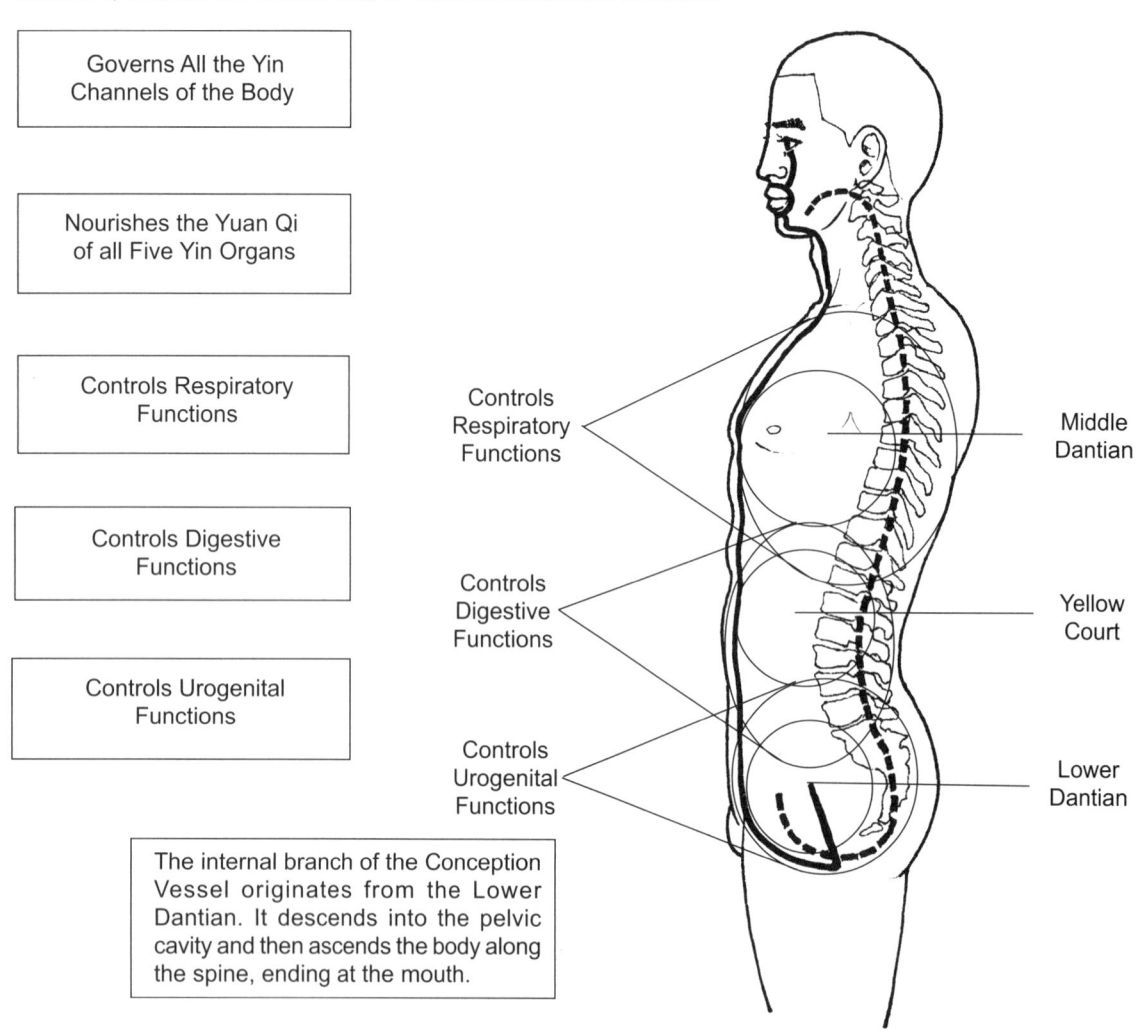

Figure 6.16. The Conception Vessel: Sea of All Yin Vessels (Side View)

the sternum controls respiratory functions
- The middle third of the Conception Vessel on the epigastrium controls digestive functions
- The lower third of the Conception Vessel on the abdomen controls the urogenital functions

In women, the Conception Vessel is primarily responsible for nourishing the Uterus and the genital system, and determines the seven-year life cycles. It links the Yin energy with all aspects of conception and reproduction. The Conception Vessel, along with the Thrusting Vessels, has an important relationship with obstetric diseases that are related to the development of the fetus, delivery, and menstruation.

Energetic Pathway

The Conception Vessel originates in the Lower Dantian in both men and women. It is composed of many energetic branches, described as follows (Figure 6.16 and Figure 6.17):

- The Primary Channel of the Conception Vessel originates in the Lower Dantian (the center of the Uterus in women) and emerges at the Huiyin CV-1 point of the perineum (bottom gate of the Lower Dantian). From the perineum it runs through the anterior aspect of the pubic region, ascends along the middle of the abdomen and passes through the umbilicus at the CV-8 point, the front gate of the Lower Dantian.

Chapter 6: The Eight Extraordinary Vessels

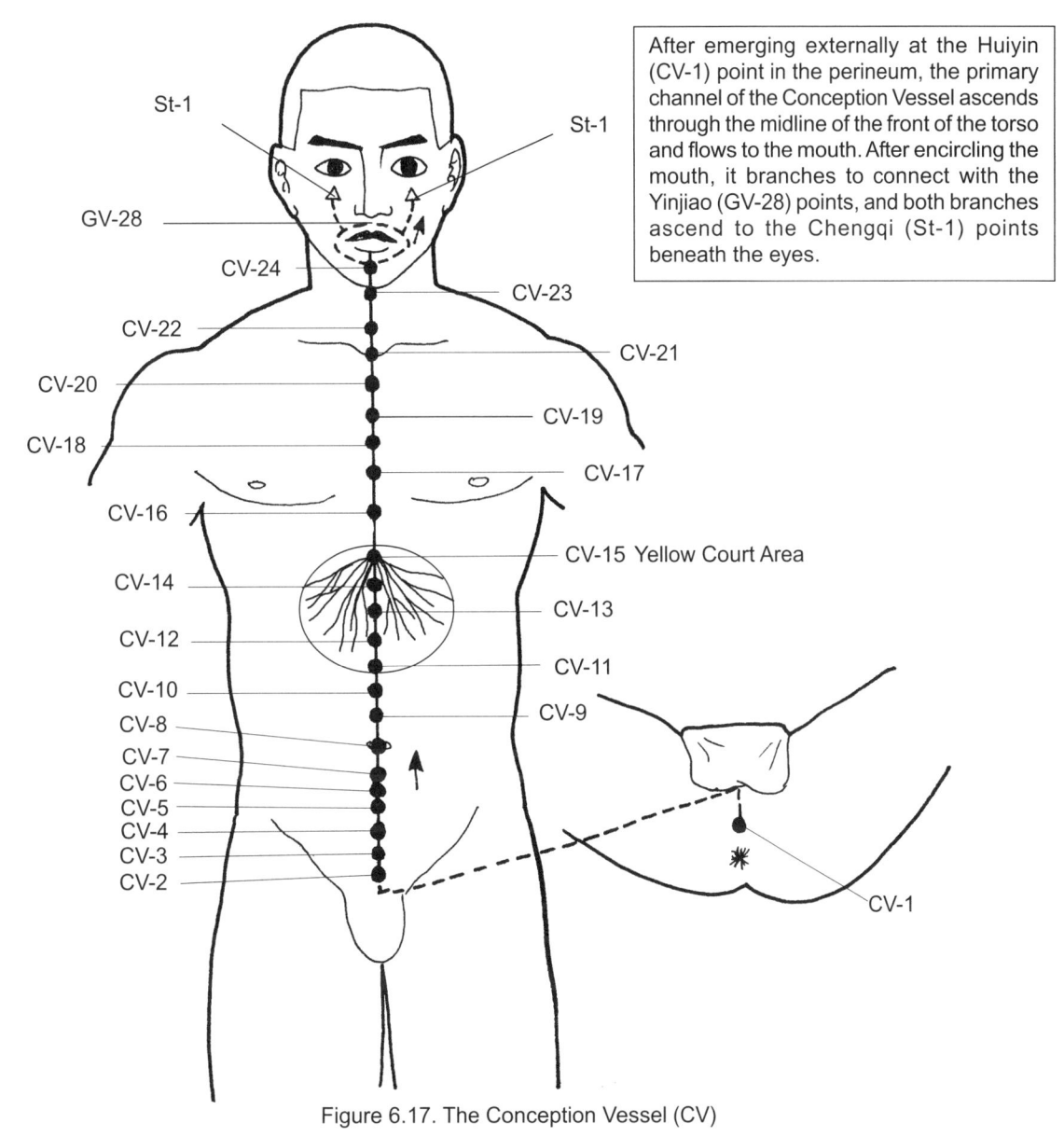

After emerging externally at the Huiyin (CV-1) point in the perineum, the primary channel of the Conception Vessel ascends through the midline of the front of the torso and flows to the mouth. After encircling the mouth, it branches to connect with the Yinjiao (GV-28) points, and both branches ascend to the Chengqi (St-1) points beneath the eyes.

Figure 6.17. The Conception Vessel (CV)

From the umbilicus it ascends the midline of the chest, passes through the Heart and Middle Dantian at the CV-17 point, ascending through the throat and jaw to reach the bottom of the lip and circle the mouth. After circling the mouth, it connects with the Governing Vessel at the top of the lip and gum area (GV-28) and further ascends in two branches to each of the eyes, terminating just below the middle of the eyes at the Chengqi St-1 point.

- The First Branch of the Conception Vessel originates in the Lower Dantian (the center of the Uterus in women), descends to the genitals and the Huiyin CV-1 point of the perineum (bottom gate of the Lower Dantian), encircles the anus and ascends into the center of the spinal column. Following the spinal column, it ascends through the back gates of the Lower and

255

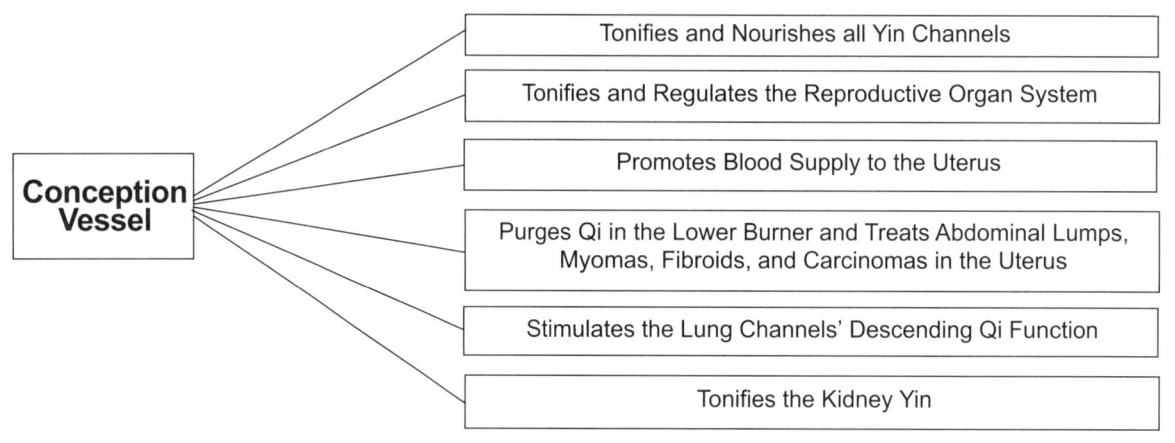

Figure 6.18. The Functions and Clinical Uses of the Conception Vessel (CV)

Conception Vessel:
- Tonifies and Nourishes all Yin Channels
- Tonifies and Regulates the Reproductive Organ System
- Promotes Blood Supply to the Uterus
- Purges Qi in the Lower Burner and Treats Abdominal Lumps, Myomas, Fibroids, and Carcinomas in the Uterus
- Stimulates the Lung Channels' Descending Qi Function
- Tonifies the Kidney Yin

Middle Dantians, entering into the mouth and medulla oblongata of the Brain.
- The Luo-Connecting Vessel of the Conception Vessel originates from the Jiuwei CV-15 point (Bottom Gate of the Middle Dantian) and disperses over the Yellow Court region.

Clinical Manifestations

The functions and clinical uses of the patient's Conception Vessel are described as follows (Figure 6.18).

1. Tonifies and nourishes Yin energy (especially in women after menopause) and harmonizes the Lungs and Kidneys.
2. Regulates the energy of the reproductive system, tonifies the Blood and Yin, and reduces the effects of Heart Empty-Heat symptoms (night sweating, hot flashes, anxiety, irritability, insomnia, and dizziness, etc.) developed from Kidney Yin Deficiency after menopause.
3. Promotes Blood supply to the Uterus and regulates menstrual disorders (dysmenorrhea, menorrhagia, amenorrhea, and metrorrhagia).
4. Moves the Qi in the Lower Burner and treats abdominal lumps, as well as myomas, fibroids, and carcinoma in the woman's Uterus, and hernia in men.
5. Stimulates the energetic interaction of the Lung Channels' descending Qi function and the Kidneys' function of receiving and holding the Lung Qi. Asthma, for example, is a common symptom of this type of imbalance.
6. Tonifies and nourishes Kidney Yin

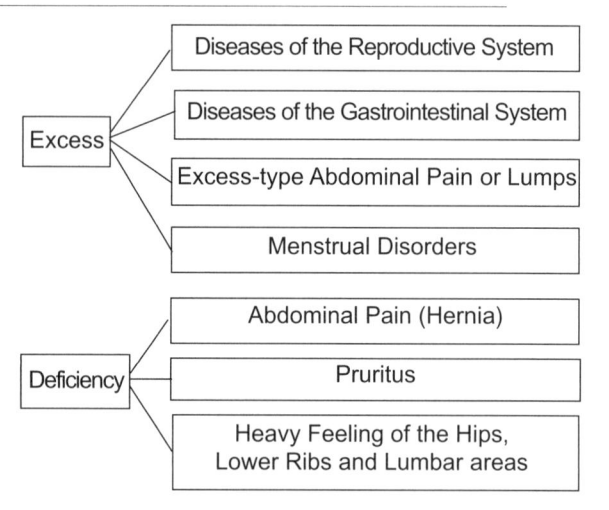

Figure 6.19. Pathological Manifestations of the Conception Vessel (CV)

Excess:
- Diseases of the Reproductive System
- Diseases of the Gastrointestinal System
- Excess-type Abdominal Pain or Lumps
- Menstrual Disorders

Deficiency:
- Abdominal Pain (Hernia)
- Pruritus
- Heavy Feeling of the Hips, Lower Ribs and Lumbar areas

Pathological Manifestations

The main diseases associated with energetic imbalances in the Conception Vessel are described as follows (Figure 6.19):

1. **Symptoms of Excess** include diseases of the reproductive and gastrointestinal systems such as hemorrhoids, diarrhea, decreased urination, abdominal hernia.
   - In men, problems in the Conception Vessel can lead to impotence and sterility.
   - In women, problems in the Conception Vessel can cause menstrual difficulties such as menoxenia, profuse leukorrhea, and dysmen-

orrhea. Other female problems associated with Excess energy in the Conception Vessel include breast pain, sterility, miscarriage, paralysis after delivery, and emaciation, as well as disorders of the external genitalia, vulva, vagina, and cervix.

2. **Symptoms of Deficiency** include abdominal pains (hernia) and pruritus, as well as a heavy feeling in the hips, lower ribs, and lumbar area.

THRUSTING AND BELT VESSELS: CHONG AND DAI MAI

The Thrusting (Chong) and Belt (Dai) Vessels balance the energies of the external tissues, internal organs, and Taiji Pole. The Thrusting and Belt Vessels maintain internal and external energetic balance, and harmonize excess or deficient conditions by evenly dispersing the Qi throughout the body.

The Thrusting Vessel can be likened to a magnet wrapped with the copper wire of the Belt Vessel. In this way, the body is like an electromagnet, connecting the positive and negative ends of the Taiji Pole to the energetic generators of Heaven and Earth. The power of the human energetic field is thus increased exponentially.

THE THRUSTING VESSELS: CHONG MAI

The word Chong translates as "street" and expresses the idea of passing or penetrating through something. In ancient China, the character meant to march, surge, rush against, clash, pour out, infuse, flush and soar. The ideograph for Chong Mai is described as follows (Figure 6.20):

- The first ideograph is the Chinese character "Chong," is composed of one radical "Xing," which can be divided into two parts. Positioned on the left is the character for walking. Positioned on the right is the character for "person" or "human." The translation for this character is to walk or step forward. Positioned in the center of the ideograph is the phonics radical for "chong," composed of three parts: "Earth", positioned on the bottom; "field", located at the center; and "dry" on top. As a whole, the character can be translated to mean "passing or

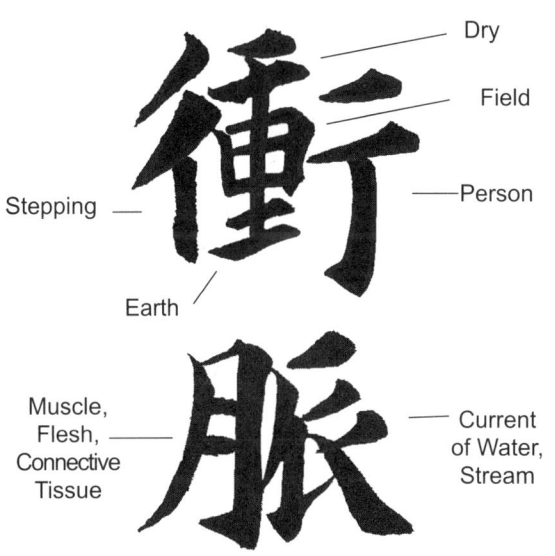

Figure 6.20. Chinese Ideograph for "Chong Mai," the Thrusting Vessel

penetrating through a dry field."

- The second character is the Chinese ideograph "Mai," which is generally translated as "vessel." It is composed of two characters: the character to the left, "Ji" depicts the Chinese ideogram for body tissue, muscle or flesh (all of which are forms of connective tissue). The character on the right "Mai" depicts a current of water, stream, or branch of a river. As a whole, the character can be translated as arteries, veins or pulse, indicating a form of energetic circulation.

DEVELOPMENT

The Thrusting Vessels' action of "passing through" refers to their function as the vital pathway for alchemical transformation. The Thrusting Vessels are the primary channels used to produce the energetic transformations constantly occurring between Jing, Qi and Shen. The Thrusting Vessels are also called the "Penetrating Channel," and it is regarded as both the Sea of Blood and the Sea of the Twelve Primary (Regulating) Channels. It regulates both the Qi and Blood of all Twelve Primary Channels and extends to the anterior, posterior, upper, and lower parts of the body. The Thrusting Vessel possess the function of blending the energetic influences of Heaven (Yang) and Earth (Yin). During the development of the embryo, the Thrusting Vessels are responsible for the development of the adrenal glands and the adrenal cortex.

The Thrusting Vessels originate in the Lower Dantian. The Qi of the Thrusting Vessels travels upwards to the head and face, and also penetrates into the lower limbs, irrigating the body's Yin. According to some doctors of Chinese medicine, all energetic points that have Chong in their names relate to the Thrusting Vessels (i.e., Qichong St-30, Taichong St-42, and Shaochong Ht-9).

Along with the Conception Vessel, the Thrusting Vessels are responsible for regulating the changes in an individual's life cycles. These life cycles occur every eight years in men and every seven years in women. Abnormalities of the Thrusting Vessels during the beginning of pregnancy can result in the spontaneous abortion of the fetus. Abnormalities of the Thrusting Vessels during the end of pregnancy may result in an inability to expel the placenta.

The Thrusting Vessels control all aspects of menstruation, influencing the supply and amount of Blood in the Uterus, as well as nourishing the woman's Jing. They flow along the Kidney Channels and are responsible for tightening the abdominal muscles and the penis.

Together, the Governing, Conception and Thrusting Vessels are considered to be the energetic gateway of an individual's ancestry, and the link to his or her ancestral skills and knowledge.

ENERGETIC PATHWAY

The Thrusting Vessels originate from the Lower Dantian, and specifically in the Uterus in females. It is composed of five energetic branches, described as follows (Figure 6.21):

- The Primary Channels of the Thrusting Vessels originates in the Lower Dantian (the center of the Uterus in women) and emerges at the Huiyin CV-1 point of the perineum (bottom gate of the Lower Dantian). From the perineum, the Primary Channel ascends the bottom of the abdomen to the top of the inner thighs (level with of the superior border of the pubic symphysis), surfacing at the Qichong St-30 points. From there, the Primary Channel travels upwards alongside the Kidney Channels, doubling the energetic potential. It then surrounds and enters into the umbilicus (front gate of the Lower Dantian). The channel further ascends from the abdomen alongside the chest, flowing into the Yellow Court and disperses into the Sea of Qi and into the Upper Burner located in the center of the chest.

- The First Branches of the Thrusting Vessels originate from the Yellow Court and ascend in two columns upwards through the Heart and Middle Dantian areas. They continue to ascend through the throat, encircle the lips and energetically connect with the Governing and Conception Vessels. The first branches of the Thrusting Vessels terminate on each side of the nasal cavity. The *Yellow Emperor's Magical Pivot* states that "the energy rising in the Thrusting Vessels emerges from the nasopharynx, and filters into all the Yang, irrigating all of the essences." When the Thrusting Vessels are full and overflowing, as happens through prayer and meditation, they radiate a sparkling white-light energy, which extends from the upper chest to the eyes.

- The Second Branch of the Thrusting Vessels originates in the Lower Dantian (the center of the Uterus in women), and travels to the lower aspect of the Kidneys. From the Kidneys, it descends, fusing into a single channel and terminates into the perineum (bottom gate of the Lower Dantian). From the perineum, it again divides into two branches and descends along the medial aspect of the thighs and into the popliteal fossa behind the knees. From behind the knees it buries itself and circulates to the tibias, where together with the Kidney channels, it descends to penetrate behind the internal aspect of the medial malleolus at the ankles. At the junction of the ankles it branches again, terminating along the Kidney channels at the bottom of the feet. This detachment, along with the Kidney channels, filters into the three Yin channels of the legs.

- The Third Branches of the Thrusting Vessels originate from the Second Branches along the tibias and obliquely penetrate the malleolus, where they connect and move along the top

CHAPTER 6: THE EIGHT EXTRAORDINARY VESSELS

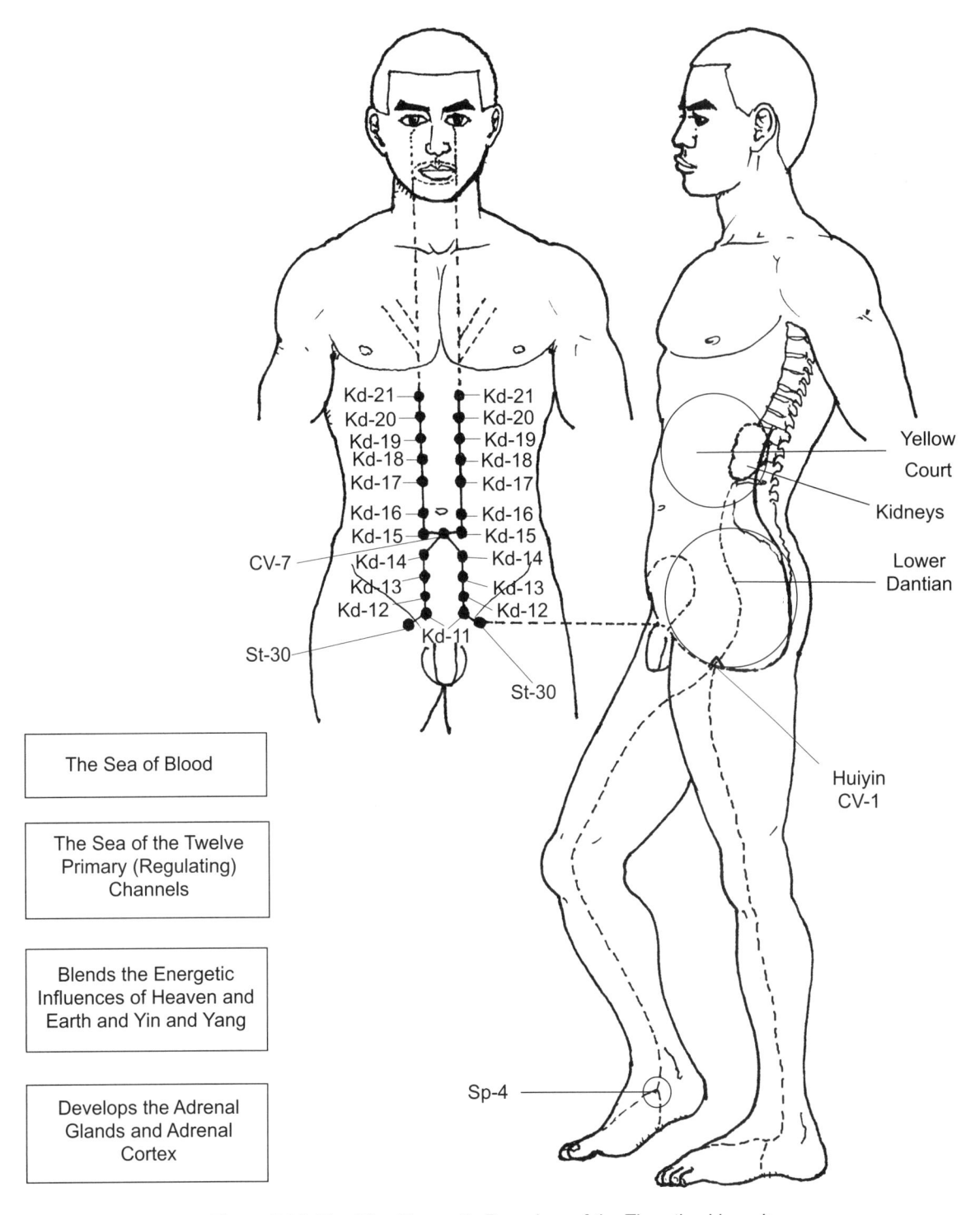

Figure 6.21. The Five Energetic Branches of the Thrusting Vessels

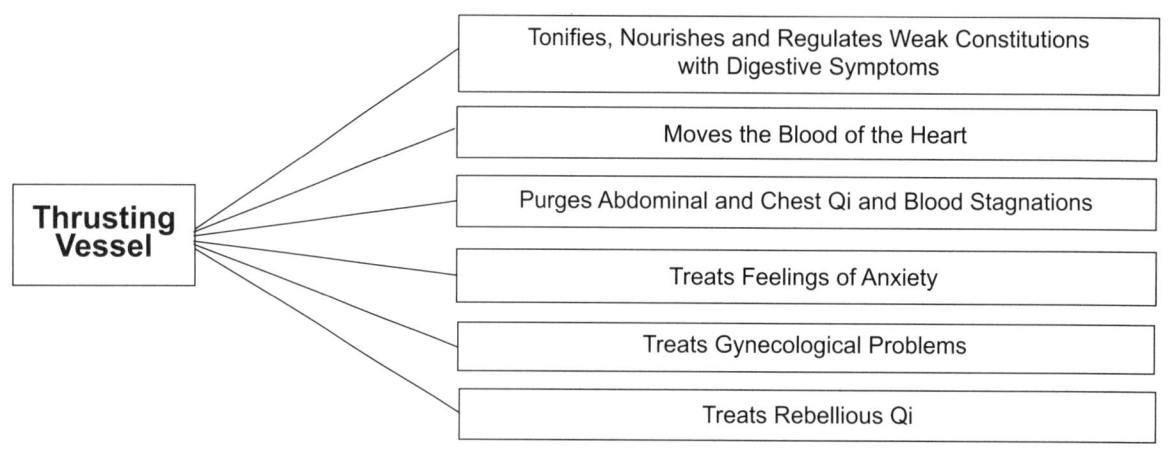

Figure 6.22. The Functions and Clinical Uses of the Thrusting Vessel

of the feet, terminating between the big toes.
- The Fourth Branch of the Thrusting Vessel originates from the Primary Channel in the pelvic cavity. It moves backwards along the lower perineum to enter the spinal column, traveling up the back, intersecting with the Mingmen (back gate of the Lower Dantian) and Shendao (back gate of the Middle Dantian).

Clinical Manifestations

The functions and clinical uses of the Thrusting Vessels are described as follows (Figure 6.22):
1. Tonifies, nourishes, and regulates weak constitutions with digestive symptoms (such as abdominal distension, poor appetite, and poor assimilation of food).
2. Moves the Blood of the Heart and relieves symptoms of pain and stiffness of the chest. This function is due to the Thrusting Vessels ability to control all of the Blood in the connecting channels.
3. Purges Abdominal and Chest Qi and Blood Stagnation.
4. Treats feelings of anxiety (within the chest) caused by Rebellious Qi. One of the Thrusting Vessels' most important pathologies is Rebellious Qi, which is Qi that moves in the wrong direction, going upwards instead of downwards. Feelings of anxiety that arise in the patient's abdomen and ascend to the chest are especially indicative of this imbalance.
5. Treats gynecological problems (hot flashes),

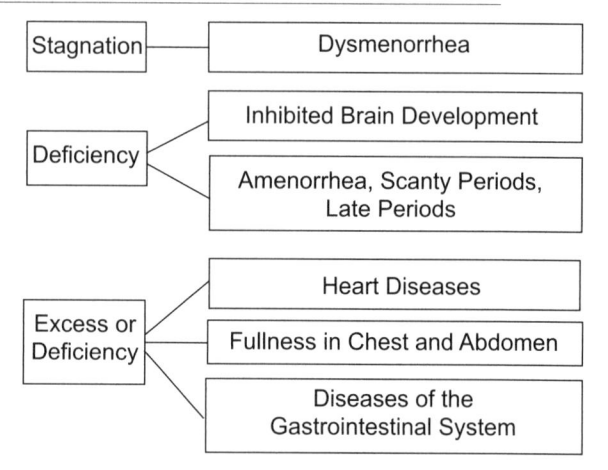

Figure 6.23. Pathological Manifestations of the Thrusting Vessel

when the Qi of the Thrusting Vessels rises upwards. This ascension of Qi can cause the patient's hands and feet to become cold, the face to get hot, and leads to a feeling of fullness in the chest. In such cases, the treatment goal is to regulate the Thrusting Vessels and subdue the Rebellious Qi. If there are accompanying emotional problems and Liver Qi stagnation, then the patient's Lv-3 points are also treated.
6. Treats Rebellious Qi caused by the upward moving energy of the Thrusting Vessels. In this type of condition, the symptoms manifest as oppressive feelings in the chest, as well as dizziness, nausea, and vomiting.

PATHOLOGICAL MANIFESTATIONS

The main diseases associated with the Thrusting Vessel are described as follows (Figure 6.23):

1. **Symptoms of Excess:** the main diseases associated with the patient's Thrusting Vessel include diseases of the Heart, fullness in the chest and abdomen, gastritis, abdominal pain, and convulsive diseases.
2. **Symptoms of Deficiency:** If the energy from the Thrusting Vessel to the cortex becomes deficient, it can inhibit the development of the Brain. If a woman's Thrusting Vessel is deficient or empty, she may develop such conditions as amenorrhea, scanty periods, or late periods.
3. **Symptoms of Stagnation:** If there is stagnant Qi and/or Blood in the Thrusting Vessel, a woman may experience dysmenorrhea. Abnormalities of the Thrusting Vessel may also result in the mother having a miscarriage.

THE BELT VESSEL: DAI MAI

The word Dai translates as a "belt" or "girdle" and refers to the action of supporting something. The ideograph for Dai Mai is described as follows (Figure 6.24):

- The first character is the Chinese ideograph "Dai," which is generally translated as "belt" or "girdle." It is composed of two parts: the top radical depicts a robe, cloak or garment. The lower radical portrays the meaning of several valuable items (usually coins and jade) being held together by a belt, ribbon or strap. The overall image of valuable items being wrapped and held together within a robe or garment suggests the meaning of a current or belt of energy binding and covering the body like a coil. This character further communicates the idea that this energetic belt is securing valuable items (energy centers, internal organs and channels) within the body.
- The second character is the Chinese ideograph "Mai," which is generally translated as "vessel." It is composed of two characters: the character to the left, "Ji" depicts the Chinese ideogram for body tissue, muscle or flesh (all

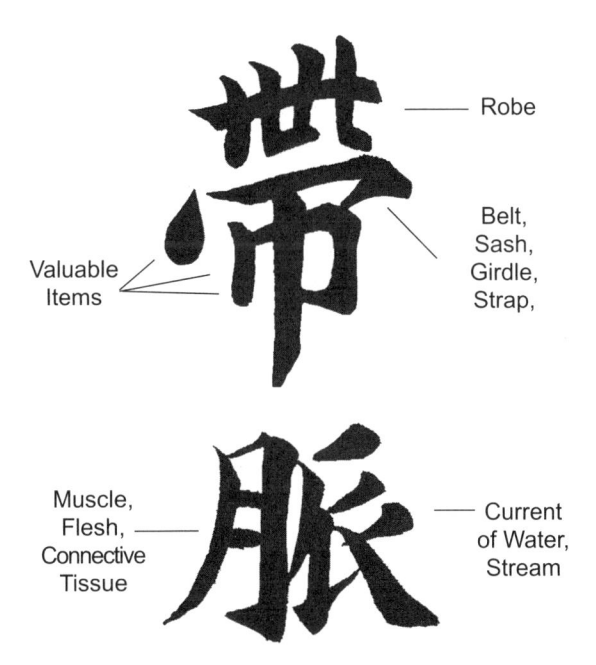

Figure 6.24. The Chinese Ideograph for "Dai Mai," the Belt Vessel

of which are forms of connective tissue). The character on the right "Mai" depicts a current of water, stream, or branch of a river. As a whole, the character can be translated as arteries, veins or pulse, indicating a form of energetic circulation.

DEVELOPMENT

The Belt Vessel is responsible for the second cellular division of the fertilized ovum in embryological development (see Chapter 2). The Belt Vessel's energetic function is to bind, join, and control all of the channels of the body, exerting an influence upon the circulation of the body's Governing and Conception Vessels. According to post-communist Traditional Chinese Medicine, the Belt Vessel is a single horizontal vessel circling the body at the waist (Figure 6.25). During the Han Dynasty (206 B.C. - 220 A.D.) it was taught that the Belt Vessel originated at the Mingmen (GV-4 point) area, and encircled the waist like a belt, dipping down into the lower abdominal region anteriorly and running across the lumbar region posteriorly. This channel connects with the GB-26, GB-

VOLUME 1, SECTION 1: FOUNDATIONS OF CHINESE ENERGETIC MEDICINE

Controls the Yin and Yang Channels

Connects and Envelops all of the leg Yin and Yang Channels

Influences the energetic actions of the genitals, waist, and hips

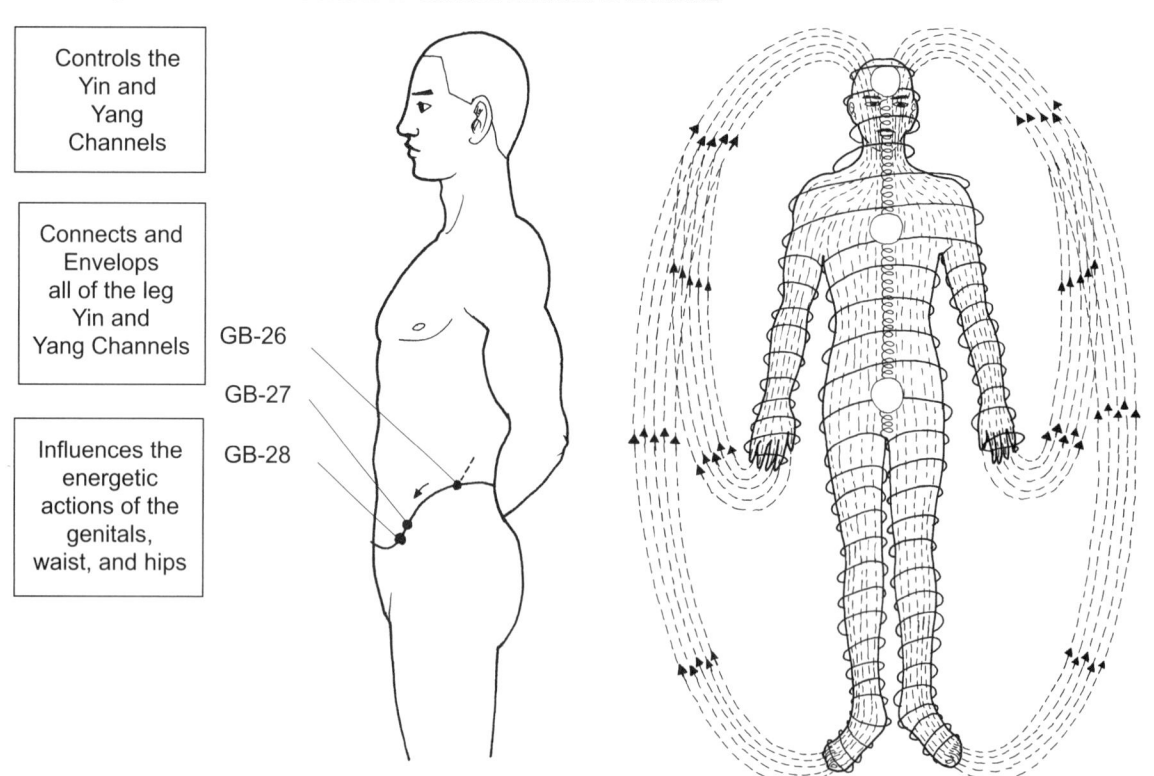

GB-26
GB-27
GB-28

Figure 6.25. During the Han Dynasty, The Belt Vessel was reduced to encircling only the center of the waist.

Figure 6.26. The ancient Daoist version of the Belt Vessel winds the body like an energetic coil.

27, and GB-28 points and crosses the Conception Vessel at CV-4. Many sources say that the Belt Channel also connects with the Liver -13 points at the free end of each 12th rib.

ENERGETIC PATHWAY

The ancient Daoist schools of Qigong training traditionally teach that the Belt Vessel originates from the Lower Dantian (Shenque CV-8 and Mingmen GV-4) and wraps the entire body like a silk cocoon or an enveloping whirlpool, flowing from the feet to the head (Figure 6.26).

The Belt Vessel can be likened to a copper wire wrapping the internal magnet of the Thrusting Vessel. In this way, the body is like an electromagnet, by connecting the positive and negative ends of the Taiji Pole to the energetic generators of Heaven and Earth. The power of the human energetic field is thus increased exponentially.

At one time, this knowledge of the horizontal energetic flow was a well-guarded secret. The ancient Daoist books on horizontal energetic flow all focused on the alchemical aspects of energetic and spiritual transformation. The main focus of these teachings concentrated on the ability of dissolving the body's Qi and Shen into the various dimensions of infinite space (Wuji) which envelop the energetic fields of Heaven, Earth and Man. These ancient books were nearly all destroyed when the Qin emperor (221 - 206 B.C.) ordered the burning of all writings containing this knowledge.

During the following Han Dynasty, only Confucianism was honored because of its focus on being obedient to the government as a means of obtaining spiritual propriety. Therefore, the "vertical" Confucian classics on energy flow were preserved while the significance of the "horizontal" energetic flow was diminished.

To the ancient Chinese, the body's waist was considered to be the hub of the energetic wheel of

262

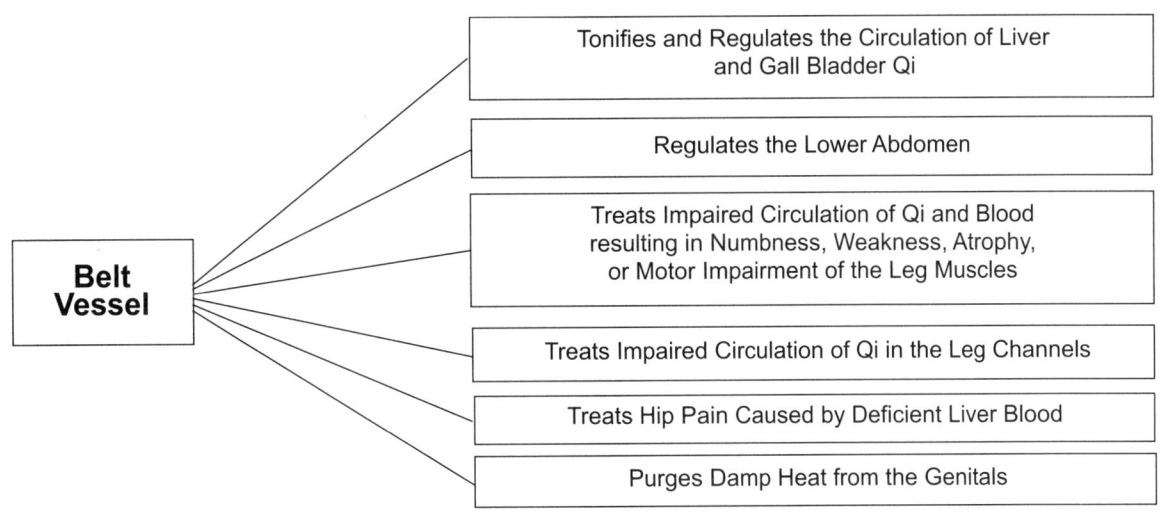

Figure 6.27. The Functions and Clinical Uses of the Belt Vessel

Belt Vessel:
- Tonifies and Regulates the Circulation of Liver and Gall Bladder Qi
- Regulates the Lower Abdomen
- Treats Impaired Circulation of Qi and Blood resulting in Numbness, Weakness, Atrophy, or Motor Impairment of the Leg Muscles
- Treats Impaired Circulation of Qi in the Leg Channels
- Treats Hip Pain Caused by Deficient Liver Blood
- Purges Damp Heat from the Genitals

the body. The access points of the Belt Vessel's center channel, which circles the waist, are commonly used to control the entire vessel, and thus the entire body. As the energy of the body increases (through Qi and Shen cultivation), the Qi within the entire Belt Vessel increases, wrapping the tissues from feet to head, and increasing the body's Wei Qi fields.

The Belt Vessel exerts an important influence on the body's physiology by encircling the leg channels. This influences the circulation of energy to and from the legs, as well as influencing the energetic actions of the genitals, waist, and hips. The Belt Vessel keeps the body's Yin and Yang channels under control, connecting all of the leg Yin and Yang channels as they traverse the body's trunk. As a result, the Belt Vessel is said to assist in regulating the circulation of Qi in all of the Yin and Yang channels of the body, especially those from the waist downward.

The Belt Vessel harmonizes the ascending and descending flow of energy from the Kidneys and Spleen through its connection with the Kidney Divergent Channel. The Belt Vessel also restrains the flow of the body's Liver and Gall Bladder Qi.

In ancient China, the Belt Vessel was used for energetically armoring and protecting the body against environmental and emotional pathogenic invasions. It was also believed to inform the individual when something was energetically or spiritually wrong, especially if he or she is out of harmony with the Dao. Thus, the loss of "life purpose" was spiritually and psychologically related to disorders of the Belt Vessel.

CLINICAL MANIFESTATIONS

The functions and clinical uses of the Belt Vessel are described as follows (Figure 6.27):

1. Tonifies and Regulates the circulation of Liver and Gall Bladder Qi due to patterns of Excess Liver Qi.
2. Regulates the lower abdomen due to a Belt Vessel imbalances that cause such symptoms as a sagging waist or bloated abdomen.
3. Treats impaired circulation of Qi and Blood that cause numbness, weakness, atrophy, or motor impairment of the leg muscles. This can be due to a deficiency of energy in the Stomach and Spleen Channels.
4. Treats impaired circulation of Qi in the leg channels resulting in such symptoms as cold legs and feet or tense leg muscles (gastrocnemius and tibiales). This condition is due to Liver Blood not moistening the sinews of the legs, and is thus improved through the Belt Vessel's influence on the Liver, as well as its influence on the flow of Qi in the legs.

5. Treats hip pain caused by Deficient Liver Blood (leading to sinew and joint malnourishment and Excess Liver Yang).
6. Purges Damp Heat from the genitals that results in symptoms such as difficulty urinating or burning during urination.

PATHOLOGICAL MANIFESTATIONS

The main diseases associated with the Belt Vessel are described as follows (Figure 6.28):

1. **Symptoms of Excess** include pain in the back (lumbar region) and sides of the lower abdomen, as well as weakness in the shoulders, upper extremities, and lower limbs. Symptoms may also include weakness in the opposite sides of the body (e.g., eye, breast, ovary, etc.) and a feeling of heaviness in the body and abdomen ("as if carrying 5,000 coins") all due to exposure to Dampness.
2. **Symptoms of Deficiency** include physical sensations similar to that of "sitting in cold water" up to the waist. This description generally refers to pain, weakness, and a cold or heavy sensation in the lumbar and sacral regions. Other symptoms include umbilical, abdominal, and lumbar pain, as well as a feeling of something like a stick pressing against the groin. There can also be abdominal fullness and distention. Symptoms in women may include abnormal white vaginal discharge, or a prolapse of the Uterus.

YIN AND YANG HEEL VESSELS: QIAO VESSELS

The word Qiao translates as "the heel" or "to stand on the toes" and refers to the action of kicking one's foot as high as possible. One text from the Shanghai College of Traditional Chinese Medicine states that the word Qiao should be translated as "nimble."

The left Yang Heel Vessel controls the Yang of the left side of the body, and the right Yang Heel Vessel controls the Yang of the right side of the body. Consequently, the left Yin Heel Vessel controls the Yin of the left side of the body, while the right Yin Heel Vessel controls the Yin of the right side of the body.

Both Yin and Yang Heel Vessels flow along the medial and lateral aspects of the lower legs and torso, connecting at the inner canthus of the eyes. They are responsible for connecting the energy of the body's Yin and Yang channels and for regulating the movement of all four limbs. They also control the amount of energy used by all the other channels in the body. Once these vessels are full, they relax the tissues, enabling the limbs to become more dexterous.

The Yin and Yang Heel Vessels are sometimes called Bridge Channels because they act like a bridge, linking the areas of the body in which Qi is stored to the areas of the body that are in need of Qi. When any channel uses more than its share of energy, other channels become deficient. Thus the Heel Vessels seek to ensure that energy is always distributed in a balanced way throughout all of the Yin and Yang channels of the body.

The Yin Heel Vessels are an offshoot of the Kidney Channels at the front of the body, while the Yang Heel Vessels are an offshoot of the Uri-

Excess
- Pain in the Back (Lumbar Region)
- Pain in Sides of the Lower Abdomen
- Weakness in the Shoulders, Upper Extremities, and Lower Limbs

Deficiency
- Pain, Weakness, and a Cold or Heavy Sensation in the Lumbar and Sacral Regions
- Umbilical, Abdominal, and Lumbar Pain
- Abdominal Fullness and Distention
- Abnormal White Vaginal Discharge and a Prolapse of the Uterus

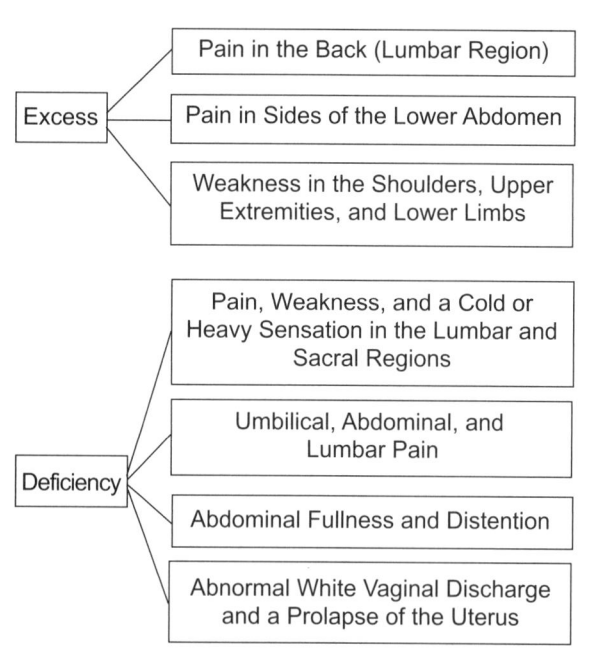

Figure 6.28. Pathological Manifestations of the Belt Vessel

nary Bladder Channels at the back of the body. Together, the Yin and Yang Heel Vessels can be used to treat structural imbalances and to harmonize the right and left sides of the body.

It is interesting to note that in ancient China, both the Kidney Channels and Urinary Bladder Channels were jointly referred to as the body's "vest." This was because the (Yang) Urinary Bladder Channels surround the (Yang) Governing Vessel, and the (Yin) Kidney Channels surround the (Yin) Conception Vessel, similar to an energetic vest.

Because the Heel Vessels cause the motor nerves to develop during the formative stages of the embryo, Traditional Chinese Medicine maintains that the Yang Heel Vessels cause boys to be more physically active (running, jumping, etc.), while the Yin Heel Vessels cause girls to be less physically active. This, in turn, suggests that the Yin and Yang Heel Vessels play a major role in establishing the secondary sex characteristics during the formative years of puberty.

In ancient China, the Heel Vessels were thought to psychologically determine who and what you are in the world. The Yang Heel Vessel relates to how you see the world (external, Yang), while the Yin Heel Vessel relates to how you see yourself (internal, Yin).

THE YIN HEEL VESSELS: YIN QIAO MAI

The ideograph depicting the Chinese characters for "Yin Qiao Mai" is described as follows (Figure 6.29):

- The first character is the Chinese ideogram "Yin," which is composed of four parts. In this particular ideograph, the character positioned on the left is generally used to describe the shady, northern watershed of a valley, hill or mound. The ideograph positioned to the right is translated as "Yin," and is composed of three parts. The character positioned on the bottom is "Yun" meaning "clouds." Located at the center is the ancient character for "Qi" meaning "energy" or "mist." Positioned at the top is the character meaning "covering." Etymologically speaking, the ideograph can be translated to mean "the dark, shady side of a hill or river bank."

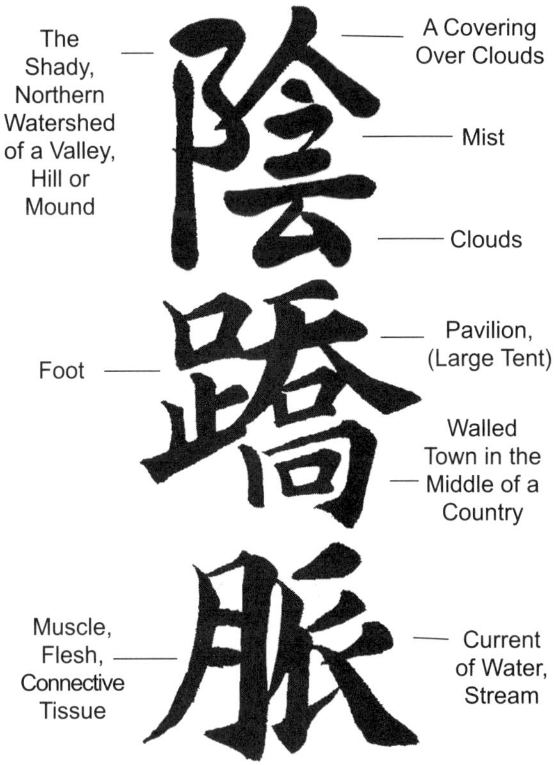

Figure 6.29. The Chinese Ideograph for "Yin Qiao Mai," the Yin Heel Vessel

- The second character is the Chinese ideogram for "Qiao," which is generally translated as Heel. It is composed of two parts. The first part positioned on the left, is the character "Zu" meaning "foot." The second part positioned on the right, is the character "Qiao" which describes a kind of pavilion (a large tent used for shelter or entertainment) and a walled town in the middle of a country.
- The third character is the Chinese ideogram "Mai," which is generally translated as "vessel." It is composed of two characters: the character to the left, "Ji" depicts the Chinese ideogram for body tissue, muscle or flesh (all of which are forms of connective tissue). The character on the right "Mai" depicts a current of water, stream, or branch of a river. As a whole, the character can be translated as arteries, veins or pulse, indicating a form of energetic circulation.

DEVELOPMENT

The Yin Heel Vessels control the Yin of the left and right sides of the body, and the motion of the lower limbs. They also nourish the eyes and control the opening and closing of the eyelids. The Yin Heel Vessels are an offshoot of the Kidney Channels at the front of the body and influence the reproductive system in both males and females, as well as the entire lower abdominal area in women.

ENERGETIC PATHWAY

The Yin Heel Vessels diverge from the Kidney Channels and begin on the medial side of the foot, distal and inferior to the medial malleolus at the Rangu Kd-2 points. They flow through the Zhaohai Kd-6 and Jiaoxin Kd-8 points before ascending to the inside of the inguinal crease and entering the reproductive organs. From the reproductive organs, the Yin Heel Vessels continue up the front of the body, through the chest to connect with the Quepen St-12 point at the throat before entering into the Renying St-9 points. From the St-9 points the vessels traverse the cheek, flowing alongside the nose to terminate at the Jingming UB-1 points (located on the inner canthus of the eyes), where they join the Urinary Bladder Channel and Yang Heel Vessels (Figure 6.30).

CLINICAL MANIFESTATIONS

The functions and clinical uses of the Yin Heel Vessels are described as follows (Figure 6.31):

1. Regulates the left and right sides of the body.
2. Treats disturbances of sleep, such as insomnia or somnolence.
3. Treats certain cases of atrophy, when the muscles of the inner aspect of the leg are loose and the outer leg muscles are tight.
4. Treats symptoms of excess conditions in the Lower Burner in women. These conditions manifest in symptoms such as abdominal distension, difficult delivery, retention of the placenta, abdominal masses or lumps, and uterine fibroids.

PATHOLOGICAL MANIFESTATIONS

The main diseases associated with the Yin Heel Vessel are describes as follows (Figure 6.32):

1. **Symptoms of Excess of the Yin Heel Vessels** occurs when Yang energy is slowed down in

- Controls the Yin of Both Sides of the Body
- Nourishes the Eyes
- Controls the Opening and Closing of the Eyelids
- Controls the Motion of the Lower Limbs
- Influences the Reproductive System
- Influences the Lower Abdomen in Women

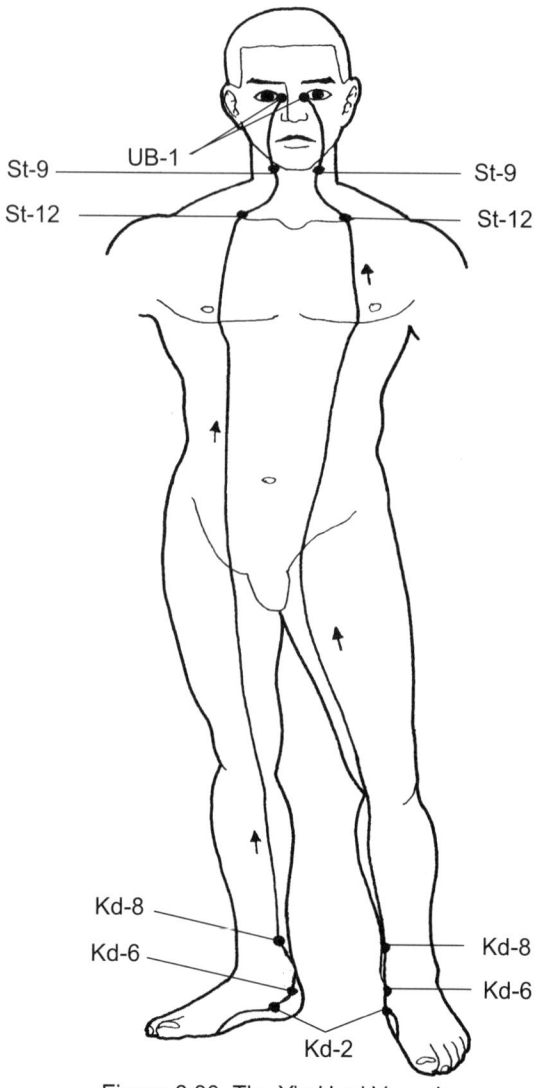

Figure 6.30. The Yin Heel Vessels

CHAPTER 6: THE EIGHT EXTRAORDINARY VESSELS

Yin Heel Vessel
- Regulates the Left and Right Sides of the Body
- Treats Disturbances of Sleep
- Treats Certain Cases of Atrophy
- Treats Symptoms of Excess Conditions in the Lower Burner in Women

Figure 6.31. The Functions and Clinical Uses of the Yin Heel Vessel

Excess
- Pain in the Lower Abdomen
- Vomiting
- Difficult Bowel Movements
- Spasms on the Medial Aspect of the Legs
- Migraine Headaches, Congestive Headaches, and Hypersomnia
- Feet and Ankles Rotate Towards the Intside of the Body

Deficiency
- Nocturnal Headaches
- Insomnia
- Cramps or Convulsions
- Feet and Ankles Rotate Towards the Outside of the Body

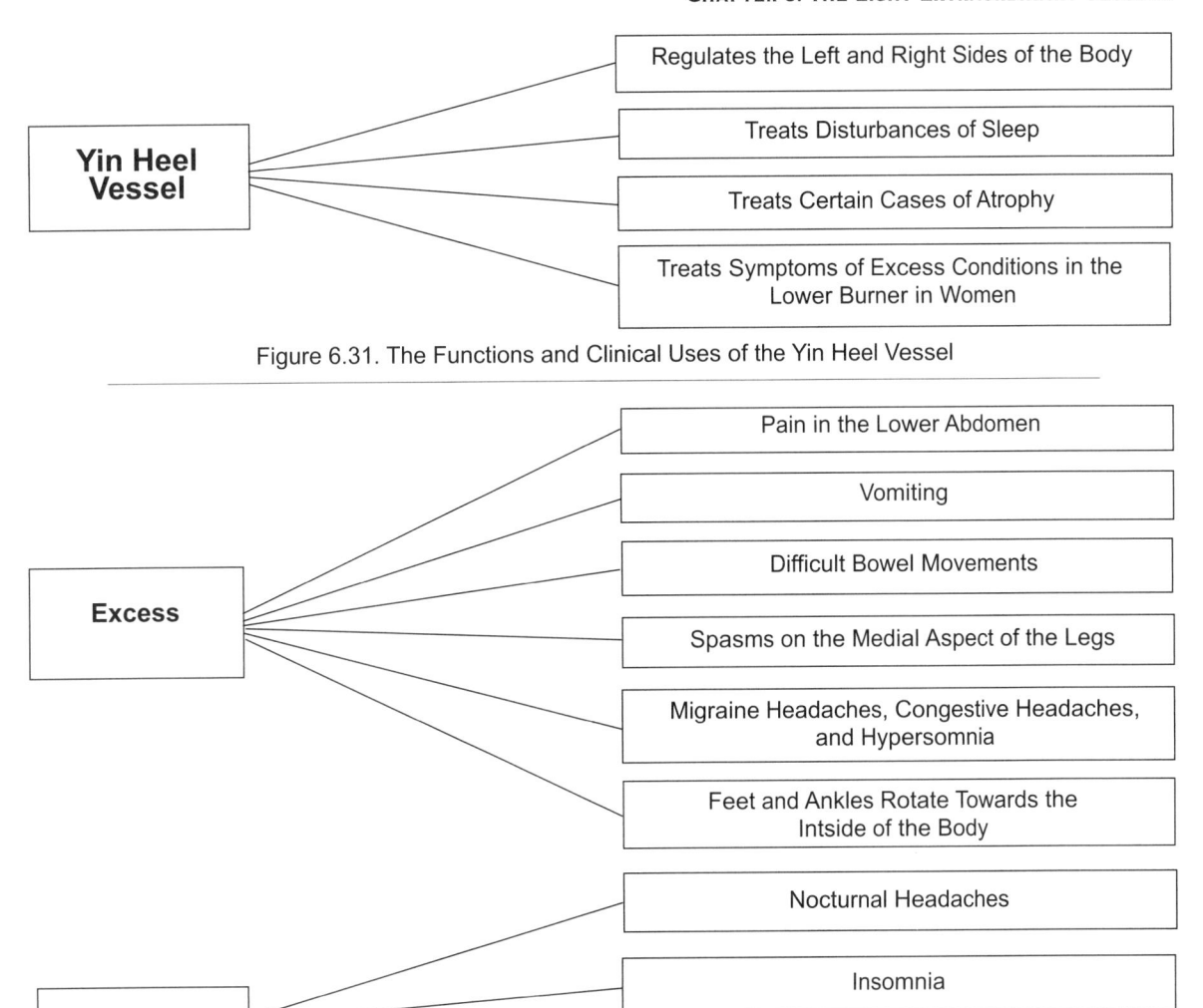

Figure 6.32. Pathological Manifestations of the Yin Heel Vessel

the Heel Vessels and the Yin energy moves more rapidly. This Excess Yin condition causes the following problems: sleepiness, hypotension, choking, painful urination, stomach rumbling, vomiting, diarrhea, difficult bowel movements, unconsciousness, lower abdominal pain and spasms on the medial aspect of the legs. Excess energy of the Yin Heel Vessels is also associated with diseases of the eyes, such as watery eyes, heavy sensations of the eyelids or an inability to open the eyes. Disorders of the Yin Heel Vessels may also result in migraine headaches, congestive headaches, and hypersomnia. Excess Yin or other abnormalities of the Yin Heel Vessels may cause pregnant women to have difficult labor. When the Yin Heel Vessels

267

are in excess, the inner leg muscles are tight, while the outer leg muscles are loose. An excess condition in the Yin Heel Vessels can cause the feet and ankles to rotate towards the inside of the body.

2. **Symptoms of Deficiency** include aggravations of symptoms during the evening time, nocturnal headaches, insomnia, cramps, or convulsions. Weakness in the Yin Heel Vessels can cause the feet and ankles to rotate towards the outside of the body.

THE YANG HEEL VESSELS: YANG QIAO MAI

The ideograph depicting the Chinese characters for "Yang Qiao Mai" is described as follows (Figure 6.33):

- The first character is the Chinese ideogram "Yang," which is composed of three parts. In this particular ideograph, the character positioned on the left is generally used to describe the sunny, southern watershed of a valley, hill or mound. The ideograph positioned to the right is translated as "Yang," and is composed of two parts. On the top right is the character "Tan" meaning "sun" above the horizon at dawn. On the bottom right is the character "Wu" meaning "sudden rays or light." The ideograph can be translated to mean "the bright, sunny side of a hill or river bank."
- The second character is the Chinese ideogram for "Qiao," which is generally translated as "heel." It is composed of two parts. The first part positioned on the left, is the character "Zu" meaning "foot." The second part position, on the right, is the character "Qiao" which describes a kind of pavilion (a large tent used for shelter or entertainment) and a walled town in the middle of a country.
- The third character is the Chinese ideogram "Mai," which is generally translated as "vessel." It is composed of two characters: the character to the left, "Ji" depicts the Chinese ideogram for body tissue, muscle or flesh (all of which are forms of connective tissue). The character on the right "Mai" depicts a current of water, stream, or branch of a river. As a whole, the

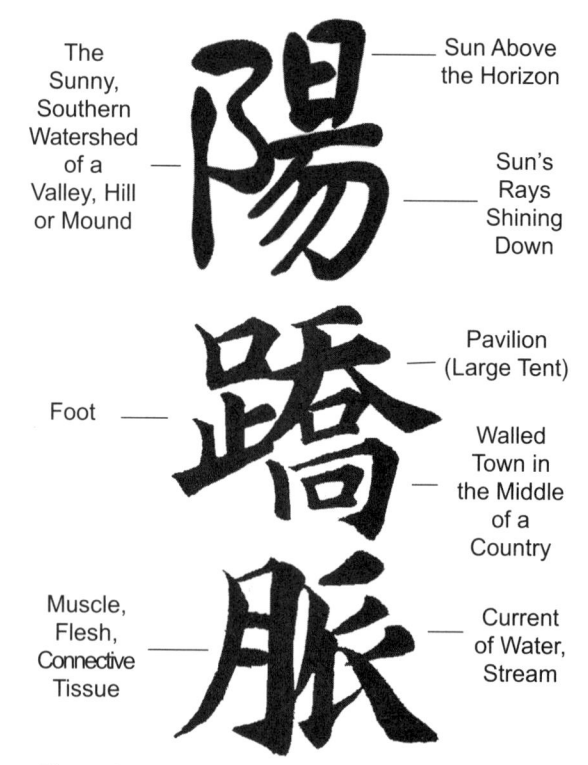

Figure 6.33. The Chinese Ideograph for the "Yang Qiao Mai," the Yang Heel Vessel

character can be translated as arteries, veins or pulse, indicating a form of energetic circulation.

DEVELOPMENT

The Yang Heel Vessels control the Yang of the left and right sides of the body. Abnormalities of the Yang Heel Vessels in newborns can cause vomiting of milk. The Yang Heel Vessels are an offshoot of the Urinary Bladder Channels which flow along the back of the body.

ENERGETIC PATHWAY

The Yang Heel Vessels divide from the Urinary Bladder Channels and begin on the lateral sides of the heels below the lateral malleolus, at the Shenmai UB-62 points. From there, the vessels travel down to the Pushen UB-61 points and then begin to ascend along the external malleolus, passing the posterior border of the fibula to transverse the lateral aspects of the thighs to connect with the Thigh-Juliao GB-29 points. They then ascend past the posterior aspects of the hypochondrium to the poste-

CHAPTER 6: THE EIGHT EXTRAORDINARY VESSELS

```
                    ┌─ Treats Acute Excess
                    │  Conditions of the Lower Back
   Yang Heel ───────┼─ Purges Internal or External
   Vessel           │  Wind from the Head
                    └─ Purges
                       Wind-Heat and Wind-Cold
```

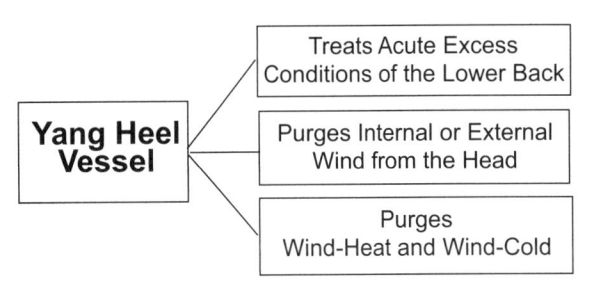

Figure 6.35. The Functions and Clinical Uses of the Yang Heel Vessel

rior axillary folds and continue to wind over the shoulders, connecting with the Naoshu SI-10, Jianyu LI-15 and Jugu LI-16 points. The Yang Heel Vessels ascend from the shoulders, passing from the lateral to the medial aspects of the neck, to enter the face where they connect with the Dicang St-4, Nose-Juliao St-3, and Chengqi St-1 points. From the St-1 points, the vessels enter the inner canthus of the eyes at the Jingming UB-1 points, where they communicate with the Yin Heel Vessels. From the UB-1 points at eyes, they join the flow of the Urinary Bladder Channels, traveling upwards to terminate at the forehead and join the Gall Bladder Channels at Fengchi GB-20 located at the back of the head, below the occiput (Figure 6.34).

CLINICAL MANIFESTATIONS

The functions and clinical uses of the patient's Yang Heel Vessel are described as follows (Figure 6.35):

1. Treats acute excess conditions of the lower back, manifesting in symptoms, such as aches due to spasm or invasion of Cold and pain along the Urinary Bladder Channels of the legs.
2. Purges Internal Wind or External Wind from the head, manifesting in symptoms such as facial paralysis, severe dizziness, and aphasia).
3. Purges Wind-Heat and Wind-Cold manifesting in symptoms such as sneezing, headache, runny nose, and stiff neck.

PATHOLOGICAL MANIFESTATIONS

The main diseases associated with the Yang Heel Vessels are described as follows (Figure 6.36):
1. **Symptoms of Excess in the Yang Heel Vessels** occurs when Yin energy is slowed within the Heel Vessels and the Yang energy moves more

```
Controls the Yang of Both Sides of the Body

Controls the Motion of the Foot and Ankle
```

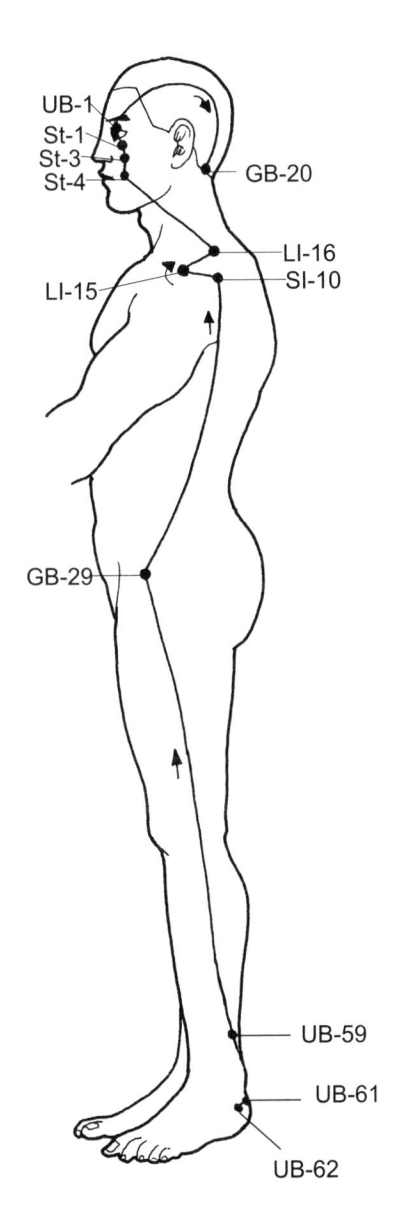

Figure 6.34. Side View of the Left Yang Heel Vessel

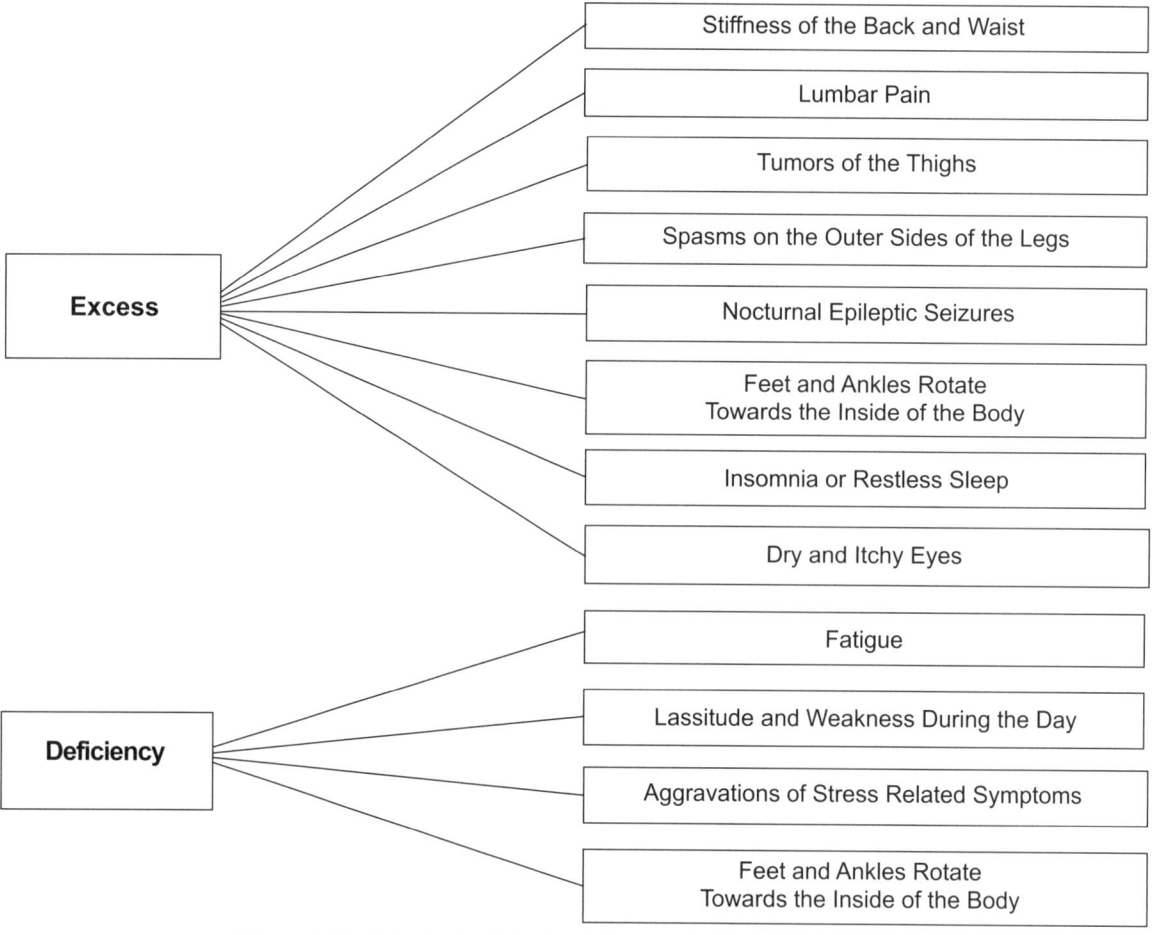

Figure 6.36. Pathological Manifestations of the Yang Heel Vessel

Excess:
- Stiffness of the Back and Waist
- Lumbar Pain
- Tumors of the Thighs
- Spasms on the Outer Sides of the Legs
- Nocturnal Epileptic Seizures
- Feet and Ankles Rotate Towards the Inside of the Body
- Insomnia or Restless Sleep
- Dry and Itchy Eyes

Deficiency:
- Fatigue
- Lassitude and Weakness During the Day
- Aggravations of Stress Related Symptoms
- Feet and Ankles Rotate Towards the Inside of the Body

rapidly. The Excess Yang causes the following problems: hypertension, lumbar pain, spasms on the outer sides of the legs, stiff back and waist (inability to bend down), tumors of the thighs, sever colds, spontaneous sweating, headaches, head sweating, nose bleeding, deafness, nocturnal epileptic seizures, insomnia or restless sleep, swelling of the body, pain in the joints, and paralysis of the arms and legs. Excess energy in the Yang Heel Vessels can also cause the vomiting of milk in infants. The Yang Heel Vessels are also involved with diseases of the eyes such as dry eyes, difficulty in closing the eyes, painful eyes and itchy eyes. When the Yang Heel Vessel is in excess, the inner leg muscles are loose and the outer leg muscles are tight. Excess in the Yang Heel Vessels can cause the feet and ankles to rotate laterally.

2. **Symptoms of Deficiency in the Yang Heel Vessels** include fatigue, lassitude and weakness during the day, and aggravated stress related symptoms during the day. These symptoms improve as the night progresses. Weakness in the Yang Heel Vessels can cause feet and ankles to rotate medially.

According to some Traditional Chinese Medical Classics, if epilepsy occurs during the daytime, Qigong and moxa are given on the Yang Heel Vessels; however, if epilepsy occurs at night, Qigong and moxa are given on the Yin Heel Vessels.

Yin and Yang Linking Vessels: Wei Vessels

The Linking Vessels are sometimes called the Wei Mai or Regulator Channels. The Linking Vessels are divided into Yin and Yang energetic pathways.

The Yin Linking Vessel maintains and communicates with all of the Yin channels of the body, while the Yang Linking Vessel maintains and communicates with all of the Yang channels of the body.

Both Yin and Yang Linking Vessels start at the lower legs and flow upwards to the head, along the medial and lateral aspects of the lower legs and torso. When the Yin and Yang Linking Vessels reach the neck and back of the head, they join the Conception and Governing Vessels, respectively.

Secondary vessels, called the Yu (surplus) Mai, branch away from each Yin and Yang Linking Vessel to connect the energetic flow of each vessel with the hands.

Instead of serving as streams transporting Qi and Blood, these two vessels act as lakes, storing the Qi and Blood that overflow from other vessels. Together, these four vessels help regulate the entire body's circulation of Qi and Blood, store the overflowing Qi and Blood, and release the Qi and Blood into the channels in the event of deficiencies.

In ancient China, the Yin and Yang Linking Vessels were considered to be responsible for the energetic and spiritual manifestations of the Jing Shen being reflected in an individual's life.

The Yin Linking Vessel: Yin Wei Mai

The ideograph depicting the Chinese characters for "Yin Wei Mai" is described as follows (Figure 6.37):

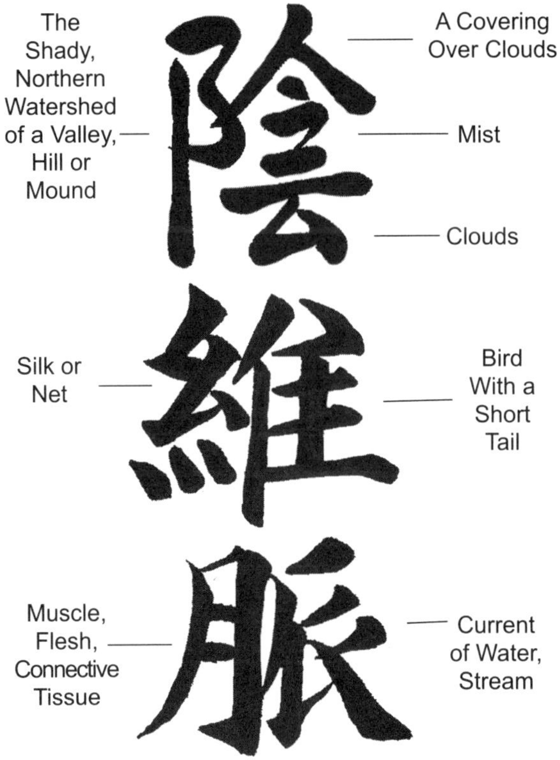

- The first character is the Chinese ideogram "Yin," which is composed of four parts. In this particular ideograph, the character positioned on the left is generally used to describe the shady, northern watershed of a valley, hill or mound. The ideograph positioned to the right is translated as "Yin," and is composed of three parts. On the bottom is "Yun" meaning

Figure 6.37. The Chinese Ideograph for "Yin Wei Mai," the Yin Linking Vessel

"clouds." Located at the center is the ancient character for "Qi" meaning "energy" or "mist," and positioned on top is the character meaning "covering." The ideograph can be translated to mean "the dark, shady side of a hill or river bank."

- The second character is the Chinese ideogram "Wei," which is generally translated as "to link or bind." Wei is composed of two parts: positioned to the left is the radical "Mi," used for silk, net or string-like objects. It depicts threads that have been twisted together to form a net, and refers to a silk rope that is tied around something, pulling and securing it, or the wrapping and enveloping of a silk net. On the right is the character "Zhui." This radical was used in ancient China to describe a particular type of bird with a short tail. In ancient China, this character originally represented the enveloping of a bird caught in a net, and by extension, came to

mean the containment of the "four limbs" and "four directions."
- The third character is the Chinese ideograph "Mai," which is generally translated as "vessel." It is composed of two characters: the character to the left, "Ji" means body tissue, muscle or flesh (all of which are forms of connective tissue). The character on the right, "Mai" depicts a current of water, stream, or branch of a river. As a whole, the character can be translated as arteries, veins or pulse, indicating a form of energetic circulation.

DEVELOPMENT

The Yin Linking Vessels (Yin Wei Mai) lie on the medial axis of the body. They help maintain the connection between all of the Yin Channels.

The Yin Linking Vessels are responsible for moving the Yin energy, regulating the Blood, and regulating the internal parts of the body. They connect with all of the body's Primary Yin Channels: Liver, Heart, Spleen, Lung, Kidney, and Pericardium.

ENERGETIC PATHWAY

The Yin Linking Vessels originate in the Kidney Channels. They are composed of two main energetic branches, described as follows (Figure 6.38):

- The Primary Channels of the Yin Linking Vessels originate in the Kidney Channels from the medial sides of the legs, at the Zhubin Kd-9 points. From there they ascend along the medial aspect of the thighs to the abdomen where they communicate with the Spleen Channels at the Fushe Sp-13, Daheng Sp-15 and Fuai Sp-16 points at the chest. They ascend to the Qimen Lv-14 points and move toward the front of the body along the sides of the chest to the center of the nipples at the Ruzhong St-17 points where the vessels split into two sets of branches. The Primary Channels continue to ascend, connecting with the Conception Vessel at the Tiantu CV-22 point at the base of the throat and terminating at the Liangquan CV23 point located on the midline of the neck.
- The First Branches of the Yin Linking Vessels (sometimes called the Yin Yu Vessels) origi-

| Moves the Yin Energy |
| Regulates the Blood |
| Regulates the Internal Parts of the Body |
| Maintains Connections with All the Body's Primary Yin Channels |

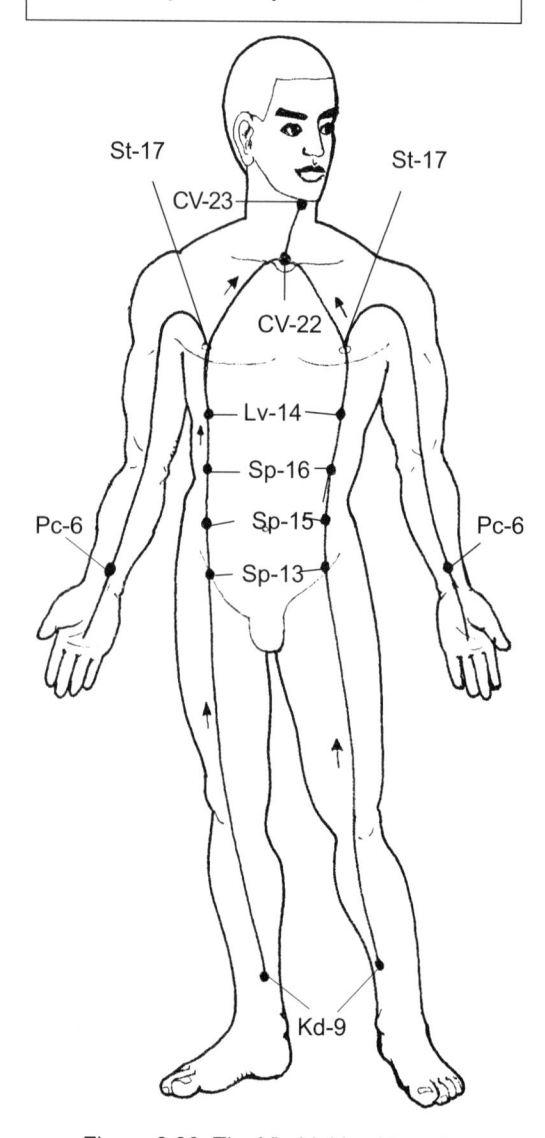

Figure 6.38. The Yin Linking Vessels

nate at the Ruzhong St-17 points located at the center of the nipples. They ascend from the chest, winding over the shoulders, and down the inside of the arms following the route of the Pericardium Channels. Each branch energetically pools at the Neiguan Pc-6 points just above the wrist folds on each arm, before flowing into the palms. The Neiguan Pc-6 points are therefore considered to be the Master Points for the Yin Linking Vessels.

CLINICAL MANIFESTATIONS

The functions and clinical uses of the patient's Yin Linking Vessel are described as follows (Figure 6.39):

1. Tonifies the Heart and is especially effective for symptoms of pain, stiffness, tightness and oppression in the chest, as well as depression, anxiety, apprehension, and nightmares.
2. Treats Deficient Yin and Blood conditions, especially if accompanied by psychological symptoms such as mental restlessness, anxiety, and insomnia.
3. Treats headaches that are located in the back of the neck due to Blood Deficiency.

PATHOLOGICAL MANIFESTATIONS

The main diseases associated with the Yin Linking Vessel are describes as follows (Figure 6.40):

1. **Symptoms of Excess in the Yin Linking Vessels** occur when the Yin energy is slowed within the Linking Vessels and the Yang energy moves more rapidly. Therefore, if the Yin Linking Vessels become unbalanced, the Excess Yang condition can cause the patient to suffer from diseases of the Heart, such as hypertension, delirium, cardialgia (tightness and oppression in the chest) and nightmares. Imbalances in the Yin Linking Vessels can also lead to dyspnea, difficulty in swallowing, convulsive diseases, contracted feeling in the lungs, prolapse of the rectum, and diarrhea.
2. **Symptoms of Deficiency in the Yin Linking Vessels** include timidity or fear, apprehension, nervous laughter, depression, hypotension, and weak respiration.

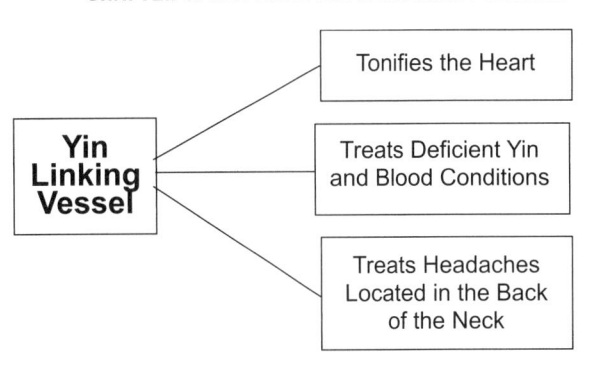

Figure 6.39. The Functions and Clinical Uses of the Yin Linking Vessel

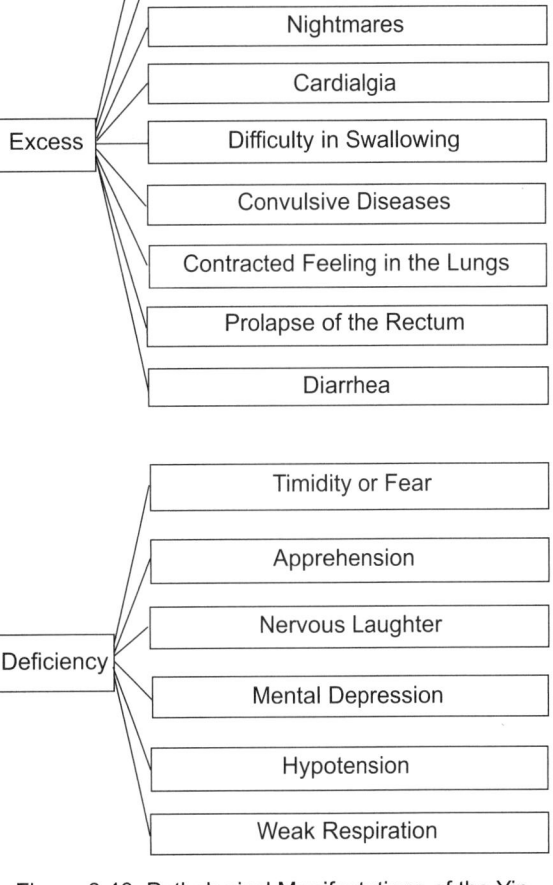

Figure 6.40. Pathological Manifestations of the Yin Linking Vessel

The Yang Linking Vessels: Yang Wei Mai

The ideograph depicting the Chinese characters for "Yang Wei Mai" is described as follows (Figure 6.41):

- The first character is the Chinese ideogram "Yang," which is composed of three parts. In this particular ideograph, the character positioned on the left is generally used to describe the sunny, southern watershed of a valley, hill or mound. The character positioned to the right is translated as "Yang," and is composed of two parts. On the top right is the character "Tan" meaning "sun above the horizon at dawn." On the bottom right is the character "Wu" meaning "sudden rays or light." The ideograph can be translated as "the bright, sunny side of a hill or river bank."

- The second character is the Chinese ideogram "Wei," which is generally translated as "to link or bind." Wei is composed of two parts: positioned to the left is the radical "Mi," meaning silk, net or string-like objects. It depicts threads that have been twisted together to form a net, and refers to a silk rope that is tied around something, pulling and securing it; or the wrapping and enveloping of a silk net. On the right, is the character "Zhui," this radical was used in ancient China to describe particular type of bird with a short tail. This character originally represented the enveloping of a bird caught in a net, and by extension, came to mean the containment of the "four limbs" and "four directions."

- The third character is the Chinese ideogram "Mai," which is generally translated as "Vessel." It is composed of two characters: the character to the left, "Ji" depicts the Chinese ideogram for body tissue, muscle or flesh (all of which are forms of connective tissue). The character on the right, "Mai" depicts a current of water, stream, or branch of a river. As a whole, the character can be translated as arteries, veins or pulse, indicating a form of energetic circulation.

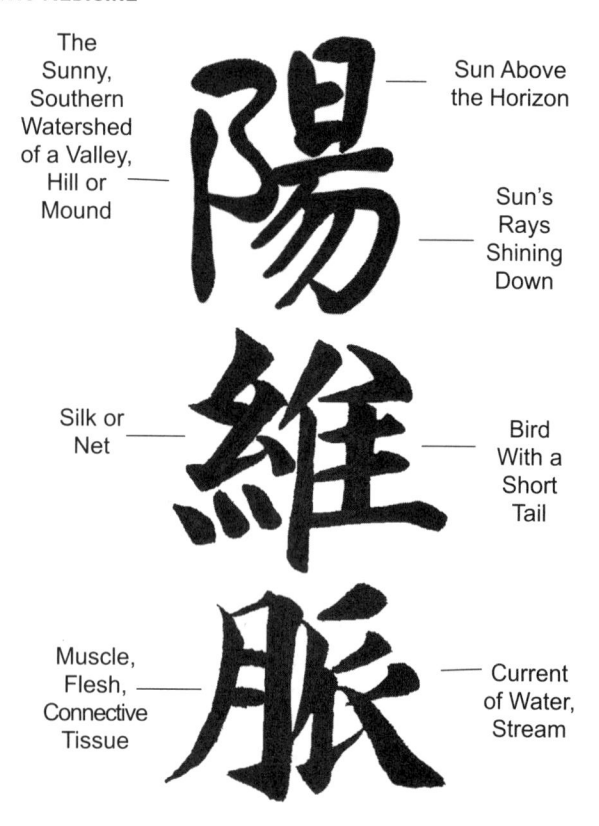

Figure 6.41. The Chinese Ideograph for "Yang Wei Mai," the Yang Linking Vessel

Development

The Yang Linking Vessels lie on the lateral aspects of the body. They serve to maintain and communicate with all of the Yang Channels on the exterior portion of the lateral aspects of the body.

The Yang Linking Vessels are responsible for moving the Yang energy and controlling the Protective (Wei) Qi by regulating its resistance to external infections, and regulating the external parts of the body. They connect with all of the body's Primary Yang Channels: Gall Bladder, Small Intestine, Stomach, Large Intestine, Urinary Bladder, and Triple Burners.

Energetic Pathway

The Yang Linking Vessels originate in the Urinary Bladder Channel. They are composed of two main energetic branches, described as follows (Figure 6.42):

- The Primary Channels of the Yang Linking Vessels originate in the Urinary Bladder Channels at the external part of the ankles, just below the lateral malleolus at the Jinmen UB-63 points. From UB-63 they join with the leg Gall Bladder Channels, and ascend into the Yangjiao GB-35 points. They continue ascending the lateral aspect of each leg, passing through the outside of the hips, and moving upward along the lateral aspect of the back. From there the Yang Linking Vessels flow through the hypochondriac and costal regions, to the Naoshu SI-10 points located at the posterior aspect of the axilla to the shoulders.

  The SI-10 points are the intersecting points of the Yang Linking Vessels and the Yang Heel Vessels (located on the Small Intestine Channels). From the SI-10 points, the Yang Linking Vessels split into two sets of branches. The Primary Channels flow up the sides of the neck communicating with the Tianliao TB-15 points before connecting with the Gall Bladder Channels at the Jianjing GB-21 points. From GB-21, the vessels intersect with the Touwei St-8 points above the temples and then continue to follow the Gall Bladder Channels from Benshen GB-13, Yangbai GB-14, Head-Linqi GB-15, Muchuang GB-16, Zhengying GB-17 Chengling GB-18, Naokong GB-19 and Fengchi GB-20 points (located at the lateral aspect of the head). Here, they join together to communicate with the Governing Vessel at the Back Gate of the Upper Dantian located at the Fengfu GV-16 point before terminating at the Yamen GV-15 point located at the lower occipital region of the head.

- The First Branches of the Yang Linking Vessels (sometimes called the Yang Yu Vessels) originate at the SI-10 points located on the posterior aspect of the shoulders. They extend from the shoulders down the back sides of the arms following the route of the Triple Burner Channels. Just above both wrists on the outside of each arm, each branch pools at the Weiguan TB-5 points before flowing into the back of the hands. The TB-5 points are there-

Moves the Yang Energy

Controls and Regulates the Wei Qi

Regulates the External Parts of the Body

Maintains Connections with All the Primary Yang Channels

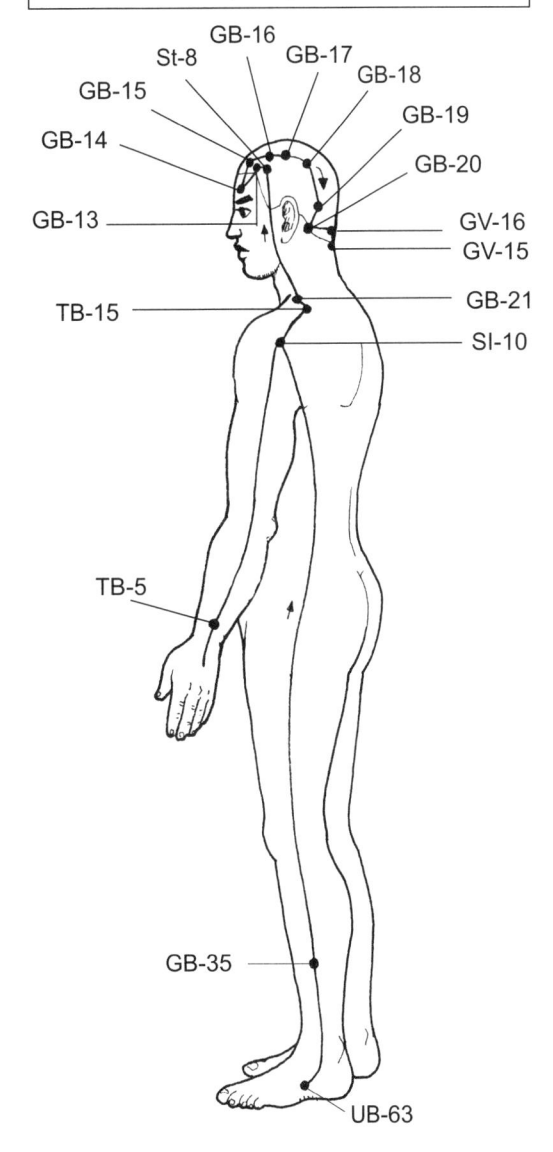

Figure 6.42. Side View of the Left Yang Linking Vessel

```
                    ┌─────────────────────────────────────────────────────┐
                  ┌─│ Treats Ear Problems Due to Rising Liver Fire        │
                  │ └─────────────────────────────────────────────────────┘
                  │ ┌─────────────────────────────────────────────────────┐
                  ├─│ Treats Ear Diseases Due to Gall Bladder Disharmony  │
                  │ └─────────────────────────────────────────────────────┘
┌──────────┐      │ ┌─────────────────────────────────────────────────────┐
│  Yang    │      ├─│ Treats Hypochondriac Pain                           │
│ Linking  │──────┤ └─────────────────────────────────────────────────────┘
│  Vessel  │      │ ┌─────────────────────────────────────────────────────┐
└──────────┘      ├─│ Treats Sciatic Pain in the Lateral Aspects of the Legs │
                  │ └─────────────────────────────────────────────────────┘
                  │ ┌─────────────────────────────────────────────────────┐
                  └─│ Treats Intermittent Fevers That Alternate Between   │
                    │ Chills and Fever                                    │
                    └─────────────────────────────────────────────────────┘
```

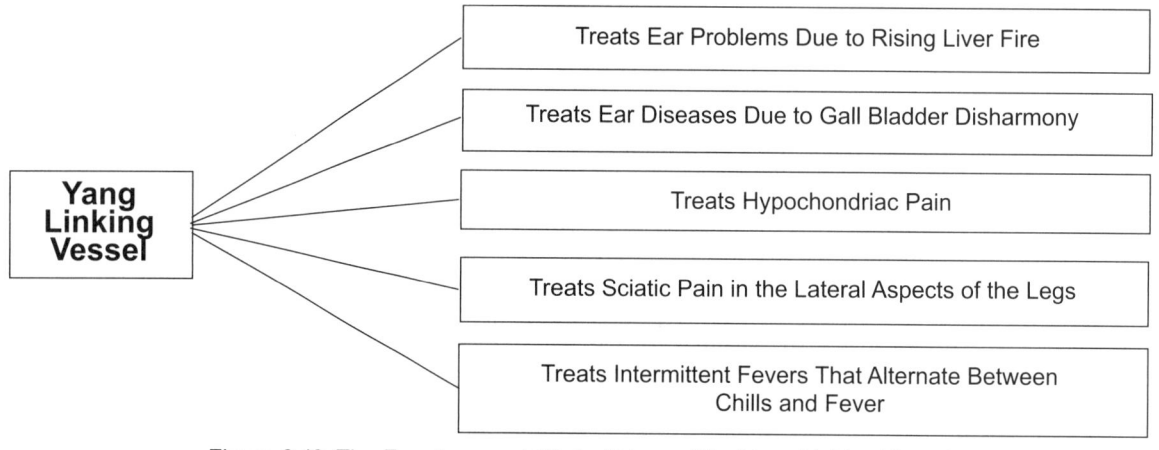

Figure 6.43. The Functions and Clinical Uses of the Yang Linking Vessel

fore considered the Master Points for the Yang Linking Vessels.

CLINICAL MANIFESTATIONS

The functions and clinical uses of the patient's Yang Linking Vessels are described as follows (Figure 6.43):

1. Treats ear problems such as tinnitus and deafness due to Liver Fire rising.
2. Treats ear diseases that are caused from a Gall Bladder disharmony.
3. Treats hypochondriac pain.
4. Treats sciatic pain in the lateral aspects of the legs (along the Gall Bladder Channels).
5. Treats intermittent fevers that alternate between chills and fever.

PATHOLOGICAL MANIFESTATIONS

The main diseases associated with disorders of the Yang Linking Vessel are describes as follows (Figure 6.44):

1. **Symptoms of Excess in the Yang Linking Vessels** occur when the Yang energy is slowed down in the Linking Vessels and the Yin energy moves more rapidly. Therefore, if the Yang Linking Vessels become unbalanced, the Excess Yin condition may cause the patient to catch colds and fevers more easily. Symptoms can manifest as alternating chills and fever and pain in the lateral sides of the head, neck, trunk, and legs. Symptoms can also include pains and skin problems that arise or worsen during weather changes, sensitivity to changes in climate (aching muscles, skin rashes, etc.), swelling, pain and fever in the joints, diarrhea, and night sweats.
2. **Symptoms of Deficiency in the Yang Linking Vessels** include coldness, loss of energy, and a lack of physical strength. Symptoms also include cold knees, stiffness, and fatigue (especially during cold or rainy weather).

SUMMARY OF EIGHT EXTRAORDINARY VESSELS

The Eight Extraordinary Vessels link together all of the Yin and Yang Channels in the body, and are thus able to regulate the flow of energy in these channels to maintain a state of balance. The clinical significance of the Eight Extraordinary Vessels manifests through certain pathological indications that are specific to the vessels' intersection with their particular Primary Channel. Their symptomatology is therefore not distinct from, but rather a composite of, the pathological symptoms associated with their joining primary channel.

A summery of the combined functions of the Eight Extraordinary Vessel Master-Couple Points is listed in Figure 6.45.

The Eight Extraordinary Vessels' energetic pathways used in certain esoteric Qigong meditations are somewhat different from those found in Traditional Chinese Medical texts and acupunc-

CHAPTER 6: THE EIGHT EXTRAORDINARY VESSELS

Excess
- Alternating Chills and Fever
- Pain on the Lateral Side of the Head Neck, Trunk, and Legs
- Pain and Skin Problems During Weather Changes
- Swelling, Pain and Fever in the Joints
- Diarrhea
- Night Sweats

Deficiency
- Lack of Body Heat
- Loss of Energy and Physical Strength
- Cold Knees
- Stiffness
- Fatigue

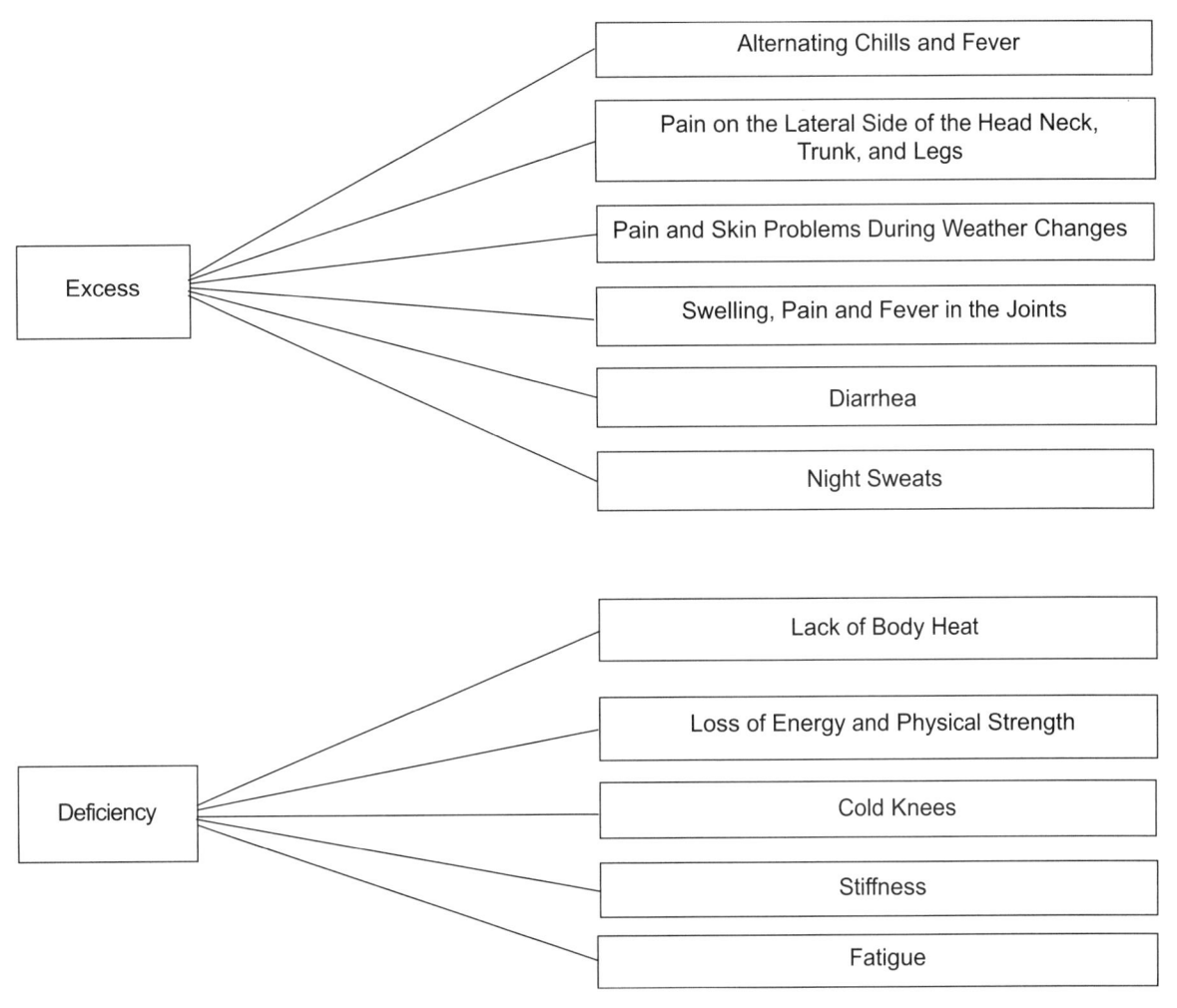

Figure 6.44. Pathological Manifestations of the Yang Linking Vessel

ture charts. The reason for this uniqueness is that their purposes are different. The goal of acupuncture is to restore sick people to health. The energetic points treated by an acupuncturist must be along the superficial channels, so that they can be activated by acupuncture needles. Medical Qigong exercises and meditations aim to maximize physical vitality and take the individual beyond physical health and toward spiritual enlightenment. In Medical Qigong treatment and training, the specific channels and points that one uses can initially be located deep within the body's tissues, since the energy is guided by the mind, postures, and movements, rather than by needles.

277

Eight Extraordinary Vessels	Pathologies
Belt (GB-41 - TB-5)	• Pain in the back, lumbar region, and sides of the navel • Weakness in the lower limbs
Conception (Lu--7 - Kd-6)	• Diseases of the reproductive and gastrointestinal systems (hemorrhoids, diarrhea, decreased urination, etc.) • In the male: sterility • In the female: menstruation problems such as leukorrhea and dysmenorrhea, breast pain, paralysis after delivery, emaciation, and sterility. All problems of the reproductive system, including internal and external genitalia (vulva, vagina, and cervix)
Governing (SI-3 - UB-62)	• Diseases of the head (apoplexy, aphasia, epilepsy, headaches, tetanus, etc.), back, neck, and Kidneys • Stiffness in the spinal column, spastic muscle movements of the extremities, night sweating, and circulatory disturbances around the anus
Thrusting (Sp-4 - Pc-6)	• Diseases of the Heart, fullness in the chest and abdomen, gastritis, abdominal pain, convulsive diseases • Brain dysfunctions of physiological origin • In womem: amenorrhea, scanty periods or late periods, dysmenorrhea, spontaneous abortion, inability to expel the placenta, menopause problems
Yang Heel (UB-62 - SI-3)	• Stiffness of the back and waist, lumbar pain, spasms on the outer side of the legs, and tumors of the thighs • Diseases of the eyes • Vomiting of milk (in newborns)
Yang Linking (TB-5 - GB-41)	• Diseases from Cold: fevers resulting in a sensitivity to changes in climate, cold knees, stiffness and fatigue; swelling, pain, and fever in the joints and extremities, and night sweating
Yin Heel (Kd-6 - Lu-7)	• Lower abdominal pain, vomiting, difficult bowel movements, and spasms on the medial side of the legs • Diseases of the eyes • Difficult labor in women
Yin Linking (Pc-6 - Sp-4)	• Diseases of the Heart (cardialgia), tightness of the chest, difficulty swallowing, and convulsive diseases • Prolapse of the rectum and diarrhea

Figure 6.45. Pathologies of the Eight Extraordinary Vessels

Chapter 7
The Six Extraordinary Organs

Introduction

The Stomach, Large Intestine, Small Intestine, Triple Burners, and Urinary Bladder are produced by the "Qi of Heaven." These five bowels and their Qi reflect the "image of Heaven." According to the *Yellow Emperor's Inner Cannon: Su Wen*, "They (the five bowels) do not store, but make outward flow." In other words, these five "hollow" Yang organs function as temporary repositories where food is transformed and its essence is absorbed as nourishment. The clean, usable essences are directed towards the five "solid" Yin organs (Liver, Heart, Spleen, Lungs and Kidneys) and body's inner core. The turbid wastes are then discharged to the exterior of the body.

The ancient Chinese Daoists believed that the Heavens govern all forms of energetic movement by controlling the transformation, development, circulation and distribution of energy. These energetic actions allow for the expansion and ascension of Qi. Once the energy has reached a crescendo, the Heavens then express their energetic form by descending through the manifestation of "rain" allowing for the development and formation of Jing, Qi and Shen.

The *Yellow Emperor's Inner Cannon: Su Wen* states, "The Brain, Marrow, Bones, Blood Vessels, Gall Bladder and the Uterus are produced by the "Qi of the Earth." These six organs store the Yin. They are produced by and reflect the "image of the Earth;" therefore, they store and do not dispel. Their name is "Qi Heng Zhi Fu." In other words, these Six Extraordinary Organs function as Yin organs in their capacity to store Jing, Qi, Shen, Blood, Marrow and Body Fluids.

The ancient Daoists believed that the Earth governs all energetic movement by keeping, storing, binding and condensing. The Earth then manifests and expresses its energetic form by releasing Qi, allowing it to rise upwards like a mist to form clouds within the Heavens. Similarly, the Six Extraordinary Organs keep, store, bind, and condense the Jing, Qi, Shen, Blood, Marrow and Body Fluids, later distributing them like a mist throughout the body to nourish the tissues.

Chinese Characters for the Extraordinary Organs: Qi Heng Zhi Fu

The ideographs depicting the Chinese characters for the Extraordinary Organs "Qi Heng Zhi Fu" are described as follows (Figure 7.1):

- The first character depicts the Chinese ideogram for Qi, which in this instance means "extraordinary." It can also be translated as surprising, strange and marvellous. It is depicted

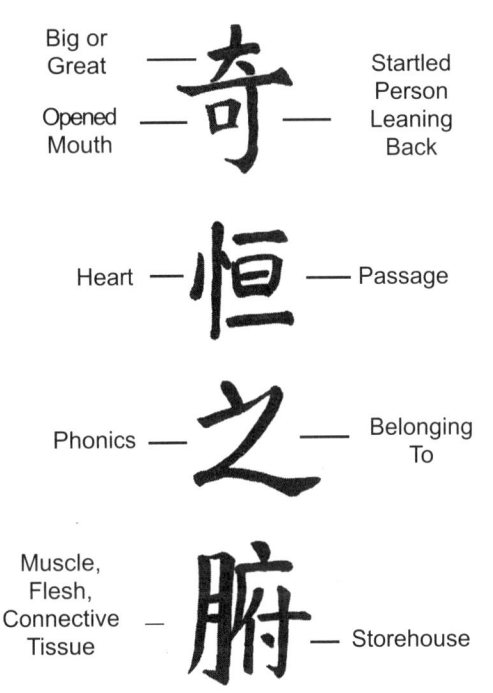

Figure 7.1. The Chinese characters for "Qi Heng Zhi Fu," the Extraordinary Organs

- Big or Great — Startled Person Leaning Back
- Opened Mouth
- Heart — Passage
- Phonics — Belonging To
- Muscle, Flesh, Connective Tissue — Storehouse

by two characters: positioned on the top is a character depicting big or great. The bottom character has two parts, with a character depicting a startled person falling backwards (bottom right) with their mouth open (bottom left), uttering an exclamation of surprise. The complete ideograph depicts a startled person discovering something strange yet wonderful.

- The second character is the Chinese ideogram "Heng," which can be translated as permanent or lasting. It is depicted by two characters. Positioned on the left is the Heart radical. The right portion of the ideograph depicts a passage, or something crossing between two sides. The combined meaning of these two radicals suggests the Heart's perpetual movement between two things of balance, and are expressed as perseverance.
- The third character is "Zhi," which can be translated as "belonging to."
- The fourth character depicts the Chinese ideogram for "Fu," and is composed of two characters. The character to the left, "Ji" means body tissue, muscle or flesh (all of which are forms of connective tissue). The character on the right can be translated as storehouse, treasury, palace or mansion. Together, both characters represent the body's internal organs as treasure houses within the flesh.

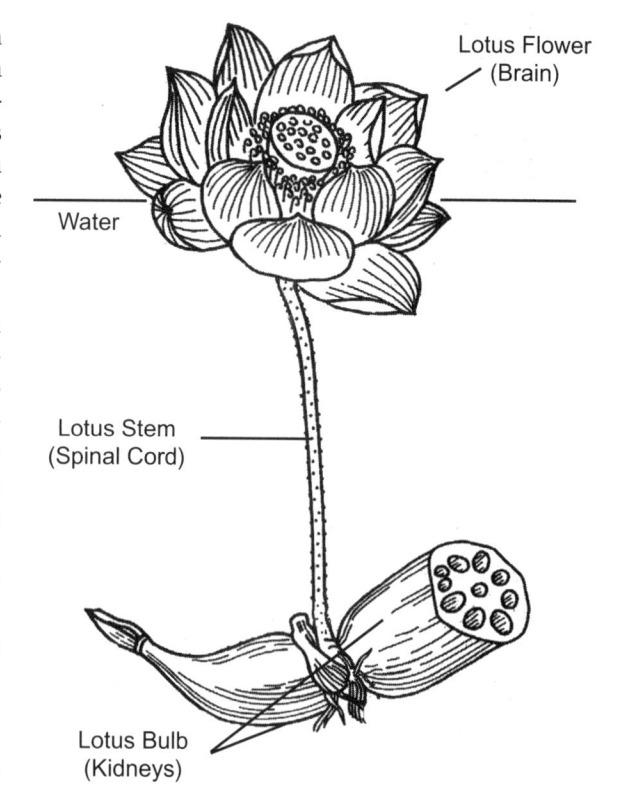

Figure 7.2. The mother's and father's essence compose the formation of the Kidneys (Lotus Bulb), Sea of Marrow, which includes the spinal cord (Lotus Stem) and brain (Lotus Flower).
(Inspired by the original artwork of Lilian Lai Bensky).

FUNCTIONS OF THE SIX EXTRAORDINARY ORGANS

The Six Extraordinary Organs are constantly functioning to maintain health, and are an essential aspect of the body's energetic matrix. Similar to the Eight Extraordinary Vessels, they regulate the specific activities needed to stabilize and harmonize the body's vitality when:

- The body's energetic structures become deficient
- The body has been attacked by External Pathogenic Factors

The energetic matrix of the Six Extraordinary Organs also functions as a entry portal to the body's "original pattern," or the DNA blueprint contained within the body's Jing. For centuries, the ancient Daoists used these energetic structures to communicate with the "original female," accessing different states of consciousness and leading to advanced energetic and spiritual transformations.

The ancient Daoists taught that as the human body forms, two spirits (the composite of the mother's Jing, Qi and Shen and the composite of the father's Jing, Qi and Shen) interlock, uniting to form Prenatal Jing. This Prenatal Essence leads to the formation of the Kidneys (Lotus Bulb), Sea of Marrow, which includes the spinal cord (Lotus Stem) and Brain (Lotus Flower) (Figure 7.2). During embryonic development, the Bones form the structural framework of the body, and the Blood Vessels begin to nourish the developing tissues.

CHAPTER 7: THE SIX EXTRAORDINARY ORGANS

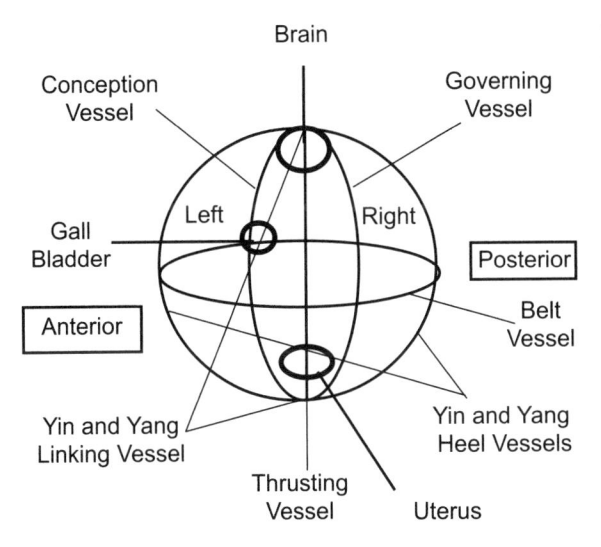

As the tissues form, the Eight Extraordinary Vessels regulate the energetic functions of the body's Six Extraordinary Organs (Figure 7.3). Because the Eight Extraordinary Vessels are the first vessels (or channels) to form in the developing fetus, they are responsible for saturating the Six Extraordinary Organs with the energy of the Four Seas, even after the baby is born (Figure 7.4).

THE EIGHT EXTRAORDINARY VESSELS AND THE SIX EXTRAORDINARY ORGANS

The body's Eight Extraordinary Vessels (Governing Vessel, Conception Vessel, Thrusting Vessel, Belt Vessel, Yin and Yang Heel Vessels, and Yin and Yang Linking Vessels) integrate the Six Extraordinary Organs with the body's six main Yang organs, and with the Kidneys. The Eight Extraordinary Vessels draw their energy from the Kidneys, and are responsible for storing and circulating the body's Jing Qi throughout the tissues, particularly to the skin, hair and Six Extraordinary Organs.

Figure 7.3. As the tissues form, the Eight Extraordinary Vessels regulate the energetic functions of the body's Six Extraordinary Organs.

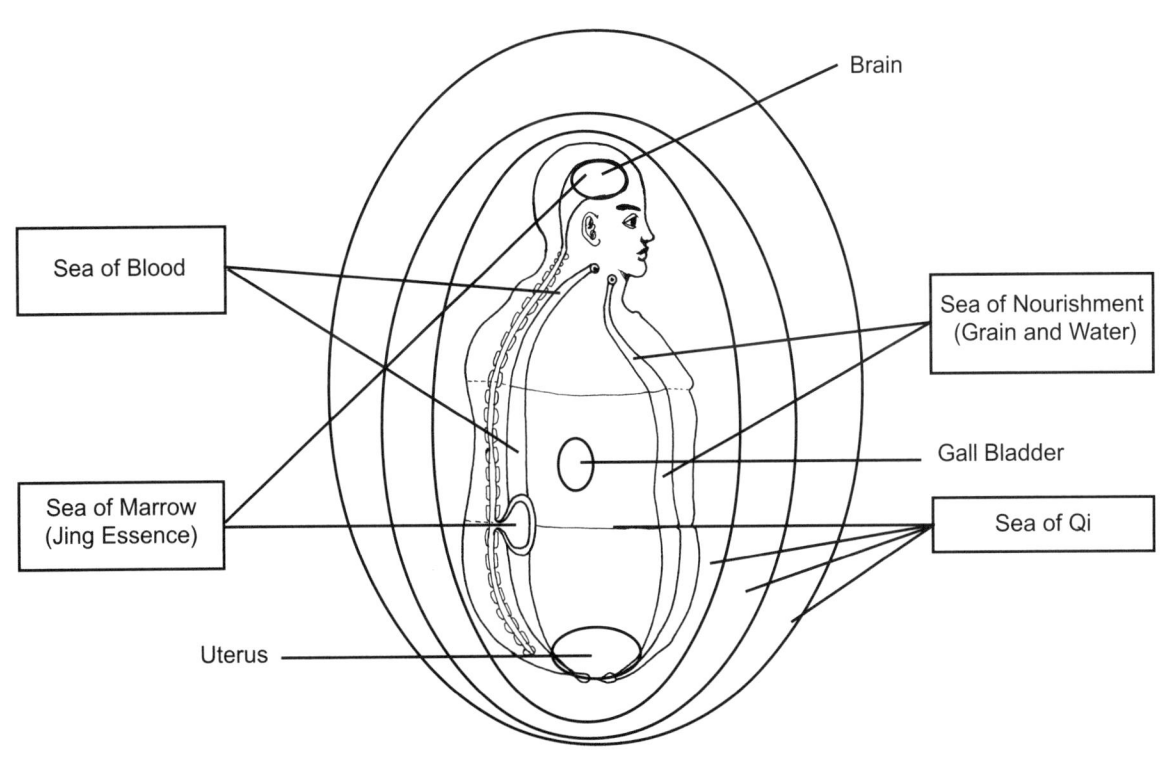

Figure 7.4. The Six Extraordinary Organs are Absorbed into the Four Seas

The Yin aspect of the body's Kidney Jing gives rise to the formation of Marrow. The Marrow flows through the body like a thick sea, pulsating slowly between the lower sacrum and the cranium. Part of the energy of the Sea of Marrow stays within the confines of the Kidney's energetic system, congealing to form the cerebral spinal fluid and Brain. Another portion of the Marrow extends outward from the spine, congealing to form the Bone Marrow, and eventually contributing to the formation of the Blood. Since the Marrow, Bones and Brain are all formed and maintained by the Kidney's Jing, they all are governed by the Kidneys.

The energy of the Six Extraordinary organs is linked to the body's internal energy systems via the Eight Extraordinary Vessels, described as follows (Figure 7.5):

1. The Uterus is regulated by the Thrusting and Conception Vessels.
2. The Brain is regulated by the Governing Vessel and the Yin and Yang Heel Vessels.
3. The Gall Bladder is regulated by the Belt Vessel.
4. The Marrow is regulated by the Thrusting Vessels.
5. The Bones are regulated by the Thrusting and Conception Vessels.
6. The Blood Vessels are regulated by the Thrusting Vessels.

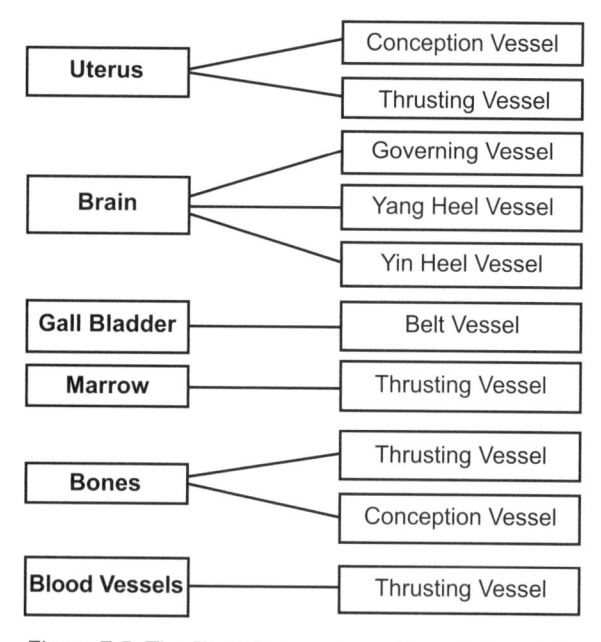

Figure 7.5. The Eight Extraordinary Vessels Regulate the Internal Energy Flow of the Six Extraordinary Organs

THE UTERUS: BAO

Several classical dictionaries translate "Bao" as the Uterus. However, the word Bao in Chinese Medicine refers to both the physical and energetic structure within which the embryo develops.

CHINESE CHARACTER FOR UTERUS

The ideograph depicting the Chinese characters for the Uterus "Bao" is described as follows (Figure 7.6):

- The Chinese character "Bao" is composed of two images. To the left, "Ji" depicts the Chinese ideogram for body tissue, muscle or flesh (all of which are forms of connective tissue). The character on the right means to wrap, and refers to a bag or sack. Together these characters depict the Uterus and represent an embryo

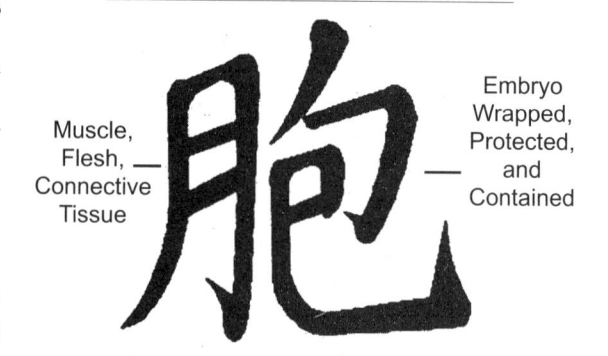

Figure 7.6. The Chinese character for "Bao," Uterus

wrapped, protected, and contained inside the mother's abdomen. In ancient China, the character for Bao was occasionally used to refer to the urinary bladder, placenta, or Uterus.

FUNCTION OF THE UTERUS

The Uterus is shaped like an inverted pear and is anatomically located in the lower abdomen of the female, behind the Urinary Bladder and in front of the rectum. It is a female reproductive organ, with its lower opening connected to the

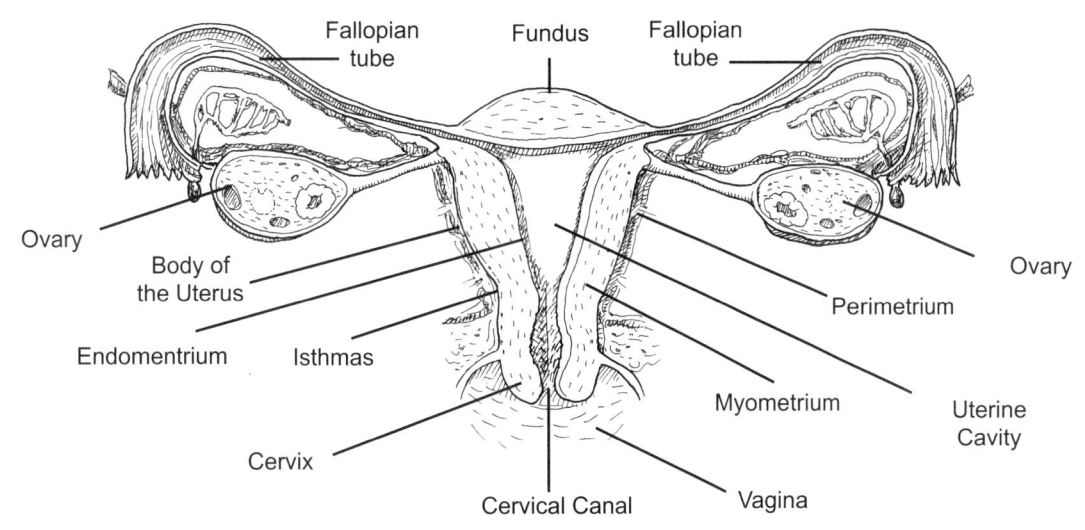

Figure 7.7. The Female Reproductive Organs, including the Uterus, Fallopian Tubes, and Ovaries (Inspired by the original artwork of Dr. Frank H. Netter).

vagina via the cervix (Figure 7.7).

In Chinese medicine, the term Uterus encompasses the woman's entire internal genital system including the fallopian tubes and ovaries. Its main physiological functions, that of regulating menstruation, conception, and pregnancy, are described as follows (Figure 7.8):

1. **Regulating Menstruation:** The Uterus is the organ by which a woman forms her menses. In ancient China, is was believed that a girl's Kidney Qi nourishes the Uterus, increasing the size of her womb into full maturation by the time she reaches the age of 14. Under the influence of "Tian Gui" (the tenth Heavenly Stem), her Conception Vessel flourishes to become more unobstructed, her Thrusting Vessel flourishes, her Sea of Blood becomes fuller and she begins her menses. It was also believed that at the time when the Kidney Jing became rich in essence, the energetic influence of "Tian Gui" (the tenth Heavenly Stem) would promote the discharge of the ovum and Blood. Tian Gui is the "Yin Water" Heavenly Stem of "Earlier Heaven," and represents the energetic regathering of new life-force associated with Kidney Yin. Tian Gui energetically moves "underground" and is considered to be the Yin Water of the congenital constitution. Being invisibly cultivated, it awaits

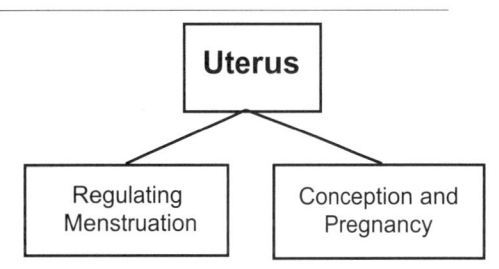

Figure 7.8. The Two Functions of the Uterus

a new breakthrough. In old age, as the Qi of the Kidneys begins to weaken, the Tian Gui begins to dry, causing menopause in women.

The three Yin organs of the Heart, Liver, and Spleen also energetically connect to the Uterus through their relationships with the Blood. The Heart governs the Blood. The Liver stores the Blood and regulates the volume of circulating Blood, which is responsible for normal menstruation. The Spleen controls the Blood.

Generally, when a woman reaches the approximate age of 49 her Kidney Qi has weakened because the "Tian Gui" in her body has become exhausted. At this point, both her Conception and Thrusting Vessels close and become obstructed creating menstrual irregularities until menopause occurs.

2. **Conception and Pregnancy:** Once a woman's Uterus becomes fully developed and she be-

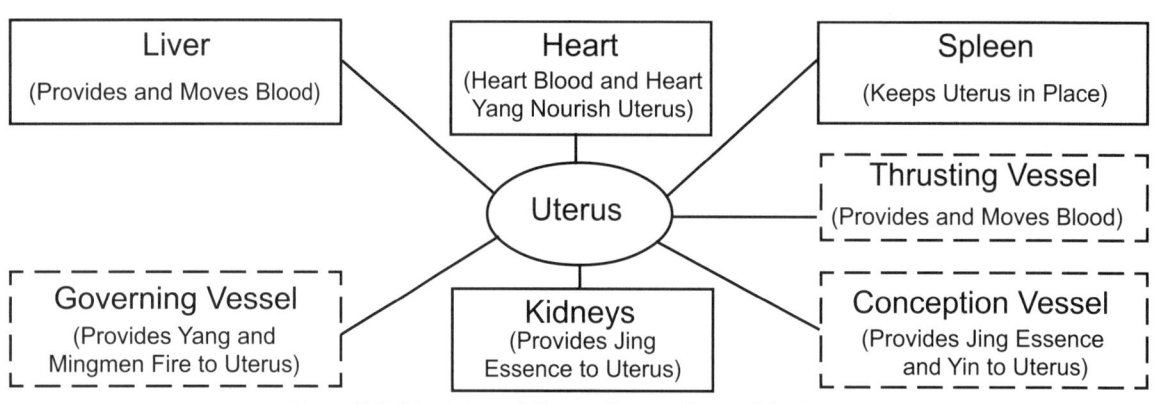

```
┌─────────────────┐    ┌──────────────────────┐    ┌─────────────────┐
│      Liver      │    │        Heart         │    │     Spleen      │
│ (Provides and   │    │ (Heart Blood and Heart│   │ (Keeps Uterus   │
│  Moves Blood)   │    │  Yang Nourish Uterus)│    │   in Place)     │
└─────────────────┘    └──────────────────────┘    └─────────────────┘
                                  │
                              ╭───────╮           ┌─ ─ ─ ─ ─ ─ ─ ─ ─ ─┐
                              │Uterus │           │ Thrusting Vessel  │
                              ╰───────╯           │ (Provides and     │
                                                  │  Moves Blood)     │
                                                  └─ ─ ─ ─ ─ ─ ─ ─ ─ ─┘
┌─ ─ ─ ─ ─ ─ ─ ─ ─ ─┐  ┌──────────────────┐      ┌─ ─ ─ ─ ─ ─ ─ ─ ─ ─┐
│ Governing Vessel  │  │     Kidneys      │      │ Conception Vessel │
│ (Provides Yang and│  │ (Provides Jing   │      │ (Provides Jing    │
│ Mingmen Fire to   │  │  Essence to      │      │  Essence and Yin  │
│    Uterus)        │  │    Uterus)       │      │    to Uterus)     │
└─ ─ ─ ─ ─ ─ ─ ─ ─ ─┘  └──────────────────┘      └─ ─ ─ ─ ─ ─ ─ ─ ─ ─┘
```

Figure 7.9. The Internal Organ Connections of the Uterus

gins her menses, an egg is released from her ovary and she can become pregnant. With each ovulation, either the right or left ovary will release a fertile egg. This release generally alternates, with the right ovary releasing an egg one month and the left ovary the next.

The physiological functions of a woman's Uterus are connected to the energetic functions of the Heart, Liver, Spleen, and Kidneys, as well as to the Conception and Thrusting Vessels (Figure 7.9). The Uterus connects to the Kidneys (which provide the Uterus with Jing), the Conception Vessel (which provides the Uterus with Qi and nourishes the fetus), and the Thrusting Channel (which provides the Uterus with Blood). When the Jing of the Kidneys becomes sufficient, the menstrual period occurs regularly, the woman can become pregnant, and her womb is capable of nourishing a fetus. The Qi and Blood of the Twelve Primary Channels pass into the Uterus through the Thrusting and Conception Vessels, affecting the quality and regularity of menstrual cycle.

THE UTERUS AS THE HEART OF THE LOWER DANTIAN

It is important to realize that every individual was conceived and developed in the center of the Uterus, which is considered the heart of a woman's Lower Dantian. Therefore, when an individual meditates and enters the Wuji (considered the womb of the universe), it is a symbolic recreation of the process of his or her original physical and energetic formation.

From a Medical Qigong perspective (and in Daoist internal alchemy), the Earth energy is gathered in the Uterus and Lower Dantian area. The Uterus is associated with the development and formation of the fetus' tissues, thereby allowing the Eternal Soul the ability to acquire familiarity with lower vibrational resonances in order to experience life on the material plane. The Uterus is, in a very real sense, a temple for the entrance of the human soul into embodied life on this plane. The quiescent state in which the fetus developed is attainable after birth through prayer, meditation, and sleep. These three states form the foundation for the creation and tonification of Prenatal Jing, Qi, and Shen.

Given its Yin nature and close proximity to the Earth, the Lower Dantian is considered a kinesthetic or physical center of consciousness. Inside the Lower Dantian, the Uterus interacts with the energetic fields of the first three lower chakra gates. Together, the three lower chakra gates of the Lower Dantian form a downward pointing triangle energetically structured to absorb and store Earth Qi into the uterine area.

The Uterus and Lower Dantian area is the major storage area for the various types of Kidney energies (i.e., Qi of the ovaries), and it is often called the Sea of Qi. It is the place where Qi is housed, the body's Mingmen Fire is aroused, the Kidney Yin and Yang Qi is gathered, and the Yuan Qi is stored. As mentioned earlier, Yuan Qi is also known as Source Qi and is the foundation of all the other types of Qi in the body. The Yuan Qi is closely linked with the Prenatal Essence (Yuan Jing). Together, the Yuan Qi and Yuan Jing determine the individual's overall health, vitality, stamina, and life span.

THE UTERUS AND DAOIST MYSTICISM

In certain ancient Daoist texts, both men and women are described as having a Bao (or Uterus). In this context, the Bao refers to the area in which the individual energetically and spiritually grows the "primordial embryo" or "golden fetus," used for the purpose of entering other energetic and spiritual realms via soul travel. The ancient Daoists used the Bao as the primary internal organ in which to nourish and store the "golden fetus." The golden fetus is constructed of refined Ling Qi and Ling Shen, developed through specific Shengong meditations. In males, the Bao area is located within the inner chambers of the Lower Dantian.

THE BRAIN: NAO

According to the *Yellow Emperor's Inner Cannon: Su Wen*, "The Brain is Yin." Being Yin, it is the end pool and junction of all Yang Qi. The Brain functions like a lid, allowing all the vapors of Yang Qi and essence to gather and be retained within the Sea of Marrow. In ancient China, the Brain was viewed as a canopy (Gai) and was believed to attract and receive the subtle emanations of Heaven.

The body's Jing, Qi, and Shen travel from the five Zang (Yin) and six Fu (Yang) organs into the Brain, allowing the seven upper orifices (eyes, ears, nostrils, and mouth) to work. The ancient Chinese believed that the Brain was the Fu (bowel) of the Yuan Shen, allowing the influence of the Shen of the Heart and the Hun of the Liver to be present in the upper orifices and the Brain.

The Brain depends on the Heart's Blood for its nourishment. Because the Kidneys store the Jing and the Heart governs the Blood, the Brain depends on a balanced state of the Heart and Kidneys for its vitality. The Brain is considered a chamber of transformation for both Prenatal and Postnatal Essence (Jing) and Energy (Qi). The Brain is regulated by the Governing Vessel, as well as the Yin Heel Vessels and the Yang Heel Vessels.

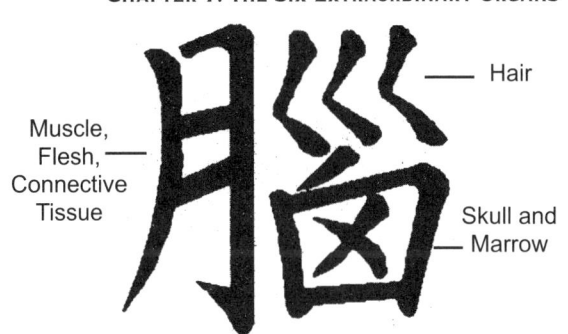

Figure 7.10. The Chinese character for "Nao," Brain

CHINESE CHARACTERS FOR BRAIN

The ideograph depicting the Chinese characters for the Brain "Nao" is described as follows (Figure 7.10):

- The Chinese character for "Nao" is composed of three images. The character to the left, "Ji" depicts the Chinese ideogram for body tissue, muscle, or flesh (all of which are forms of connective tissue). The character on the right is itself composed of two characters. The upper right hand portion depicts head hair and reflects the manifestation of the Kidney's Jing. The bottom right hand portion depicts a box with something inside, representing the skull filled with Marrow. Together, these characters are used to represent the Brain. In ancient China, the character for Brain did not have the "flesh" radical on the left, but instead had another radical that depicted the two halves of the symmetrical structure of the Brain.

THE BRAIN AS THE SEA OF MARROW

In Traditional Chinese Medicine, the Brain is also called the Sea of Marrow, and it is considered to extend from the top of the head to the Fengfu GV-16 (Wind Palace) point, just below the external occipital protuberance. There is an old Chinese saying, "The Marrow returns to the Brain." Kidney Jing flows from the Kidneys producing Marrow, a unique semifluid substance (different from the marrow of Western Medicine) that fills the spinal cord (cerebrospinal fluid) and the Brain. In Chinese Medicine, the Sea of Marrow flows into the cranial cavity and congeals to form the Brain.

The main functions of the Brain are controlling

mental and thinking activities, and guiding sense and language activities, which are described as follows (Figure 7.11):

1. **Controlling Mental and Thinking Activities:** The Brain is considered to be the house of the innate intelligence (Yuan Shen) and the seat of mental function. The ancient Chinese believed that the spine and spinal cord extend consciousness into the body from the Brain. The thinking ability is strengthened when Qi and Blood in the cerebral cortex, are abundant. The "memory zone," and the "thought center," are also located in the cerebral cortex. These regions will not develop until the Kidney Channels travel through the spine (along with the Liver Channels) to reach the cortex. When the Qi of these two channels is abundant, the memory function is strong.

2. **Guiding Sense and Language Activities:** Chinese Medicine maintains that the senses and the control of the body's physical movements are related to the Brain. The Brain is functionally related to the Kidneys and controls memory, concentration, hearing, touch, sight, and smell. Auditory and visual associations are especially emphasized.

THE BRAIN AND DAOIST MYSTICISM

The ancient Daoists believed that with the increase in thinking activity, a circle of light develops within the body's Taiji Pole. The individual's innate spirit (Yuan Shen) is represented by the intensity of light reflected from within the Taiji Pole. The degree of accumulated spiritual energy is reflected by the number of light circles developed within the Taiji Pole.

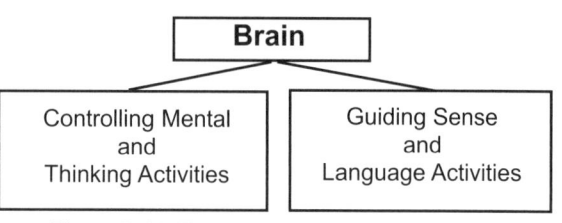

Figure 7.11. The Two Functions of the Brain

These circles of light can be best observed upon awakening after sleep. By placing slight pressure on the external eye lids, the inner light of the Taiji Pole is projected onto the optic nerves, reflecting an image of this circle of light (known as a phosphene in Western Medicine). If the circle of light is complete, it reflects a strong, healthy condition. If the circle of light is dark within its center (similar to a doughnut), this reflects a deficient condition. If the circle of light is broken or interrupted, it reflects an extreme deficiency (Figure 7.12).

WESTERN MEDICAL VIEWPOINT

The Chinese energetic viewpoint is quite different from the Western approach which views the brain's anatomy as consisting of five regions, including (Figure 7.13):

1. The cerebral hemispheres, or cerebrum (the neocortex, neopallium)
2. The thalamus, hypothalamus, and epithalamus (pineal)
3. The midbrain/mesencephalon (the colliculi and cerebral peduncles)
4. The pons and cerebellum
5. The medullae oblongata

The cerebral cortex of the brain is divided into two hemispheres that communicate with each other via a large bundle of fibers known as the corpus

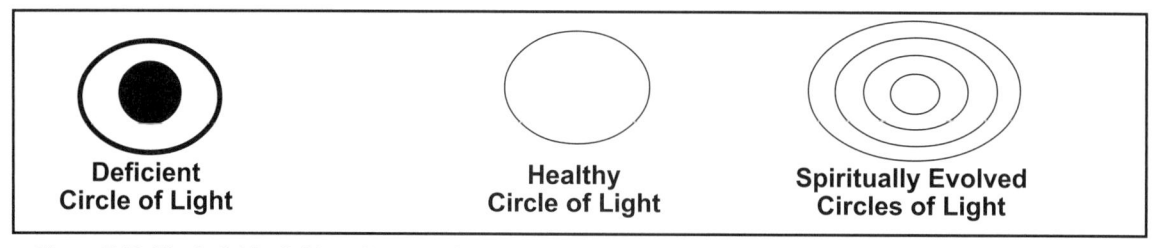

Figure 7.12. The individual's Yuan Shen is reflected in the intensity of the light present in the Taiji Pole. The degree of accumulated spiritual energy can be seen in the number and quality of light circles within the Taiji Pole.

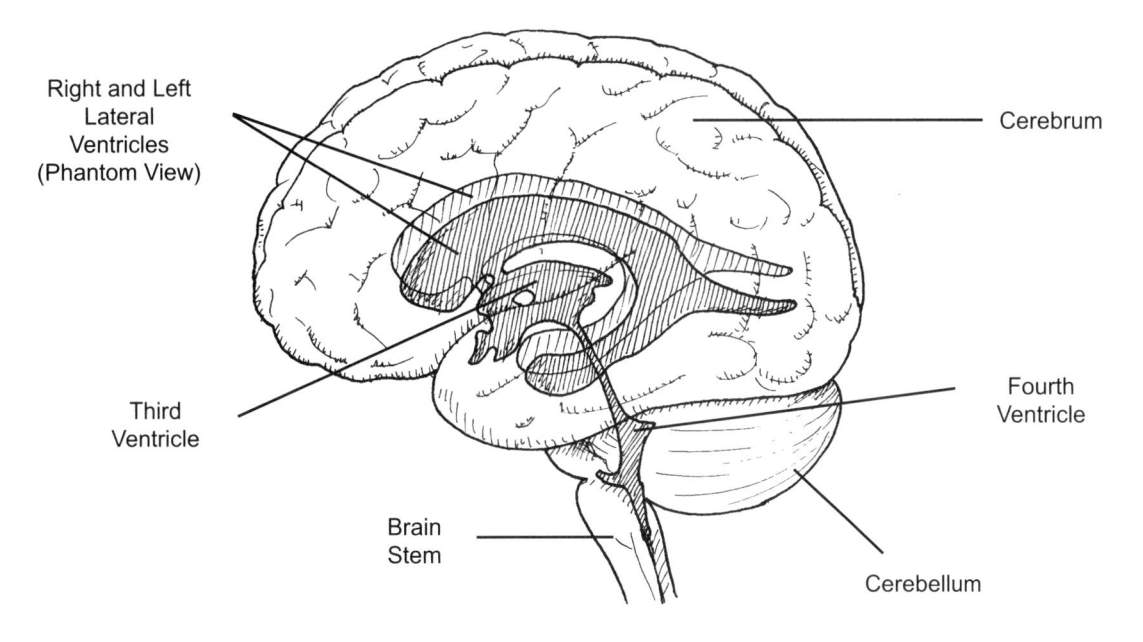

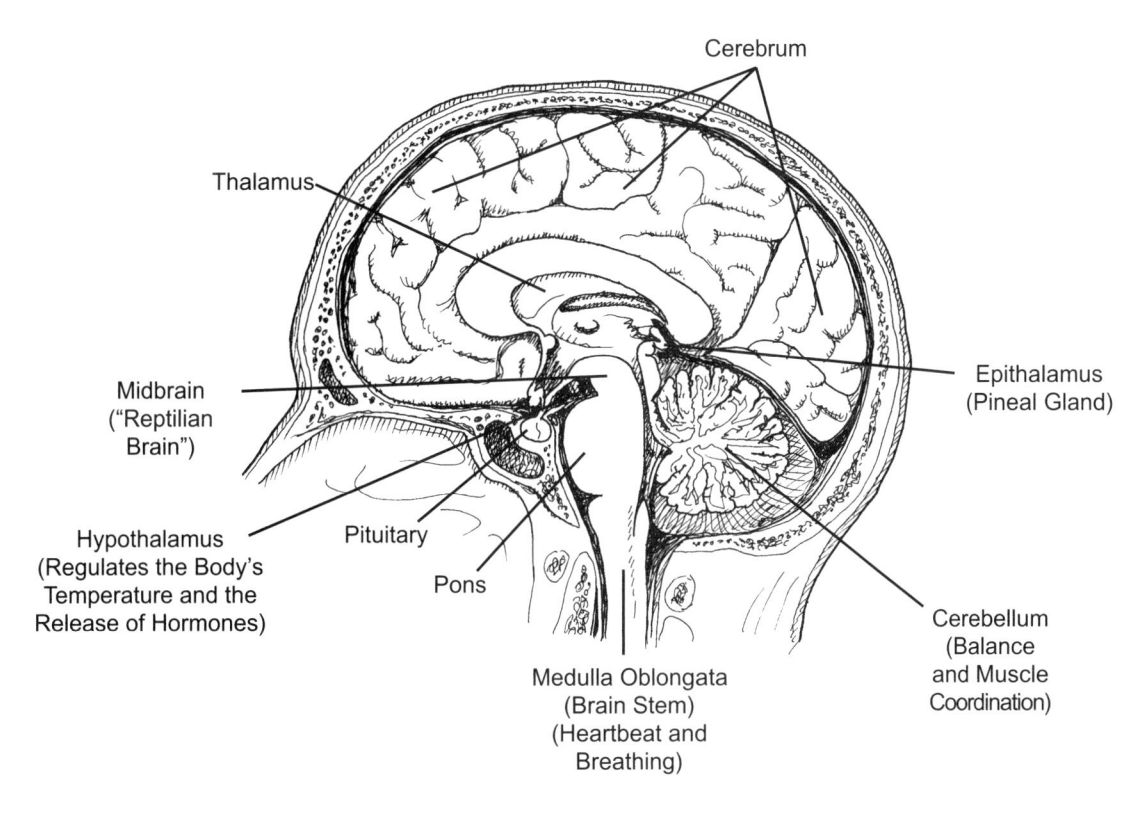

Figure 7.13. The Human Brain (Inspired by the original artwork of Dr. Frank H. Netter).

Stage	State of Consciousness	Psychological Dimension	Brainwave Pattern	Realm of Expierience
1st	Awake	Conscious Mind	Beta (13-26 Hertz)	Consciousness: waking consciousness, sensory awareness receiving external information
2nd	Prayer, Meditation	Superconscious Mind	Alpha (8-12 Hertz)	Day dreaming: calm, relaxation, hypnagogic state between being awake and asleep, visionary states, archetypal imagery
3rd	Dreaming Sleep	Subconscious Mind	Theta (4-7 Hertz)	Deep Relaxation: deep relaxation, drowsiness (the beginning hypnagogic state before sleep), and release of suppressed emotions
4th	Deep Sleep	Unconscious Mind	Delta (0.5-4 Hertz)	Sleep or Unconsciousness: the awakening of primal instincts and primitive drives

Figure 7.14. The four main frequencies of an individual's Brain-Wave Patterns

callosum. The left side of the body is controlled mainly by the right side of the cortex, and the right side of the body is controlled by the left cortex. The left hemisphere is predominantly responsible for the individual's analytical and logical thinking, as well as verbal skills, reading, writing, and the ability to make complex mathematical calculations. The right hemisphere is predominantly responsible for the individual's artistic and musical abilities, as well as the recognition of faces, body language, nonverbal (symbolic) ideas, and creativity.

The frontal lobes of the brain govern functions such as our analytical decision making. The cerebral hemispheres are responsible for the body's sense and movement. The brain stem controls the heartbeat and breathing. The cerebellum directs the balance and muscle coordination, and the hypothalamus regulates the body's temperature and the release of hormones.

In Western medicine, the oldest part (evolutionarily speaking) of the brain is often called the "reptilian brain" because its anatomical formation is similar to that found in lizards, alligators, and turtles. The reptilian brain is situated at the top of the brain stem and is surrounded by the limbic system, which itself is known as the mammalian brain. The third part of the brain is called the neocortex which wraps itself around the limbic system. All three parts of the brain (reptilian, mammalian, and neocortex) are viewed as biologically distinct, both in chemistry and in structure. The older formations of the brain are responsible for the autonomic nervous system, whereas the neocortex (being the most recent to evolve) is responsible for thinking and voluntary movement. It is interesting to note that ninety-eight percent of the protein-based tissue in the brain is replaced once a month.

Brain-Wave Patterns

Normal brain function involves the continual electrical activity of the neurons. This electrical brain-wave activity is measured in patterns or cycles per second, known as "hertz." Traditionally, Western medical science divides brain-wave activity into four main frequency domains: beta, alpha, theta and delta, described as follows (Figure 7.14):

- **Beta (13-26 Hertz):** The beta state is associated with an active, waking consciousness, and open eyes.
- **Alpha (8-12 Hertz):** The alpha state is associated with a calm, relaxed body, with the eyes closed (or day dreaming with the eyes open).
- **Theta (4-7 Hertz):** The theta state is associated with a deep relaxation, and drowsiness (the hypnagogic state before sleep). This state is common in children and in adults during the early stages of sleep.
- **Delta (0.5-4 Hertz):** The delta state is associated with sleep or unconsciousness.

At the borderline between any two states (e.g., between the beta and alpha state), the brain-waves generally manifest as a combination of both patterns. Research conducted in England by C. Maxwell Cade on brain-wave patterns revealed a hierarchy of states of consciousness, each with physiological correlations. State "four" is comparable to the "relaxation response" state associated with traditional meditation. States "five" and beyond are considered to be "mystical" states. While in these deeper states, Cade's subjects began to speak like mystics, while others, with no previous artistic talent, produced beautiful drawings or ecstatic poetry. It was noted that the subjects experienced new patterns of neural activity, in these mystical states, which affected both hemispheres of the brain, as well as both parts of the limbic system and brain-stem. The research concluded that mystical states of awareness can be induced by balancing the right and left hemispheres of the brain.

Research involving EEG studies on the brain-waves of children under the age of five has shown that they habitually function in an alpha mode of consciousness (the first state of altered consciousness), rather then the beta mode.

SCIENCE, THE BRAIN AND MEMORY

Scientists have discovered that the Brain primarily "talks to itself" through the language of wave interference (phase, amplitude, and frequency) and patterns, as opposed to images or chemical impulses. Within this model, we can understand that the electrical and chemical structures and impulses within the Brain are governed by the more subtle energetic wave form patterns of the Upper Dantian. The Brain perceives and analyzes an object by first "resonating" with its energetic wave pattern, then breaking it down into wave frequencies and transmitting this wave-pattern to the rest of the body.

Each set of human Brain cells absorbs and records sets of vibrations. The Brain primarily receives these vibrations through the skin, eyes, ears, nose, and mouth, and it records them as patterns of resonance within its cells. The mind interprets these incoming vibrations as images, sounds, smells, and sensations, and then organizes these into memories. The accuracy and extent of the interpretation of this incoming data depends upon the level of consciousness of the individual at the time of the interaction.

By applying the model of wave interference patterns to the process of memory, it has been conservatively estimated that the average human Brain has the potential to accumulate more than 280 quintillion (280,000,000,000,000,000,000) bits of information during a lifetime. The Brain retrieves "old" information the same way it processes "new" information, through the holographic transformation of wave interference patterns.

The Brain contains a certain mechanism that acts as a highly sensitive frequency analyzer, sorting perceptions and incoming knowledge in order to prevent "information overload." Without this, the infinite waves of information contained within the Wuji would overwhelm the individual. Normally, the Brain is "tuned in" to only a limited range of frequencies; however, through prayer, meditation, and quiescent relaxation, the receptive areas in the Brain become increasingly open to the near infinite spectrum of wavelengths existing within the Wuji. In this way, the individual personality is capable of expanding into a greater awareness and harmony with the Dao.

Scientists believe that the part of the brain that creates wave-interference patterns might not be located in only one particular area or group of cells, but rather it exists in the spaces between the cells. The Brain simply retrieves and relates the information of the Wuji. What we think of as perception and memory is simply a coherent emission of signals stemming from the Wuji; the stronger memories are but a structured grouping of this type of wave information.

FOUR MAJOR CHANGES OCCURRING IN THE BRAIN DURING MEDITATION

According to current research conducted by Dr. Gregg Jacobs of Harvard Medical School, scientists have now discovered that four major changes occur within the Brain during meditation, described as follows (Figure 7.15):

1. **Meditation and the Frontal Lobe of the Cerebral Cortex:** The frontal cortex is the most

highly evolved part of the Brain. It is responsible for intellectual functions such as reason and abstract thinking, aggressive and sexual behavior, smell, speech, language, and the initiation of movement. During meditation, the normal active processes of the frontal cortex shut down.

2. **Meditation and the Parietal Lobe of the Cerebral Cortex:** The parietal lobe is concerned with the recognition of specific sensory stimuli concerning the surrounding environment; the ability to use symbols as a means of communication; the ability to develop ideas and the motor responses to carry them out; and the ability to orientate in space and time. During meditation, the activity in the parietal lobe slows down.

3. **Meditation and the Thalamus:** The thalamus is considered to be part of the diencephalon (the smaller of the two derivatives of the early forebrain), consisting of several groups of cell bodies and processes that function mostly as a complex relay center. The relay nuclei of the thalamus receives input indirectly from most of the sensory neurons of the cranial and spinal nerves. Acting as the "gate keeper" of the senses, it primarily focuses the mind's attention by funneling sensory data deeper into the Brain and stopping other signals from overloading the system. During meditation, the flow of information flowing into the thalamus is reduced to a trickle.

4. **Meditation and the Reticular Formation of the Brain-stem:** The reticular formation is a massive but vaguely defined neural apparatus composed of closely intermingled gray and white matter extending throughout the central core of the brain-stem into the diencephalon. It acts as the Brain's sentry. Always receiving incoming stimuli, it puts the Brain on alert, ready to respond. During meditation, the arousal signals lessen significantly.

Subjects showed a pronounced change in brain-wave patterns, shifting from the beta waves (the conscious thought wave pattern) to alpha waves (the relaxation wave pattern) after training in meditation for only eight weeks.

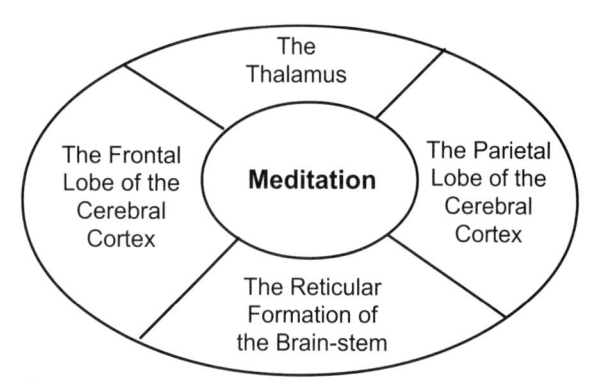

Figure 7.15. The four major areas in the brain affected during meditation.

CHINESE ENERGETIC MEDICINE

In Chinese energetic medicine, the central nervous system governs both conscious and unconscious actions. The lower brain stem and spinal cord are connected to the Yin energetic field, while the cerebral cortex is connected to the Yang energetic field.

When a Qigong doctor attunes his or her vibrations to the patient's energetic field and emits Qi, this activates the patient's Brain cells responsible for receiving and storing vibrational patterns. When these vibrational patterns are accessed by the Qigong doctor's projected energy, the patient's tissues respond and reproduce an energetic pattern similar to the original pattern used to record the patient's physical, mental, emotional, energetic, and spiritual experiences. This energetic reaction occurs physically due to the fact that the patient's tissues and cells conform to the subtle vibrational patterning of the energy body.

BRAIN CELLS RECEIVE, RECORD, AND MAINTAIN THE VIBRATIONS OF THOUGHTS

One set of Brain cells receives, records, and maintains the vibrational patterns that make up thoughts, pictures, actions, and movements of various forms of energy and matter. These vibrational patterns can be perceived and registered within the mind of the Qigong doctor. Once perceived and registered, these vibrational patterns can then be reproduced and projected.

The Qigong doctor can arrange the energetic patterns of his or her cells in such a way as to reproduce the sounds and movements of these forms or objects, and even the thoughts of the individuals that sent them. Through these energetically activated cells, the doctor can assist the patient, as well as him or herself, in controlling thoughts.

The Brain's vibrational patterns have a direct influence on the external environment, and routinely play a significant role in one's social interactions. For example, when someone either observes or imagines the occurrence of a specific event, that particular vibrational pattern becomes registered and fixed within the cells. When this pattern is energetically fed through focused intention (whether consciously or unconsciously), it develops a powerful charge. The vibrational pattern is then projected outward to be imprinted on the corresponding cells of another's Brain, which is then projected back until the incident is so fixed that the event actually occurs. This is known as a self-fulfilling prophecy. Similarly, it is thought that accidents and disease are brought into existence through the resonant influence of the cells' energetic patterns.

Another set of Brain cells receives, records, and maintains the vibrations of the thoughts and activities of the divine. The divine energy vibration pervades every substance and is constantly sending out divine knowledge in the form of true wisdom. All of the cells within the body naturally receive and project the vibrations of the "divine mind." If the doctor separates him or herself from the divine in thought, he or she will also separate from the divine in manifestation.

PATHOLOGY OF THE BRAIN

According to the *Yellow Emperor's Inner Cannon: Su Wen*, "An excess of the Sea of Marrow allows one to become alert and robust, with much strength. It permits the individual to fulfill the number of his or her allotted years. A deficiency of the Sea of Marrow causes the Brain to spin (vertigo), the ears to buzz (tinnitus), the legs to become weak with a form of lower back paralysis (lumbago) and causes the eyes to lose their sight. One becomes slow and lazy, and desires to lay down quietly."

"Hot" diseases can also affect the Brain and Marrow, especially when combined with either Wind or Cold invasion.

THE BRAIN DETECTS EMITTED QI

The following is an excerpt from clinical research on Qi emission and its effects on the human Brain gathered by Richard Lee, Director of China Healthways Institute in California, and Professor Lu Yan Fang of the National Institute of Electro-Acoustics in Beijing, China, and the Beijing College of Traditional Chinese Medicine:

I had learned in my many years of research with the Electro-Encephalograph (EEG) that the human Brain responds to even the most subtle of stimuli to the body, so I reasoned that, if there were really any scientific basis to emitted Qi, it would show up in the Brain waves of test subjects who were placed in the path of these emissions. I expected to see no difference between the resting states and the Qi emission states.

What we saw was extraordinary. Within a few seconds after the Qigong master began to emit Qi, the subject's EEG would begin to shift. The EEG power spectrum was enhanced on all channels while the most pronounced increase was in the frontal lobe. Also, there was an enhancement and synchronization of the alpha rhythm in all channels. When the Qigong master stopped emitting Qi, the EEG would gradually shift back toward the baseline readings.

To determine whether infrasonic energy was a significant part of the emitted Qi, we used the infrasonic Qigong prototypes in the same experiment. It was located 18 inches away, directly behind the back of the head of the test subject. The EEG electrodes were attached as before. The simulator was activated for short periods of time and the results recorded. We found that the effects on the receiver's EEG were quite similar to those of the emitted Qi.

Our further research involved monitoring the various sensory-cortical evoked potentials during Qigong meditation, emitted Qi, and infrasonic Qigong simulation. We again found very similar results from all three stimuli. We found that a large portion of the cerebral cortex was inhibited while other somatosensory cortex were excited. One of the significant findings of this study is that the inhibition of the cerebral cortex during Qigong meditation is clearly different from the excitation of the cerebral cortex that is measurable during sleep.

Through Acoustical Brainstem Evoked Response (ABER), it was found that the brainstem structures from the medulla to the hypothalamus were significantly facilitated. The brainstem plays an important role in regulating the functions of the inner organs, motor function, and emotion.

The implications of these studies were startling. Qigong masters can, without touch, voice, eye contact or any other traditional communication means, induce a clear, strong, and highly measurable change in a subject's Brain functioning. A synchronization of alpha rhythm indicates deep relaxation, and is closely associated with accelerated healing. Enhanced power spectrum in the frontal lobe is especially significant because the association cortex of the frontal lobe is concerned with higher motor action, higher sensory function, emotional and motivational aspects of behavior, and integration of autonomic function. Facilitation of the brain stem, with its regulation of internal organs, may be a mechanism by which physical healing is induced or accelerated.

Despite these highly significant changes in EEG and evoked potentials, the subjects had felt nothing and had no idea of the profound changes taking place within them.

The findings of these studies are solid evidence that a Qigong master can induce real physiological changes in a subject from several feet away, and further, may help to explain the high rate of recovery from chronic degenerative diseases in groups of hospital patients under the care of Qigong masters (Figure 7.16). These studies also show that the infrasonic Qigong simulator can induce similar changes in Brain function and that, through Qigong meditation, a Qigong master can induce these same changes in his own Brain.

Scientific Controls

There is much disagreement on how emitted Qi affects the Brain. Many doctors insist that Brain changes are psychologically induced, and that verbal suggestion, impressive hand motion, and the subject's expectations account for the observed phenomena surrounding Qi emission.

To test this, we had several people pretending to be Qigong masters treat the test subjects. The subjects

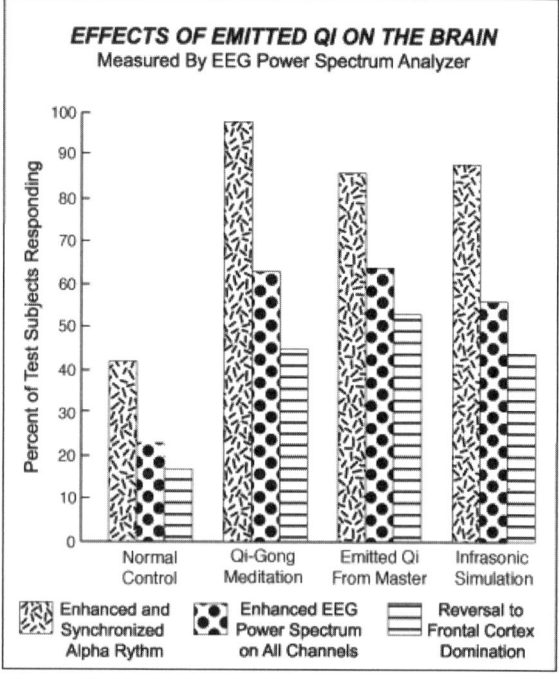

Figure 7.16. Emitted Qi has a pronounced and repeatable effect on EEG measurements. It enhances frontal and occipital EEG power spectra, and often enhances the frontal to the extent that it becomes the dominant EEG activity (whereas occipital dominance is more common). Emitted Qi also enhances and synchronizes the alpha rhythm.

were told that all were Qigong doctors, and all moved their hands in similar ways. We saw no significant changes in Brain wave patterns with the fake Qigong masters, but when the real doctors emitted their Qi, we repeatedly observed highly significant changes.

Even this did not satisfy many of the doctors who reviewed our work, so we repeated the study with animals. We monitored EEG in awake rabbits and ABER (Acoustical Brainstem Evoked Response) in anesthetized cats as Qigong masters emitted Qi toward them. Even though there was no voice or eye contact between the Qigong masters and the animals, and the masters emitted Qi from several feet away, we saw shifts in EEG and ABER similar to those observed in the human subjects. This is a highly convincing result because all kinds of placebo effects are eliminated, yet modification of Brain function at a distance remains constant.

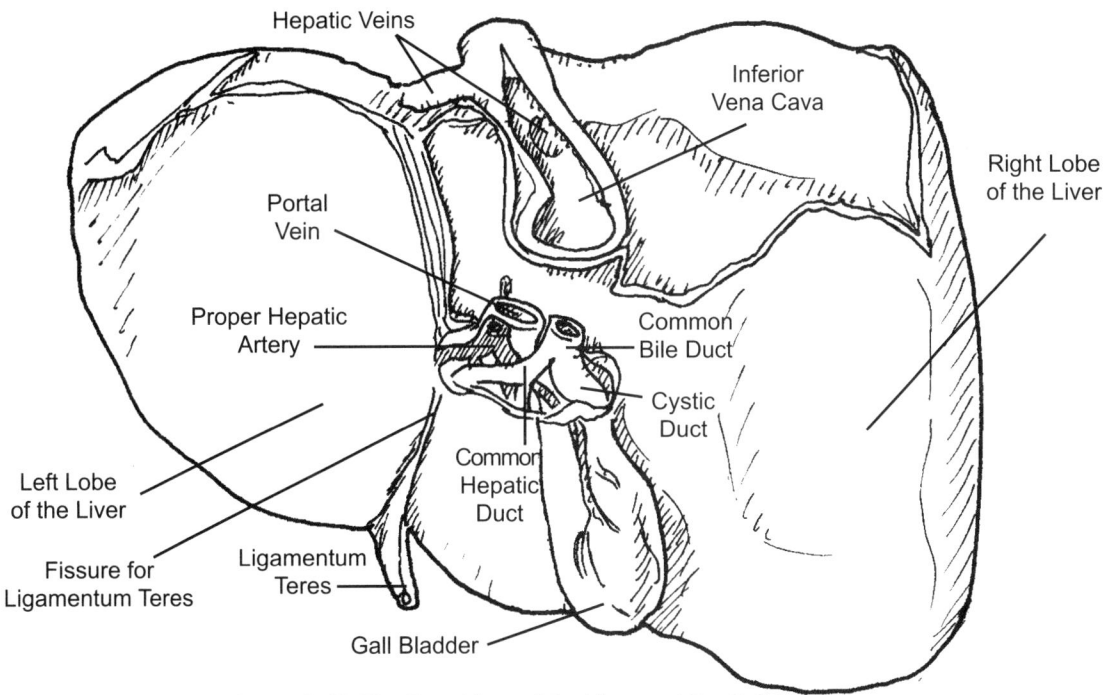

Figure 7.17. The Rear View of the Liver and the Gall Bladder (Inspired by the original artwork of Dr. Frank H. Netter).

THE GALL BLADDER: DAN

The Gall Bladder is a green colored, hollow, thin-walled, capsule-shaped Yang organ. It is about three to four inches long, and is located in a shallow fossa on the visceral surface of the liver (Figure 7.17). It is categorized as an "Extraordinary Organ" because it is the only Yang organ that neither receives "turbid" food and drink nor produces digestive waste products. Instead, it stores a refined "clean" substance (the bile), thus making it functionally similar to the Yin organs. Another reason that the Gall Bladder is considered "extraordinary," is that it does not communicate with the exterior directly, as the other Yang organs do, via the mouth, rectum or urethra. The Gall Bladder Channels, however, travel into the sensory organs (eyes, ears, nose and mouth) via its trajectories, allowing the sensory organs to become more rooted and grounded.

Energetically, the Gall Bladder is in charge of making the right decisions and determinations and acting accordingly. It has the responsibility of being stable, quiet, tranquil and unshakable.

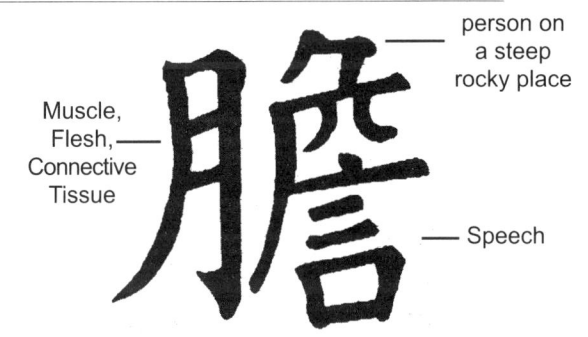

Figure 7.18. The Chinese character for "Dan," Gall Bladder

CHINESE CHARACTERS FOR GALL BLADDER

The ideograph depicting the Chinese characters for the Gall Bladder "Dan" is described as follows (Figure 7.18):

- The Chinese "Dan" is composed of three images: The character to the left, "Ji" depicts the Chinese ideogram for body tissue, muscle or flesh (all of which are forms of connective tissue). The character on the right is divided into two characters: the upper right hand side de-

Figure 7.19. The Energetic Functions of the Gall Bladder

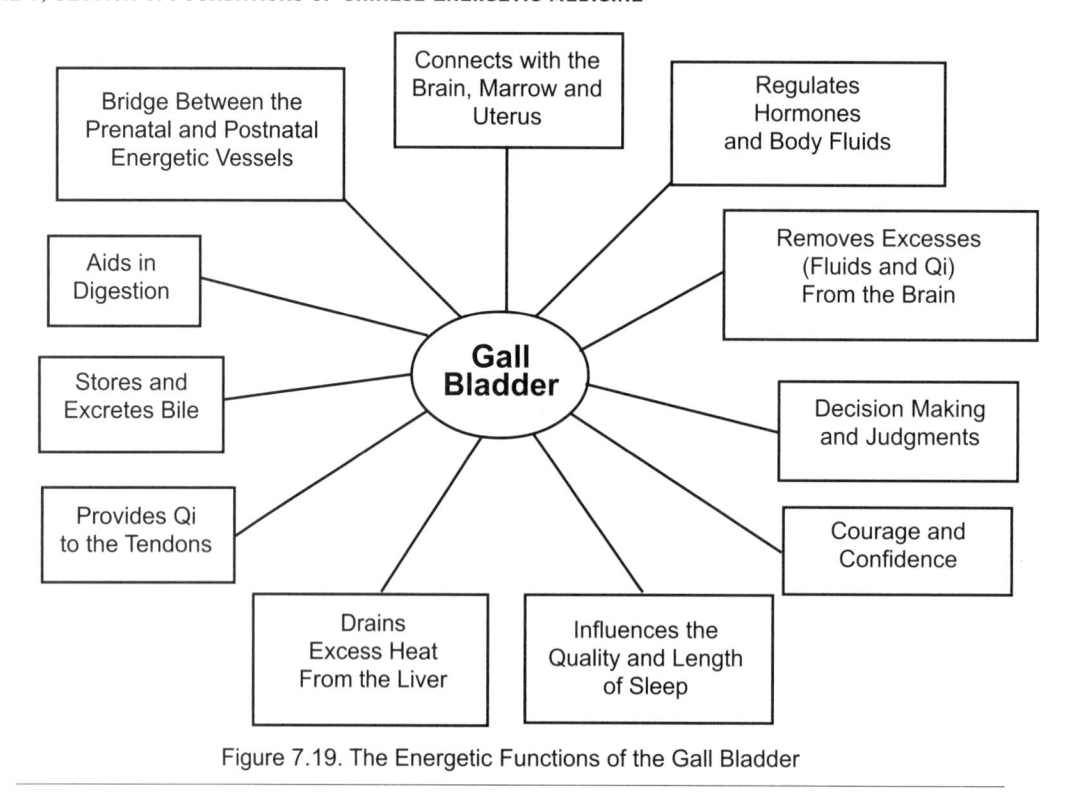

- Bridge Between the Prenatal and Postnatal Energetic Vessels
- Connects with the Brain, Marrow and Uterus
- Regulates Hormones and Body Fluids
- Aids in Digestion
- Removes Excesses (Fluids and Qi) From the Brain
- Stores and Excretes Bile
- Decision Making and Judgments
- Provides Qi to the Tendons
- Courage and Confidence
- Drains Excess Heat From the Liver
- Influences the Quality and Length of Sleep

picts a person on a steep rocky place bent over and afraid of falling. The bottom right hand side is the character "Yan," meaning speech. Together, these characters are used to represent a person in a hazardous position who cannot make a decision. This expresses the Gall Bladder's role in making difficult decisions and initiating courage.

FUNCTION OF THE GALL BLADDER

The Gall Bladder's associated Yin organ is the Liver and its element is Wood. In Traditional Chinese Medicine, the Gall Bladder functions the same way as described in Western Medicine, except that in Chinese medicine it also incurs some partial functions of the nervous system. The main functions of the Gall Bladder are that it: stores and excretes bile, provides Qi to the tendons, and the psycho-emotional aspects of courage and decision making, which are described as follows (Figure 7.19):

1. **Stores and Excretes Bile:** Bile is created and secreted by the Liver and stored and concentrated in the Gall Bladder. The Gall Bladder then releases the bile into the Small Intestine as needed to aid in the digestion and absorption of food.

2. **Provides Qi to the Tendons:** The Gall Bladder also helps the Liver control the tendons. The Liver provides Blood to the tendons, while the Gall Bladder provides Qi to the tendons in order to ensure proper movement and agility. These combined functions of the Liver and Gall Bladder ensure that the sinews are soft and pliant and supplied with an abundance of energy.

3. **Psycho-Emotional Aspects:** The Gall Bladder is sometimes called "the court of justice," or "the general's advisor," as it is responsible for making decisions and judgments, overseeing and empowering discernment, as well as providing bravery, courage, confidence, and meeting challenges. Although the Kidneys control drive and vitality, the Gall Bladder

provides the capacity to turn this drive and vitality into decisive action.

The Gall Bladder travels into the sensory organs (eyes, ears, nose and mouth) via its channels, allowing the sensory organs to become more rooted and grounded. The Gall Bladder is also responsible for the regulation of hormones and body fluids (bile and Ye).

The Gall Bladder Channels are often used to drain toxic energy from an overheated or excess Liver condition. The internal flow of the Liver Channel moves Qi into the Brain and Sea of Marrow; consequently, the Gall Bladder Channel can be used to remove excesses (such as fluids and Qi) from the Brain.

The Gall Bladder Channels link to the Brain, Marrow and Uterus and act as a bridge between the prenatal and postnatal energetic vessels.

THE GALL BLADDER AND DAOIST MYSTICISM

The ancient Mao Shan Daoists used the Gall Bladder as the primary internal organ in which to store the Qi of thunder (gathered during the Spring thunder storms). The Liver is responsible for containing the Hun (the individual's Ethereal Soul), and the Gall Bladder is the Liver's paired organ. Therefore, during meditation, the ancient Daoists would dispatch their Hun to gather the power of thunder (considered to be divine arrows, and weapons of the Dao) and store them in their Gall Bladder. These divine Yang arrows of light and heat were then stored within the quiver of the Gall Bladder, so as not to disturb the dwelling place of the Hun inside the Liver. The emanation of Yang light and heat contained within the thunder was then sealed with an incantation inside the Gall Bladder organ, and later released, used as a powerful spiritual weapon (i.e., infused into specific talismans or incantations for protection against the dark, Yin, demonic forces).

THE MARROW: SUI

In Traditional Chinese Medicine, the term Marrow (Sui) is different from the concept of bone

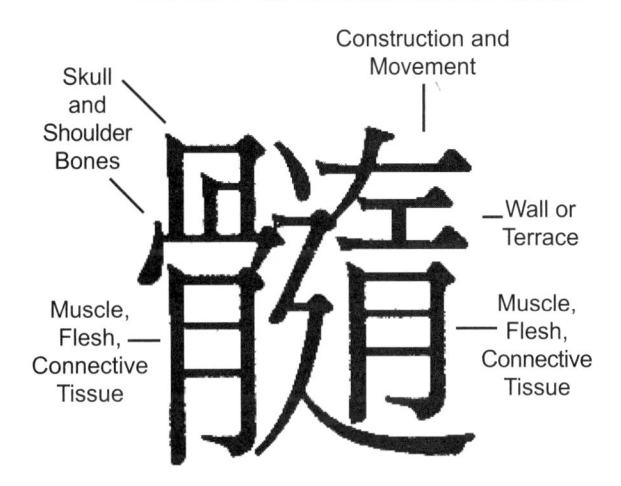

Figure 7.20. The Chinese character for "Sui," Marrow

marrow as defined in Western medicine. Marrow in Chinese medicine is considered the substance that is the common matrix of the Bones, Bone Marrow, spinal cord, and Brain. One of the main functions of the Marrow is to circulate, flow into and irrigate the Bones, hollows, skull and orifices, like "water flowing through a riverbed."

CHINESE CHARACTERS FOR MARROW

The ideograph depicting the Chinese characters for the Marrow, "Sui," is described as follows (Figure 7.20):

- The Chinese character for "Sui" is composed of two images: the character on the top left can be translated as Bone (Gu), and it depicts the framework of the body's Bones above the bottom left character "Ji," which means muscle, flesh, connective tissue, and flesh. The character on the right is comprised of several characters. The "Ji" character appears again, this time below the upper portion of a character that depicts the idea of building a wall or terrace, and something walking beside the wall or terrace. Together, these characters are used to represent the movement of the body's Marrow, flowing inside the Bones, and constructing or building something.

THE MARROW AND JING

In ancient Chinese medical texts, it is stated that the Marrow is rooted in the Kidney's Jing and is connected to the Lower Dantian through the Governing Vessel (Figure 7.21). It is regulated by the energy of the body's Thrusting Vessels.

Kidney Jing is the origin of Marrow. Marrow functions to form the Bone Marrow, as well as to nourish the Brain and spinal cord. When the Mingmen warms and nourishes the body, the Marrow becomes full. This sustains the body's vertical posture and gives strength to both the Brain and the Bones. When the Marrow is full, thinking is clear and the individual expresses fearlessness.

Western medical physiology shows that both red and white blood cells are produced in the marrow of the bones. The red blood cells (which circulate oxygen and eliminate carbon dioxide) are produced within the body's long bones (humerus, femur, tibia, etc.). The white blood cells (vital to the body's immune system) are produced within the body's flat bones (skull, sternum, scapulae, pelvis, etc.). The type of blood cells that are produced depends on the type of marrow that predominates.

THE MARROW AND DAOIST MYSTICISM

The ancient Daoists believed that when all of the postnatal energy acquired from the combination of physical (air, food, and drink), mental and emotional (thoughts and emotions), and spiritual (prayer, meditation, and sleep) cultivations is circulated through the Microcosmic Orbit (Fire Cycle), the Prenatal Qi stored in the Bone Marrow and Brain become stimulated, and the spiritual consciousness is awakened. This circulation of combined physical, mental, emotional, and spiritual energies is why the brain Marrow is considered to be constructed from the finest and most subtle essences, manifesting the original and hidden power of the Kidneys.

PATHOLOGY OF THE MARROW

The Marrow's energetic constitution is particularly vulnerable to Heat and Dryness. In conditions of Marrow deficiency, symptoms can manifest such as pain in the Bones and insomnia may arise.

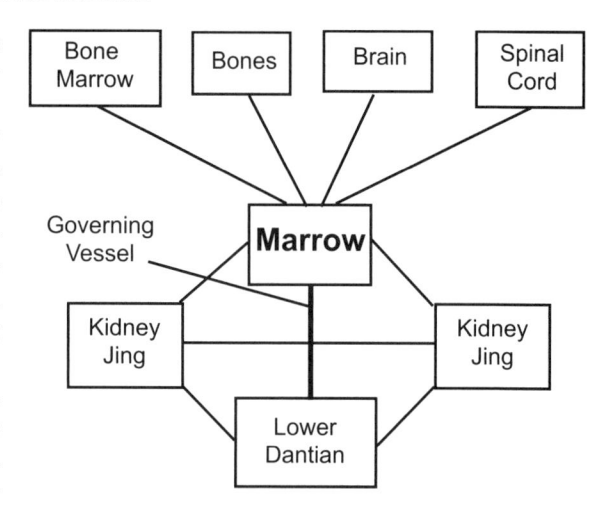

Figure 7.21. The Energetic Connections of the Marrow

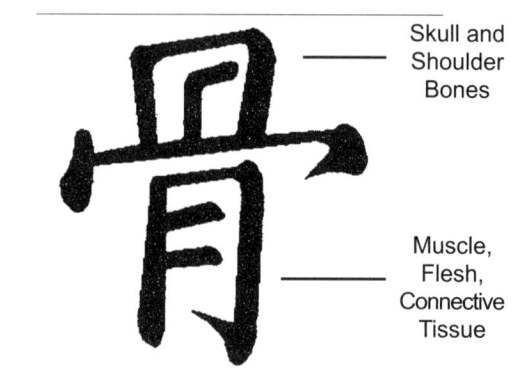

Figure 7.23. The Chinese character for "Gu," Bone

THE BONES: GU

In Traditional Chinese Medicine, the Bones are considered to be the structural framework of the body (Figure 7.22).

CHINESE CHARACTERS FOR BONES

The ideograph depicting the Chinese character for Bone, "Gu," is described as follows (Figure 7.23):

- The Chinese character for "Gu" is composed of two images: the character to the left, "Ji," depicts the Chinese ideogram for body tissue, muscle or flesh (all of which are forms of connective tissue). The character on the top is composed of two characters: the upper por-

CHAPTER 7: THE SIX EXTRAORDINARY ORGANS

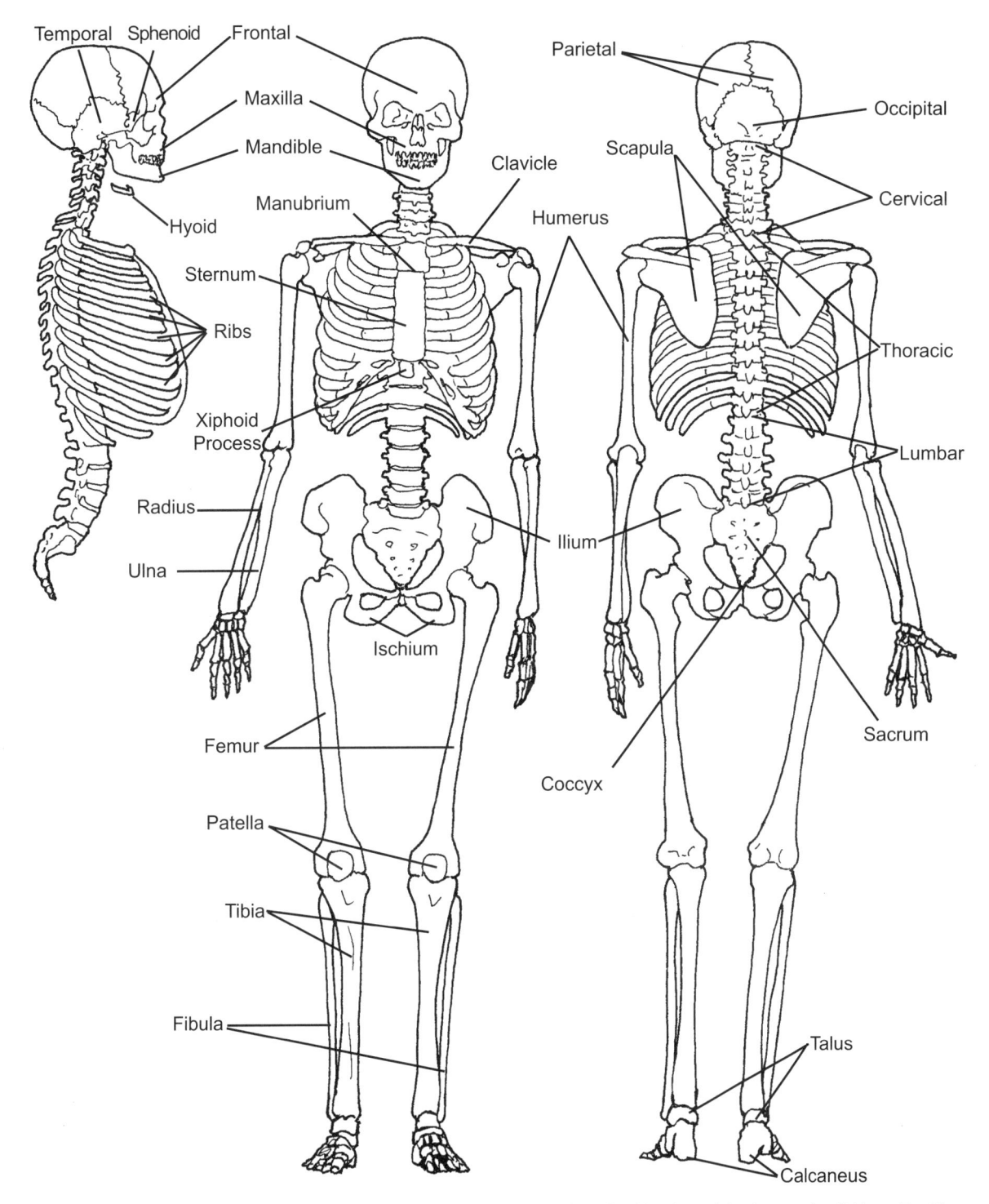

Figure 7.22. The human skeleton consists of roughly 200 bones (Inspired by the original artwork of Wynn Kapit).

tion depicts a box with something inside of it, representing the skull. The center portion of the box and crossbar represents the shoulder blade. Together, these characters depict the framework of the body's Bones.

BONES AND MARROW

There is an inherent correspondence between the energetic function of Marrow and that of the Bones. The Marrow held within the Bones assures the power, strength, and suppleness of the Bones. The Bones, in return, prevent the dissipation of the essential richness of the Marrow.

Bones are related to the Kidney's Jing. Bones support the body's structure, strength, and mobility, as well as store the Bone Marrow. Bones are extremely porous and are always "breathing." The porous quality of Bones allows for the absorption and release of Qi and Blood, similar to the way a sponge absorbs and releases water. Energetically, Bones are regulated by the body's Conception and Thrusting Vessels.

BONES AND DAOIST MYSTICISM

The ancient Daoists believed that Bones function within the human body similar to the way that the mountains function on the Earth. Just as the mountains naturally guide the flow and circulation of water, Bones guide the circulation and movement of the body's Jing, Qi, Shen, Blood, Marrow, and Body Fluids.

Additionally, Bones are believed to vibrate like hollow reeds, especially when the divine wind (Qi) flows over and through them. These living reeds (or tuning forks) were thought to be responsible for vibrating celestial and environmental Qi throughout the body's entire physical structure, extending this energy outward into the body's external Wei Qi fields.

BONES PRODUCE PIEZOELECTRIC CHARGES

Bones are the only substance in the body capable of generating piezoelectric charges. Due to their solid crystalline structure, a piezoelectric charge is created when pressure is applied to the Bones. These electromagnetic charges generate

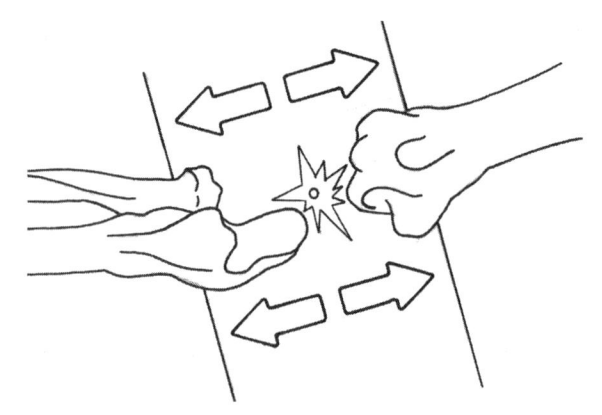

Figure 7.24. Stretching the Tendons and Ligaments while Relaxing the Muscles to Produce Increased Vibrational Resonance

fields of energy that receive and send impulses to the body's cells, tissues, organs, Blood, and channels. The Brain, nervous system, Heart, and lower abdomen also generate electromagnetic fields that resonate with the Bones. The crystalline structures of the Bones amplify, radiate, and transmit energy and information to the rest of the body. The rhythmic oscillation of these Bone-generated electromagnetic fields is further amplified and released through the body due to the tuning fork-like organization of the skeletal structure. The stretching of the tendons and ligaments while relaxing the muscles also produces increased vibrational resonance within Bone tissue (Figure 7.24).

WESTERN MEDICAL PERSPECTIVE

Bone (osseous) tissue forms most of the body's skeletal system and is the framework that supports and protects the internal organs. The main functions of the skeletal system are: to store energy and marrow; to allow for mineral homeostasis, blood cell production and physical movement; and to provide protection and structural support.

The skeletal system is composed of bone tissue, bone marrow, periosteum (the membrane surrounding the bones), and cartilage. Like other connective tissue, bone tissue contains an abundant matrix of various types of cells, such as osteoprogenitor cells, osteoblasts, osteocytes, and osteoclasts.

Bones are constantly being "remodeled" in order to maintain the integrity of the skeletal system. The osteoclasts break down the bones, while the osteoblasts build them up. The osteoclasts and osteoblasts signal to each other, via the bone marrow, when to start and stop each action in order to maintain balance.

Pathology of the Bones

In the Tang Dynasty (618-907 A.D.), the famous physician Sun Simiao wrote that in cases of deficiency of the Bones, "symptoms such as continuous aches and pains will manifest, and the patient will be tired and stiff. In cases of excess of the Bones, the patient will have no pain, but will experience uneasiness." This type of agitation is initiated from Heat in the chest.

The Blood Vessels: Mai

Through associative diagnosis, observation, and the study of clinical bloodletting, the ancient Chinese developed an advanced understanding of the vascular system and Blood circulation. Much effort was spent in understanding the organizational structure, pathways, and various branches of the internal Blood Vessels.

The early Chinese physicians observed the body's arterial and venous circulation, identifying the flow of Blood within all of the major Blood Vessels (Mai). Critical junctures, known as "Jie" (meaning joint, node, or knot) were believed to be formed where the finer branches of the Mai (arterioles, venules, and capillaries) intersected with related nerves and collateral vessels. These finer branches of the Mai supplied Blood and nutrients to the various regions of the body.

The ancient Chinese physicians had many reasons for placing great emphasis on understanding the flow of Blood and the pathways of the body's Blood Vessels. To the ancient Chinese, Blood circulation was one of the most important physiological manifestations of the energetic body. Impeded Blood flow to any region of the body resulted in pain, tissue dysfunction, and cellular degeneration. Additionally, the five Yin organs (Liver, Heart, Spleen, Lungs and Kidneys) were believed to store and circulate the refined substances of the body's Wu Jing Shen (Five Essence Spirits: Hun, Shen, Yi, Po and Zhi) within the bloodstream.

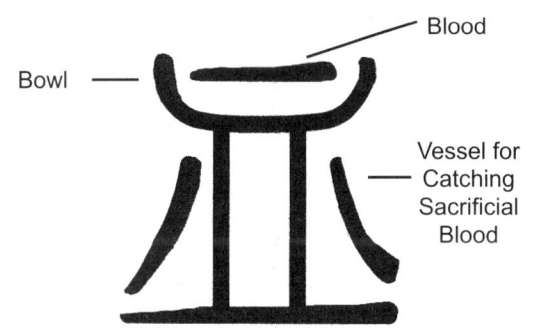

Figure 7.25. The ancient Chinese character for "Xue," Blood

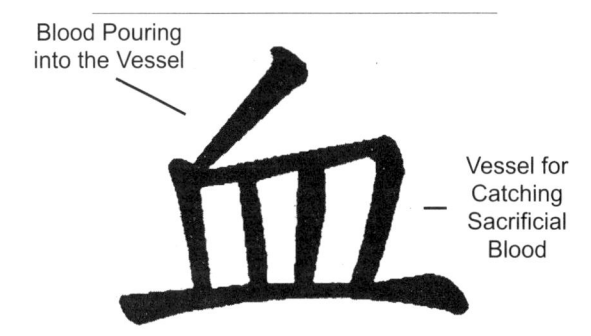

Figure 7.26. The modern Chinese character for "Xue," Blood

Chinese Characters for Blood

The Chinese word "Xue" translates as "Blood." Its ancient character is composed of a pictograph representing a small, wide-lipped, clay vessel used for collecting Blood (during the Shang Dynasty these vessels were crafted out of bronze). Contained within the bowl is a horizontal line representing Blood (Figure 7.25).

Its modern character is composed of two parts: positioned on the top is a line representing the flow of Blood as it pours into a sacrificial vessel; positioned to the bottom is the radical "Min," meaning a vessel for catching sacrificial Blood (Figure 7.26).

In Traditional Chinese Medicine, the concept of Blood is different, both in characteristics and in function, from the concept of blood in Western medicine. In the Chinese model (see Volume 3,

Chapter 23), Blood originates from the transformation of food and drink by the Spleen, and from Kidney Jing. The Spleen then transfers this refined food energy upwards to be further enhanced by the Heart Qi and Lung Qi to form Blood.

In ancient China, it was believed that the Lungs were responsible for energizing the Blood, and the Spleen and Kidneys assisted in the formation of the basic composition of the Blood. The Blood in its natural form is a precious liquid, composed of Body Fluids and nutrition for the body's tissues.

Chinese Characters for Blood Vessels

The ideograph depicting the Chinese characters for Blood Vessels "Mai" is described as follows (Figure 7.27):

- The Chinese character for "Mai" is composed of two images: the character to the left, "Ji" depicts the Chinese ideogram for body tissue, muscle or flesh (all of which are forms of connective tissue). The character on the right depicts a current of water or a stream. In ancient China, the right side of the Mai character was "Yong," which is a current of water flowing deep within the Earth. Together, the character can be translated as vein or pulse, depicting a form of energetic circulation.

The word "Mai" has two meanings; it can refer to the pulse, and it can also be used to denote the Blood Vessels. When used as "pulse," the word Mai refers to the rhythmic, energetic pulsating movement of the "substances" within the Blood Vessels. When the word "Mai" is used to denote Blood Vessels, it describes the vascular network of the arteries, arterioles, capillaries, venules and veins. The energetic functions and interactions of Qi, Blood and Mai, described as follows:

- **Qi:** The Qi (Commander of Blood) provides the dynamic force associated with the movement of the "substances" through the Vessels.
- **Blood:** The Blood (Mother of Qi) provides vital nourishment and moistens the body, thus providing a Yin substance and foundation that allows for the proper functioning of Qi. The Blood also fills the vessels and is the foundation for mental activity.

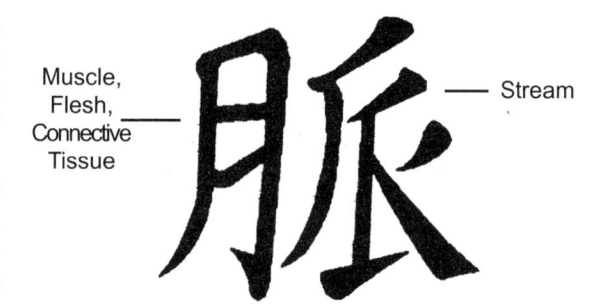

Figure 7.27. The Chinese character for "Mai," Blood Vessels

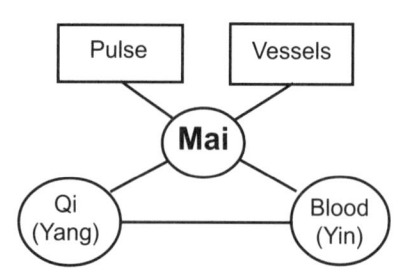

Figure 7.28. The Energetic Relations of the Blood Vessels

- **Mai:** The Mai is both the network of the vessels and the rhythmic pulsations from the movement of the "substances" within the vessels.

Qi and Blood

Both Qi and Blood flow within the channels and Blood Vessels (Mai), continuously circulating throughout the body to nourish, maintain, and moisten the tissues. Qi and Blood flow together, with Qi being both the active force that makes the Blood circulate and the force that keeps it within the Blood Vessels. Qi is an energetic form, and is considered to be a Yang substance, while Blood (Volume 3, Chapter 23) is a liquid form of energy and is considered to be a Yin substance (Figure 7.28).

The Energetic Channels and Streams of the Blood Vessels

The ancient Chinese divided the various Blood Vessels into twelve primary pairs of longitudinal arteries and veins. The reason for viewing the Blood circulation as flowing along a linear pathway of the body can be explained by understanding the Chinese emphasis of the Yin and Yang energetic aspects of Qi and Blood distribution. The energetic cycle of Yin and Yang moves from the extremities and superficial regions to the deep internal organs, and back, flowing along the pathway of the veins and arteries.

The twelve primary pairs of arteries and veins were known as the "Jing Mai," meaning "channel streams" (Figure 7.29). There were thus six primary pairs of Blood Vessels positioned on each side of the body (making a total of twelve pairs) flowing along the energetic pathways of the Twelve Primary Channels.

The collateral branches of the twelve primary pairs of arteries and veins supply nutrients to the body's tissues, either surfacing along the superficial areas of the Twelve Skin Zones, or descending internally into the deeper tissue areas of the body. These collateral branches are known as "Luo Mai," meaning "Connecting Streams" (Figure 7.30).

The names of the twelve primary pairs of arteries and veins (Jing) and their collateral branches (Luo) are often combined to form the word "Jingluo," a term that is used in the modern T.C.M. colleges to describe the vascular system.

The collateral branches further divide into the Minute Vessels which comprise the body's arterioles, capillaries, and venules. These Minute Vessels were known as "Sun Mai," meaning "Grandson Streams." The Minute Vessels communicate between the arteries, which direct Blood flow outward, and the veins, which return Blood flow to the Heart. The Minute Vessels are thus the smallest link in the body's continuous flow of Blood circulation.

The Chinese medical understanding of the internal structure and function of the vascular system is nearly identical to that of Western Medicine. The Chinese system, however, places a different emphasis on the deep and superficial branching of the vessels' energetic flow. The Chinese system of differential diagnosis relies heavily on understanding the flow of energy within the individual Blood Vessels and the relationships between them.

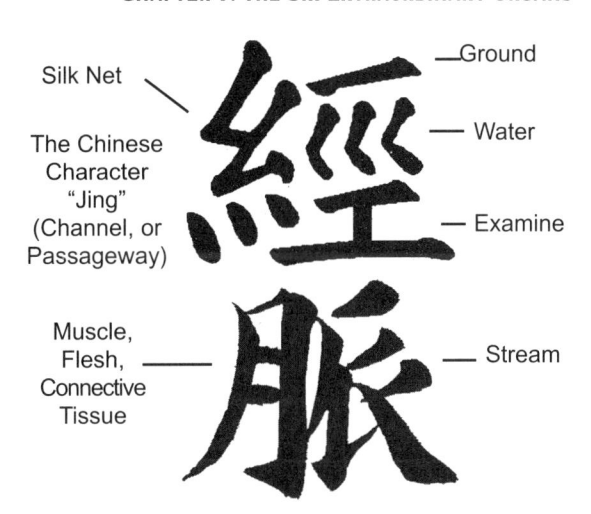

Figure 7.29. The Chinese characters for "Jing Mai," the body's Twelve Major Blood Vessels

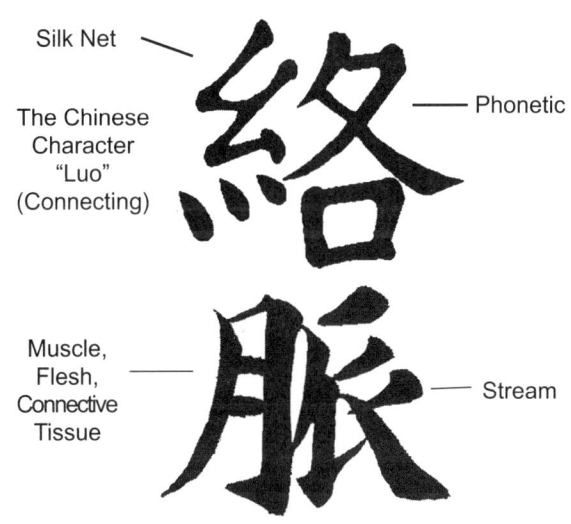

Figure 7.30. The Chinese characters for "Luo Mai," the body's Connecting Streams

THE ENERGETIC PATHWAYS OF THE BLOOD VESSELS

The ancient Chinese divided the Twelve Primary Blood Vessels into various out-flowing arteries and returning veins, each being differentiated by the presence of a pulse. The following is a list of the Twelve Primary Blood Vessels and their venous and arterial associations:

1. Gall Bladder: Artery
2. Liver: Vein
3. Lungs: Artery
4. Large Intestine: Vein
5. Stomach: Artery
6. Spleen: Vein
7. Heart: Artery
8. Small Intestine: Vein
9. Urinary Bladder: Artery
10. Kidneys: Vein
11. Pericardium: Artery
12. Triple Burners: Vein

FUNCTION OF THE BLOOD VESSELS

The Blood Vessels serve as the primary reservoir of Blood. In Traditional Chinese Medicine the Heart is considered to be the master of the Blood Vessels (Figure 7.31). The Blood Vessels contain Blood and are indirectly related to the Kidneys in that the Kidney Essence (Jing) produces Marrow, which contributes to the production of Blood. The function of the Blood Vessels is to transport Qi and Blood throughout the body for nutrition and regeneration.

The Blood Vessels are regulated by the energy of the body's Thrusting Vessels, and Blood is held within the Blood Vessels by the Spleen Qi. The Zong Qi (Pectoral Qi), stored within the chest, incorporates Lung Qi to assist the Heart in moving the Blood through the channel network, to nourish the tissues of the body.

According to the *Yellow Emperor's Inner Cannon: Su Wen*, "the Ying Qi (Nutritive Qi) circulates inside of the Blood Vessels, and the Wei Qi (Defensive Qi) circulates outside the Blood Vessels."

THE BLOOD VESSELS AND ANCIENT DAOIST MYSTICISM

In ancient China, red blood was believed to be the seat of the soul, and that magical powers could be imbued into any object that was ritually smeared with Blood. This is why when statues or pictures of gods or goddesses are being consecrated, the eyes are painted over with Blood. In this way, the picture or statue is energetically animated and given a soul.

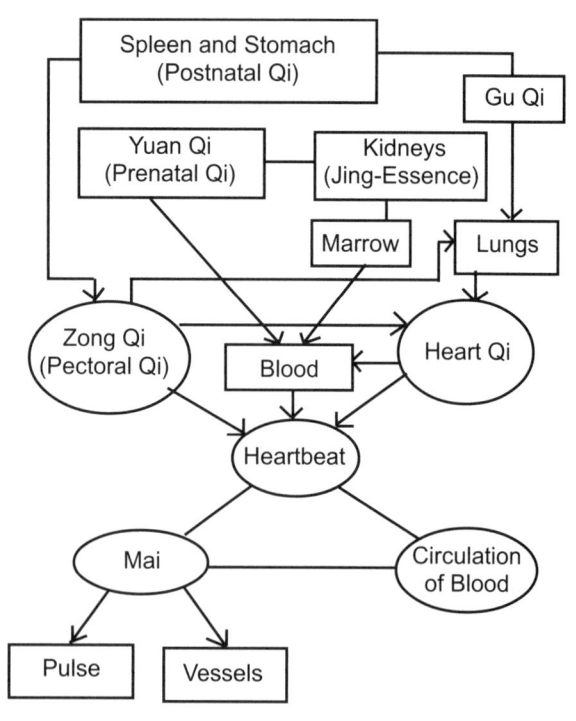

Figure 7.31. The Energetic Connections of the Blood and Blood Vessels

It was also believed that although the Lungs were responsible for the oxygenation of the Blood (and the Spleen and Kidneys have the function of assisting in forming the basic composition of the Blood), Blood in its natural form is only liquid, composed of Body Fluids and nutritive juices. Blood only becomes red because the Heart puts its "imperial stamp" onto the liquids, which penetrates the Body Fluids with the power of the Heart's Shen. This "imperial" action transforms the liquids into Blood. The energetic and spiritual component Blood now receives its red color of fire and has the ability to bring life to the body.

Additionally, male semen is believed to be transformed Blood, and if too much semen is expended, the man's health suffers. Likewise, a mother's milk is also considered Blood in a different form.

Finally, it was believed that if a demon could be successfully smeared with Blood, it would forced to assume its true form during an exorcism.

PATHOLOGY OF THE BLOOD VESSELS

According to the *Magical Pivot*: "When the Blood is deficient, the complexion is pale and there is insufficient irrigation in the layers of the skin, the Blood Vessels in this area (of the skin) are completely empty."

WESTERN MEDICAL PERSPECTIVE

The blood, heart and blood vessels (arteries, capillaries and veins) form the cardiovascular system. The general function of the cardiovascular system is the circulation of the blood. As a whole, blood is composed of two components: 55% is formed from blood plasma (a watery liquid containing dissolved substances), while the remaining 45% is formed from cells and cell fragments.

Arteries conduct oxygenated blood away from the heart to the internal organs and the extremities, while the veins circulate the blood back to the heart. The capillaries are simple endothelial tubes from which nutrients and gases diffuse into and out from the tissues. The hollow center, through which the blood flows, is called the lumen.

The unique structure of the arteries allows them two important properties: elasticity and contractility. The arterial wall is composed of three coats or "tunics," described as follows:

- **Tunic Interna:** The tunic interna is the inner coat of the arteries, and is composed of a lining of endothelium (a skin-like tissue that stays in contact with the blood), a basement membrane, and a layer of elastic tissue called the internal elastic lamina.
- **Tunic Media:** The tunic media is the middle coating of the arteries, and is composed of both elastic fibers and smooth muscle fibers. It is usually the thickest layer.
- **Tunic Externa:** The tunic externa is the outer coating of the arteries, and is composed of both elastic and collagen fibers. An external elastic lamina sometimes separates the tunic externa from the tunic media.

CIRCULATORY SYSTEM

As outlined above, the Chinese concept of the Mai includes more than just the physical structure of the Blood Vessels. The integrated roles of Qi, Blood, and Mai do not conflict with, but rather augment the western medical understanding of the circulatory system. The circulatory system includes the Heart, the Blood Vessels, and the Blood. Chapter eight explains in detail the structure and function of the Heart as a Yin organ, though certain subtle aspects of the pulse that are ascribed to the Heart in Western physiology are equivalent to aspects of the Blood Vessels in Chinese medicine. The term Blood Vessels refers to the entire closed network of vessels that begins and ends at the Heart. The Blood is the essential substance that is energized by the Lungs, pumped outwards by the Heart, and distributed throughout the body via the Blood Vessels.

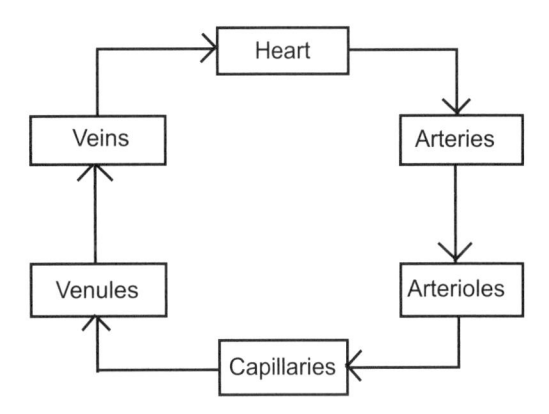

Figure 7.32. Blood Flow Within the Circulatory System

There are over 60,000 miles of Blood Vessels in the average adult human body. The various types of Blood Vessels include arteries, arterioles, capillaries, venules, and veins (Figure 7.32). Blood is carried away from the Heart through a network of vessels called arteries. The arteries distribute Blood throughout the body by branching into smaller vessels, termed arterioles. The arterioles then branch further into tiny vessels, called capillaries, the walls of which are thin enough to allow for the essential exchange of energy and nutrients between the Blood and the individual cells. After distributing Blood through all the tissues of the body, the capillaries begin to merge together, forming into progressively larger vessels called venules. The venules then form the larger vessels, called veins, which return the Blood back to the Heart.

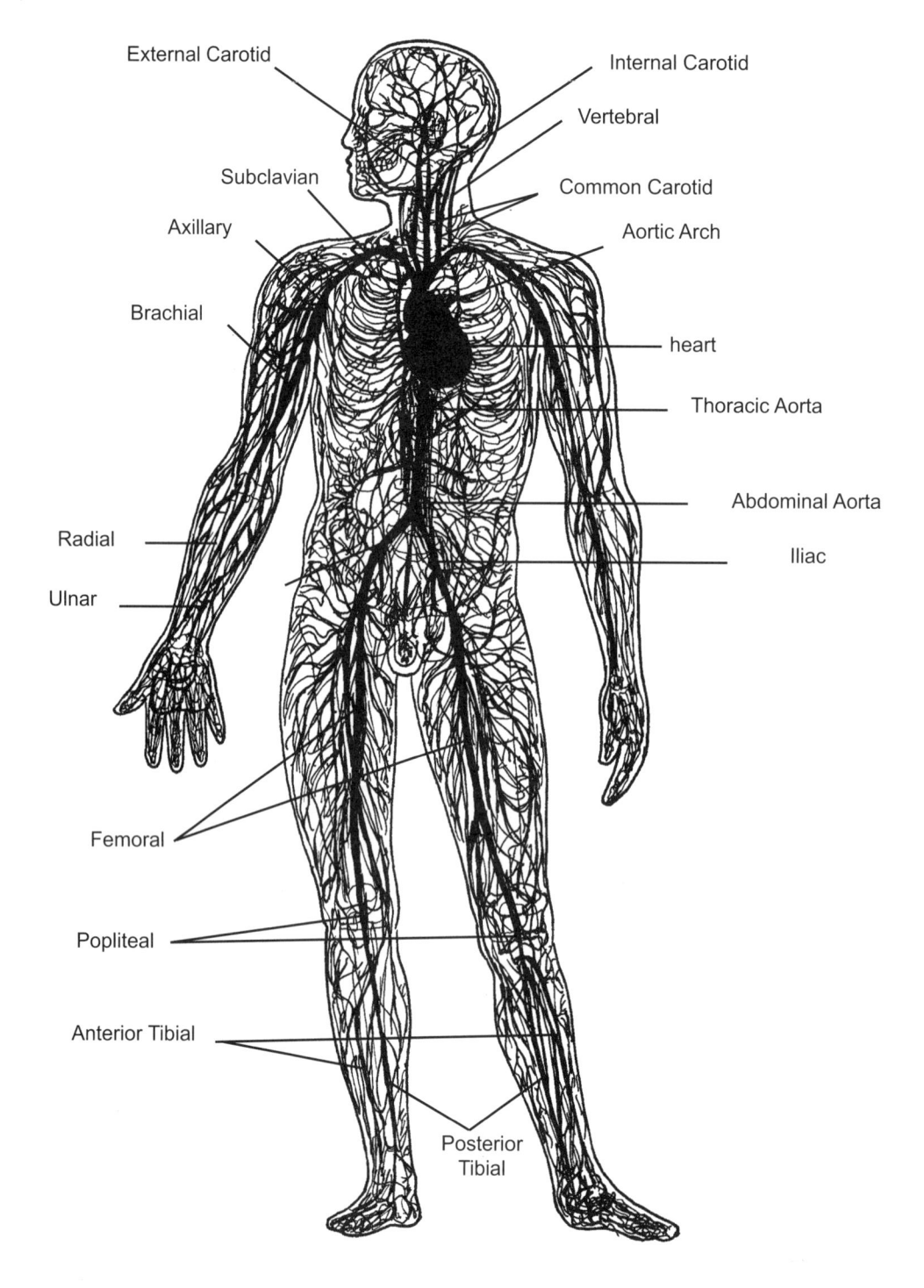

VOLUME 1, SECTION 1: FOUNDATIONS OF CHINESE ENERGETIC MEDICINE

Figure 7.33. The Arterial Network of the Circulatory System

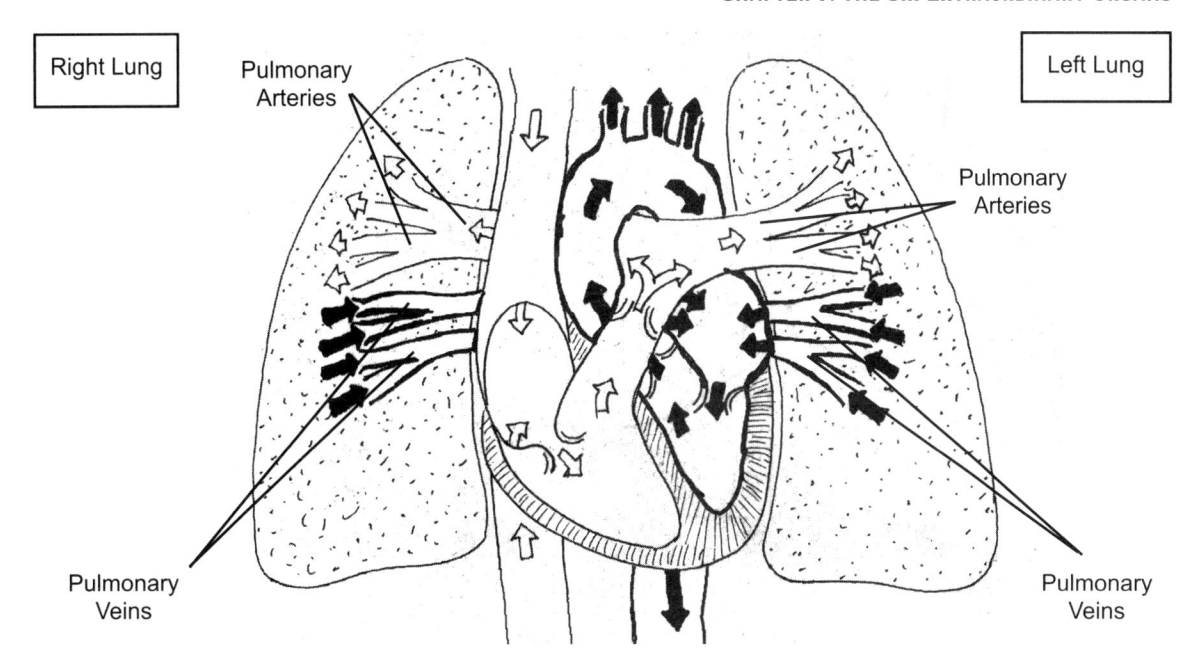

Figure 7.34. Pulmonary Circulation (Inspired by the original artwork of Wynn Kapit).

THREE CIRCULATORY ROUTES

Each individual will develop and utilize a total of three circulatory routes: fetal circulation, pulmonary circulation and systemic circulation. The circulatory system of a fetus is slightly different than that of an adult, and is termed fetal circulation. The two circulatory routes within the adult body are termed systemic circulation, and pulmonary circulation. These two routes begin and end at the Heart.

SYSTEMIC CIRCULATION

The systemic circulatory route delivers oxygenated Blood (red) to the entire body by pumping it outwards from the left ventricle of the Heart through a vast network of arteries, arterioles, and capillaries. At the level of the capillaries, oxygen and nutrition are delivered to all the tissues of the body, passing from the Blood through the thin capillary walls and into the cells. The capillaries also allow for the Blood to absorb carbon dioxide and other waste products of cellular metabolism from the cells. The Blood (now blue) flows from the capillaries through venules and veins, eventually returning to the right atrium of the Heart (Figure 7.33).

PULMONARY CIRCULATION

Pulmonary circulation refers to the circulatory loop the leads blood from the Heart into the Lungs to be oxygenated, and then back to the Heart again. The pulmonary arteries lead deoxygenated Blood (blue) away from the right ventricle of the Heart and into the right and left Lungs. Arterioles and pulmonary capillaries lead the Blood into contact with the alveoli of the Lungs, where carbon dioxide and other wastes are released from the Blood, and oxygen is reabsorbed into the Blood. The pulmonary capillaries then gather to form venules and veins, eventually forming the pulmonary veins which return oxygenated Blood (now red) to the left atrium of the Heart. The pulmonary veins are the only postnatal veins that carry oxygenated Blood back to the Heart (Figure 7.34).

FETAL CIRCULATION

The blood-vascular system of a fetus constantly changes throughout embryonic development and differs functionally from that of an adult. During fetal development, the fetus receives and releases material from its Blood via the vascular network of the placenta. Umbilical arteries direct

Blood from the fetus along the umbilical cord and into the placenta. The Blood Vessels of the placenta contain tiny villi that allow for oxygen, nutrition, and wastes to be exchanged between the Blood of the fetus and the Blood of the mother. Purified Blood returns into the fetus from the placenta via the umbilical vein.

Fetal circulation also differs from that of an adult because the gastrointestinal tract, Lungs, and Kidneys of a fetus are nonfunctional, and therefore do not play a role in energizing or detoxifying the Blood. Because the fetus is dependant on the placenta (and not its own internal organs) for the maintenance of its Blood, there are numerous peculiarities to the internal anatomy of the network of Blood Vessels and veins within the fetus, though these peculiarities normally disappear after birth. It is important to note that the circulatory system of the fetus does not flow directly into the circulatory system of the mother. The Blood of the mother flows into and out of the placenta via a network of arteries and veins that stems from her Uterus.

THE PULSE

The pulse, one meaning of the Chinese word "Mai," can be understood in western terms as a combined function of the Heart and the arteries. While the left ventricle of the Heart is the primary force for pumping oxygenated Blood throughout the body, the arteries and arterioles create an additional pumping action as the Blood flows outward and into the capillaries. This pumping action is due to the unique structure of the arteries that allows them to expand and contract passively (elasticity), and also to actively contract (contractility).

The arteries have a much more developed layer of smooth muscle than do the veins, allowing for the arteries to play an active role in the distribution of Blood.

As Blood is pumped from the Heart, the arteries passively expand, allowing the extra Blood to flow outward. This is followed by a peristaltic muscular contraction within the arteries that continues to push the Blood outward towards the capillaries. The veins do not have this property of contractility, nor do they have the same degree of elasticity as do the arteries. Instead, the venous network contains numerous one way valves, making return of Blood along the veins to the Heart relatively passive in comparison to the flow of Blood within the arteries. Venous circulation is thus greatly influenced by the pull of gravity and by the contraction of skeletal muscles.

CHAPTER 8
THE TWELVE PRIMARY ORGANS, CHANNELS AND COLLATERALS

THE INTERNAL ORGANS AND CHINESE INTERNAL MEDICINE

In ancient China, various medical graphs and anatomical drawings were used to assist the doctor in clinical practice. The oldest of these detailed charts can be traced back to the Han Dynasty (206 B.C.-220 A.D.). Since that time, textbooks on internal medicine have used two primarily different methods to depict the human body. One method was similar to Western anatomy in that the internal organs were conceptualized as having shape, form and function. The illustrations depicting the internal organs in this manner were traditionally known as either the "Charts of Inner Lights" or the "Charts for Visualizing the True Ones" (Figure 8.1). In their most ancient form, such charts would depict the body's internal organ "pools of energy" along with their "energetic presence." The subtle energetic presence of an internal organ was sometimes referred to as the "Radiant One," which was said to reside within the organ itself. The internal organs and their associated systems were sometimes known in ancient times as "orbs" or "spheres of influence."

The second common method of illustrating human anatomy involves maps which showed the routes of the body fluids, arteries and energetic channels. They were traditionally called the "Charts of the Halls of Light" (Figure 8.2), and focused on the body's "rivers of energy." These ancient maps of the channels of the human energy system are the predecessors of today's modern acupuncture charts. Doctors in ancient China focused their attention on the circulation and movement of energy and fluids moving throughout the body rather than just the physical functions of each of the internal organs.

A thorough comprehension of energetic anatomy and physiology is necessary in order to

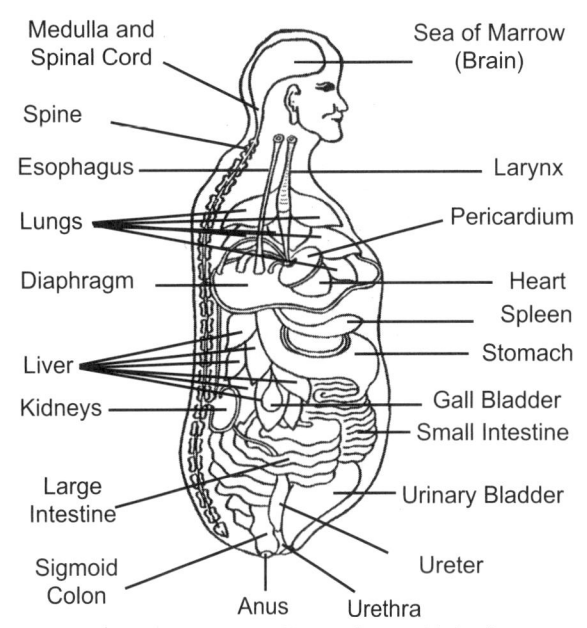

Figure 8.1. The Ancient "Chart of Inner Lights"

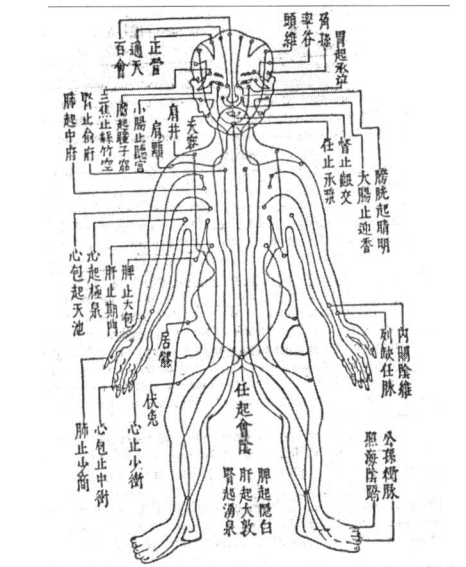

Figure 8.2. The Ancient "Chart of the Halls of Lights"

understand the fundamental characteristics of each internal organ and each energy channel, as well as the complex interactions between the two. This understanding is a prerequisite for learning differential diagnosis, which is necessary in order to categorize various symptoms into meaningful (clinically useful) patterns of disharmony. The ability to categorize various symptoms enables the Qigong doctor to recognize and treat pathologies unique to specific organs and channel energies.

ENERGETIC ANATOMY

In order to gain a deeper understanding of the anatomy of human tissue and the causes of death, ancient Chinese physicians studied the internal formation and structures of the human body through postmortem examination. Initially, the size and weight of all of the body's internal organs were measured and recorded by these ancient physicians. Historians speculate that postmortem autopsies were practiced in ancient China during the Zhou Dynasty (1028-221 B.C.), but were prohibited during later dynasties because of Confucianistic beliefs, several hundred years later.

There are many ancient records in Chinese literature describing dissections. For example, it is recorded that during the Han Dynasty (206 B.C.-220 A.D.), the Emperor Wang Mang ordered his court physicians to dissect the body of a captured revolutionary. During the procedure, measurements were made of the internal viscera, bowels and vessels by inserting fine bamboo rods into the individual's dissected body.

The *Huangdi Neijing* (Yellow Emperors Inner Classic) contains details on postmortem dissection, and refers to standard procedures for performing autopsies. In the *Neijing Ling Shu*, it states, "upon death, a dissection study can be performed to examine, reveal and disclose the condition of the internal organs. There are great standard measures used to determine the strength or fragility of the viscera, the size of the bowels and the contents of the digestive system, being plentiful or sparse. The length of the vessels can be measured, the Blood examined being either clear or turbid, and the Qi observed being plentiful or sparse."

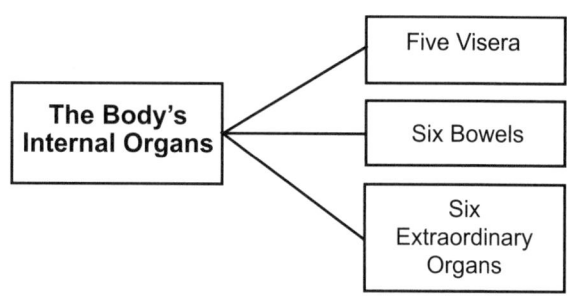

Figure 8.3. The Three Groups of Internal Organs

ENERGETIC PHYSIOLOGY

In Chinese medical science, the study of energetic physiology is called Zhang Xiang Xue Shou, which literally translates as "the theory of the phenomena of internal organs." Here, the word "phenomena" means visible external manifestations. As all of the major internal organs had already been identified by the postmortem examinations of the past, Chinese physicians placed little importance on the internal organ's physical structure, focusing instead on each organ's energetic function. While Western anatomy and physiology is primarily concerned with the physical body in its most concrete forms (investigating the structures of the major body organs and systems, etc.), energetic anatomy and physiology focus mainly on the underlying patterns of energy that animate and sustain the physical form.

The ancient Chinese physicians noted that when diagnosing illness, all of the body's viscera reflect disease conditions related to functional disorders that were the result of pathogenic factors. Disruptions within the energetic function of any organ system manifest clinically through various physiological and psychological symptoms.

In Traditional Chinese Medicine, the internal organs are divided into three main groups: the five viscera, the six bowels, and the six Extraordinary organs, described as follows (Figure 8.3):

1. **The Five Viscera (Wu Zang):** These Yin organs include the Liver, Heart, Spleen, Lungs and Kidneys. These organs function to preserve the body's vital substances (Jing, Qi, Shen, Blood, Marrow and Body Fluids), and are important for their role in the distribution and dispersion of the body's nutrients. Each of the five

viscera is capable of containing and storing a particular refined substance known as the body's Jing Shen (Spirit Essence). There is a spirit essence unique to each internal organ. The spirit essence of the five Yin organs are collectively known as the Wu Jing Shen, or "Five Essence Spirits."

It is important to clarify that in modern T.C.M., there are only five Yin organs or viscera (Zang). The Pericardium, which is sometimes categorized as a sixth Yin viscera, is not actually considered to be an independent Yin organ, but rather a protective covering of the Heart organ.

- The Chinese ideogram for "Zang," is composed of two characters (Figure 8.4). The character to the left, "Ji" depicts the Chinese ideogram for body tissue, muscle or flesh (all of which are forms of connective tissue). The character on the right can be translated as to gather, conceal, hold, hoard and hide in a safe place (as a treasure). Together, both characters depict the body's internal viscera as the organs that gather and hoard the energetic Jing, Qi and Shen within the flesh.

2. **The Six Bowels (Liu Fu):** These Yang bowels include the Gall Bladder, Small Intestine, Stomach, Large Intestine, Urinary Bladder and Triple Burners. Their function is to transmit and digest food and water, and to eliminate the body's waste products.

    In ancient times, the Chinese considered the Triple Burners as a hollow Yang organ (Fu) containing the body's vapors (Qi and Shen), fluids (Jing, Blood, Marrow, Jin and Ye) and "Fire" (Heart Fire, Mingmen Fire and Urinary Bladder Fire). Extending through the torso, the Triple Burners do not have an anatomical equivalent in Western Medicine.

- The Chinese ideogram for "Fu," is composed of two characters (Figure 8.5). The character to the left, "Ji" depicts the Chinese ideogram for body tissue, muscle or flesh (all of which are forms of connective tissue). The character on the right can be translated as a storehouse for precious objects, treasury, palace, mansion

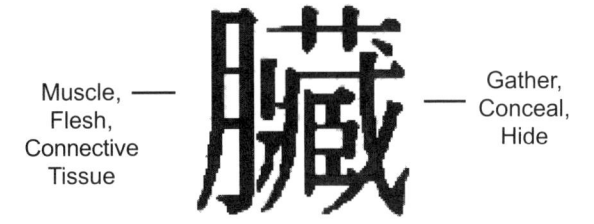

Figure 8.4. The Chinese character for "Zang," Viscera

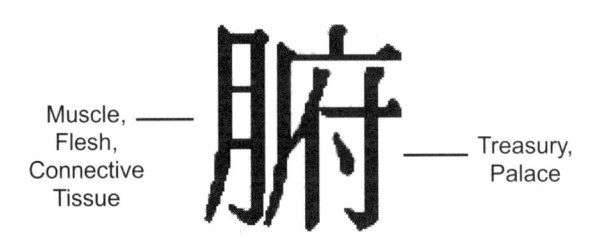

Figure 8.5. The Chinese Ideograph for "Fu," Bowel

or officer. Together, both characters depict the body's internal bowels as treasure house organs within the flesh. In ancient China, the concept of a storehouse or treasury related to short-term storage, since the items were constantly moving in and out.

3. **The Six Extraordinary Organs:** The Extraordinary Organs include the Uterus, Brain, Gall Bladder, Marrow, Bones and Blood Vessels. They function like Yin organs in storing the body's vital substances, but are hollow and resemble Yang organs.

Medical Qigong students study the physiological functions and the pathological changes of the internal organs, in addition to their relationship with the universal and environmental energies. Chinese medicine groups the body's Zang/Fu internal organs into five discrete functional systems. Each Zang/Fu system has specific interior (internal organs) and exterior (superficial muscles, tissues, skin and senses) correspondences and is assigned a specific physical, energetic, and spiritual attribute. By observing the physiological features of the internal organs, the ancient Chinese established a consistent model for describing the functions of each organ. This model was then applied to diagnose and treat organ pathologies.

THE INTERNAL ORGANS AND YIN AND YANG

The Yin organ (Zang) and Yang organ (Fu) systems were considered officials, each in charge of specific duties in the governing of the human body. In defining the Zang Fu organs, the Chinese character "Zang" may be translated as "viscera," while the character "Fu" may be translated as "archives," "treasury," "storehouse," or "palace."

In ancient times, each Zang Fu organ signified a place where "human records" in the form of emotions, thoughts and experiences were stored. The celestial counterparts of these twelve internal organs were believed to reside in Heaven, located within the twelve spirits that reside within the Big Dipper constellation. The job of these twelve spirits was to oversee the individual's health and destiny, and to guide the individual in the cultivation of virtue. The five virtues (or Five Agents) of the Zang organs (kindness, order, trust, integrity and wisdom) influence the individual through the spiritual insight of the three Hun, and through the Dao. By acting as a vessel for the Dao, the individual is capable of bringing the heart of Heaven into the world, thereby fulfilling his or her destiny.

Each of the internal Zang Fu organs is paired according to their energetic actions of transforming, transporting and storing. Each Yin (Zang) organ is thus paired with a Yang (Fu) organ. The relationship between the Yin and Yang paired internal organs represents an energetic correspondence in both structure and function. Each of the Yin organs has a corresponding energetic function of storing one of the body's vital substances, while each of the Yang organs corresponds to a particular aspect of the process of transportation and transformation.

The two primary types of internal organs (Yin and Yang) are described as follows:
- **Yin (Zang Organs):** These are solid organs and are responsible for storing the pure, refined vital substances (Qi, Blood, Essence and Body Fluids), which they receive from the Yang organs after the transformation of food.
- **Yang (Fu Organs):** These are hollow organs and are responsible for receiving, moving, transforming, digesting and excreting food substances.

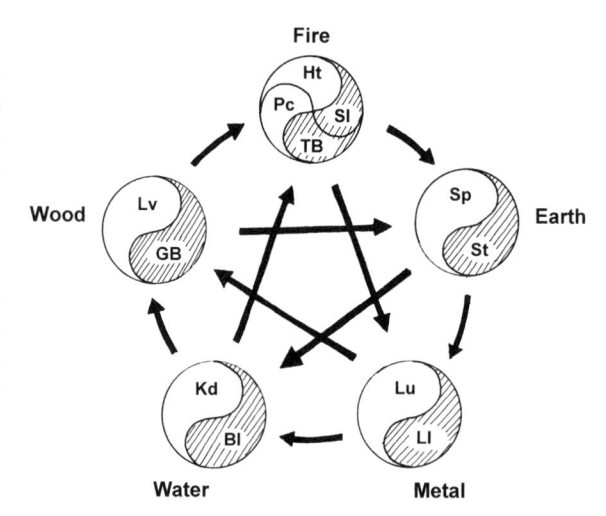

Figure 8.6. The Energetic Movement of the Five Element Correspondences

The body's ten internal organs (Zang Fu) and their Yin and Yang divisions are described as follows:
- The Liver (Yin) is paired with the Gall Bladder (Yang)
- The Heart (Yin) is paired with the Small Intestine (Yang)
- The Spleen (Yin) is paired with the Stomach (Yang)
- The Lungs (Yin) are paired with the Large Intestine (Yang)
- The Kidneys (Yin) are paired with the Urinary Bladder (Yang)

THE INTERNAL ORGANS AND FIVE ELEMENTS

Traditional Chinese Medicine utilizes the concept of the Five Elements, or Five Phases as an integral part of both diagnosis and treatment. The Five Element theory (Chapter 25, Volume 3) was an essential aspect of virtually every discipline in ancient China (medicine, martial arts, military strategy, politics, painting, poetry, architecture). This theory allowed the Chinese to classify tangible and intangible substances, internal organs, and herbs into five interrelating categories (i.e., five senses, five viscera, five emotions, five virtues, five flavors, etc.) for observation and study, as well as for diagnosis and treatment. The complex interactions between the body's internal organs could be understood and

simplified by identifying the various patterns of relationship between the Five Elements. The Five Element Theory is applied to the internal organs as follows (Figure 8.6):
- The Liver and Gall Bladder are associated with the Wood Element.
- The Heart and Small Intestine (as well as the Pericardium and Triple Burners) are associated with the Fire Element.
- The Spleen and Stomach are associated with the Earth Element.
- The Lungs and Large Intestine are associated with the Metal Element.
- The Kidneys and Urinary Bladder are associated with the Water Element.

INTERNAL ORGANS AND THE VITAL SUBSTANCES

The human body essentially consists of fluids and energy. In Chinese medical science, the body's internal organs are responsible for creating and distributing Jing, Qi, Shen, Blood and Body Fluids. Clinical diagnosis in Medical Qigong is based on observing the smooth flow or stagnation of the body's Jing, Qi and Shen; the excess or deficiency of Qi, Shen, Blood and Body Fluids; and their influence on internal organ functions (Figure 8.7).

The external orifices of the body serve as the gates and windows of the Jing and Shen, which are themselves ultimately rooted in the energy of the Blood. The body's Qi and Zhi (Will) serve as the messengers of the Five Orbs (the five Yin organs) and are used for sense reception, respiration and excretion. The physical and psychological associations of each of the orifices are governed by the Jing and Shen of the organ's orb with which they are connected.

The internal organs create and distribute Qi, Blood and Body Fluids. These actions occur regularly throughout the body's tissues, and manifest in the Blood Heat Cycle. The Blood Heat Cycle is the alternation of peaks (high-tide) and ebbs (low-tide) of each of the internal organs and channels, which occurs over a 24 hour time period. Each internal organ and channel has either a Yin or Yang characteristic and is grouped and paired according to its Five Element nature.

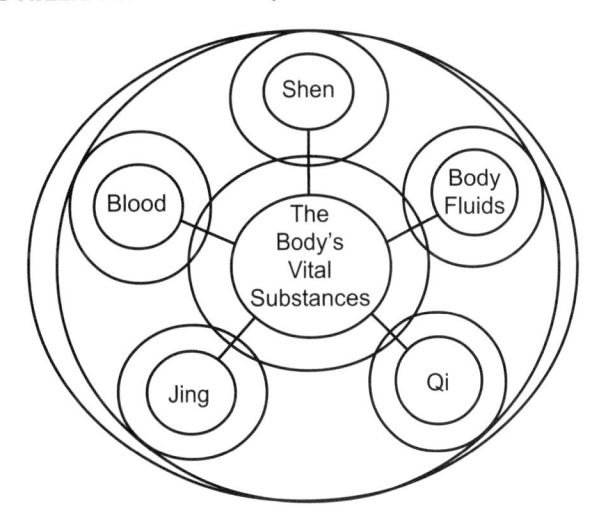

Figure 8.7. The Body's Vital Substances

One of the main functions of the internal organs is to ensure the production, storage, replenishment, transformation and movement of vital substances. Each of the body's vital substances (Qi, Blood, Jing, Body Fluids and Shen) is related to one or more of the internal organs. For example:
- The Liver stores the Blood and is responsible for the body's metabolic process and the dispersal of nutrients.
- The Heart governs the Blood and provides the energetic force for Blood circulation.
- The Spleen holds the Blood, governs Gu Qi (energy derived from food and drink), and influences Body Fluids. Additionally, it is also responsible for governing the body's lymph system, functions as part of the immune system, and the controls Blood coagulation.
- The Lungs govern Qi, influence Body Fluids, and are responsible for the absorption of oxygen and expulsion of respiratory gases.
- The Kidneys store Jing, influence Body Fluids, and are responsible for filtering metabolic waste products from the Blood through the process of urine formation.

THE INTERNAL ORGANS AND THE TISSUES

Each internal organ has a direct influence over specific tissues of the body. The health of a particular body tissue is indicative of the state of health of the internal organ with which it is associated. A summery of the internal organs and their associated tissues is described as follows:

- The Liver controls the nerves and tendons, and manifests through the body's fingernails and toenails.
- The Heart controls the Blood and the Blood Vessels, and manifests through the body's complexion.
- The Spleen controls the muscles and flesh, and manifests through the lips.
- The Lungs control the skin, and manifest through body hair.
- The Kidneys control the Bones, and manifest through the head hair and eyebrows.

THE INTERNAL ORGANS AND THE EMOTIONS

Each of the internal organs is related to a particular emotional and mental state. These emotional and mental states are divided into two main categories of congenital emotional patterns (due to the Five Agents) and acquired emotional patterns (due to external contact with the environment). The congenital emotional patterns of the five Yin organs are representative of an individual's natural state of spiritual harmony. The acquired emotions become a cause of imbalance when they are chronic or excessive. The energetic state of an internal organ (balanced, excess or deficient) will affect the individual's emotions. Likewise, external exposure to certain emotions and experiences will affect the energetic state of the individual's internal organs. A summary of the emotional and mental states correlated with the internal organs is described as follows:

- The Liver: Congenital state relates to love and kindness; Acquired state relates to anger and rage.
- The Heart: Congenital state relates to peace and order; Acquired state relates to excitement and nervousness.
- The Spleen: Congenital state relates to trust and honesty; Acquired state relates to worry and obsession.
- The Lungs: Congenital state relates to integrity and righteousness; Acquired state relates to grief and sadness.
- The Kidneys: Congenital state relates to wisdom and self-understanding; Acquired state relates to fear and insecurity.

THE INTERNAL ORGANS AND THEIR SPIRITUAL ASPECTS

The five Yin organs (Liver, Heart, Spleen, Lungs, and Kidneys) store and protect the Jing essence. The five Yin organs are considered to be the command centers responsible for all energetic and spiritual movement. The specific movements are governed and directed by Wu Jing Shen (Five Essence Spirits: Hun, Shen, Yi, Po, and Zhi), which are physically represented in the five Yin organs.

Each of the internal organs is responsible for creating and maintaining certain spiritual energetic states. This manifests in a multidimensional correspondence between the internal organs and all of the body's physiological, energetic, mental, emotional and spiritual states (Figure 8.8). The correspondence between the five Yin organ and the Wu Jing Shen is described as follows:

- The Liver stores the Hun (Ethereal Soul)
- The Heart stores the Shen (Spirit)
- The Spleen stores the Yi (Intention)
- The Lungs store the Po (Corporeal Soul)
- The Kidneys store the Zhi (Will)

THE INTERNAL ORGANS AND CLIMATE

Each internal organ is particularly susceptible to the influence of a different climatic condition, described as follows:

- The Liver is influenced by Wind
- The Heart is influenced by Heat
- The Spleen is influenced by Dampness
- The Lungs are influenced by Dryness
- The Kidneys are influenced by Cold

THE INTERNAL ORGANS AND THEIR SENSE ORGAN OPENINGS

Each of the internal organs is functionally related to one of the sense organs. The physical health and function of a particular sense organ relies specifically on the nourishment that it receives from the internal organ with which it is linked. Each of the internal organs "opens" into a particular sense organ orifice, allowing for communication between the external and the internal environments. The Chinese character for "to open" also carries the meaning "to move," suggesting this movement of

Chapter 8: The Twelve Primary Organs, Channels and Collaterals

Organ	Jing			Qi			Shen	
	Yin/Yang	Element	Tissue	Sense	Taste	Climate	Color	Spirit
G.B.	Yang	Wood	Nerve/Tendons	Sight	Sour	Wind	Green/Blue	Hun
Lv.	Yin	Wood	Nerve/Tendons	Sight	Sour	Wind	Green/Blue	Hun
Lu.	Yin	Metal	Skin/Body Hair	Smell	Pungent	Dry	White	Po
L.I.	Yang	Metal	Skin/Body Hair	Smell	Pungent	Dry	White	Po
St.	Yang	Earth	Muscles/Flesh	Taste	Sweet	Damp	Yellow/Brown	Yi
Sp.	Yin	Earth	Muscles/Flesh	Taste	Sweet	Damp	Yellow/Brown	Yi
Ht.	Yin	Fire	Blood/Vessels	Touch	Bitter	Heat	Red	Shen
S.I.	Yang	Fire	Blood/Vessels	Touch	Bitter	Heat	Red	Shen
U.B.	Yang	Water	Bones/Head Hair	Hearing	Salty	Cold	Black/Dark Blue	Zhi
Kd.	Yin	Water	Bones/Head Hair	Hearing	Salty	Cold	Black/Dark Blue	Zhi
Pc.	Yin	Fire	Blood/Vessels	Touch	Bitter	Heat	Red	Shen
T.B.	Yang	Fire	Blood/Vessels	Touch	Bitter	Heat	Red	Shen

Figure 8.8. The Internal Organs and their Jing, Qi, and Shen Associations

energy between the internal organs and external organs. The internal organs open into the senses, and are described as follows:
- The Liver "opens" into the eyes, controlling both the eyes and sight. This allows sight to influence the energetic nature of the Hun (Ethereal Soul).
- The Heart "opens" into the tongue, controlling both the tongue and speech. This allows speech to influence the Shen (Spirit).
- The Spleen "opens" into the mouth, controlling both the mouth and taste. This allows taste to influence the Yi (Intention).
- The Lungs "open" into the nose, controlling both the nose and smell. This allows smell to influence the Po (Corporeal Soul).
- The Kidneys "open" into the ears, controlling both the ears and hearing. This allows hearing to influence the Zhi (Will).

THE INTERNAL ORGANS AND TASTE

Each of the internal organs responds to a certain flavor. A moderate amount of the corresponding flavor has a tonifying effect on that particular organ system, described as follows:
- The Liver (Yin) and the Gall Bladder respond to the sour flavor
- The Heart (Yin) and the Small Intestine respond to the bitter flavor
- The Spleen (Yin) and the Stomach respond to the sweet flavor
- The Lungs (Yin) and the Large Intestine respond to the pungent flavor
- The Kidneys (Yin) and the Urinary Bladder respond to the salty flavor

THE INTERNAL ORGANS AND SOUNDS

Each of the internal organs responds to a particular sound. An organ's associated sound will cause a strong resonant vibration within that organ and organ system, and is generally used in the Medical Qigong clinic for purgation, described as follows:
- The Liver (Yin) and the Gall Bladder respond to the sound Jue and the note E
- The Heart (Yin) and the Small Intestine re-

spond to the sound Zhi and the note G
- The Spleen (Yin) and the Stomach respond to the sound Gong and the note C
- The Lungs (Yin) and the Large Intestine respond to the sound Shang and the note D
- The Kidneys (Yin) and the Urinary Bladder respond to the sound Yu and the note A

The Internal Organs and Color

Each of the internal organs responds to a particular color, which has a tonifying effect on that particular organ and its internal and external systems, described as follows:
- The Liver (Yin) and the Gall Bladder respond to the color green/blue (Qing)
- The Heart (Yin) and the Small Intestine respond to the color red (Chi)
- The Spleen (Yin) and the Stomach respond to the color yellow/light brown (Huang)
- The Lungs (Yin) and the Large Intestine respond to the color white (Bai)
- The Kidneys (Yin) and the Urinary Bladder respond to the color black (Hei)

Introduction to Channels

According to Traditional Chinese Medicine, a system of channels exists that integrates all the body's separate parts and functions into a unified organism. The study of these channels, their energetic functions, and the interactions between them provides the Qigong doctor with a basis for understanding the relationships among various physiological and pathological disorders which occur within the patient's tissues.

Extensive research conducted by Dr. Kim Bong Han of the University of Pyongang in North Korea, found that the energetic channels are composed of a special type of histological tissue, an association yet to be explored by Western science. Dr. Kim has also discovered that the channels have a thin membranous wall which contains a type of transparent and colorless liquid which provides a pathway for Qi (Figure 8.9)

The study of Chinese medicine rests on the understanding of the patterns and cycles of Qi circulation (Figure 8.10). Through the observation

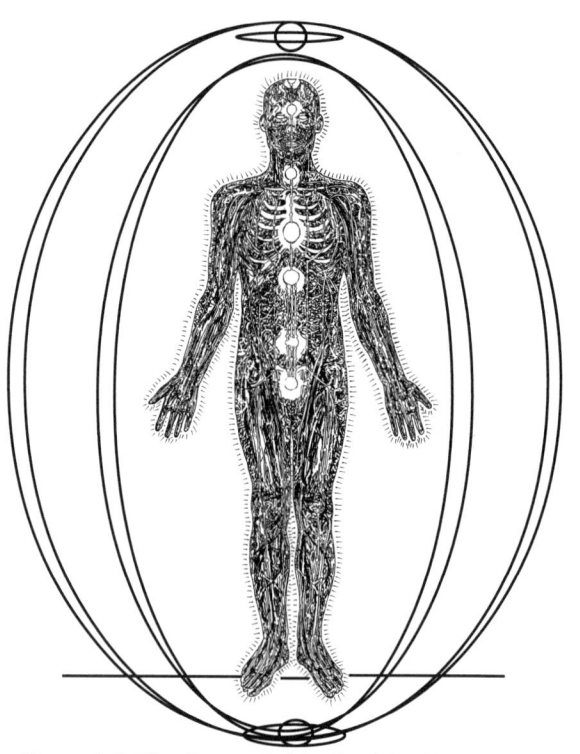

Figure 8.9. The Energetic Matrix of the Human Body (Inspired by the original artwork of Alex Grey).

and study of these patterns, it becomes apparent that many diseases follow a predictable course of development. The pathology of an internal organ will often manifest in specific symptoms, which can be diagnosed and linked to the organ or channel of origin through the previously mentioned set of correspondences. Therefore, understanding the circulation of Qi flow allows the doctor to control each organ's energetic function and the health of its entire orb. By stimulating specific sites on the body's surface, diseases in both the superficial tissues and internal organs can be treated.

A doctor of Medical Qigong uses various techniques to facilitate the purgation, tonification and regulation of the body's major energetic pathways responsible for carrying energy and nutrition to the internal organs. These energetic pathways function as channels and vessels, and are responsible for connecting the flow of Qi throughout the whole body to transfer energy and nutrition both internally and externally.

The channels are also known as meridians or Jing-luo. The Chinese character commonly used for this type of Jing means "to move through" (not to be confused with the Chinese character Jing, commonly used for "essence"). The character "Luo" means "a net" (the body's inner fascia). Along these channels are major trunks and lesser branches that connect internally with the vital organs and externally with the major channels, limbs, sensory organs, and orifices.

The smaller branches are known as collaterals. The tiny areas where the Qi pools along these channels and collaterals are called points. These points are the spots where the patient's spirit and energy enter and leave the body. When stimulated, these channel points (also called "acupuncture points") cause an energetic response from within the internal organs and channels, thus changing the flow of Qi within the body. The Qi flowing within these channels can be directed by the Qigong doctor to flow from organ to channel, from channel to channel, or from point to point along the same channel.

The channels unite and bind the body into an energetic whole. Channel theory is related to organ theory. Traditionally, the internal organs were not regarded simply as independent anatomical entities. Rather, Traditional Chinese Medicine focuses on the functional and pathological interrelationships between the channel network and the internal organs.

For example, although Chinese herbalists emphasize the internal organs, acupuncturists primarily focus on the use of the channels. When combined, both acupuncture and herbs make a powerful contribution towards healing. This is why acupuncturists will commonly prescribe herbs to further a treatment's effect.

Qi travels throughout the physical body along the channels and collaterals in much the same way as water flows through rivers and streams. An ancient Chinese medical text explains this concept as follows: "Heaven is covered with the constellations, Earth with the waterways, and Man with channels." The Qigong doctors of ancient China paid much more attention to the body fluids and energies circulating through the body than to the

Channel Name	Yin or Yang	Associated Organ	Element	Blood Heat Cycle	Qi Blood Cycle	Abbreviation
Gall Bladder	Yang	Liver	Wood	11 p.m.– 1 a.m.	More Qi Less Blood	G.B.
Liver	Yin	Gall Bladder	Wood	1 a.m.– 3 a.m.	Less Qi More Blood	Lv.
Lungs	Yin	Large Intestine	Metal	3 a.m.– 5 a.m.	More Qi Less Blood	Lu.
Large Intestine	Yang	Lung	Metal	5 a.m.– 7 a.m.	Balanced Qi and Blood	L.I.
Stomach	Yang	Spleen	Earth	7 a.m.– 9 a.m.	Balanced Qi and Blood	St.
Spleen	Yin	Stomach	Earth	9 a.m.– 11 a.m.	More Qi Less Blood	Sp.
Heart	Yin	Small Intestine	Fire	11 a.m.– 1 pm.	More Qi Less Blood	Ht.
Small Intestine	Yang	Heart	Fire	1 p.m.– 3 p.m.	Less Qi More Blood	S.I.
Urinary Bladder	Yang	Kidney	Water	3 p.m.– 5 p.m.	Less Qi More Blood	UB.
Kidney	Yin	Bladder	Water	5 p.m.– 7 p.m.	More Qi Less Blood	Kd.
Pericardium	Yin	Triple Burner	Fire	7 p.m.– 9 p.m.	Less Qi More Blood	Pc.
Triple Burner	Yang	Pericardium	Fire	9 p.m.– 11 p.m.	More Qi Less Blood	T.B.

Figure 8.10. The Twelve Primary Channels are divided into Yin channels (connected to the solid organs) and Yang channels (connected to the hollow organs).

physical anatomical structures, as the body's fluids and energies were considered to be much more fundamental.

The channels serve as the link between the energies (such as Jing, Qi, Shen) and the ingredients (such as Blood and Body Fluids) that enliven and feed the tissues. The human body's main energetic rivers are the Twelve Primary Channels and Eight Extraordinary Vessels (see Chapter 7).

CLASSIFICATION OF CHANNELS

The energetic pathways of the body are classified into four main categories: Jing (Channels), Luo Mai (Collaterals), Jing Jin (Muscle and Tendon), and Pi Fu (Skin Zones), and are described as follows (Figure 8.11):

1. **Jing:** The Jing are the Primary Channels. These channels include the Eight Extraordinary Vessels, the Twelve Primary Channels, and the Twelve Divergent Channels.
2. **Luo:** The Luo are the Collaterals. These collaterals include the Fifteen Major Collaterals, the Minute Collaterals, and the Superficial Collaterals.

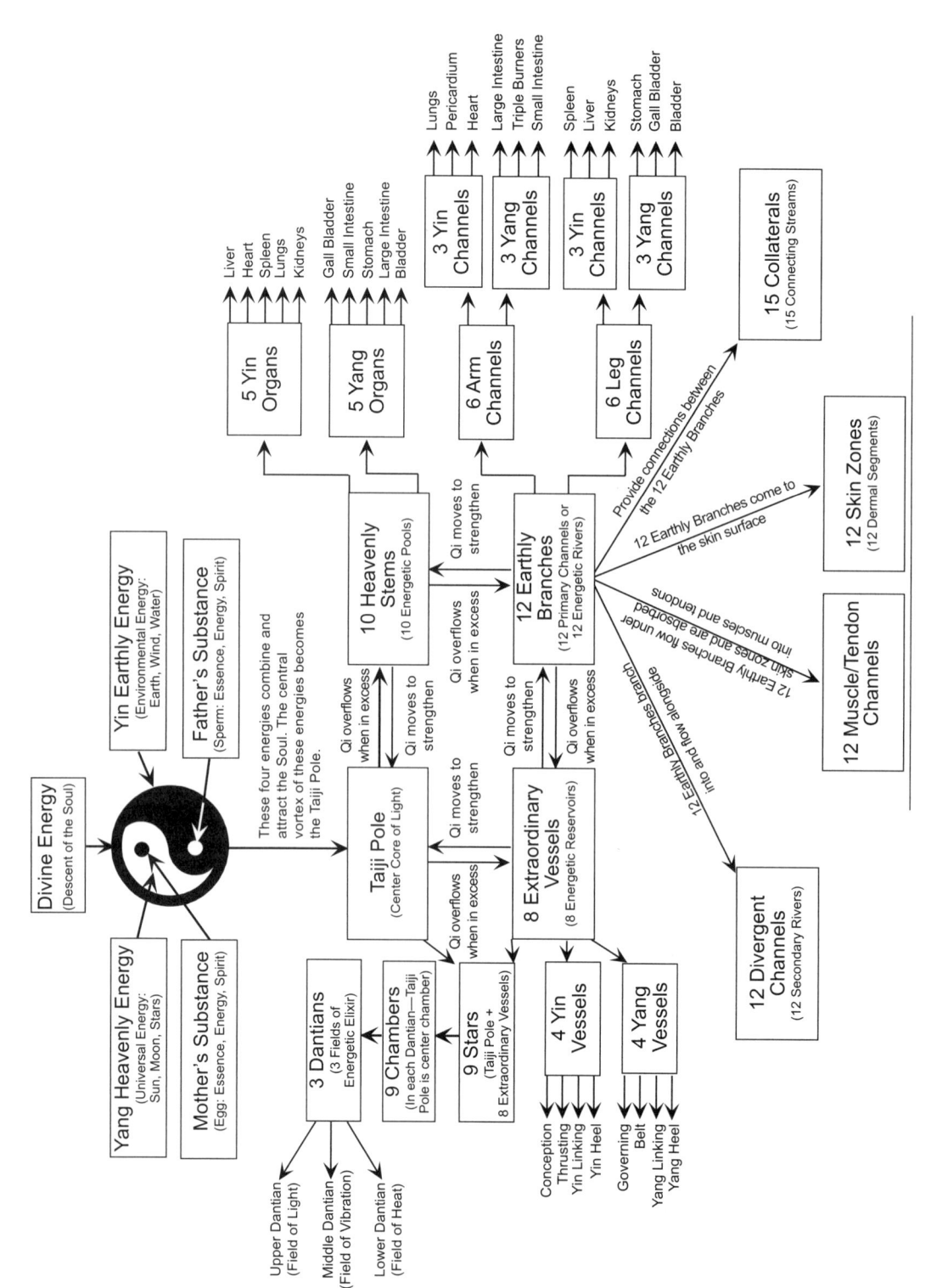

VOLUME 1, SECTION 1: FOUNDATIONS OF CHINESE ENERGETIC MEDICINE

Figure 8.11. The Energetic Connections and Multidimensional Interactions of the Body's Internal Organ and Channel Systems

3. **Jing Jin:** The Jing Jin are the Muscle and Tendon Channels. These channels consist of twelve channels that serve as external connections to the major channels, flowing through the body's muscles, tendons, and ligaments.
4. **Pi Fu:** The Pi Fu are the Cutaneous Regions. These regions are the skin zones where the channels surface on the external tissues.

THE CHANNELS: JING

The character for channel is depicted by the Chinese ideogram "Jing," which can also be translated as meridian, to pass through, and the wrapping of a silk fiber or net (Figure 8.12). The word Jing carries a multitude of meanings, reflected by the many components of the character. Positioned to the left is the radical "Mi," used for silk, net or string-like objects; the right side of the character is the phonetic "Jing," and is sometimes used to denote the flow of water underground. The top right character represents the ground, while the three curved lines beneath it represent the flow of water. Positioned to the bottom-right is the modification for the ancient phonetic "Ting," meaning to examine the underground veins. Together, the ideograph describes the deep aquatic passageways or subterranean rivers which energetically knit together the internal fabric of the human body.

The Jing channels are the major trunks of the body's circulatory tree and are considered to be the underlying energetic support of the internal organs. They generally flow vertically through the body connecting all the deep tissues. They traverse the limbs and penetrate the body cavities to connect with the internal organs. They are the body's main interior and exterior rivers of Qi, and are described as follows:

1. **The Eight Extraordinary Vessels** (see Chapter 6) connect with and regulate the Qi and Blood of the Twelve Primary Channels by either absorbing the energetic overflow in times of channel excess, or by replenishing energy in times of deficiency.
2. **The Twelve Primary Channels** are bilateral and symmetrical. They can be identified in three specific ways: (1) according to the Yin or Yang organ to which they are connected, (2) by the arms or legs in which the channels originate or end, and (3) according to the six divisions of Yin or Yang Qi (i.e., Tai Yang, Yang Ming, Shao Yang, Tai Yin, Shao Yin, and Jue Yin) to which the channels relate.

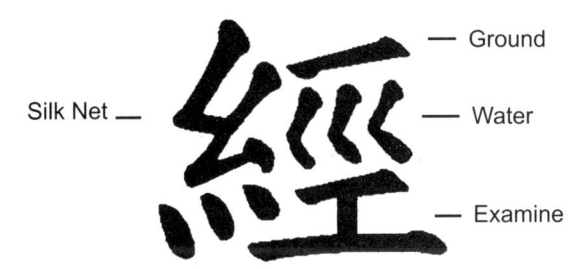

Figure 8.12. The Chinese character for "Jing," Channel, or Passageway

The Yin channels run along the medial and anterior aspects of the body. They are associated with the solid Yin organs although they also connect with the hollow Yang organs. The three Yin channels of the legs (Kidneys, Spleen, and Liver) flow from the feet to the torso, while the three Yin channels of the arms (Heart, Pericardium, and Lung) flow from the torso to the hands.

The Yang channels run along the lateral aspect of the body. They belong to the hollow Yang organs although they also connect with the solid Yin organs. The three Yang channels of the arms (Small Intestine, Triple Burners, and Large Intestine) flow from the hands to the head, while the three Yang channels of the legs (Urinary Bladder, Gall Bladder and Stomach) flow from the head to the feet. The Yin/Yang, internal/external, and substantial/insubstantial relationships of the organs and channels allow for numerous alchemical interactions, and provide the foundation for the transformation of matter and energy within the body.

3. **The Twelve Divergent Channels** (see Chapter 9) branch off from the Twelve Primary Channels. They are mainly distributed on the chest, abdomen, and head. The Divergent channels have the energetic functions of connecting various internally and externally re-

lated channels, strengthening the connection of the Twelve Primary Channels to their related organs, and serving as extensions of the Twelve Primary Channels.

THE COLLATERALS: LUO

Also known as the "collaterals," the literal translation of the Chinese term "Luo Mai" is "the Connecting Vessels" (see Chapter 9).

The character "Luo" depicts the Chinese ideogram for connecting, which can also be translated as a net, cord, a fibrous mesh or a fine silk thread. This character is composed of two radicals. Positioned to the left is the radical "Mi," used for silk, net or string-like objects; the right side of the character is the phonetic sound. The word Luo carries the meaning of energetically enveloping something in a net (Figure 8.13).

The character "Mai" is generally translated as "vessel." It is composed of two characters. The character to the left, "Ji" depicts the Chinese ideogram for body tissue, muscle or flesh (all of which are forms of connective tissue); the character on the right "Mai" depicts a current of water, stream, or branch of a river. As a whole, the character can be translated as arteries, veins or pulse, indicating a form of energetic circulation (Figure 8.14).

The Twelve Primary Channels are interconnected by collaterals, which are small inter-linking streams. These collaterals are the connecting branches of the energetic circulatory system, and are considered to be a the underlying energetic support of the Twelve Primary Channels. They generally flow superficially in both horizontal and vertical directions. They are the body's secondary streams of Qi, and form an intricate network that traverses the body's surface and interconnects the main rivers, connective tissues, and cutaneous regions (Skin Zones). The three types of collaterals are described as follows:

1. **The Fifteen Major Collaterals (Luo)** transfer Qi and Blood from the Twelve Primary Channels to all parts of the body. These collaterals link together the interior and exterior aspects of the body by connecting the body's internal and superficial channels. They also link together the Governing and Conception Vessels and the Great Luo of the Spleen (see Chapter 7).

2. **The Minute Collaterals** are smaller branches of the Fifteen Major Collaterals. They are countless in number.

3. **The Superficial Collaterals** are smaller branches of the Minute Collaterals. They are also countless in number.

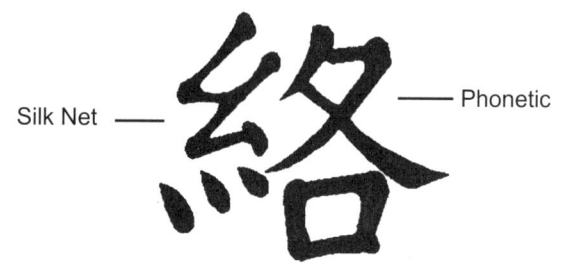

Figure 8.13. The Chinese character for "Luo," Connecting

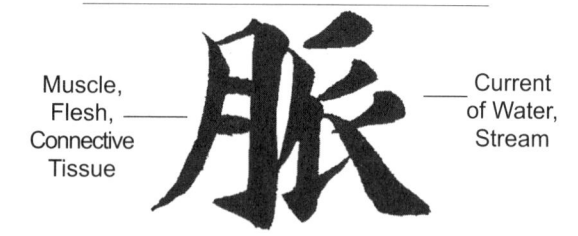

Figure 8.14. The Chinese character for "Mai," Vessel

MUSCLE TENDON CHANNELS: JING JIN

The Twelve Muscle and Tendon Channels (see Chapter 9) are the external connections of the major channels. They generally flow superficially along the body's surface and join the main rivers, connective tissues, and Cutaneous Regions. The Twelve Muscle and Tendon Channels are also regions of the body where the Qi and Blood of the Twelve Primary Channels nourish the muscles, tendons, and ligaments.

The character "Jing" depicts the Chinese ideogram for "channel," which can also be translated as meridians, to pass through, and the wrapping of a silk fiber or net. The word Jing carries a multitude of meanings, reflected by the many components of the character. Positioned to the left is the radical "Mi," used for silk, net or string-like objects. The right side of the character is the phonetic "Jing," and is sometimes used to denote the flow of water underground. The top right character represents the ground, while the three curved lines beneath it represent the flow of water. Positioned to the bottom-right is the modification for the ancient phonetic "Ting," meaning to examine the underground veins. Together, the ideograph describes the deep aquatic passageways or subterranean rivers which energetically knit together the internal fabric of the human body (Figure 8.15).

The character "Jin" depicts the Chinese ideogram for "tendon." One of the earliest Chinese medical dictionaries, the *"Shou Wen Jie Zi,"* explains the term "Jin" (translated as sinew, tendon or ligament) as "the strength of the flesh," and explains that the ancient character is composed of the bamboo radical "Zhu" above two other radicals. The character to the left, "Ji" depicts the Chinese ideogram for body tissue, muscle or flesh (all of which are forms of connective tissue), and on the right is the character "Li" meaning "strength" (Figure 8.16). Therefore, the word "Jin" compares the resilient fibrous qualities of the tendons to the flexible fibrous, intertwining quality of bamboo.

Cutaneous Regions: Pi Fu

The Twelve Cutaneous Regions (also called Twelve Skin Zones) (see Chapter 9) are the areas of the body where the Blood and Qi of the Twelve Primary Channels surface and connect to the body's skin tissues. These cutaneous regions have a direct contact with the external environment.

The character "Pi" depicts the Chinese ideogram for "skin." The second character "Fu" is composed of two radicals. The character to the left, "Ji" depicts the Chinese ideogram for body tissue, muscle or flesh (all of which are forms of connective tissue). The right side of the character is the phonetic for Fu. Together the words Pi Fu translate as skin (Figure 8.17).

The body resonates in a continuous interplay of Yin and Yang harmony, balancing the energy flow within and between the channels and organs. The network of channels creates the energetic matrix of the body, giving form and structure to the body's Yin and Yang polarities (internal/external, inferior/superior, etc.). This energetic ma-

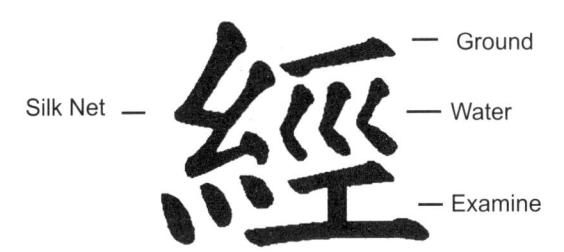

Figure 8.15. The Chinese character for "Jing," Channel, or Passageway

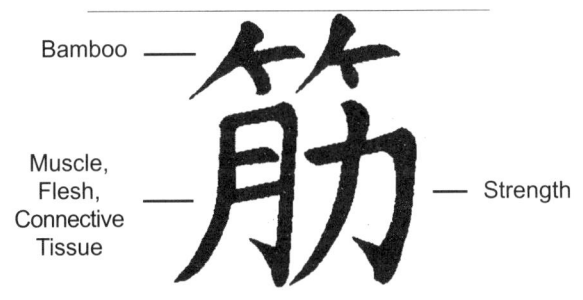

Figure 8.16. The Chinese character for "Jin," Sinew, Tendon or Ligament

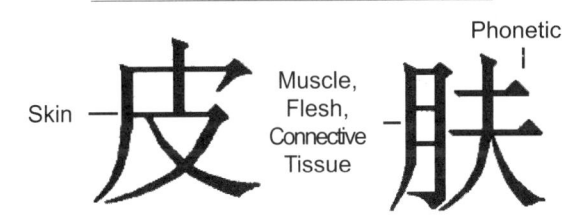

Figure 8.17. The Chinese characters for "Pi Fu," Skin

trix defines the Qi fields surrounding and penetrating the physical body, thus providing an energetic foundation for the creation and sustenance of all of the body's tissues.

The Channels' Relationship to Qi and Blood

The channels transport Qi and Blood to nourish, moisten, and vitalize the entire body. Healthy body function depends on the balanced circulation of Qi and Blood. Qi is Yang and provides the energy or force necessary for the body's functional activity (i.e., moving and transporting, warming, containing, transforming, and defending). Blood is Yin and is the source of the body's moisture, nourishment, and lubrication.

Blood, Qi, and heat circulate through all of the Twelve Primary Channels within a twenty-four hour cycle. The maximum peak of a channel's Qi and Blood flow (commonly known as "high-tide") occurs for a period of two hours during the time of day or night when the Qi and Blood within that channel is at its fullest. The weakest period of a channel's Qi and Blood flow (commonly known as "low tide") occurs twelve hours opposite of its peak time period (Figure 8.18).

There is some speculation that the energy of the channels is transmitted through the body's vast fascial network. The body's connective tissues (also known as fascia) provide a network of semi-flexible structural support for all the tissues of the body.

Nearly every cell and tissue in the body is linked to every other cell and tissue in the body by indirect fascial connection. The inner fascia can be thought of as lubricated layers of living plastic wrap that cover and connect all of the muscles and internal organs, allowing the tissues to slide and move easily while maintaining structural integrity. The primary channels are woven within the lining of the superficial fasciae, while the deeper channels (e.g., Collaterals, Extraordinary Vessels, and Divergent Channels) exist deeper within the internal fascia matrix. This webbed network conducts energy in the form of electron, proton, and ion transmission, and is also influenced by light and sound. The fascia is responsible for transmitting a variety of biological energies. When stretched, for example, the fascia creates a Stress Generated Electrical Potential (SGEP). Although the fascia represents the primary physical tissue associated with the body's channels, the channels are also associated with numerous other tissues and their energetic functions.

According to Traditional Chinese Medicine theory, each of the Twelve Primary Channels has its own individual reservoirs of Qi and Blood; however, the energetic quality of each channel varies in accordance with the amount of Qi and Blood available in each organ and its corresponding organ channel (Figure 8.19).

From a Traditional Chinese Medical perspec-

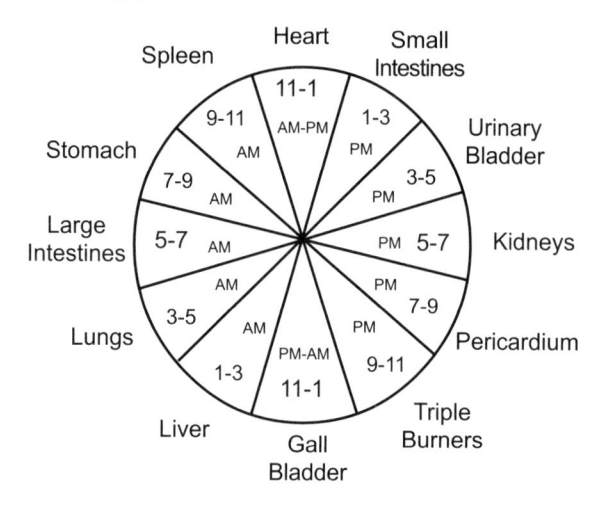

Figure 8.18. The Blood Heat Cycle (24 Hour Cycle) of the Body's Twelve Internal Organs can be divided into High and Low Energetic Tides

Organs & Channels	Qi	Blood
Gall Bladder	More	Less
Liver	Less	More
Lungs	More	Less
Large Intestine	Balanced	Balanced
Stomach	Balanced	Balanced
Spleen	More	Less
Heart	More	Less
Small Intestine	Less	More
Urinary Bladder	Less	More
Kidney	More	Less
Pericardium	Less	More
Triple Burners	More	Less

Figure 8.19. The Body's Organs and Channels Contain Different Proportions of Qi to Blood

tive, the Spleen plays two important roles in relationship to Qi and Blood. First, it converts food and drink into Gu Qi which, when further refined by the Liver and Kidneys, becomes Ying (Nutritive) Qi. Second, it manages the Blood by keeping it within the channels. Ying Qi nourishes Body Fluids that enter into the Blood Vessels and are transformed into Blood by the Heart. The Heart both creates and governs the Blood; whereas, the Liver stores the Blood and spreads Qi throughout the body. Blood is considered to be a denser, more material form of Qi. Qi and Blood are interdependent: Qi moves the Blood, and the Blood nourishes Qi. Both flow together.

FUNCTION OF THE CHANNELS

The channel system has four major functions: promotes, regulates, distributes and protects, described as follows:

1. To promote communication between the internal organs and the exterior of the body, thus connecting the individual to the environmental (Earth) and universal (Heaven) rhythms of life.
2. To regulate and harmonize the activity of the body's Yin and Yang energy within the internal organs and within the Five Primary Substances (Jing, Qi, Shen, Blood and Body Fluid).
3. To distribute the Qi of the internal organs throughout the body.
4. To protect the body by creating an energetic shield in order to deflect foreign pathogens, as well as to fortify the body's internal organ system (Figure 8.20).

The channels are responsible for reacting to any malfunction in the body, though they can also be disseminators of energetic dysfunction and disease. Disease passes into the internal organs, or from one organ to another, via the channel system. Exogenous diseases progress from the body's skin pores to the tiny collaterals, then to primary channels, and finally to the internal organs. The channels are affected by and respond to disease in predictable patterns described as follows (Figure 8.21):

1. Diseases and symptoms manifest along the channel pathway.

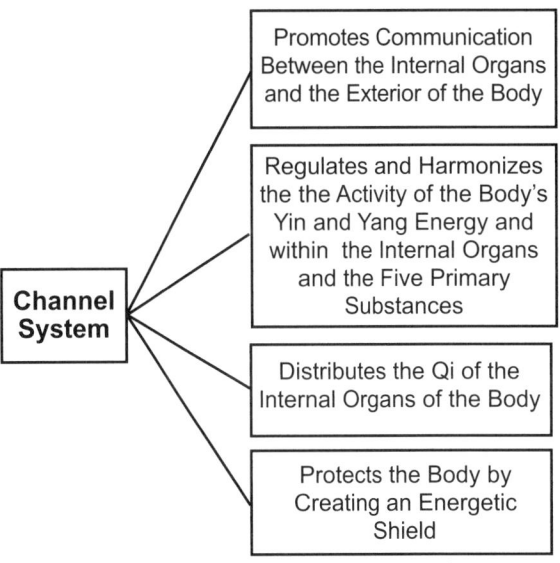

Figure 8.20. The Four Major Functions of the Channel System

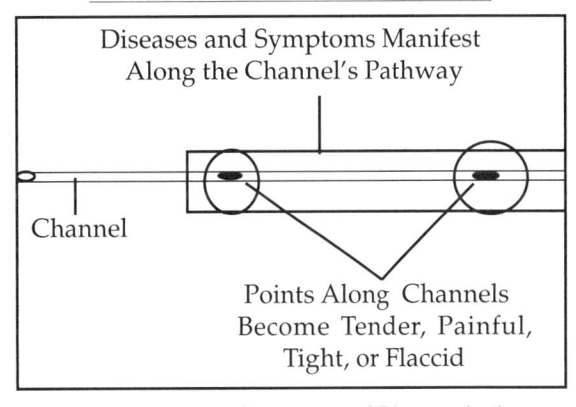

Figure 8.21. The Symptoms of Disease in the Channels

2. Points along the channels become tender, painful, tight, or flaccid.
3. When in a deficient state, the electrical resistance and heat tolerance diminish on the skin at the diseased point(s).
4. The body's sensory organs and senses (sight, smell, taste, hearing and touch) are affected through channel relationships.

From a Traditional Chinese Medical perspective, the functions and flow of the channels and collaterals, as well as the health of the internal organs, can be influenced by Medical Qigong, acupuncture, Chinese massage, and herbal medicine. Each of the above Traditional Chinese Medicine modalities utilize the channel system to disperse excess, to move stagnation, to stimulate and nourish the Qi, to tonify deficiency, and to stimulate the Wei Qi in fighting external pathogens. When the body's channels and collaterals are trained or regulated, they become thicker with Qi.

Centrifugal and Centripetal Energy Flow

The energy of the body's channels normally flows in only one direction, while the polarity of the channel's points normally alternates between Yang (centrifugal spirals) and Yin (centripetal spirals) energetic movements. These two energy currents are described as follows:

1. Some channels possess an outward centrifugal flow of Qi that moves from the organ, through the channel, to the extremities. The primary channels with this centrifugal flow of energy are: Heart, Pericardium, Lung, Stomach, Gall Bladder, and Urinary Bladder. This outward flow of energy is expressed or intensified during the exhalation (Figure 8.22). The outward centrifugal flow of energy manifests in points along the channel, or in other areas of the body where there are conditions of excess.

2. Some channels posses an inward centripetal flow of Qi that moves from the extremities, through the channel, to the organ. The primary channels with this centripetal flow of energy are: Small Intestine, Triple Burner, Large Intestine, Spleen, Liver and Kidney. This inward flow of energy is expressed or intensified during the inhalation (Figure 8.23). The inward centripetal flow of energy manifests in points along the channel, or in other areas of the body where there are conditions of deficiency.

Internal and External Channel Flow

As the Qi of an internal channel flows into or away from its primary organ, it generates a current that is similar to either a river rushing back

The outward centrifugal flow of the channel moves Qi and Blood from the internal organs through the channel towards the extremities	The Arm Yin Channels (Heart, Pericardium and Lungs) flow from the chest to the hands
	The Leg Yang Channels (Stomach, Gall Bladder, and Urinary Bladder flow from the head to the feet

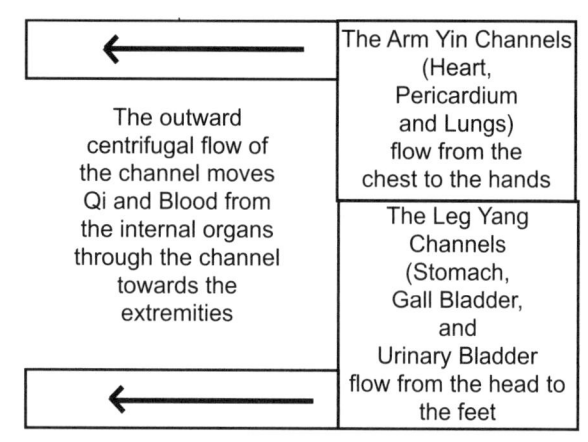

Figure 8.22. Internal and External Channel Flow

The inward centripetal flow of the channel moves Qi and Blood from the extremities through the channel towards the internal organs	The Arm Yang Channels (Small Intestine, Triple Burner, and Large Intestine) flow from the hands to the head
	The Leg Yin Channels (Spleen, Liver and Kidney) flow from the feet to the chest

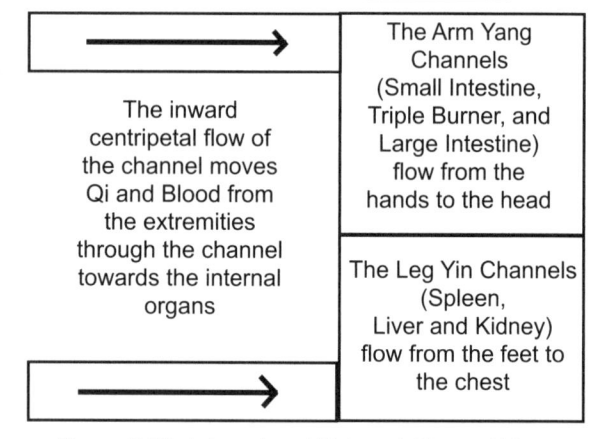

Figure 8.23. Internal and External Channel Flow

into the sea, or a river flowing out of the sea into deep caverns of the Earth. As the Qi flows through the energetic cavern of an internal channel, it stimulates the energy of its primary organ. This reaction initiates a spontaneous energetic connection that is immediately created and felt within the organ's tissues.

However, when the Qi from a primary organ's internal channel flows into its "paired" or "associated organ," the energetic reaction is quite different. Instead of immediately permeating the associated organ, the channel's energy "spirally wraps" the associated organ's tissues through the internal fascia that envelops the associated organ. The tissues of the associated organ then absorb the energy through and from the surrounding fascia (Figure 8.24).

This difference in energetic penetration and absorption rate is an important factor to consider when working with the body's internal energetic channels. When Qigong doctors extend their energy into a patient's channels, they must be aware that the absorption rate will be immediately felt in the channel's primary organ, and will also have a gradual effect on the associated organ.

HUN AND PO CHANNEL INFLUENCE

Each of the Twelve Primary Channels correspond to one of the Five Elements, and are additionally aligned within their channel progressions according to the energetic and spiritual influence of the Hun (Ethereal Soul) and Po (Corporeal Soul). According to Energetic Anatomy, the creation of the channel progression via the Heavenly influence of the Hun and Earthly influence of the Po occurs during prenatal formation (Figure 8.25).

In postnatal manifestation, each of the primary Yin channels begins with the Wood Element, and is connected to its primary organ by the Hun's Heavenly influence. This alignment allows for the flow of Qi through the Yin channels in the Five Element Creative Cycle progression; starting with Wood, then Fire, Earth, Metal, and finally Water.

Each of the primary Yang channels begins with the Metal Element, and is connected to its primary organ through the Po's Earthly influence. This alignment allows for the flow of Qi through the Yang channels in the Five Element Creative Cycle progression; starting with Metal, then Water, Wood, Fire, and Earth.

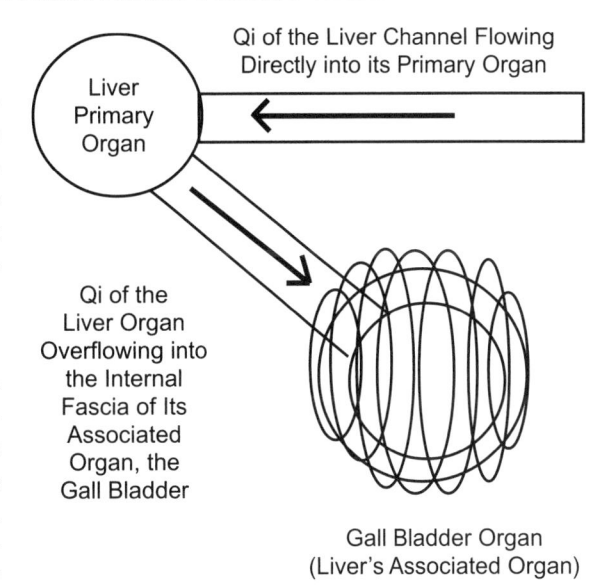

Figure 8.24. Internal and External Channel Flow

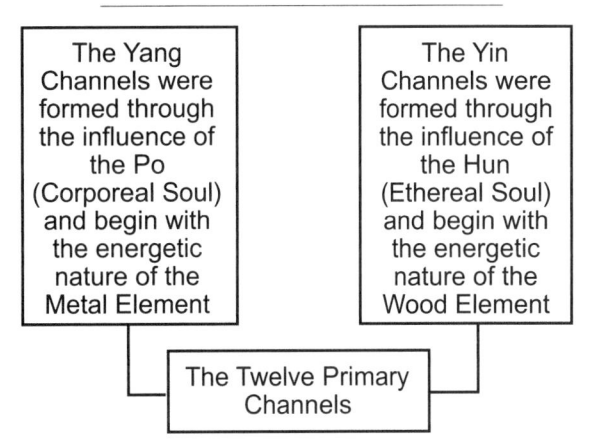

Figure 8.25. The Correspondence of the Hun and Po with Channel Flow

THE GALL BLADDER: DAN

The Gall Bladder belongs to the Wood Element, and its associated Yin organ is the Liver (Figure 8.26). The Gall Bladder is categorized as both a Yang organ and an "Extraordinary Organ." It is the only Yang organ that does not receive "turbid" food or drink, but instead stores a refined "clean" substance (the bile), similar to the way a Yin organ functions. Another reason that the Gall Bladder is considered "extraordinary" is that it does not communicate with the exterior directly (via the mouth, rectum or urethra), as do the other Yang organs. The Gall Bladder channels travel into the sensory organs (eyes, ears, nose and mouth) and thus serve to root and ground the senses.

CHINESE CHARACTER FOR THE GALL BLADDER: DAN

The Chinese character "Dan" translates as "Gall Bladder." It refers to a general description of the image of the Gall Bladder organ, and is composed of three images. The character to the left, "Ji" depicts the Chinese ideogram for body tissue, muscle or flesh (all of which are forms of connective tissue). The character on the right is divided into two characters: the upper right side depicts a person on a steep rocky place bent over and afraid of falling; the bottom right hand side is the character "Yan" meaning speech. Together, these characters are used to represent a person in a hazardous position who cannot make a decision. This expresses the Gall Bladder's role in making difficult decisions (Figure 8.27).

THE GALL BLADDER IN CHINESE MEDICINE

The functions of the Gall Bladder described in Traditional Chinese Medicine are similar to those that are described in Western Medicine. In Chinese Medicine, however, the Gall Bladder is also associated with certain functions that are attributed to the nervous system in Western Medicine. Additionally, Chinese Medicine places an special emphasis on specific psychological, emotional and spiritual states that correspond to the condition of the Gall Bladder.

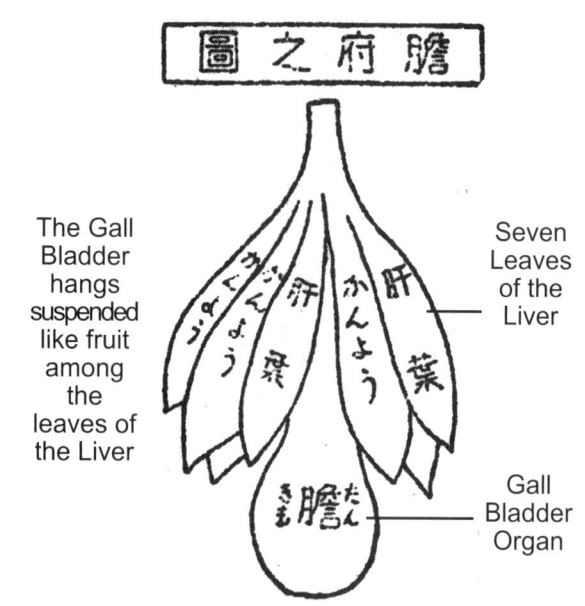

Figure 8.26. The ancient Chinese anatomical diagram of the Gall Bladder (GB) Organ, as it appeared in "Important Useful Notes on Acupuncture and Moxibustion," published in Japan in 1718, by Masatoyo Hongo

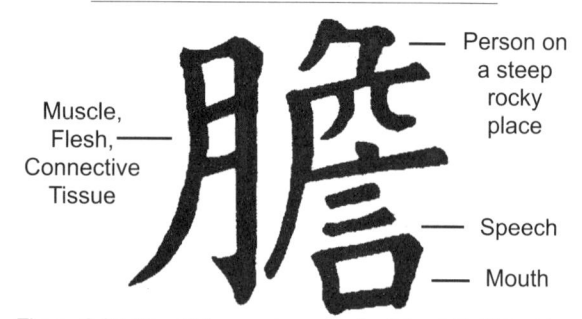

Figure 8.27. The Chinese character for "Dan," Gall Bladder

According to Traditional Chinese Medicine, the main functions of the Gall Bladder are to: store and excrete bile, control the tendons, and express itself through the pyscho-emotional aspects of courage and decision making. These main functions are described as follows (Figure 8.28):

1. **Stores and Excretes Bile:** Bile is created and secreted by the Liver and stored and concentrated in the Gall Bladder. From there it is pumped into the Small Intestine for promoting the digestion and absorption of food via the Liver's function of smoothing and regu-

```
┌─────────────┐      ┌──────────────────────┐      ┌──────────────────────┐
│             │─────▶│Stores and Excretes   │─────▶│  Aids in Digestion   │
│             │      │        Bile          │      │                      │
│   The       │      └──────────────────────┘      └──────────────────────┘
│   Main      │      ┌──────────────────────┐      ┌──────────────────────┐
│ Functions   │─────▶│ Controls the Tendons │─────▶│Provides Qi to the    │
│  of the     │      │                      │      │       Tendons        │
│   Gall      │      └──────────────────────┘      └──────────────────────┘
│  Bladder    │                                    ┌──────────────────────┐
│   Organ     │                                 ┌─▶│Influences the Quality│
│    and      │                                 │  │   and Length of Sleep│
│  Channels   │      ┌──────────────────────┐   │  └──────────────────────┘
│             │─────▶│Psycho-Emotional      │───┤  ┌──────────────────────┐
│             │      │     Aspects          │   ├─▶│Makes Decisions and   │
│             │      │                      │   │  │      Judgments       │
└─────────────┘      └──────────────────────┘   │  └──────────────────────┘
                                                │  ┌──────────────────────┐
                                                └─▶│Courage and Initiative│
                                                   │       Insight        │
                                                   └──────────────────────┘
```

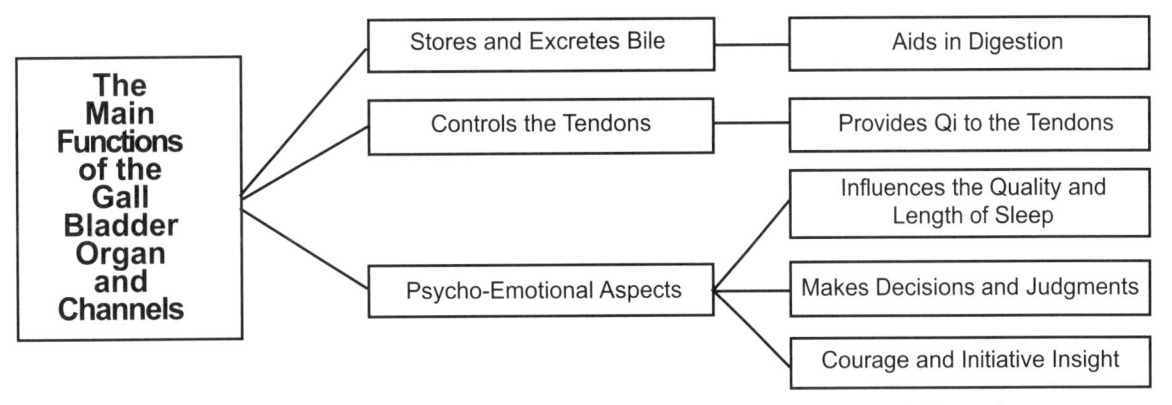

Figure 8.28. The Main Energetic Functions of the Gall Bladder Organ and Channels

lating the flow of Qi. The Gall Bladder is also said to be responsible for hormonal regulation and bodily fluids (bile and Ye).

2. **Controls the Tendons:** The Gall Bladder aids the Liver in controlling the tendons. The Gall Bladder provides Qi to the tendons in order to ensure proper movement and agility, while the Liver provides Blood to the tendons.

3. **Psycho-Emotional Aspects:** The Gall Bladder is sometimes called "The Court of Justice," or "The General's Advisor." As such, it plays a role in making decisions and judgments, overseeing discernment, providing bravery, courage, and confidence, meeting challenges, and initiating perceptions. Although the Kidneys control drive and vitality, it is the Gall Bladder that provides the capacity to turn this drive and vitality into decisive action.

THE GALL BLADDER CHANNELS

The Gall Bladder Channels are Yang channels. The external branches flow from the head to the feet on both sides of the body (Figure 8.29). The internal branches of the Gall Bladder Channels flow from the head to the Gall Bladder. Both the internal and the external branches of these two rivers originate from the outer canthus of the eyes. The external branches zigzag around the side of the head, and then flow down the sides of the torso. The internal branches leave the outer canthus of the eye and descend the neck, entering the supraclavicular fossa where they meet the main channels at the St-12 and Pc-1 points. From these points, the internal branches pass through the diaphragm, to spirally wrap the Liver, before permeating the Gall Bladder. From the Gall Bladder organ the internal channels descend deep into the lower torso and encircle the genitals, before emerging at the sacrum.

The external rivers continue to descend the lateral aspects of the torso and legs, ending at the lateral sides of the bases of the fourth toenails.

CHANNELS' ENERGY FLOW

The Gall Bladder travels into the sensory organs (eyes, ears, nose and mouth) via its trajectories, allowing the sensory organs to become more rooted and grounded.

The Gall Bladder Channels act on the skin, muscles, and nerves that are found along their pathways. Therefore, the Gall Bladder Channels are often used to drain Heat gathered within the head area, as well as remove energy stagnation due to an overheated or excess Liver condition. The internal flow of the Liver Channel moves Qi into the Brain and Sea of Marrow; consequently, the Gall Bladder Channel can be used to remove excesses (fluids, Marrow, Qi) from the Brain.

The Gall Bladder Channels link to the Brain, Marrow and Uterus and act as a bridge between the prenatal and postnatal energetic vessels.

Energetically, the Gall Bladder Channels store more Qi than Blood, affecting energetic and nervous functions more than physical substances and

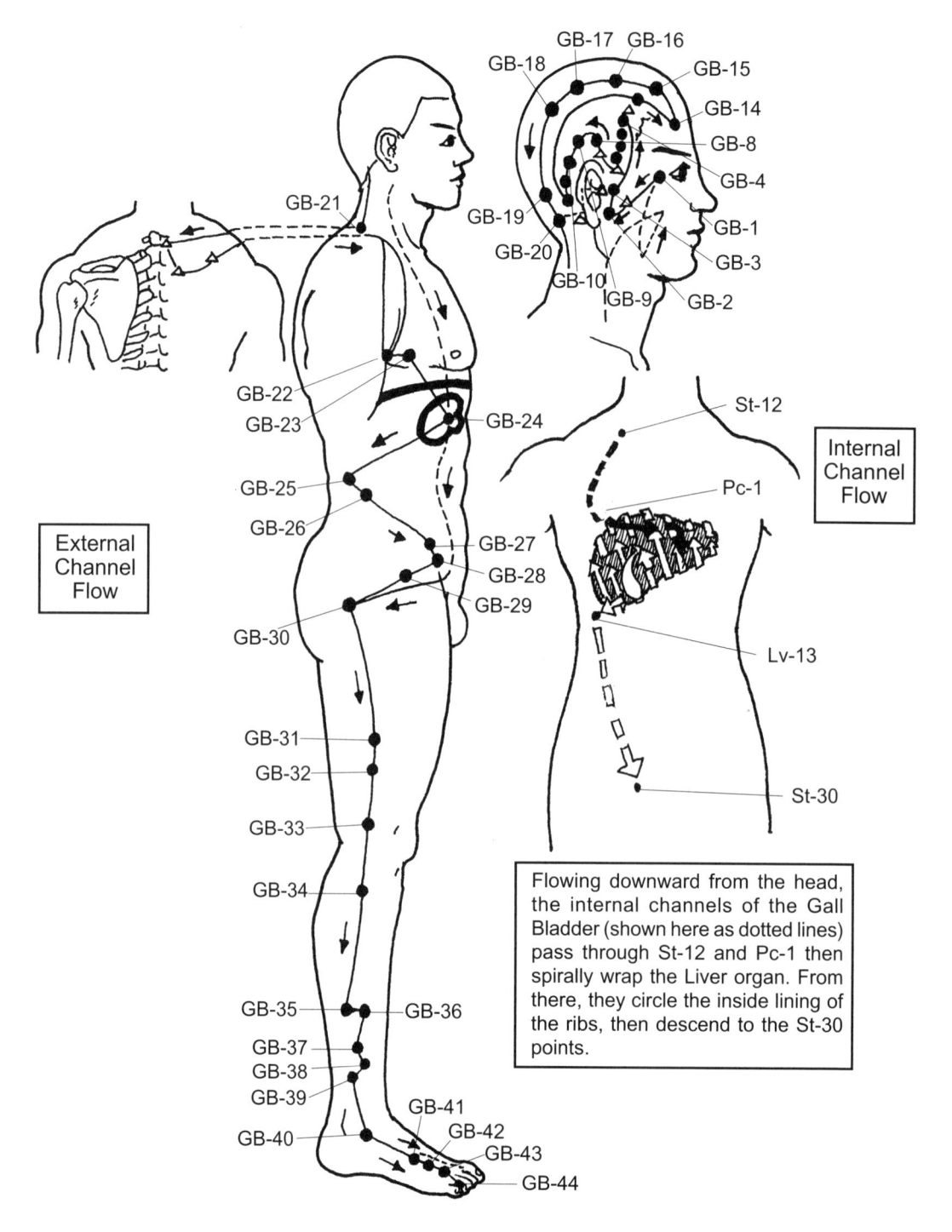

VOLUME 1, SECTION 1: FOUNDATIONS OF CHINESE ENERGETIC MEDICINE

Figure 8.29. The Internal and External Qi Flow of the Gall Bladder (GB) Channels

Flowing downward from the head, the internal channels of the Gall Bladder (shown here as dotted lines) pass through St-12 and Pc-1 then spirally wrap the Liver organ. From there, they circle the inside lining of the ribs, then descend to the St-30 points.

```
Gall Bladder ─┬─ Deficient Gall Bladder Heat ── Insomnia, nightmares and dream disturbed sleep
              ├─ Deficient Gall Bladder Qi ──── Indecisive, scared, timid, fearful of confrontation or being attacked, easily discouraged by slight adversity, or panic easily
              └─ Excess Gall Bladder Heat ───── Irritability, headaches, and thirst
```

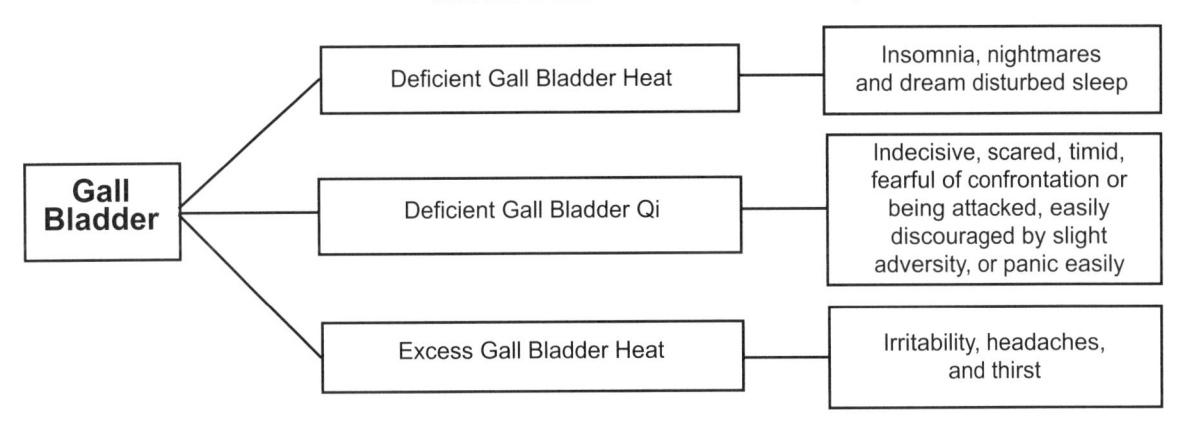

Figure 8.30. Chart of Liver-Gall Bladder Disharmonies

the functions of the Blood. At the high-tide time period (11 p.m. to 1 a.m.), Qi and Blood abound in the Gall Bladder and Gall Bladder channels. At this time period, the Gall Bladder organ and channels can be more easily dispersed and purged; whereas during low tide (11 a.m. to 1 p.m.), they can be more readily tonified.

The Influence of Climate

An External Damp Heat climate (such as that found in tropical and sub-tropical regions) can aggravate a Damp Heat condition within the Gall Bladder.

The Influence of Taste, Color, and Sound

- The sour taste can be used to tonify both the Gall Bladder and Liver
- The light green/blue color is used to tonify the Gall Bladder
- The "Shu" and "Guo" sounds are used to purge both the Gall Bladder and Liver

Gall Bladder Pathology

The main symptoms associated with imbalances of the Gall Bladder organ and channels are described as follows:

- pain in the right and left upper quadrants of the abdomen, abdominal distension, jaundice, hepatitis, cholecystitis, cholelithiasis and digestive disorders including belching, vomiting of sour material, bitter taste in the mouth and flatulence.
- disorders of the head, which include the eyes, ears, and face; poor concentration, dizziness and insomnia with tossing and turning.
- disorders of the external sides of the legs along the channel's pathways.

T.C.M. Patterns of Disharmony

In Traditional Chinese Medicine, disharmonies of the Gall Bladder are generally included within the category of Liver disharmonies. There are, however, minor disharmonies particular to the Gall Bladder organ such as deficient Gall Bladder Heat, deficient Gall Bladder Qi and excess Gall Bladder Heat, the symptoms of which are described as follows (Figure 8.30):

- **Deficient Gall Bladder Heat:** The Gall Bladder has an influence on the quality and length of sleep. If the Gall Bladder is deficient, the patient will often wake up suddenly, very early in the morning, and be unable to fall asleep again. The Gall Bladder is often treated for insomnia, nightmares and dream disturbed sleep.
- **Deficient Gall Bladder Qi:** Patients who are indecisive, scared, timid, fearful of confrontation or being attacked, are easily discouraged by slight adversity, or who panic easily are said to have a weak Gall Bladder. Conversely, decisive, courageous, and determined patients are said to have a strong Gall Bladder.
- **Excess Gall Bladder Heat:** Like its paired Yin

organ the Liver, the Gall Bladder is affected by frustration, anger, rage and resentment. These emotional states give rise to Liver Qi Stagnation, and thus produce heat, which affects the Gall Bladder. When Fire is created within the Liver and Gall Bladder, the symptoms are similar (irritability, headaches, thirst, etc.).

THE GALLBLADDER IN WESTERN MEDICINE

The gallbladder is a small pear-shaped organ lodged in an indentation (fossa) immediately beneath the right lobe of the liver. It is three to four inches long, and is situated with its widest section (the fundus) slightly beneath and forward to its neck, which is angled upwards and slightly to the left (Figure 8.31).

The gallbladder is wrapped in a layer of fascial tissue that is derived from the peritoneum. Within this is a layer of smooth muscle fibers that form the body of the gallbladder; it is the contractions of these fibers that expel bile from the gallbladder into the cystic duct. Like the stomach, the internal structure of the gallbladder contains many folds (rugae), allowing it to expand and contract as it receives and condenses the bile fluid. Its inner surface is protected by a layer of mucous, which insulates it from the effects of the bile.

Parasympathetic impulses delivered by the vagus nerves have a minor impact on stimulating gall bladder contraction. The major stimulus comes from an intestinal hormone known as cholecystokinin (CCK), which is released into the blood when acidic, fatty chyme enters the duodenum. This also stimulates the secretion of the pancreatic juice into the duodenum.

The gallbladder serves to store and condense bile, which it receives from the liver via the cystic duct. Bile, also called gall, is a bitter yellowish substance secreted from the liver to aid in digestion. It consists mainly of water, bile acids, bile salts, bile pigments, lecithin, cholesterol, electrolytes, and various fatty acids. Bile is transferred into the duodenum (uppermost portion of the small intestine) via a system of ducts. The bile secretions of the liver are directed through several

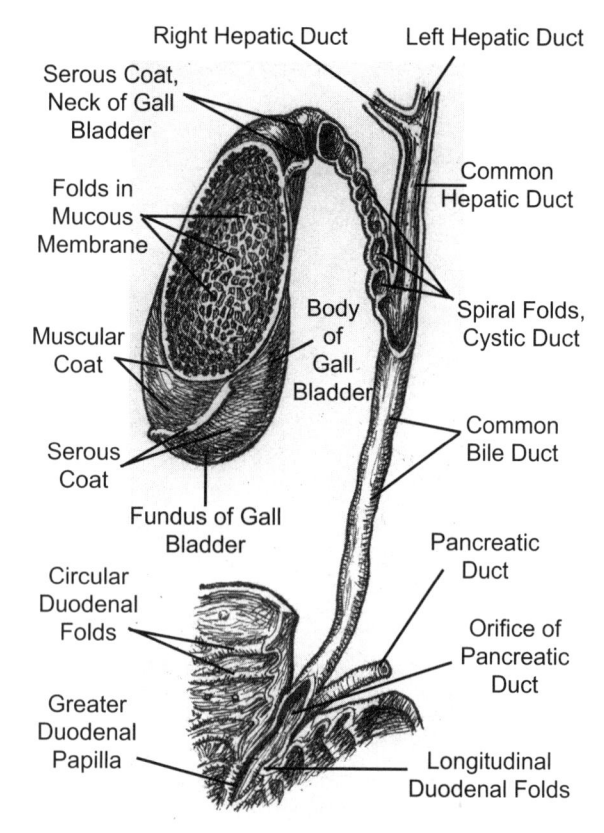

Figure 8.31. The Gall Bladder (GB) Organ

ducts that ultimately join together to form the hepatic duct, which carries bile away from the liver. The cystic duct connects the gallbladder to the hepatic duct, and is the common duct through which bile enters and exits the gallbladder. The common bile duct flows from the junction of the cystic and hepatic ducts into the duodenum.

When chyme enters the small intestine, a complex system of chemical and nervous impulses directs the gallbladder to contract, expelling bile through the cystic duct, along the common bile duct and into the duodenum to aid in the process of digestion. When digestion is not taking place, a valve (sphincter of the hepatopancreatic ampulla) closes the connection of the common bile duct to the duodenum, and bile is redirected into the gallbladder for storage. The gallbladder concentrates the bile by absorbing water and ions from the bile while it is being stored. In some cases the bile released from the gallbladder is ten times more concentrated than the bile secreted by the liver (Figure 8.32).

COMMON DISORDERS OF THE GALL BLADDER

Gallstones, or biliary calculi, are the result of an imbalance among the components of bile. Bile is the primary vehicle through which the body excretes cholesterol. When the amount or concentration of bile salts contained in the bile is insufficient to dissolve all of the cholesterol within the bile, the remaining cholesterol can crystallize and form into balls, commonly known as gallstones. Large or numerous gallstones can partially or completely obstruct the flow of bile. Gallstones may be composed entirely of cholesterol, entirely of pigment, entirely of minerals, or contain a crystallized mixture of various bile components.

Disorders of the bile duct system include: cholestasis (blockage of bile flow), cholangitis (inflammation of the bile duct system), and cholecystitis (inflammation of the gallbladder wall).

When blockages within the common bile duct

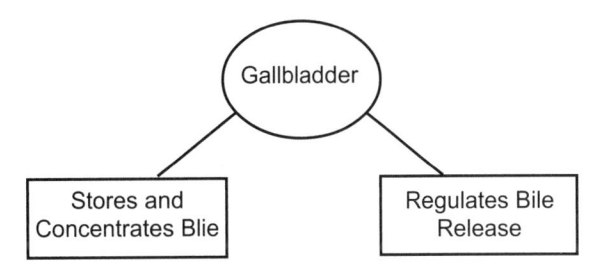

Figure 8.32. The Functions of the Gallbladder (Western Medical Perspective)

prevent the excretion of bile, the excess bile salts and pigments (primarily bilirubin) are absorbed into the blood, giving the body a yellow color. This is known as obstructive jaundice. If the blockage is total, the gallbladder may rupture and leak its contents into the peritoneum, causing peritonitis.

Because it is possible for an individual to survive without the gallbladder organ, the gallbladder is sometimes surgically removed in western medical treatments of gallbladder dysfunction. In patients who have undergone the removal of the gallbladder, the bile is secreted from the liver directly into the duodenum.

THE LIVER: GAN

The Liver belongs to the Wood Element, and its associated Yang organ is the Gall Bladder (Figure 8.33). In Chinese Medicine, the Liver is responsible for the circulation and smooth movement of the body's internal Qi. The Liver is sometimes referred to as the "Green Emperor." It is a solid (Zang) organ which stores the Blood.

The Liver governs the Belt (Dai) and Thrusting (Chong) Vessels, as well as the flow and circulation of Qi throughout the body. The smooth flow of Qi ensures balanced mental and emotional activity, as well as normal secretion of bile.

Although the Liver is anatomically situated on the right side of the body, its energetic movements and flow originate on the left side of the body. To understand this function, it is helpful to think of the Liver as a living bellows, in which the right side compresses, causing the Qi to flow out through the left side.

CHINESE CHARACTER FOR THE LIVER: GAN

The Chinese character "Gan" translates as "Liver." It refers to a general description of the image of the Liver organ, and is divided into two sections. The character to the left, "Ji" depicts the Chinese ideogram for body tissue, muscle or flesh (all of which are forms of connective tissue). The character to the right depicts an ideogram that is a representation of a raised pestle, ready to pound, grind and destroy. Some translators maintain that the raised pestle image is actually a warrior's shield, thrust into the ground in front in order to defend, protect and support, hence the Liver's ability to control the body's aggressive warrior spirit (Figure 8.34).

THE YIN AND YANG OF THE LIVER

Traditional Chinese Medicine defines the Liver as having two energetic aspects, Yin and Yang, described as follows:
- **The Yin of the Liver:** This pertains to the material structures of the Liver, including the Blood stored within it.
- **The Yang of the Liver:** This pertains to the Liver's function of heating and moving the Qi.

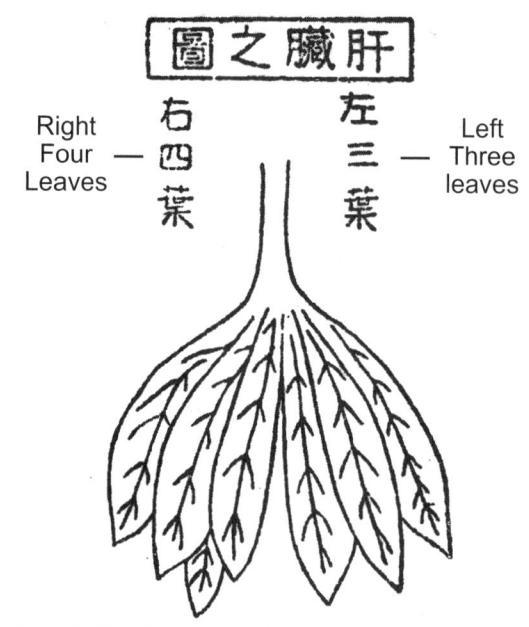

Figure 8.33. The ancient Chinese anatomical diagram of the Liver (Lv) Organ, as it appeared in "Important Useful Notes on Acupuncture and Moxibustion," published in Japan in 1718, by Masatoyo Hongo

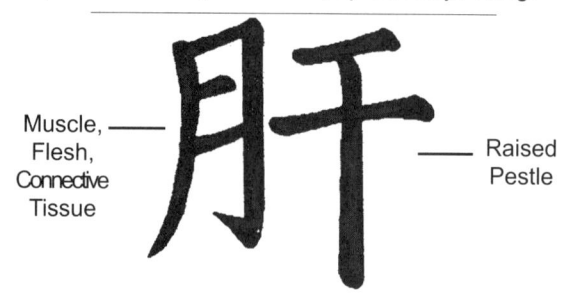

Figure 8.34. The Chinese character for "Gan," Liver

THE LIVER'S WOOD JING FORMATION

During the seventh lunar month of a woman's pregnancy, the Wood Jing begins to be accepted by the fetus' body. The Wood Jing energy supervises the direction of the emotional and spiritual aspects of the fetus. Any faltering of the Wood Jing energy during embryonic formation is associated with serious psychological problems (i.e., passive-aggressive personality disorder, etc.).

After birth, the Wood Jing can be affected through the color green, the sour taste, and the "Shu" and "Guo" sounds.

```
                                          ┌─ Physical Activity
                   ┌─ Stores and Regulates ┤
                   │   the Blood           └─ Menstruation
                   │
                   │                       ┌─ Secretion of Bile
                   │   Smooths and Regulates│
                   ├─  the Flow of Qi      ├─ Digestion
The Main           │                       └─ Emotional State
Functions          │
of the             ├─ Rules the Tendons ─── Controls Physical Strength
Liver              │
Organ and          ├─ Manifests in the Nails
Channels           │
                   ├─ Opens at the Eyes
                   │
                   ├─ Psycho-Emotional Aspects ─── Love and Anger
                   │
                   └─ Spiritual Influence ─── Seven Functions of the Hun
```

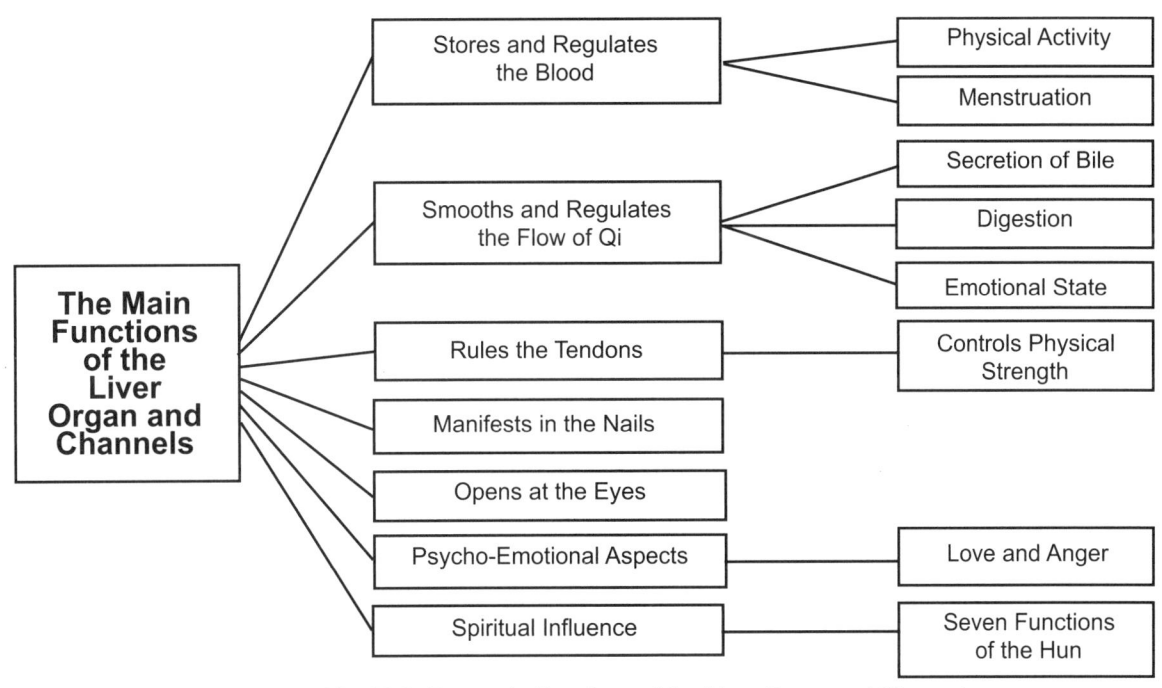

Figure 8.35. The Main Energetic Functions of the Liver Organ and Channels

THE LIVER IN CHINESE MEDICINE

The functions of the Liver described in Traditional Chinese Medicine are similar to those that are described in Western Medicine. In Traditional Chinese Medicine, however, the Liver also assumes various functions of the Blood, visual organs, central nervous system, and autonomic nervous system. The Liver also governs various psycho-emotional aspects and has specific spiritual influences. According to Traditional Chinese Medicine, the main functions of the Liver are to: store and regulate the Blood, smooth and regulate the flow of Qi, rule the tendons, manifest in the nails, open at the eyes, express itself through the psycho-emotional aspects of love and hate, and exert certain important spiritual influences via the Hun (Ethereal Soul). These main functions are described as follows (Figure 8.35):

1. **Stores and Regulates the Blood:** The Liver is the most important organ for storing the Blood and serves as a reservoir to regulate the circulation of Blood volume. The Liver's responsibility of storing the Blood manifests in two ways:

- **The Liver stores and releases the Blood according to physical activity:** When the body is active, the Blood flows into the muscles to nourish and moisten the muscle tissues, and to warm and moisten the tendons, allowing them to become more supple. When the skin and muscles are well-nourished by the Blood, the body maintains a stronger resistance to attacks from external pathogenic factors. When the body rests, the Blood flows back into the Liver, allowing the body to restore and recharge its energy.

- **The Liver regulates the Blood in menstruation:** The Liver assists the Uterus, regulates the menses and is responsible for nourishing the growth of the embryo during the first month of pregnancy. The Liver's function of storing Blood also influences the way the Governing and Conception Vessels regulate Blood in the Uterus. During pregnancy, the mother's Blood is transformed into Jing-Essence, which nourishes the mother's body as well as the embryo's. The mother's Liver Channels cause Essence and Blood to coagulate in her womb. This Blood coagulation continues after the initial cellular division.

An imbalance of the Liver is often reflected in a woman's menstrual cycle. In the gynecology of Traditional Chinese Medicine, the Liver's function of storing Blood is a major factor in determining the state of a woman's reproductive physiology and pathology. Problems due to malfunctions of Liver Qi and Blood can manifest in symptoms such as premenstrual tension, amenorrhea, dysmenorrhea, depression, etc.

2. **Smooths and Regulates the Flow of Qi:** The Liver is responsible for the "free and easy wandering" of Qi throughout the entire body (through all organs and in all directions). This is considered to be the Liver's most important function. The Liver makes the Qi flow smoothly in and around the body. It governs the energy within the Belt and Thrusting Vessels, and is in charge of the circulation of Qi through all of the body's internal organs. An impairment of this function is one of the most common patterns observed in the clinic. The movement of Liver Qi affects the body in three primary ways. It affects the secretion of bile, digestion and the emotional state.

- **Secretion of Bile:** The smooth flow of Qi ensures normal secretion of bile. If the Liver Qi becomes stagnant, the flow of bile may become obstructed, resulting in symptoms such as belching with bitter taste and jaundice.

- **Digestion:** The smooth flow of Qi ensures the normal digestive functions of the Stomach and Spleen, thus allowing for a harmonious movement of Qi within the Middle Burner. If the Liver Qi becomes stagnant, or "invades the Stomach or Spleen" it will adversely affect the digestive functions.

- **Emotional State:** The Liver's function of ensuring the free and easy wandering of Qi has an influence on the body's mental and emotional activity, affecting the emotional states that each organ generates. Impairment of this function can lead to a "binding depression of Liver Qi" associated with impatience, hasty decisions, impulsive actions, and anger.

3. Rules the Tendons: The Liver regulates the function and control of the tendons and ligaments via the contraction and relaxation of the muscles, and is the source of the body's physical strength. In ancient Chinese Martial Neigong training, it is said that, "For power, it is better to stretch the tendons half an inch, than to increase the muscle mass three inches." The stretching of the tendons (called "reeling and pulling the silk" in Chinese martial arts training) allows an individual the ability to increase his or her strength, as well as produce a powerful vibrational resonance used to maximize full striking potential. This vibrational skill is used in the Medical Qigong clinic (in techniques such as Vibrating Palm and Thunder Fingers) for dispersing stagnations.

If the Liver Blood becomes deficient, the body will be unable to moisten and nourish the tendons. This often results in symptoms such as muscle cramps, tremors, spasms, numbness of the limbs, impaired extension or flexion ability and an overall lack of strength. Internal Liver Wind can adversely affect the tendons, and in some cases cause contractions of the tendons resulting in convulsions and tremors.

4. Manifests in the Nails: In Traditional Chinese Medicine, the fingernails and toenails are considered to be an offshoot of the tendons, and as such are also influenced by the flow of Liver Blood. The condition of the nails reflect the quality of nourishment that the tendons are receiving and can be used to determine the state of Liver Blood. If the Liver Blood is abundant, the finger and toenails will be flexible, smooth and healthy, with no ridges or spots.

5. Opens at the Eyes: The Liver is connected to the eyes and the sense of sight. The Liver Blood moistens the eyes and gives them the capacity to see. When the Liver Blood is deficient, there will be blurry vision, myopia, color blindness or dry eyes.

The images absorbed into the body through the eyes are filtered through the Liver by the spiritual influences of the Hun (Ethereal Souls) or Po (Corporeal Souls), which then generate emotional responses according to the individual's current state of mind.

6. **Psycho-Emotional Aspects:** The Liver is responsible for planning and creating, and is also responsible for instantaneous solutions or sudden insights. It is for this reason that the Liver is sometimes called "The General in Charge of Strategy."

   The Liver's positive psycho-emotional attributes are all influenced by the Hun, and are expressed as love, kindness, benevolence, compassion, and generosity. In normal function, these psycho-emotional aspects of the Hun influence the Liver, allowing the individual to experience love and compassion in thoughts and actions.

   The Liver's negative attributes are influenced by the Po, and are expressed as anger, irritability, frustration, resentment, hate, jealousy, rage, and depression. If the circulation of Qi becomes obstructed, the resulting Liver Qi stagnation gives rise to emotional turmoil. This emotional turmoil may sometimes manifest through energetic outbursts of anger (Yang) or sinking into depression (Yin), and is initiated by the Po's effect on the Liver.

7. **Spiritual Influence:** The Liver stores the Three Ethereal Souls, also called the Hun (see Chapter 2). In the context of classical Chinese theology, the Eternal Soul (Shen Xian) is different from the Ethereal Souls (Hun), in that the Eternal Soul is seen as the more personal of the two; whereas, the Ethereal Souls are seen as more universal temperaments or as archetypes. The ancient medical classics say that there are Three Ethereal Souls (Hun) and Seven Corporeal Souls (Po) that symbolize different attributes of the human being. The Hun's spiritual energy is said to be able to leave the body and then return, thus indicating a relationship with out-of-body travel into the spirit world.

Chinese Ideogram of the Hun

The Chinese ideogram for the Hun has two parts (Figure 8.36). The character to the right represents the Earthly spirits "Gui" (Ghost), depicted

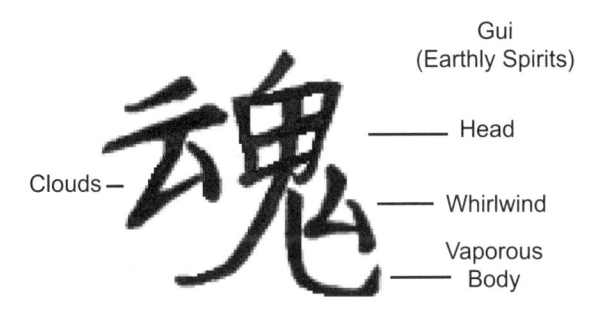

Figure 8.36. The Chinese character for "Hun," Three Ethereal Souls

by a head suspended above a vaporous form of a body with an appendage (symbolizing the whirlwind that accompanies the movements of the Earthly spirits). The character to the left is the image for clouds, that are seen as vapor rising from the Earth and gathering in the Heavens. The cloud character represents a more "ethereal" aspect of the spirit. From the ideogram we also get a distinct picture of the spirit rising to the Heavens.

The ancient Chinese believed that the Hun move within the body as freely as clouds, following the Yi (intent) of the "Heavenly Breath (Eternal Soul), within the celestial vault" (within the Heart, originating within the Taiji Pole).

The Liver and the Hun

The Hun have many functions. They are responsible for controlling sleep and dreaming, assisting the Shen in mental activities, maintaining balance in one's emotional life (under the leadership of the Shen), governing the eyes, influencing a person's courage, controlling planning with the aid of the Shen, and spirit travel (Figure 8.37).

The Hun, or Three Ethereal Souls, are rooted in the Liver Yin (which includes the Liver Blood). The Hun influence the sense of spiritual direction in one's life. The Hun are responsible for providing vision, either through the physical eyes (observing colors, patterns and forms) or through the spiritual eyes (observing spiritual visions and clairvoyance). When the Liver Blood and Liver Yin are flourishing, the Hun become firmly rooted, giving the individual insights and spiritual perceptions. Mental confusion and a lack of direction

```
Liver stores the Hun → Controls Sleep and Dreaming
                     → Assists the Shen in Mental Activities
                     → Maintains Balance in One's Emotional Life
                     → Are Responsible for the Eyes
                     → Influences a Person's Courage
                     → Controls Planning and the Sense of Direction
                     → Controls Spirit Travel
```

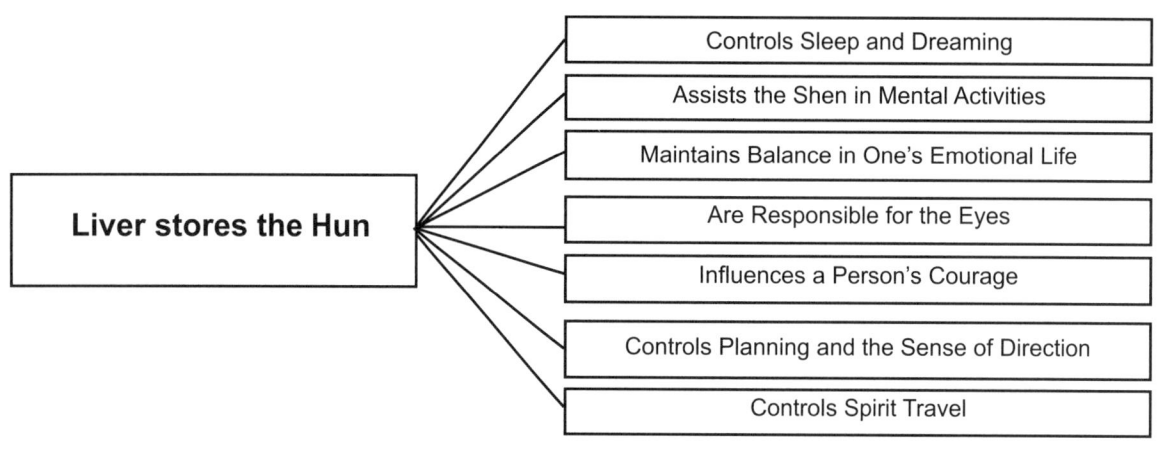

Figure 8.37. The Seven Energetic and Spiritual Functions of the Three Hun

(disassociated syndrome) is often considered to be a state in which the Hun have left the body (wandering in other energetic dimensions) and usually occurs when the Liver Blood and Liver Yin are deficient. If the body's Liver Yin is depleted, the Liver is unable to hold the Hun. Deprived of their residence, the Hun begin to wander. This can result in such conditions such as fear, excessive day dreaming, insomnia, and a lack of sense of direction or purpose in life (one of the main features of depression).

The Hun store the sum total of past experiences. The expressions of the Hun are manifested through images, symbols and ideas from the divine and through the energetic state of the Wuji. These images, symbols, and ideas emerge from the individual's spiritual life influencing his or her mental, emotional and physical life. Without this interaction, the individual's mental and emotional life would be deficient in images, ideas, and dreams, resulting in a lack of life purpose.

- **The Hun Control Sleep and Dreaming:** The Hun represent the "giving of images" and the "function of imaging." There is an interesting correlation between the Hun controlling sleep and dreaming, and the Hun being rooted in the Liver Blood and Yin. The Hun's moving in and out of the Liver governs the free flow of Liver Qi and vice-versa; the free flow of Liver Qi is a manifestation of the swimming energy of the Hun moving in and out of the tissues. The Hun reside in the eyes during the day to see, and at night they lodge in the Liver to create dreams. Dreams are the roaming of the body's Hun. It is the nature of the Hun to wander. Dreams are an example of the information gathered during the Hun's travels. The ancient Chinese understood and believed that the body's Hun traverse through the Nine Levels of Heaven or Nine Levels of Earth instantaneously.

- **The Hun Assist the Shen in Mental Activities:** Like the emperor and his chief counsel, the Shen and the Hun are always interacting and must be in constant harmony. The Shen is related to rational thinking and inspiration. The Hun give the Shen a sense of direction by projecting intentions outward to interrelate with people. The Hun gives the Shen its movement and direction, encouraging the Shen to relate with people, to socialize and to bond. The Hun, however, also need to be gathered and restrained by the Shen. Otherwise, if the Shen is weak and does not control the Hun, then the Hun will overload the Shen with too many ideas, which leads to frustration.

It is important that the Shen allow the Hun to move in and out of the body, but in so doing must give the Hun direction and purpose. That is why the words "movement," "coming and going," and "swimming" are often used in connection with the Hun. In fact, many doctors say that the Hun are the coming and going of the body's Shen.

The Hun inspire us and give us dreams. In mediumistic trances, when the spirit of one person enters the body of another, the host's Shen is disabled, and the energetic form of the spirit's Hun comes inside the host body to communicate.

Because knowledge is dependent on the awareness of the Hun, the Hun are therefore considered to be the collectors of information. The Hun however, do not interpret, rationalize, or analyze the knowledge; they just receive information and pass it on to the Shen. In this context, the Shen is responsible for rational thinking, intuition, and inspiration. The Shen also helps to distinguish between the useful and irrelevant information.

- **The Hun Maintain Balance in One's Emotional Life:** The Hun are responsible for keeping the emotions balanced, preventing any one emotion from becoming excessive and from causing disease. The Hun have a regulatory function closely related to the balance between Liver Blood (Yin) and Liver Qi (Yang). The Hun's function here is the mental equivalent of the Liver's emotional regulating and harmonizing function.

Because of its acquired nature, the Shen Zhi discriminates, while the Hun does not. The relationship between the Shen and the Hun is very similar to the Jungian concepts of the conscious and the unconscious aspects of mind. The Hun are a repository of images and archetypes connecting the (personal) subconscious mind with the collective unconscious. If the Hun are unsettled, then the Shen (consciousness) is cut off, confused, isolated, aimless, sterile, and without dreams. The movement of ideas within the body has to be controlled, otherwise it gets out of hand and leads to madness. This irrational behavior occurs to the degree that the Shen is unable to control the Hun which is causing the individual to receive an uncontrolled amount of emotional, mental, and spiritual input. All of the energies and symbols coming through the Hun have to be integrated and assimilated. A lack of the assimilation can lead to serious mental illness and possibly psychosis. An exception being the active perceptions of young children, who are continually full of ideas and have active imaginations. In a child, the Hun are very active, and the Shen is not as restraining; so, there is a continual flow of energies streaming from the unconscious world of symbols without resulting in insanity.

- **The Hun are Responsible for the Eyes:** When the Hun wander in through the eyes, the eyes can see. The Hun are responsible for physical, mental and spiritual vision. Since the Hun are related both to dreaming and to the eyes, some Qigong masters believe that the Rapid Eye Movement (REM) associated with dreaming is the Hun's way of downloading the day's lessons into the Shen (Heart) via the subconscious mind.

- **The Hun Influence a Person's Courage:** The Liver houses the body's Hun and governs fright. If the Hun are not strong, the person is timid and fearful. If the Hun are strong, the person is fearless, can face up to the difficulties in life, and dares to take action even in difficult or confusing circumstances. A patient with weak Hun will have difficulty gathering information and making decisions; he or she will lack courage, and become easily discouraged and apathetic.

- **The Hun Control Planning and the Sense of Direction:** With the aid of the Shen, the mental and spiritual confusion about one's role in life, what to do, what goals to set, can be compared to the aimless wandering of the Hun. This is a strong feature of major depression. If the Liver is strong and the Hun are strong and rooted, the person will have a powerful sense of direction.

- **The Hun Control Spirit Travel:** While deep in meditation, the Hun can leave the body for spirit travel, causing the physical body to enter into a vegetative state. By performing Shengong Meditations, the Qigong doctor can "house the Shen" for spirit travel, allowing the spirit to journey outside of the physical body, consciously directing the Hun's travelling. Spirit travel is different from soul travel, which is the human soul journeying outside of the physical body connected to the Middle Dantian by a silver "cord of life." The three Ethereal Souls accompanied by the individual's consciousness, act as one unit which is sometimes referred to as the spirit-soul. The spirit-soul allows the individual to know the exact location of the "spirit routes" travelled, as well as which path and direction it takes when it leaves the body. Otherwise, when the Hun wander, the individual will "Shen out" (disassociates) and have no recollection of where he or she has been in the spiritual realms.

THE LIVER CHANNELS

The Liver Channels are Yin channels that flow externally from the feet to the torso (Figure 8.38). These two rivers originate externally from the lateral side of the big toes and flow upward on the medial side of the legs to encircle the groin. From there they continue to ascend externally to the lateral aspects of the torso, where they enter internally and penetrate the Liver. They then connect to, and spirally wrap around the Gall Bladder. From there, they flow to the Lungs, ascend internally through the thorax, and into the head to connect with the eyes, cheeks, and inner surfaces of the lips. The Liver channel then emerges at the forehead and flows upwards to connect with the Governing Vessel at the Baihui (GV-20) point.

CHANNELS' ENERGY FLOW

From the external and internal pathways of Qi flowing from the Liver organ, the circulating movement of the Qi washes over the whole body, assisting the tissues in storing and distributing the Blood. The Liver Channels contain more Blood than Qi; they therefore affect physical substances more than they affect energetic functions.

The internal energetic flow of the Liver follows the path of the Microcosmic Orbit Water Cycle (Figure 8.39). This is the natural energetic path used for stimulating the intuitive perceptions of the Hun, and it is used in advanced meditation

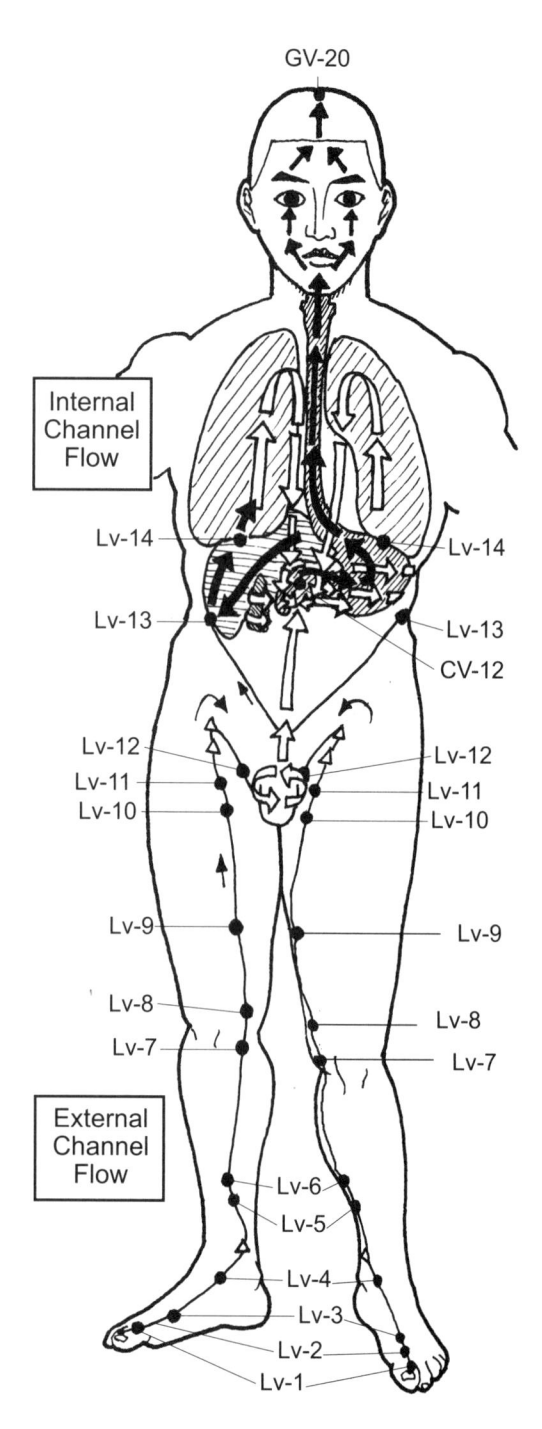

Figure 8.38. The Internal and External Qi Flow of the Liver (Lv) Channels

practices for cultivating deep spiritual states.

At the high-tide time period (1 a.m. to 3 a.m.), Qi and Blood abound in the Liver organ and Liver channels. At this time, the Liver organ and channels can more easily be dispersed and purged; whereas during low tide (1 p.m. to 3 p.m.), they can be more readily tonified. The energy of the Liver Channels acts on the skin, muscles, tendons and nerves that are found along the channels' pathway.

The Influence of Climate

In the springtime, Liver conditions become more pronounced. Liver Qi becomes more active in individuals with strong Liver Qi. Likewise, it may become deficient in those with weak Liver Qi. When Liver Qi is deficient, the patient becomes withdrawn and fearful; when the Liver Qi is in excess, the patient becomes consumed by anger and irritability.

During this season, the excessive consumption of foods containing preservatives, foods that have been contaminated with pesticides, and the excessive drinking of alcohol can deplete the Liver.

An external Windy climate, which is typically stronger during the spring time, can interfere with the functions of the Liver by aggravating a preexisting Internal Liver Wind condition. Symptoms relating the External Wind invasion aggravating internal Liver Wind include headaches, stiff neck, skin rashes that start suddenly and move quickly, and Wind Stroke.

The Influence of Taste, Color, and Sound

- The sour taste can be used to tonify both the Liver and Gall Bladder
- The dark green/blue color is used to tonify the Liver
- The descending "Shu" and "Guo" sounds are used to purge the Liver and Gall Bladder

Liver Pathology

As the Liver supplies the tendons with the energy and nutrients necessary for the development and maintenance of physical strength, Liver impairment is the cause of many disorders of physi-

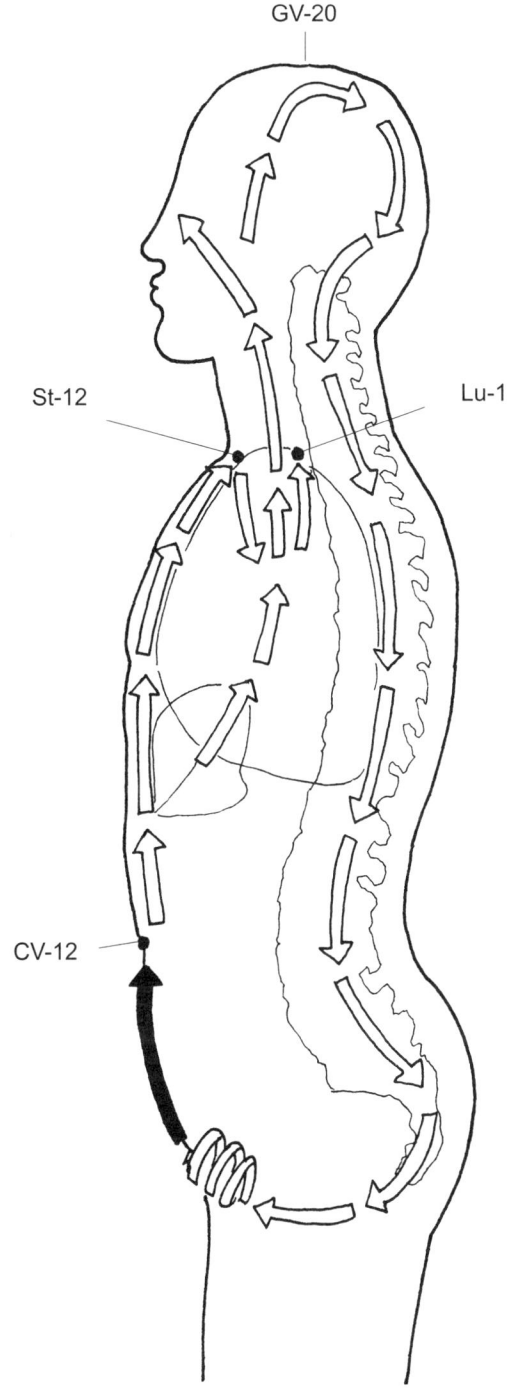

Figure 8.39. Side View of the Liver Channels' Internal Flow of Energy Following the Energetic Path of the Microcosmic Water Cycle

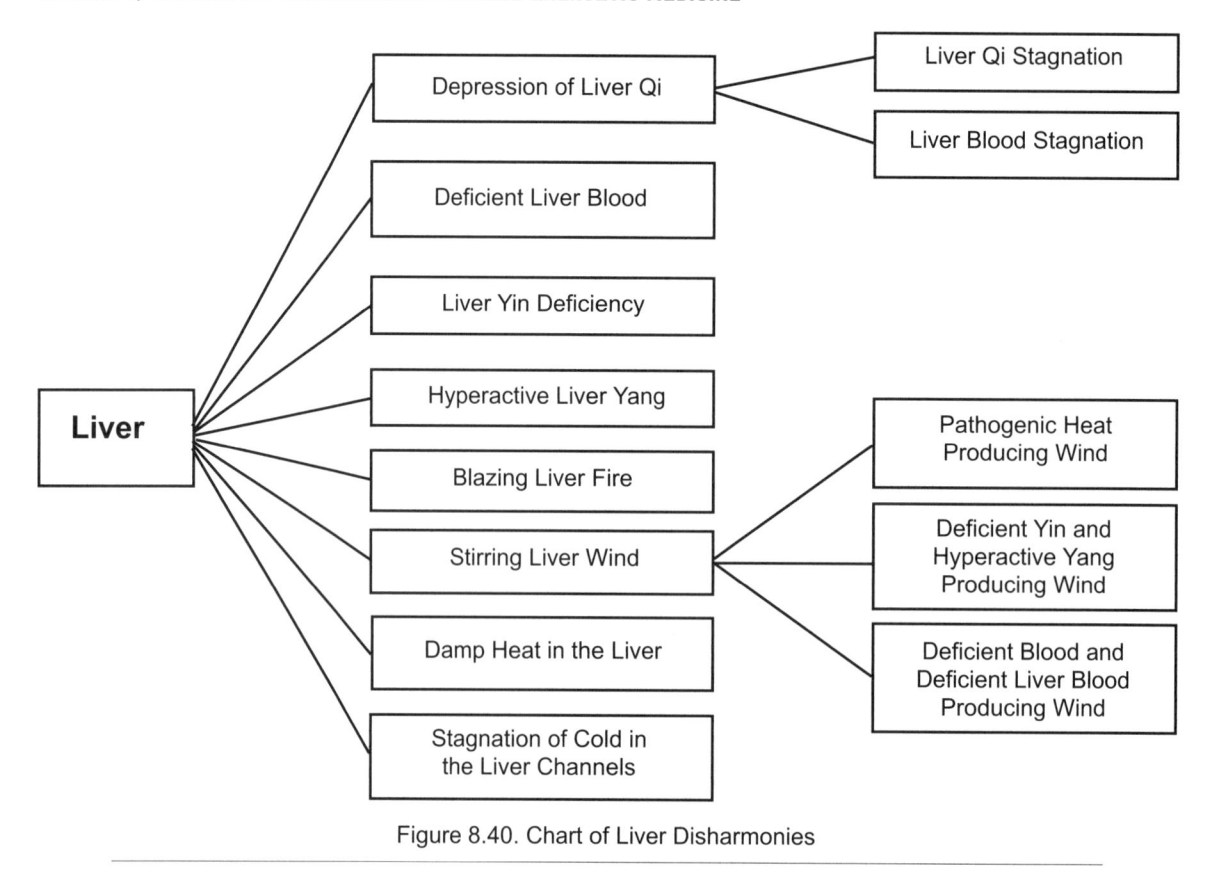

```
                           ┌─────────────────────┐     ┌─────────────────────┐
                           │ Depression of Liver Qi │────▶│  Liver Qi Stagnation  │
                           └─────────────────────┘  ╲   └─────────────────────┘
                                                     ╲  ┌─────────────────────┐
                                                      ▶│ Liver Blood Stagnation│
                                                       └─────────────────────┘
                           ┌─────────────────────┐
                           │  Deficient Liver Blood │
                           └─────────────────────┘
                           ┌─────────────────────┐
                           │  Liver Yin Deficiency │
                           └─────────────────────┘
                           ┌─────────────────────┐     ┌─────────────────────┐
                           │ Hyperactive Liver Yang │   │   Pathogenic Heat    │
                           └─────────────────────┘     │    Producing Wind     │
┌───────┐                  ┌─────────────────────┐     └─────────────────────┘
│ Liver │─────────────────▶│   Blazing Liver Fire  │     ┌─────────────────────┐
└───────┘                  └─────────────────────┘     │  Deficient Yin and    │
                           ┌─────────────────────┐────▶│  Hyperactive Yang     │
                           │  Stirring Liver Wind  │     │   Producing Wind     │
                           └─────────────────────┘     └─────────────────────┘
                           ┌─────────────────────┐     ┌─────────────────────┐
                           │ Damp Heat in the Liver │   │  Deficient Blood and  │
                           └─────────────────────┘     │  Deficient Liver Blood│
                           ┌─────────────────────┐     │   Producing Wind      │
                           │  Stagnation of Cold in │   └─────────────────────┘
                           │   the Liver Channels  │
                           └─────────────────────┘
```

Figure 8.40. Chart of Liver Disharmonies

cal strength and movement. These disorders include tremors or spasms of the muscles, tiredness, numbness, and sluggishness in joint movements. Diseases of the Liver Channels can also cause swelling and a distended sensation of the hypochondrium. The Liver Channels also correspond to diseases of the lower abdomen and genital organs.

The Liver and Kidneys are mutually dependent upon each other. The Liver stores the Blood that nourishes the Kidney Jing; whereas the Kidneys store Jing that helps produce the Blood. Deficient Kidneys may lead to Blood Deficiency, and Deficient Liver Blood may cause weakness of the Kidney Jing due to lack of nourishment from the Blood. The hair on top of the head is also nourished by the Blood. When the hair turns grey, it is often said to be caused by insufficient Blood stored in the Liver, as well as a Kidney Jing deficiency.

T.C.M. PATTERNS OF DISHARMONY

In Traditional Chinese Medicine, Liver disharmonies originate from Deficient Liver Blood, Deficient Liver Yin, Blazing Liver Fire, Internal Liver Wind, or Liver Qi Stagnation. For clinical purposes, Liver dysfunctions can be categorized into eight major pathological conditions. These pathological conditions are described as follows (Figure 8.40): Depression of Liver Qi, Deficient Liver Blood, Liver Yin Deficiency, Hyperactive Liver Yang, Blazing Liver Fire, Liver Wind, Damp Heat in the Liver and Gall Bladder, and Stagnation of Cold in the Liver Channels, which are described as follows (Figure 8.41):

1. **Depression of Liver Qi:** This is one of the most common patterns of disharmony observed in the clinic. Depression of Liver Qi is usually due to emotional disharmony such as frustration, irritation, anger or depression.

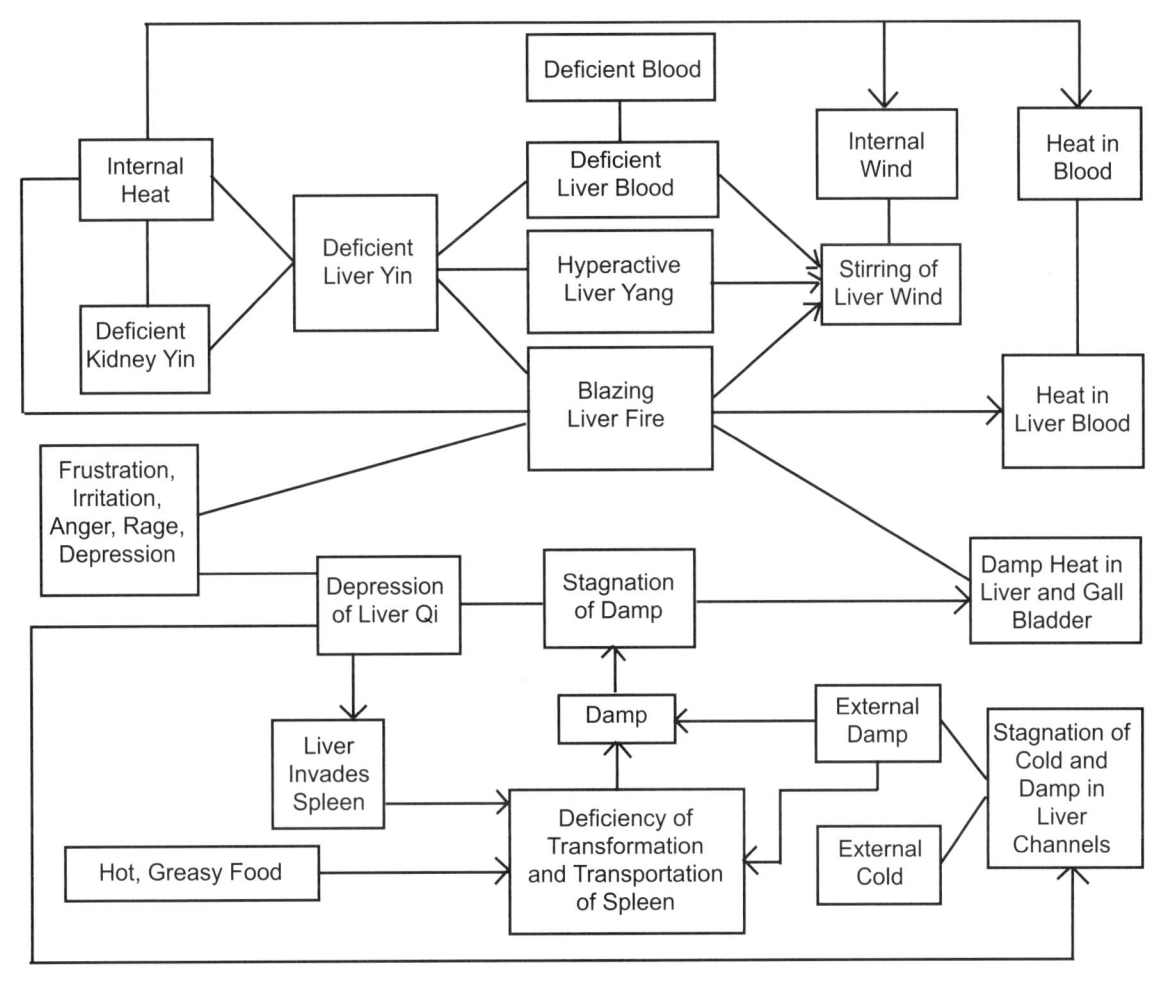

Figure 8.41. The Origins of Liver Disharmony

This condition results in stagnation of both Qi and Blood throughout the body. It can create a disharmony within the patient's digestive system, affect menstruation, and influence the patient's emotional and behavioral patterns (Figure 8.42).

- **Liver Qi Stagnation:** When Liver Qi is stagnant, it may invade other internal organs and cause further disharmony. Symptoms can manifest as irritability, impatience, headaches, plum-pit stagnation in the throat, depression, abdominal pain, abdominal masses, diarrhea, constipation, pain and distension of the hypochondrium, epigastric pain, poor appetite, belching, nausea, vomiting, irregular menses,

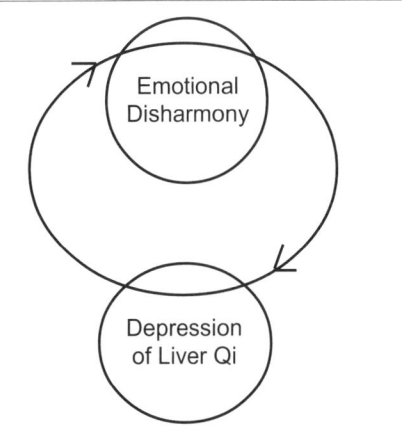

Figure 8.42. Depression of Liver Qi

premenstrual tension, dysmenorrhea and painful urination. Stagnant Liver Qi invading the Stomach can result in epigastric pain, nausea and vomiting. Stagnant Liver Qi invading the Lungs can cause wheezing and asthma.
- **Liver Blood Stagnation:** Stasis of Liver Blood is usually a consequence of chronic Liver Qi stagnation. When Liver Blood is stagnant, symptoms can manifest as irritability, impatience, depression, hypochondriac pain, nose bleeds, vomiting blood, abdominal masses, abdominal pain, dysmenorrhea, painful periods, irregular periods, dark blood and clotted menses.

2. **Deficient Liver Blood:** Poor nourishment can weaken the Spleen, resulting in an insufficient production of Blood. When not enough Blood is produced by the Spleen, insufficient Blood is stored by the Liver. Additional pathogenic factors creating deficient Blood or Liver disharmony can give rise to Deficient Liver Blood (e.g., loss of Blood due to hemorrhage; injury to Yin, injury to Body Fluids, injury to Liver due to Heat caused by fever or Blazing Liver Fire). Deficient Liver Blood can cause such symptoms as headaches, numbness of the limbs, insomnia, blurry vision, dry brittle nails, tiredness, hypochondriac pain, constipation, irritability, impatience, depression, scanty menstruation, and amenorrhea (Figure 8.43).

3. **Liver Yin Deficiency:** Can cause such symptoms as insomnia, dry eyes, tiredness, irritability, impatience, depression and pain in the hypochondriac region.

4. **Hyperactive Liver Yang:** Deficient Liver Yin can give rise to conditions of excess Dryness and Heat. Excessive Dryness and Heat can easily lead to conditions of Hyperactive Liver Yang, or the more extreme condition of Blazing Liver Fire. In ancient China, the Liver is sometimes called the "root of resistance to fatigue." Whenever the Liver is not functioning properly (stagnant, deficient, or excessively hot) the patient can experience fatigue as well as physical weakness (Figure 8.44).

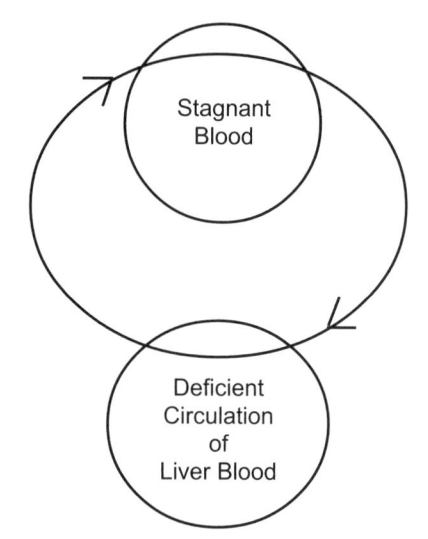

Figure 8.43. Deficient Liver Blood

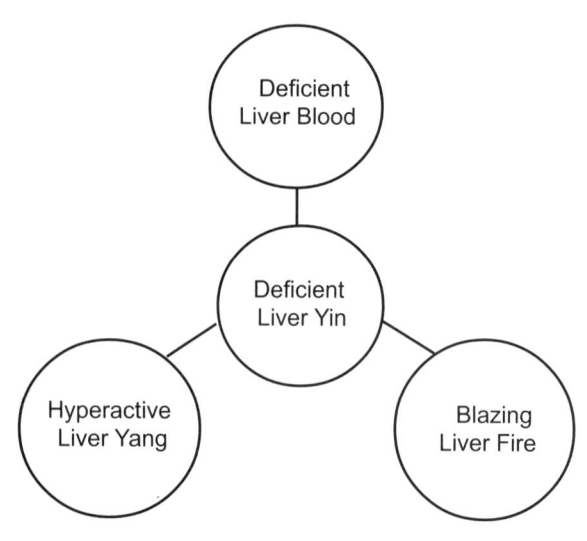

Figure 8.44. Interrelationship of Hyperactive Liver Yang Patterns

Liver Yang Rising can cause such symptoms as: irritability, headaches, dizziness, high blood pressure, and tiredness.

5. **Blazing Liver Fire:** A chronic condition of Internal Heat or Deficient Liver Yin may predispose the patient to Blazing Liver Fire. Blazing Liver Fire can be caused by suppressed anger or rage, or by excessive consumption of alcohol, tobacco, spicy and greasy food, or

drugs. If extreme or chronic in nature, Deficient Liver Blood, and Hyperactive Liver Yang can also result in Blazing Liver Fire. This energetic pattern can also arise from chronic depression of Liver Qi. Stagnation can eventually give rise to Internal Heat and ultimately flare up as Fire. Blazing Liver Fire can cause such symptoms as red eyes and face, angry outbursts, tinnitus, temporal headaches, dizziness, dream-disturbed sleep and insomnia.

6. **Stirring Liver Wind:** Deficient Liver Blood, Hyperactive Liver Yang, Blazing Liver Fire or severe fever can result in the stirring of Liver Wind. Liver Wind is considered Yang and light in nature. It generally rises within the body, affecting the upper torso, and especially the head. It manifests through sudden or irregular movements primarily affecting the upper body, and is associated with Liver disharmony. Pathogenic Liver Wind manifests as tics, tremors, spasms, convulsions and stroke, as well as a shaking and vibrating in the tongue. The upward movement of Liver Wind affects the circulation of Qi and Blood and can cause dizziness or loss of consciousness. There are three main energetic patterns of Stirring Liver Wind: Pathogenic Heat Producing Wind, Deficient Yin and Hyperactive Yang Producing Wind and Deficient Blood and Deficient Liver Blood producing Wind.

- **Pathogenic Heat Producing Wind:** This is a sudden, acute condition that only occurs in severe febrile diseases. In this condition, the Yin and Blood are damaged by the extreme Heat generated from the fever.
- **Deficient Yin and Hyperactive Yang Producing Wind:** Deficient Yin and Hyperactive Yang, stemming from chronic Liver Yin Deficiency, can cause the rising of Liver Yang. This condition can sometimes give rise to Liver Wind, resulting in such symptoms as weakness, sudden loss of consciousness and mental disorders.
- **Deficient Liver Blood Producing Wind:** Deficient Yin and Deficient Blood result from a lack of nourishment and moisture of the body's muscles and tendons. This pattern of deficiency creates an emptiness within the Blood Vessels, which become "filled" with Internal Wind. This condition of Internal Wind results in such symptoms as blurred vision, dizziness, aphasia, weakness, numbness, trembling, stiffness and spasms of the head and extremities.

7. **Damp Heat in the Liver:** A combination of External or Internal Dampness and Heat (with a tendency towards Liver Stagnation) can result in the condition of Damp Heat in the Liver and/or Gall Bladder. If the transformation and transportation functions of the Spleen are impaired (caused from Liver invasion or External Dampness), Internal Dampness can be produced. If there is depression of Liver Qi, this Dampness may stagnate and create Heat. Symptoms of Damp Heat in the Liver include: abdominal distension, fullness and pain in the chest and hypochondrium, loss of appetite, bitter taste in the mouth, nausea, vomiting, and a sour taste. Damp Heat in the Liver and Gall Bladder can cause such symptoms as jaundice, headaches, bitter taste in the mouth, nausea, abdominal fullness, leukorrhea, painful and inflamed scrotum, loss of appetite, irritability, impatience, depression, hypochondriac pain, and abdominal pain.

8. **Stagnation of Cold in the Liver Channels:** Stagnation due to Liver Qi Depression in combination with stagnation of Cold can result in stagnation of Cold in the Liver Channels. Cold concentrates in the lower part of the body, therefore symptoms generated from a stagnation of Cold in the Liver Channels include disharmonies of the lower body, such as hernia, pain and distension in the lower abdomen, testes and scrotum. As these pathologies are due to stagnation of Cold, they are alleviated by movement and warmth.

THE LIVER IN WESTERN MEDICINE

The liver is situated on the right side of the torso immediately beneath the diaphragm, and is surrounded by the rib cage. It is the largest gland in the body, weighing about 3 pounds in the average adult, and is slightly smaller in women than

Figure 8.45. The Liver Organ.

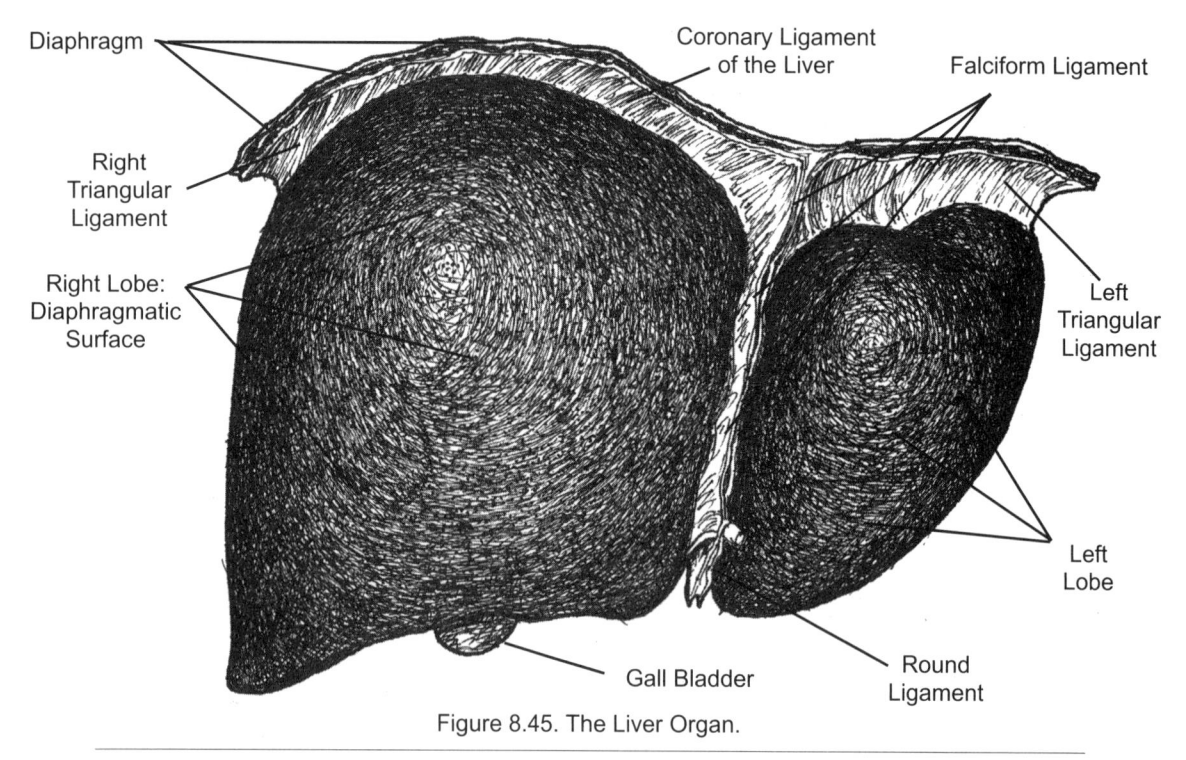

in men. The liver is also the second largest organ of the human body, with the skin being the largest. The liver is responsible for a wide range of metabolic and regulatory functions, and is one of the most important organs in the body for maintaining the health of the blood. The bile produced by the liver plays an important role in the digestion of fats and the excretion of wastes.

ANATOMY OF THE LIVER

The liver is a roughly wedge-shaped organ, with its base directed towards the right of the rib cage, and its edge angled to the left (Figure 8.45). Except for the superior aspect of the liver, which is fused to the diaphragm, the entire liver is surrounded by a layer of visceral peritoneum. Within this peritoneum the liver is enveloped in a further layer of dense irregular connective tissue.

The liver organ is divided into two primary lobes: the right lobe, which comprises the majority of the liver's mass; and the left lobe, which is smaller and extends slightly across the midline of the body. Two smaller lobes, the caudate lobe and the quadrate lobe, lie along the vertical border of the left and right lobes. The right and left lobes are separated by the falciform (sickle-shaped) ligament, which also connects to the diaphragm above, and to the right rectus-abdominis muscle in front. The round ligament (or ligamentum teres) is a remnant of the fetal umbilical vein, and it spans the distance between the liver and the navel, enmeshing itself into the falciform ligament. The liver is further anchored to the abdomen by the coronary ligament, and by two lateral ligaments.

In the average adult, the liver receives roughly 2 pints of blood every minute, equal to about 28% of the total cardiac output of blood. This blood supply enters the liver through both the hepatic artery and the hepatic portal vein (Figure 8.46). The hepatic artery divides into right and left branches which nourish the tissues of the right and left lobes of the liver respectively. The hepatic portal vein carries venous blood from the abdominal organs into the liver to be processed. It is important to note that the liver is the first internal

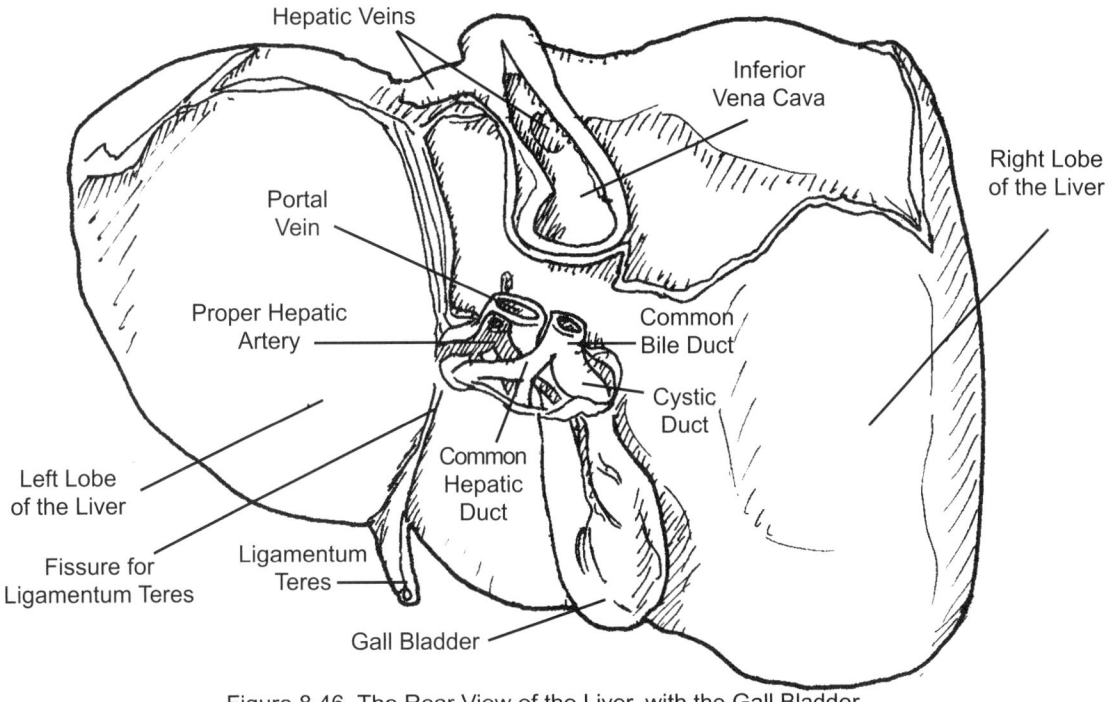

Figure 8.46. The Rear View of the Liver, with the Gall Bladder
(Inspired by the original artwork of Dr. Frank H. Netter).

organ to receive blood that has been exposed to the intestinal capillaries; for this reason the liver is especially susceptible to diseases originating in the digestive tract. Entering the underside of the liver, the hepatic portal vein then quickly divides into a network of capillaries that disperse blood throughout the liver.

The lobes of the liver are composed of numerous sesame seed sized lobules, which are the essential structural and functional units of the liver organ. Each lobule consists of numerous hepatic (liver) cells organized around a central vein. On a horizontal plane, a liver lobule gives the appearance of a roughly hexagonal plate of hepatic cells. These cells are arranged in branching, irregular, interconnected plates which are irrigated by venous capillaries, and which essentially stack together to give the lobule a somewhat oblong vertical dimension.

A portal triad flows vertically along each of the six corners of the lobule, and consists of a branch of the hepatic artery (carrying fresh blood into the liver tissue), a branch of the hepatic portal vein (carrying venous blood from the digestive system), and a bile duct. Blood from both the hepatic artery and the hepatic portal vein flow through large capillaries (termed sinusoids) within the liver lobule. These sinusoids are surrounded by hepatic cells that essentially clean the blood as it flows past them. Sinusoids also contain hepatic macrophages (called Kupffer cells) which remove bacteria, old blood cells, and other debris from the blood. Each sinusoid empties into the vein at the center of each lobule. These veins then join together into interlobular veins which eventually flow into the hepatic veins. Cleansed blood is drained from the liver by the hepatic veins, which converge with the inferior vena cava before reaching the heart.

BILE SECRETION

Bile is secreted from the hepatic cells into tiny canals (called bile canaculi) that flow between every other row of cells, such that each row of hepatic cells has a bile canaculi on one side, and a sinusoid on the other. Bile is directed away from the center of the lobule, and on reaching the bile duct at the lobule's corner, it flows downwards.

The bile secretions of the liver are directed through several ducts that ultimately join together to form the hepatic duct, which carries bile away from the liver. The cystic duct connects the gallbladder to the hepatic duct, and is the common duct through which bile enters and exits the gallbladder. The common bile duct flows from the junction of the cystic and hepatic ducts, and it is this duct that eventually delivers bile into the duodenum.

PHYSIOLOGY OF THE LIVER

The various functions of the liver can be categorized into the following areas: metabolism of carbohydrates, proteins, and lipids; storage of vitamins and minerals; phagocytosis; removal of poisons, drugs, and certain hormones; and the synthesis and excretion of bile (Figure 8.47). The Liver metabolism has the capacity to convert one nutrient into another nutrient, or to change the form of a nutrient to make it more appropriate for activation, storage, or excretion.

1. **Metabolism of Carbohydrates:** in combination with the pancreas, the liver helps to maintain a steady glucose level in the blood. When blood sugar levels are too high, the liver can draw glucose from the blood and convert it into glycogen (a molecule that is a composition of numerous smaller glucose molecules) for storage. The liver can also convert glucose into triglycerides for storage within liver or muscle tissue. If there is a decrease in the blood-glucose level, the liver then converts glycogen (or other available sugars such as lactose and galactose) it has stored back into the glucose form to be used by the cells. In a process known as gluconeogenesis, the liver is also capable of making glucose from lactic acid or from certain amino acids.
2. **Metabolism of Proteins:** the liver alters amino acids so that they can be used for ATP production or changed into fats or carbohydrates. The liver also removes ammonia (produced by bacteria in the GI tract, and also as a by-product of protein metabolism) and other nitrogenous wastes from the system by converting it into the much less toxic urea, which is then later excreted through the urine. Certain enzymes within the liver are capable of converting one amino acid into another, or converting one amino acid into an entirely different nutrient. Liver cells also synthesize heparin and most plasma proteins, such as albumin, alpha and beta globules, fibrinogen (used in blood coagulation), and prothrombin
3. **Metabolism of Lipids:** the liver manufactures cholesterol, some of which is then used in the production of bile. Among other things, cholesterol plays an important role in the creation of certain hormones and is necessary for the

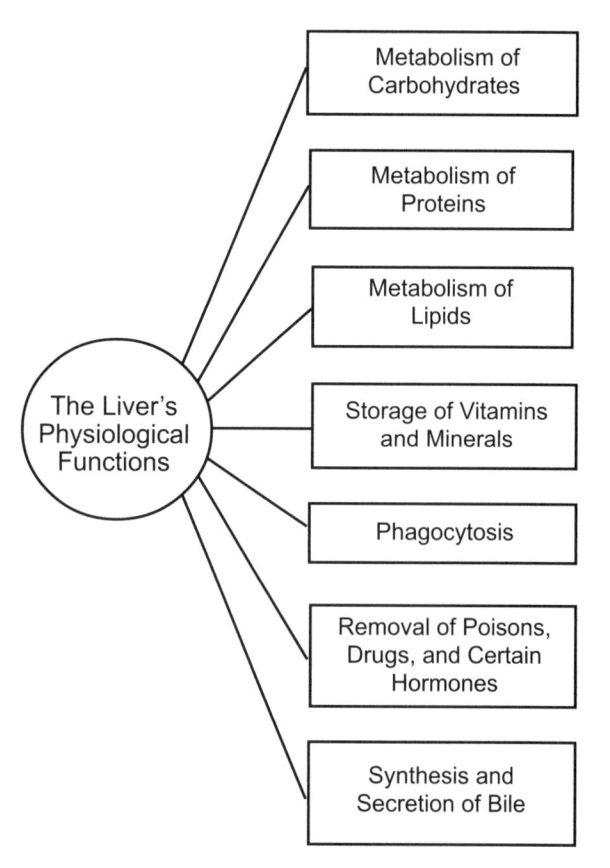

Figure 8.47. The Functions of the Liver (Western Medical Perspective)

The Liver's Physiological Functions:
- Metabolism of Carbohydrates
- Metabolism of Proteins
- Metabolism of Lipids
- Storage of Vitamins and Minerals
- Phagocytosis
- Removal of Poisons, Drugs, and Certain Hormones
- Synthesis and Secretion of Bile

production of vitamin D. The liver also synthesizes various lipoproteins, which include both high-density lipoproteins (HDL) and low-density lipoproteins (LDL). Lipoproteins also combine with cholesterol, fatty acids, and triglycerides in order to transport hem through the blood. Certain cells within the liver also store triglycerides, which are the body's most concentrated source of energy. The liver breaks down fatty acids into acetyl coenzyme A, the excess of which is converted into ketone bodies. Other examples of lipids that are metabolized within the liver include phospholipids, steroids, and prostaglandins.

4. **Storage of Vitamins and Minerals:** The liver stores vitamins A, B-12, E, and K, and plays and important role in both the activation and storage of vitamin D. Minerals such as copper, iron (in the form of ferritin), and cobalt are also stored within the liver. These stored nutrients are later released into the bloodstream whenever they are needed by the body.

5. **Phagocytosis:** Within the liver, the Kupffer cells phagocytize (engulf or consume) worn out white and red blood cells as well as some bacteria. This process aids the immune system by removing unwanted material from the blood. The iron and globulin thus extracted from the breakdown of erythrocytes is recycled, while the bilirubin (derived from heme) is excreted into the bile ducts. Resident bacteria within the GI tract further breakdown bilirubin after the bile is excreted into the intestines, giving the feces their normal brown color.

6. **Removal of Poisons, Drugs, and Certain Hormones:** The liver serves to detoxify the body by chemically altering or excreting certain drugs and organic compounds such as penicillin, sulfonamides, and erythromycin. The liver can also alter or excrete hormones such as estrogen, aldosterone, thyroid hormones, and steroid hormones. Various poisons such as DDT and other pesticides are removed from the bloodstream and stored within the liver. The liver also produces numerous protective, antitoxic substances.

7. **Synthesis and Excretion of Bile:** The liver's only digestive function is the creation and secretion of bile, which is released into the small intestine via the hepatic duct. When considered as a part of the digestive system, both the liver and gallbladder are thus seen as being accessory organs associated with the small intestine.

Bile, is a bitter yellowish substance consisting mainly of water, bile acids, bile salts, bile pigments, lecithin, cholesterol, electrolytes, and various fatty acids. Once delivered into the small intestine, bile salts and acids play an important role in the digestion of fats; though the secretion of bile is also a vehicle for the excretion of unwanted materials from the liver. Nearly one quart of bile is secreted each day by the liver. Secreted bile is stored and concentrated in the gallbladder, and when needed for digestion, it is transferred into the duodenum (uppermost portion of the small intestine) via a system of ducts. The bile secretions of the liver are directed through several ducts that ultimately join together to form the hepatic duct, which carries bile away from the liver. The cystic duct connects the gallbladder to the hepatic duct, and is the common duct through which bile enters and exits the gallbladder. The common bile duct flows from the junction of the cystic and hepatic ducts into the duodenum.

COMMON DISORDERS OF THE LIVER

Impairment of liver function can be at the root of a wide range of symptoms and functional disorders. Some of the most widely recognized disorders of the liver are jaundice, hepatitis, and cirrhosis. Jaundice is a condition in which there is a buildup of bilirubin in the system, giving the eyes and skin a yellowish discoloration. The three main types of jaundice are: prehepatic jaundice (including neonatal jaundice), in which there is an excess production of bilirubin; hepatic jaundice (due to liver dysfunction); and extrahepatic (or obstructive) jaundice (caused by a blockage of bile drainage). Hepatitis, of which jaundice can be a symptom, refers to either an acute or chronic inflammation of the liver. Acute hepatitis is usually nonviral, and can be caused by an overtaxing of the liver due to drug toxicity, oral-fecal contamination, or wild mushroom poisoning. Chronic hepatitis, of which there are now more than a dozen types, is generally attributed to a virus. Liver cirrhosis is a chronic inflammation and scarring of the liver usually resulting from chronic hepatitis, or from long term alcohol or drug abuse. Eventually, cirrhosis of the liver can lead to liver fibrosis, in which the liver has an excess of scar tissue inhibiting its proper functioning.

Other liver disorders include liver enlargement, portal hypertension, ascites (fluid buildup in the abdomen due to liver leakage), liver encephalopathy (brain deterioration due to blood toxicity), liver failure, and metabolic disorders such as hemochromatosis and Wilson's disease. Hepatocellular adenoma and hemangioma are examples of benign liver tumors, while liver cancers include hepatoma (primary liver cancer), cholangiocarcinoma, hepatoblastoma, and angiosarcoma. Congenital liver disorders include neonatal jaundice, biliary atresia, and choledochal cysts.

The Lungs: Fei

The Lungs are solid Yin organs. Their associated Yang organ is the Large Intestine. They correspond to the Metal Element. Since the Lungs are the uppermost organs, they are compared to canopies, in that they shelter and protect all the other internal organs. The Lungs control the cycle of Qi circulation in the body, and are sometimes referred to as the "White Emperor" (Figure 8.48).

Chinese Character for the Lung: Fei

The Chinese character "Fei" translates as "Lungs." It refers to the image of the Lung organs, and is divided into two sections. The character to the left, "Ji" depicts the Chinese ideogram for body tissue, muscle or flesh (all of which are forms of connective tissue). The character to the right depicts an ideogram that is a representation of a creeping type of plant, branching upward from the soil of the Earth, like a fibrous vine. Together, both ideographs express the idea that the Lung organs are responsible for connecting into and enveloping the tissues, as well as spreading the Qi (Ying Qi and Wei Qi) throughout the interior and exterior aspects of the torso (Figure 8.49).

The Yin and Yang of the Lungs

Traditional Chinese Medicine describes the Lungs as having two energetic aspects, Yin and Qi:

- **The Yin of the Lungs:** This pertains to the material structures of the Lungs.
- **The Qi of the Lungs:** This pertains to the physiological functions of the Lungs.

The Lungs' Metal Jing Formation

The Metal Jing is established in the fetus' body during the sixth lunar month of pregnancy, and serves to stabilize the sinews and connective tissues. The Metal Jing energy is also responsible for fetal formation and for the ability to form and maintain emotional bonding with others. Faltering of the Metal Jing energy is commonly associated with problems of emotional attachment (e.g., autism).

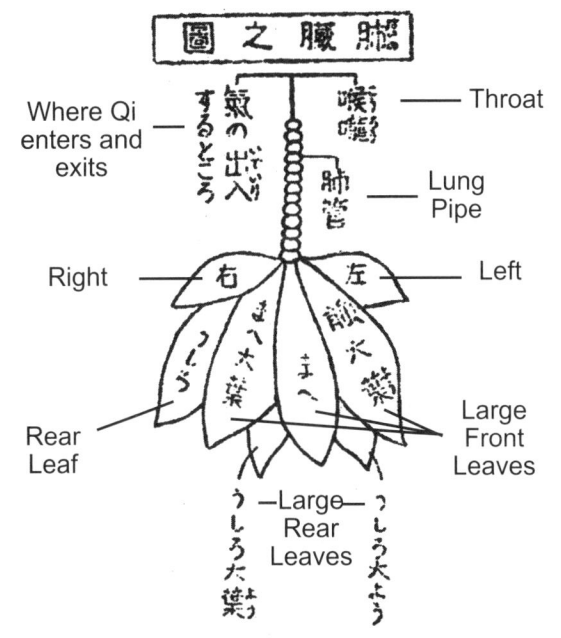

Figure 8.48. The ancient Chinese anatomical diagram of the Lungs (Lu) Organ, as it appeared in "Important Useful Notes on Acupuncture and Moxibustion," published in Japan in 1718, by Masatoyo Hongo

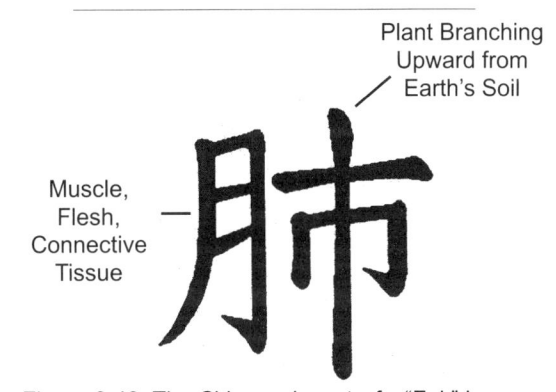

Figure 8.49. The Chinese character for "Fei," Lungs

After birth, the Metal Jing can be affected through the color white, the pungent taste and the "Shh," "Sss," and "Shang" sounds.

The Lungs in Chinese Medicine

In Traditional Chinese Medicine, the Lungs function much in the same way as described in Western Medicine. The Lungs are viewed as part of the respiratory system and are related to water metabolism, Blood circulation, the autonomic ner-

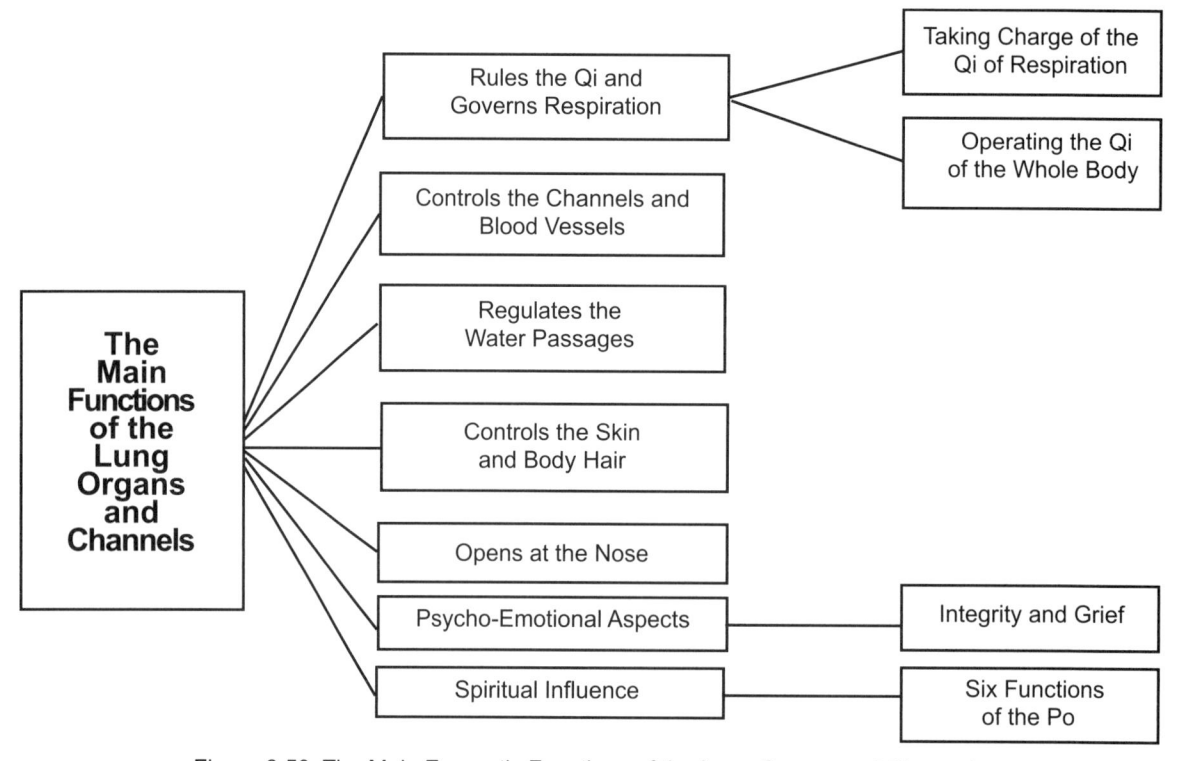

Figure 8.50. The Main Energetic Functions of the Lung Organs and Channels

The Main Functions of the Lung Organs and Channels:
- Rules the Qi and Governs Respiration
  - Taking Charge of the Qi of Respiration
  - Operating the Qi of the Whole Body
- Controls the Channels and Blood Vessels
- Regulates the Water Passages
- Controls the Skin and Body Hair
- Opens at the Nose
- Psycho-Emotional Aspects
  - Integrity and Grief
- Spiritual Influence
  - Six Functions of the Po

vous system, and the immune system. Traditional Chinese Medicine, however, expands the role of the Lungs to include the psycho-emotional aspects of integrity, attachment and grief. The Lungs also exert a powerful spiritual influence on the individual due to their relationship with the Corporeal Souls, or Po.

The Lungs, located in the Upper Burner, are viewed as the internal representation of our connection to Heaven, and contain the most rarefied form of our essential Qi. The Large Intestine, located in the Lower Burner, is seen as the internal representation of our connection to Earth, and contain the most turbid form of our essential Qi. In the upper thorax of the chest, the Lungs surround the Heart energetically as well as physically. In the abdomen, the Lungs' associated Yang organ, the Large Intestine, is energetically as well as physically surrounded by the Heart's associated organ, the Small Intestine.

Prior to the nineteenth century, certain Chinese medical texts expressed the belief that the Lungs were the first internal organs to complete their structural formation, occurring when a baby is born (this energetic completion enables the child to breath and cry). In the same texts, it states that at the end of life, the Lungs are the last internal organ to expire (this is because if the Brain is dead, but the Qi is not interrupted and the respiration continues, the individual is still considered alive).

According to Traditional Chinese Medicine, the main functions of the Lungs are to: govern the Qi and respiration, control the channels and Blood Vessels, regulate the water passages, control the skin and hair, open to the nose, express itself through the psycho-emotional aspects of integrity and grief, and exert an important spiritual influence via the Po (Corporeal Soul). These main functions are described as follows (Figure 8.50):

1. **Rules the Qi and Governs Respiration:** The Lungs are responsible for controlling the formation and movement of Qi and function in

two specific ways: taking charge of the Qi of respiration, and operating the Qi of the whole body.

- **Taking Charge of the Qi of Respiration:** The main function of the Lungs is to regulate breath, controlling both pulmonary and cellular respiration. The Lungs are the main organ responsible for respiration and for the gathering Heaven Qi. For this reason, the chest is sometimes called the "Upper Sea of Qi." According to the *Ling Shu* (Magical Pivot), "the Sea of Qi, which comes out of the Lungs, goes into the throat and facilies inhalation and exhalation." It is through the action of the Lungs' respiration that Qi (energy) and gases (subtle substances) of the body are exchanged between the interior and exterior of the body. The taking in of fresh oxygen from the air during inhalation and the expelling of waste gas in the form of carbon dioxide during exhalation function to maintain healthy internal organ regulation. This healthy exchange helps to keep the body's energetic and physical metabolism functioning smoothly.
- **Operating the Qi of the Whole Body:** The Lungs operate the Qi of the whole body through two ways: forming Zong Qi (Pectoral Qi), and controlling the ascending and descending, entering and exiting aspects of the body's life-force energy.
- **Forming Zong Qi (Pectoral Qi):** When Heaven (Universal) Qi and Earthly (Environmental) Qi are absorbed into the body in the form of fresh air and food essence (Gu Qi), they accumulate within the chest to create what is known in Traditional Chinese Medicine as Zong (Pectoral) Qi. Zong Qi exits the body from the larynx, promoting the Lung's respiratory activities. Zong Qi is responsible for the heartbeat, assisting the Lungs in the circulation of Qi, and assisting the Heart in the circulation of Blood. The Zong Qi also functions to warm the tissues of the torso, including all the viscera and the bowels, and in this way serves to regulate the physiology of the whole body.
- **Controlling the Ascending and Descending, Entering and Exiting:** The Lungs have the responsibility of causing the Qi and Body Fluids to flow throughout the whole body via the True Qi. The True Qi (Zhen Qi) formed by the Lungs has two components; Wei Qi (Protective Qi) and Ying Qi (Nourishing Qi). The Wei Qi flows through the muscles and skin, mainly outside the channels; the Ying Qi flows throughout the body within the channels and Blood Vessels. The dispersing action of the Lungs assists the spreading of the thin Body Fluids (Jin) throughout the skin and muscles via the Wei Qi; and the distribution of the thick Body Fluids (Ye) to the Zang Fu Organs, Brain, joints and orifices via the Ying Qi. At the surface of the body, the Lungs govern the "entering and exiting" of energy to and from the body (a function of the Wei Qi). Internally, the Lungs are in charge of the "ascending and descending" movements of Qi and Body Fluids.
- **Circulation of Qi:** The Lungs send Qi downward throughout the body. In particular, Qi is sent from the Lungs to the Heart, which receives and holds onto this Qi, transforming it into Blood and Body Fluids. Qi is also sent down to the Kidneys, which receive and hold onto it in order to maintain and strengthen the inhalation.
- **Circulation of Body Fluid (Jin and Ye):** The Lungs receive the vaporous form of the Body Fluids from the Spleen, and then separate them for circulation throughout the body. The Lungs liquefy the impure fluids and send them to the Heart. The Heart receives and holds these impure fluids, vaporizing and further separating part of the Body Fluids, sending them back to the Lungs. The Lungs then spread the vaporized Body Fluids to the skin in the form of a mist, which moistens the tissues and regulates sweating and the opening and closing of the pores.
- **The Entering and Exiting of Qi:** Like a fog descending from Heaven, the Lungs ensure the free movement of Qi throughout the body. In this aspect, the Lungs ensure that all of the organs receive the nourishment that they need via the distribution of Qi, Blood and Body Fluids. The Lungs also prevent excess or de-

ficient accumulation of fluids.

2. **Controls the Channels and Blood Vessels:** There is a Chinese saying, "all Blood Vessels lead to the Lungs," meaning that all of the Blood within the body must pass through the Lungs. The Lungs also control the circulation of Qi in both the vessels and the channels, in addition to being in charge of the dispersing or spreading of the body's Wei Qi (Protective Energy).

    According to the *Su Wen*, "the Lungs receive the 100 vessels in the morning audience." In order to understand this statement, the reader should know that every morning, in ancient China, all of the palace officials would go to the court to be assigned specific tasks. Likewise, every morning, in the human body, the 100 vessels go to the Lungs' "courtyard" in order to be regulated and recharged to start the new day.

3. **Regulates the Water Passages:** The Lungs regulate the body's water passages (sweat and Body Fluids), the opening and closing of the pores, the skin, and the texture of the body's hair. The Lungs receive the vaporous form of the Body Fluids (Jin and Ye) from the Spleen, and further separate them via the Heart for circulation throughout the body organs, tissues, and skin. The Kidneys also receive the Body Fluids from the Lungs and vaporize a portion of them, sending this refined mist back to the Lungs in order to keep the Lung organs moist.

4. **Controls the Skin and Body Hair:** The Lungs are directly exposed to the air through the organs of the respiratory tract (nose, mouth, larynx and trachea). The Lungs are indirectly exposed to the air through their association with the skin (including pores, sweat glands and body hair). The Lungs receive the vaporous form of the Body Fluids from the Spleen, and then separate them for circulation throughout the body. The skin and body hair derive both their nourishment and their moisture directly from this function of the Lungs.

    The ancient Chinese Qigong masters believed that the hair follicles of the body contained both Fa Men (Dharma Gates) and Gui Men (Ghost Gates). Each of these Gates are connected in pairs and find their expression in the respiration (inhalation and exhalation) of the body's pores, described as follows:

    - **Fa Men:** There are 84,000 "Fa Men" (Dharma Gates) contained within the hair follicles of the body. Dharma Gates are defined by the Daoists as a way of resolving things for the good of the individual. The Fa Men act as talismanic controls, gathering and releasing Qi and Shen within the body's energetic fields, according to the direction of the Shen.
    - **Gui Men:** There are 84,000 "Gui Men" (Ghost Gates) contained within the hair follicles of the body. Ghost Gates are defined by the Daoists as a way for the dark aspects of the Po to initiate control.

5. **Opens at the Nose:** The Lung Qi opens externally at the nose via the throat, and is considered a "phonic-organ," energetically manifesting itself through the voice. When the Lung Qi is in excess the voice is too loud; when it is deficient the voice is too soft. The nose's function of smelling is dependent mainly on the action of the Qi within the Lungs.

    According to the *Su Wen*, "Heaven nourishes Man through the Five Qi." These Five Qi pertain to the five odors from Earth (rancid, scorched, sweet, fishy and rotten) and the Five Climatic conditions from Heaven (Wind, Warmth, Cold, Dampness and Dryness). These Five Qi enter the body's tissues via respiration and environmental osmosis. Once absorbed into the body, the Five Qi penetrate into the Lungs and expand outward towards the Five Yin Organs, affecting the Qi circulation.

6. **Psycho-Emotional Aspects:** The Lungs are said to be "the priest" or "Minister of Heaven," and are responsible for establishing the foundation of Qi for the entire body. The effects of the Hun and Po on the Lungs allow the individual to experience integrity and dignity in thoughts and actions (influenced by the Hun) or healthy grief (influenced by the Po). However, if the circulation of Qi becomes obstructed for long periods of time, the Lung Qi stagnation can give rise to chronic emotional turmoil, sometimes manifesting

through energetic outbursts of crying or sinking into despair, (again influenced by the Po). The Lungs' positive psycho-emotional attributes are righteousness, dignity, integrity, and high self-esteem. The negative psycho-emotional attributes of the Lungs are disappointment, sadness, grief, despair, shame, and sorrow.

7. **Spiritual Influence:** The Lungs house the body's Seven Corporeal Souls (Po) which are responsible for self-protection and self-preservation. The Po are physical in nature and are attached to the body's Jing and Qi. The Po are defined as the driving force of the individual's passions, expressed through his or her desires and animation in life.

CHINESE IDEOGRAM OF THE PO

There are two parts to the Po ideogram. The character to the right represents the Earthly spirits called Gui (ghost), depicted by a head suspended above a vaporous form of a body with an appendage (symbolizing the whirlwind that accompanies the movements of the Earthly spirits). The character to the left is the image for the color white. The white color represents the more tangible, concentrated form of the corporeal spirit. The color white can also be represented by the image of dried Bones lying on the Earth (Figure 8.51). Thus, the Po are linked with a descending movement of energy and with the Jing.

THE LUNGS AND THE PO

In Medical Qigong therapy, the human soul (Shen Xian) is seen as being strongly influenced by the two main internal spiritual energies, the Hun and the Po. The Hun are the three Ethereal Souls and represent the positively charged aspects of the human soul; while the Po are the seven Corporeal Souls and are considered the physical, negative, Yin, heavy, and Earthly aspects of the human soul. The Po are the counterpart of the Hun, and they manifest through six energetic and spiritual functions, which are described as follows (Figure 8.52):

- **The Po are the Somatic Expressions of the Human Soul:** They are related to the reflexive nervous system and limbic system, the oldest part of the Brain, which is sometimes referred to as

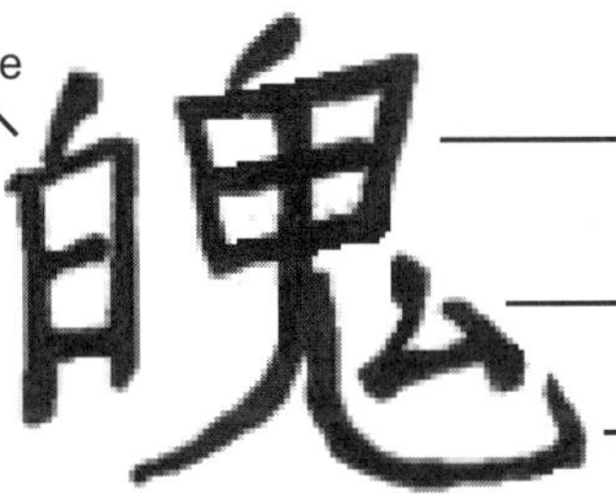

Figure 8.51. The Chinese character for "Po," Seven Corporeal Souls

the "reptilian brain." The Po manifest through the body's senses of feeling (tactile), hearing, and seeing. The Po have an impulsive tendency towards movement and action, rather than logic or careful consideration. They correspond to automatic reflexes, animal instincts, and the innate pre-programmed responses of the individual's subconscious mind. The Po also provide us with the raw animal strength and resources necessary to immediately mobilize and supercharge the body in times of extreme need, and to perform incredible feats of power. The "animal within" is driven by the Po. The Po are considered to be the manifestation of the body's Jing in the realm of sensations and feelings. Just as the Hun provide the individual with the energetic movements of the Shen, the Po provide the individual with the energetic movements of the body's Jing (see Chapter 2).

- **The Po are Responsible for All Physiological Processes in Childhood:** During the formative years of life, the Po are responsible for the sensations of pain and itching known as "growing pains." The Po serve as the intermediary between the Jing of the body and the body's other vital substances. At conception, the interaction of the mother's and father's Jing forms the embryo and establishes the Po within the body. Although the Po are primarily stored in the Lungs, they also remain connected to the entire physical body until death, when they return their energy back to the Earth within a few days.

- **The Po are Related to Weeping and Crying:** The interconnection between the Po and Lungs

Lungs Store the Po
- The Po are the Somatic Expressions of the Human Soul
- The Po are Responsible for All Physiological Processes in Childhood
- The Po are Related to Weeping and Crying
- The Po are Closely Linked to Breathing
- The Po are Connected to Sexuality on the Sensation Level
- The Anus is Considered the "Po Men" or "Door of the Po"

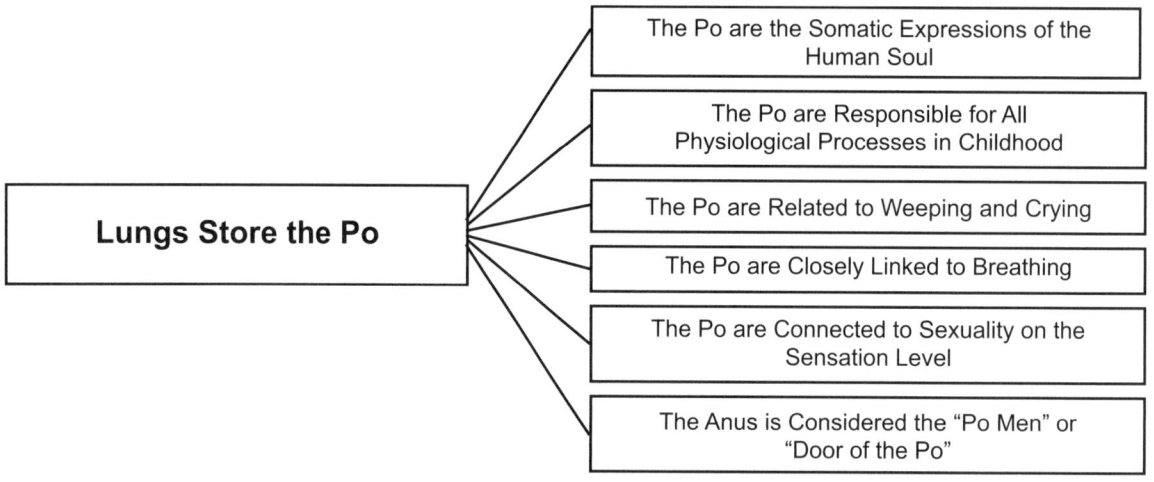

Figure 8.52. The Six Energetic and Spiritual Functions of the Seven Po

is very important in emotional anatomy. When the movement of the Po in the Lungs is inhibited, the emotions of grief and sadness are suppressed, there is constriction within the chest, and breathing becomes shallow.

In the morning time when waking, if the patient feels dull and depressed, it is a sign that his or her Shen is clinging to the body. This indicates that the Shen is being dominated by an excessive of Po energy, while the Hun are in a state of deficiency.

- **The Po are Closely Linked to Breathing:** Breathing is the pulsation of the Po. Each emotional change that takes place within the body is related to a shift in the body's respiratory pattern. The breath (air from Heaven) interacts with the Po in the Lungs, and plays a significant role in applying the Heaven-Man-Earth concept for balancing the emotions. Because breath control relies on the Lungs, and the Lungs influence the sympathetic and parasympathetic nervous systems, the quality of Qi and Qi circulation are dependent upon the method, depth, speed, and quality of the breath.

Because the Po reside in the Lungs, the condition of the Po manifests itself in the breath. Any modification of the breath will have a corresponding influence on the condition of the Po. Understanding this, it can be seen that all forms of physical exercise, breath control and meditation that utilize the breath are methods of training and calming the Po. This in turn, helps to calm the Shen, allowing access to the higher spiritual states of the Hun.

To support the greatest longevity possible, it is important to breathe with a long, slow, and even quality to the breath. Slow, deep breathing maximizes the beneficial exchange of Qi, gases, and subtle elements between the body and the environment, increases available energy, and prolongs life. Conversely, fast or inhibited breaths deplete the Qi, and decrease the individual's life span.

The Lungs' spiritual virtues are integrity, honesty, righteousness and truth. These virtues give a person the drive and strength to do the "right thing." These virtues manifest and promote good health when a correct energetic alignment with the Po is achieved. This balance can be initiated by slow gentle breathing patterns which calm and stabilize the Po.

- **The Po are Connected to Sexuality on the Sensation Level:** The Po are related to the physical sensations and responses associated with sex and sexuality. All instinctive sexual reactions and passions come under the authority of the Po. The Po provide the fundamental biological energy necessary for survival, and are the source of biological needs and impulses. They are driven by basic instincts and urges, and their sole concern is the immediate gratification of biological needs and drives. This is expressed through reproductive urges and impulses concerning emotional or physical survival. Most self destructive behavior, such as an attraction to unhealthy or dangerous habits and life-styles, is due to an imbalance of the Po. Sexual dreams and perverse sexual fantasies are associated with the unrestrained traveling of the Po while asleep or daydreaming.

- **The Anus is Considered the "Po Men" or "Door of the Po:"** The Corporeal Souls have a relationship with both the Lungs and Large Intestine. The anus is therefore considered to be the "Po Men" or "door of the Po." It acts as a doorway for the elimination of the waste by-products of the five Yin organs from the body through draining off the impure liquids and waste.

THE LUNG CHANNELS

The Lung Channels are Yin channels and flow externally from the torso to the hands. The main river originates internally from the Middle Burner in the middle of the chest (extending from the navel to the respiratory diaphragm) and descends downward connecting with and spirally wrapping the Large Intestine. From there, it ascends along the upper surface of the Stomach and through the diaphragm, where it branches to connect with both Lungs (Figure 8.53).

From the Lungs, the two rivers of Qi merge together and ascend into the pit of the throat, where they separate again into two channels. These channels travel beneath the clavicles. These two main channels then travel externally, descending the arms to end on the lateral side of each thumb. A small stream of energy branches from each wrist at the Lu-7 point and runs directly to the radial side of the tip of the index finger, where it connects with a branch of the Large Intestine Channels.

CHANNELS' ENERGY FLOW

The energy of the Lung Channels acts on the Lungs, bronchi, throat, and larynx. If the Lung Qi combines with Liver Qi and stagnates in the throat area, a condition known as a "plum pit" (a knot in the throat) will develop. The Lung Channels store more Qi than Blood, and thus have a greater effect on energetic and nervous functions than on physical substances and Blood functions. At the high-tide time period (3 a.m. to 5 a.m.), Qi and Blood abound in the Lung organs and Lung channels. At this time period the Lungs and Lung channels can more easily be dispersed and purged. During low-tide (3 p.m. to 5 p.m.), they can more readily be tonified. The energy of the Lung Channels acts on the skin, muscles, and nerves found along the channel pathways.

THE INFLUENCE OF CLIMATE

In the fall months, the Lung Qi becomes more active in individuals who already possess strong Lung Qi but becomes deficient in those who already have weak Lung Qi. During this season, the excessive consumption of pungent food or beverages and overexposure to Dryness can further impede Lung Qi.

Exposure to External Wind Cold, Wind Heat, Damp and overly Dry climates can interfere with the proper functioning of the Lungs. Because the Lungs need a certain amount of moisture to function, they are easily injured by Dryness. Therefore, a Dry climate (the climate associated with autumn in T.C.M.) can interfere with the functions of the Lungs.

THE INFLUENCE OF TASTE, COLOR, AND SOUND

- The pungent taste (garlic, green onions, etc.) can be used to tonify both the Lungs and Large Intestine, though excessive consumption can weaken them.
- The white color is used to tonify the Lungs and Large Intestine.
- The "Shhh", "Sss" and "Shang" sounds are used to purge the Lungs and Large Intestine.

LUNG PATHOLOGY

Dysfunctions of the Lung organs and channels can result in diseases of the chest or Lungs, and diseases on the radial side of the upper arm and palmar area of the hand. Since the Lungs have their

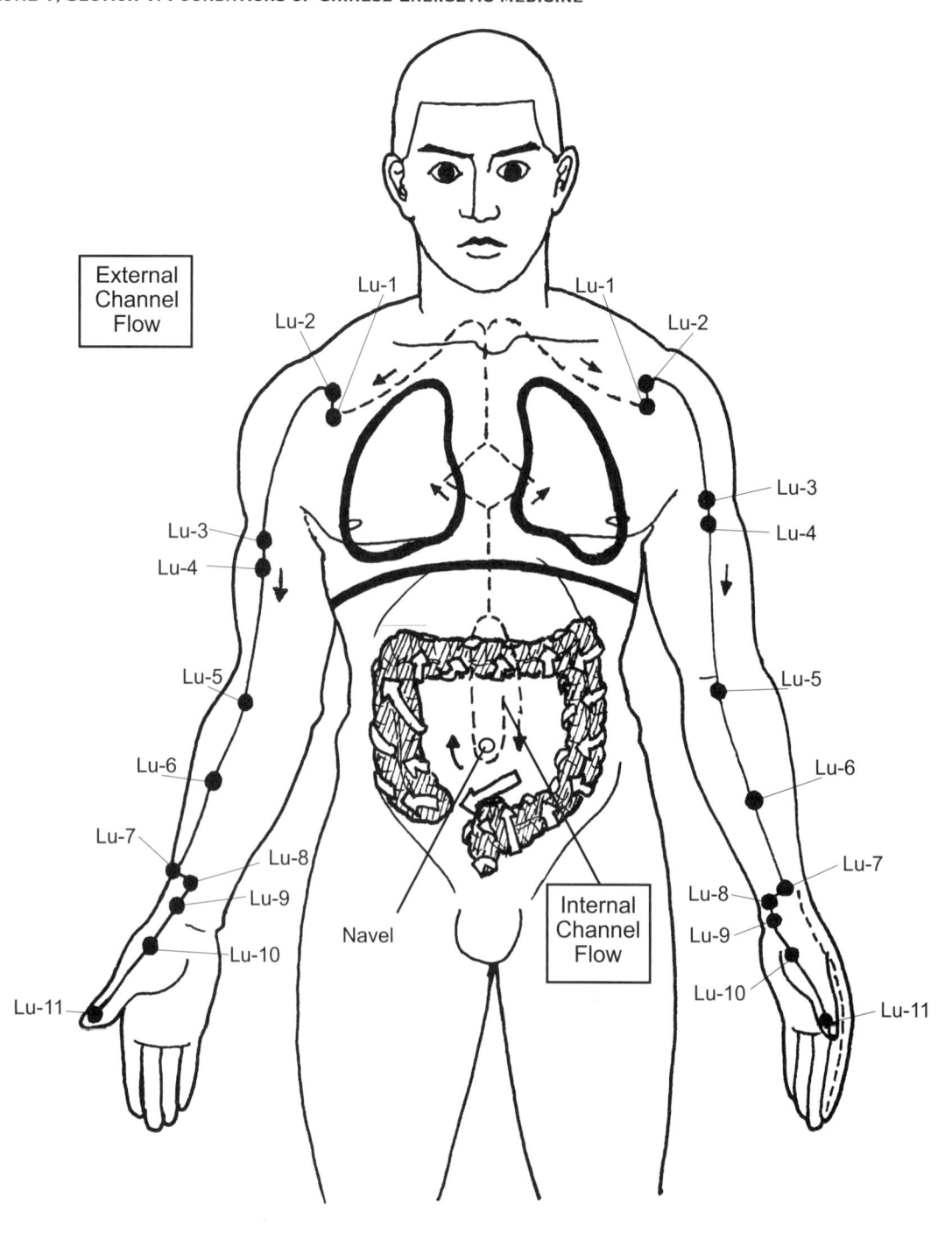

Figure 8.53. The Internal and External Qi Flow of the Lung (Lu) Channels

```
                    ┌─ Deficient Lung Qi
                    │
                    ├─ Deficient Lung Yin
                    │
                    ├─ Lung Heat
                    │                              ┌─ Wind Cold
                    │                              │
                    │                              ├─ Wind Heat
  Lungs ────────────┼─ Invasion of the ────────────┤
                    │  Lungs by Wind               ├─ Wind Dampness
                    │                              │
                    │                              └─ Wind Dryness
                    │
                    │  Retention of Phlegm in      ┌─ Hot Phlegm
                    └─ the Lungs ──────────────────┤
                                                   └─ Cold Phlegm
```

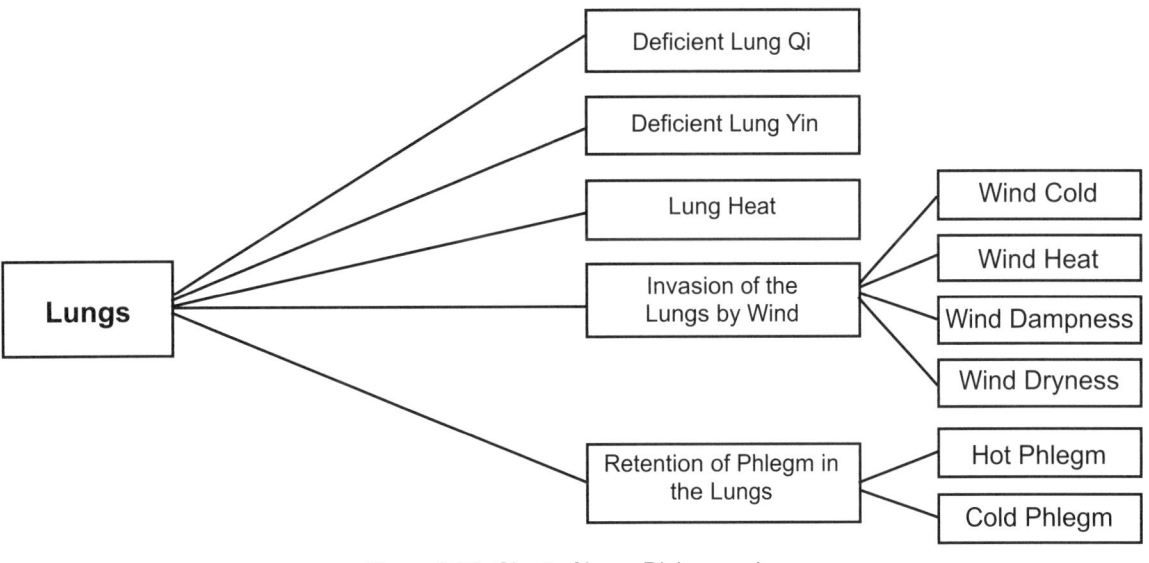

Figure 8.54. Chart of Lung Disharmonies

external orifice at the nose, stuffy nose, nasal discharge, and impairment of the sense of smell are common symptoms when the Lungs are being attacked by a pathogenic invasion of Wind and Cold.

The Lungs keep the respiratory passages open and disseminate vital Qi throughout the body. If these functions are impeded, obstructions of the nose, coughing, dyspnea, and fullness of the chest may occur.

The Lungs also function to cleanse the inhaled air and to keep the Qi flowing downward. If these functions are impeded, coughing, asthma, oliguria (scanty urine production), and edema may occur.

T.C.M. Patterns of Disharmony

Patterns of Lung disharmony are divided into syndromes of Deficient Lung Qi, Deficient Lung Yin, Lung Heat, Invasion of the Lungs by Wind, and the Retention of Phlegm in the Lungs, described as follows (Figure 8.54 - 8.55):

1. **Deficient Lung Qi:** Because the Lungs rule the body's Qi, they play an important role in patterns of Qi Deficiency. Deficient Lung Qi can manifest from a prenatal condition, an invasion of the Lungs by Wind, or the retention of Phlegm in the Lungs. Symptoms can manifest as fatigue, weak cough, weak voice, lack of desire to speak, shortness of breath, weak respiration, wheezing, asthma, spontaneous daytime perspiration, slight cough with no phlegm, allergic rhinitis, and enuresis or incontinence.

2. **Deficient Lung Yin:** Deficient Lung Yin may manifest through symptoms such as dry unproductive cough, dry cough in short bursts, asthma, emaciation, malar flush, afternoon fever and "Five Palms Heat." In the condition of Five Palms Heat (also known as "Five Center Heat," or "Sweating of the Five Palms") the patient experiences Heat in the palms of the hands and soles of the feet, accompanied by Heat and agitation in the chest or head area.

3. **Lung Heat:** Heat within the Lungs can cause the following symptoms: a feeling of Heat and restlessness, common cold, influenza, cough, sinusitis, breathlessness, and atrophy syndrome.

4. **Invasion of the Lungs by Wind:** Of all the Yin organs, the Lungs are the most susceptible to invasion of external pathogenic factors. The Lungs are especially vulnerable to Wind, especially Wind Cold and Wind Heat, which can transform into each other. Symptoms of Wind Invasion in the Lungs differ according to the specific nature of the invading pathogenic Wind (Cold, Hot, Damp, Dry), but generally

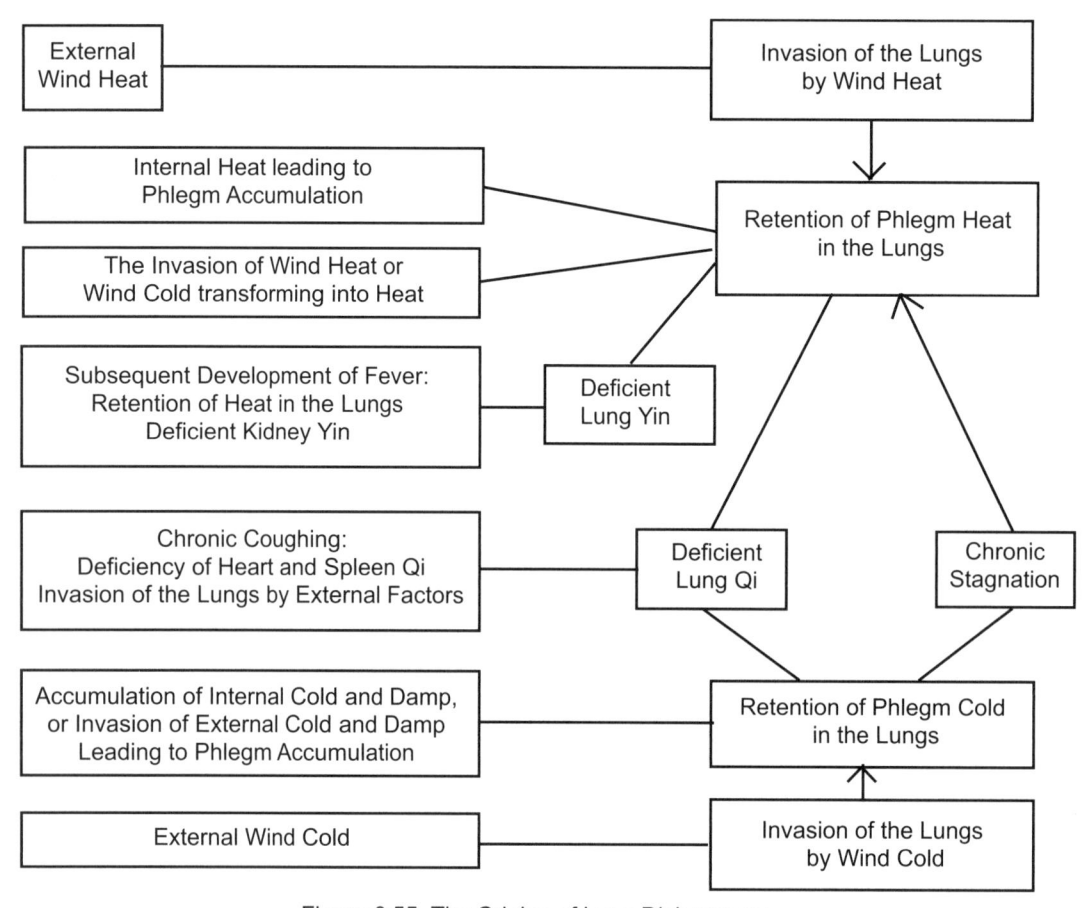

```
┌─────────────┐                                    ┌──────────────────┐
│  External   │────────────────────────────────────│ Invasion of the Lungs │
│ Wind Heat   │                                    │   by Wind Heat   │
└─────────────┘                                    └──────────────────┘
                                                            │
┌──────────────────────────┐                                ▼
│ Internal Heat leading to │                      ┌──────────────────┐
│   Phlegm Accumulation    │──────────────────────│ Retention of Phlegm Heat │
└──────────────────────────┘                      │   in the Lungs   │
┌──────────────────────────┐                      └──────────────────┘
│ The Invasion of Wind Heat or │──────────────────
│ Wind Cold transforming into Heat │
└──────────────────────────┘

┌──────────────────────────────┐    ┌──────────┐
│ Subsequent Development of Fever: │    │ Deficient │
│  Retention of Heat in the Lungs  │────│ Lung Yin │
│     Deficient Kidney Yin         │    └──────────┘
└──────────────────────────────┘

┌──────────────────────────────┐    ┌──────────┐    ┌──────────┐
│     Chronic Coughing:        │    │ Deficient │    │ Chronic  │
│ Deficiency of Heart and Spleen Qi │────│ Lung Qi  │    │Stagnation│
│ Invasion of the Lungs by External Factors │    └──────────┘    └──────────┘
└──────────────────────────────┘

┌──────────────────────────────────┐    ┌──────────────────┐
│ Accumulation of Internal Cold and Damp, │    │ Retention of Phlegm Cold │
│ or Invasion of External Cold and Damp   │────│   in the Lungs   │
│   Leading to Phlegm Accumulation       │    └──────────────────┘
└──────────────────────────────────┘              ▲
┌─────────────────┐                      ┌──────────────────┐
│ External Wind Cold │──────────────────│ Invasion of the Lungs │
└─────────────────┘                      │   by Wind Cold   │
                                         └──────────────────┘
```

Figure 8.55. The Origins of Lung Disharmony

include itchy throat, cough, nasal drip, headaches, chills, fever, sweating and aversion to wind.

- **Wind Cold invading the Lungs** usually enters the patient through the pores of the skin and body hair, both of which are ruled by the Lungs. If the Lungs' energetic field is invaded by Wind Cold, this can cause the Lung Qi to become impure. The impure Lung Qi then ascends, causing obstructions in the pores, resulting in a Wind Cold syndrome. This can cause the following symptoms: headache, cough, aches at the nape of the neck, chills and fever, the common cold, influenza, breathlessness, asthma, allergic rhinitis and aversion to cold.
- **Wind Heat invading the Lungs** usually enters the body by way of the mouth and nose. The nose is the orifice of the Lungs and the direct opening into the Lung organ. If the Lungs' energetic field is invaded by Wind Heat, it can cause the Lung Qi to become impure, ascend, and impede the ability of the pores to expel pathogenic evils, resulting in a Wind Heat syndrome. This can cause the following symptoms: chills and fever, headache, sore throat, cough, the common cold, influenza, asthma, allergic rhinitis, sinusitis, and slight aversion to cold.
- **Wind Dampness is a type of Wind Cold syndrome.** It consists of both Wind and Dampness invading either the skin (causing itching and rashes) or the channels and joints (causing painful obstruction syndrome). If the Lungs' energetic field is invaded by Wind

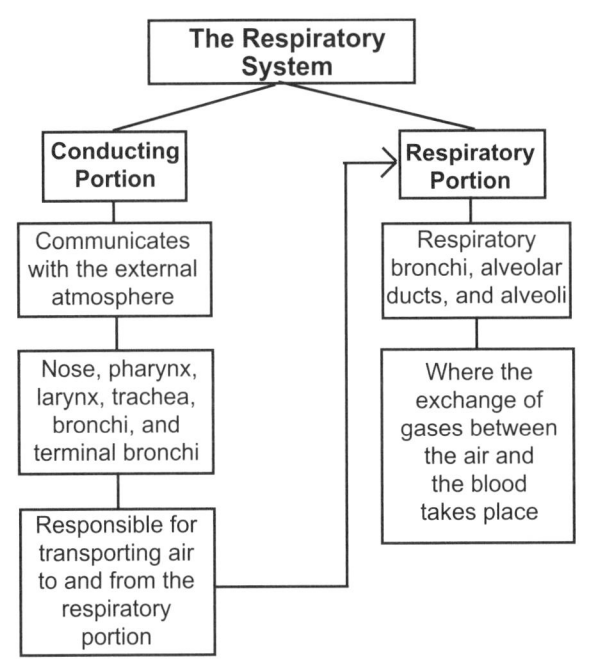

CHAPTER 8: THE TWELVE PRIMARY ORGANS, CHANNELS AND COLLATERALS

Figure 8.56. The Two Divisions of the Respiratory System

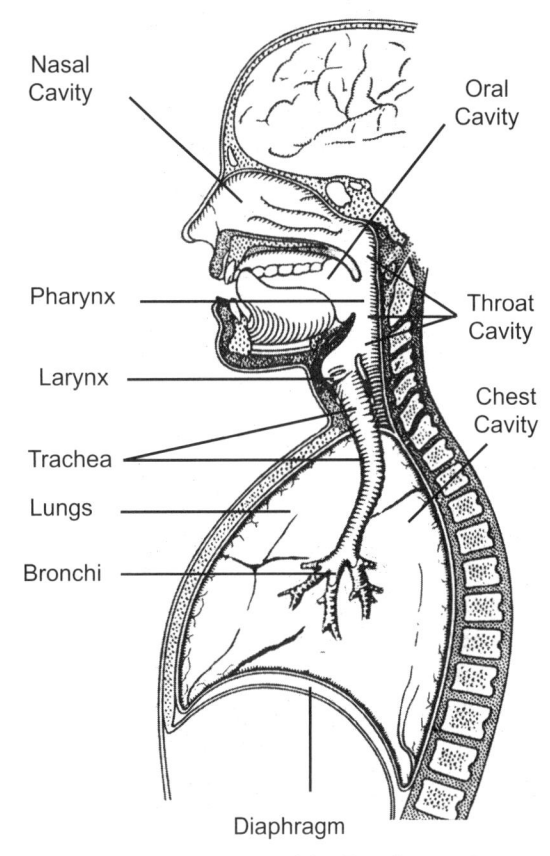

Figure 8.57. The Anatomy of the Respiratory System

Dampness, the following symptoms may arise: skin rashes, swollen joints, body aches, headaches, the common cold, and influenza.
- Wind Dryness invading the Lungs can cause the following symptoms: dryness, itchy sore throat, dry lips, dry mouth, the common cold, influenza, cough, and nose bleeds.

5. **Retention of Phlegm in the Lungs:** Phlegm is considered a secondary disease factor, derived from either Internal or External Dampness. The Spleen forms the Phlegm, and the Lungs store it. As a Lung disease progresses from a Cold to a Hot condition, the patient's mucus (Phlegm) changes color. The pathological condition of the Phlegm progresses from clear watery, to yellow and thick, to green and pussy, and finally to brown and red as heat increases. Internal conditions leading to the retention of Phlegm in the Lungs can arise due to chronic Qi Deficiency, Kidney Yang Deficiency, Spleen Deficiency or Lung Deficiency. External conditions leading to the retention of Phlegm in the Lungs can arise from excess conditions that are due to invasions of Wind Heat, Wind Cold, or Dampness.
- **Lung Phlegm Heat** can cause the following symptoms: influenza, the common cold, cough with yellow or green expectoration, breathlessness, and a sensation of oppression in the chest.
- **Cold-Damp Phlegm invading the Lungs** can cause the following symptoms: a feeling of heaviness, cough with clear or white profuse expectoration, wheezing, nausea, poor appetite, and breathlessness.

ANATOMY OF THE RESPIRATORY SYSTEM

The lungs are the primary organs of respiration. The lungs are paired organs, roughly cone-shaped, located on both sides of the chest and immediately surrounded by the pleural membrane. Between the right and left lungs lies the mediastinum, which contains the heart, its main Blood ves-

```
Lungs ──┬── The Upper Respiratory System ─── Nose (Nostrils and Nasal Cavity) and Pharynx
        └── The Lower Respiratory System ─── Larynx, Trachea, Bronchi, and Lungs
```

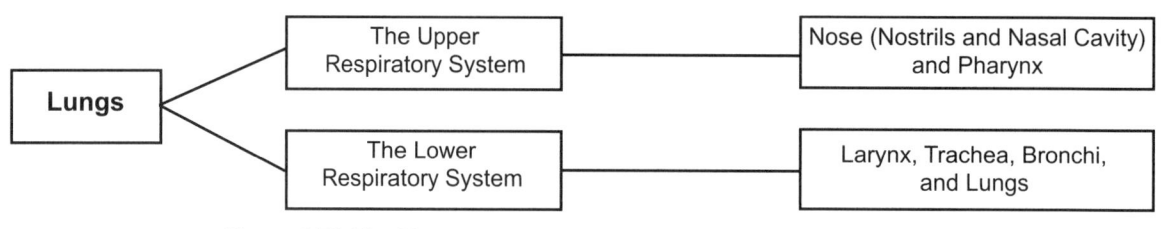

Figure 8.58. The Upper and Lower Respiratory Systems of the Lungs

sels, the esophagus, and the bronchi. The lungs have their base at the diaphragm, and extend upwards to their apex, which (for each lung) is located just above and deep to the clavicles. The lungs lie closely against the ribs along their lateral, anterior, and posterior surfaces.

The respiratory system can functionally be divided into two portions: the conducting portion, and the respiratory portion (Figure 8.56). The lungs communicate with the external atmosphere via the conducting portion of the respiratory system, which consists of the nose, pharynx, larynx, trachea, bronchi, and terminal bronchi (Figure 8.57). These interconnecting tubes and cavities serve to transport air to and from the respiratory portion, which is where the exchange of gases between the air and the blood takes place. The respiratory portion consists of the respiratory bronchi, alveolar ducts, and alveoli. Anatomically, the respiratory system is sometimes also divided into the Upper Respiratory System (nose and pharynx) and the Lower Respiratory System (larynx, trachea, bronchi, and lungs) (Figure 8.58).

The entire respiratory tract is covered with a thin layer of protective mucous that serves to keep the tissue moist, and to protect it from airborne particles such as dust and bacteria. This mucous contains numerous immune cells (i.e. macrophages and antibacterial enzymes). Pathogens are continuously being swept towards the pharynx (and eventually into the stomach) by the tiny hair-like cilia that line the respiratory passages. Common examples of this mucous movement are sniffling and the clearing of the throat.

THE UPPER RESPIRATORY SYSTEM

The upper respiratory system consists of the nose (nostrils and nasal cavity) and the pharynx, which is described as follows:

The Nose: Nostrils and Nasal Cavity

The external portion of the nose connects the nasal cavity to the external atmosphere, and includes the nasal Bones (the bridge of the nose), a supportive and semi-flexible structure of cartilage, and the soft tissue of the nostrils. The internal portion of the nose (also known as the sinuses) is a large cavity in the skull immediately superior to the mouth and inferior to the cranium.

The nasal cavity includes the entire area inside of the external and internal nose, and is divided into right and left sides by a midline nasal septum. The structure of the nasal cavity contains several shelf-like projections (conchae) that serve to create turbulence within the sinuses. The arrangement of these lateral shelves causes the inhaled air to twist and whirl, thus increasing the internal surface area exposed to the air. The tissues of the nasal cavity are richly supplied with blood vessels, and the exposed surface area is covered with countless tiny hairs and lined with olfactory and respiratory mucosa. As the incoming air is directed through the sinuses, nongaseous particles are filtered out by these tiny hairs and trapped in the mucous lining, the excess of which drains downward into the stomach. Every day the nasal cavity produces roughly a quart of this essential mucous.

The internal structure of the nose allows for three important functions:
- Filtering, moistening, and warming the incoming air
- Receiving olfactory stimuli (smell)
- Modifying speech sounds

The Pharynx

The pharynx, commonly called the throat, connects the nasal cavity and the mouth to the larynx.

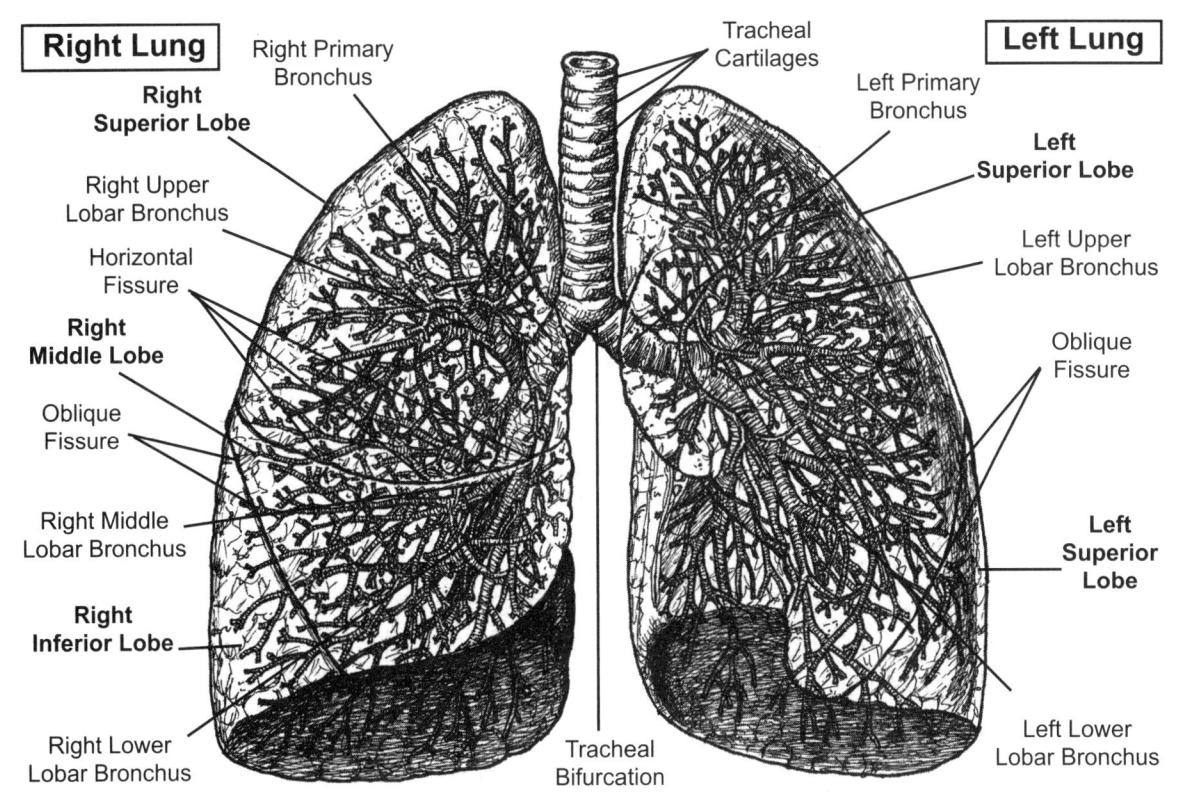

Figure 8.59. The Lung (Lu) Organ

The auditory (eustachian) tubes open from the lateral walls of the pharynx, and serve to equalize atmospheric pressure within the ear. Pairs of tonsils are located throughout the pharynx.

THE LOWER RESPIRATORY SYSTEM

The lower respiratory system consists of the larynx, trachea, bronchi, and lungs, described as follows:

The Larynx: Voice Box

The larynx, or voice box, connects the pharynx with the trachea and has two important functions. The first of these functions is accomplished by the epiglottis, a leaf-shaped flap of cartilage that serves to insure that only the passageway from the throat to the trachea or the passageway from the throat to the esophagus is open at any one time. The second important function of the larynx is voice production, involving the combined action of several pairs of cartilaginous vocal cords. Another cartilage formation within the larynx forms the externally visible "Adam's apple."

The Trachea: Windpipe

The trachea, or windpipe, is a tubular passageway that descends from the larynx. Its structure consists of numerous interconnected C-shaped rings of cartilage, providing a passageway that is both rigid and flexible. The posterior portion of the trachea lies immediately against the esophagus. The trachea ends within the mediastinum, where it splits into the two primary bronchi.

The Bronchi

The right and left primary bronchi are formed by the division of the trachea at the level of the sternum, and are the beginnings of the internal branch-like structures of the right and left lungs. This branching pattern of the lungs is known as the bronchial (or respiratory) tree, and can be effectively compared to the branching pattern of the vascular system.

THE LUNGS IN WESTERN MEDICINE

The external borders of the lungs are defined by the pleural membrane, which consists of two layers of serous (watery) membrane and the lubricated cavity between them (Figure 8.59). The outer membrane (parietal pleura) is attached to the wall of the thoracic cavity, while the inner layer (visceral pleura) covers the lungs themselves. The space between them is known as the pleural cavity, and is filled with a lubricating substance that decreases the friction between the parietal and visceral pleura as they slide against each other during the expansive and contractive phases of the breathing process. Thus it is the pleural membranes that allow the lungs to move freely within the thorax.

The two lungs differ slightly in both size and shape. The left lung is slightly smaller than the right, as there is a notch-like indentation on the medial aspect of the left lung that is molded to accommodate the heart. Because the diaphragm is higher on the right side (to accommodate the liver), the right lung is shorter than the left lung is. The right lung is also thicker and broader than the left lung, and it consists of three lobes, while the left lung has only two. Within each lung, these lobes are separated from each other by fissures.

Each lung receives a primary bronchus that further divides within the lung into secondary and tertiary bronchi, which themselves divide into bronchioles, terminal bronchioles (smaller), and respiratory bronchioles (microscopic). The respiratory bronchioles further subdivide into alveolar ducts, which lead directly into the alveoli, and alveolar sacs (two or more alveoli that share a common opening) where the bulk of gas exchange takes place (Figure 8.60).

Each lobe of the lungs receives a secondary bronchus and contains a number of pyramid-shaped structures called bronchopulmonary segments. There are ten bronchopulmonary segments in each lung, and each of these receives a single tertiary bronchus. Each of the bronchopulmonary segments has many smaller compartments, termed lobules, that are each fed by a branch from a terminal bronchiole. Each lobule is wrapped in a layer of elastic connective tissue, and also contains an arteriole, a venule, and a lymphatic vessel. It is within these lobules that the smallest bronchioles subdivide into alveolar ducts, which are themselves covered with the essential respiratory structures: the balloon-like alveoli. The alveoli serve to maximize the amount of surface area of the respiratory membrane that is exposed to the incoming air. The average adult has over 300 million alveoli, creating a total respiratory surface area of over 70 square meters.

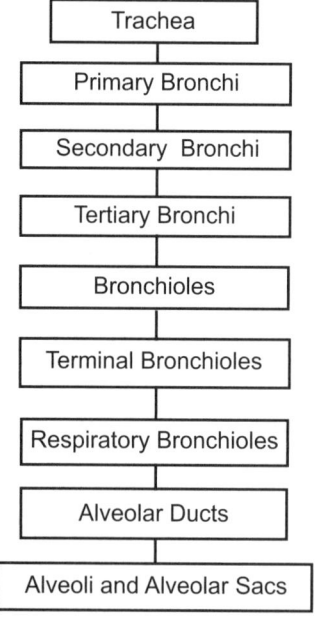

Figure 8.60. The Bronchial Tree

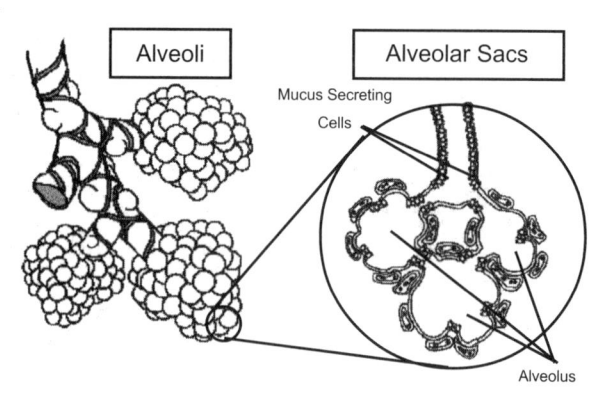

Figure 8.61. The Alveoli and Alveolar Sacs

The alveoli are densely clustered together into sacs which lie along the alveolar ducts, giving the appearance of bunches of grapes opening into a common chamber (Figure 8.61). The alveoli are separated from the capillaries by a very thin membrane known as the respiratory or alveolar-capillary membrane. This respiratory membrane is thin enough to allow for the exchange of oxygen (absorbed from the air by the red blood cells) and carbon dioxide (released by the red blood cells into the air within the alveoli) between the air-filled alveoli and the blood. Trace amounts of other gases and fine particles are also exchanged. Most of the alveoli perform this function of diffusing respiratory gases through the thin alveolar-capillary membrane that defines the border between them and the capillaries. However, a few alveoli (type II alveoli) have the function of secreting a liquid surfactant that prevents the collapse of the other alveoli.

Blood Supply to the Lungs

The lungs receive a double blood supply. One route brings blood into the lungs for the nourishment and maintenance of lung tissue, while another route brings deoxygenated blood into contact with the alveoli before sending it out to the rest of the body. The tissue of the lungs receives oxygenated blood from the bronchial arteries, while deoxygenated blood flows out primarily by way of the bronchial veins. Blood that is to be oxygenated by the lungs is pumped out from the right ventricle of the heart and is delivered by the pulmonary arteries, which accompany the primary bronchi into the lungs. The pulmonary arteries quickly branch out within each lung, eventually forming the pulmonary capillary networks that surround the alveoli. Oxygen-rich blood is then carried away from the lungs by the pulmonary veins, which lead to the left atrium of the heart. The left ventricle of the heart then pumps this fresh blood throughout the body.

Respiration

The primary purpose of respiration is to deliver oxygen to the cells and to remove carbon dioxide from them. The actual process of respiration can effectively be divided into three stages:

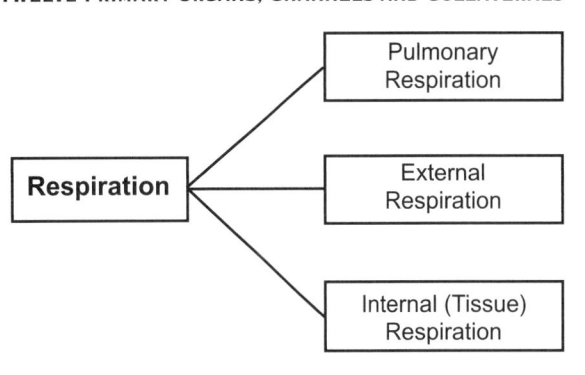

Figure 8.62. The Three Stages of Respiration

pulmonary ventilation, external (or pulmonary) respiration, and internal (or tissue) respiration. Both pulmonary respiration and tissue respiration are intimately connected with the distribution and content of the blood. The three stages of breathing are described as follows (Figure 8.62):

- **Pulmonary Respiration:** This is what is normally referred to as breathing, and consists of the inhalation and exhalation of air arising from the exchange of gases between the inside of the body and the external atmosphere.
- **External Respiration:** This refers to the diffusion of gases across the respiratory membrane. This involves both the oxygenation of the blood, and the diffusion of carbon dioxide (and trace amounts of other material) from the blood into the alveoli of the lungs.
- **Internal (Tissue) Respiration:** This is the exchange of gases between the blood and the cells that takes place throughout the body at the level of the capillaries. In addition to being dependent on the two previous stages of respiration, this last phase of respiration is completely reliant on the ability of the heart and blood vessels to deliver a continuous supply of fresh blood to all areas of the body.

Physiology of Respiration: Inhalation

In order for inhalation to occur, the lungs must expand. This is primarily caused by the contraction of the diaphragm in conjunction with the external intercostals, though numerous other muscles surrounding the rib cage (erector spinae, sternocleidomastoid, pectoralis minor, and scalenes) are involved to a lesser extent, particularly during abnormally deep or labored breathing. Of all the muscles involved in the breathing process, the diaphragm is the most important. The diaphragm is a dome shaped skeletal muscle that is attached to the inferior portions of the rib cage, thus separating the abdominal and thoracic cavities. The diaphragm exerts a downward pull on the pleural cavity as it contracts, while contraction of the external intercostals pulls the chest upwards and outwards. The resulting expansion of the thoracic cavity creates a negative internal pressure (relative to the atmospheric pressure outside the body) that causes air to flow in through the respiratory passages and fill the lungs.

PHYSIOLOGY OF RESPIRATION: EXHALATION

Normal exhalation is a passive process that takes place when the diaphragm and the muscles of the rib cage relax. The passive recoil action of the elastic connective tissues surrounding and supporting the rib cage, in conjunction with the elastic qualities of the lung tissue itself, creates a positive internal pressure (relative to the atmospheric pressure outside the body) while gently pulling the thoracic cavity inwards; this causes the lungs to expel air while contracting to return to their resting size. Forced exhalation (due to obstruction or labored breathing) requires an additional and active muscular contraction that further reduces the size of the thoracic cavity. This contraction involves the action of certain muscles around the ribs (primarily the internal intercostals) that contract to decrease the size of the rib cage, and also the action of various abdominal muscles (rectus abdominis, transverse abdominis, internal obliques, and external obliques) that compress the abdominal viscera and thus exert an upward force on the diaphragm as they contract.

DIAPHRAGMATIC AND COSTAL BREATHING

Diaphragmatic breathing, often called abdominal breathing, involves the near exclusive use of the diaphragm for the process of inhalation. This is almost always associated with the outward expansion of the abdomen that takes place as the diaphragm pushes downwards on the abdominal viscera during the process of inhalation. Costal breathing, also known as chest (or thoracic) breathing, refers to a breathing pattern that relies primarily on the contraction and release of various intercostals and other muscles surrounding the rib cage.

RESPIRATORY VOLUMES

The total amount of inhaled or exhaled air varies according to many different factors. In order to describe the capacities in different stages of respiration, several descriptive terms have been developed. About 500 ml of air enters and leaves the respiratory passages with each normal breath; this amount is known as the tidal volume. Nearly 150 ml of this air remains within anatomical dead space of the respiratory passages, leaving about 350 ml that actually reaches the alveoli. During deep breathing, the amount of inhaled air can be up to 3100 ml or more above the average tidal volume of 500 ml; this is known as the inspiratory reserve volume. Similarly, a forced exhalation can expel an average of 1200 ml more air than the 500 ml released during a passive exhalation; this amount of exhaled air is known as the expiratory reserve capacity. Even after a forced exhalation, an amount of air known as the residual volume, about 1200 ml on average, remains in the lungs to prevent lung collapse, and to insure that the alveoli stay slightly inflated.

RESPIRATORY CAPACITIES

The average healthy male has a total lung capacity of about 6 liters, while the capacity of the average female is slightly less due to her smaller size. Because of the differences in atmospheric pressure, an individual living at sea level will develop a relatively smaller total lung capacity then that of an individual living at a high altitude. As noted above, not all of this air can be exhaled at any one time. The vital capacity, about 4,800 ml, represents maximum amount of exchangeable air. Vital capacity decreases with age, and is decisively less in smokers than in nonsmokers. The inspiratory capacity, about 3,600 ml, refers to the amount of air that can be inhaled after a tidal inhalation. Similarly, the functional residual capacity, roughly 2,400 ml, refers to the amount of air remaining in the lungs after a tidal exhalation.

It is estimated that a normal adult breathes about 12 times a minute, 720 times per hour, 17,280 times per day. This translates as an average exchanged air volume (excluding the air held in the dead air space of the respiratory passages), known as the alveolar ventilation rate, of 4200 ml per minute, 252,000 ml (252 liters) per hour, and 6,048,000 ml (6,048 liters) per day. Rapid shallow breathing does little to increase the alveolar ventilation rate, because of the amount of inspired air that remains in the dead air space within the respiratory passages. Slow deep breathing, on the other hand, can drastically increase the amount of gaseous exchange within the lungs, as the amount of available air increases much further above the 150 ml of dead air space than occurs during tidal or shallow breathing.

The average content of the inhaled air is as follows (Figure 8.63): nitrogen - 78.6%, oxygen - 20.9%, carbon dioxide 0.04%, water - 0.46%. The atmosphere also contains trace amounts of other inert gases such as argon and helium. Exhaled air contains less oxygen (about 16%), and significantly more carbon dioxide (4.5%) and water vapor. About 200 ml of oxygen is diffused across the respiratory membrane and absorbed into the blood each minute.

Common Disorders of the Lungs and Respiratory System

Common disorders of the lungs include: rhinitis (inflammation of the mucous membrane of the nose), sinusitis (sinus infection), sore throat, laryngitis, coryza (common cold), influenza (flu), tuberculosis, cystic fibrosis, pulmonary embolism (the presence of a blood clot that obstructs pulmonary circulation), pulmonary edema (accumulation of interstitial fluid in and around the alveoli), pneumonia, pleurisy (inflammation of the pleura), pneumothorax (air in the plural cavity), hemothorax (blood in the pleural cavity), and atelectasis (collapsed lung). Diseases that involve some degree of obstruction of the air passages, such as asthma, diphtheria (enlarged respiratory mucous membranes), bronchitis, and emphysema (disintegration of the alveolar walls), come under the category of chronic obstructive pulmonary disease, or COPD.

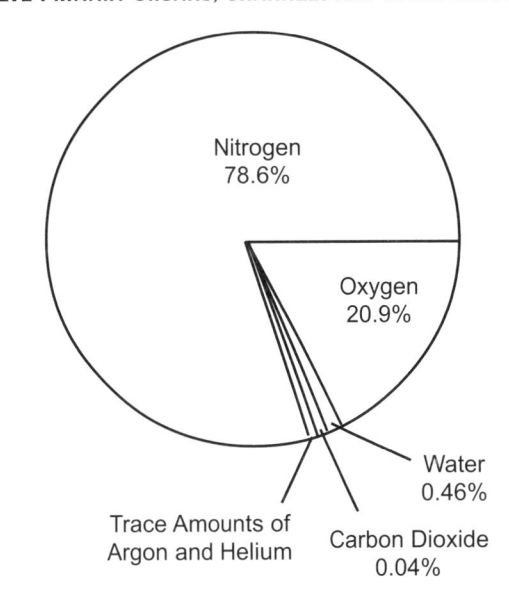

Figure 8.63. The Average Content of Inhaled Air

Disorders involving respiratory failure at the level of tissue respiration include various types of hypoxia, a condition in which there is a low level of oxygen available to the cells. The major classes of hypoxia are described as follows: hypoxic (or hypoxemic) hypoxia, in which there is a low relative pressure of oxygen in the arterial blood; anemic hypoxia, caused by hypofunction of hemoglobin; stagnant hypoxia, in which the blood is unable to deliver oxygen to the cells fast enough; and histionic hypoxia, in which the cells are unable to properly utilize the delivered oxygen. Elevated levels of carbon monoxide in the atmosphere can also lead to hypoxia, as even small amounts of inhaled carbon monoxide (as little as 1%) can drastically reduce the ability of hemoglobin to carry oxygen.

Apnea is a term used to describe the cessation of respiration (such as sleep apnea). Dyspnea refers to any condition in which breathing is painful or difficult, and tachypnea refers to rapid breathing. Respiratory distress syndrome, also called glassy lung disease, is a lung disease that affects newborns. Sudden infant death syndrome (SIDS) has also been linked to several respiratory disorders.

THE LARGE INTESTINE: DA CHANG

The Large Intestine is a tubular Yang organ, belongs to the Metal Element, and its associated Yin organ is the Lungs. The Large Intestine communicates with the skin and the anus, and is responsible for controlling the departure of the Po from the anus through the "Po Men" (Gate of the Po) after the time of death (Figure 8.64).

CHINESE CHARACTER FOR LARGE INTESTINE: DA CHANG

The Chinese character "Da Chang" translates as "Large Intestine." It refers to a general description of the image of the Large Intestine organ, and is composed of two images:
- The first character "Da" translates as "large," "great," or "big."
- The second character "Chang" translates as "Intestine," and is divided into two ideographs. The character to the left, "Ji" depicts the Chinese ideogram for body tissue, muscle or flesh (all of which are forms of connective tissue). The character on the right depicts the image of the sun above the horizon, with its rays shinning downward. It expresses the Heavenly Yang influence on this particular bowel. The ideograph expresses the image of the sun enriching and transforming something within the flesh and conveys the Large Intestines digestive process.

Together, the Chinese characters "Da Chang" can be translated as, "the large Heavenly transformation occurring within the flesh." The Large Intestines command the "Jin," the flowing intestinal fluids (Figure 8.65).

THE LARGE INTESTINE IN CHINESE MEDICINE

The functions of the Large Intestine described in Traditional Chinese Medicine are similar to those found in Western Medicine. However, some of the functions that are attributed to the Large Intestine in Western Medicine (such as controlling the transformation and transportation of food and fluids throughout the digestive system) are

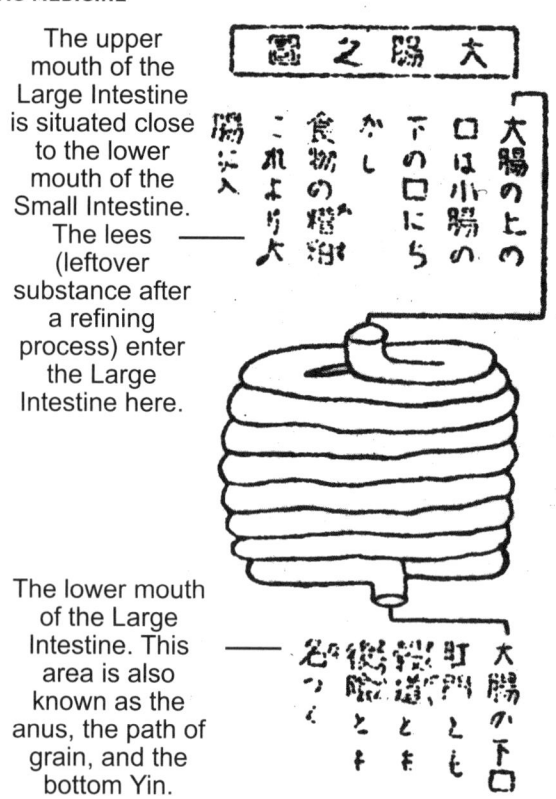

The upper mouth of the Large Intestine is situated close to the lower mouth of the Small Intestine. The lees (leftover substance after a refining process) enter the Large Intestine here.

The lower mouth of the Large Intestine. This area is also known as the anus, the path of grain, and the bottom Yin.

Figure 8.64. The ancient Chinese anatomical diagram of the Large Intestine (LI) Organ, as it appeared in "Important Useful Notes on Acupuncture and Moxibustion," published in Japan in 1718, by Masatoyo Hongo

Large

Muscle, Flesh, Connective Tissue

Sun Above the Horizon

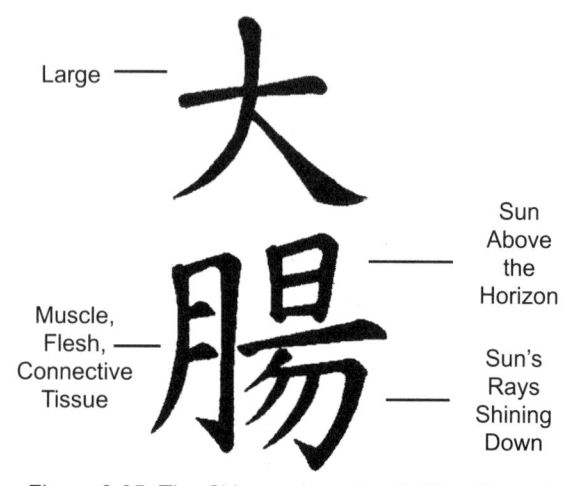

Sun's Rays Shining Down

Figure 8.65. The Chinese characters for "Da Chang," Large Intestine

```
                           ┌─ Governs Fluids
                           │
                           ├─ Controls Transformation ──── Reabsorbs Fluid from
                           │  and Transportation of       Indigestible Food
The Main                   │  Solid Waste
Functions                  │
of the      ───────────────┤                              Eliminates Indigestible
Large                      ├─ Controls Waste Removal ──── Food in the
Intestine                  │  and Defecation              Form of Semi-solid Feces
Organ and                  │
Channels                   ├─ Controls the Throat and
                           │  Lower Teeth
                           │
                           ├─ Controls Nasal Drainage
                           │                              Emotional Release
                           └─ Psycho-Emotional Aspects ── and
                                                          Introversion
```

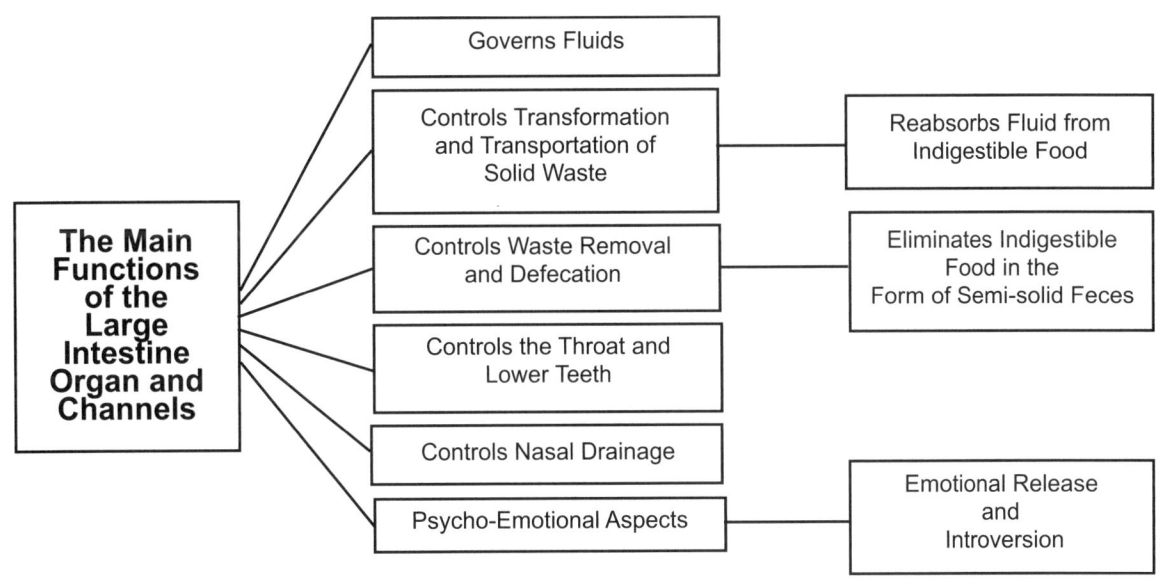

Figure 8.66. The Main Energetic Functions of the Large Intestine Organ and Channels

assigned to the Spleen from a Chinese medical perspective. In Chinese Medicine, the Large Intestine also has a number of psycho-emotional components which exert an influence on the body's functions.

According to Traditional Chinese Medicine, the main functions of the Large Intestine are to: govern fluids, control transformation and transportation of solid waste, control waste removal and defecation, control the throat and lower teeth, control nasal drainage, and express itself through the psycho-emotional aspects of emotional release and introversion (Figure 8.66). These functions are described as follows:

1. **Governs Fluids:** The Large Intestine organ is said to govern Body Fluids (any fluid or semi-fluid substance in the body). The Large Intestine reabsorbs the fluid from indigestible food and then eliminates waste from the body in the form of semi-solid feces.

2. **Controls Transformation and Transportation of Solid Waste:** The Large Intestine's main function is to receive the fluid form of food essence from the Small Intestine. After it absorbs this food essence, the Large Intestine is responsible for the transformation and transportation of solid waste in the body, absorbing water and eliminating the waste as fecal matter.

3. **Controls Waste Removal and Defecation:** The Lungs ability to send Qi downwards depends on the Large Intestine's role in excreting waste. Consequently, the descending Lung Qi supplies the Large Intestine with the necessary Qi needed for defecation.

4. **Controls the Throat and Lower Teeth:** The Large Intestine controls the throat and lower teeth.

5. **Controls Nasal Drainage:** The Large Intestine controls the drainage of the nose.

6. **Psycho-Emotional Aspects:** The Large Intestine is both energetically and physically associated with letting go of impurity. Emotional imbalances such as unhealthy attachments, or the inability to let go of past people, places and things often have their root in the Large Intestine. Because the Large Intestine is associated with the Lungs, it is equally affected by the emotions of sadness, grief, and worry. An energetic imbalance in the Large Intestine can result in physical weakness and provoke emotional introversion, accompanied by feelings of depression, irritability, discouragement, distress, and apathy. Strong emotions of fear or panic can produce an energetic

stool reflex reaction in the Large Intestine resulting in a spontaneous defecation.

THE LARGE INTESTINE CHANNELS

The Large Intestine Channels are Yang channels that flow externally from the hands to the head (Figure 8.67). The Large Intestine Channels originate externally from the tips of the index fingers, ascend the arms, and cross the shoulders, where they connect with the 7th cervical vertebra before splitting into two branches.

One set of branches (one branch from the left Lung and its corresponding branch from the right Lung) descends internally and spirally wraps the Lungs before flowing downwards to permeate the Large Intestine. The other two branches ascend externally through the neck and cheek to the gums of the lower teeth. Here each branch curves around the upper lip before flowing to the opposite side of the nose, to connect with the Stomach Channels.

CHANNELS' ENERGY FLOW

The Large Intestine Channels contain equally abundant amounts of both Qi and Blood. Thus the Large Intestine Channels influence the body's energetic and nervous functions, as well as affect the Blood and physical substances of the body.

At the high-tide time period (5 a.m. to 7 a.m.), Qi and Blood abound in the Large Intestine organ and Large Intestine channels. At this time, the Large Intestine organ and channels can more easily be dispersed and purged. During low tide (5 p.m. to 7 p.m.), they can be more readily tonified. The energy of the Large Intestine Channels acts on the skin, muscles, and nerves found along the channel pathways.

THE INFLUENCE OF CLIMATE

An External Cold, Damp Cold or Dry climate can interfere with the proper functioning of the Large Intestine. The Large Intestine requires a certain amount of moisture in order to function efficiently, and is therefore easily injured by Dryness. The Dry climate (generally active in the autumn time) can interfere with the functions of the Large Intestine.

THE INFLUENCE OF TASTE, COLOR, AND SOUND

- The pungent taste (garlic, green onions, etc.) can be used to tonify both the Large Intestine and Lungs, though excessive use can weaken them.
- The color of white is used to tonify the Large Intestine and Lungs.
- The "Shhh," "Sss," and "Shang" sounds are used to purge the Large Intestine and Lungs.

LARGE INTESTINE PATHOLOGY

Dysfunctions in the Large Intestine organ and channels can result in diseases of the lower part of the face (including the nose, oral cavity, and teeth), throat, and front part of the neck, as well as disease of the back and radial sides of the upper extremities.

Tonification of the Large Intestine can be used to eradicate eye pain, toothache, ear ache, to prevent hemorrhages, and to greatly reduce excessive menstrual bleeding.

Because of its relationship to the Lungs, the Large Intestine can be purged to treat coughing and asthma caused from excessive Heat in the Lungs. Similarly, replenishing the vital Qi of the Lungs can cure constipation in debilitated patients.

Patterns of energetic imbalances in the Large Intestine generally relate to disturbances in bowel movements. Energetic dysfunctions in the Large Intestine can be categorized as either excess or deficient conditions, described as follows:

1. **Excess conditions of the Large Intestines** can result in symptoms of: Heat, Heat obstruction, Damp Heat, or Cold invading the Large Intestine.
2. **Deficient conditions of the Large Intestines** can lead to an invasion of Cold or Dryness, and in severe cases of Deficiency, to the Collapse of the Large Intestine.

T.C.M. PATTERNS OF DISHARMONY

Patterns of disharmony associated with the Large Intestine are generally related to the conditions of the other internal organs of digestive system (Spleen, Stomach and Small Intestine). The most common Large Intestine disharmonies arise from deficient Qi of the Large Intestine, Damp

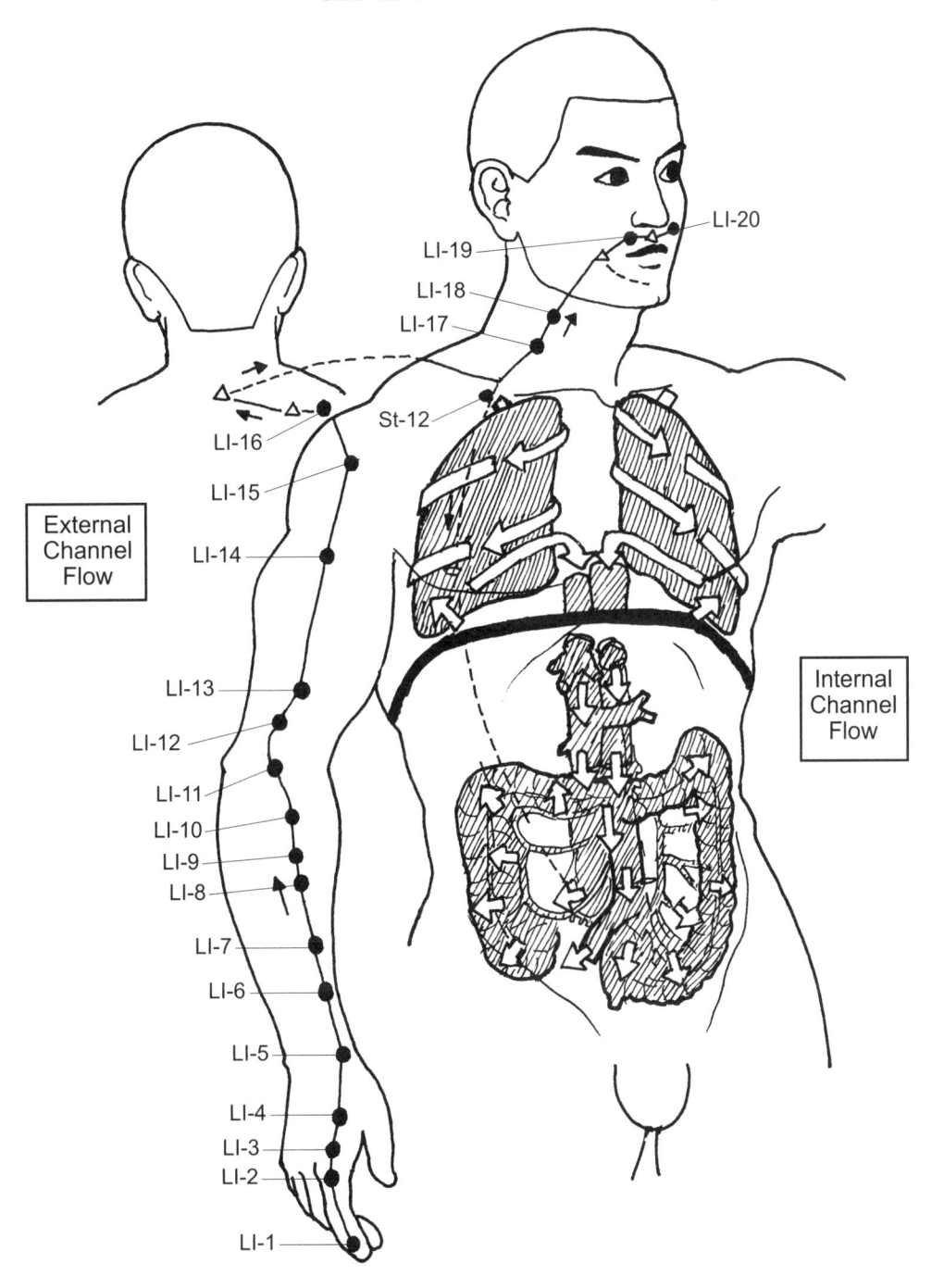

Figure 8.67. The Internal and External Qi Flow of the Large Intestine (LI) Channels

Large Intestine	Disharmony	Manifestations
	Deficient Qi of the Large Intestine (Deficient Spleen Yang)	This type of Large Intestine disharmony is often called Deficient Spleen Yang Disharmony
	Cold Damp in the Large Intestine	Sudden abdominal pain, painful diarrhea, a cold sensation in the abdomen, and a feeling of cold
	Damp Heat Invading the Large Intestine	Fever, sweating, a heavy feeling in the body and limbs, abdominal pain, diarrhea with mucus and blood in the stools, smelly stool, and burning in the anus
	Exhausted Fluid of the Large Intestine	Constipation, dry stool, burning and swelling in the anus, abdominal distention, high fever, sweating (especially on the limbs), thirst, and delirium
	Intestinal Abscess	Sharp pain in the lower right abdominal area and possible fever

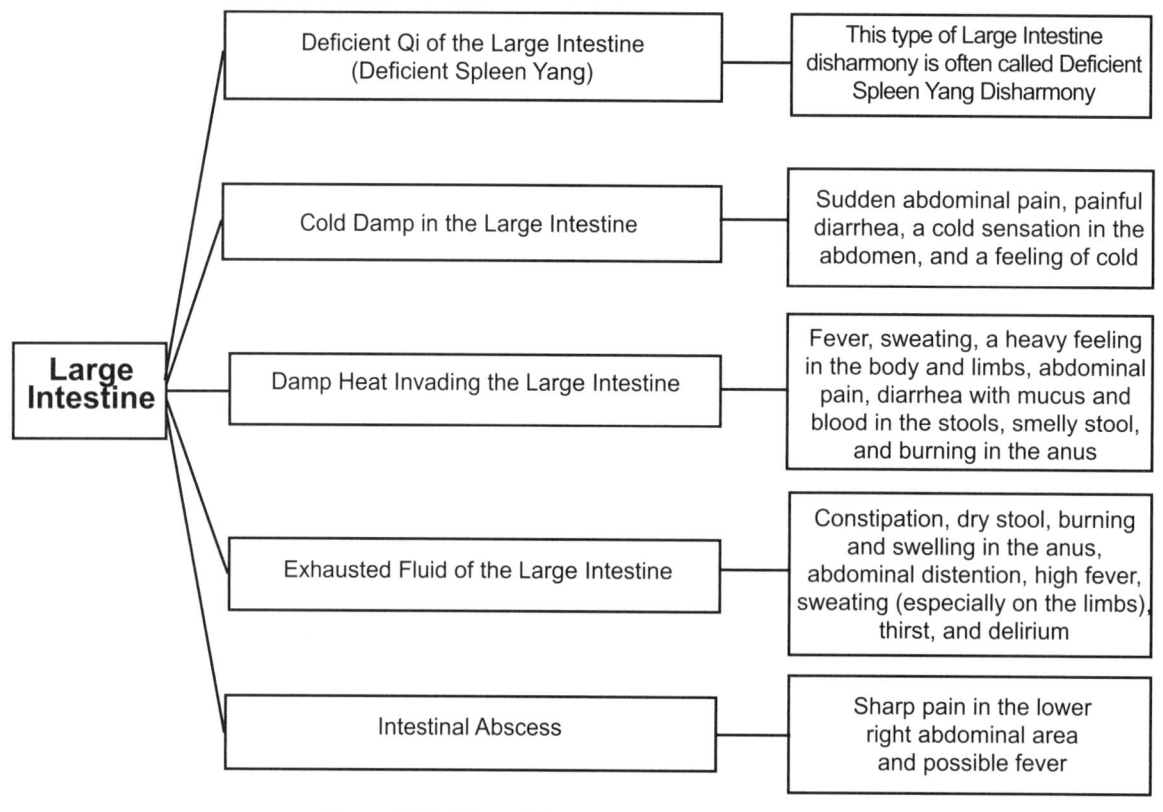

Figure 8.68. Chart of Large Intestine Disharmonies

Cold in the Large Intestine, Damp Heat Invading the Large Intestine, Exhausted Fluid of the Large Intestine and Intestinal Abscess, described as follows (Figure 8.68):

1. **Deficient Qi of the Large Intestine:** This type of Large Intestine disharmony is often called Deficient Spleen Yang Disharmony.

2. **Damp Cold in the Large Intestine:** This type of Large Intestine disharmony often occurs in conjunction with invasion of the Spleen by Cold and Damp. Cold invading the Large Intestine is considered to be an excess pattern, and its clinical manifestations include sudden abdominal pain, painful diarrhea, a cold sensation in the abdomen, and a feeling of cold.

3. **Damp Heat Invading the Large Intestine:** This type of Large Intestine disharmony is often associated with Damp Heat accumulating in the Spleen. Damp Heat invading the Large Intestine is considered to be an excess pattern. Its clinical manifestations include fever, sweating, a heavy feeling in the body and limbs, abdominal pain, diarrhea with mucus, blood in the stool, smelly stool, and burning around the anus.

4. **Exhausted Fluid of the Large Intestine:** This type of disharmony occurs when Heat within the Large Intestine consumes the fluids necessary for the organ to function properly. This can result in constipation, dry stool, burning and swelling in the anus, abdominal distention, high fever, sweating (especially on the limbs), thirst, and delirium.

5. **Intestinal Abscess:** This type of Large Intestine disharmony is similar to the Western syndrome of acute appendicitis. It can originate from irregular (or otherwise unhealthy) eating habits, excess physical activity too soon after eating, or an imbalance of Cold and Heat in the abdomen (affecting the Spleen and Stomach's abil-

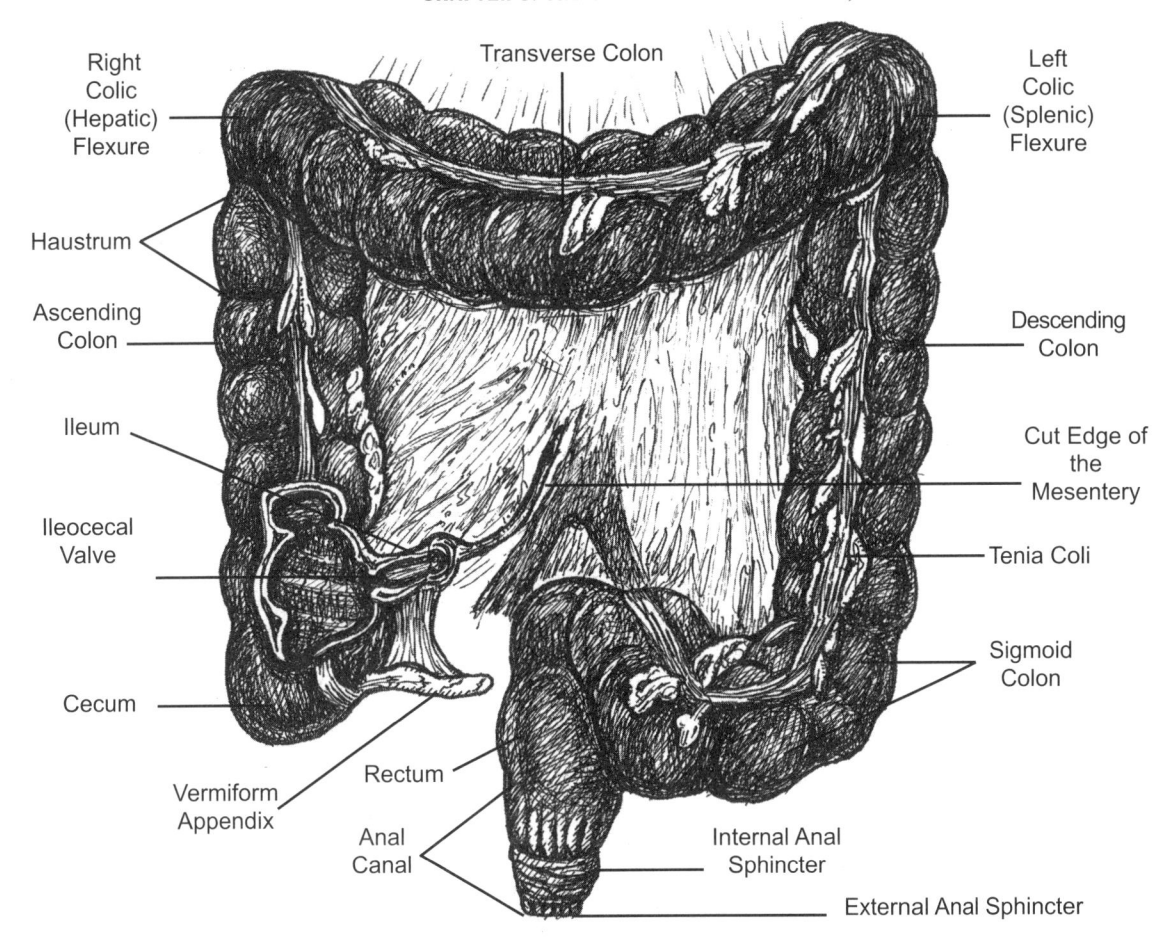

Figure 8.69. The Large Intestine (LI) Organ (Inspired by the original artwork of Dr. Frank H. Netter).

ity to transform and transport). Symptoms include sharp pain in the lower right abdominal area and possible fever.

The Large Intestine in Western Medicine

Situated in the lower abdomen, the large intestine is a tubular organ about 5 feet in length that comprises the terminal portion of the gastrointestinal tract. It has the name large intestine due to the fact that it has a greater diameter (2.5 inches) than that of the small intestine (one inch), while the small intestine actually has a greater length (approximately 21 feet). The large intestine is attached to the posterior abdominal wall by its mesocolon of visceral peritoneum.

The walls of the large intestine are also structurally different from the walls of the small intestine, corresponding to the differing functions of each organ. The large intestine stretches from its connection with the small intestine (at the ileocecal valve) to the anus, and is shaped roughly like an upside-down "U". The large intestine can be structurally divided into four parts: the cecum, the colon (ascending, transverse, descending, and sigmoid), the rectum, and the anal canal. These four sections are described as follows (Figure 8.69):

1. **Cecum:** The cecum is a small pouch about 2.5 inches in length, and is the first part of the large intestine to receive chyme (via the ileocecal valve) from the small intestine. The ileocecal valve (also called the ileocecal sphinc-

ter) is a small fold of mucous membrane that acts as a valve between the ileum of the small intestine and the cecum of the large intestine. The vermiform appendix, a small convoluted tube about three inches in length, is attached at the medial portion of the cecum and extends roughly in the direction of the rectum.

2. **Colon:** The colon makes up the majority of the large intestine, and is itself divided into four parts: the ascending colon, the transverse colon, the descending colon, and the sigmoid colon. The colon weaves itself through several layers of the abdomen, though not all of the colon is situated behind the peritoneum. It is anchored to the walls of the abdominal cavity by sheet-like layers of connective tissue called mesentery colons.

- **The ascending colon** is attached to the open end of the cecum and extends upwards on the right side of the abdomen. At about the height of the under-surface of the liver, the colon turns abruptly, forming the right colic (hepatic) flexure that marks the end of the ascending colon and the beginning of the transverse colon.
- **The transverse colon** begins at the right colic flexure and extends horizontally across the abdomen towards the left. Near the lower left end of the spleen, there is another acute turn in the colon, known as the left colic (splenic) flexure. This marks the end of the transverse colon and the beginning of the descending colon.
- **The descending colon** begins at the left colic flexure and extends downwards along the left side of the abdomen. Upon entering the pelvis, the descending colon becomes the S-shaped sigmoid colon.
- **The sigmoid colon** begins near the iliac crest of the pelvis, extends inwards towards the midline, then joins the rectum at the level of the third sacral vertebrae.

3. **Rectum:** The rectum, roughly eight inches in length, is the next to last portion of the gastrointestinal tract. Situated anterior to the sacrum and coccyx, the rectum extends downwards from the sigmoid colon to join the anal canal. The rectum has three transverse folds, called rectal valves, that serve to separate feces from flatus. The nature of the location of the rectum allows for a number of lower-abdominal organs to be examined digitally through its anterior wall.

4. **Anal Canal:** The anal canal forms the last inch of the gastrointestinal tract. The anal canal contains an internal sphincter (involuntary - composed of smooth muscle) and an external sphincter (voluntary - composed of skeletal muscle); these lie between the rectum and the anus and control the expulsion or retention of feces. Within the anal canal are longitudinal fold of mucous membrane (anal columns) that contain a number of arteries and veins. It is these veins and the rectal veins that can, when put under excessive pressure, overstretch and cause the condition known as hemorrhoids or piles.

Physiology

The primary functions of the large intestine can be divided into the following four basic categories (Figure 8.70): completion of the digestive process, manufacture and absorption of certain nutrients, formation of feces, and the expulsion of feces.

By the time the chyme reaches the large intestine, most of the available water and nutrients have already been absorbed into the bloodstream. Though the large intestine possesses no villi to enable any large scale absorption of nutrients, it plays and important role in maintaining the bodies water balance, absorbing all but 100 to 200 ml of the liter or so of water that it receives. It also absorbs small but essential amounts of various electrolytes. The resident bacteria within the large intestine serve to complete the process of digestion by fermenting and breaking down the proteins and carbohydrates that are still present within the chyme. Once the bacteria have completed the process of breaking down the chyme, the undigested material is now known as feces.

The process of fermenting carbohydrates releases hydrogen, carbon dioxide, and methane gas; while the proteins are broken down and con-

```
                    Large Intestine
                    ┌──→ Completion of Food Digestion
                    ├──→ Manufacture and Absorption of Certain Nutrients
                    │       (a function of the intestinal bacteria)
                    ├──→ Formation of Feces
                    └──→ Expulsion of Feces
```

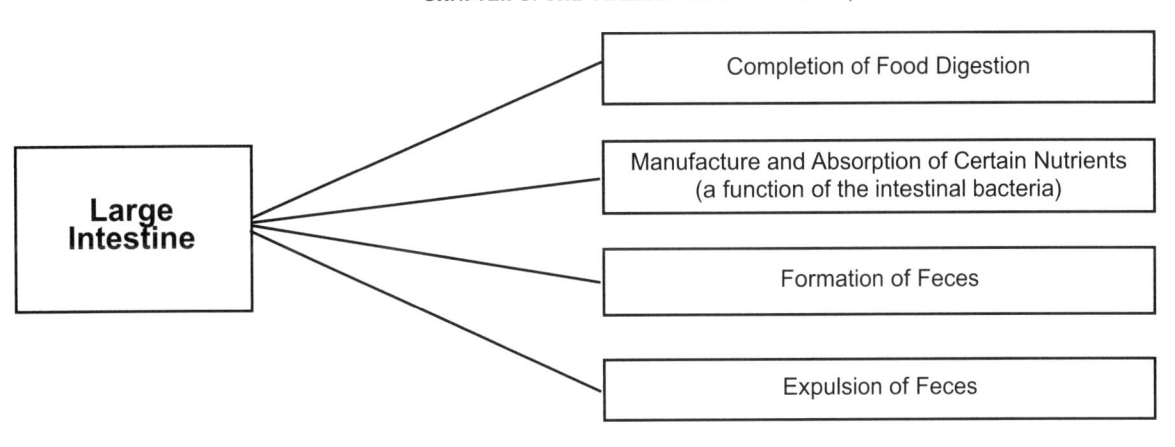

Figure 8.70. The Functions of the Large Intestine (Western Medical Perspective)

verted into amino acids and their fatty acid components. Protein fermentation in the large intestine also releases indole and skatole, which contribute to the odor of the feces. Bacteria also decompose the bilirubin released by the liver, giving feces their characteristic brown color. Several vitamins (e.g., vitamin K and some B vitamins) are also created as bacterial by-products, and are absorbed into the body through the colon. Depending on the composition of the chyme, the bacteria in the large intestine may also release large or small amounts of toxic materials; once absorbed into the body, these are generally converted into less toxic substances by the liver and then released in the form of urine.

The large intestine has a thick layer of mucosa to ease the passage of feces towards the end of the digestive tract. This thick mucous layer also protects the walls of the large intestine from the irritating acids and gases produced by the resident bacteria. A gastrocolic reflex, initiated by introduction of food into the stomach, causes peristaltic waves in the large intestine. While feces travels along the colon by peristaltic contractions it is also churned about by haustral churning, in which alternate sides (haustra) of the large intestine expand and contract. Mass peristalsis, which begins at the middle of the transverse colon, pushes feces downwards and into the rectum. When the rectal wall is adequately distended, stretch receptors then initiate a reflex for defecation; in defecation, the rectum is emptied through a combined contraction of the diaphragm, abdominal muscles, and increased peristalsis in the other portions of the colon. If defecation is postponed, due to the voluntary contraction of the external anal sphincter, the feces backs up into the sigmoid colon. Upon the next wave of peristaltic contractions, the intensity of the defecation reflex increases.

THE STOMACH: WEI

The Stomach's associated Yin organ is the Spleen, and its Element is Earth. The Stomach is considered to be the origin of the Body's Fluids. The Stomach and the Spleen are the primary organs through which the body acquires Postnatal Qi. These organs are often called the "Ministers of Food Storage" (Figure 8.71).

CHINESE CHARACTER FOR THE STOMACH: WEI

The Chinese character "Wei" translates as "Stomach." It refers to the image of the Stomach organ, and is divided into two sections. The character on the top "Tian," represents a field or farmland. The character on the bottom, "Ji" depicts the Chinese ideogram for body tissue, muscle or flesh (all of which are forms of connective tissue). Together, both ideographs express the idea that the Stomach organ is responsible for the harvesting of the "grains and liquids" (Figure 8.72).

THE STOMACH IN CHINESE MEDICINE

The functions of the Stomach described in Traditional Chinese Medicine are similar to those that are described in Western Medicine, except that in Traditional Chinese Medicine the Stomach is also responsible for certain psycho-emotional aspects.

According to Traditional Chinese Medicine, the main functions of the Stomach are to: control the ripening and rotting of food, control the transportation of food essence, control the descending of Qi, create the Body's Fluids, and express itself through the psycho-emotional aspects of influencing mental states. These main functions are described as follows (Figure 8.73).

1. **Controls the Rotting and Ripening of Food:** The Stomach's main function is to receive and decompose food. It receives the ingested food, churns and ferments (rots) it into a "ripe" absorbable liquid, reduces it into chyme by the fermenting and grinding action. The Stomach then separates the "clean" ("pure"), usable portion of the food from the "turbid" ("impure") portion. It then transfers the clean portion to the Spleen (where the food essence is absorbed into the body), while sending the turbid portion to the Small Intestine to be further refined.

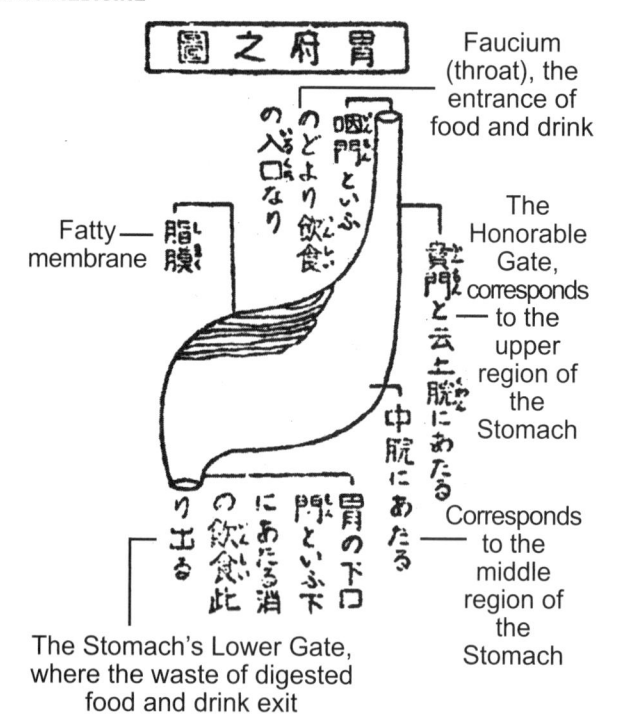

Figure 8.71. The ancient Chinese anatomical diagram of the Stomach (St) Organ, as it appeared in "Important Useful Notes on Acupuncture and Moxibustion," published in Japan in 1718, by Masatoyo Hongo

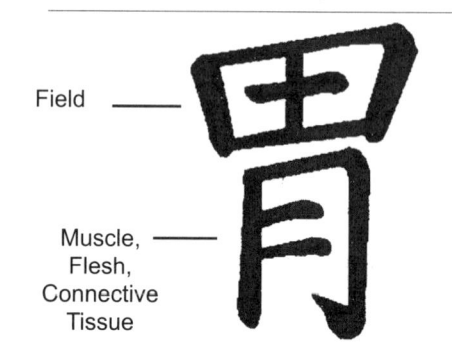

Figure 8.72. The Chinese character for "Wei," Stomach

2. **Controls the Transportation of Food Essence:** The Stomach ensures the smooth flow of Qi in the Middle Burner. Together with the Spleen, the Stomach is responsible for the transportation of food essences throughout the body.

3. **Controls the Descending of Qi:** The Stomach

```
The Main                 ┌─ Controls the Ripening and ─┬─ Creates Chyme by Fermenting and Grinding Action
Functions                │   Rotting of Food           └─ Separates "Clean" and "Turbid"
of the       ────────────┤
Stomach                  ├─ Controls the Transportation of Food Essence
Organ                    │
and                      ├─ Controls the Descending ───┬─ Ensures Smooth Flow of Qi in Middle Burner
Channels                 │   of Qi                     └─ Downward Action of Stomach Qi Aids in Digestion
                         │
                         ├─ Creates the Body's Fluids
                         │
                         └─ Psycho-Emotional Aspects ──── Influence the Mental State
```

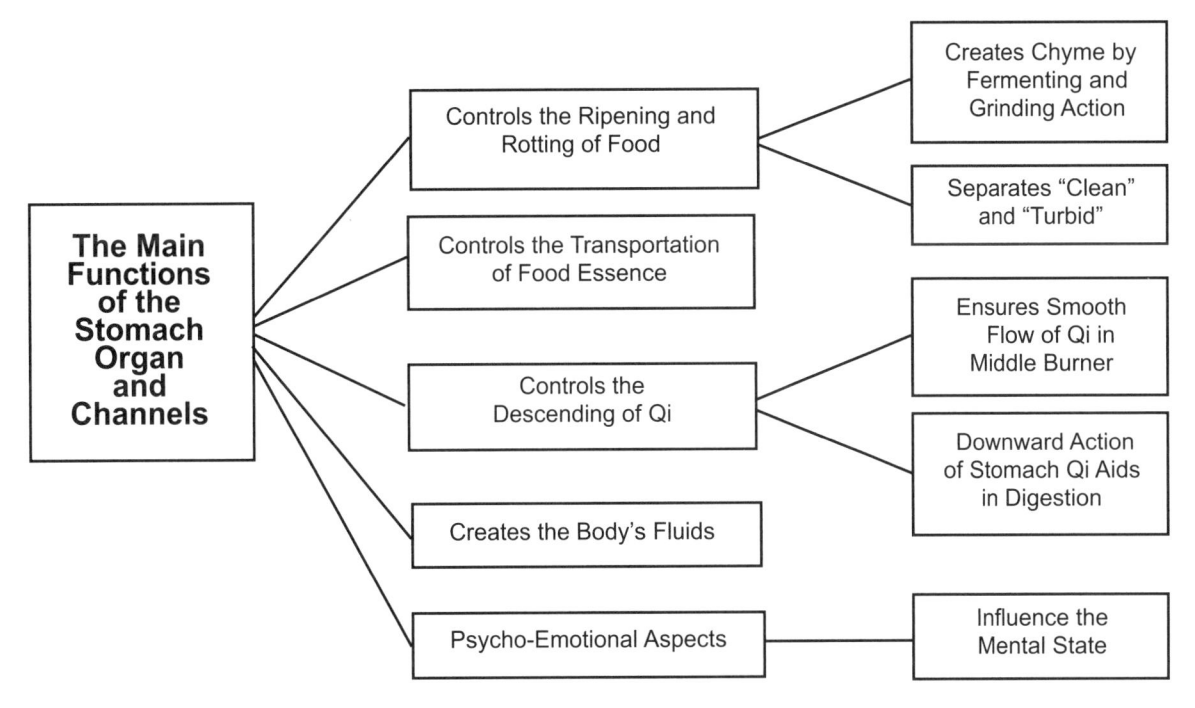

Figure 8.73. The Main Energetic Functions of the Stomach Organ and Channels

sends Qi downward, while the Spleen (its paired organ) sends "clean" Qi upward. The downward action of the Stomach Qi aids in digestion.

4. **Creates the Body's Fluids:** The Stomach requires a considerable amount of fluids in order to rotten and ripen the ingested food. To create adequate fluids for this function, the Stomach ensures that a part of the ingested food and drink does not go to make food essence, but is condensed to form Body Fluids. The Stomach is closely related to the Kidneys in its role of being the origin of the Body Fluids. The Kidneys are sometimes called the "Gate of the Stomach," because they transform the Body Fluids (which have their origin in the Stomach) in the Lower Burner.

5. **Psycho-Emotional Aspects:** The Stomach also has an influence on the mental state. Stomach Fire or Stomach Phlegm Fire can cause emotional symptoms such as manic behavior, mental confusion, severe anxiety, insomnia, and hyperactivity.

THE STOMACH CHANNELS

The Stomach Channels are Yang channels and flow externally from the head to the feet (Figure 8.74). The two Stomach Channels originate externally from the lateral sides of the nose (LI-20), ascending upward to the base of the eye and the bridge of the nose where they communicate with the Urinary Bladder Channels (UB-1). From the bridge of the nose, they then descend beneath the eyes, down the face, along the angle of the mandible (jaw), and then ascend in front of the ears, following the anterior hairline until they reach the forehead. From the St-5 point (at the curve of the jaw), the external branches on each side descend the neck and torso. These branches continue to flow externally down the torso and legs to end at the lateral sides of the second toes. Internal branches separate from the St-12 points and penetrates the Stomach before spiral wrapping the Spleen and joining the primary channel branches at the St-30 points.

VOLUME 1, SECTION 1: FOUNDATIONS OF CHINESE ENERGETIC MEDICINE

A set of branches separates from the St-12 points, then descends internally to penetrates the Stomach and spirally wrap the Spleen, before rejoining the primary channel branches at the St-30 points

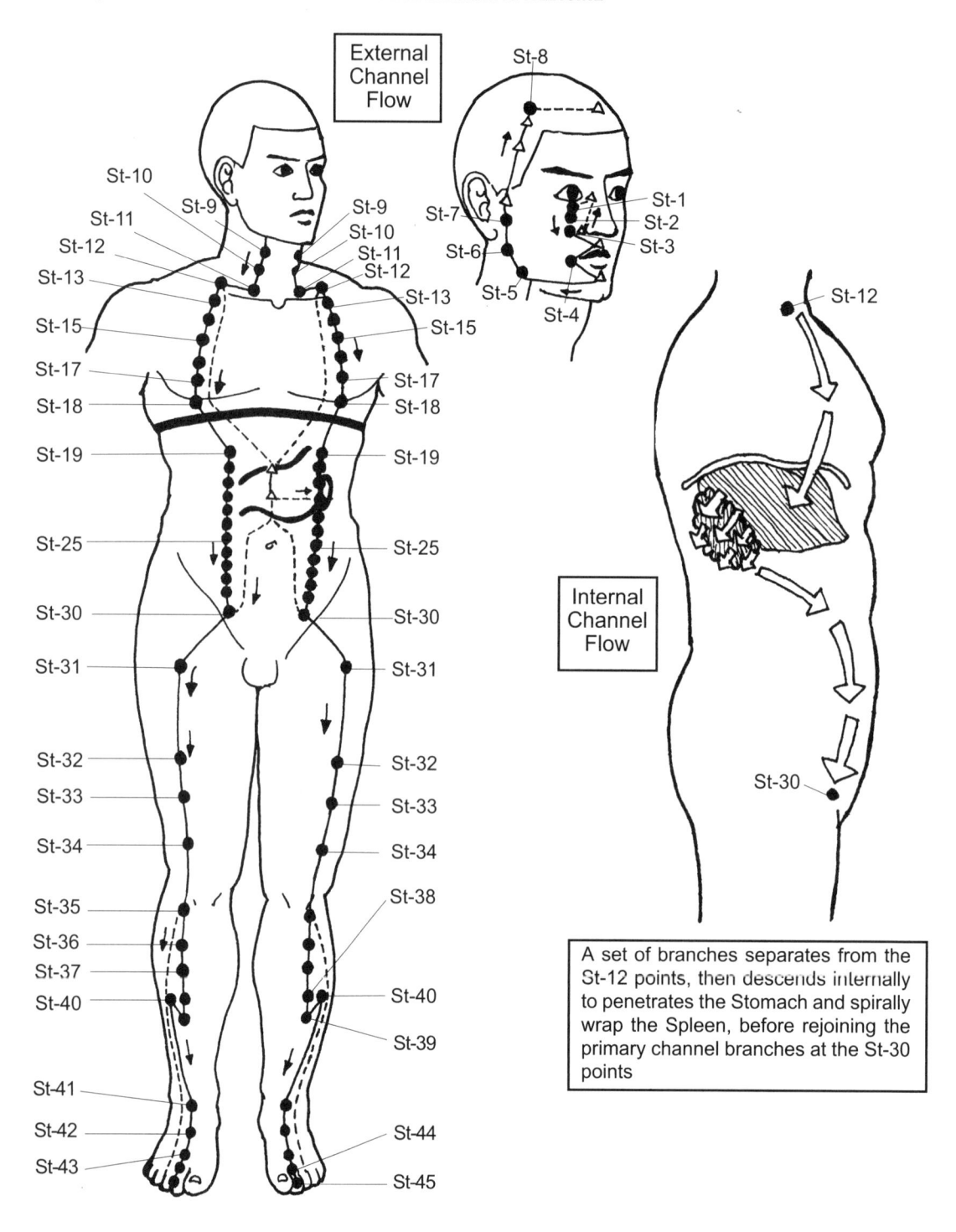

Figure 8.74. The Internal and External Qi Flow of the Stomach (St) Channels

374

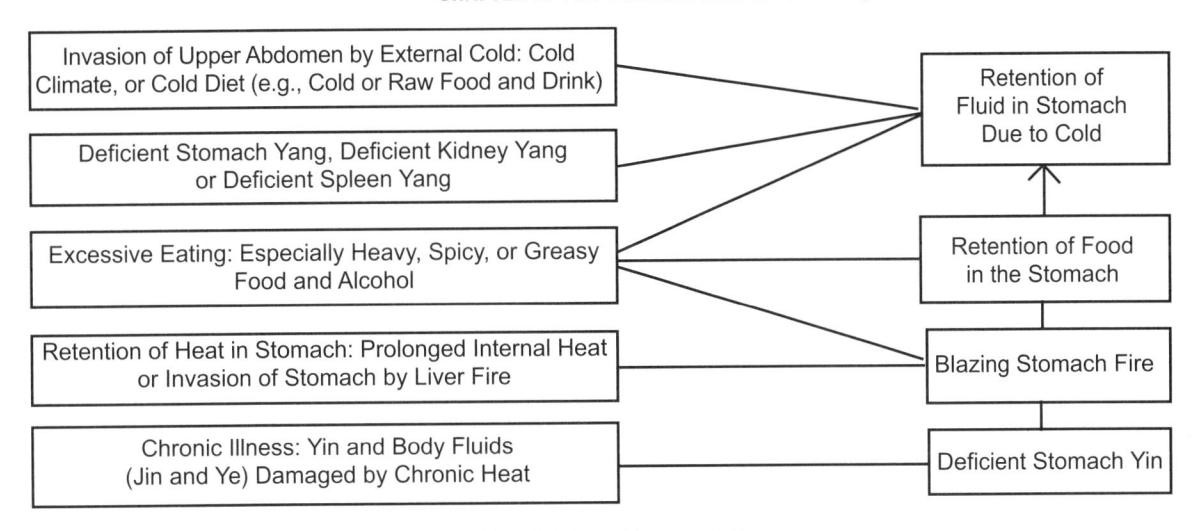

Figure 8.75. The Origins of Stomach Disharmony

Cause	Result
Invasion of Upper Abdomen by External Cold: Cold Climate, or Cold Diet (e.g., Cold or Raw Food and Drink)	Retention of Fluid in Stomach Due to Cold
Deficient Stomach Yang, Deficient Kidney Yang or Deficient Spleen Yang	Retention of Fluid in Stomach Due to Cold
Excessive Eating: Especially Heavy, Spicy, or Greasy Food and Alcohol	Retention of Food in the Stomach / Retention of Fluid in Stomach Due to Cold
Retention of Heat in Stomach: Prolonged Internal Heat or Invasion of Stomach by Liver Fire	Blazing Stomach Fire
Chronic Illness: Yin and Body Fluids (Jin and Ye) Damaged by Chronic Heat	Deficient Stomach Yin

Channels' Energy Flow

The Stomach Channels contain equally abundant amounts of both Qi and Blood, acting equally on the body's energetic and nervous functions, as well as on physical substances.

At the high-tide time period (7 a.m. to 9 a.m.), Qi and Blood abound in the Stomach organ and Stomach channels. At this time period the Stomach organ and channels can more easily be dispersed or purged. During low tide (7 p.m. to 9 p.m.), they can be more readily tonified. The Stomach Channels' energy acts on the skin, muscles, and nerves found along their pathways.

The Influence of Climate

An external Cold climate can interfere with the functions of the Stomach. The Stomach needs a certain amount of moisture to function, it is easily injured by Cold and Dryness

The Influence of Taste, Color, and Sound

- The taste of sweet can be used to tonify both the Stomach and Spleen
- The color of light yellow/light brown is used to tonify the Stomach
- The "Who" and "Dong" sounds are used to purge the Stomach

Stomach Pathology

Diseases of the Stomach organ and channels include diseases of the face (nose, oral cavity, and teeth), throat, front of the neck, the abdomen, the frontal part of the legs and gastrointestinal area (Figure 8.75).

The Stomach has the function of sending the semi-digested food downward. An impairment of this function often causes vomiting.

Diseases of the Stomach organ are primarily caused by improper diet. To determine the root of a Stomach imbalance, the following five areas are considered:

1. The patient's Five Element constitution and present state of health.
2. The type and energetic quality of the foods ingested (Hot or Cold), and whether the food is in season or out of season.
3. The scheduling of meals. This includes eating meals at regular times, eating balanced meals, allowing adequate time for eating (not eating fast), and not eating too late at night.
4. The Yin and Yang balance of the types of food digested. This includes evaluating the foods eaten in terms of Yin and Yang, the Five Tastes, and the Five Colors.
5. The emotional factors surrounding meal time. This includes avoiding emotional distresses

Stomach

- **Retention of Fluid in the Stomach Due to Cold** — Coldness and pain in the epigastric region, vomiting after eating, and the absence of thirst
- **Retention of Food in the Stomach** — Distention and pain in the epigastric region, loss of appetite, belching or regurgitation, foul stool with diarrhea, or constipation
- **Deficient Stomach Yin** — Lack of appetite, dry-heaves, dry lips and mouth, and constipation
- **Blazing Stomach Fire** — Burning in the epigastrium, thirst with a preference for cold drinks, vomiting of sour fluid or undigested food, foul breath, constipation and pain, ulceration, and bleeding of the gums

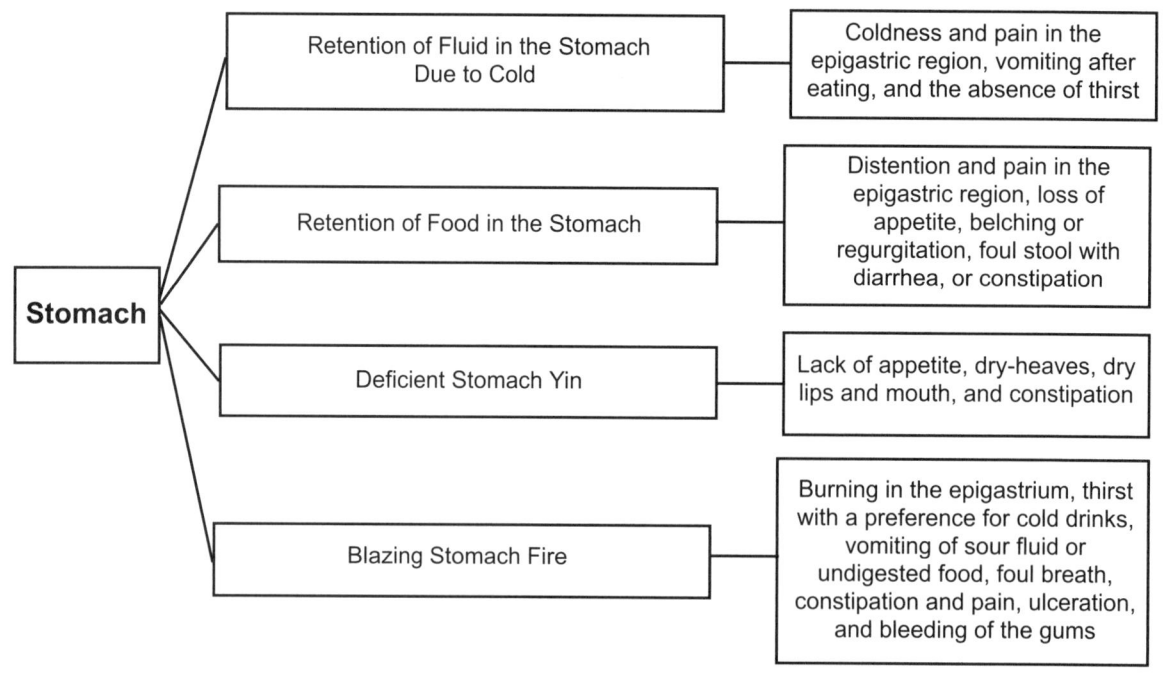

Figure 8.76. Chart of Stomach Disharmonies

(feeling rushed, upset, etc.), and having the proper mental attitude (being relaxed and calm).

The Stomach easily suffers from excess patterns (e.g., Fire or Phlegm Fire), which in turn can agitate the Shen. Due to the Stomach's association with the psycho-emotional states of worry and excessive thinking, Stomach disharmonies can often play a primary or supporting factor in numerous emotional or psychological disorders. When the Shen is disturbed, it can cause manic symptoms such as inappropriate laughter, violent or otherwise inappropriate behavior (e.g., taking off one's clothes in public), pressured speech, unconscious talking, laughing or singing. In milder cases, symptoms may include mental confusion, severe anxiety, obsessive-compulsive thinking, hyperactivity, and hypomania (a milder form of mania).

T.C.M. Patterns of Disharmony

Patterns of disharmony associated with the Stomach generally originate from: Retention of Fluid in the Stomach Due to Cold, Retention of Food in the Stomach, Deficient Stomach Yin and Blazing Stomach Fire, described as follows (Figure 8.76):

1. **Retention of Fluid in the Stomach Due to Cold:** When the Stomach's Yang Qi becomes deficient, it is prone to the accumulation of Cold and Damp. The accumulation of Cold in the Stomach can result in symptoms such as coldness and pain in the epigastric region, vomiting after eating, and the absence of thirst.

2. **Retention of Food in the Stomach:** If the Stomach's functions of receiving, storing and digesting food becomes compromised due to retention of food, the Stomach Qi becomes impaired. This can result in distention and pain in the epigastric region and a loss of appetite. As the retained food begins to rot, the Stomach Qi rebels resulting in belching or regurgitation, foul smelling stool with diarrhea, or constipation.

3. **Deficient Stomach Yin:** When the Stomach's Yin Qi becomes deficient, it is prone to patterns of Dryness and Heat. The reduction of Body Fluids in the Stomach due to Dryness

Figure 8.77. The Stomach (St) Organ

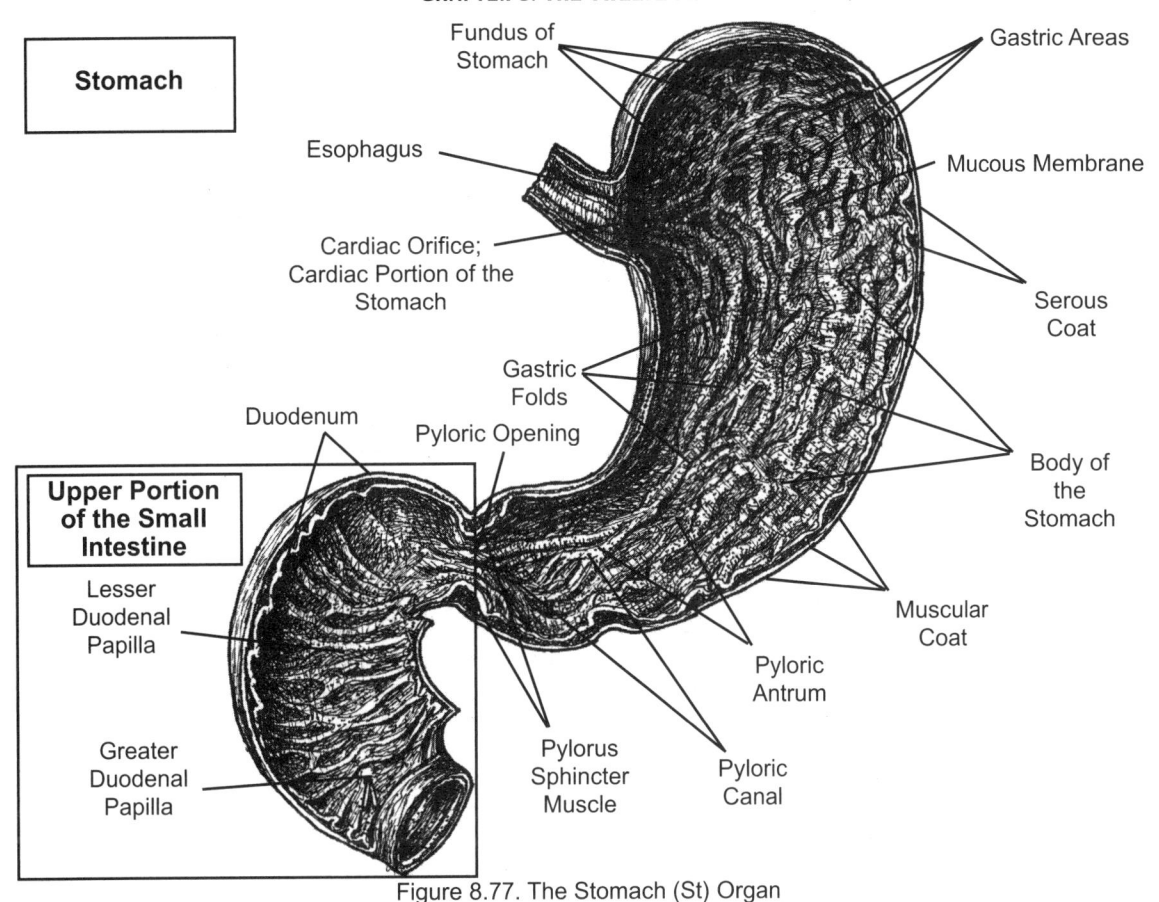

and Heat can cause symptoms such as lack of appetite, dry-heaves, dry lips and mouth, and constipation.

4. **Blazing Stomach Fire:** Excessive Internal Heat generated from the Fire in the Stomach can create symptoms such as burning in the epigastrium, thirst with a preference for cold drinks, vomiting of sour fluid or undigested food, foul breath, constipation, Stomach pain, ulceration, and bleeding of the gums.

THE STOMACH IN WESTERN MEDICINE

The stomach is a "J" shaped organ located under the diaphragm in the epigastric, umbilical, and left hypochondriac regions of the abdominal cavity. Its upper opening connects to the esophagus, while its lower opening is at the pylorus, which connects to the duodenum of the small intestine (Figure 8.77).

The adult stomach is approximately 10 inches long. However, the size and position of the stomach constantly changes, depending on the amount of food (chyme) present in the stomach at any given time. When the stomach is empty, the mucosa and submucosa lie in large, longitudinal folds called rugae. When filled with food, the rugae of the stomach unfold, increasing its holding capacity.

The diaphragm pushes the stomach downward during each inhalation; during exhalation, the stomach is pulled upwards. The concave medial border of the stomach is called the lesser curvature, while the convex lateral border is called the greater curvature. The stomach can be divided into four main areas: cardia, fundus, body, and pylorus, described as follows.

1. **Cardia:** This part of the stomach surrounds the superior opening of the stomach organ (the cardiac orifice), through which food from

the esophagus enters the stomach. Several minutes after food enters the stomach, rippling peristaltic movements known as mixing waves begin to pass over the stomach every 15 to 25 seconds. These mixing waves blend the food with the secretions of the gastric glands, dissolving it into a thin creamy liquid paste called chyme.

2. **Fundus:** The rounded dome-shaped portion of the stomach, located above and to the left of the cardia is called the fundus. The fundus is the storage area for food. When necessary food can remain in the fundus for over an hour without becoming mixed with gastric juice.

3. **Body:** Below the fundus is the large central portion of the stomach called the body of the stomach. During digestion, more vigorous mixing waves begin at the body of the stomach and intensify as they reach the pylorus.

4. **Pylorus:** At the inferior region of the stomach, where it connects to the duodenum, is a funnel-shaped area called the pylorus. The pylorus has two parts: the pylorus antrum, which is connected to the stomach; and the pylorus canal, which leads to the pyloric valve and the duodenum of the small intestine. As food reaches the pylorus, the mixing waves force several milliliters of the chyme into the duodenum through the pyloric sphincter. Most of the food is forced back into the body of the stomach, where it is again mixed with the gastric juices. Each wave pushes a little more chyme into the duodenum, while the remaining chyme continues to mix with the gastric juices of the stomach. The back and forth movements of these mixing waves are responsible for the preliminary digestive process that takes place in the stomach.

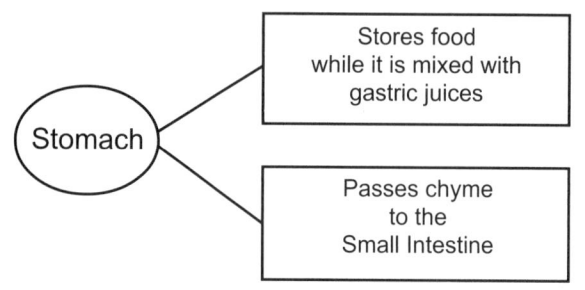

Figure 8.78. The Functions of the Stomach (Western Medical Perspective)

Physiology

The stomach functions both as a reservoir for ingesting food and as a digestive organ (Figure 8.78). The gastric glands of the stomach secrete gastric juice (hydrochloric acid and a few enzymes) for food digestion. The stomach then passes the resulting mixture, now called chyme, on to the small intestine via the pyloric sphincter. The internal surface of the stomach replenishes its cells every three days, allowing all of the cells of the stomach to be replaced over a time period of one to three months.

THE SPLEEN: PI

The Spleen is a solid (Zang) organ that stores and nourishes the body's Ying Qi. The Spleen corresponds to the Earth Element and is sometimes referred to as the "Yellow Emperor." It is energetically paired with the Stomach, which is a Yang (hollow) organ. The functions attributed to the pancreas in Western Medicine are seen in Traditional Chinese Medicine as being part of the collective functions of the Spleen and Stomach. The pancreas is an essential energetic component of the Spleen Orb, assisting in the function of processing nutrients, though it is not considered as an independent organ in Traditional Chinese Medicine. The pancreas also produces insulin, and is energetically connected to the Spleen Orb. The pancreas also shares certain Blood Vessels with the Spleen and connects with the intestinal tract at the outflow junction of the Stomach.

Because it is responsible for distributing and absorbing what the Stomach has stored and digested, the Spleen is sometimes called the "Minister of Grains." Energetically, the Spleen controls the body's central cavity and holds the internal organs in their places. It is therefore responsible for resisting the downward pull of gravity and preventing the prolapse of the internal organs.

The Spleen houses the "Yi," which contains the hereditary predisposition towards schemas. Schemas, in this sense, are energetic, biological, mental, emotional and spiritual patterns and tendencies that are passed down through the individual's biological and cultural lineages. The Yi codifies the individual's biological and psychic behavior, and permits these patterns to be repeated within the individual's lineage. The ancient Chinese also believed that the Yi represented the "music of the Heart," and therefore encouraged singing in order to purge the Spleen's acquired emotion of "worry" (Figure 8.79).

CHINESE CHARACTER FOR THE SPLEEN: PI

- The Chinese character "Pi" translates as "Spleen." It refers to a general description of the image of the Spleen organ, and is divided

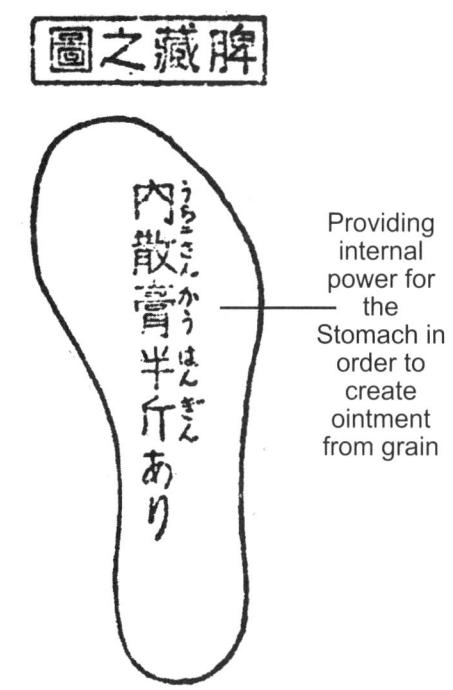

Figure 8.79. The ancient Chinese anatomical diagram of the Spleen (Sp) Organ, as it appeared in "Important Useful Notes on Acupuncture and Moxibustion," published in Japan in 1718, by Masatoyo Hongo

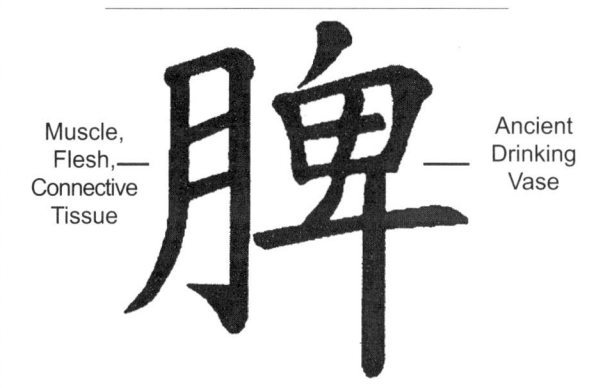

Figure 8.80. The Chinese character for "Pi," Spleen

into two sections. The character to the left, "Ji" depicts the Chinese ideogram for body tissue, muscle or flesh (all of which are forms of connective tissue). The character to the right depicts an ideogram that was originally a representation of an ancient drinking vase, provided with a handle on the left side (later, this charac-

```
                                    ┌─ Transforms, Transports and Distributes Nutrients ─┬─ The Distribution of Food Essence
                                    │                                                    └─ The Distribution of Fluids
                                    ├─ Rules the Muscles and Limbs
The Main Functions of the Spleen ───┼─ Controls the Blood ─── Keeps Blood Within Vessels
Organ and Channels                  ├─ Holds the Internal Organs in Place
                                    ├─ Opens to the Mouth and Manifest in the Lips
                                    ├─ Psycho-Emotional Aspects ─── Trust and Worry
                                    └─ Spiritual Influence ─── Spiritual Functions of the Yi
```

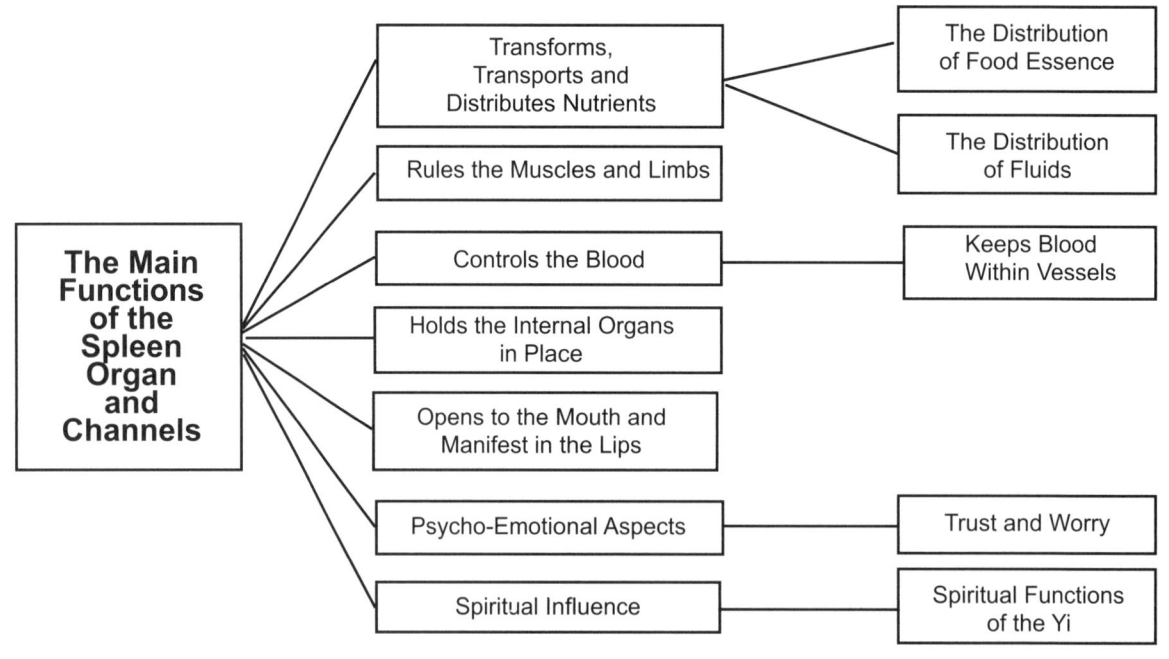

Figure 8.81. The Main Energetic Functions of the Spleen Organ and Channels

ter for wine vessel was taken in the abstract sense to mean both noble and vulgar, depending on the context in which it was used). Together, both ideographs express the idea that the Spleen organ is responsible for collecting "pure" and necessary things for the body (e.g., the collecting of Gu Qi and the gathering of ideas) (Figure 8.80).

THE YIN AND YANG OF THE SPLEEN

Traditional Chinese Medicine defines the Spleen as having two energetic aspects: a Yin aspect and a Yang aspects.
- **The Yin of the Spleen:** This pertains to the material structures of the Spleen, including the Blood stored within it.
- **The Yang of the Spleen:** This pertains to the Spleen's function of heating, transforming, holding, and moving the Qi.

THE SPLEEN'S EARTH JING FORMATION

During the eighth lunar month, the fetus receives the Zong (Essential) Qi from the mother's Spleen. The Zong Qi is the energy collected from Heaven and Earth, and it accumulates within the chest. At this time, the Earth Jing begins to be incorporated into the fetus' body, completing the formation of the skin.

The Earth Jing energy also supervises the quality and maturation of the emotional and spiritual bonding and boundaries of the fetus. Any faltering of the Earth Jing energy is associated with problems of severe psychological disturbances (e.g., schizophrenia). These psychological disturbances may be evident at birth or develop later in life.

After birth, the Earth Jing can be affected through the color yellow, the sweet taste and "Who," and "Gong" sounds.

THE SPLEEN IN CHINESE MEDICINE

In Traditional Chinese Medicine, the functions attributed to the Spleen are completely different than those identified by Western Medicine. From a Chinese energetic perspective, the Spleen is associated with most of the functions of the digestive system, Blood coagulation, and Body Fluid metabolism. It also governs certain psycho-emotional aspects and spiritual influences. Western Medicine, on the other hand, identifies the functions of the Spleen as primarily relating to the body's lymph system.

According to Traditional Chinese Medicine, the main functions of the Spleen are to: transform, transport and distribute nutrients; rule the muscles and limbs; control the Blood; hold internal organs; open into the mouth and manifest in the lips; express itself through the psycho-emotional aspects of trust and worry; and spiritually influencing the individual through the Yi (Intention). These main functions are described as follows (Figure 8.81):

1. **Transforms, Transports and Distributes Nutrients:** The Spleen is sometimes called the "Minister of Grains," as it is responsible for distributing what the Stomach has stored and digested. According to the *Simple Questions*, the "distribution of nutrients" pertains to two digestive functions originating from the energetic interactions of the Stomach and Spleen: the distribution of food essence, and the distribution of fluids.

   • **The Distribution of Food Essence:** According to the *Su Wen*, the Stomach organ is responsible for transforming food essence and separating it into pure (refined) and impure (unrefined) substances. The pure portion (Gu Qi) is absorbed by the Stomach and transported to the Liver, the excess is transported into the tendons and permeates all of the muscles with Qi. The turbid portion (it is important to note that the digestive Qi is only considered turbid in contrast to respiratory Qi) is passed to the Heart. The overflow is transported into the Blood Vessels (Figure 8.82).

   • **The Distribution of Fluids:** The Spleen organ is responsible for transforming, separating and distributing the fluid substances received from the Stomach into pure and impure substances. The pure portion (Gu Qi) is absorbed by the Spleen and transported to the Lungs where it is converted into Qi, Blood, and Body Fluids. The turbid portion is passed to the Small Intestine, Large Intestine, and Urinary Bladder for further absorption and eventual excretion. The Spleen's main function is to govern or oversee this transportation and transformation of Gu Qi (Figure 8.83).

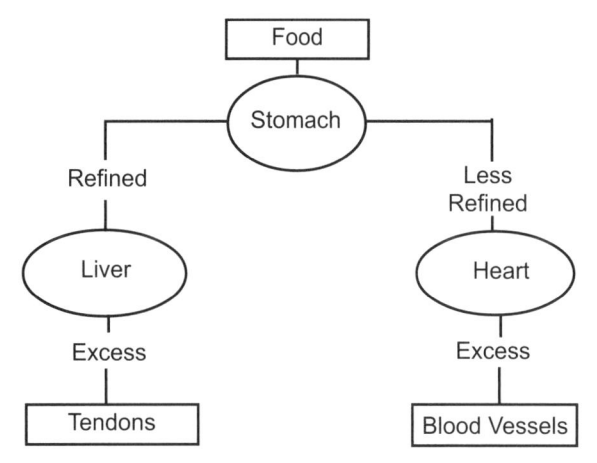

Figure 8.82. The Distribution of Food Essence

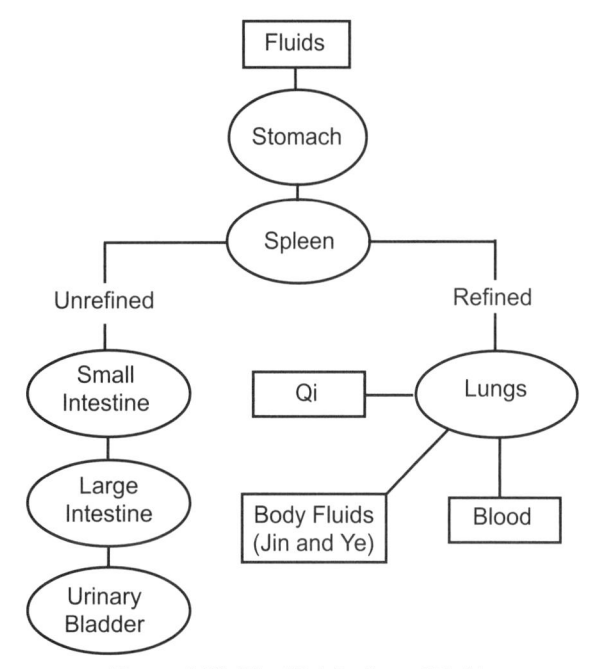

Figure 8.83. The Distribution of Fluids

2. **Rules the Muscles and Limbs:** The Spleen has the function of nourishing and governing the muscles, flesh, and limbs. According to the "Simple Questions," if the Spleen is invaded by Heat, the patient will experience thirst and his or her muscles will become weak and begin to atrophy. This atrophy occurs because all four limbs are dependent on the Stomach for Qi, and the Ying (Nourish-

ing) Qi transformed by the Stomach can only reach the extremities (via the channels) through the energetic actions of the Spleen. If the Spleen is diseased, it cannot transport the fluids of the Stomach, and thus all four limbs will not receive adequate nourishment.

3. **Controls the Blood:** The Spleen has the function of controlling the Blood by keeping it circulating normally within the Blood Vessels. If the Spleen Qi (especially the Spleen Yang) is deficient, the Blood is not held within the Blood Vessels, and the Blood will leak out, creating various forms of hemorrhaging. The energy of the Spleen, via the Blood, also plays a part in the heat regulation of the body by warming the five Yin organs.

4. **Holds the Internal Organs in Place:** Energetically, the Spleen Yang controls the body's central cavity and holds the internal organs in their places. It is therefore responsible for resisting the downward pull of gravity and controlling the prolapse of the internal organs. The ancient Chinese believed that the Spleen was responsible for influencing the "forms" (the development of the tissues' physical shapes) of the body.

5. **Opens to the Mouth and Manifesting in the Lips:** The Spleen organ's energy opens externally at the mouth, controlling taste, and manifests externally at the lips. According to the *Magical Pivot*, the Spleen Qi connects to the mouth. If the Spleen Qi is abundant, the mouth can differentiate the Five Flavors (sour, bitter, sweet, pungent and salty), and the lips will be red and moist. The word "taste" should not be confused with the Western sense of a perceived taste, as it is used here to denote the flavor's influence on the tissues (via the Spleen's energetic function of digestion and assimilation).

6. **Psycho-Emotional Aspects:** In addition to governing physical movement, the Spleen is also responsible for distributing physical, emotional and spiritual nourishment. In this respect, the Spleen digests and assimilates the more subtle aspects of life experiences, incorporating them into the individual's personality. It houses the body's thoughts and intentions (Yi) and is responsible for analytical thinking, memory, cognition, intelligence, and ideas. The Spleen is also responsible for directing memories to the Kidneys for short-term retention. The Kidneys will later transfer these memories to the Heart for long-term memory storage.

    When functioning in harmony, the influences of the Hun on the Spleen allow the individual to experience trust and honesty in both thought and action. If the circulation of Qi becomes obstructed, the resulting Spleen Qi stagnation can give rise to emotional turmoil, sometimes manifesting through obsessions (Yang), or self-doubt (Yin), both of which are influenced by the Po. The Spleen's positive psycho-emotional attributes are trust, honesty, openness, acceptance, equanimity, balance, and impartiality. Its negative attributes are worry, excessive thinking, pensiveness, obsessiveness, remorse, regret, obsessions, and self-doubt.

7. **Spiritual Influence:** The Spleen stores the "Yi," one of the Wu Jing Shen. The Chinese word Yi can be translated as mind, thought, opinion, idea, sentiment, inclination, intention, intellect, scholarly mind, analytical thinking, and memorization.

CHINESE IDEOGRAM OF THE YI

The Chinese ideogram for Yi is depicted by two characters. On the bottom is the Heart; on the top is the character for the musical note or sound "Yin." Together, both characters describe the Heart's intention to think, speak or act through sounds, thoughts or actions (Figure 8.84).

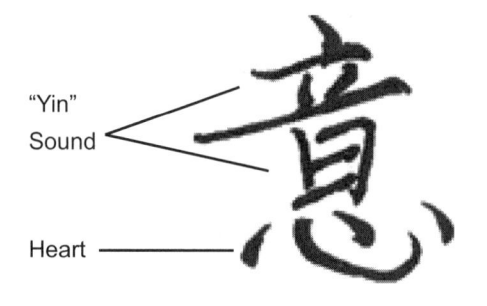

"Yin" Sound

Heart

Figure 8.84. The Chinese character for "Yi," Idea

The Spleen and the Yi

Because the Spleen stores the Yi, it is responsible for the transformation and transportation of all thoughts and ideas on an intellectual level through study, concentration, and memorization. This is different from the creative faculties of the Hun. It is the interaction between the Yi of the Spleen and the Shen of the Heart that allows an individual to place how he or she thinks, speaks, and acts to sounds, thoughts, and actions. The process of memory retention involves an integrated relationship between the functions of the Spleen (responsible for memory in terms of concentration and studying), the Kidneys (responsible for storing short term memory), and the Heart (responsible for storing the long term memory of past events).

The Postnatal Qi and Blood form the physiological basis for the intellect. A person with well-developed Yi has total recall of events experienced in the past and is able to memorize things easily. A patient with an excess of Yi will be obsessed with the past, while a patient with deficient Yi will be absentminded, suffer memory loss, be inattentive, and have problems in maintaining concentration and mental focus. These observations can be especially useful in the Medical Qigong clinic.

Although all physical pain is registered by the Po, and all psychological pain is registered by the Hun, the memory of the pain is registered by the Yi (Figure 8.85). Therefore, a deficient Yi condition can often lead to the phenomenon of transference and countertransference. Transference refers to the process whereby the patient projects onto the doctor, or any authority figure, past feelings or attitudes toward significant people in his or her life. Countertransference involves the same type of projection of one's feelings, colored by one's own expectations in response. In countertransference, the doctor or therapist is projecting back on to the patient.

Yi also has the meaning of "divine purpose" when applied to the Yuan Shen energy. Whenever the physical energy is purified by self-cultivation and connection to the divine, the intention of the Shen and the divine purpose become unified. It is

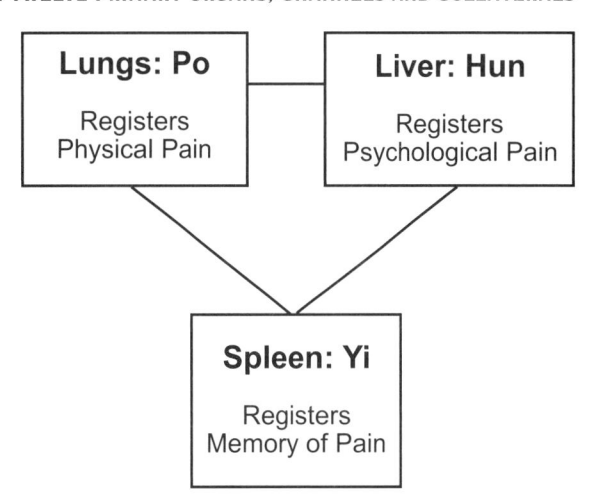

Figure 8.85. Three Ways the Body Registers Pain

said that when the Yi is conserved, it will help build the Zhi (or willpower). The Yi is filled with information from the past along with current knowledge and sensations.

The Spleen Channels

The Spleen Channels are Yin channels that flow externally from the feet to the torso. These two rivers originate externally from the medial tips of the big toes, ascending upwards along the inner thighs, before entering the abdomen (connecting to the CV-3 and CV-4 points) and travelling through the upper torso to connecting with the CV-12 point. The external Spleen Channels join at the CV-12 point and enter into the body. From the CV-12 point, a branch of the Spleen Channel descends internally to flow into the Spleen, and then spirally wraps the Stomach organ. Another internal branch ascends from the CV-12 point into the Heart. At the CV-12 point, both left and right main channels meet and separate again to ascend through the diaphragm, up the torso and throat alongside the esophagus, eventually reconnecting at the base of the tongue. From the Sp-20 points, external branches descend along the lateral aspects of the torso and terminate on the mid-axillary line in the seventh intercostal space (Figure 8.86).

VOLUME 1, SECTION 1: FOUNDATIONS OF CHINESE ENERGETIC MEDICINE

Internal Channel Flow

External Channel Flow

The external Spleen Channels join at the CV-12 point and enter into the body. From the CV-12 point, a branch of the Spleen Channel descends internally to flow into the Spleen, and then spirally wraps the Stomach organ. Another internal branch ascends from the CV-12 point into the Heart. At the CV-12 point, both left and right main channels meet and separate again to ascend through the diaphragm, up the torso and throat alongside the esophagus, eventually reconnecting at the base of the tongue.

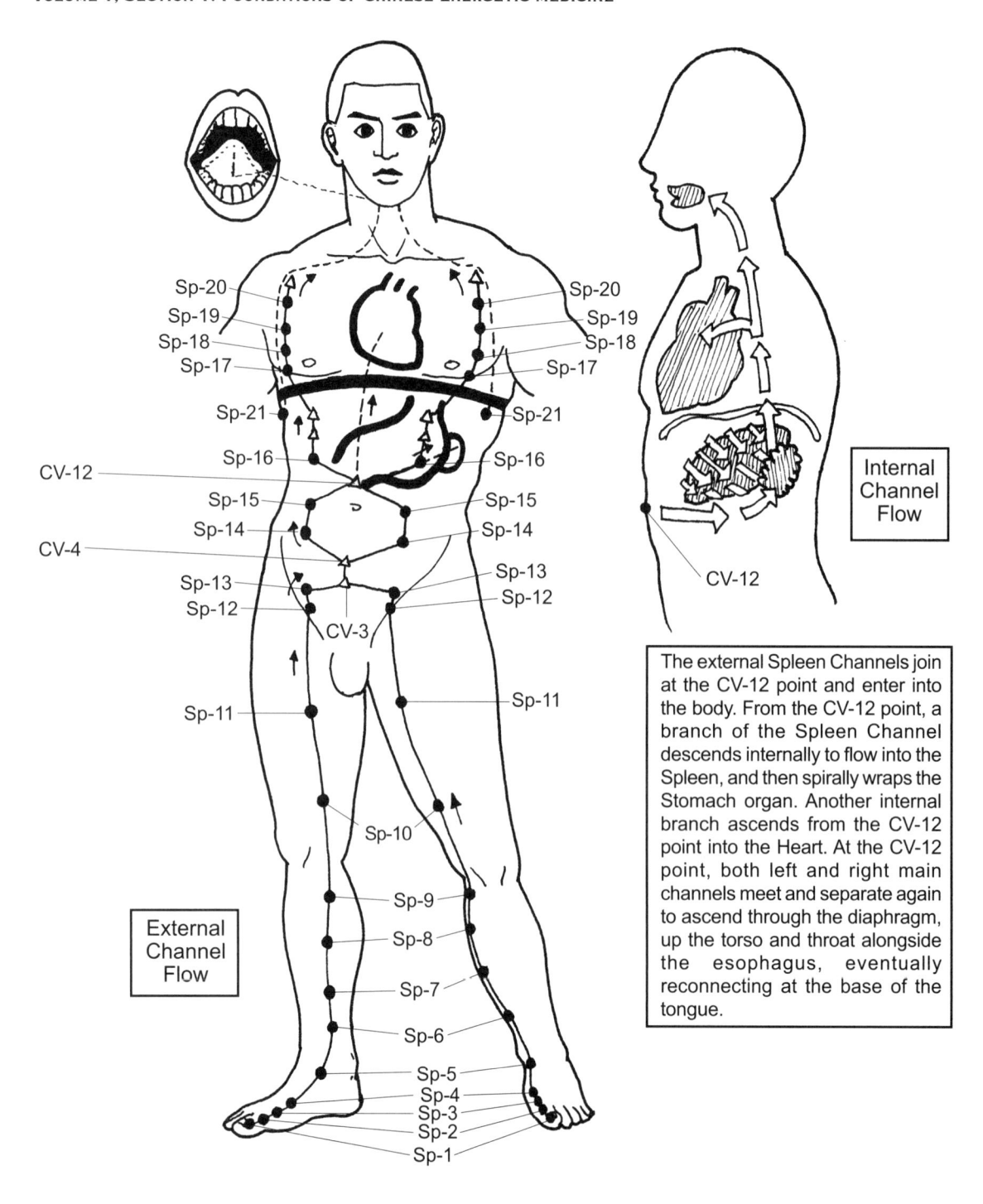

Figure 8.86. The Internal and External Qi Flow of the Spleen (Sp) Channels

Channels' Energy Flow

The Spleen Channels store more Qi and less Blood, acting more on energetic and nervous functions than on physical substance and Blood functions. At the high-tide time period (9 a.m. to 11 a.m.), Qi and Blood abound in the Spleen organ and Spleen channels. At this time period the Spleen organ and Spleen channels can more easily be dispersed and purged. During low tide (9 p.m. to 11 p.m.), they can be more readily tonified. The Spleen Channels' energy acts on the skin, muscles, and nerves found along their pathway.

The Influence of Climate

In the late summer months, Spleen Qi becomes more active in individuals who possess strong Spleen Qi, but can become deficient in those individuals who already have weak Spleen Qi. In ancient China, the Spleen was sometimes tonified during the transitional period between seasons to bring the individual back into a state of harmony. During this season, the excessive eating and drinking of sweet foods, greasy foods and overexposure to dampness can weaken the Spleen. Overexposure to a Damp climate will also have a draining effect on the Spleen.

The Influence of Taste, Color, and Sound

- An External Damp climate can interfere with the functions of the Spleen. The Spleen needs a certain amount of dryness to function. It is easily injured by Damp Heat and Damp Cold.
- The sweet taste can be used to tonify both the Spleen and Stomach.
- The dark yellow/light brown color is used to tonify the Spleen.
- The "Who" and "Gong" sounds are used to purge the Spleen.

Spleen Pathology

The main diseases associated with imbalances of the Spleen organ and channels include gastrointestinal dysfunctions (disturbances of digestion and absorption of food) and diseases of the tongue and throat. Spleen disorders also affect the inner side of the lower extremities along the Spleen's Channels.

The Spleen has the function of sending food essence upwards (to the Lungs). If this function is impeded, diarrhea or prolapse of the viscera may occur. The Spleen also has the function of keeping the Blood flowing within the Blood Vessels. Chronic Spleen Qi Deficiency can lead to hemorrhagic diseases.

The Spleen has the function of nourishing the flesh (muscles). A person with a healthy Spleen will usually have a healthy figure and a toned body. A diseased Spleen can lead to loss of muscle definition.

The Spleen nourishes the limbs. Since the strength of the limbs depends upon the nourishment produced by the normal functioning of the Spleen, a diseased Spleen usually causes weakness of the limbs.

T.C.M. Patterns of Disharmony

The foundations of Spleen disharmony stem from a tendency of the Spleen to become deficient (Qi and Yang) and its susceptibility to invasion by Damp and Cold (Figure 8.87). In the clinic, patterns of Spleen disharmonies include diseases stemming from: Deficient Spleen Qi, Deficient Spleen Yang, Spleen Blood Deficiency, Spleen Yin Deficiency, The Inability of the Spleen to Govern the Blood, The Sinking of Spleen Qi, Invasion of the Spleen by Cold and Damp, Damp Heat Accumulating Within the Spleen and Turbid Phlegm Disturbing the Head. These syndromes are described as follows:

1. **Deficient Spleen Qi:** The signs of Deficient Spleen Qi manifest as signs of Deficient Qi, Deficient Blood, Body Fluid Disharmony and a general weakness of the patient's digestive system. Symptoms of Spleen Qi Deficiency include: slight abdominal pain, abdominal distension, loss of appetite, edema, loose stools with increased frequency, general lassitude, weak limbs and thin muscles. When left unchecked, Deficient Spleen Qi can lead to other functional disorders, the most common of these are failure of transporting and transforming Qi, sinking Middle Burner Qi, and failure to control Blood circulation.

- **Failure of Transporting and Transforming**

VOLUME 1, SECTION 1: FOUNDATIONS OF CHINESE ENERGETIC MEDICINE

Figure 8.87. The Origins of Spleen Disharmonies

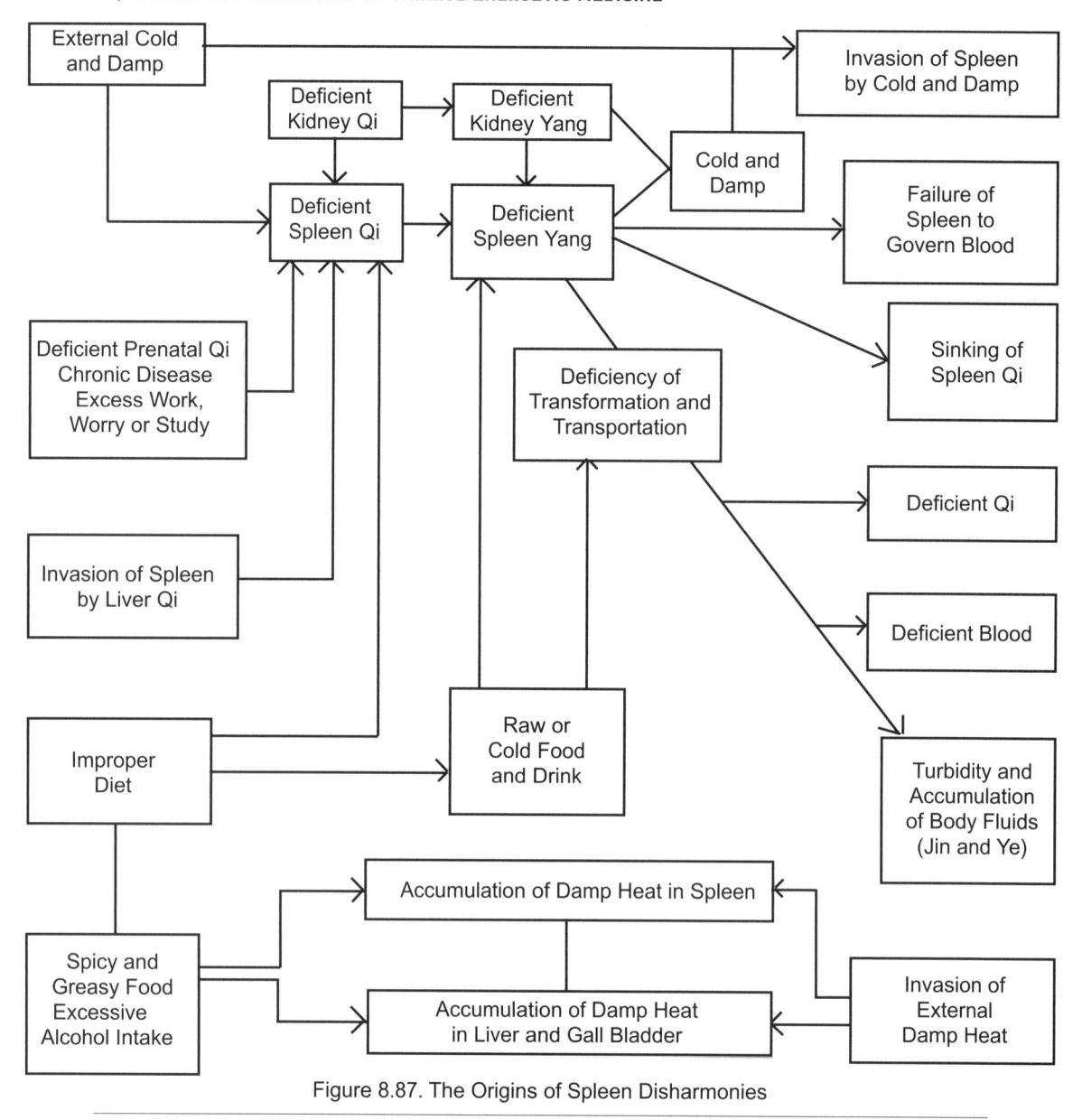

Qi: When there is insufficient Qi to support the normal transporting and transforming action of the Spleen, a patient may show symptoms such as a poor appetite, abdominal distention, or loose stools. Turbidity of Body Fluids (Jin and Ye) and their accumulation (such as edema and the retention of Phlegm) may also occur due to the Spleen's inability to "transform and transport water (fluids)."

- **Sinking Middle Burner Qi:** A failure of the Spleen's function of holding the organs in place due to Deficient Spleen Qi may cause the Qi in the Middle Burner to sink. This can result in persistent diarrhea, prolapse of the anus, prolapse of the Urinary Bladder or prolapse of the Uterus, gastroptosis (downward displacement of the Stomach), muscle atrophy, weakness, and sagging of the muscles (such as the eyelid). A Deficient Spleen Qi may also compromise the vessels creating such conditions as mitral valve prolapse, varicose veins and aneurysms.

- **Failure to Control Blood Circulation:** Spleen Qi Deficiency can result in failure of the Spleen to keep the Blood within the vessels and may manifest in the following symptoms: bloody stool, bruising easily, intermittent uterine bleeding, subcutaneous hemorrhaging, bleeding from the nose, Blood in the urine, bleeding from the Lungs, and vomiting of Blood. The patient will also show signs of general weakness due to this deficiency-related type of bleeding.

2. **Deficient Spleen Yang:** This condition is often a progression of Deficient Spleen Qi, and is considered to be a more severe type of deficiency. In addition to the signs of deficiency and weakness, there are also signs of Cold due to Deficient Yang. Symptoms of Deficient Spleen Yang include: cold limbs, aversion to cold, edema, fatigue transforming into exhaustion, no appetite, retention of urine, undigested food in a loose watery stool, and abdominal pain that is relieved by Heat and pressure.

3. **Spleen Blood Deficiency:** This condition can result in anemia due to insufficient nutrition. The Spleen's ability to transform and transport Gu Qi into Ying Qi makes the body unable to produce Blood.

4. **Spleen Yin Deficiency:** This condition can result in fatigue, emaciation, dry lips, and an inability of the Spleen to deliver nutrients to the cells.

5. **The Inability of the Spleen to Govern the Blood:** This condition results from a deficiency of Spleen Qi and Spleen Yang. This leads to an insufficiency of Qi and Yang which is necessary to hold the Blood in the Blood Vessels, resulting in hemorrhage. This type of hemorrhage is associated with deficiency and signs of Cold, and should be differentiated from the type of hemorrhage associated with excess and Heat. Symptoms include: hemorrhaging, especially in the lower part of the body, purpura (Blood spots under the skin), Blood in the stool or urine, menorrhagia or metrorrhagia, and shortness of breath.

6. **The Sinking of Spleen Qi:** The Sinking of Spleen Qi results from a failure of the holding function of Spleen Qi and Spleen Yang. Symptoms of the Sinking of Spleen Qi may be expressed through signs of Deficient Spleen Qi and Deficient Spleen Yang, and can lead to prolapse of the lower body's internal organs. Other symptoms include: severe chronic diarrhea, urinary incontinence and prolapse of the Stomach, Uterus, Urinary Bladder, vagina or anus.

7. **Invasion of the Spleen by Cold and Damp:** External Cold can enter the body through either exposure to a Cold climate or the ingestion of raw or cold food and drink. External Damp can also enter the body through exposure to a Damp climate, becoming pathological through prolonged or excessive exposure to rain, mists and fog, or from wearing damp clothes after profuse perspiration. Either Cold or Damp can give rise to Deficient Yang, which, can in turn give rise to Internal Cold (due to a lack of Yang to warm the body) or Internal Damp (caused from a deficiency in the function of transformation and transportation by the Spleen, leading to the accumulation of Body Fluids). Deficient Kidney Yang may also accompany Deficient Spleen Yang, both giving rise to Internal Cold and Damp. The patterns of Cold and Damp invasion of the Spleen can be further differentiated according to whether Cold or Damp predominates.

- **Damp:** If Damp predominates, the patterns can be further subdivided according to whether the Damp is from an internal influence (sometimes called Dampness distressing the Spleen) or external influence (sometimes called External Dampness obstructing the Spleen).

- **Cold:** If Cold predominates, there may be an acute aggravation of chronic Yang Deficiency patterns which can result in a temporary Excess Cold condition.

Symptoms arising from an invasion of the Spleen by Cold and Damp include: loss of appetite and sense of taste, lethargy, leukorrhea, a feeling of heaviness in the head and limbs, a feeling of fullness in the chest or abdominal area, copious or turbid secretions, and retention or dribbling of urine and edema.

8. **Damp Heat Accumulating Within the Spleen:** External Heat can enter the body through either exposure to a Hot climate or the ingestion of hot or spicy food and drink. External Damp can also enter the body through exposure to a Damp climate, becoming pathological through prolonged or excessive exposure to rain, mists and fog, or from wearing damp clothes after profuse perspiration. The pattern of Damp Heat accumulating within the Spleen can be subdivided according to whether Dampness or Heat predominates.

   - **Damp:** When Dampness predominates, there may be such symptoms as: no thirst, thirst with no desire to drink, loss of appetite, nausea, vomiting, loose stools, leukorrhea, diarrhea with mucous or bad smell, heaviness in the head, a headache that feels as if there is a tight head-band on the head, foggy thinking, edema, oily skin, or rashes with pus and fluid-filled cysts.
   - **Heat:** If Heat predominates, there may be such symptoms as: thirst, jaundice, loss of appetite, abdominal distention, yellow leukorrhea, nausea, vomiting, a heavy sensation in the body and mouth sores.

   The pattern of Damp Heat can be further subdivided according to whether the Damp Heat originates from an internal imbalance (generally chronic and of gradual onset) caused from a Hot, humid climate, the consumption of contaminated food, or from pathogenic evils. Damp Heat can also emerge from an external influence (generally acute and of sudden onset), caused from excess consumption of greasy foods or alcohol over long periods of time.

   Patterns of disharmony created from Damp Heat accumulating within the Spleen give rise

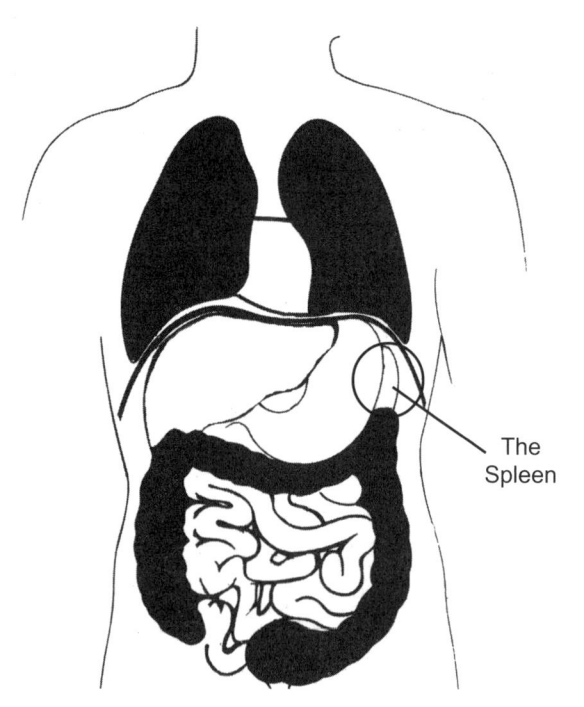

Figure 8.88. The Anatomical Location of the Spleen

to the following symptoms: no appetite, lethargy, feeling of heaviness, stiffness of the epigastrium and lower abdominal area, abdominal distension and pain, yellow leukorrhea, thirst with no desire to drink or with a desire to drink small sips, nausea, vomiting, loose stools with offensive odor, burning sensation of the anus, low-grade fever, headache, and scanty dark-yellow urination.

9. **Turbid Phlegm Disturbing the Head:** This pattern of disharmony is developed from Spleen Dampness. Long term Dampness leads to Phlegm. Because Phlegm is heavier than Dampness, a typical symptom is severe dizziness. Additionally, nodules, cysts, sinusitis, asthma, and copious sputum may also occur.

THE SPLEEN IN WESTERN MEDICINE

The spleen is a soft oval shaped organ, roughly the size of a fist, located in the left hypochondriac region of the body. With its base at the height of the 11th thoracic vertebrae, the spleen lies behind the fundus of the stomach and below the diaphragm. It also borders with the pancreas, the left flexure of the colon, and with the left kidney (Figure 8.88). The spleen is a secondary lymph organ (as are the lymph nodes), being a place where immune training and response occurs. The primary lymph organs, such as the Bone Marrow and the thymus gland, are where the majority of B and T cells (among others) are actually produced. The spleen is the largest of the body's ductless glands, and is also considered to be the largest mass of lymphatic tissue in the body.

Externally, the spleen is surrounded by a serous coat that is derived from the peritoneum. Immediately within the serous coat lies a fibroelastic coat that encapsulates the spleen while also extending into the organ in numerous tiny fibrous bands called trabeculae. These trabeculae form the primary internal framework of the spleen. The spleen receives blood through the splenic artery which, upon entering into the spleen, quickly divides into a number of smaller convoluted arterial branches that eventually serve to expose the blood to as much spleen tissue as possible. This cleansed blood then leaves the spleen via the splenic vein. Thus, one of the primary functions of the spleen is to bring the blood into contact with the lymphatic tissue contained within it. The inner tissue of the spleen (termed splenic pulp) is sponge-like, and consists of both red and white pulp (Figure 8.89).

PHYSIOLOGY

The spleen serves three primary functions in the adult human body: cleansing the blood, immune response, and storing and releasing blood. These functions are described as follows (Figure 8.90:

- **Cleansing the Blood:** The blood cleansing function of the spleen takes place within the red pulp, which consists of venous sinuses filled with blood and of cords of splenic tissue called splenic cords. These splenic cords contain erythrocytes (red blood cells), macrophages (which serve to phagocytize - or engulf - dead cells and foreign material), lymphocytes (including T and B cells), granulocytes (which contain granules filled with potent chemicals), and plasma cells (which are

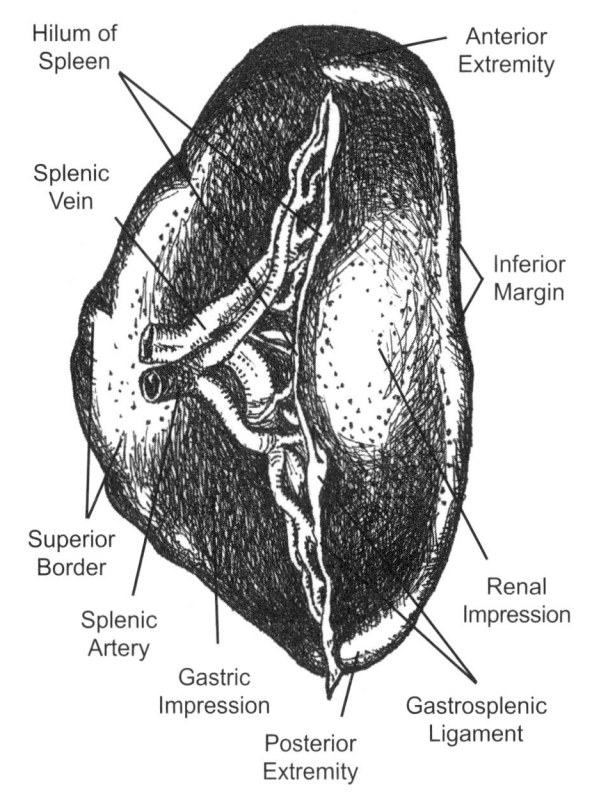

Figure 8.89. The Spleen (Sp) Organ

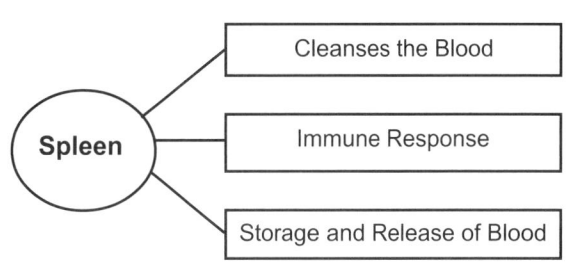

Figure 8.90. The Functions of the Spleen (Western Medical Perspective)

derived from B cells, and produce antibodies). As blood travels through the venous channels of the spleen, it is exposed to as many of these splenic cords as possible within the red pulp. Thus, the red pulp primarily serves to cleanse the blood through the phagocytosis of bacteria, viruses, and other blood-borne pathogens (including particulate matter present in the blood stream), and also through

the recycling of aged or damaged erythrocytes and platelets. As the macrophages breakdown and recycle the hemoglobin of the red blood cells, bilirubin is produced and is released back into the blood plasma to later be removed from the blood by the liver and, to a lesser extent, by the kidneys.
- **Immune Response:** The spleen's role in the immune system is generally considered to be a function of the white pulp of the spleen. The white pulp consists of lymphatic tissue (mostly lymphocytes, with some macrophages) arranged in sleeves or clusters around central arteries. This can give the appearance of islands of white pulp that are surrounded by a sea of red pulp. The spleen's functions of immune surveillance and response (e.g. the generation of antibodies) occur as a result of bringing this lymphatic tissue into contact with the blood. This contact activates the lymphocytes, which then act on any antigens or pathogens present in the blood.
- **Storage and Release of Blood:** Due to its expandable quality and the large amount of blood that passes through the spleen, this organ also serves as a reservoir of blood. When extra blood is needed in the body (as in cases of hemorrhaging), stored blood is released from the spleen through a sympathetic contraction of the smooth muscle tissue of the fibro-elastic layer. Because of its adaptability, the size and weight of the spleen vary dramatically with age. The spleen of an elderly person tends to be about half the size of that of a child or adult based on nutrition, disease status, and other factors. The spleen increases in size during and after digestion, and tends to be relatively large in well-fed animals and small in starved or malnourished animals.

In the fetus, the spleen also serves as a site for red blood cell production. This function normally disappears after birth, but can be reactivated during conditions of extreme erythrocyte depletion.

COMMON DISORDERS OF THE SPLEEN

Because its walls are very thin and it holds a great deal of blood, the spleen can be relatively easily injured as a result of local impact trauma or severe infection. In Western Medicine as a precaution in certain types of blood (leukemia) or lymphatic (lymphoma) cancers, a splenectomy is generally performed. Under such conditions, the spleen is usually removed (splenectomy) immediately to prevent the occurrence of a life-threatening hemorrhage. Once the spleen has been removed, the body is usually able to adapt quite well, as the bone marrow and the liver take over many of the spleen's previous functions.

CHAPTER 8: THE TWELVE PRIMARY ORGANS, CHANNELS AND COLLATERALS

THE HEART: XIN

The Heart is a solid (Zang) organ and is considered to be the most important internal organ of the body. It controls Blood circulation, and governs all of the viscera and bowels (Figure 8.91). The Heart corresponds to the Fire Element and it is sometimes referred to as the "Red Emperor," or as the "supreme controller of all Yin and Yang organs." It is energetically paired with the Small Intestine, which is the hollow organ in charge of separating the pure and clean energy from the impure Qi.

CHINESE CHARACTER FOR HEART: XIN

The word "Xin" translates as "Heart." It refers to a general description of the image of a Heart organ, and is divided into three sections (Figure 8.92). The upper half depicts the aorta and major arteries. The Heart itself is depicted in the center, and the lower left part of the character depicts the Pericardium. In Traditional Chinese Medicine, the character "Xin" also refers as much to the Mind (thoughts and emotions) as it does to the actual Heart organ.

THE YIN AND YANG OF THE HEART

Traditional Chinese Medicine defines the Heart as having two energetic aspects: a Yin aspect and a Yang aspect:
- **The Yin of the Heart:** this pertains to the vital essence of the Heart, including the Blood stored within it.
- **The Yang of the Heart:** this pertains to the Heart's function of heating and moving the Qi and Blood.

THE HEART'S FIRE JING FORMATION

During the fifth lunar month, the Fire Jing energy generates, controls, protects, integrates, divides, and harmonizes the fetus' internal energies in order to promote emotional and spiritual well-being. Any faltering of the Fire Jing energy is associated with problems of right (Yin) and left (Yang) Brain communication (e.g., the correct balance of male/rational and female/intuitive energies).

After birth, the Fire Jing can be affected through the red color, the bitter taste and the "Ha," "Ke" and "Zheng" (Jong) sounds.

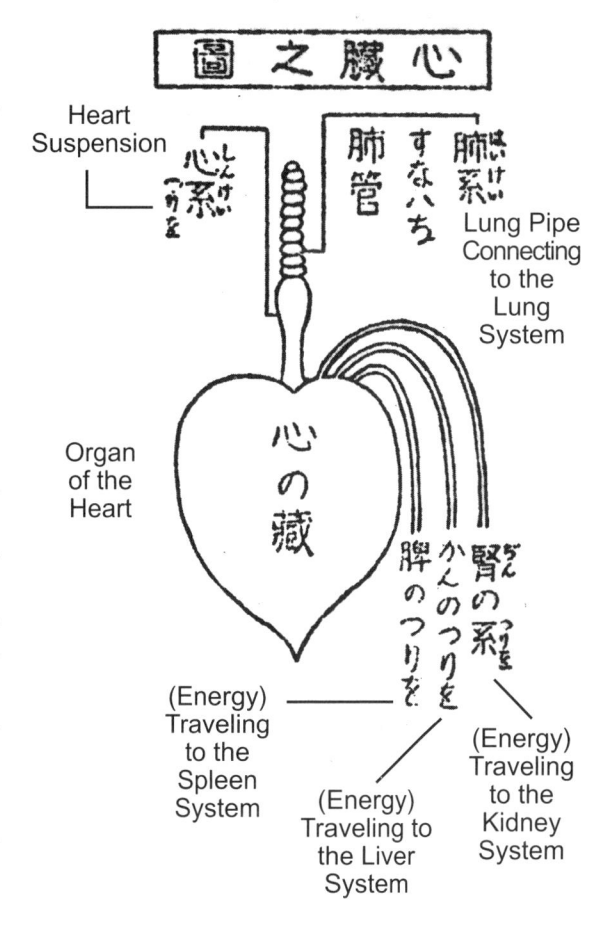

Figure 8.91. The ancient Chinese anatomical diagram of the Heart (Ht) Organ, as it appeared in "Important Useful Notes on Acupuncture and Moxibustion," published in Japan in 1718, by Masatoyo Hongo

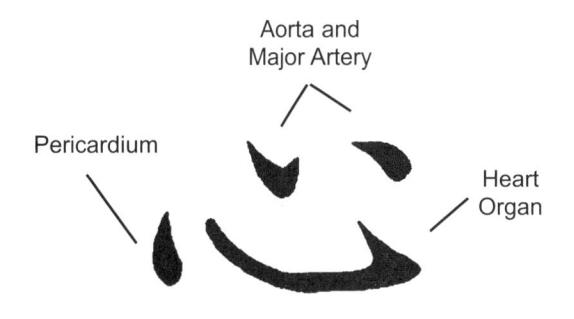

Figure 8.92. The Chinese character for "Xin," Heart

THE HEART IN ANCIENT CHINESE MEDICINE

The *Suwen*, from the *Yellow Emperor's Inner Classics* states, "the Heart is the trunk where life takes root." This phrase expresses the belief that the Eternal Soul (Shen Xian) takes its residence in the core of the Heart, residing within the Taiji Pole.

In ancient China, it was once believed that tissues of both the Heart and its associated organ the Small Intestine were Yang, of the Fire Element, and were Hot and expansive. Because of this, the color red is traditionally ascribed to these organs.

In anatomical placement, the Lungs surround the Heart in the upper thoracic cavity of the chest, while the Large Intestine surrounds the Heart's associated organ, the Small Intestines in the abdominal region.

It was also believed that tissues of both the Lungs and its associated organ the Large Intestines were Yin, of the Metal Element, and were Cold and contractive. Because of this, the color white is traditionally ascribed to these organs.

The continuous interaction of expansion and contraction emanating from the Yin (Cold) and Yang (Hot) energetic properties of these internal organs develops the rhythmic patterns of the cardiopulmonary and digestive systems (Figure 8.93).

THE HEART IN CHINESE MEDICINE

The functions ascribed to the Heart in Traditional Chinese Medicine differ from the functions of the Heart that are described in Western Medicine. Chinese energetic functions of the Heart include the functions associated with the circulatory system, nervous system, the psycho-emotional aspects, and spiritual influences.

According to Traditional Chinese Medicine, the main functions of the Heart are to: govern the Blood, control the Blood Vessels, manifest through the complexion, house the Mind, open into the tongue, control perspiration, express itself through the psycho-emotional aspects of order and excitement, and exert certain important spiritual influences via the Shen (Spirit). These main functions are described as follows (Figure 8.94).

1. **Governs the Blood:** Within the Heart, Heart Qi and Heart Blood are mutually dependent.

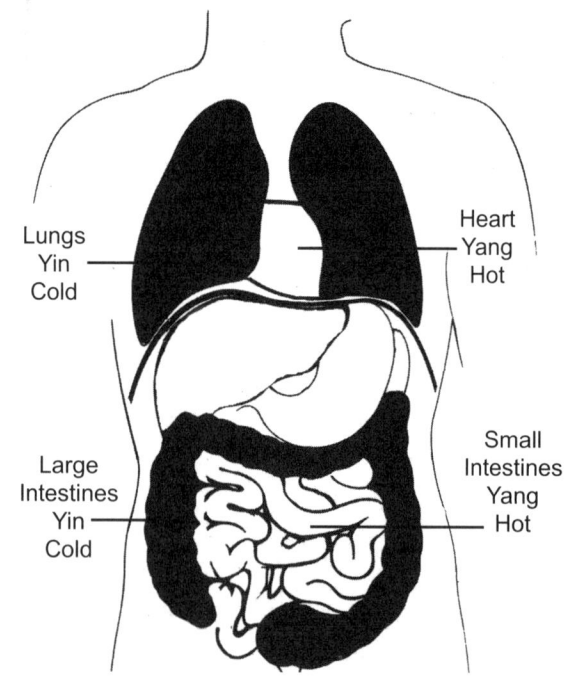

Figure 8.93. The ancient Chinese Yin and Yang relationship between the rhythmical patterns of the body's cardiopulmonary and digestive systems

The Qi of the Heart is the driving force for the Heart's beat, rhythm, rate and strength. The Heart governs the Blood in two ways: the transformation of Gu Qi into Blood and Blood Circulation.

- **Transformation of Gu Qi into Blood:** Blood is considered to be a dense, material form of Qi. Within the Heart, the food essence from the Lungs along with the Yuan Qi from the Kidneys is transformed into Blood.
- **Blood Circulation:** The Heart is responsible for the circulation of Blood. The Lungs, Spleen and Liver also play a role in Blood circulation.

2. **Controls the Blood Vessels:** The Heart distributes the Blood throughout the body through the driving pulse of the Heart. The state of the Blood Vessels depends on the harmony of Heart's Qi and Blood.

3. **Manifests Through the Complexion:** The Heart has its outward manifestation in the face and complexion, therefore the state of the Heart and the Heart's Blood are reflected in the complexion.

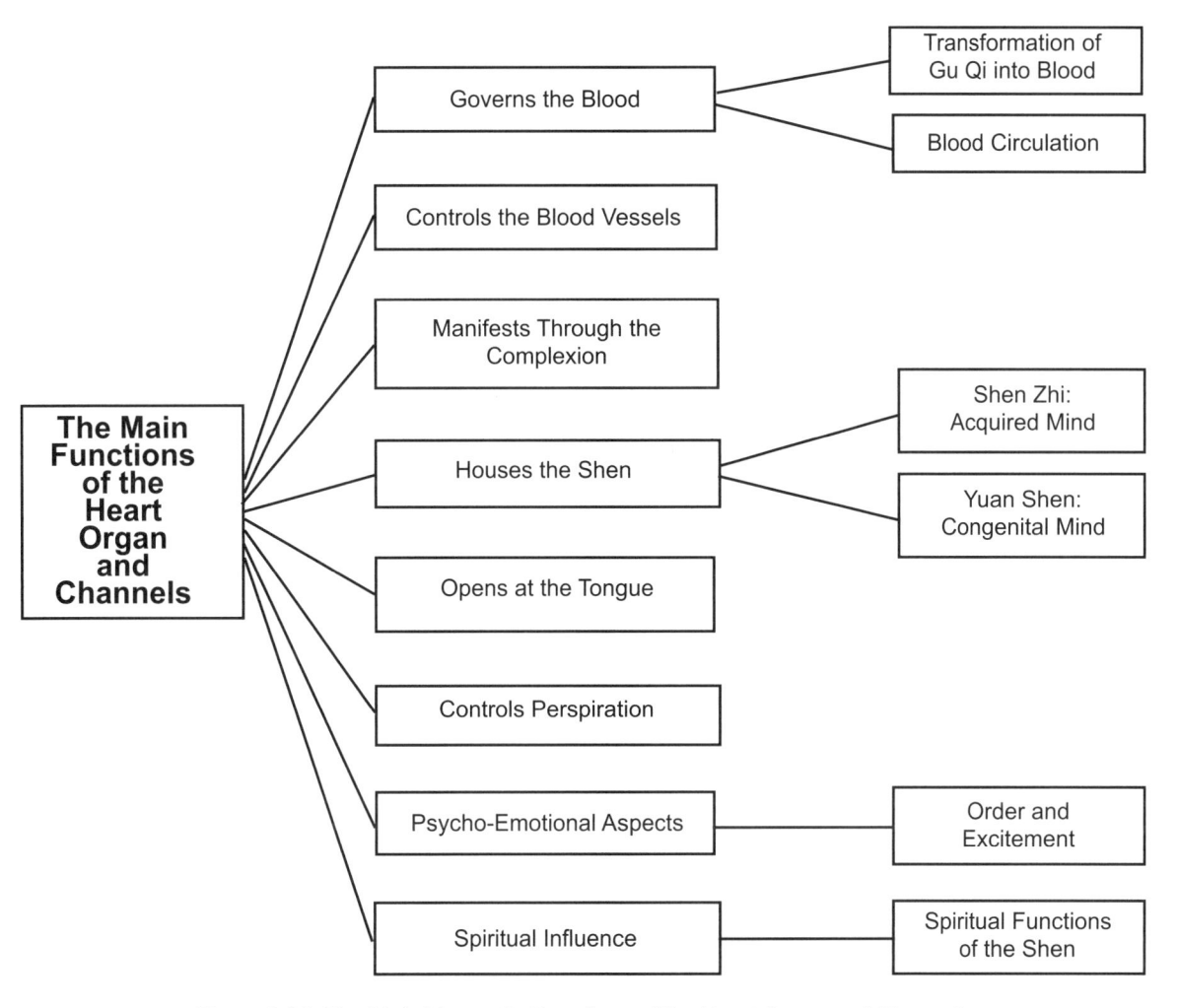

Figure 8.94. The Main Energetic Functions of the Heart Organ and Channels

The Main Functions of the Heart Organ and Channels
- Governs the Blood
  - Transformation of Gu Qi into Blood
  - Blood Circulation
- Controls the Blood Vessels
- Manifests Through the Complexion
- Houses the Shen
  - Shen Zhi: Acquired Mind
  - Yuan Shen: Congenital Mind
- Opens at the Tongue
- Controls Perspiration
- Psycho-Emotional Aspects
  - Order and Excitement
- Spiritual Influence
  - Spiritual Functions of the Shen

---

4. **Houses the Shen:** The Heart stores the Mind and Spirit, traditionally called the "Shen." The functions of the Shen are divided into two main components: The Shen Zhi or Acquired Mind, developed from the analytical senses, and the Yuan Shen or Congenital (Original) Mind, existing as the body's innate intuitive intelligence. Therefore, the ancient Chinese believed the Heart's Shen was responsible for mental and emotional activities, intimacy, cognition, intelligent consciousness, and long term memory. The Shen also has the capacity to judge, and influences sleep.

In Traditional Chinese Medicine, conscious mental thinking activities are considered to be a function of the Heart's Acquired Mind (Shen Zhi) as opposed to the brain in Western Medicine. Dreaming, spirit projection, and spirit travel are considered to be functions of the Heart's Congenital Mind (Yuan Shen). There are five functions of the Heart's Shen Zhi: mental activities, emotional activities, consciousness, memory, and sleep.

There are two ways in which the Shen is nourished. One way is through the dreams, along with the intuitive or unconscious information that comes from the Hun of the Liver. The other way is through the thoughts and ideas that stem from the Yi of the Spleen (Figure 8.95).

5. **Opens into the Tongue:** The tongue is said to be the external branch of the Heart and therefore it is seen as a "mirror of the Heart." The condition of the Heart's Qi manifests through the subtle variations in the color, form, and appearance of the tongue. In tongue diagnosis, the tip of the tongue in particular is said to reveal the state of the Heart.

6. **Controls Perspiration:** Perspiration is considered to be one of the fluids of the Heart. In Traditional Chinese Medicine, Blood and Body Fluids have the same origin, and sweat comes from Body Fluids. Body Fluids are considered to be a very important aspect of Blood. Blood and Body Fluids also mutually interchange; for example, if the Blood is too thick, Body Fluids will enter the Blood Vessels to thin it.

7. **The Psycho-Emotional Aspects:** The Heart is sometimes called "The Emperor," or the "Supreme Controller of all Yin and Yang Organs," and it coordinates all of the energetic and emotional functions of the body. When functioning normally, the effects of the Hun on the Heart allow the individual to experience peace and joy in thoughts and actions. If the circulation of Qi becomes obstructed, Heart Qi stagnation can give rise to emotional turmoil, sometimes manifesting through excitement (Yang), or longing (Yin), both influenced by the Po. The Heart's positive psycho-emotional attributes are joy, peace, contentment, tranquillity, propriety, insight, wisdom, order, forgiveness, and courtesy. Its negative attributes are nervousness, restlessness, excitement, anxiety, panic, shock, longing, craving and guilt.

8. **The Spiritual Influence:** The Heart houses the body's Yuan Shen (Congenital or Original Spirit). An individual's psychic abilities and intuitive faculties are brought about through the influence, cultivation, and training of the Yuan Shen. Extraordinary abilities that can be developed from the cultivated spiritual consciousness of the Yuan Shen include: telepathy, clairvoyance, clairaudience, precognition, time travel, levitation, and teleportation.

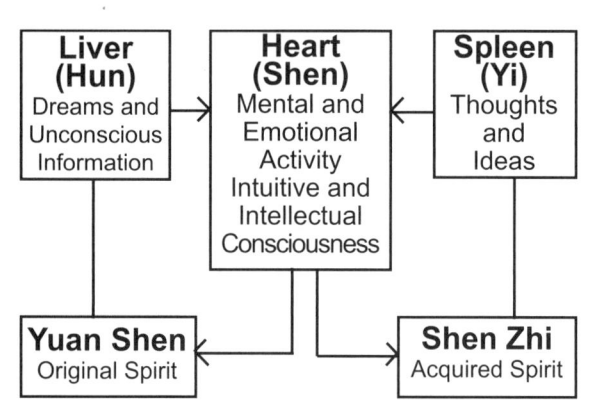

Figure 8.95. Two Ways in which the Shen is Fed

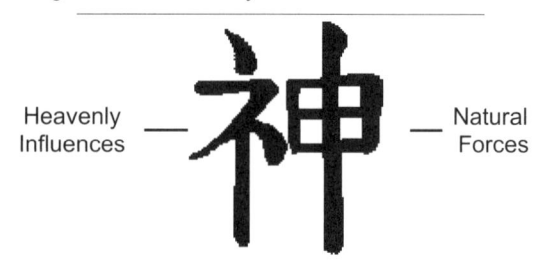

Figure 8.96. The Chinese character for "Shen," Spirit

CHINESE IDEOGRAM OF THE SHEN

The Chinese ideogram for Shen (Spirit) is depicted by two characters. Positioned on the right is a character representing the alternating expression of natural forces. On the left is a character representing the unfolding of things under the authority and influence of Heaven. The ideograph depicts the Heavenly influence that penetrates and instructs the core of the Heart (Figure 8.96).

THE HEART AND THE SHEN

Shen is subdivided into the two categories: Prenatal Shen (Yuan Shen) and Postnatal Shen (Shen Zhi). The term Yuan Shen is sometimes translated as Prenatal Mind (Prenatal Spirit), Original Mind (Original Spirit), Congenital Mind (Congenital Spirit), Original Personality, etc. The term Shen Zhi is alternately translated as Postnatal Mind (Postnatal Spirit), Willful Mind (Willful Spirit), Acquired Mind (Acquired Spirit), Acquired Personality, etc.

```
                    ┌─ Observing the Present
                    │
                    ├─ Comprehending the Past and
                    │   Observing the Future
  The Six           │
Transportations ────┼─ Knowing a Person's Thoughts
  of Shen           │
                    ├─ Perceiving a Person's Destiny
                    │
                    ├─ Hearing the Sounds of the Universe
                    │
                    └─ Examining the Universe
```

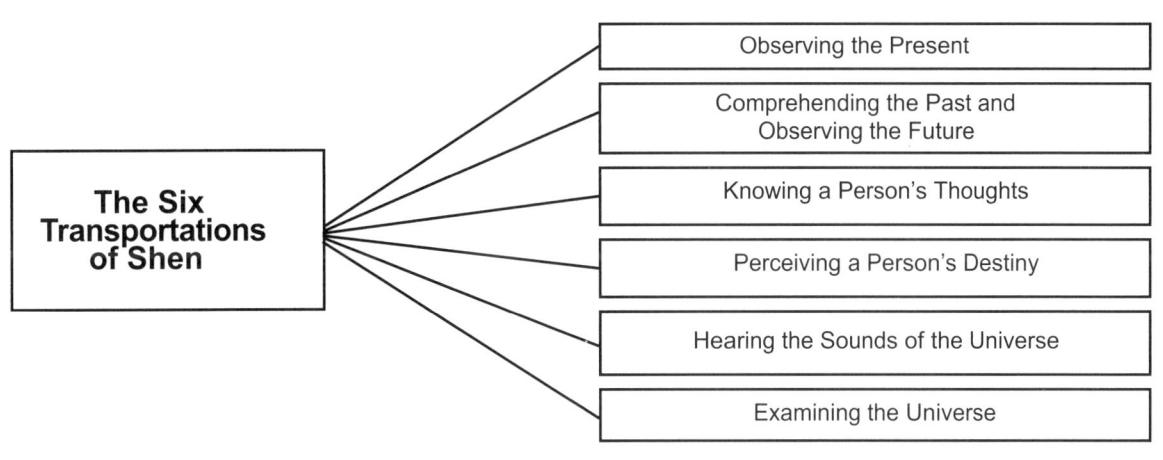

Figure 8.97. The Six Transportations of Shen

The Yuan Shen is associated with the congenital spiritual energy, the Shen Xian or Eternal Soul, that descends from Heaven. This is the universal divine spirit that is implanted in each person, connecting the individual to the spiritual reality that exists beyond the physical and mental realms. This has been referred to as the "higher self." The Postnatal (Acquired) Shen is associated with the wisdom of the five senses and the knowledge acquired through the individual's accumulated experiences.

Each individual's Yuan Shen can be taught to transcend the space-time continuum, as both space and time are multidirectional and interconnected. However, when intuitive perceptions begin to flow, the conscious analytical mind of the Shen Zhi acts as a filter, seeking to analyze every energetic movement and attempting to identify and categorize each perception. Once the Shen Zhi is engaged, the flow of intuitive perception arising from the Yuan Shen usually stops or becomes unconscious. The ancient Qigong masters explained this process of accessing the Yuan Shen with the following aphorism: "by rooting the Acquired Mind (Shen Zhi), the Heart (Yuan Shen) opens to 10,000 voices (the infinite knowledge of the Wuji)." This can be understood to mean that when the "chattering mind" is anchored through focused intention, the Heart is able to perceive the spiritual realm (the 10,000 voices), and to be aware of its connectedness to the multidirectional space-time continuum.

Once the Yuan Shen has been sufficiently cultivated, focused and trained, it reaches a higher level of subtlety and power, and the result is a gradual unveiling of six supernatural diagnostic powers known as the Six Transportations of Shen. These six metaphysical abilities enable the Qigong doctor to evaluate a patient's physical, energetic and spiritual states with accuracy, and by extension, predict the probable future progressions of the patient's life, as well as states or natures of disease. The Six Transportations of Shen are: observing the present, comprehending the past and observing the future, knowing a person's thoughts, perceiving a person's destiny, hearing the sounds of the universe, and examining the universe (Figure 8.97).

THE HEART CHANNELS

The Heart Channels are Yin channels that flow externally from the torso to the hand (Figure 8.98). Three rivers originate internally from the Heart on each side of the body. The first pair of these channels ascends from the Heart and flows into the tissues connecting the eyeball. The second pair first penetrates the Pericardium, and then descends to connect with and spirally wrap the Small Intestine. The third pair of channels flows upwards from the Heart into the Lungs, and emerges externally at the armpits. It then descends along the medial aspect of the arms and ends on the inside of the little fingers.

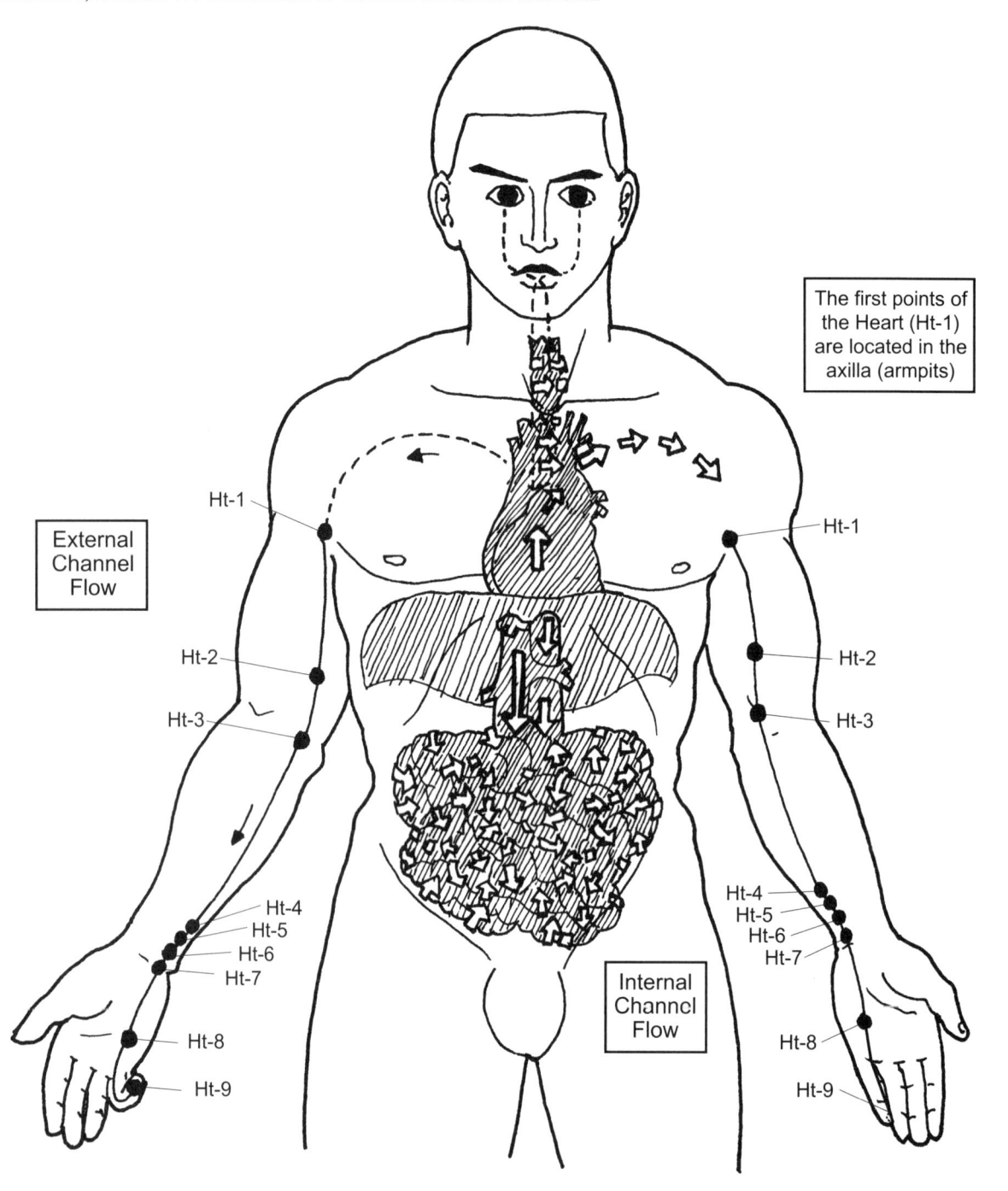

Figure 8.98. The Internal and External Qi Flow of the Heart (Ht) Channels

CHANNELS' ENERGY FLOW

Qi and Blood flow within the channels and Blood Vessels (Mai), continuously circulating throughout the body to nourish, maintain, and moisten the tissues. Qi is an energetic form and is considered a Yang substance, while Blood is a liquid form of energy and is considered a Yin substance (Figure 8.99).

Qi and Blood flow together. Qi is the active energetic force that makes the Blood circulate and keeps it within the Blood Vessels. Blood is a liquid substance that grounds ("roots") the Qi and distributes it along with nutrients to all of the body's tissues. The vessels serve as the reservoir of Blood.

The concept of Blood in Traditional Chinese Medicine is different both in characteristics and in function than the concept of blood in Western medicine. In Traditional Chinese Medicine, Blood originates from the transformation of food and drink by the Spleen. The Spleen transfers the refined food energy to be further enhanced by the Heart Qi and Lung Qi.

The Heart Channels store more Qi than Blood; that is to say, their dominant action affects the energy of the body. This energetic action controls the morale and the spirit of enterprise. The Heart channels also provide the energy required for respiration. At the high-tide time period (11 a.m. to 1 p.m.), Qi and Blood abound in the Heart organ and Heart channels. At this time, the Heart organ and channels can more easily be dispersed and purged. During low tide (11 p.m. to 1 a.m.), they can be more readily tonified. The Heart Channel's energy acts on the skin, muscles, and nerves found along their pathways.

THE INFLUENCE OF CLIMATE

In the early summer months, the Heart energy becomes more active in individuals who already have strong Heart Qi, but can become deficient in those who already have weak Heart Qi. During this season, excessive eating and drinking of bitter foods and the overexposure to Heat depletes the Heart. Overexposure to Hot climate will also have a draining effect on the Heart.

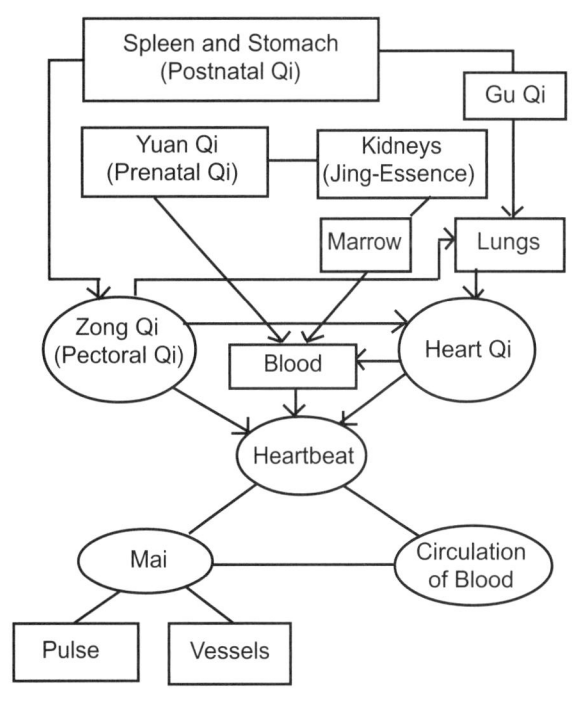

Figure 8.99. The Energetic Functions of the Heart, Blood and Blood Vessels

THE INFLUENCE OF TASTE, COLOR, AND SOUND

- External climate factors do not affect the Heart directly but influence the Pericardium instead. The Heart can be easily injured, however, by Heat and Fire.
- The bitter taste can be used to tonify both the Heart and Small Intestine, and is also used to drain Excess Heat.
- The dark red color is used to tonify the Heart.
- The "Ha," "Ke" and "Zheng" sounds are used to purge the Heart and the Small Intestine.

HEART PATHOLOGY

The Heart is responsible for governing the flow of Blood through the body's arteries and veins. Coronary artery disease (CAD) is a disease in which the patient's coronary arteries begin to harden or impede adequate vascular flow to the myocardium, resulting in an insufficient supply of Qi and Blood throughout the body. This causes such diseases as hypertension, vasculitis, myocarditis, congenital Heart disease, rheumatic Heart disease, nervous malfunctioning of the Heart, organic pathological changes of the Heart, and arteriosclerosis of the Brain.

The main diseases of the Heart organ and channels include diseases that exert pressure on the Brain, eyes, pharyngeal wall, or the lateral side of the chest, as well as diseases of the Heart itself. The Heart also relates to diseases of the ulnar side of the arm.

The Heart is in charge of mental activities, including consciousness and thinking. Dysfunctions of the Heart can thus lead to insomnia, impairment of consciousness, stuttering, amnesia, and psychosis.

The Heart and Kidneys have a mutual energetic relationship of both supporting and checking each other. The Heart controls the body's Fire, while the Kidneys control the body's Water. Normally, the Fire of the Heart is sent down to warm the Kidneys, and the Water of the Kidneys is sent up to irrigate the Heart. If this balanced relationship breaks down (especially when the Kidney Water is insufficient to check the Heart Fire), a series of Fire symptoms such as hypertension, hyperactivity, palpitations, and insomnia may result.

Since the Heart has its external opening in the tongue, the condition of the Heart is reflected in the tongue. Further distinctions can be made as follows:
- A red-tipped tongue indicates Heart Fire
- A dark purple tongue indicates Blood Stasis of the Heart
- A pale tongue reveals Deficient Blood of the Heart
- An ulcer on the tongue reveals Excess Fire of the Heart or Small Intestine

T.C.M. Patterns of Disharmony

Heart pathologies have their origin in the Heart's functions of ruling the Blood and the Blood Vessels, and of housing the Shen. The main patterns of Heart disharmony can be divided into two categories: those associated with Yang Deficiencies (such as Deficient Heart Qi, Deficient Heart Yang, Stagnant Heart Blood and Cold Phlegm Misting the Heart), and those associated with Yin Deficiencies (such as Deficient Heart Blood, Deficient Heart Yin, Blazing Heart Fire and Phlegm Fire Agitating the Heart). These Heart disharmonies are described as follows (Figure 8.100):

1. **Yang Deficiency:**
   - **Deficient Heart Qi:** The pattern of Deficient Heart Qi can arise from malnutrition, chronic illness, prolonged hemorrhaging, and can also be caused by various emotional imbalances such as chronic worry or sadness. Symptoms of Heart Qi Deficiency can manifest as palpitations, spontaneous sweating, listlessness, facial pallor, fatigue and shortness of breath on exertion.
   - **Deficient Heart Yang:** The patterns and pathology of Deficient Heart Yang are similar to, and therefore can arise from, the pathologies of Deficient Heart Qi. Symptoms of Deficient Heart Yang include conditions of Cold: aversion to cold, cold limbs, edema and stuffiness in the chest. If the deficiency is severe, the Yang may collapse, manifesting as profuse sweating, extreme cold in the limbs or in the entire body, and loss of consciousness. If the Yin and Yang separate entirely, the patient may die.
   - **Stagnant Heart Blood:** Deficient Heart Yang can progress to Stagnant Heart Blood, just as Deficient Heart Qi can progress to Deficient Heart Yang. Sometimes all three conditions can occur together, creating common disease patterns such as angina pectoris and myocardial infarction. Other symptoms can manifest as palpitations, shortness of breath, purple facial color, cyanosis of the lips and nails, cold extremities, lassitude, stabbing pain in the chest, tightness in the chest and Heart region, or along the Heart Channel.
   - **Cold Phlegm Misting the Heart:** This is a Yin Excess pattern in which the Heart is obstructed by Phlegm. However, in this pattern, the Phlegm is associated with signs of Cold rather than with signs of Heat. Seen occasionally in children, the pattern of Cold Phlegm Misting the Heart can cause mental retardation or speech difficulties. In adults, the pattern of Cold Phlegm Misting the Heart often occurs after an attack of Wind Stroke. In such cases, the Wind associated with the obstruction of Phlegm can

Figure 8.100. The Origins of Heart Disharmony

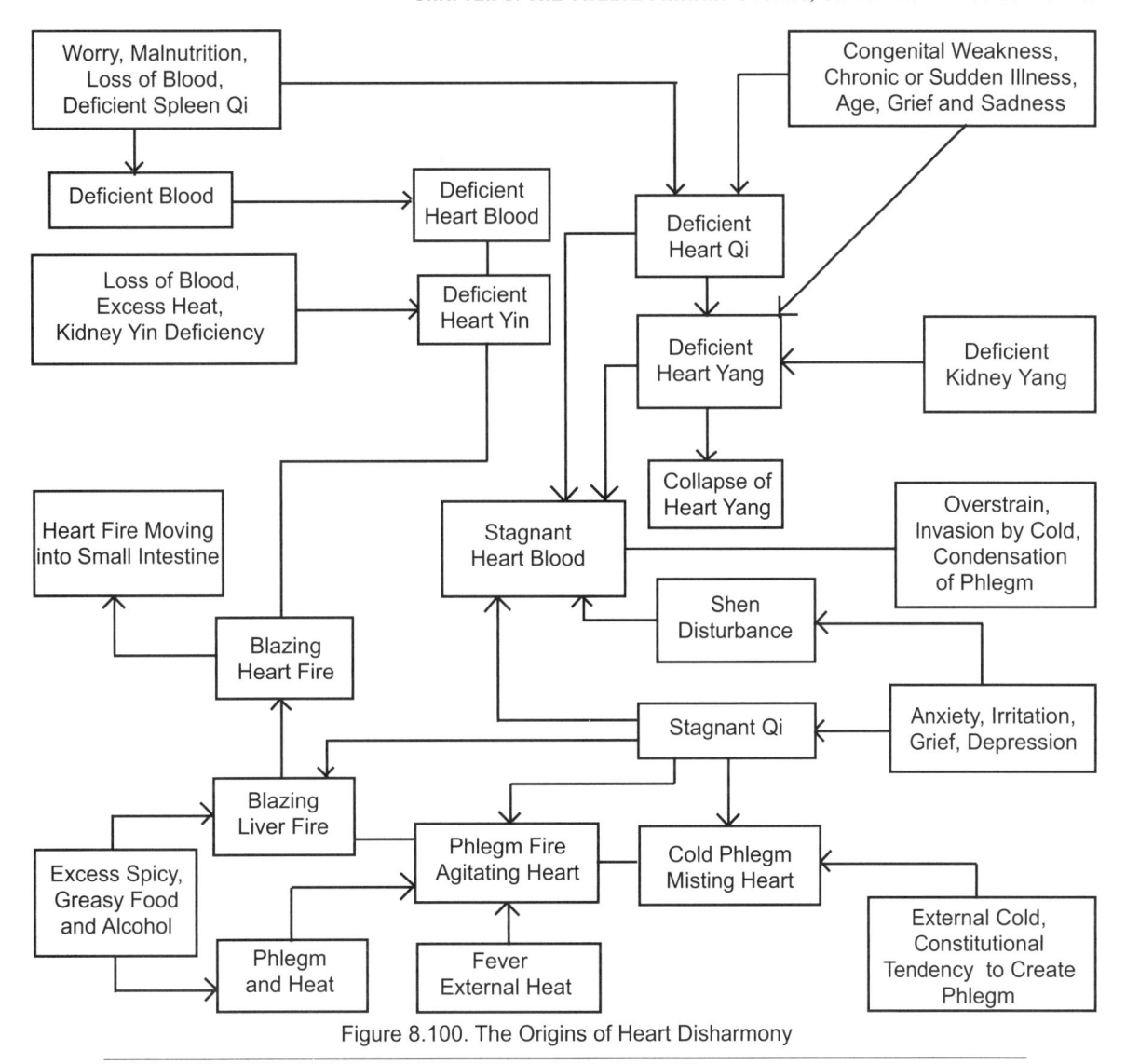

cause aphasia, paralysis and coma. The pathological patterns of Cold Phlegm Misting the Heart generally manifest through Yin (inward) imbalances, such as aphasia, depression, muttering to oneself, staring at the walls, lethargic stupor, rattling sound in the throat, or the sudden loss of consciousness.

2. **Yin Deficiency:**
   - **Deficient Heart Blood:** The pattern and pathology of Deficient Heart Blood can arise from severe hemorrhaging, chronic stress, or a poor diet (i.e., a deficiency of nourishment or lack of Blood producing foods which leads to Spleen Qi Deficiency). Symptoms of Deficient Heart Blood include palpitations, vertigo, dizziness, insomnia, poor memory, dream disturbed sleep, restlessness, headaches, anxiety, being easily startled, and general tiredness.
   - **Deficient Heart Yin:** The pattern of Deficient Heart Yin can arise either from chronic emotional stress or from an invasion of Exterior

Heat that consumes the Body Fluids and exhausts the Yin of the Heart. Symptoms of Deficient Heart Yin can manifest as low fever, palpitations, insomnia, poor concentration, poor memory, fatigue, anxiety, mental restlessness, feelings of heat, malar flush, night sweats, dry mouth and throat, and Five Palms Heat.

- **Blazing Heart Fire:** This is a Yang Excess pattern of Full Heat in the Heart, and can arise from patterns of Deficient Heart Yin. Blazing Heart Fire can form during a severe fever caused by pathological Heat invading the Pericardium. It can also originate from chronic emotional problems that lead to long term Qi Stagnation, which can eventually turn into Fire and disturb the patient's Shen. The patterns of Blazing Heart Fire are associated with mental depression. Symptoms of Blazing Heart Fire include irritability, restlessness, insomnia, feelings of heat, flushed face, tongue ulcers, bitter taste in the mouth, thirst, palpitations, dark urine, or Blood in the urine.

- **Phlegm Fire Agitating the Heart:** This is a Yang Excess pattern with similar origins to that of Blazing Heart Fire. However, in the pattern of Phlegm Fire Agitating the Heart, the pathogenic Fire and Phlegm obstruct the Heart orifices causing disturbances in the patient's Shen. When severe, these disturbances can result in violent behavior and insanity. The main manifestations of Phlegm Fire Agitating the Heart are Heart dysfunctions, often occurring in addition to pathological patterns (such as allowing Phlegm to accumulate) that are derived from Spleen Qi Deficiency. The Internal Heat aspect of Phlegm Fire Agitating the Heart, can develop during fevers caused by External Heat invading the Pericardium, or from chronic emotional problems that lead to long term Qi Stagnation. The Qi stagnation turns into Fire and disturbs the patient's Shen. The Excess consumption of hot greasy foods creates both Heat and Phlegm, and can lead to or exacerbate conditions of Phlegm Fire Agitating the Heart. The pathological patterns of Phlegm Fire Agitating the Heart generally manifest through Yang (outward) imbalances, such as palpitations, mental restlessness, confusion, agitation, violent behavior (shouting or hitting people), uncontrolled laughter or crying, mental depression, talking to oneself, aphasia, and coma (Figure 8.101).

Type of Phlegm	Cold Phlegm Misting Heart	Phlegm Fire Agitating Heart
Yin and Yang	Yin, Cold Signs, Slow Pulse, White Tongue Coat	Yang, Heat Signs, Rapid Pulse, Yellow Tongue Coat
Mental Signs	Introverted, Depressed, Staring at Walls	Extroverted, Laughing & Crying, Incoherent Talking
Disease Patterns	Wind Stroke, Depressive Psychosis	Violent Insanity, Manic Psychosis

Figure 8.101. Difference Between Cold Phlegm Misting the Heart and Phlegm Fire Agitating the Heart

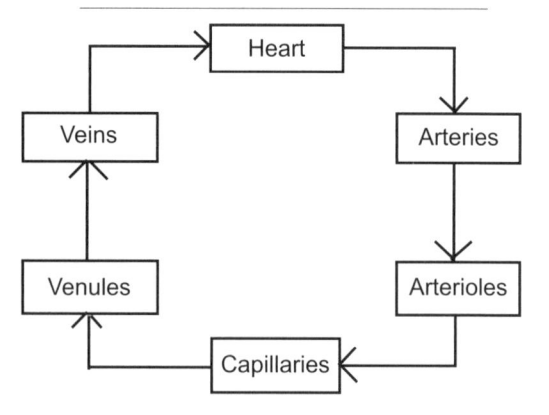

Figure 8.102. The Blood Flow within the Cardiovascular System

THE HEART IN WESTERN MEDICINE

The heart is a hollow muscular organ, located roughly in the center of the chest, It serves to pump blood throughout the body via the body's vast network of blood vessels. This network of vessels includes all the veins and arteries of the body, and

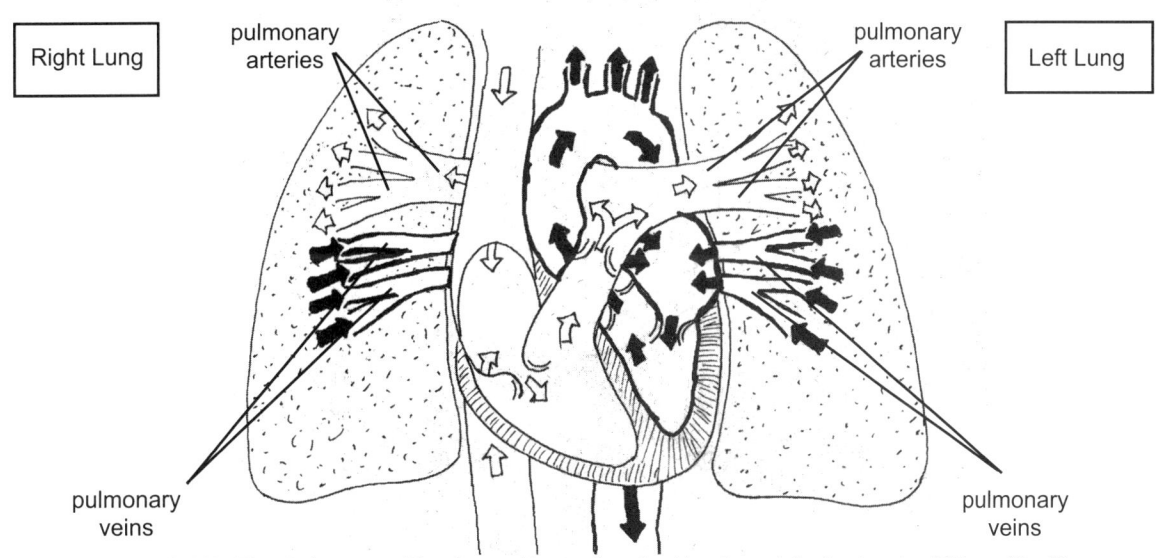

Figure 8.103. The Pulmonary Circulatory Route (Inspired by the original artwork of Wynn Kapit).

is known as the vascular system (Figure 8.102). Together, the heart and the vascular system are collectively known as the cardiovascular system. The cardiovascular system distributes blood throughout the body so that the blood may deliver nourishment directly to the cells, and remove waste from them. Though it is only about the size of a fist, and weighs an average of ten ounces, the heart is the structural and functional center of the cardiovascular system.

The heart is the hardest working muscle in the human body, beating more than 100,000 times each day. Every minute the heart pumps roughly of 10 liters of blood through approximately 96,000 kilometers (60,000 miles) of blood vessels. In trained athletes the amount of blood pumped by the heart in one minute can exceed 70 liters per minute. There are two major circulatory routes in the adult human body, each of which begins and ends with the heart. In the pulmonary circulatory route, the heart delivers deoxygenated venous blood to the lungs, and retrieves oxygenated blood from them (Figure 8.103). The systemic circulatory route then delivers this vitalized blood to all the tissues of the body, and retrieves devitalized blood from them (Figure 8.104). In systemic circulation, the heart is responsible primarily for pumping vitalized blood to the cells, while the

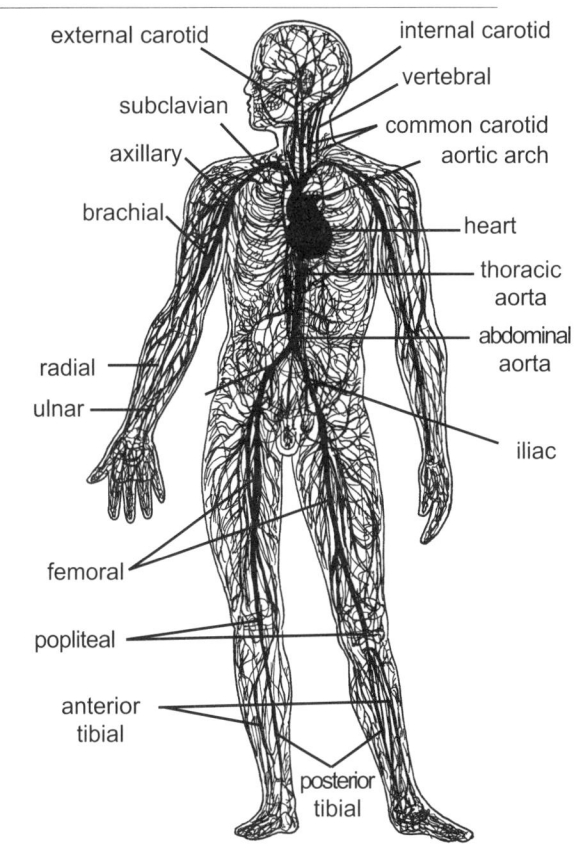

Figure 8.104. The Arterial Flow of the Systemic Circulatory System

body must rely mainly on skeletal muscular contractions and gravity for the return of venous blood to the heart.

Anatomy of the Heart

The heart organ is situated in the center of the thoracic cavity, behind and slightly to the left of the sternum, and in front of the vertebral column. Flanked by the lungs, the heart is enclosed in the mediastinum, which also contains the esophagus, the trachea, and the major blood vessels. Vertically, the heart extends from height of the second rib down to the fifth intercostal space, and it projects horizontally more to the left than to the right, due to the large size of the left ventricle. It is roughly conical in shape, with its base directed upwards and to the right, and its apex directed downward and to the left.

The heart is wrapped in a multilayered sac of connective tissue known as the pericardium. The inner layer of the pericardium is called the serous pericardium, and is itself divided into two layers. An inner visceral layer known as the epicardium covers the heart and the initial sections of the major blood vessels and is and integral part of the heart wall. The outer layer of the serous pericardium is called the parietal layer, and it surrounds the epicardium, but is separated from it by a fluid (pericardial fluid) that serves to reduce friction around the heart as it beats. This fluid-filled space between the two layers of the serous pericardium is known as the pericardial cavity. The outer (parietal) layer of the serous pericardium connects into the fibrous pericardium which surrounds it, and which is the pericardium's outermost layer.

The fibrous pericardium is a strong and dense sheath of connective tissue that surrounds the heart and firmly anchors within the thorax. It surrounds the major blood vessels (the superior and inferior vena cava, the right and left pulmonary arteries, the pulmonary veins, and the aorta), which extend outward from superior aspects of the heart, and continues upward to anchor into the cervical fascia. In front, the fibrous pericardium attaches to the internal aspect of the sternum, while it also extends downward to anchor firmly into the diaphragm below.

The wall of the heart is itself composed of three layers. The outer layer of the heart is the epicardium, described above. The myocardium is the middle layer, while the innermost layer of the heart is called the endocardium. The muscular contractions that are the beating of the heart take place at the level of the myocardium. The myocardium forms the bulk of the heart, and is composed mainly of heart muscle tissue. Within the cardiac muscle tissue of the myocardium, crisscrossing bundles of connective tissue wrap around the heart in a dense network that both reinforces the heart internally and provides additional support for the major vessels that connect with the heart. The endocardium is a sheet of endothelial tissue that lines all the inside of all the chambers of the heart; the tissue of the endocardium is continuous with the endothelium (inner lining) of the blood vessels.

The Four Chambers of the Heart

Structurally, the heart is divided into four chambers: two atria (right and left) that receive blood into the heart, and the two comparatively larger ventricles (right and left) that pump blood away from the heart. Within the heart, blood flows in one direction only. Atrioventricular valves (the tricuspid valve and the bicuspid valve) act as one-way valves that prevent the blood pumped by the atria into the ventricles from flowing backwards into the atria again. Semilunar valves (the pulmonary semilunar valve and the aortic semilunar valve) prevent arterial blood from flowing backwards into the ventricles.

The sequence of blood flow within the heart is as follows: superior and inferior vena cava - right atrium - (tricuspid valve) - right ventricle - (pulmonary semilunar valve) - pulmonary trunk - right and left pulmonary arteries - (lungs) - pulmonary veins - left atrium - (bicuspid valve) - left ventricle - (aortic semilunar valve) - aorta - whole body. The four chambers of the heart are described as follows (Figure 8.105):

1. **Right Atrium:** The right atrium receives deoxygenated venous blood via the superior vena cava, which drains the upper body; and the inferior vena cava, which drains the lower

body. The coronary sinus, which drains venous blood from the heart organ itself, also flows into the right atrium. After expanding to receive this blood, the right atrium contracts and pumps the blood into the right ventricle.

2. **Right Ventricle:** the right ventricle receives the deoxygenated blood pumped from the right atrium. As the right ventricle contracts, a valve known as the tricuspid valve prevents blood from flowing back into the right atrium. The right ventricle pumps blood to the lungs via a major vessel known as the pulmonary trunk, which quickly branches into the right and left pulmonary arteries. After contracting, the left ventricle expands, and the pulmonary semilunar valve closes to prevent the back-flow of blood from the pulmonary trunk. The pulmonary arteries are the only arteries in the body that carry deoxygenated (blue) blood.

3. **Left Atrium:** Four pulmonary veins return blood that has been oxygenated by the lungs, delivering it into the left atrium. The left atrium pumps this blood into the left ventricle. The bicuspid (mitral) valve, which is situated between the left atrium and the left ventricle, immediately closes as the left atrium finishes its contraction, and thus serves to prevent a back-flow of blood as the left ventricle contracts.

4. **Left Ventricle:** The left ventricle is the largest and strongest of the heart's four chambers, and it has the function of pumping vitalized blood through the whole body. For this reason, the muscular walls of the left ventricle are thicker than those of the heart's other chambers. After receiving blood from the left atrium, the left ventricle contracts to pump blood out into the aorta. Back-flow into the left ventricle from the aorta is prevented by the aortic semilunar valve. The aorta is the largest blood vessel in the body, and it quickly divides into the other major arteries (left and right subclavian arteries, left and right carotid arteries, descending aorta, and the coronary arteries) that distribute oxygenated blood to the tissues.

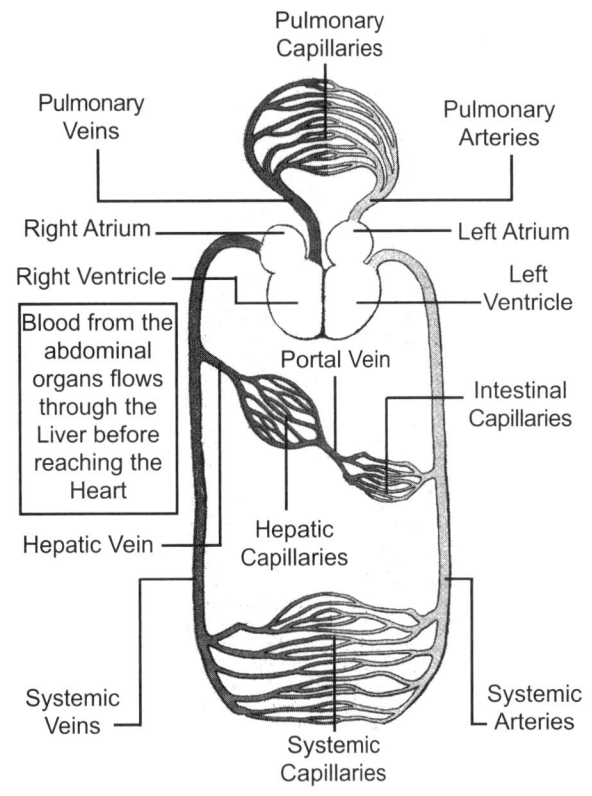

Figure 8.105. The sequence of arterial and venous blood flow (Inspired from the original artwork of H.V. Carter).

THE HEARTBEAT: CARDIAC CYCLE

Each heartbeat, or cardiac cycle, is divided into two phases in which both sides of the heart contract and relax simultaneously. The term systole is used to denote the contractive phase of the cardiac cycle, while the term diastole refers to the relaxation period. The two ventricles contract (ventricular systole) as the atria relax (atrial diastole), then the two atria contract (atrial systole) as the ventricles relax (ventricular diastole).

Listening through a physician's stethoscope, the "lub" sound of the heartbeat is produced as the tricuspid and bicuspid valves snap shut during ventricular contraction, while the "dub" sound is the result of the closing of the aortic and pulmonary semilunar valves during ventricular diastole. Ventricular diastole takes slightly longer than ventricular systole, hence the pause between heartbeats. Heart rate in the average adult is around 72 beats per minute. It is usually about 80 beats per minute in children, while in infants a normal heart rate may be as high as 120 beats per minute.

THE HEART'S ELECTRICAL SYSTEM

The heart produces its own electrical impulses independent of nervous stimulation from the central nervous system. Communication between the heart and the central nervous system takes place through the both sympathetic and parasympathetic nerve impulses. The electrical stimulus that initiates the contractions of the heart originates within the sinoatrial node (SA node). The SA node is alternately known as the sinus node, or the pacemaker, and it is located in the right atrium of the heart (Figure 8.106). The electrical impulse it produces travels into the atria, causing them to contact, while also continuing through conductive pathways to the atrioventricular node (AV node). Located in the septum between the two atria, the AV node rapidly conducts this charge into the ventricles (via the AV bundle, then the Purkinje fibers), causing them to contract immediately after the atrial contraction. Other areas of the heart contain electrically insulating tissue to insure the proper conduction of this essential electrical impulse. An electrocardiogram (ECG) is the most common method of recording the electrical activity of the heart.

COMMON DISORDERS OF THE HEART

Common disorders of the heart include the following: heart failure (inability of the heart to supply adequate blood flow to the tissues), artherosclerosis (hardening or narrowing of the vessels), valve disorders (such as valve prolapse), fibrosis of the cardiac muscle, myocarditis, pericarditis, hypertension, hypotension (low blood pressure), and congenital heart defects. In coronary artery disease, sometimes known as ischemic heart disease, there is inadequate blood flow to the heart tissues, often resulting in hypoxia and

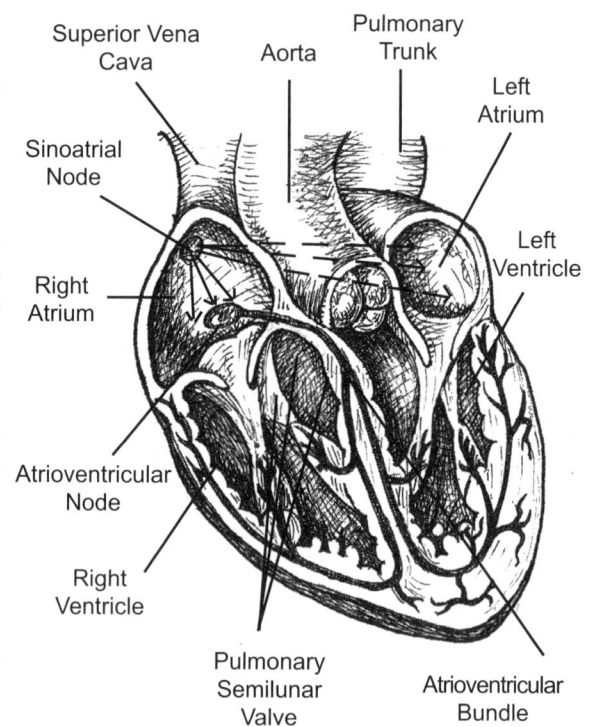

Figure 8.106. The Sinoatrial (SA) Node is located in the right atrium of the heart

angina. A heart attack, or myocardial infarction, generally involves severely reduced blood flow to the heart tissue resulting in irreversible damage to myocardial tissues. Cardiac arrhythmias include dysrhythmia, heart block, heart flutters, atrial or ventricular fibrillation, and ventricular premature contraction. A heart palpitation is a heartbeat that is unusually fast, strong, or otherwise irregular enough to be noticed by a patient. Tachycardia is any abnormally fast heart rate (over 100 BPM), while bradycardia describes an unusually slow heart rate (lower than 60 BPM). The term murmurs refers to unusual or abnormal heart sounds, angina pectoris refers to general chest pain in the area of the heart (usually due to hypoxia), and cardiac arrest refers to the cessation of an effective heartbeat.

CHAPTER 8: THE TWELVE PRIMARY ORGANS, CHANNELS AND COLLATERALS

THE SMALL INTESTINE:
XIAO CHANG

The Small Intestine is the Yang (hollow) organ paired with the Heart, and is associated with the Fire Element. The ancient Chinese understood the role of the Small Intestine in digestion and observed that the veins of the organ provided the means of absorbing nutrients into the Blood stream (Figure 8.107).

CHINESE CHARACTER FOR SMALL INTESTINE: XIAO CHANG

- The first character "Xiao" describes an object that has been split in two, and translates as "small or little."
- The second character "Chang" translates as "intestine," and is divided into two ideographs. The character to the left, "Ji" depicts the Chinese ideogram for body tissue, muscle or flesh (all of which are forms of connective tissue). The character on the right depicts the image of the sun above the horizon, with its rays shining downward. It expresses the Heavenly Yang influence on this particular organ. The ideograph represents the image of the sun enriching and transforming something within the flesh and conveys the Small Intestine's role in the digestive process.

Together, the Chinese characters "Xiao Chang" can be translated as, "the small Heavenly transformation occurring within the flesh." The Small Intestines command the "Ye," the thicker aspect of the intestinal fluids (Figure 8.108).

THE SMALL INTESTINE IN CHINESE MEDICINE

The functions of the Small Intestine described in Traditional Chinese Medicine are similar to those that are described in Western Medicine. According to Traditional Chinese Medicine, the main functions of the Small Intestine are to: control the reception, transformation and absorption of food content; separate the clear from the turbid; and express itself through the psycho-emotional aspects of mental clarity and powers of discernment. These main

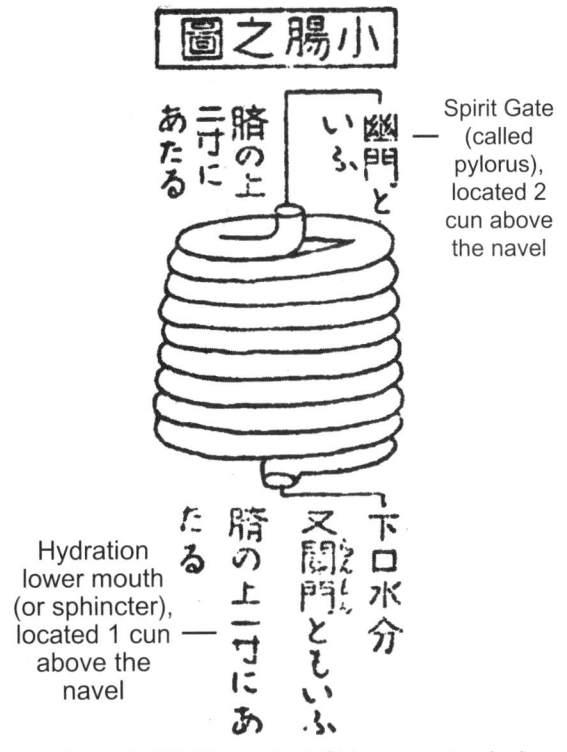

Spirit Gate (called pylorus), located 2 cun above the navel

Hydration lower mouth (or sphincter), located 1 cun above the navel

Figure 8.107. The ancient Chinese anatomical diagram of the Small Intestine (SI) Organ, as it appeared in "Important Useful Notes on Acupuncture and Moxibustion," published in Japan in 1718, by Masatoyo Hongo

An Object Being Split in Two

Sun Above the Horizon

Muscle, Flesh, Connective Tissue

Sun's Rays Shining Down

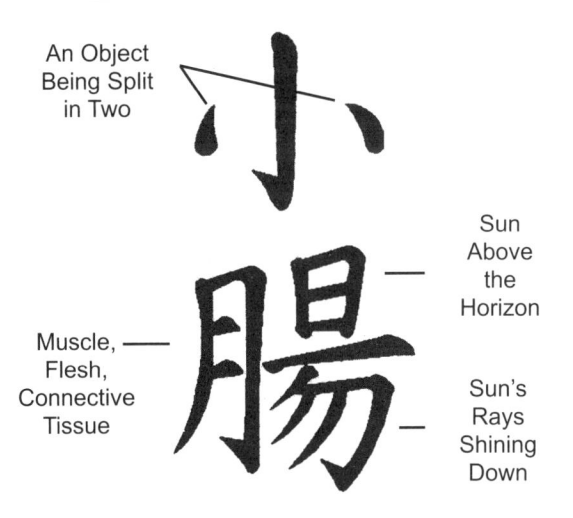

Figure 8.108. The Chinese characters for "Xiao Chang," Small Intestine

405

```
                    ┌─ Controls the Reception, Transformation and Absorption of Food Content
The Main Functions  │
of the Small        ├─ Separates the Clear from the Turbid ── Separating the Pure From the Impure
Intestine Organ     │
and Channels        └─ Psycho-Emotional Aspects ── Influences Mental Clarity, Judgment, and Powers of Discernment
```

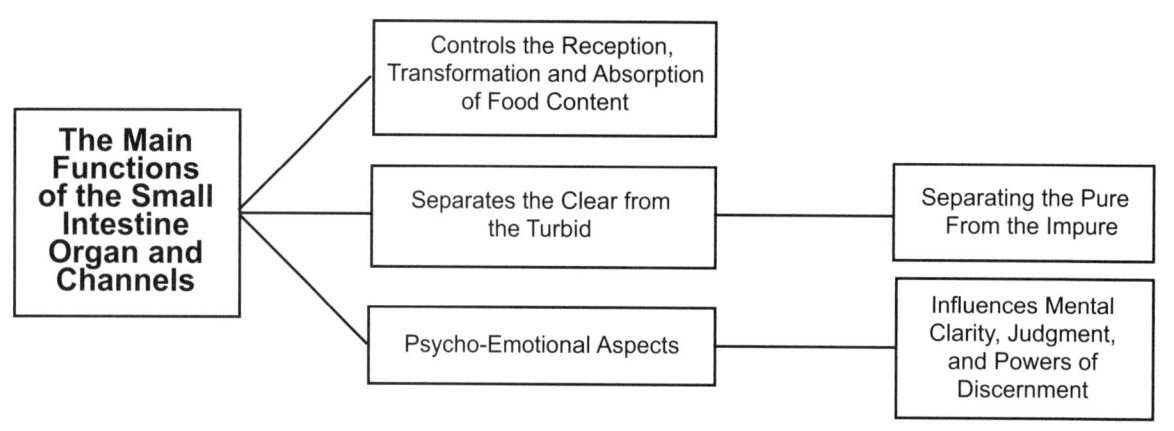

Figure 8.109. The Main Energetic Functions of the Small Intestine Organ and Channels

functions are described as follows (Figure 8.109):

1. **Controls the Reception, Transformation and Absorption of Food Content:** The Small Intestine temporarily stores partially digested food, allowing for the absorption of the essential substances of the undigested food and a portion of the liquid content. It later transfers the remaining residue (along with a considerable amount of liquid) to the Large Intestine. It is for this reason that the Small Intestine is said to "govern liquid."

2. **Separates the Clear from the Turbid:** The Small Intestine is sometimes called "the official in charge of separating the pure from the impure" because it separates the "clean" (usable) food essence (Gu Qi) from the "dirty, turbid" (unusable) food essence. The clean Gu Qi is sent to the Spleen, which transports and distributes it throughout the body to nourish the tissues. The waste (turbid) portion is transported to the Large Intestine and Urinary Bladder organs to be further processed. The unwanted liquid is directed into the Urinary Bladder which further refines the liquid into pure and impure portions; the pure portion is sent to moisten the skin and muscles, and the impure portion is excreted from the body in the form of urine.

3. **Psycho-Emotional Aspects:** The Small Intestine is also in charge of sorting the pure from the impure on the level of thoughts and emotions, influencing the individual's mental clarity, judgment, and powers of discernment. Thus, the ability to effectively distinguish relevant issues with clarity before making a decision is attributed to the Small Intestine.

The Small Intestine is also known as "the minister who guards the emperor's inner quarters," and it can act as a filtering lens that focuses the intention of the Heart. The Small Intestine helps the Heart to maintain clarity of Mind, and to distinguish right from wrong. It is believed that sarcasm and sexual perversion may be the result of the Small Intestine not being able to receive or transmit Heart essence properly.

THE SMALL INTESTINE CHANNELS

The Small Intestine Channels are Yang channels that flow externally from the hands to the head. These two rivers originate externally from the lateral tips (ulnar side) of the little fingers, then ascend the arms to the shoulders where they divide into two pairs of branches. At the SI-16 points, one pair of branches descends the supraclavicular fossa internally, spiral wraps the Heart, then continues down the esophagus, diaphragm, and Stomach before penetrating the Small Intestine (Figure 8.110).

The other pair of branches ascends from the SI-16 point, travelling externally up the sides of the neck, before dividing into two more pairs of branches at the cheek. One pair of these branches ends at the ears, while the other pair ends at the lateral sides of the nose and inner canthus of the eyes.

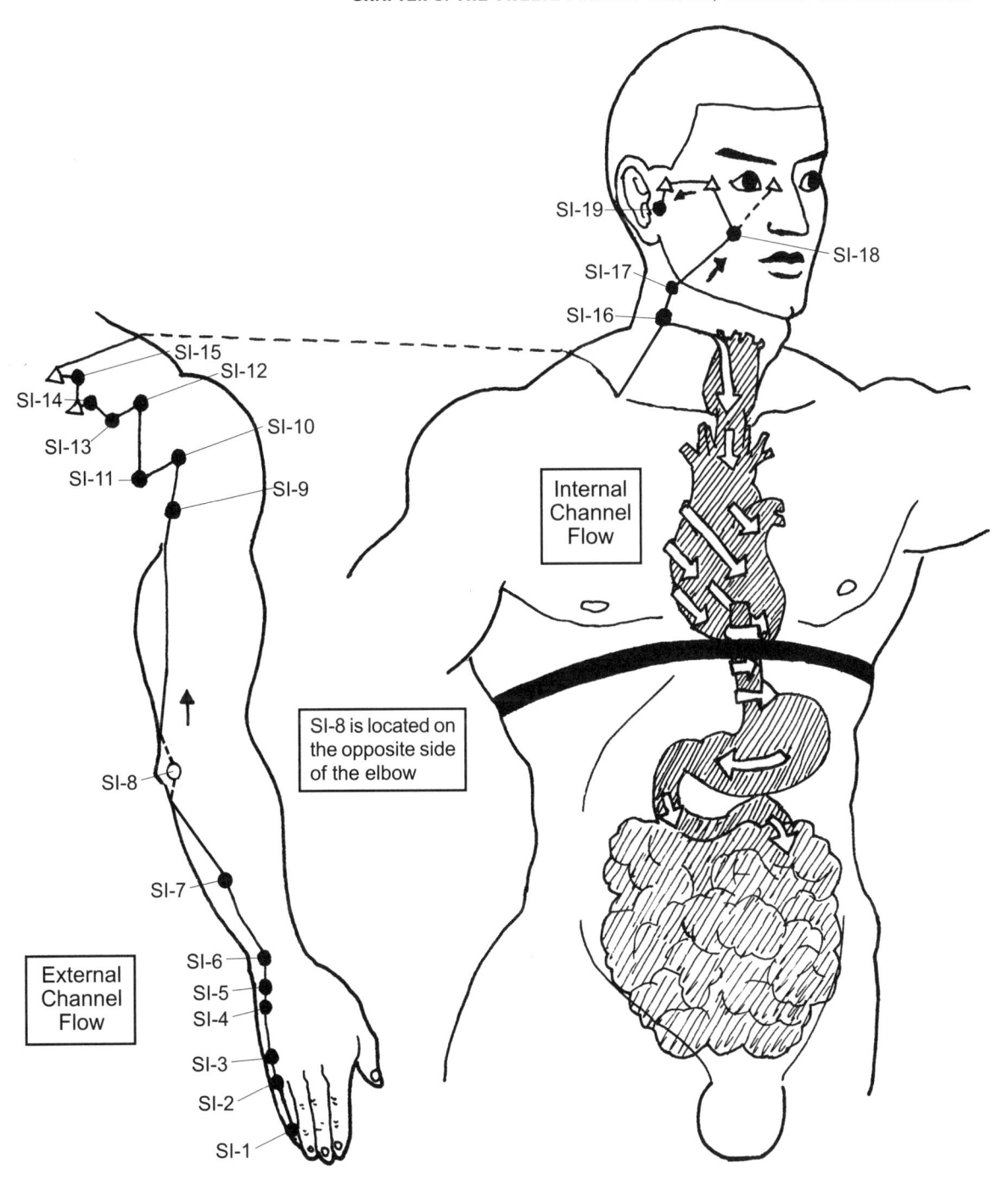

CHAPTER 8: THE TWELVE PRIMARY ORGANS, CHANNELS AND COLLATERALS

Figure 8.110. The Internal and External Qi Flow of the Small Intestine (SI) Channels

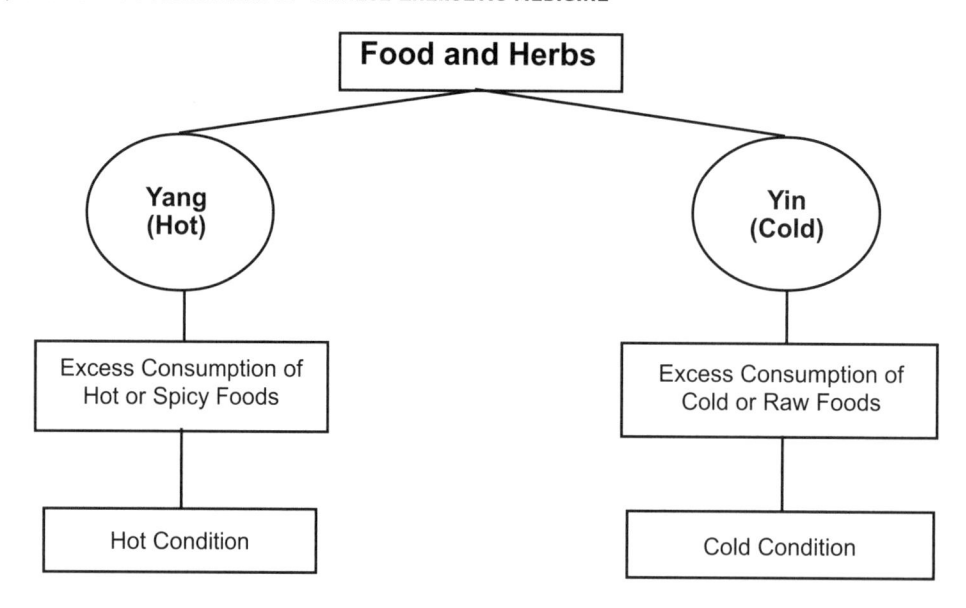

Figure 8.111. The Small Intestine is easily affected by the type and temperature of food eaten

Channels' Energy Flow

The Small Intestine Channels store more Blood than Qi and act more on the physical substances and Blood functions than on energy. At the high-tide time period (1 p.m. to 3 p.m.), Qi and Blood abound in the Small Intestine organ and Small Intestine channels. At this time, the Small Intestine organ and channels can more easily be dispersed and purged. During low tide (1 a.m. to 3 a.m.), they can be more readily tonified. The energy of the Small Intestine Channels acts on the skin, muscles, and nerves found along their pathway.

The Influence of Food Temperature

The Small Intestine can be easily injured by specific types and "temperatures" of food. In Traditional Chinese Medicine, food and herbs are categorized as having either Yin (Cold) or Yang (Hot) properties. An excess consumption of Cold or raw foods, for example, can create a Cold condition within the Small Intestine, while an excess consumption of Hot or spicy foods can create a Hot condition (Figure 8.111).

The Influence of Taste, Color, and Sound

- The bitter taste can be used to tonify both the Small Intestine and Heart
- The light red color is used to tonify the Small Intestine.
- The "Ha," "Ke" and "Zheng" sounds are used to purge the Small Intestine and the Heart.

Small Intestine Pathology

Diseases of the Small Intestine organ and channels include diseases of the face, ear, cheek, lower jaw, neck, throat, and the dorsal ulnar side of the upper extremities.

Pathologic Heat in the Heart may be transmitted to the Small Intestine, resulting in urodynia (painful urination) and hematuria (blood in the urine). Herbal prescriptions used to dispel Heat from the Heart are sometimes employed in treating these urinary symptoms when they contribute to a dysfunction of the Small Intestine.

T.C.M. Patterns of Disharmony

Patterns of disharmony associated with the Small Intestine organ and channels are classified

```
                           ┌─────────────────────────────────────┐
                         ┌─│   Full Heat in the Small Intestine  │
                         │ └─────────────────────────────────────┘
                         │ ┌─────────────────────────────────────┐
                    ┌────┤ │     Pain in the Small Intestine     │
                    │Excess─┤─────────────────────────────────────┘
                    │Patterns ┌─────────────────────────────────────┐
                    │    │ │  Obstructed Qi in the Small Intestine │
Small ──────────────┤    │ └─────────────────────────────────────┘
Intestine           │    │ ┌─────────────────────────────────────┐
Disorders           │    └─│ Infestation of Worms within the Small Intestine │
                    │      └─────────────────────────────────────┘
                    │ ┌─────────┐ ┌─────────────────────────────────────┐
                    └─│Deficient│─│  Deficient and Cold in the Small Intestine │
                      │Patterns │ └─────────────────────────────────────┘
                      └─────────┘
```

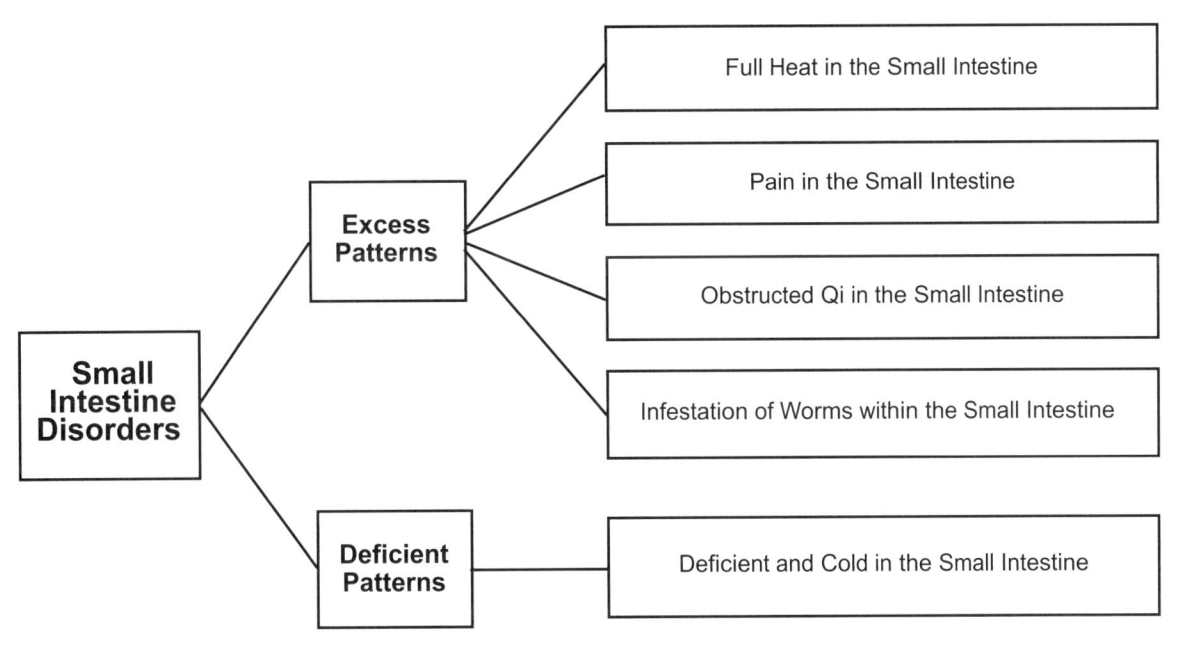

Figure 8.112. The Origins of Small Intestine Disharmony

as either excess or deficient patterns, described as follows (Figure 8.112):

1. **Excess Patterns of the Small Intestine:**
   - **Full Heat in the Small Intestine:** This pattern is closely associated with Blazing Heart Fire and Internal Full Heat, and can be created through chronic emotional stress. Symptoms can manifest as mental restlessness, irritability, abdominal pain, uncomfortable feelings of heat in the chest, thirst, tongue ulcers, painful urination, and Blood in the urine.
   - **Pain in the Small Intestine:** This pattern is a type of Qi Stagnation, and is usually associated with Liver Qi invading the Spleen. This condition can either be acute or chronic. Symptoms can manifest as abdominal distension, borborygmus (intestinal rumbling caused by moving gas), flatulence, lower abdominal "twisting" pain (which may extend into the patient's back), and pain in the testes.
   - **Obstructed Qi in the Small Intestine:** This pattern is closely associated with the Western syndrome of acute intestinal obstruction, and can resemble an acute appendicitis. Obstructed Qi in the Small Intestine can be caused from an excessive consumption of Cold or raw foods, which can impede the Small Intestine's function of transforming food essence. Symptoms of obstructed Qi in the Small Intestine can manifest as violent abdominal pain, abdominal distension, borborygmus, flatulence, constipation, and vomiting of faecal material.
   - **Infestation of Worms within the Small Intestine:** This type of obstruction of the Small Intestine is due to the infestation of intestinal parasites that cause abdominal pain and distension. According to ancient Chinese medicine, the infestation of worms was believed to be caused by a Cold condition occurring within the Small Intestines and the Spleen, which allows the worms to live. Different worms manifest through various symptoms: roundworms can cause abdominal pain, cold limbs, and the vomiting of the roundworm parasites; hookworms may cause the patient to eat unnatural objects such as dirt, leaves, and various uncooked foods; tapeworms often cause the patient to experience a state of

constant hunger; and pinworms can cause the patient to experience itching in or around the anus which worsens at night.
2. **Deficient Patterns of the Small Intestine:**
- **Deficiency and Cold in the Small Intestine:** This is an internal pattern of deficiency (usually of Spleen Yang) and Cold. It can be caused from an excessive consumption of Cold and raw foods. Symptoms can manifest as abdominal pain, borborygmus, diarrhea, and a desire for hot drinks.

THE SMALL INTESTINE IN WESTERN MEDICINE

The small intestine is a convoluted tube, 1 inch in diameter, with an average length of 21 feet (Figure 8.113). It begins at the pyloric sphincter of the stomach and coils through the central and lower aspect of the abdominal cavity, terminating at the ileocecal valve, which connects to the large intestine. The entire length of the small intestine is anchored to the peritoneum by sheetlike extensions of connective tissues called mesentery.

The small intestine is the body's primary organ of digestion and assimilation. Nearly all of the digestion and absorption of nutrients takes place within the small intestine. In order to facilitate this function, the small intestine is lined with nearly 500 million villi which greatly increase the surface area available for food absorption. These intestinal villi are tiny hairlike projections of epithelium (skin-like tissue) that extend outwards from the internal wall of the small intestine. The villi contain a rich network of capillaries that serve to expose the blood to the nutrients available in the chyme contained within the small intestine. Combined with the microvilli, the villi of the small intestine expose about 300 square meters (roughly the size of tennis court) of surface area to the chyme.

The mucosa and submucosa within the walls of the small intestine are designed to allow for the ability to efficiently digest and absorb chyme. The epithelial cells in the mucosa consist of simple columnar epithelium, and contain absorptive cells, enteroendocrine cells, Paneth cells, and goblet cells. The goblet cells secrete additional mucus.

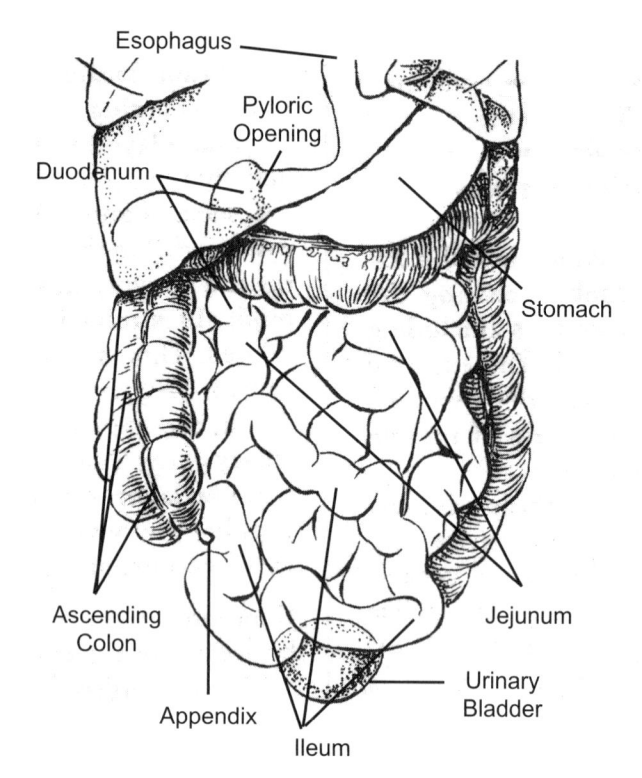

Figure 8.113. The Small Intestine (SI) Organ (Inspired by the original artwork of Wynn Kapit).

The small intestine is divided into three segments: the duodenum, the jejunum, and the ileum, which are described as follows:

1. **Duodenum:** Originating from the pyloric sphincter of the stomach, the duodenum is the shortest piece of the small intestine, extending only 10 inches before merging with the jejunum. The duodenum is relatively immovable and mostly retroperitoneal, curving around the head of the pancreas. Within the duodenum, secretions from the liver and pancreas, in addition to certain secretions from the small intestine, are introduced into the chyme, causing it to break down and become more absorbable. The submucosa of the duodenum also contain duodenal glands, that secrete an alkaline mucus that helps to neutralize the gastric acid within the chyme.
2. **Jejunum:** The jejunum is an intraperitoneal (contained within the peritoneum) organ.

Originating from the duodenum, the jejunum coils and winds through the abdomen, extending a distance of about 8 feet before it merges with the ileum.

3. **Ileum:** The ileum is also an intraperitoneal organ, and is the longest portion of the small intestine. Originating from the jejunum, the ileum coils and winds through the abdomen, extending for a distance of about 12 feet. It terminates at the ileocecal valve, which separates the small intestine from the large intestine.

Physiology

The small intestine has two primary functions, digestion and assimilation (Figure 8.114). Digestion refers to the process of breaking down the chyme to make it absorbable, while assimilation refers to the process whereby nutrients are absorbed into the blood through the intestinal wall. Wavelike peristaltic contractions ripple along the entire length of the gastrointestinal tract, propelling the food mass through the esophagus, stomach, small intestine, and large intestine. Chyme travels from the stomach and through the small intestine in this way, before being introduced into the cecum of the large intestine via the ileocecal valve.

Chyme from the stomach is released a little at a time into the small intestine via the pyloric sphincter. At this point, the chyme has already been partially broken down by the hydrochloric acid, intrinsic factor, and pepsin that were released into it within the stomach. Secretions of bile (from the liver and gallbladder) are released into the chyme in the duodenum via the bile duct, while the pancreatic duct introduces into the chyme various enzymes (amylase, trypsin, lipase, etc.) secreted by the pancreas. The pancreas also releases sodium bicarbonate into the duodenum to neutralize the acidity of the chyme, changing the PH of the chyme in the small intestine to slightly basic.

The bile released into the small intestine serves mainly to emulsify (cause large molecules to break down into smaller ones) fats, thereby making it possible for them to be absorbed into the blood through the thin cell walls of the villi (Figure 8.115). Pancreatic amylase combines starches with water and converts them into the

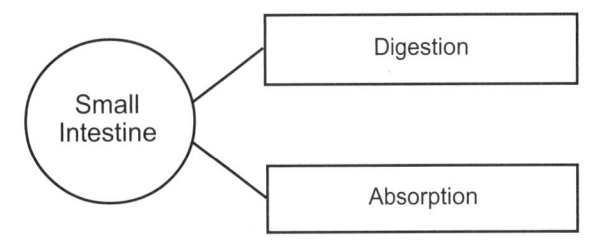

Figure 8.114. The Functions of the Small Intestine (Western Medical Perspective)

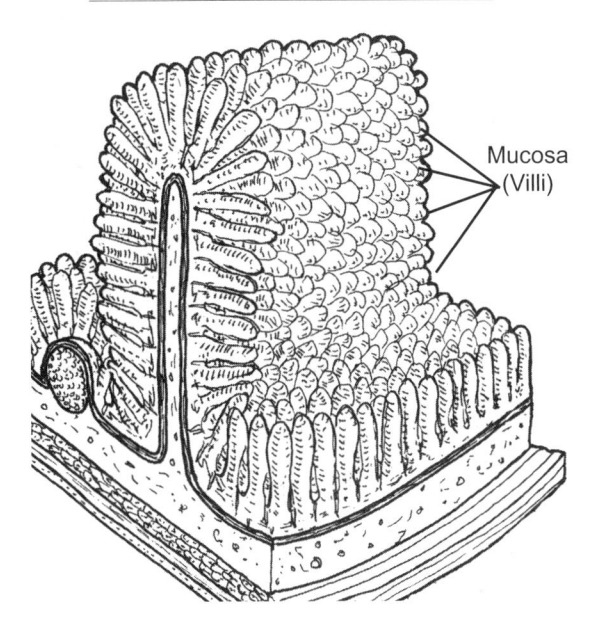

Figure 8.115. The Small Intestine Mucosa (Villi) (Inspired by the original artwork of Wynn Kapit).

absorbable sugar maltose. Trypsin combines proteins with water to form peptides, which are then absorbed through the intestinal wall. Lipase digests fat droplets and converts them into absorbable glycerol and various fatty acids. The cells of the small intestine also secrete various enzymes (maltase, sucrase, lactase, peptidases, etc.) into the chyme, thus breaking it down still further.

By the time the chyme reaches the ileocecal valve, nearly all available nutrients (e.g., carbohydrates, proteins, and fats) have been absorbed into the bloodstream. The remainder of the food mass then passes into the large intestine, at which point it is referred to as feces.

The Urinary Bladder: Pang Guang

The Urinary Bladder is a Yang (hollow) organ that is paired with the Kidneys, and is associated with the Water Element (Figure 8.116).

Chinese Character for Urinary Bladder: Pang Guang

The Chinese characters "Pang Guang" can be translated as the internal organ that operates as "the roadside place of brightness." This expresses the Urinary Bladder's function as the keeper of the "Bladder Fire" or "Common Peoples Fire," which is responsible for transforming Jing (Essence) into Qi (Energy).

- The first character "Pang" translates as "Urinary Bladder." It is composed of two characters: the character to the left, "Ji" depicts the Chinese ideogram for body tissue, muscle or flesh (all of which are forms of connective tissue); on the right upper half is the radical for roadside, the bottom half is the radical for place (Figure 8.117).
- The second character "Guang" is composed of two characters: the character to the left, "Ji" depicts the Chinese ideogram for body tissue, muscle or flesh (all of which are forms of connective tissue). On the right is the radical for brightness, light and illumination. In ancient China, the character Guang was composed of two separate characters: the radical twenty placed at the top of the ideograph, and the fire radical placed at the bottom. Together the characters stood for the brightness of twenty fires.

The Urinary Bladder in Chinese Medicine

The functions of the Urinary Bladder in Traditional Chinese Medicine are almost the same as those described in Western Medicine. However, Chinese energetic medicine also considers the functions of the Urinary Bladder to include the transforming fluids, the storing of the Urinary Bladder Fire, and the governing of various psycho-emotional aspects.

According to Traditional Chinese Medicine,

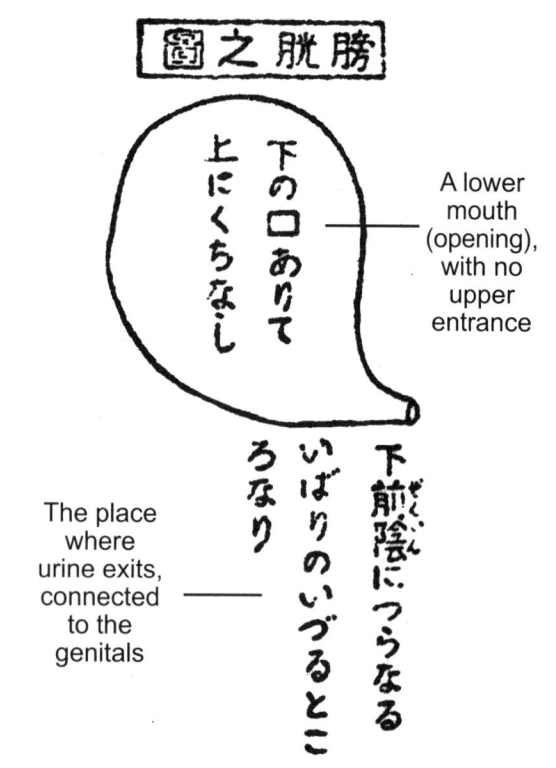

Figure 8.116. The ancient Chinese anatomical diagram of the Urinary Bladder (UB) Organ, as it appeared in "Important Useful Notes on Acupuncture and Moxibustion," published in Japan in 1718, by Masatoyo Hongo

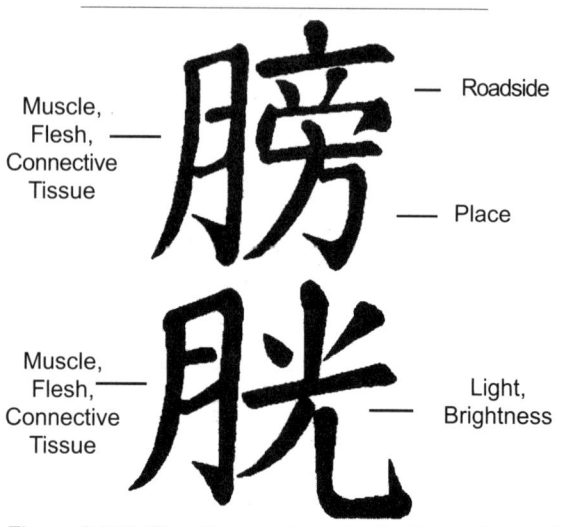

Figure 8.117. The Chinese character for "Pang Guang," Urinary Bladder

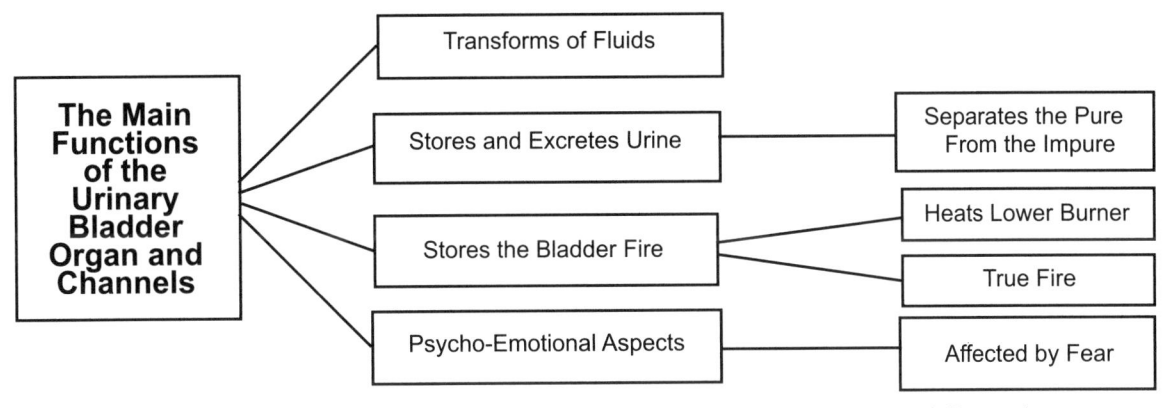

Figure 8.118. The Main Energetic Functions of the Urinary Bladder Organ and Channels

the main functions of the Urinary Bladder are to: store and excrete urine, store the Urinary Bladder Fire, transform fluids, and express itself through the psycho-emotional aspects of fear and lack of decision making. These main functions are described as follows (Figure 8.118):

1. **Transforms Fluids:** One function of the Urinary Bladder is to remove water by Qi transformation. The Urinary Bladder receives the "impure" portion of the fluids that have been separated by the Kidneys from the Lungs, and from the Small Intestine and Large Intestine. The Urinary Bladder temporarily stores and transforms these fluids into urine, and then discharges the urine when the Urinary Bladder is full.

2. **Stores and Excretes Urine:** The Urinary Bladder is sometimes called "the water district officials (or controllers) of the storage of waste water." The Urinary Bladder's function of storing and excreting urine is dependent on the Qi and Heat that is provided by Kidney Yang.

   Because the primary function of the Triple Burner is Body Fluid movement and metabolism, there is a functional link between the Urinary Bladder and the Lower Burner. The Urinary Bladder and the Small Intestine work together to remove fluids from the Lower Burner.

3. **Stores the Urinary Bladder Fire:** The Bladder Fire, also called the Common People's Fire, is located in the lower abdominal area near the perineum. It is responsible for evaporating water, heating the Lower Burner, the transforming Jing into Qi; it is also an aspect of the body's "True Fire" (see Triple Burners).

4. **Psycho-Emotional Aspects:** The Urinary Bladder stores and utilizes the body's energetic reserves, and like the Kidneys, it is affected by fear. An imbalance in the Urinary Bladder can cause such psychological symptoms as habitual fear, lack of ability to make decisions, and diminished moral character. If the imbalance becomes chronic, it can result in emotional responses such as jealousy, suspicion, and holding on to long-standing grudges.

THE URINARY BLADDER CHANNELS

The Urinary Bladder Channels are Yang channels that flow externally from the head to the feet (Figure 8.119). The two rivers of the Urinary Bladder Channels originate externally from the inner canthus of the eyes. From the inner canthus of the eyes they ascend upward over the head to join the Governing Vessel at the GV-20 point where they divide into two additional branches that flow into each temple and into the Brain. From the GV-20 point, the main channels flow down the back of the head to the UB-10 points, where they again divide into two sets of branches that descend the lateral aspect of the back and connect to the Kidneys at the UB-23 points. From the UB-23 points, the internal flow of the Urinary Bladder Channels rushes into the lower back and lumbar area, passing through the renal arteries, and spirally wrapping the Kidneys. From the Kidneys, the energy flows downward, along the ureter, and penetrates

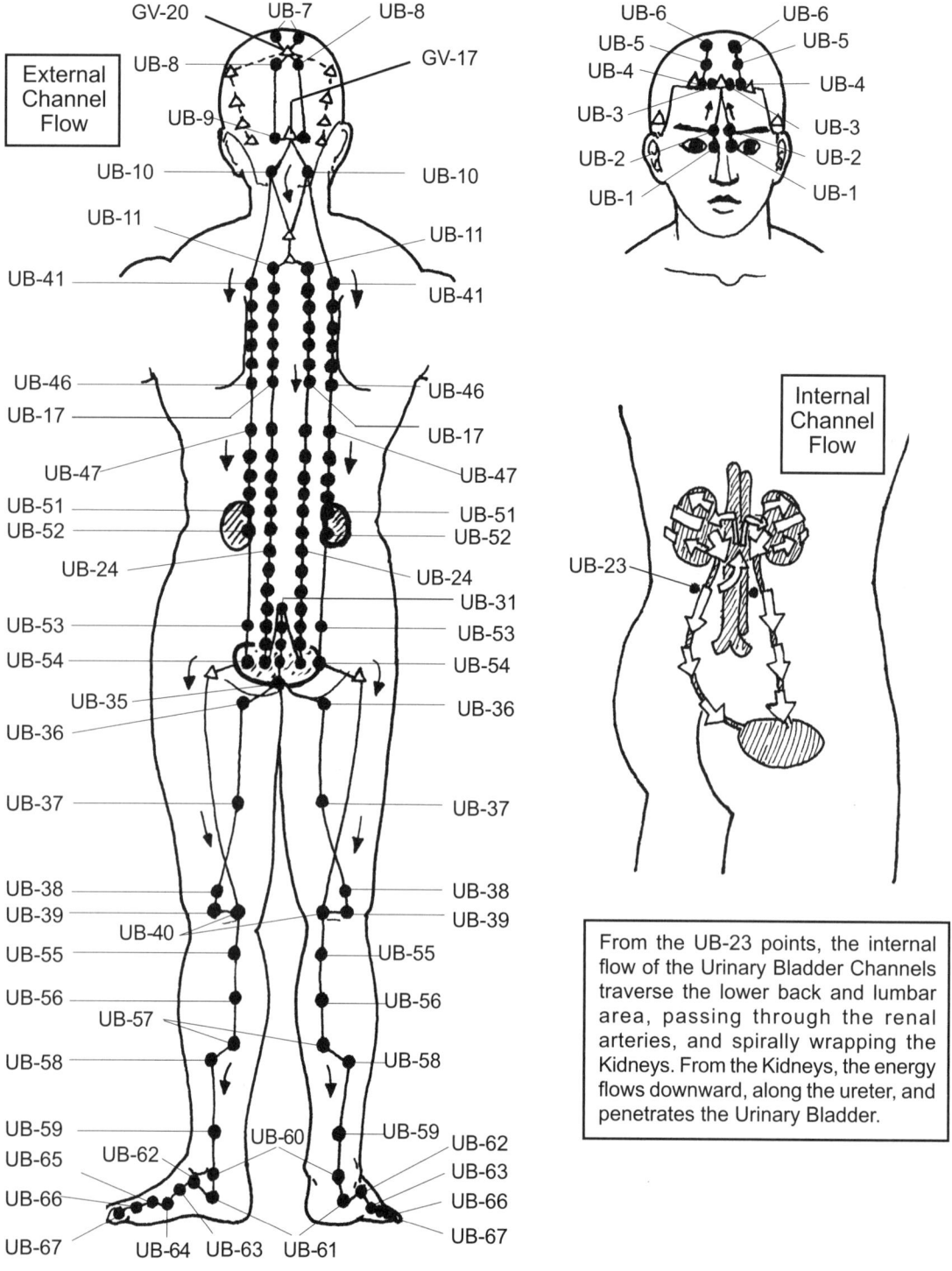

Figure 8.119. The Internal and External Qi Flow of the Urinary Bladder (UB) Channels

From the UB-23 points, the internal flow of the Urinary Bladder Channels traverse the lower back and lumbar area, passing through the renal arteries, and spirally wrapping the Kidneys. From the Kidneys, the energy flows downward, along the ureter, and penetrates the Urinary Bladder.

the Urinary Bladder. From the Urinary Bladder the main branches continue externally down the medial aspect of the thighs, pooling at the popliteal fossa located at the back of the knees. From the popliteal fossa the main channels further descend the calf and foot, ending on the lateral sides of the tips of the little toes.

Channels' Energy Flow

The Urinary Bladder Channels regulate the functions of the Kidneys. The Urinary Bladder Channels store more Blood than Qi, and act more on the physical substances and the Blood functions than on energy. At the high-tide time period (3 p.m. to 5 p.m.), Qi and Blood abound in the Urinary Bladder organ and Urinary Bladder channels. At this time period the Urinary Bladder organ and channels can more easily be dispersed and purged. During low tide (3 a.m. to 5 a.m.), they can be more readily tonified. The Urinary Bladder Channels' energy also acts on the skin, muscles, and nerves found along their pathway.

The Eighteen Back-Shu Points

The Eighteen Back-Shu points are all located on the back along the Urinary Bladder Channel. They correspond to the twelve Zang Fu organs and are used both for diagnosis and for treatment. These points transport Qi very effectively and directly to the internal organs. They can also be used for treating disorders of the corresponding sense organs. The Eighteen Back Transporting points are: Lungs UB-13, Pericardium UB-14, Heart UB-15, Governing Vessel UB-16, Diaphragm UB-17, Liver UB-18, Gall Bladder UB-19, Spleen UB-20, Stomach UB-21, Triple Burners UB-22, Kidneys UB-23, Sea of Qi UB-24, Large Intestine UB-25, Gate to the Yuan Qi (Guan Yuan) UB-26, Small Intestine UB-27, Bladder UB-28, Sacrum UB-29, and Anus UB-30.

The Influence of Climate

The Urinary Bladder can be easily injured by chronic or excessive exposure to Cold and Damp environments. This can lead to the accumulation of Dampness in the Urinary Bladder, which manifests as Damp Cold or Damp Heat syndromes.

The Influence of Taste, Color, and Sound

- The salty taste can be used to tonify both the Urinary Bladder and the Kidneys.
- The light blue color is used to tonify the Urinary Bladder.
- The "Chree," "Fuu" and "Yuu" sounds are used to purge the Urinary Bladder and the Kidneys.

Urinary Bladder Pathology

The main diseases of the Urinary Bladder organ and channels include: diseases located at the top of the head, brain disorders, disorders of the neck and back (especially the lumbar and sacral regions), disorders of the back of the legs and thighs, and disorders of the lateral sides of the feet.

Diseases of the Urinary Bladder Organ manifest in changes in urine and urination; these changes will reflect either a deficient or excess condition of the Urinary Bladder, described as follows:

1. **Deficient Conditions** are attributed to a condition of Deficient Kidney Qi which then affects the Urinary Bladder's ability to transform Qi. This dysfunction causes frequent urination, dribbling, or enuresis (involuntary discharge of urine).
2. **Excess Conditions** are attributed to Damp Heat in the Urinary Bladder, and may manifest in symptoms such as: heat and pain during urination, the short release of murky or reddish urine, frequent difficulty in urination, pus or Blood in the urine, and Bladder stones which cause a urinary block and painful distention of the lower abdomen.

Most pathological diseases of the Urinary Bladder organ are due to the accumulation of Dampness (Damp Heat or Damp Cold). The most common pattern of Urinary Bladder disharmony is Damp Heat in the Urinary Bladder (Figure 8.120).

T.C.M. Patterns of Disharmony

Generally, patterns of disharmony associated with the Urinary Bladder originate either from Damp Heat in the Urinary Bladder or Damp Cold in the Urinary Bladder, and are described as follows:

Figure 8.120. The Origins of Damp Heat in the Urinary Bladder Disharmony

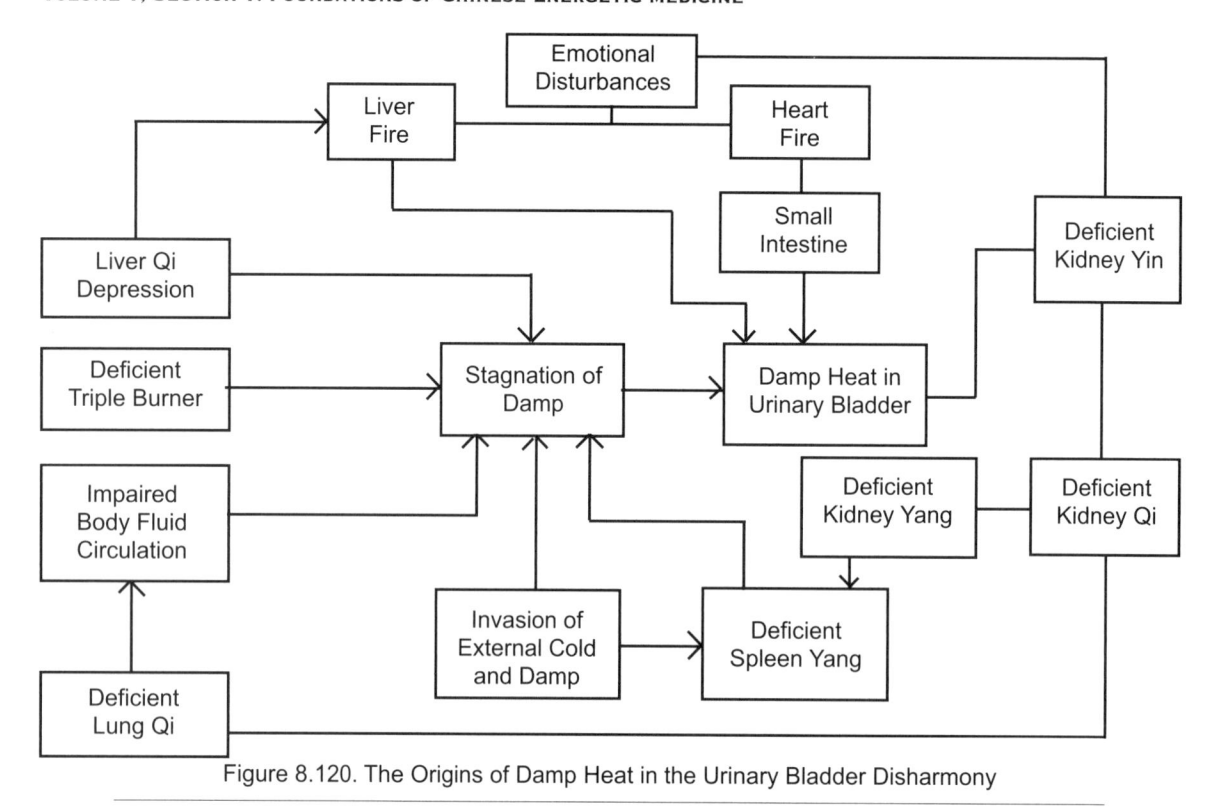

1. **Damp Heat in the Urinary Bladder:** The pattern of Damp Heat in the Urinary Bladder can be caused from several factors: Depressed Liver Qi, Deficient Lung Qi, Deficient Spleen Qi, Deficient Triple Burner Qi, External Dampness and the invasion of pathogenic evils, or an invasion of External Cold and Damp. Symptoms include frequent and urgent urination, burning during urination, turbid urine, Blood or "sand" in the urine, fever, and thirst.
   - **Depressed Liver Qi:** Depressed Liver Qi can give rise to Liver Fire, which then causes emotional disturbances that aggravate both Liver Fire and Heart Fire. This pathogenic pattern can create Deficient Kidney Yin, Deficient Liver Yin, and Deficient Heart Yin. If the Toxic Heat moves downward, it can affect the Urinary Bladder and aggravate a condition of Damp Heat.
   - **Deficient Lung Qi:** Deficient Kidney Qi may interact with Deficient Lung Qi.
   - **Deficient Spleen Qi:** Deficient Kidney Yang can contribute to Deficient Spleen Yang and facilitate the invasion of Cold and Damp.
   - **Deficient Triple Burner Qi:** Chronic retention of Cold and damp in the Lower Burner can injure Kidney Yang.
   - **Invasion of External Cold and Damp:** An invasion of External Cold and Damp may lead to the stagnation of Dampness.
2. **Damp Cold in the Urinary Bladder:** The pattern of Damp Cold in the Urinary Bladder can be caused from excessive exposure to External Dampness and Cold, characterized by the presence of dampness and Cold in the Lower Burner. Symptoms include frequent and urgent urination, heaviness in the hypogastrium and urethra and turbid urine.

THE URINARY BLADDER IN WESTERN MEDICINE

The urinary bladder is a smooth, collapsible, muscular sac, located on the pelvic floor just posterior to the pubic symphysis. The interior of the

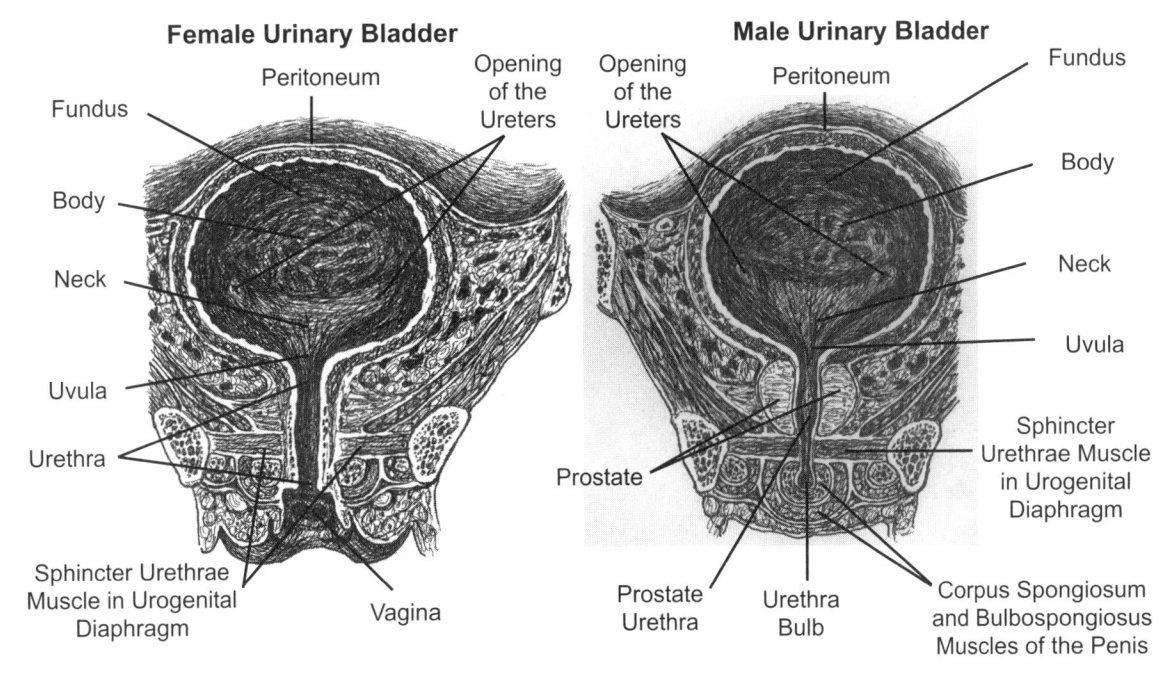

CHAPTER 8: THE TWELVE PRIMARY ORGANS, CHANNELS AND COLLATERALS

Figure 8.121. The Female and Male Urinary Bladder (UB) Organs
(Inspired by the original artwork of Dr. Frank H. Netter).

urinary bladder has three openings. The upper part of the urinary bladder communicates with the kidneys via the two ureters. Its lower part is connected to the urethra, which opens externally by means of the urinary orifice. In males, the urinary bladder lies immediately anterior to the rectum, and surrounded by the prostate gland before it empties into the urethra. In females, the urinary bladder lies anterior to the vagina and inferior to the Uterus (Figure 121).

Though somewhat movable, the urinary bladder is held in position by folds of the peritoneum. Its size and shape fluctuate, depending on how much urine it contains. As the urine volume increases, the urinary bladder expands into a pear-shape and rises inside the abdominal cavity.

The urinary bladder wall has three layers. The innermost coat, known as the mucosa, is a mucous membrane composed of transitional epithelium (which allows the urinary bladder to stretch) and an underlying lamina propria (connective tissue). These inner walls of the urinary bladder are thick, and contain folds known as rugae that allow it to expand and contract (similar to the stomach).

The middle layer of the urinary bladder consists of a muscular layer which itself is composed of three layers of interwoven smooth muscle tissues. The entire urinary bladder organ is surrounded by a protective adventitia that merges with the parietal peritoneum.

Physiology

The urinary bladder is a temporary reservoir for the urine produced by the kidneys; it discharges urine from the body through the urethra (Figure 8.122).

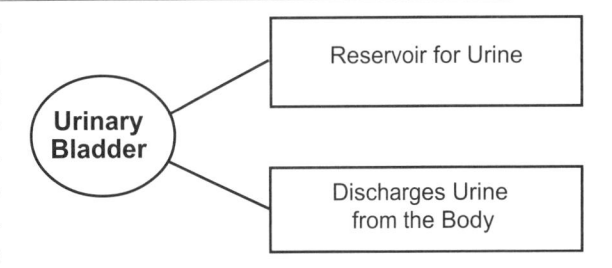

Figure 8.122. The Functions of the Urinary Bladder
(Western Medical Perspective)

417

VOLUME 1, SECTION 1: FOUNDATIONS OF CHINESE ENERGETIC MEDICINE

THE KIDNEY: SHEN

The Kidneys are a Yin organ, and their paired Yang organ is the Urinary Bladder. Their Element is Water. The Kidneys are different from the other Yin organs in that they are the foundation of all of the Yin and Yang energies within the body. It is for this reason that the Kidneys are sometimes called the "Black Emperor." They are also said to be the origin of Fire and Water in the body (Figure 8.123).

CHINESE CHARACTER FOR THE KIDNEY: SHEN

The Chinese character "Shen" translates as "Kidneys," (not to be confused with the "Shen" which translates as Mind or Spirit). It refers to the image of a Kidney organ, and is divided into two sections. The upper left hand side of the character depicts the radical for a slave or servant prostrating and bowing before the Emperor. The upper right hand side of the character depicts the radical for the right hand, signifying someone who has power and authority. The character to the bottom, "Ji" depicts the Chinese ideogram for body tissue, muscle or flesh (all of which are forms of connective tissue). Together, the Chinese ideograph for "Shen" can be translated as, "that which pushes the organism to the actualization of all its potentialities" (Figure 8.124).

THE YIN AND YANG OF THE KIDNEYS

Traditional Chinese Medicine defines the Kidneys as having two energetic aspects: A Yin aspect and a Yang aspect.

- **The Yin of the Kidneys (Primary Yin):** This pertains to the vital essence of the Kidneys, including its material structures. The Kidney Yin is the foundation and fundamental substance of all the Yin in the body. It is responsible for nourishing the tissues and providing them with fluid-like moistening and cooling essences. It rules the cycles of birth, growth, maturation, and reproduction. Kidney Yin is the foundation of all the Yin energies of the body, including the Yin of the Liver, Heart and Lungs. According to the *Nan Jing: Classic of Difficulties*, the left Kidney is Yin and is connected with the "Water of Life," and is associated with the wa-

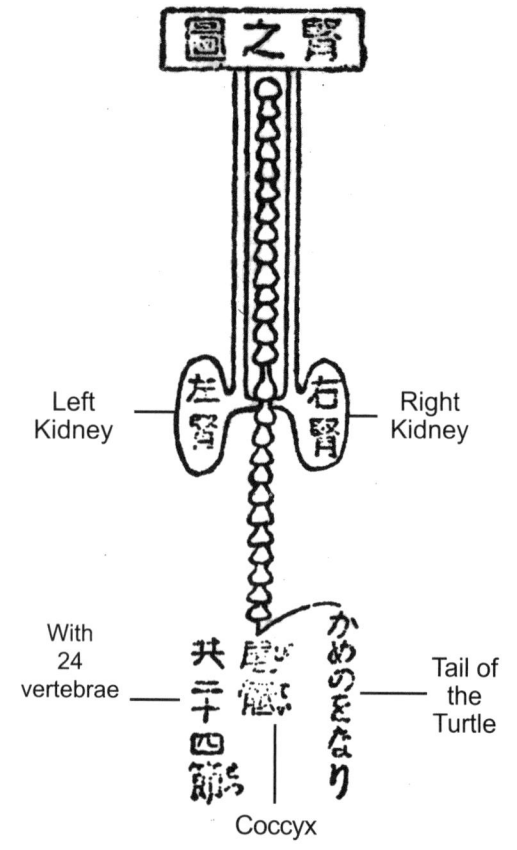

Figure 8.123. The ancient Chinese anatomical diagram of the Kidney (Kd) Organ, as it appeared in "Important Useful Notes on Acupuncture and Moxibustion," published in Japan in 1718, by Masatoyo Hongo

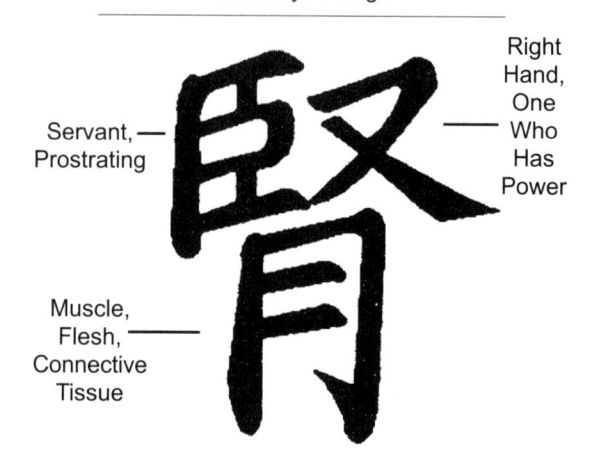

Figure 8.124. The Chinese character for "Shen," Kidney

ter metabolism functions of the Urinary Bladder.

- **The Yang of the Kidneys (Primary Yang):** This pertains to the Kidney's function of heating and moving the Qi. The Kidney Yang is the primary motivating force behind all of the body's physiological processes. Kidney Yang is the foundation of all the Yang energies of the body, including the Yang of the Spleen, Heart, and Lungs. According to the *Nan Jing: Classic of Difficulties*, the right Kidney is Yang and is connected with the "Fire of Life" and the Ming Men (Gate of Destiny), and is associated with the energetic functions of the Triple Burners (Figure 8.125).

Since the Ming Dynasty (1368 - 1644 A.D.), Chinese doctors have no longer considered the Mingmen to be a part of the right Kidney, but rather believed that it was energetically situated between both Kidneys, continually pulsating under the influence of the Ancestral Qi (Figure 8.126).

THE KIDNEY'S WATER JING FORMATION

The Water Jing energy is the first Jing to be introduced into the body of the fetus. Its energy becomes active during the fourth lunar month of fetal development. The water supervises the genetic developmental phase of the fetal growth. This energy encompasses the fetus' unconscious reservoir of innate and intuitive intelligence, will, and other life-force energies relating to divine love, power, and spirit. Any faltering of this energy (e.g., due to the influence of fetal toxins or trauma) is associated with both pervasive and subtle neurological disorders, and with a predisposition to psychological disorders (e.g., schizophrenia). Symptoms of possible Deficient Kidney Jing disorders are described as follows:

- **Signs of Deficient Kidney Jing in children** can manifest as slow physical development, poor Bone development, slow mental development, mental dullness, poor memory, retardation, and the late or incomplete closure of the child's cranial fontanels. Deficient Kidney Jing can also lead to Congenital Qi Deficiency (i.e., Deficiency in the Sea of Marrow),

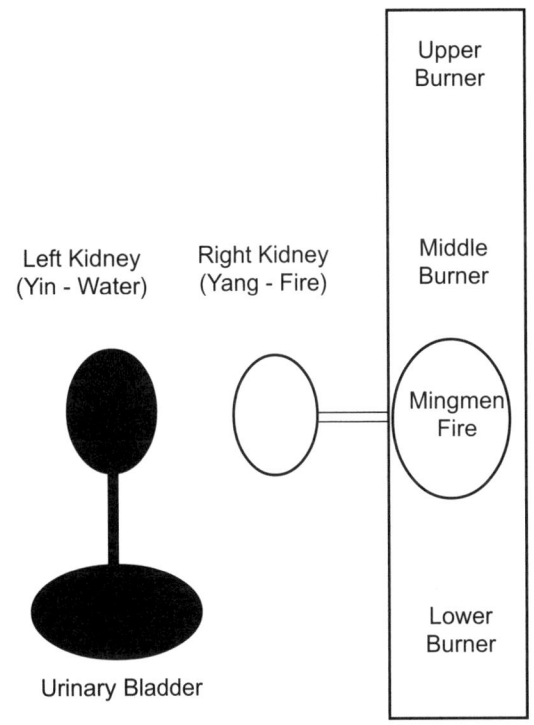

Figure 8.125. In the Nan Jing, the left Kidney is presented as the "Water of Life" and is connected to the energetic functions of the Urinary Bladder. The right Kidney is Yang, is connected with the "Fire of Life" and the Ming Men (Gate of Destiny), and is associated with the energetic functions of the Triple Burners.

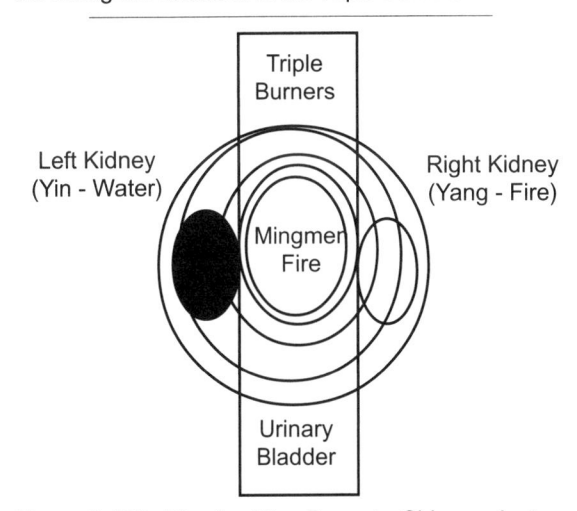

Figure 8.126. After the Ming Dynasty, Chinese doctors no longer saw the Mingmen as part of the right Kidney, but rather as existing between both Kidneys.

which can lead to Down Syndrome, Attention Deficit Disorder (ADD) and learning disabilities.
- **Signs of Deficient Kidney Jing in adults** include brittle Bones, weak knees and legs, loose teeth, poor memory, premature senility, premature graying, premature hair loss, soreness in the lumbar, dizziness, deafness, tinnitus, and a weakness of sexual activity (impotence, infertility, low sex drive, an inability to conceive or carry a baby to full-term, etc.).

After birth, the Water Jing can be affected through the colors black and dark navy-blue, the salty taste, and the "Chree," "Fuu" and "Yu" sounds.

THE KIDNEYS IN ANCIENT CHINESE MEDICINE

To the ancient Chinese, the Kidneys represented "that which pushes the organism to the actualization of all its potentialities." It was further believed that the Kidneys were the "trunk where the gathered treasure takes root." These sayings can better be understood by examining the energetic nature of the Kidneys, and the role they play in body functions.

THE KIDNEYS IN CHINESE MEDICINE

In Traditional Chinese Medicine, the functions ascribed to the Kidneys are different from those defined in Western Medicine. The Chinese energetic functions of the Kidneys also include the functions of the urinary system, reproductive system, aspects of the endocrine system, the nervous system, production of Bone Marrow, development of Bones, various psycho-emotional aspects, and spiritual influences.

According to Traditional Chinese Medicine, the main functions of the Kidneys are to: store Jing (Essence); provide the foundation of body's Yin and Yang, produce Marrow, fill the Brain and control the Bones; govern water; control and promote inhalation; open at the ears; manifest in the head hair; control the two lower orifices; house the Gate of Destiny (Mingmen); express itself through the psycho-emotional aspects of wisdom and fear; and exert certain important spiritual influences via the Zhi (Will). These main functions are described as follows (Figure 8.127):

1. **Stores Jing (Essence):** The Kidneys store both the body's Prenatal (congenital) Jing and Postnatal (acquired) Jing.
   - **Storing the Prenatal (congenital) Jing:** The Kidneys are called the "Root of Life," because they store the Prenatal Jing. The Prenatal Jing is the body's innate and inherited Original Essence (Yuan Jing) which determines the individual's basic constitutional makeup, strength, and vitality. Before birth, the Prenatal Jing nourishes the fetus. After birth, the Prenatal Jing controls the child's growth, sexual maturation, and development.

   In ancient China, it was believed that at the time when the Kidney Jing became rich in essence, the energetic influence of "Tian Gui" (the tenth Heavenly Stem) would promote the development of sperm in boys, and initiate the discharge of ovum and the beginning of menstruation in girls. Tian Gui is known as the "Yin Water" Heavenly Stem of "Earlier Heaven." Tian Gui represents the energetic regathering of new life-force, associated with Kidney Yin. It energetically moves "underground" and is considered to be the Yin Water of the congenital constitution. Being invisibly cultivated, it awaits a new breakthrough. In old age, as the Qi of the Kidneys begins to weaken, the Tian Gui begins to dry up, causing menopause in women and diminished sexual activity in men.
   - **The Postnatal (acquired) Jing:** Postnatal Jing (Zhi Jing) is the body's refined essence, extracted from food essence via the Spleen and Stomach's transformational digestion functions.
2. **Provides the Foundation of Body's Yin and Yang:** The Kidneys are the root of all the Yin and Yang Qi within the body's organs and tissues.
3. **Produces Marrow, Fills the Brain, and Controls the Bones:** The Kidneys produce Marrow and control the development of the Bones. The Chinese concept of "Marrow" does not correspond to marrow as defined in Western Medi-

```
The Main Functions of the Kidney Organs and Channels
├── Stores Jing (Essence of Life)
│   ├── Prenatal Jing
│   └── Postnatal Jing
├── Provides the Foundation of Body's Yin and Yang
├── Produces Marrow, Fills the Brain and Controls the Bones
├── Governs the Water
│   ├── Disseminating Body Fluids
│   └── Discharging Waste Fluid
├── Controls and Promotes Inhalation
├── Opens at the Ears
├── Manifests in the Head Hair
├── Controls the Two Lower Orifices
│   ├── Urethra and Vas Deferens
│   └── Anus
├── Houses the Mingmen Fire
│   ├── Heat Middle Burner
│   └── True Fire
├── Psycho-Emotional Aspects
│   └── Wisdom and Fear
└── Spiritual Influence
    └── Spiritual Functions of the Zhi
```

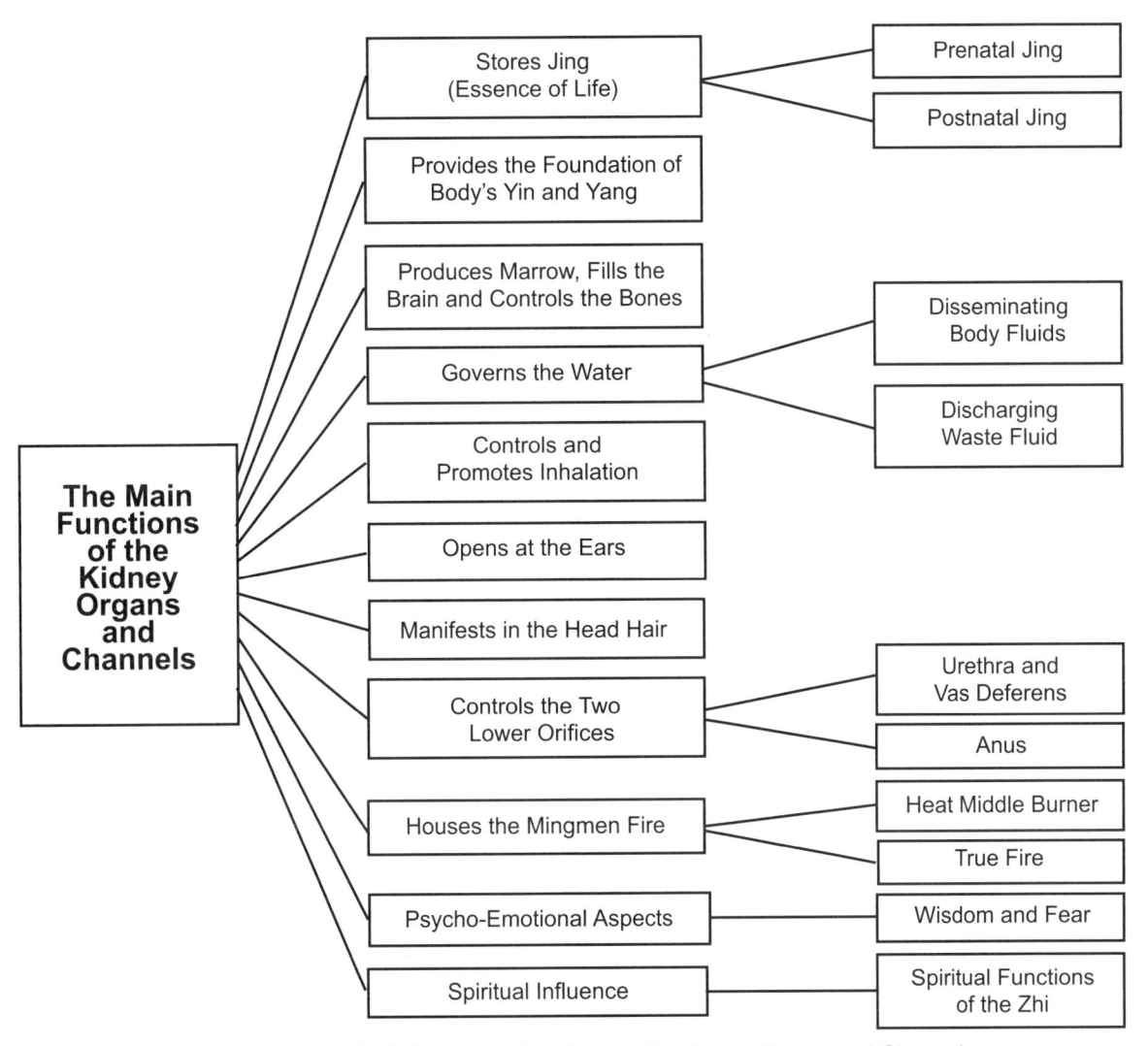

Figure 8.127. The Main Energetic Functions of the Kidney Organs and Channels

cine. In Chinese Energetic Medicine, Marrow is considered a substance which provides the common tissue of the body's Bones, Bone Marrow, spinal cord, and Brain. The "Sea of Marrow" is also considered to be the energetic essence that flows from the Kidneys through the spinal cord and into the Brain.

4. **Governs Water:** The Kidneys govern Body Fluids and water metabolism, and for this reason are sometimes called the "controller of water." They act as a gate, opening and closing the circulation and flow of Body Fluids in the Lower Burner. The Kidneys' function of governing the body's water metabolism has two aspects: disseminating body fluids and discharging waste fluid.

- **Disseminating Body Fluids:** Disseminating the Body Fluids involves dispersing and distributing throughout the body those fluids which have been derived from food essence. The Kidneys are thus responsible for delivering nutritive and nourishing liquid energy to all of the internal organs and tissues of the body.

- **Discharging Waste Fluid:** The Kidneys also separate and discharge from the body all the turbid waste fluid that is produced by the internal organs as a by-product of fluid metabolism.

5. **Controls and Promotes Inhalation:** The Kidneys' Yang Qi has the function of controlling and promoting the inhalation of the air, moving the Qi downwards and "holding" it. One type of asthma is associated with Kidney Yang Qi Deficiency.

6. **Opens at the Ears:** The Kidneys energetically open externally through the ears and rely on the nourishment of the Jing for proper hearing.

7. **Manifests in the Head Hair:** Although the nutrients for the head hair come from the Blood, its life energy originates in the Kidney's Jing. The quality and color of the head hair is related to the state of the body's Kidney Jing. If the Kidney Jing is strong, the head hair will be thick and of good color.

8. **Controls the Two Lower Orifices:** The Kidney Jing controls the function of the lower front and rear Yin orifices: the genitalia and the anus.

- **Genitalia:** The front Yin orifice includes the vas deferens in men and urethra in women.
- **Anus:** The rear Yin orifice is the anus. Although the anus is anatomically related to the Large Intestine, it is functionally related to the Kidneys.

9. **Houses the Mingmen Fire:** During the Ming Dynasty (1386-1644 A.D.), the popular theory was that the location of the Mingmen Fire was positioned between the two Kidneys rather than in the right Kidney alone (refer back to Figure 8.108 and Figure 8.109). The Mingmen is the embodiment of the Fire within the Kidneys. It is the "Root of Yuan Qi," and one of the body's "Three Fires." The Three Fires are together responsible for creating the "True Fire," needed for warming the body's internal organs and tissues and must be differentiated from the Triple Burner. The Mingmen Fire heats the Qi within the Middle and Lower Burners and assists the body in causing the Jing to transform into Qi (see Triple Burners section).

10. **Psycho-Emotional Aspects:** The Kidneys provide the capacity and drive for strength, skill, and hard work, and for this reason are sometimes called the "minister of ingenuity and vitality." An individual with strong Kidneys can work hard and purposefully for long periods of time. The Hun influence the energetic nature of the Kidneys, allowing the individual to experience clear perception and gentleness in thoughts and actions. If the circulation of Qi in the Kidneys becomes obstructed, this Kidney Qi stagnation can give rise to emotional turmoil, sometimes manifesting through fear (Yang), or loneliness (Yin), influenced by the Po. The Kidney's positive psycho-emotional attributes are wisdom, rationality, clear perception, gentleness, and self-understanding. The negative attributes are fear, loneliness, insecurity, and shock (which attacks the Heart then descends into the Kidneys). When the Kidneys are in a state of disharmony, the patient can sometimes be driven to a state of obsessive-compulsive working habits (e.g., a workaholic). A patient with weak Kidneys can lack strength, endurance, confidence, and will power.

11. **Spiritual Influence:** The Kidneys house the body's willpower (Zhi) and store the individual's inherited constitution. The Chinese term Zhi is translated as "will," "ambition" and "determination" (not to be confused with the "Zhi" which translates as acquired wisdom and intelligence, and is used to describe the Postnatal Mind). The Zhi is the Prenatal spiritual entity (Jing Shen) associated with the Kidneys. The willpower of the Kidney's Zhi is not the personal will of the ego that is driven by our desires. The term Zhi has two common meanings: memory and willpower, both of which are primary features of the Zhi. The word Zhi can also be used to mean the Mind (whole body consciousness and awareness). The five mental aspects of the Spirit (Wu Jing Shen), the Hun, Po, Shen, Yi, and Zhi are sometimes referred to as the Five Zhi, eluding to the fact that each of the five Yin organs has a physio-spiritual will of its own, but each is expressed differently.

CHINESE IDEOGRAM OF THE ZHI

The Chinese ideogram for Zhi is composed of two characters. The character on the bottom is the Heart. The character above depicts a plant beginning to rise upward from the soil. Together, both characters represent the continuous, persistent intention of the Heart, developing towards an intended goal. The plant represents the process of life's development through the uniting of both will and intention (Figure 8.128).

The word Zhi can also be used to mean the Mind (whole body consciousness and awareness). The five mental aspects of the Mind, the Ethereal Soul, Corporeal Soul, Shen, Intention and the "Willpower" are sometimes referred to as the Five Zhi.

THE KIDNEYS AND THE WILLPOWER

The willpower is the most important aspect of the Zhi, and includes elements of the individual's mental drive, willpower, determination, and the single-minded pursuit of goals and aspirations. It enables the realization of ambitions by providing the focused energy necessary to carry ideas to fruition. A powerful Zhi creates the magnetism and charisma necessary to manifest and materialize our dreams.

Even if a person has acquired all the information available via the Hun, Po, and Yi, without the Zhi there can be no action. The Hun give an individual the inspiration and goal, but the Zhi is needed to accomplish it (committing to the decision and following through with constant action). A person with a well-developed Zhi demonstrates perseverance, determination, and a tenacity to complete personal goals. Patients with a deficient Zhi become indecisive, fearful, submissive (often with a blind obedience to authority), and have a tendency to procrastinate. Patients with excess Zhi often tend to be fanatics, forcing their power, rules or philosophy onto others.

The goal of the Qigong doctor is to reach a level of atonement in which his or her personal will merges with Heaven's will (Tian Zhi) and the two become one and the same. Tian Zhi is considered to be the movement of the divine expressed in man as his personal virtue (De).

The ancient Daoists taught that a man's vir-

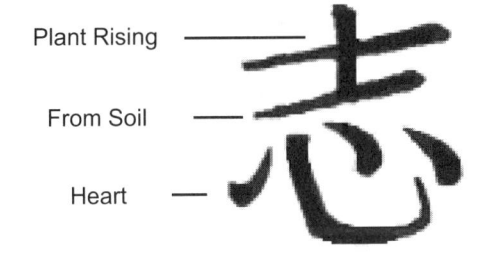

Figure 8.128. The Chinese character for "Zhi," Will

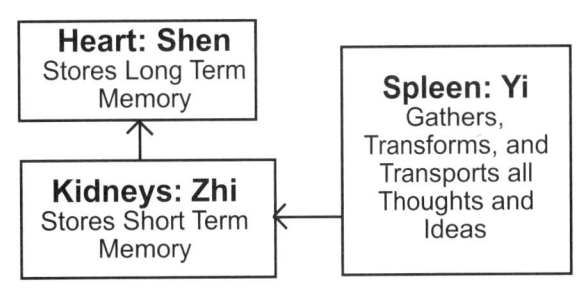

Figure 8.129. Three Ways the Body Stores Memory

tue is defined as his spiritual righteousness, and the authenticity of his Heart and actions. It is through the acquisition of virtue that man finds and possesses his true nature. If a man's virtue is initiated into the "mysterious" (embracing Heaven's will), his intuitive evolution will lead him towards limitless perception.

Tian Zhi is a divine inner prompting that guides us on our spiritual quest if we are open to its message. Tian Zhi is what we can call the divine will and carries within it man's purpose in life.

MEMORY

The Kidneys control short-term memory and store data. Memory, another meaning for the word "Zhi," is defined as the ability to remember information when studying or learning a particular subject or pattern. The Kidneys help to maintain a determined focus on our goals, and help us to remember where we are going and what we are working to achieve. In other words, the Kidneys maintain a certain vital mindfulness. The Kidneys are associated with short term memory, whereas the Heart is associated with the long term memory (Figure 8.129). This is why elderly patients (whose Kidney energy is declining), often cannot remember what day or year it is but can remember events long past.

From the Kd-16 points, the Qi follows the Belt Vessel and enters into and penetrates the Kidneys. From the Kidneys, the Qi descends along the ureters, before spirally wrapping the Urinary Bladder

Internal Channel Flow

The internal flow of the Kidney Qi passes the GV-1 point, moving up and down the spine, and exiting the body at the Kd-11 points. From Kd-11, the energy ascends superficially up to the Kd-16 points

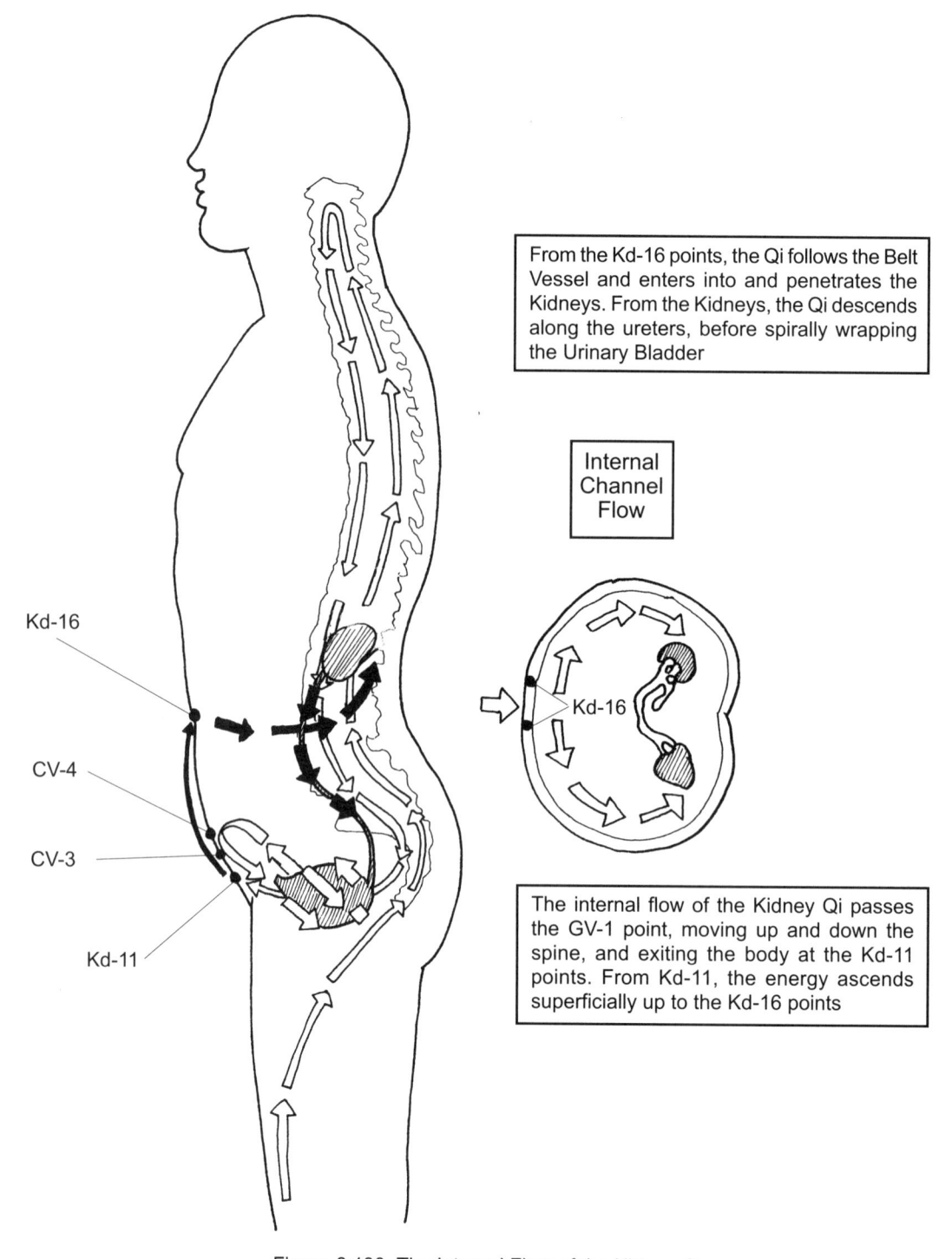

Figure 8.130. The Internal Flow of the Kidney Qi

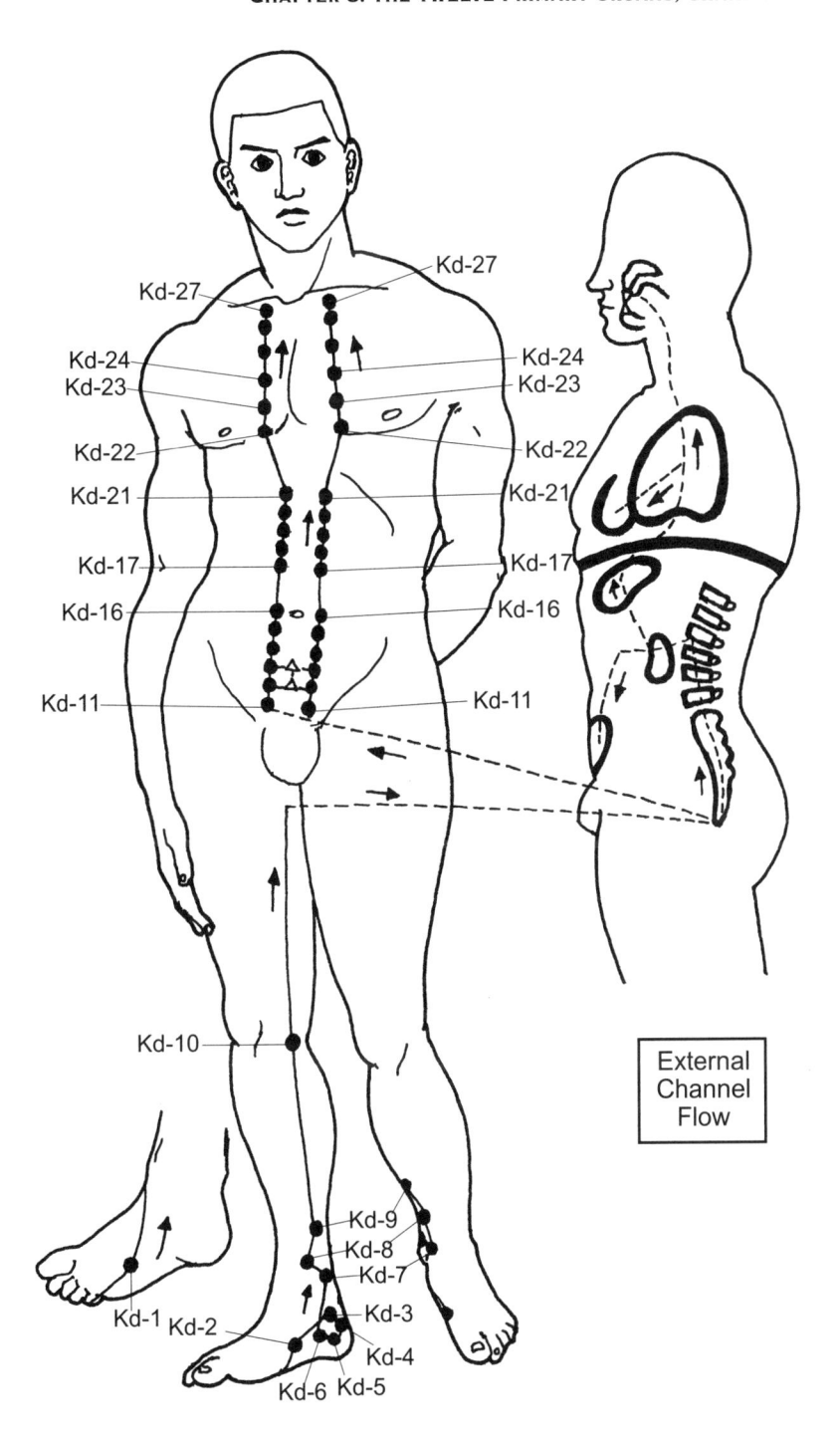

CHAPTER 8: THE TWELVE PRIMARY ORGANS, CHANNELS AND COLLATERALS

Figure 8.131. The Internal and External Qi Flow of the Kidney (Kd) Channels

THE KIDNEY CHANNELS

The Kidney Channels are Yin channels that flow externally from the feet to the torso (Figure 8.130). These two main rivers of Kidney energy originate externally from underneath the little toes before circling the inside of the heels and ascending the medial aspect of the legs, where they then merge and enter into the coccyx and lower lumbar vertebrae. The internal flow of the Kidney Qi passes through the GV-1 point, moving up and down the spine, and exiting the body at the Kd-11 points. From the Kd-11 points, the energy ascends superficially up to the Kd-16 points.

From the Kd-16 points, the Qi follows the Belt Vessel and enters into and penetrates the Kidneys. At the Kd-16 points, the channels divide into two branches. One branch penetrates the Kidneys, while the other branch continues to ascend within the spine before entering into the cerebral cortex. From the Kidney organs, two additional pairs of channels emerge internally. One pair descends along the ureters before spirally wrapping the Urinary Bladder. The other set ascends into the Liver, diaphragm, and Lungs. It then spirally wraps the Heart and travels up through the throat, stopping at the root of the tongue (Figure 8.131).

CHANNELS' ENERGETIC FLOW

The Kidney Channels store more Qi than Blood, acting more on energetic and nervous functions than on physical substances and Blood functions. At the high-tide time period (5 p.m. to 7 p.m.), Qi and Blood abound in the Kidney organ and Kidney channels. At this time period the Kidney organ and channels can more easily be dispersed and purged. During low tide (5 a.m. to 7 am.), they can be more readily tonified. The energy of the Kidney Channels also acts on the skin, muscles, and nerves found along their pathways.

The Kidney Yin Qi flows to the Liver, Heart, and Lungs. It is responsible for the body's Jing, and rules the cycles of the birth, growth, maturation, and reproduction. The Kidney Yang Qi flows to the Spleen, Liver, Heart, and Lungs. It supports the Yang of all the body's organs via the energy of the Mingmen (Figure 8.132).

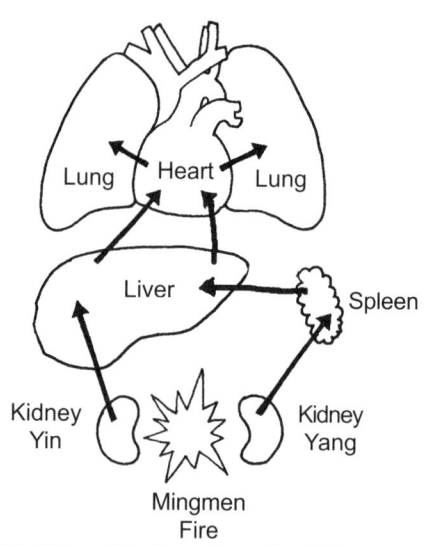

Figure 8.132. Kidney Yin flows from the Kidneys to the Liver, and then to the Heart and Lungs. Kidney Yang flows from the Kidneys to the Spleen, Liver, Heart, and Lungs.

THE INFLUENCE OF CLIMATE

In the winter months the Kidneys become more active in individuals who already possess strong Kidney Qi, but become deficient in those with weak Kidney Qi. The Kidneys are injured by irregular sleep patterns, fear, excessive caffeine, sex, drugs, alcohol, or smoking. During this season, the excess consumption of salty or Cold foods has a draining effect on the Kidneys. Overexposure to a cold climate will also have a draining effect on the Kidneys.

THE INFLUENCE OF TASTE, COLOR, AND SOUND

- The Kidneys can be easily injured by excessive exposure to cold and damp weather and environments. This can lead to the accumulation of Dampness in the Kidneys, manifesting as either Damp Cold or Damp Heat syndromes.
- The salty taste can be used to tonify both the Kidneys and the Urinary Bladder.
- The black, dark navy-blue, or purple color is used to tonify both the Kidneys and the Urinary Bladder.
- The "Chree," "Fuu," and "Yuu" sounds are used to purge both the Kidneys and the Urinary Bladder.

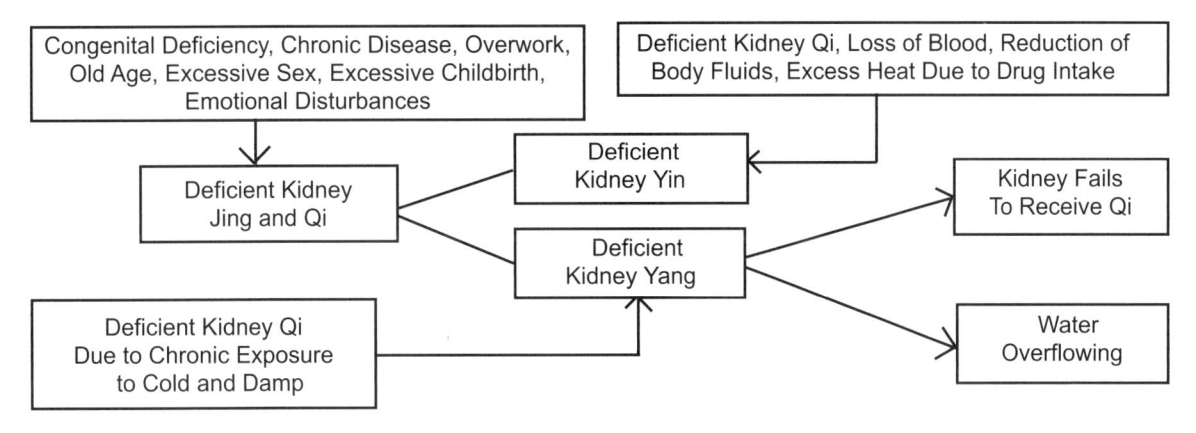

Figure 8.133. The Origins of Kidney Disharmonies

Flow chart:
- Congenital Deficiency, Chronic Disease, Overwork, Old Age, Excessive Sex, Excessive Childbirth, Emotional Disturbances → Deficient Kidney Jing and Qi
- Deficient Kidney Jing and Qi → Deficient Kidney Yin, Deficient Kidney Yang
- Deficient Kidney Qi, Loss of Blood, Reduction of Body Fluids, Excess Heat Due to Drug Intake → Deficient Kidney Yin
- Deficient Kidney Qi Due to Chronic Exposure to Cold and Damp → Deficient Kidney Yang
- Deficient Kidney Yang → Kidney Fails To Receive Qi, Water Overflowing

KIDNEY PATHOLOGY

Kidney organ and channel diseases may cause general deterioration of the entire body, weakness in the lower extremities, lumbar pain, or hot sensations deep inside the feet.

The Kidneys open through the urogenital orifices and the anus. The energetic condition of the Kidneys can be partially reflected by the condition of the patient's urination and defecation; in males this includes the ejaculation process.

Since the Kidneys are responsible for concentration and memory retention, poor concentration and loss of memory are common symptoms of Kidney Deficiency.

T.C.M. PATTERNS OF DISHARMONY

Patterns of disharmony associated with the Kidneys include: Deficient Kidney Jing, Deficient Kidney Yang, Deficient Kidney Yin, The Kidneys Fail to Receive Qi and Water Overflowing (Figure 8.133).

1. **Deficient Kidney Jing:** This pattern of disharmony can be due to hereditary factors, fetal toxins, or old age. Signs of Deficient Kidney Jing include problems that appear during birth, development, reproduction and aging; especially when these problems relate to the formation and function of the Marrow, Bones, Brain, ears and hair.
   - **Deficient Kidney Jing in children** can be due to hereditary factors or fetal toxins, and will result in a poor congenital constitution. Symptoms of Deficient Kidney Jing can manifest as slow physical development, poor Bone development, slow mental development, mental dullness, poor memory, retardation, and the late or incomplete closure of the child's cranial fontanelles. Deficient Kidney Jing can also lead to Congenital Qi Deficiency (i.e., Deficiency in the Sea of Marrow), which in turn can lead to Down Syndrome, Attention Deficit Disorder (ADD) and learning disabilities.
   - **Deficient Kidney Jing in adults** can develop from an excess of sexual activity, constant stress, chronic exposure to pathogens, or from old age. Symptoms of Deficient Kidney Jing can manifest as brittle bones, weak knees and legs, loose teeth, poor memory, premature senility, premature graying, premature hair loss, lumbago, dizziness, deafness, tinnitus, impotence, infertility, low sex drive, and an inability to conceive or carry a baby to full-term.

2. **Deficient Kidney Yang:** This pattern of disharmony can be the result of a chronic illness, old age, excessive sexual activity, excess exposure to Cold, or a chronic retention of Dampness that obstructs the movement of fluids. Deficient Yang results in deficient warmth, with symptoms such as a sensation of cold or soreness in the back, cold knees,

cold limbs, and aversion to cold. Other symptoms of Deficient Kidney Yang include weak knees and legs, lassitude, edema of the legs, poor appetite, headaches, breathlessness, wheezing, asthma, tiredness, mental and emotional problems, diarrhea, painful urination, enuresis, edema, loose stools, abundant clear urination, impotence, premature ejaculation, menorrhagia, and infertility.

3. **Deficient Kidney Yin:** This pattern of disharmony can be the result of overwork, excessive Blood loss, chronic illness affecting the Liver, Heart and Lungs, a depletion of Body Fluids due to consumption by Heat after a fever, or an overdose of Chinese medicine used to strengthen Kidney Yang (thus accidentally injuring the Kidney Yin). Symptoms of Deficient Kidney Yin can manifest as dizziness, vertigo, poor memory, tinnitus, deafness, malar flush, night sweating, Five Palms Heat, dry throat and mouth, thirst, tiredness, chest tightness, asthma, breathlessness, mental and emotional problems, sore knees and back, ache in the bones, nocturnal emissions, enuresis, premature ejaculation, menorrhagia, constipation, and dark scanty urine.

4. **Kidneys Fail to Receive Qi:** This pattern of disharmony manifests when the Kidneys fail to hold the Qi that is sent down by the Lungs during respiration. The Qi rebels upward resulting in a difficulty inhalation and shortness of breath, cough and asthma (aggravated by exertion). This pattern can originate from a long standing chronic disease which inevitably affects the Kidneys, excessive physical strain on the body, or from a hereditary weakness of the Lungs and Kidneys. Symptoms of the Kidneys failing to receive the Qi include rapid and weak breathing, difficulty in inhaling, shortness of breath on exertion, cough, asthma, sweating, cold limbs, cold limbs after sweating, mental listlessness, sore back, and the release of clear urination during an asthma attack.

5. **Water Overflowing:** This pattern of disharmony is considered to be a severe form of Kidney Yang Deficiency, and can develop from chronic retention of Dampness that interferes with the Kidney's function of transforming the body's fluids. It can also be caused by Spleen Yang Deficiency due to excessive consumption of Cold raw foods, Water overflowing the Heart due to Heart Yang Deficiency, Water overflowing the Lungs due to Lung Qi Deficiency, and a retention of External Cold within the Lungs. Symptoms of Water overflowing include edema in the legs and ankles, feeling cold, lumbago, coldness in the legs and back, and abdominal distension.

THE KIDNEYS IN WESTERN MEDICINE

The kidneys are paired organs that are located on the sides of the spine, just above the waist and half hidden under the rib cage. The kidneys can be included in a group of organs whose function is to eliminate wastes from the body. The other major eliminative organs are the lungs, skin, and gastrointestinal tract.

The primary function of the kidneys is to filter out by-products of cellular metabolism, bacterial toxins, and other wastes from the blood. The kidneys are the major channels through which nitrogenous wastes and drugs are eliminated. In addition to simply filtering the blood, the kidneys also help control the concentration of the various elements (glucose, electrolytes, etc.) contained within the blood. The Kidneys help control blood pressure (through the production of renin), stimulate red blood cell production (through the production of erythropoietin), and regulate the PH of the blood. The kidneys also assist in metabolizing vitamin D, thus allowing the bones and teeth to calcify, while also normalizing the functions of the heart, nervous system, and blood coagulation (Figure 8.134).

FILTERING FLUIDS FROM THE BLOODSTREAM

The kidneys normally filter the entire volume of blood in the body every 45 minutes. To accomplish this, they filter out nearly 48 gallons (180 liters) of fluid every day, though only a small amount of this fluid (1%) actually leaves the body as urine; the rest is reabsorbed into the blood. The function of the kidneys is regulated by the pituitary gland and the hypothalamus.

Kidneys

- Regulate Water and Electrolytes — Filter Fluids from the Bloodstream
- Detoxify Ingested Drugs — Eliminate Nitrogenous Wastes, Toxins and Drugs from the Body
- Reprocess Nutrients — Return Needed Substances to the Blood
- Process the Body's Urine
- Regulate the Volume and Chemical Makeup of the Blood — Maintain Balance Between Water and Salts, Acids and Bases
- Produce Renin — Regulate Blood Pressure
- Produce Erythropoietin — Stimulate Red Blood Cell Production in Bone Marrow
- Metabolize Vitamin D — Bone and Teeth Calcification, Stabilize Nervous System, Normalize Heart Function, Normalize Blood Coagulation

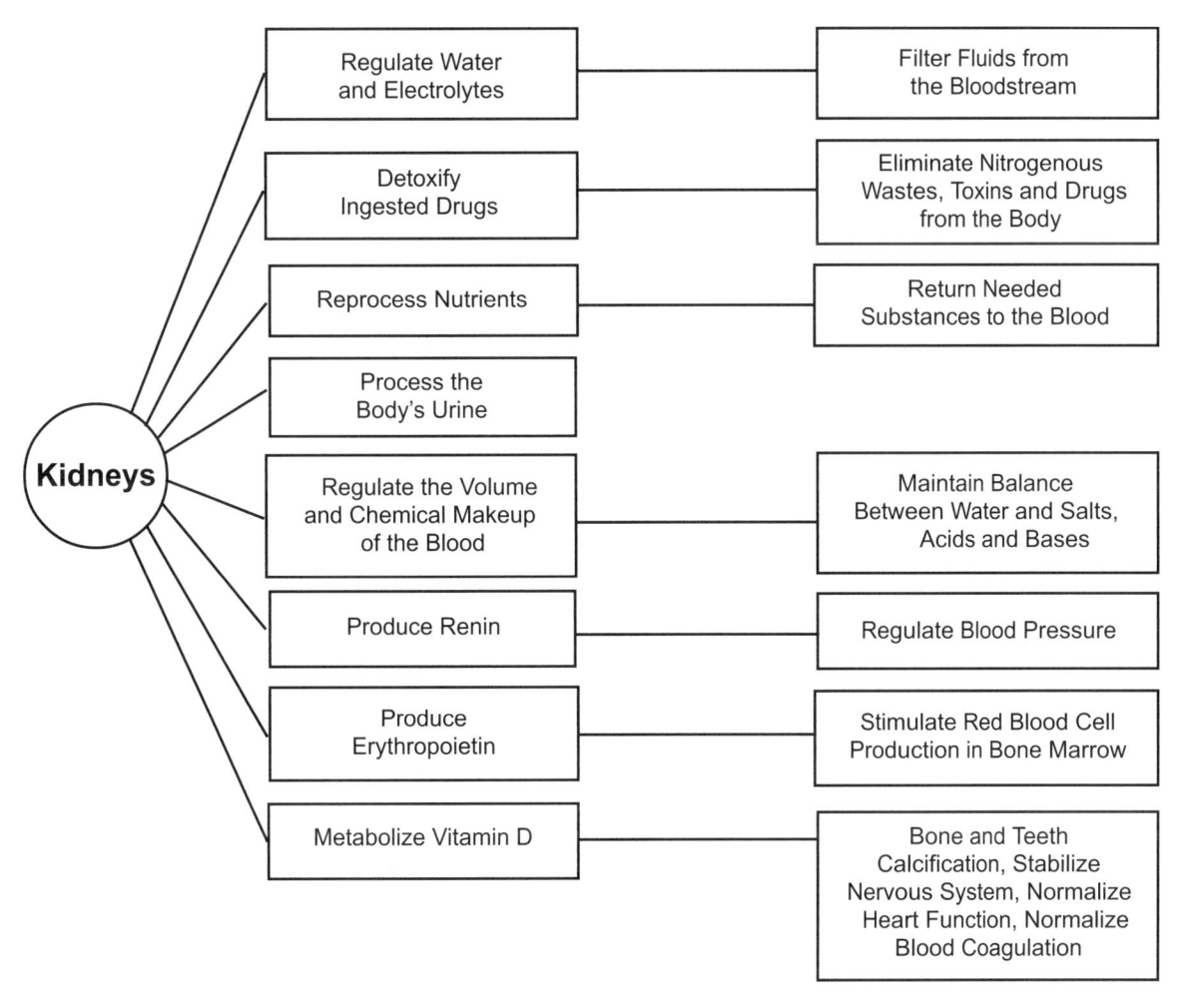

Figure 8.134. The Functions of the Kidney (Western Medical Perspective)

Urinary System

The kidneys are the essential organs of the urinary system. The other organs of the urinary system are the ureters, the urinary bladder, and the urethra. Urine is the end product of the kidneys' function of blood filtration. Urine is composed of various toxic or unneeded materials that are released by the cells into the bloodstream, then extracted from the blood by the kidneys. From the kidneys, urine passes downwards along two ureters (one from each kidney) and into the bladder. Situated behind the pubic bone, the urinary bladder stores urine, and then releases it from the body via the pathway of the urethra. Urine is generally slightly acidic, but can range in PH from 4.5 to 8.0, depending on the condition of the blood.

Anatomy of the Kidneys

Nestled against the musculature of the back body, the kidneys sit behind the peritoneum (abdominal cavity), extending vertically from the height of T-12 down to L-3.

Each kidney is approximately the size of a fist, being 4 to 5 inches long, 2 to 3 inches wide, and 1 inch thick. The kidneys are shaped like two beans with their concave edges directed internally towards the spine. The central area of this concave curvature is called the hilus, and the kidneys are open to the rest of the body only through this area (Figure 8.135).

The kidneys collectively receive about one quarter of the total cardiac output of blood, which travels into them from the descending aorta via the renal arteries. Purified venous blood flows out of the kidneys into the inferior vena cava via the renal veins. As each renal artery enters the kidney it branches into smaller and smaller arteries and arterioles, which eventually extend into the nephrons in capillary formations that allow for maximum exposure to the filtration membrane. The path of the veins as they leave the kidney are generally side by side with the path of the arteries that bring blood into the kidney. The ureter also exits the kidney at the hilus, before traveling downwards to meet with the bladder.

Externally, each kidney is wrapped in three protective layers. The outermost of these is a dense layer of connective tissue, called the renal fascia, that surrounds not only the kidney, but also the adrenal gland located on top of the kidney. The renal fascia anchors itself to the surrounding tissue areas, thus keeping the kidneys in place. The middle protective layer, termed the adipose capsule, is composed primarily of fatty adipose tissue that holds both the kidneys in place and serves to insulate them from impact trauma. The innermost layer, called the renal capsule, is a clear smooth membrane that also wraps the ureter and lines the renal sinus.

THREE REGIONS OF THE KIDNEYS

Internally, each kidney is divided into three distinct parts or regions. From the outermost (convex) portion of the kidney to the innermost (concave) portion, the three regions of the kidney are: the renal cortex, the renal medulla, and the renal pelvis. These three layers are described as follows:

Renal Cortex: The renal cortex is the outermost tissue area of the kidney organ; it is immediately deep to the renal capsule described above. The renal cortex lies between the renal capsule and the base of the medullary pyramids, and it also fills the space between one medullary pyramid and the next. The renal cortex and the renal pyramids constitute

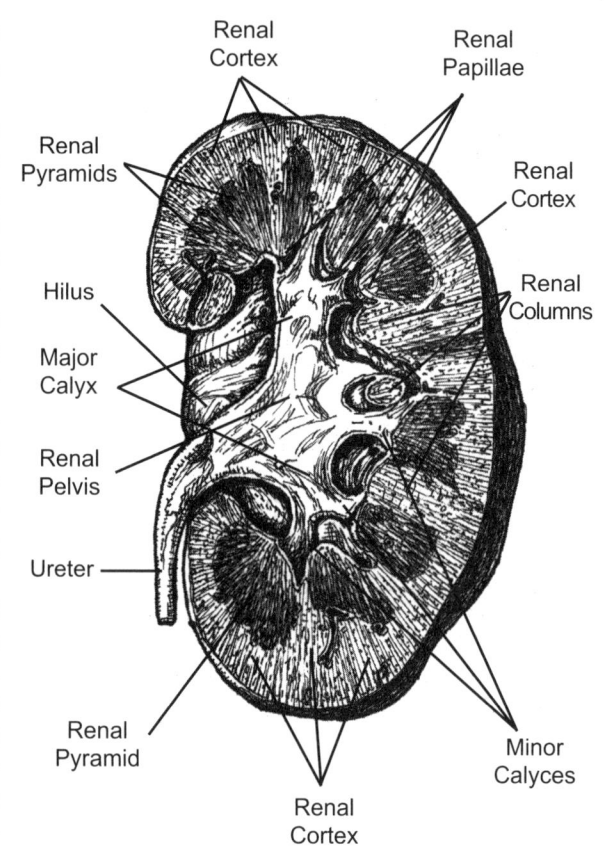

Figure 8.135. The Kidney (Kd) Organ

the functional portions of the kidneys, and are collectively called the parenchyma.

Renal Medulla: The renal medulla is of a reddish brown color and contains eight or more cone shaped medullary (or renal) pyramids. These pyramids have their base directed towards the cortex and their apex pointing towards the center of the kidney. Because they are filled with parallel bundles of straight tubes and blood vessels, the renal pyramids have a striped appearance. Tissue from the renal cortex extends between the medullary pyramids to form what are called renal columns.

Renal Pelvis: The renal pelvis is a funnel shaped structure situated in the central portion of the kidney. Its serves to collect the final filtrate of the nephrons (urine) from the calyces and collecting ducts. To accomplish this, the renal pelvis branches to penetrate into the renal pyramids through several major calyces, each of which then branches into minor calyces that enclose the area around the renal pyramids. Peristaltic contractions of the smooth muscles along the length of the calyces, renal pelvis, and the ureter are responsible for propelling the urine out of the kidneys and into the urinary bladder. The renal pelvis is continuous with the ureter, which serves to transport urine downwards into the bladder.

Nephrons

The functional units of the kidneys are the microscopic nephrons, which carry out the basic processes of cleansing the blood. Each kidney contains roughly 1 million nephrons, the majority of which (85%) are located in the renal cortex. The three essential functions of nephrons are filtration, secretion, and reabsorption, which take place at different areas within the nephron.

Each nephron is made up of a renal corpuscle and a renal tubule. The renal corpuscle is a convoluted bundle of capillaries (glomerulus) surrounded by a capsule called the glomerular (or Bowman's) capsule. The glomerulus is a looping tuft of capillaries extending from one of the arteriole branches of the renal artery. It is almost completely surrounded by the filtrate-collecting glomerular capsule. The glomerulus and the glomerular capsule meet to form a filtration membrane, the endothelial-capsular membrane, that serves to filter certain materials (e.g. water, salts, glucose, amino acids, vitamins, and nitrogenous wastes such as ammonia) from the blood. This process, called glomerular filtration, takes place because of a unique pressure differential between the glomerular capillaries and the glomerular capsule. Thus in the first stage of urine formation, the filtrate contains both desirable and undesirable materials.

The renal tubule carries this filtrate away and is continuous with the glomerular capsule. Along the length of the renal tubule, the majority of filtrate is reabsorbed into the blood through a series of complex passive and active transport mechanisms including: diffusion, facilitated diffusion, primary active transport, secondary active transport, and osmosis.

Three Main Sections of the Renal Tubule

The three main sections of the renal tubule are the proximal convoluted tubule, the loop of Henle (nephron loop), and the distal convoluted tubule, described as follows (Figure 8.136):

Proximal Convoluted Tubule: Leading away from the glomerular capsule, the proximal convoluted tubule serves to allow the body to reabsorb the desirable portion of the filtrate. The materials recovered into the blood from the proximal convoluted tubule include: water, glucose, amino acids, vitamins, sodium, chlorine, carbonic acid, and potassium, in addition to other substances.

Loop of Henle: The loop of Henle is continuous with both the proximal convoluted tubule and the distal convoluted tubule, and is the connection between them. In the loop of Henle, water, potassium, sodium, and chlorine are reabsorbed into the blood.

Distal Convoluted Tubule: By the time filtrate reaches the distal convoluted tubule, it is fairly concentrated. Here nearly all of the remaining water is reabsorbed, along with further amounts of sodium and chlorine.

The distal convoluted tubule empties into a collecting tube, which receives this concentrated filtrate from several neurons before emptying into a papillary duct. The last phases of water, sodium, and chlorine reabsorption take place along the collecting tube. The resulting filtrate flows down through a papillary duct into one of the minor calyces, then into a major calyce, and eventually into the renal pelvis. The renal pelvis then empties into the urinary bladder via the ureter.

Common Disorders of the Kidneys

Common disorders of the kidneys include: pyelonephritis (kidney infection), pyelitis (inflammation of renal pelvis and calyces), azotemia (caused by excessive wastes in the blood), hydronephrosis (obstruction of urine flow due to the enlargement of one or both kidneys), nephritic syndrome (protein lost into the urine), polycystic disease (deformities in the nephrons), kidney tumors (e.g. renal cell carcinoma), acute or chronic renal failure, nephrotosis (floating kidney), dia-

VOLUME 1, SECTION 1: FOUNDATIONS OF CHINESE ENERGETIC MEDICINE

betes insipidus (excessive glucose secretion), and kidney stones. Kidney stones are composed primarily of calcium salts, uric acid, and various other crystals such as struvite. Anuria is a condition in which the kidneys produce less than 50 ml of urine per day, and be caused by several internal dysfunctions.

In end-stage renal failure, one of the kidneys may be removed without causing the death of the patient. In cases where the remaining kidney is healthy, it may eventually be able to function at 80% of the original combined capacity of both kidneys. If both kidneys are functioning inadequately, kidney dialysis (in which the blood is filtered by a machine outside the body) is often performed. Another increasingly common procedure is a kidney transplant.

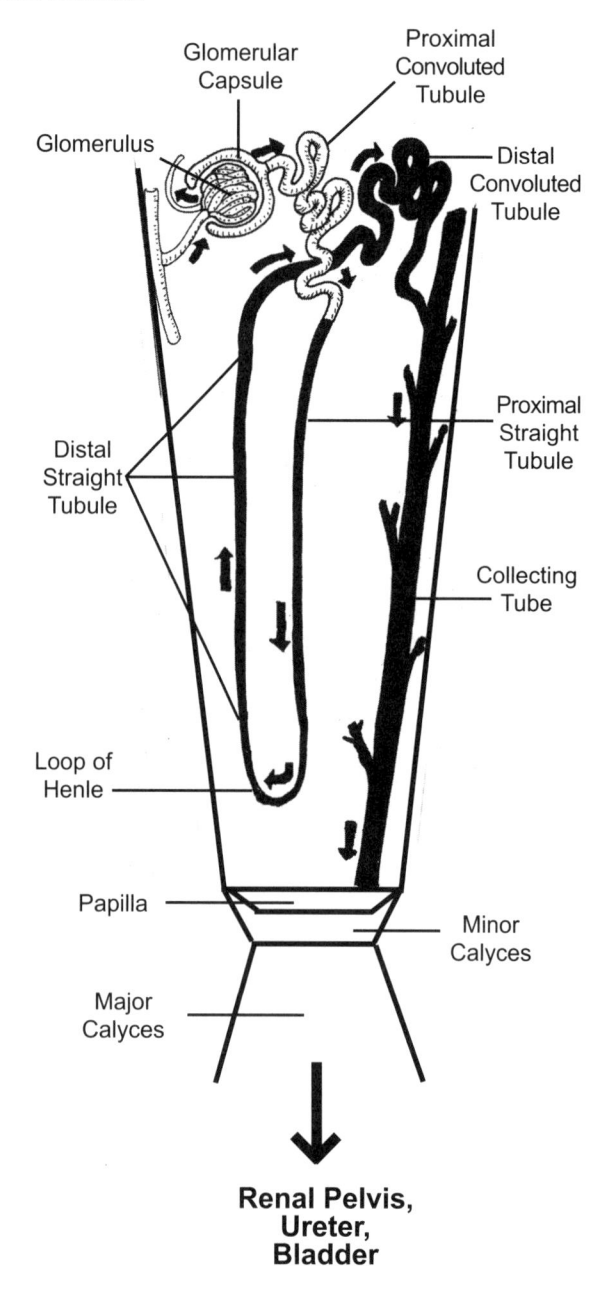

Figure 8.136. Order of Kidneys Filtration Mechanisms: Glomerulus, Glomerular Capsule, Proximal Tubule, Loop of Henle, Distal Tubule, Collecting Tube, Minor then Major Calyces, Renal Pelvis, Ureter, Bladder (storage), and then discharged through the Urethra. (Inspired by the original artwork of Wynn Kapit).

432

CHAPTER 8: THE TWELVE PRIMARY ORGANS, CHANNELS AND COLLATERALS

PERICARDIUM: XIN ZHU

The Pericardium is a Yin organ, and its associated Yang organ is the Triple Burner. Its Element is Fire. In Chinese Energetic medicine, the Pericardium is not considered to be an independent organ, but rather serves as a protective covering for the Heart. Thus the Pericardium's primary responsibility is to protect the Heart from pathogenic factors.

The Pericardium activates, energizes, and controls the Yin channel's distribution of the Kidney Yang Qi to the Yin organs. The Pericardium assists the Heart in governing the Blood and housing the Shen. The Pericardium is also known as the "prime minister," and is the official who protects the Heart.

The Pericardium is sometimes known as the "Heart Protector," and its channel is sometimes referred to as the "circulation-sex meridian." The Pericardium is also responsible for housing the Shen, maintaining the "Emperor's Fire," and for setting emotional boundaries (Figure 8.137).

CHINESE CHARACTER FOR PERICARDIUM: XIN ZHU

The ancient Chinese ideograph for the Pericardium "Xin Zhu," can be translated as the "Heart Master," which expresses the Pericardium's responsibility of assisting the Heart in governing the body's Qi and Shen.

- The first character "Xin" translates as "Heart." It refers to a the image of a Heart organ, and is divided into three sections. The upper half of the character depicts the aorta and major arteries. The Heart itself is depicted in the center. The lower left part of the character depicts the Pericardium. In Traditional Chinese Medicine, the character "Xin" also refers as much to the Mind (thoughts and emotions) as it does to the actual internal organ (Figure 8.138).
- The second character "Zhu" translates as "Overlord" or "Master." It depicts the image of a lamp-stand with flames rising upward. The character gives us the image of a man who spreads "light, illumination, brilliance," expressing the clarity of the divine spirit, or the

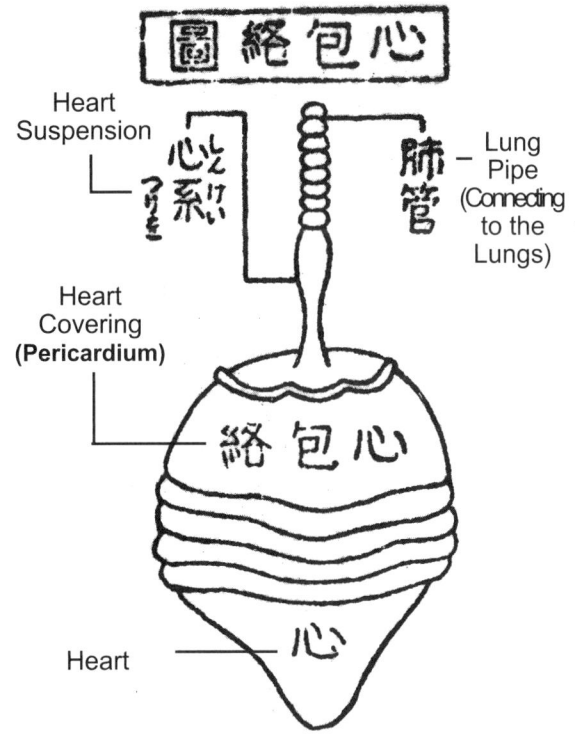

Figure 8.137. The ancient Chinese anatomical diagram of the Pericardium (Pc) Organ, as it appeared in "Important Useful Notes on Acupuncture and Moxibustion," published in Japan in 1718, by Masatoyo Hongo

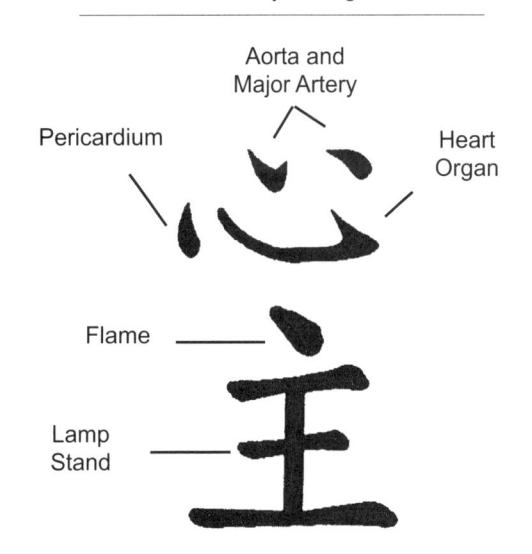

Figure 8.138. The Chinese character for "Xin Zhu," Heart Master (Pericardium)

433

```
                                    ┌─ From Invasion of External Pathogens
                  ┌─ Protects the Heart ─┤
                  │                 └─ From Invasion of Toxic Emotions
The Main          │
Functions         ├─ Houses the Mind
of the            │
Pericardium       │                      ┌─ Warms Qi in the Upper Burner
Organ and         ├─ Houses the Emperor's Fire ─┤
Channels          │                      └─ True Fire
                  │
                  └─ Psycho-Emotional Aspects ─── Boundary Setting
```

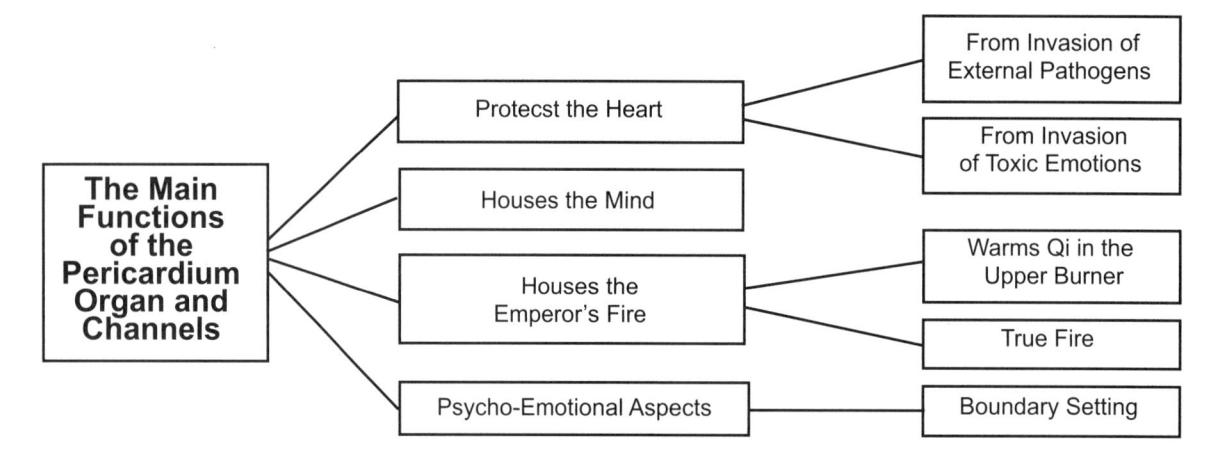

Figure 8.139. The Main Energetic Functions of the Pericardium Organ and Channels

expression of the individual's "Shen Ming." The "Shen Ming" is a special type of spiritual brightness with transformative powers.

THE PERICARDIUM IN CHINESE MEDICINE

In Traditional Chinese Medicine, the functions ascribed to the Pericardium are different from the physiological functions described in Western Medicine. Some of the major differences in the Chinese energetic interpretation of the Pericardium are that it also includes certain functions that are ascribed to the nervous system in Western Medicine, and governs important psycho-emotional aspects.

According to Traditional Chinese Medicine, the main functions of the Pericardium are to: protect the Heart, house the Mind, house the "Emperor's Fire," and express itself through the psycho-emotional aspects of relationship and boundaries. These main functions are described as follows (Figure 8.139):

1. **Protects the Heart:** The Pericardium protects the Heart from external invasion of pathogens and the external invasion of toxic emotions.
   - **External Invasion of Pathogens:** When a pathogenic factor attacks the Heart, it is diverted to the Pericardium instead.
   - **External Invasion of Toxic Emotions:** The Pericardium is considered the Heart's advisor, assisting the Heart in bringing order and peace. It intercepts the emotional discharges directed to the Heart, released from the Zang Fu organs via respiration. The Pericardium restrains the emotional charge by energetically neutralizing it and temporarily placing it into the Heart's courtyard (also known as the Yellow Court) to be later investigated at a more opportune time, when the individual is ready.
2. **Houses the Mind:** The Pericardium is considered to be the "center of the thorax," and it assists the Heart in circulating the Blood and in housing the mental, emotional, and sexual states of the Mind.
3. **Houses the Emperor's Fire:** The Heart Fire is located in the center of the chest, and is also called the "Commanding Fire" or "Emperor's Fire." The Heart Fire is an essential component of the body's True Fire, and is responsible for transforming the body's energy (Qi) into spirit (Shen).
4. **Psycho-Emotional Aspects:** The Pericardium is responsible for setting the emotional boundaries for the Heart, and has a powerful influence on the patient's mental and emotional states. It governs energetic circulation, sexuality and intimacy. In ancient times, the purpose of the Pericardium was viewed as a

"minister of council" designed to protect the "emperor" (Heart) and to help create feelings of security, joy, happiness and pleasure. In this respect, an important function of the Pericardium is to energetically intercept strong emotions that may overwhelm the Heart, and then place them in the courtyard (solar plexus area) until the Heart is ready to deal with such matters (Figure 8.140).

In ancient times, the Heart was also known by the name of the "Yellow Emperor" or "Suspended Gold" and the courtyard of the Heart (located in the solar plexus area) was known as the "Yellow Emperor's Court," more commonly called the "Yellow Court." The Yellow Court stores the emotional experiences such as being rejected, betrayed or abandoned. The stored belief structures of these emotions are later absorbed by the specific energetic natures of the body's other Yin organs (Liver, Spleen, Lungs and Kidneys).

One example of the Pericardium protecting the Heart at the formative years of childhood can be observed when a newborn baby is startled. When startled (as the baby cries), a baby will automatically thrust its chest upward in order to discharge the emotional shock away from the Heart. The emotions are then instinctively released outward through the child's extremities (hands and feet). Later, as the baby grows older, the experienced traumatic feelings that are not released from his or her tissues will be stored in the Yellow Court away from the child's Heart, and distributed according to the corresponding Yin organ relationships (fear to the Kidneys, anger to the Liver, etc.).

A patient with Deficient Pericardium Qi will have very weak emotional boundaries and will allow the Heart to constantly and indiscriminately connect, bond and fall in love with other individuals, even when it is not appropriate. A patient with Excessive Pericardium Qi will be emotionally armored, pushing others away, feeling no need for emotional connection.

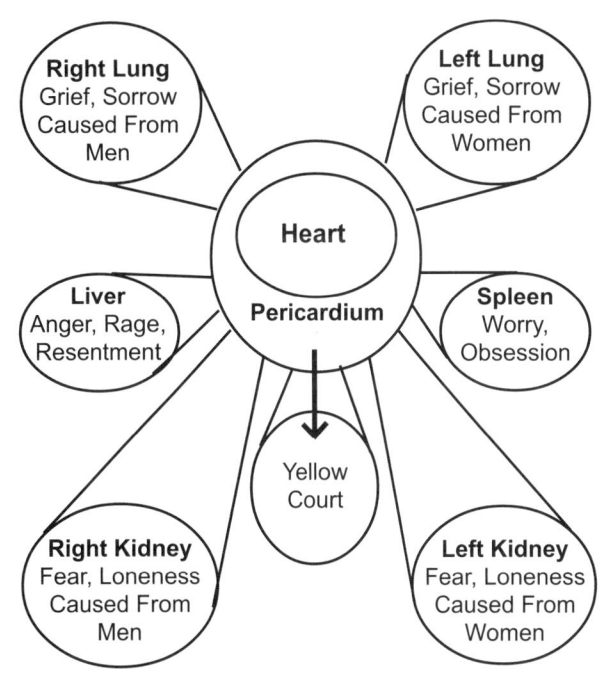

Figure 8.140. The Relationships of the Pericardium

THE PERICARDIUM CHANNELS

The Pericardium Channels are Yin channels that flow externally from the torso to the hands. The two main energetic rivers originate internally from the center of the chest, flowing from the Pericardium. They descend through the center of the body, spirally wrapping the Upper, Middle, and Lower Burners. The two main energetic rivers then surface and branch externally near the nipples before proceeding down the center of each arm to end at the tips of the middle fingers. A second branch arises from the Pc-8 points at the center of each palm and flows into the ring fingers to connect with the Triple Burner Channels (Figure 8.141).

CHANNELS' ENERGY FLOW

The Pericardium Channels affect the body's circulation of Blood. They are considered to be the "mother of Yin," and are also connected to the Mingmen. The Pericardium Channels store more Blood than Qi, acting more on the physical substance and Blood functions than on the energy. At

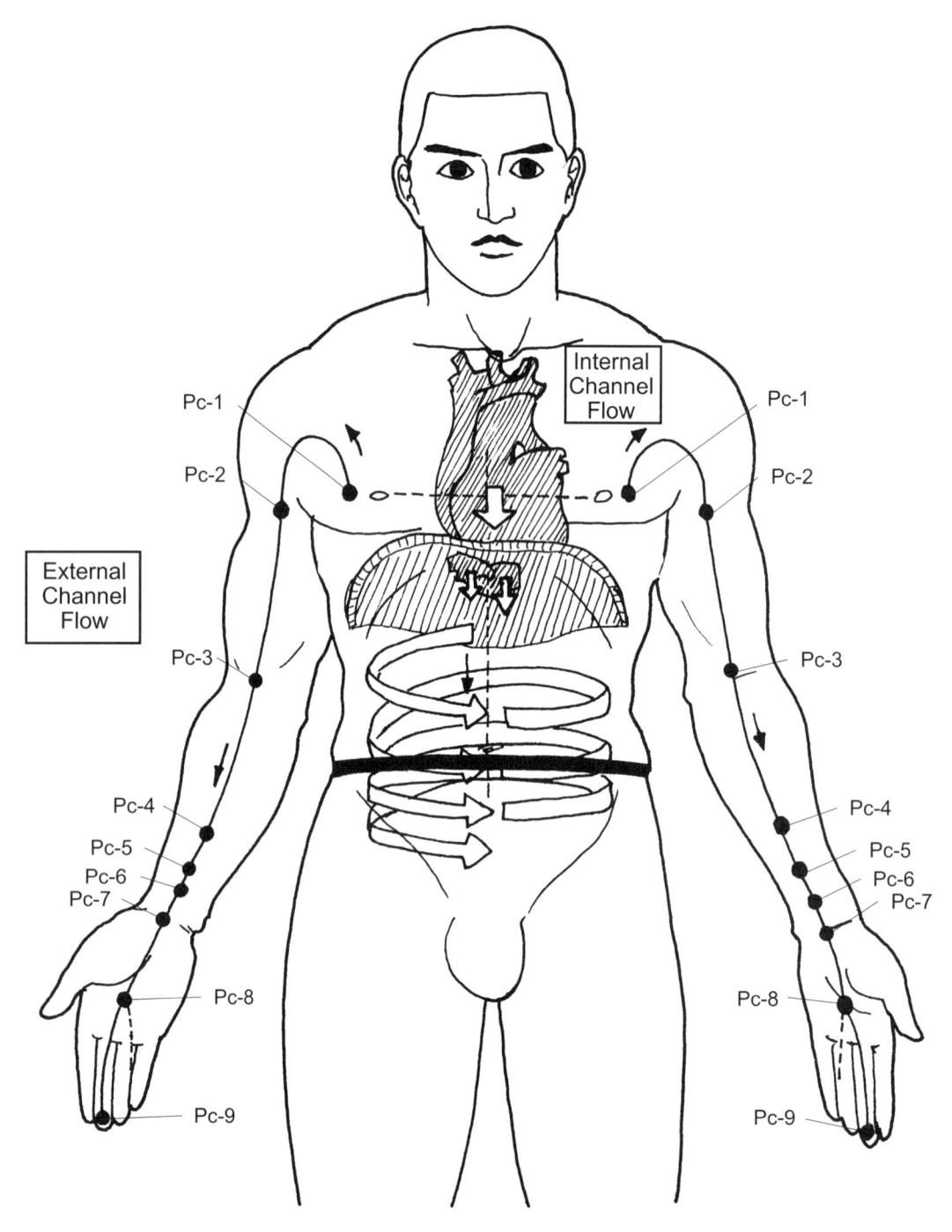

Figure 8.141. The Internal and External Qi Flow of the Pericardium (Pc) Channels

```
Pericardium ─┬─ Heat Affecting the Pericardium ───── Heat misting the Mind: manifesting in symptoms such as a very high temperature, delirium, and in severe cases coma
             │
             └─ Phlegm Affecting the Pericardium ── Turbidity clouding the Pericardium: manifesting in symptoms such as mental depression and dementia
```

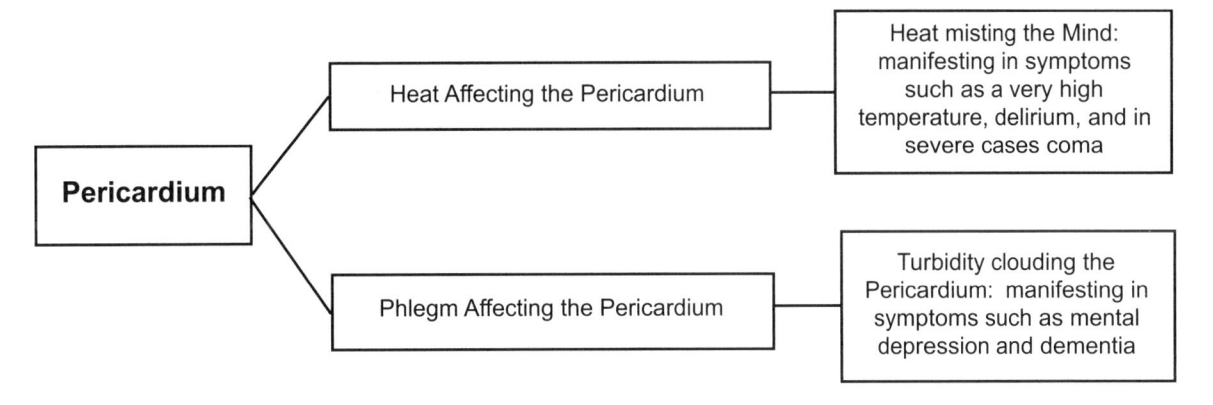

Figure 8.142. Chart of Pericardium Disharmonies

the high-tide time period (7 p.m. to 9 p.m.), Qi and Blood abound in the Pericardium organ and Pericardium channels. At this time period the Pericardium organ and channels can more easily be dispersed and purged. During low tide (7 a.m. to 9 a.m.), they can be more readily tonified. The energy of the Pericardium Channel also acts on the skin, muscles, and nerves found along their pathways.

THE INFLUENCE OF CLIMATE

The Pericardium is primarily affected by the invasion of external pathogenic Heat and Phlegm, which together obstruct the Pericardium.

THE INFLUENCE OF TASTE, COLOR, AND SOUND

- The bitter taste can be used to tonify the Pericardium, or clear Excess Heat.
- The red color is used to tonify the Pericardium.
- The "Shee" sound is used to purge toxic Heat from both the Pericardium and the Triple Burners.

PERICARDIUM PATHOLOGY

The main diseases of the Pericardium organ and channels include Heat and Phlegm affecting the Heart, resulting in symptoms that cause discomfort in the front of the chest, disorders of the major Blood Vessels, and diseases on the midline to upper palmar side of the upper extremities.

Mental abnormalities may also manifest. Disharmonies of the Pericardium are associated with the last two levels, "Ying or Xue," of diagnosis according to the "Four Levels" patterns of disease, and are also associated with the "Upper Burner Phase" of the diagnosis according to the Triple Burners patterns of disease (see Volume 3, Chapter 25).

T.C.M. PATTERNS OF DISHARMONY

There are two main patterns of Pericardium Disharmony, both of which originate from an invasion by external factors: heat affecting the Pericardium and Phlegm affecting the Pericardium. These two patterns have similar symptoms to that of the Heart Disharmony patterns caused from internal disease factors of Phlegm Fire Agitating the Heart and Cold Phlegm Misting the Heart (see Heart Section), which are described as follows (Figure 8.142):

1. **Heat Affecting the Pericardium:** The main pattern of disharmony associated with the Pericardium organ is that of Heat invasion. Heat invading the Pericardium is said to mist the Mind, and can manifest in symptoms such as a very high temperature, anxiety, insomnia, delirium, and in severe cases coma.
2. **Phlegm Affecting the Pericardium:** This pattern of disharmony associated with Phlegm turbidity clouding the Pericardium. The main symptoms are mental depression, unclear speech, Phlegm Stroke, and dementia.

The Pericardium in Western Medicine

The pericardium is a double-walled (triple-layered) fibroserous sac that surrounds and protects the heart (Figure 8.143).

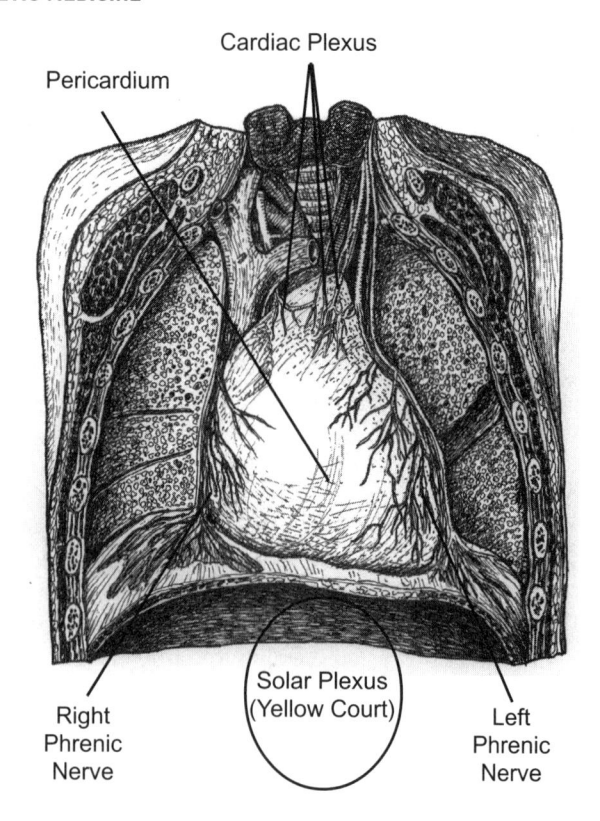

The pericardium confines the heart to its position in the mediastinum, and also creates a lubricated space that allows sufficient freedom of movement for the heart's vigorous and rapid contractions. The pericardium is divided into two main sections, the fibrous pericardium and the serous pericardium, described as follows:

- **Fibrous Pericardium:** The bag shaped, tough outer layer of inelastic fibrous connective tissue is called the fibrous pericardium. It provides protection and prevents the overstretching of the heart. The fibrous pericardium attaches to the diaphragm and sternum, with its open end fused to the connective tissues of the blood vessels that enter and exit the heart.

- **Serous Pericardium:** The thinner, more delicate serous pericardium forms a double layer around the heart. The outer portion, known as the "parietal layer," is fused with the fibrous pericardium. The inner portion, known as the "visceral layer" or "epicardium," adheres tightly to the outermost layer of the heart. The space between the parietal and visceral pericardium is known as the pericardial cavity, and is filled with a thin slippery film of serous fluid known as the pericardial fluid. The pericardial fluid reduces friction between the serous membranes allowing the heart to move in a relatively friction-free environment.

Physiology

The function of the pericardium is to provide a protective covering for the heart, and reduce the friction caused by the heart's pumping action (Figure 8.144).

Figure 8.143. The Pericardium (Pc)

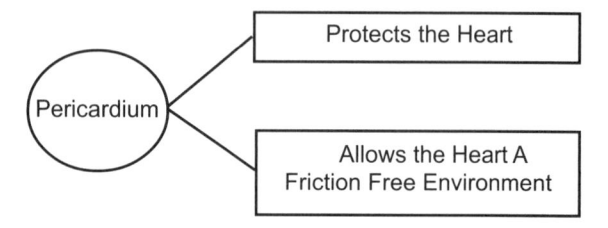

Figure 8.144. The Functions of the Pericardium (Western Medical Perspective)

CHAPTER 8: THE TWELVE PRIMARY ORGANS, CHANNELS AND COLLATERALS

TRIPLE BURNERS: SAN JIAO

The Triple Burners (San Jiao) are considered a Yang Organ, their associated Yin organ is the Pericardium, and their Element is Fire. The Triple Burners are also known as the Triple Heaters and Triple Warmers, and are called the "Father of Yang Qi," because they are responsible for commanding the circulation of Yang Qi. In ancient China, the Triple Burners were conceptualized as being a large bowel that contained all of the body's internal organs (Figure 8.145).

CHINESE CHARACTER FOR TRIPLE BURNERS: SAN JIAO

The Chinese characters for Triple Burners, "San Jiao" can be translated as, "the three fires (or ovens) that cook and process food" (Figure 8.146).
- The first character "San" translates as the number "three or triple."
- The second character "Jiao" translates as "burners, cauldrons or combustion oven," and is divided into two ideographs. The character on the top is the ideogram of a bird without a tail being cooked by the action of fire. The character on the bottom depicts the small flames of fire rising upward. The ideograph expresses the image of a bird in the process of being cooked or roasted.

THE TRIPLE BURNERS IN ANCIENT CHINESE MEDICINE

Like the other Yang organs, the Triple Burners have an energetic "form." In the Ming Dynasty (1368 - 1644 A.D.), the renowned doctor Zhang Jiebin taught that the Triple Burners were in fact the largest bowel within the body's cavity, and that they existed as an energetic field within the body, surrounding and containing the viscera and bowels.

THE TRIPLE BURNERS IN CHINESE MEDICINE

The functions of the Triple Burners are derived from observations unique to Chinese energetic medicine, as they do not possess any physical anatomical form. Therefore, the Triple Burners are not described in Western Medicine.

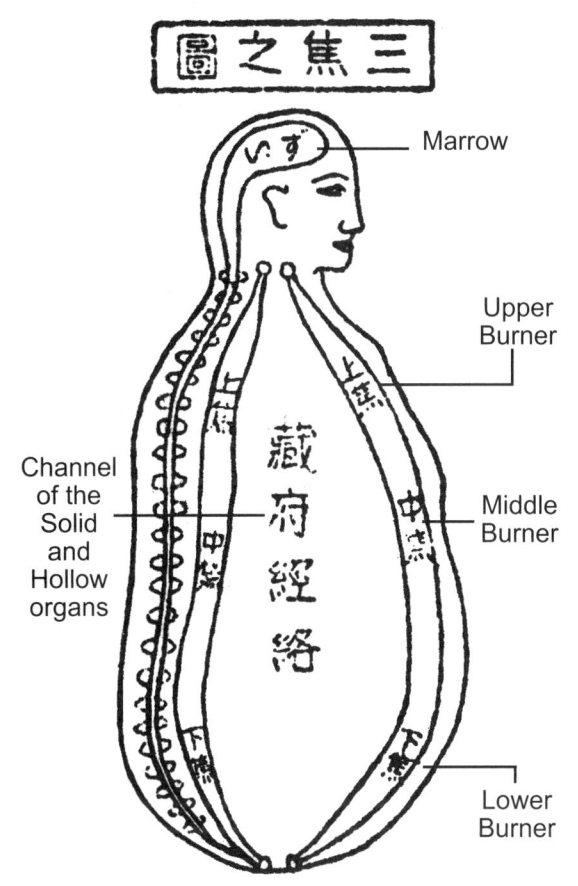

Figure 8.145. The ancient Chinese anatomical diagram of the Triple Burners (TB) Organ, as it appeared in "Important Useful Notes on Acupuncture and Moxibustion," published in Japan in 1718, by Masatoyo Hongo

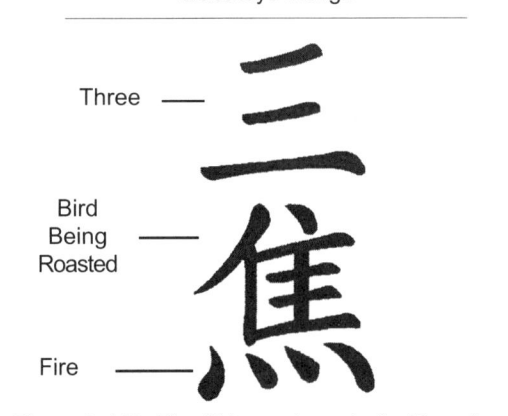

Figure 8.146. The Chinese character for "San Jiao," Three Burners

439

VOLUME 1, SECTION 1: FOUNDATIONS OF CHINESE ENERGETIC MEDICINE

```
The Main Functions of the Triple Burners
├── Controls the Activities of Qi
├── Transports and Transforms Qi and Body Fluids
├── Separates Clear Fluid From Turbid
├── Provides an Avenue For Yuan Qi
├── Regulates Balance and Harmony
│   ├── Governs Water Metabolism
│   ├── Controls Production of Wei Qi
│   └── Transports Yuan Qi
├── Regulates the Body's Auric Fields
├── Houses the Body's True Fire
│   ├── Warms Qi in the Three Burners
│   └── Transforms Jing to Qi to Shen
└── Psycho-Emotional Aspects
    └── Regulates Social Relations
```

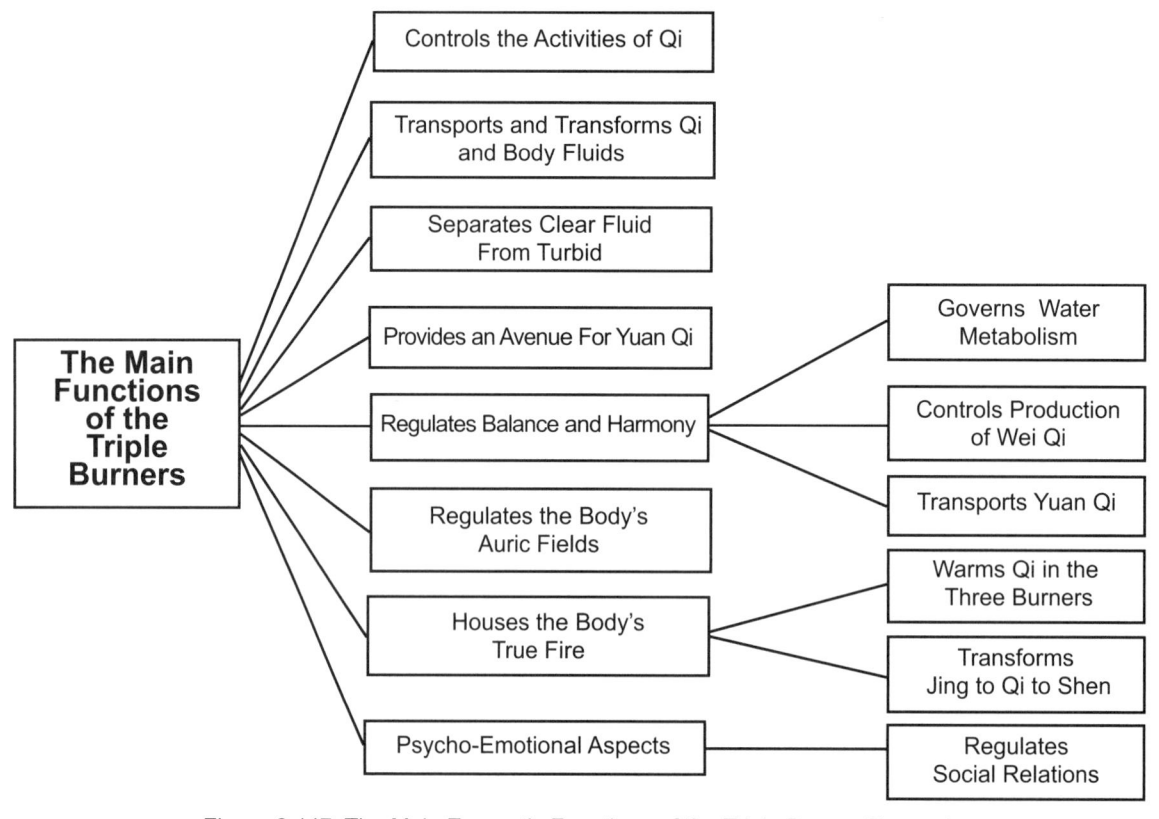

Figure 8.147. The Main Energetic Functions of the Triple Burner Channels

Because the Triple Burners relate to the internal organ membrane system of the thoracic, abdominal, and lower abdominal cavities, modern T.C.M. understands the energetic fields of the Triple Burners as including and influencing the pleura, and both the parietal and visceral peritoneum of the abdominal cavities.

The Triple Burners are regarded as an independent Yang organ. They are assigned to three specific energy areas within the body's cavity, and regulate the general ingestion and digestion of food and fluids throughout the body.

According to Traditional Chinese Medicine, the main functions of the Triple Burners are to: control the activities of Qi, transport and transform Qi and food essence, separate clear fluid from turbid, provide an avenue for Yuan Qi, regulate balance and harmony, regulate the body's aura fields, house the body's True Fire, and manifest through the psycho-emotional aspects of regulating social relations. These main functions are described as follows (Figure 8.147):

1. **Controls the Activities of Qi:** Each of the three Burners controls the movement of specific types of Qi, and various stages of energetic transformation. The Upper Burner assists in transforming Wei Qi (Defensive Energy); the Middle Burner assists in transforming Ying Qi (Nutritive Energy); and the Lower Burner assists in transforming Body Fluids. The Upper Burner also controls respiration and activates the flow of Qi, Blood, and Body Fluids.

2. **Transports and Transforms Qi and Food Essence:** The Triple Burners are considered to be the "passage through which water, food and fluid are transported." The Middle Burner, in particular, plays an essential role in the transportation and transformation of food essence to produce Qi and Blood.

3. **Separates Clears Fluid From Turbid:** In medi-

cal texts from ancient China, the Triple Burners are described as "opening up, discharging Qi, and letting Qi out." The Lower Burner separates clear fluid from turbid fluid, discharges urine and stool, and also releasing Turbid Qi in the form of gas.

4. **Provides an Avenue For Yuan Qi:** The Triple Burners are considered to be the ambassadors or "intermediaries" for the body's Yuan Qi. They transport Yuan Qi from the Kidneys to all the other organs of the body, and also provide the internal Heat for digestion. The Conception Vessel brings the Qi to the Triple Burners to assist in this process.

5. **Regulates Balance and Harmony:** The Triple Burners are known as "the official of balance and harmony," because they govern water metabolism, control the production of Wei Qi, and transport Yuan Qi from the Kidneys to all the other organs of the body. This name also refers to the Triple Burners' role in regulating the body's metabolic functions, and to their production of Qi, Blood, Body Fluids, and waste products.

6. **Regulates the Body's Auric Fields:** The Triple Burners are said to regulate the body's auric fields. The Lower Burner is connected to the first and innermost level of Wei Qi; the Middle Burner is connected to the second and middle level of Wei Qi responsible for aura field movement; and the Upper Burner is connected to the third level and outermost level of Wei Qi.

7. **Houses the Body's True Fire:** One function of the Triple Burners' energy is to produce heat, and thus to regulate the body temperature like a thermostat. The heat of the Triple Burners can be increased through meditative disciplines such as circulating energy along the Microcosmic Orbit (which connects the Governing and Conception Vessels) or the Macrocosmic Orbit (which connects all Twelve Primary Channels with the Governing and Conception Vessels).

8. **Psycho-Emotional Aspects:** The Triple Burners assist in regulating the emotional interactions of the individual's social relations. On a psycho-emotional level, the Triple Burners can be used to move Qi and lift depression derived from a stagnation of Liver Qi. When the Triple Burners (which regulate the consciousness) are full, the consciousness becomes stable, and the Mind's intent becomes benevolent and kind-hearted. The Triple Burners are especially linked with the Heart and Pericardium and are easily affected by the emotion of joy.

From and ancient Daoist perspective, it is taught that when the energy of the Heart is strong and pure (e.g., internally consistent and without guilt), and the desires and thoughts of an individual are at peace, then the energy of the body's sexual essence (Jing) will spread into the Triple Burners, and the Blood will flourish within the vessels. If the "fire of desire" (sexual passion) is allowed to heat and combine with the energy of the Triple Burners, the energy of the individual's sexual essence will overflow, mix itself with the energy of the Mingmen, and leave the body via the reproductive organs and tissues. This can lead to a depletion of both Jing and Qi.

THE TRIPLE BURNER CHANNELS

The Triple Burner Channels are Yang channels that flow externally from the hands to the head. The two main channels originate externally from the tips of the ring fingers and ascend along the lateral aspect of the arms, continuing over the shoulders to the clavicles. From the St-12 points they branch internally, dispersing into the chest to envelop and spiral wrap the Pericardium. They then circle the diaphragm and penetrate the Upper, Middle, and Lower Burners. A set of branches originate internally from the chest CV-17 point at the Heart, and the front gate of the Middle Dantian. Flowing upwards, these branches return back to the supraclavicular fossa at the St-12 points before ascending up the neck, head, and circling the ears. From the TB-20 points, another set of branches flows above the ears towards the outer canthus of the eyes; from the TB-22 points, a final set of branches flows downward to the cheek, terminating in the infraorbital region (Figure 8.148).

The internal flow of the Triple Burner Channels moves from St-12 down to CV-17, where it disperses into the chest and envelops the Pericardium. As the channel's energy flows down through the diaphragm, it circulates through the chest and penetrates the Triple Burners (a continuing branch flows upward to the St-12 points)

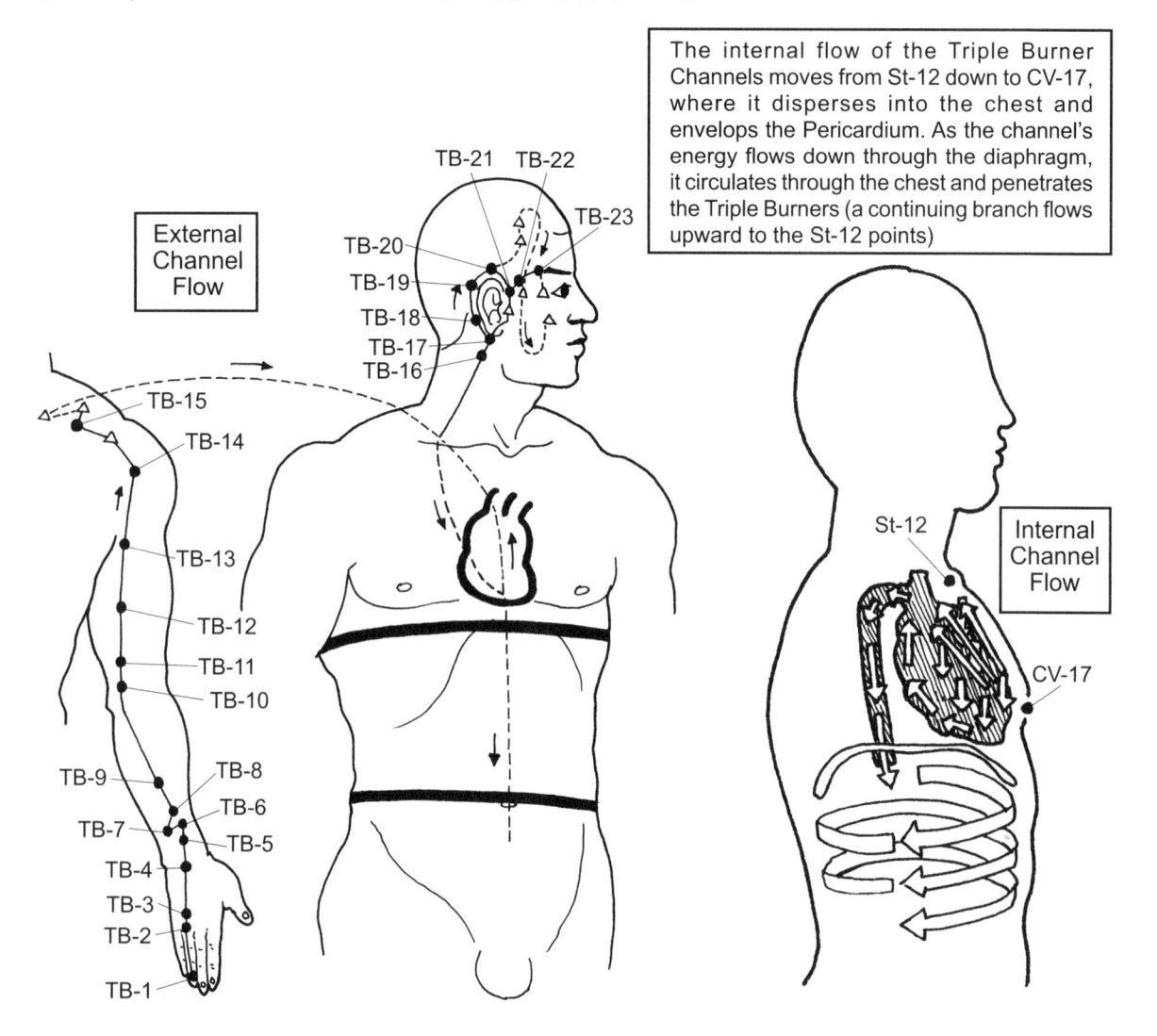

Figure 8.148. The Internal and External Qi Flow of the Triple Burners (TB) Channel

Channels' Energy Flow

The Triple Burner Channels store more Qi than Blood, and act more on the energetic and nervous functions of the body than on physical substance and Blood functions. At the high-tide time period (9 p.m. to 11 p.m.), Qi and Blood abound in the Triple Burner Channels. At this time period the Triple Burner channels can more easily be dispersed and purged. During low tide (9 a.m. to 11 a.m.), they can be more readily tonified. The energy of the Triple Burner Channels also acts on the skin, muscles, and nerves found along their pathways. The Triple Burners move the body's True Fire.

The Energetic Anatomy of the Triple Burners

The Triple Burners' energy is primarily composed of Zong Qi (Essential Qi). The Zong Qi assists the Heart in the circulation of Blood and assists the Lungs in respiration. The Zong Qi is in charge of distributing the Ying Qi (Nourishing Qi)

CHAPTER 8: THE TWELVE PRIMARY ORGANS, CHANNELS AND COLLATERALS

Receiving: the Upper Burner is also known as "Mist," and it governs the area from the diaphragm upwards, including the head, throat, Lungs, Heart and Pericardium. The Upper Burner assists the Spleen in its function of directing the body's clean fluids upwards, and also helps the Lungs in dispersing and scattering fluids to the skin and muscles.

Ripening and Rotting: the Middle Burner is also known as the "Muddy Pool," and it governs the area between the diaphragm and umbilicus, including the Stomach, Spleen, and Gall Bladder. The Middle Burner assists the Stomach in the transformation and transportation of fluids and liquids, and also in directing their impurities downwards.

Excreting: the Lower Burner is also known as the "Drainage Ditch," and it governs the area below the umbilicus, including the Liver, Kidneys, Intestines, and Urinary Bladder. The Lower Burner assists the Small Intestine, Large Intestine, the Blood, and the Kidneys in transforming and transporting liquids and wastes.

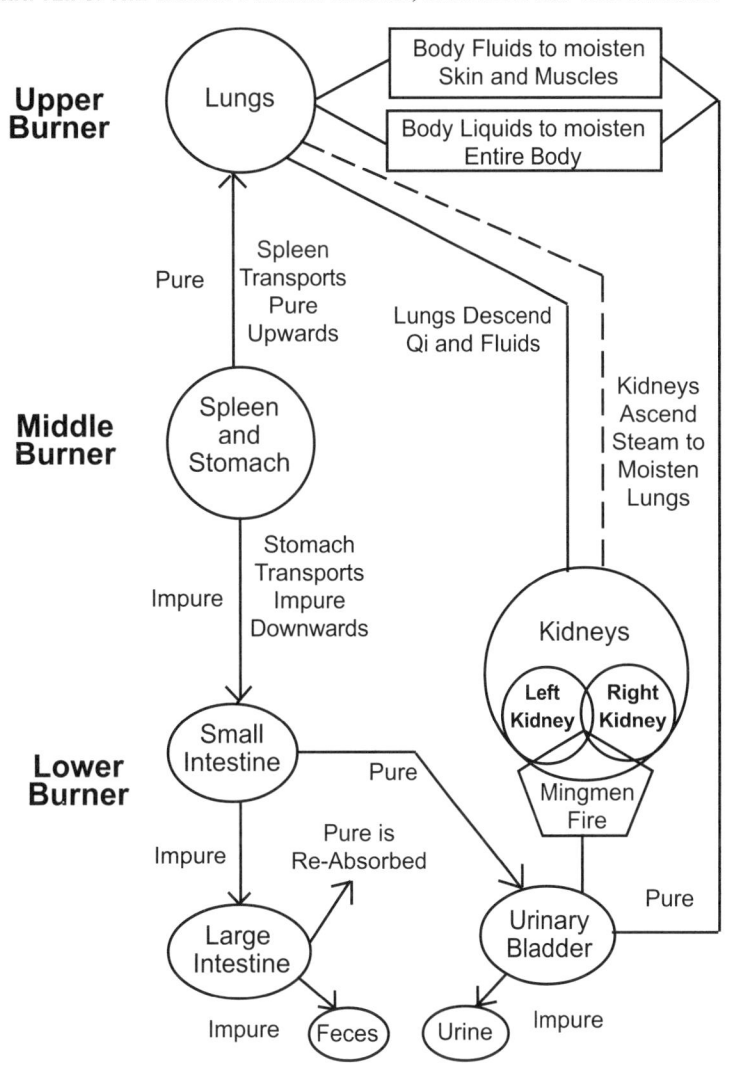

Figure 8.149. The Metabolic Functions of the Triple Burners are divided into three parts or functions: the Upper Burner, Middle Burner, and Lower Burner. These different functions of the Triple Burners control the movement of various types of Qi in the three stages of energy production

throughout the body to nourish the Blood, organs, and tissues. Another function of the Zong Qi is to strengthen the Wei Qi (Protective Qi) that protects the external body from pathogens (Figure 8.149).

1. **The Upper Burner:**

The Upper Burner is formed from the Fire that is created from the combined energies of the Heart, Pericardium, and Lungs. The Upper Burner's energy is housed within the head, throat, and upper chest, and extends down to the diaphragm. The Upper Burner is responsible for respiratory and cardiac functions. It moves the body's finer energy, circulating and distributing nutrients and Qi throughout the body like a mist.

2. **The Middle Burner:**

The Middle Burner is formed from the Fire that is created from the combined energies of the Stomach, Spleen, pancreas, and Gall Bladder. The Middle Burner's energy is housed

443

within the upper abdomen (the diaphragm) and the umbilicus.

The Middle Burner is responsible for digestion, fermentation, and the transformation of food and drink into nutrients for distribution. In the Middle Burner area, the Small Intestine connects downward to the Urinary Bladder. The Small Intestine transforms waste, then sends the unusable portion down to the Large Intestine. The Small Intestine also distills the body's fluids before sending them down to the Urinary Bladder.

The Ying Qi (Nourishing Qi) of the Middle Burner receives its substance from the Stomach and Spleen. The Spleen extracts Gu Qi from the food prepared by the Stomach, churning the food essence into "foam." The Spleen refines this energetic foam, and then sends it as processed Gu Qi to the Lungs. The Lungs (in the Upper Burner) further refine the Gu Qi and send the impure portion to the Kidneys for further refinement of the Gu Qi. The Kidneys return the clean Qi to the Lungs, while sending the turbid portion to the Urinary Bladder to be expelled from the body. In the Lungs, the Qi from the air mixes with the Gu Qi to produce Zong Qi. The Lungs circulate the refined Gu Qi in the form of a vapor (or mist) which is then housed in the Upper Burner. The Heart then utilizes this vapor in the production of Blood.

3. **The Lower Burner:**

The Lower Burner is formed from the Fire that is created from the combined energies of the Liver, Kidneys, Urinary Bladder, Intestines, and genitalia. The Lower Burner's energy is housed within the area just below the umbilicus and extends down to the lower perineum.

The Lower Burner is responsible for the reproductive functions and for the filtration and elimination of waste products. It moves the body's coarser energy, acting as a "channel for water."

The Triple Burners contribute to the process of the three stages of transformation and aid in the distribution of Ying and Wei Qi throughout the body as follows:

- After the Gu Qi (food energy) has been separated into clean and turbid Qi, the Upper Burner releases the body's clean Wei Qi, directing it to the Lungs.
- The Middle Burner releases the body's clean Ying Qi, directing it to all of the body's organs and tissues.
- The Lower Burner releases the Body Fluids, directing the turbid part to the Urinary Bladder.

THE BODY'S THREE FIRES

From a Medical Qigong perspective, and according to the ancient Daoist writings contained within the *Compendium of the Doctrine of the Mean*, heat in the body is generated from the combined action of the Three Fires, which emanate from three specific locations within the body. The Heart Fire is located within the body's chest cavity; the Kidney Fire is located within the abdominal cavity; and the Bladder Fire is located in the lower perineum. There is an ancient Daoist saying, "when the Heart Fire first awakens, the Kidney Fire responds to it; when the Kidney Fire moves, the Bladder Fire follows it."

When these Three Fires follow their normal course of energetic movement, they lead the body's life-force energy in the process of creating and sustaining life. The Three Fires are responsible for regulating the Yin and Yang energy of the body by fusing the Five Element energies (stored within the body's Wood, Fire, Earth, Metal, and Water organs) with the energy of the Three Dantians.

According to the ancient Daoist writings contained within the *Nine Levels of Improper Approaches to the Gate*, when transporting the Jing and Qi, the Three Fires return back to the navel. As the Shen from the Heart Fire is drawn into the Lower Dantian via the Yi (Intention), the Urinary Bladder Fire fuses with the Kidney Fire to create heat and form the body's True Fire. This action causes the body's Jing to transform into Qi within the Lower Dantian. Due to the influence of this Qi, the Heart Fire then transforms Qi into Shen within the Middle Dantian. Once this transformation is completed, the mind, breath, and body connection becomes regulated.

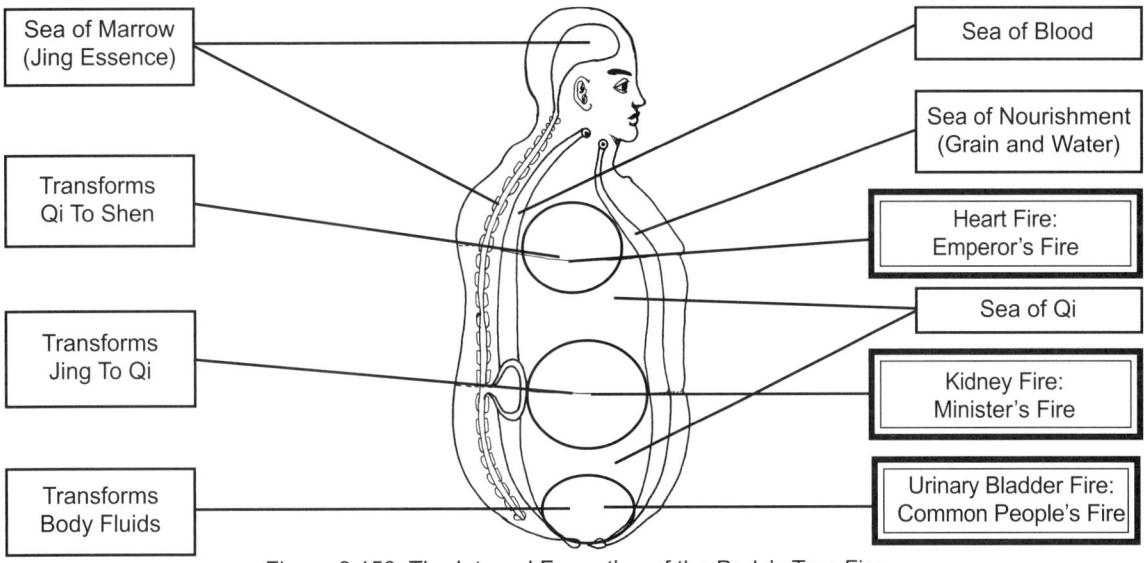

CHAPTER 8: THE TWELVE PRIMARY ORGANS, CHANNELS AND COLLATERALS

Figure 8.150. The Internal Formation of the Body's True Fire

The Three Fires also represent the regions of vital heat that are responsible for the circulation of vital energy that sustains the human soul. The energy of the Three Fires is also used for cultivation and spiritual liberation and can be accessed through Medical Qigong practice, prayer and meditation. The Three Fires are described as follows:

1. **The Heart Fire:** The Heart Fire is located in the center of the chest, and is also called the "Commanding Fire" or "Emperor's Fire." According to the *Complete Method of the Treasure of the Spirit*, "the Heart is the Emperor's Fire." The Heart Fire is responsible for transforming the body's Qi into Shen, and it heats the internal organs within the Upper Burner, energizing both thought and emotion.

2. **The Kidney Fire:** The Kidney Fire is located in the back of the body, just below the last floating rib, between the two Kidneys. It is also called the "Ministerial Fire," "Prime Minister's Fire," and "Mingmen Fire." The Kidney Fire is responsible for transforming the body's Jing into Qi, heating the internal organs in the Middle and Lower Burners, and is the "Root" of the body's Yuan Qi (Prenatal Qi). According to the *Classic of Intelligence and Destiny*, "the Ministerial Fire warms the entire body, promotes the functions of the internal organs, and improves their activity."

Qigong masters in ancient times regarded the Mingmen Fire as the motivating force of the body, and they paid special attention to its training during Qigong exercises. A deficiency of Mingmen Fire may lead to decreased sex-drive, hypogonadism, or impotency. Conversely, if the Mingmen Fire is in excess, increased sex-drive, sexual obsession, or hypergonadism can occur.

Dr. Zhao Xianke, an expert on medicine during the Ming dynasty period, states, "the Mingmen Fire dominates all Twelve Primary Channels. Without it, the Kidneys would be weak, the Spleen and Stomach could not digest food, the Liver and Gall Bladder would not give any energy to think or plan, the urine and feces would not be moved, and the Heart would malfunction causing dizziness and endangering life."

3. **The Urinary Bladder Fire:** According to the ancient Daoist text, *The Complete Method of Magical Treasure*, "the Urinary Bladder Fire is located in the lower abdominal area by the perineum." The Urinary Bladder Fire is also called the "Common People's Fire" according to Volume Eight of *Looking at the Channels*. The Urinary Bladder Fire is responsible

for heating the internal organs in the Lower Burner, evaporating water, and transforming Body Fluids.

The body's Three Fires are not the same as the Triple Burners. The purpose of the Triple Burners is to regulate the ingestion, digestion, and distribution of food and fluids throughout the body. It is considered a completely different energetic system from the Three Fires. The purpose of the Three Fires is to transform and transport the energy of Jing, Qi, and Shen throughout the body, to transform and transport the energetic natures of the Four Seas, to provide Heat to the internal organs within the Triple Burner bowel, and to assist in evaporating water and transforming Body Fluids. However, the physical locations of the Three Fires coincide with the anatomical locations of the Triple Burners (Figure 8.150).

THE INFLUENCE OF CLIMATE

The Triple Burners are especially susceptible to the invasion of external pathogens such as Wind Heat and Wind Cold in the Upper Burner, and Damp Heat and deficient conditions affecting the Lower Burner.

THE INFLUENCE OF TASTE, COLOR, AND SOUND

- The bitter taste can be used to tonify the Triple Burners.
- The red color is used to tonify the Triple Burners.
- The "Shee" sound is used to purge both the Triple Burners and Pericardium.

TRIPLE BURNER PATHOLOGY

The main diseases along the Triple Burner Channels involve the face, ear, cheek, larynx, and neck. Diseases of the Triple Burner Channels also include disorders of the back of the upper extremities from the midline to the upper arm and forearm.

When diagnosing problems due to dysfunctions of the Triple Burners, the Qigong doctor considers the following:

- **A blockage of the Wei Qi in the Upper Burner** causes an impairment of the Lungs' dispersing function. This can result in the invasion of the Lungs by External Evils (e.g., Wind and Heat) that penetrate the Pericardium, corresponding to the initial stage of externally contracted Wind Heat or Wind Cold diseases.
- **A blockage of the Ying Qi in the Middle Burner** causes an impairment of the Spleen's transporting function. This can result in gastrointestinal Heat stagnation and can cause Spleen and Stomach Damp Heat, corresponding to the second stage of externally contracted Heat diseases.
- **A blockage of the Body Fluids in the Lower Burner** causes an impairment of the Urinary Bladder's function of fluid transformation. This results in the deep penetration of Toxic Evils, which weakens the body's Kidney Yin.

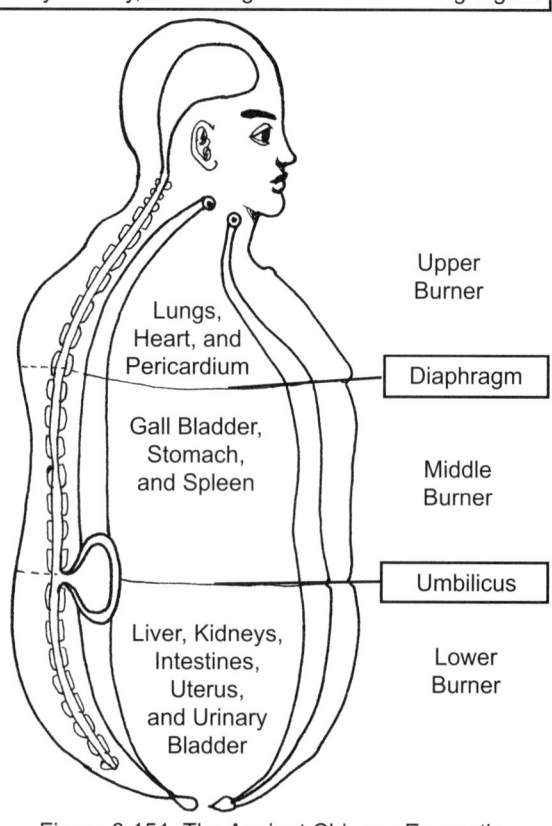

Figure 8.151. The Ancient Chinese Energetic Subdivisions of the Triple Burners

This in turn can cause Deficient Liver Blood and Wind stirring due to Empty Yin, and corresponds to the advanced stages of externally contracted Heat diseases.

T.C.M. PATTERNS OF DISHARMONY

Generally, the patterns of disharmony in the Triple Burner are related to the patterns of the internal organs located within the bowels of the Triple Burner, which are described as follows (Figure 8.151):

1. **Patterns of Disharmony in the Upper Burner:** These involve patterns of disharmony that are associated with the Lungs and Heart, and can manifest through symptoms associated with the invasion of External Wind Cold and Wind Heat invasion.
2. **Patterns of Disharmony in the Middle Burner:** These involve patterns of disharmony that are associated with the Stomach and Spleen, and can manifest through symptoms associated with stagnation and Rebellious Qi.
3. **Patterns of Disharmony in the Lower Burner:** These involve patterns of disharmony that are associated with the Urinary Bladder, Kidneys, Small Intestine and Large Intestine. Lower Burner Disharmony can manifest through symptoms associated with Damp Heat in the Urinary Bladder, Damp Cold in the Urinary Bladder, Kidney Yang Deficiency, Damp Heat in the Large Intestine, or Damp Heat in the Small Intestine.

THE TRIPLE BURNERS IN WESTERN MEDICINE

Though some attempts have been made at correlating the Triple Burner with the Western concept of the maintenance of metabolic balance in the body, Western Medicine recognizes no translation of, or reference to, the Triple Burners.

Understanding Internal Organ Pathology

In Traditional Chinese Medicine, the study of internal organ pathology is based on understanding the physiological functions of each of the body's twelve organ systems. This study also includes the internal organ relationships with the energetic function of the body's Jing, Qi, Shen, Blood, and Body Fluids.

The primary goal of an internal organ's metabolic function is to enhance the overall energetic quality of its reserves, while contributing to the support and function of the body as a whole. For example, when healthy, an internal organ will transmute the Qi, Blood, and Shen it consumes, harmonizing its energetic flow within and between the tissues. When in a diseased state, however, an internal organ will consume its source of vitality as it strives to support its own functions.

Understanding Channel Pathology

Channel pathology is the oldest of all the modes of pathological pattern classification, dating back to the Spiritual Axis from the *Yellow Emperor's Classic on Internal Medicine*. In understanding a channel's pathology, the Qigong doctor takes into consideration several aspects of the patient's energy flow (i.e., the channels are viewed as exterior; whereas, the organs are viewed as interior). Channel pathology is often related to organ disturbances, but it can also be distinct from organ pathology.

The disease of one channel may cause disease in other channels and organs. Likewise, tonification of one channel may cause a tonification of other channels and organs.

The Four Causes of Channel Pathology

There are four main causes of channel pathology: invasion of external pathogens, physical strain, injuries, and internal organ disharmonies, described as follows (Figure 8.152):

1. **The Invasion of External Pathogens:** The six external pathogens of Fire, Summer Heat,

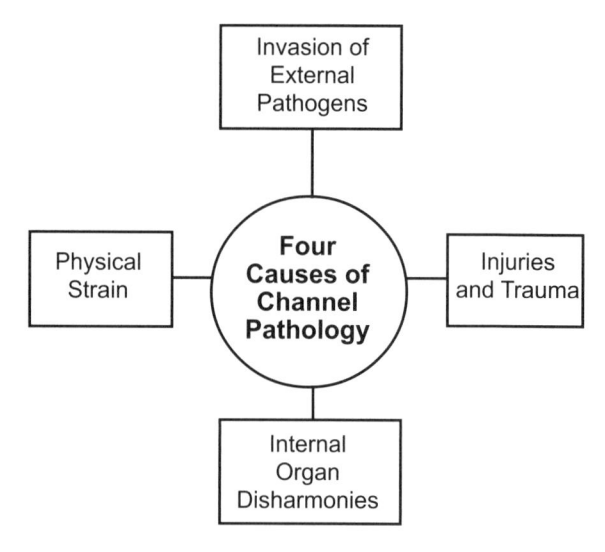

Figure 8.152. The Four Causes of Channel Pathology

Cold, Wind, Dry, and Damp can lead to channel dysfunction. These external pathogenic factors often settle in the joints, causing Bi syndrome (painful obstruction). Channel pathology is also closely related to joint pathology. In Traditional Chinese Medicine, joints play important roles in the circulation of Qi and Blood. Both Qi and Blood gather and concentrate in the joints, and Qi enters and exits the channels at the joints. The five Source points, also called Shu points (see Chapter 10), are usually located on or near the joints. It is at these points that the external pathogenic influences may enter the body and settle in the joints. These external pathogenic influences upset the balance of Yin and Yang and block the flow of Qi and Blood, causing pain and swelling. The body's joints are also affected by Deficient Qi and Blood, causing local weakness and pain from lack of movement.

2. **Physical Strain:** The overuse of joints can cause local stagnation to occur within the Muscle/Tendon Channels, which can manifest as physical pain and tissue weakness.

3. **Injuries and Trauma:** Injuries can cause local Qi and Blood stagnation. This results in the impairment of channel flow, which can manifest as stiffness, bruising, and pain.

4. **Internal Organ Disharmonies:** Excess or Deficiency occurring within the Yin and Yang organs can also affect the functional relationship of the channels.

Differentiation by Channel Full/Excess and Empty/Deficient

It is important for the Medical Qigong doctor to differentiate between conditions of channel excess and channel deficiency. Normal indicators of channel dysfunction are described as follows (Figure 8.153 and 8.154):

- When a channel is too full or in an excess condition, the symptoms include localized stiffness, contractions, cramps, or intense pain along the channel.
- When a channel is empty or in a deficient condition, the symptoms include dull aches, weakness in the muscles, numbness, and muscle atrophy along the channel.
- A red color observed along the channel pathway indicates Heat.
- A bluish color observed along the channels pathway indicates Cold.

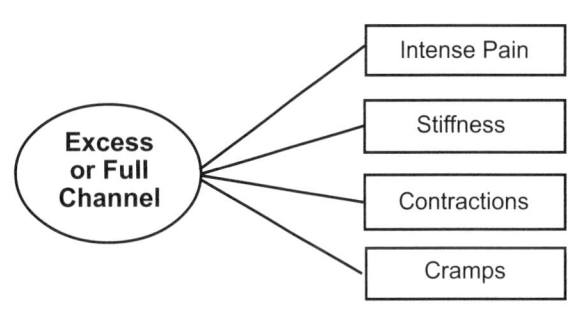

Figure 8.153. Excess or Full Channel Pathology

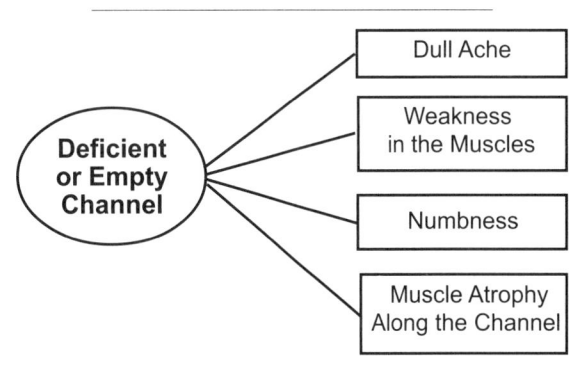

Figure 8.154. Deficient or Empty Channel Pathology

Differentiation of Channel Patterns by Specific Channels

Channel pathology was originally discussed in the *Ling Shu* (Magical Pivot). Channel pathology is described as follows (for more in-depth discussion please see *The Foundations of Chinese Medicine* by Giovanni Maciocia):

1. **Diseases of the Gall Bladder Channels** may cause alternating chills and fever, temporal headache, acute onset of deafness, pain and distention of the breasts, pain in the hip and on the sides of the body, and pain along the lateral sides of the legs.
2. **Diseases of the Liver Channels** may cause vertex headache, pain and swelling of the eyes, pain and distention of the breasts, and cramps in the legs.
3. **Diseases of the Lung Channels** may cause fever, aversion to cold, stiffness in the chest, and pain in the shoulders, clavicles or arms.
4. **Diseases of the Large Intestine Channels** may cause sore throat, toothache, nosebleed, runny nose, swollen and painful gums, swollen eyes, and pain along the channel's pathway.
5. **Diseases of the Stomach Channels** may cause pain in the eyes, nosebleed, neck swelling, facial paralysis, cold legs and feet, and pain along the channel's pathway.
6. **Diseases of the Spleen Channels** may cause vaginal discharge, weakness of the leg muscles, and a Cold feeling along the channel's pathway.
7. **Diseases of the Heart Channels** may cause pain in the eyes, pain along the scapula, and pain along the inner side of the arms.
8. **Diseases of the Small Intestine Channels** may cause pain and stiffness in the neck, and pain along the lateral side of the scapula, elbow, or arms.
9. **Diseases of the Urinary Bladder Channels** may cause fever and aversion to cold, headache, stiff neck, pain in the lower back, pain in the eyes, and pain in the back side of the leg along the channel's pathway.

Twelve Primary Channels	Channel Pathologies
Gall Bladder	Pain in the upper right and left quadrants of the abdomen Diseases of the head, face, eyes and ears Diseases of the external sides of the lower extremities
Liver	Swelling and a distended sensation of the hypochondrium Diseases of the lower abdomen and genital organs
Lungs	Chest and Lung diseases Diseases on the radial side of the upper arm and palmar area of the hand
Large Intestine	Diseases on the lower part of the face, nose, oral cavity, teeth, throat, and neck Diseases of the back and radial side of the upper extremities
Stomach	Diseases of the face, nose, oral cavity, teeth, throat, and front of the neck Diseases of the abdomen, the frontal part of the lower extremities and gastrointestinal area Certain psychiatric diseases
Spleen	Diseases of the tongue and throat Gastrointestinal diseases (disturbances of digestion and absorption of food) Diseases of the medial side of the extremities
Heart	Diseases that exert pressure on the brain, eyes, or pharyngeal wall Diseases of the Heart and lateral side of the chest Diseases of the ulnar and palmar sides of the upper extremities Insomnia, impairment of the consciousness, amnesia, and psychosis
Small Intestine	Diseases of the face, ear, cheek, lower jaw, neck, and throat Diseases of the back and ulnar side of the upper extremities
Urinary Bladder	Diseases of the top of the head, brain, neck, back, lumbar and sacral region Diseases of the back of the legs and thighs, as well as the lateral side of the foot
Kidneys	Diseases that cause the general deterioration of the entire body Weakness in the lower extremities and lumbar pain Hot sensations deep inside the feet
Pericardium	Diseases of the Heart, front of the chest, major blood vessels Diseases of the midline to palmar side of the upper extremities Mental abnormalities
Triple Burners	Diseases of the face, ears, cheeks, larynx and neck Diseases of the back of the upper extremities from the midline of the torso to the upper arm and forearm

Figure 8.155. Pathologies of the Twelve Primary Channels

10. **Diseases of the Kidney Channels** may cause lower back pain, or pain in the soles of the feet.
11. **Diseases of the Pericardium Channels** may cause stiff neck, contraction of the elbow or hand, and pain along the course of the channel's pathway.
12. **Diseases of the Triple Burner Channels** may cause alternating chills with fever, acute onset of deafness, pain and discharge from the ear, pain at the top of the shoulders, pain in the elbow, and pain along the course of the channel's pathway.

SUMMARY OF TWELVE PRIMARY CHANNEL PATHOLOGY

The clinical significance of studying the energetic pathways of the Twelve Primary Channels is made evident through observing the association of certain pathological manifestations with specific patterns peculiar to each channel and its associated internal organ. The quality, quantity, and proportions of Qi and Blood circulation through each of the Twelve Primary Channels has a vital impact on all the body's organ systems. This conceptual understanding of the flow of Qi and Blood helps to define the patterns of the reciprocal relationships that exist among the body's internal organs, channels, and energetic points. Some of the most common Twelve Primary Channel pathologies and their clinical manifestations occurring along the "roots and branches" of these channel pathways are categorized in the preceding diagram (Figure 8.155).

The term "root and branch" is used to describe the difference between either the medial and lateral, or between the upper and lower orientations of the channels and their points of origin. These terms are also used to describe the progression of a disease, and the priorities and sequence of the Qigong doctor's treatment. Specifically, the word "branch" is used to describe the channels' flow of Qi and Blood and the progression and direction of a disease. The word "root" is used to described the channels' internal organ, or the origin of a disease.

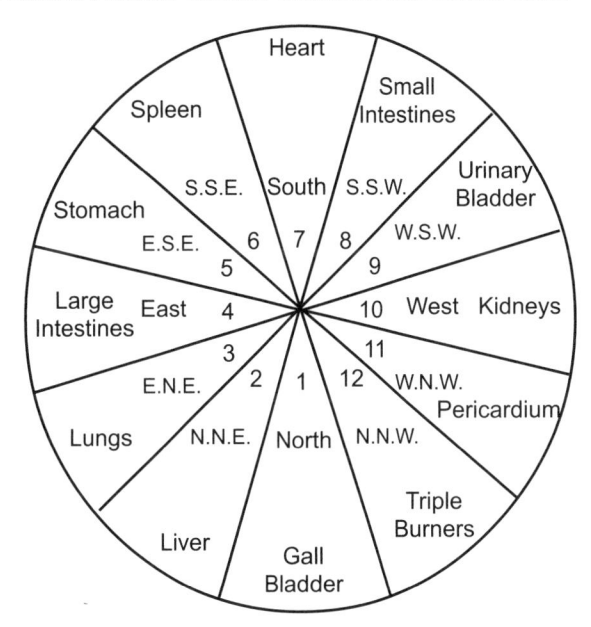

Figure 8.156. The Energy of the Body's Twelve Internal Organs Divided as the Focal Points for Ritual Summoning.

THE ANCIENT DAOIST SHAMAN'S TWELVE INTERNAL ORGANS

The ancient Chinese Daoist shamans believed that since the energy of the year is divided into twelve months, likewise, the energy of the human body's twelve internal organs could be subdivided. These twelve subdivisions were selected as the focal points for ritual summoning. That is, the body's twelve internal organs acted as terrestrial living quarters within the microcosm of man, that could be used to initiate and summon the celestial spirits of the Dao. In auspicious times, and times of trouble, these celestial spirits could be brought fourth to bless or aid mankind.

Each of the twelve internal organs was also associated with one of the twelve directions of the Lo Pan compass (Figure 8.156). This compass image was mentally imprinted as a Hand Seal (Mudra) on the left hand of the Daoist shaman, and could be used to summon a specific spirit from within his or her internal organs (Figure 8.157).

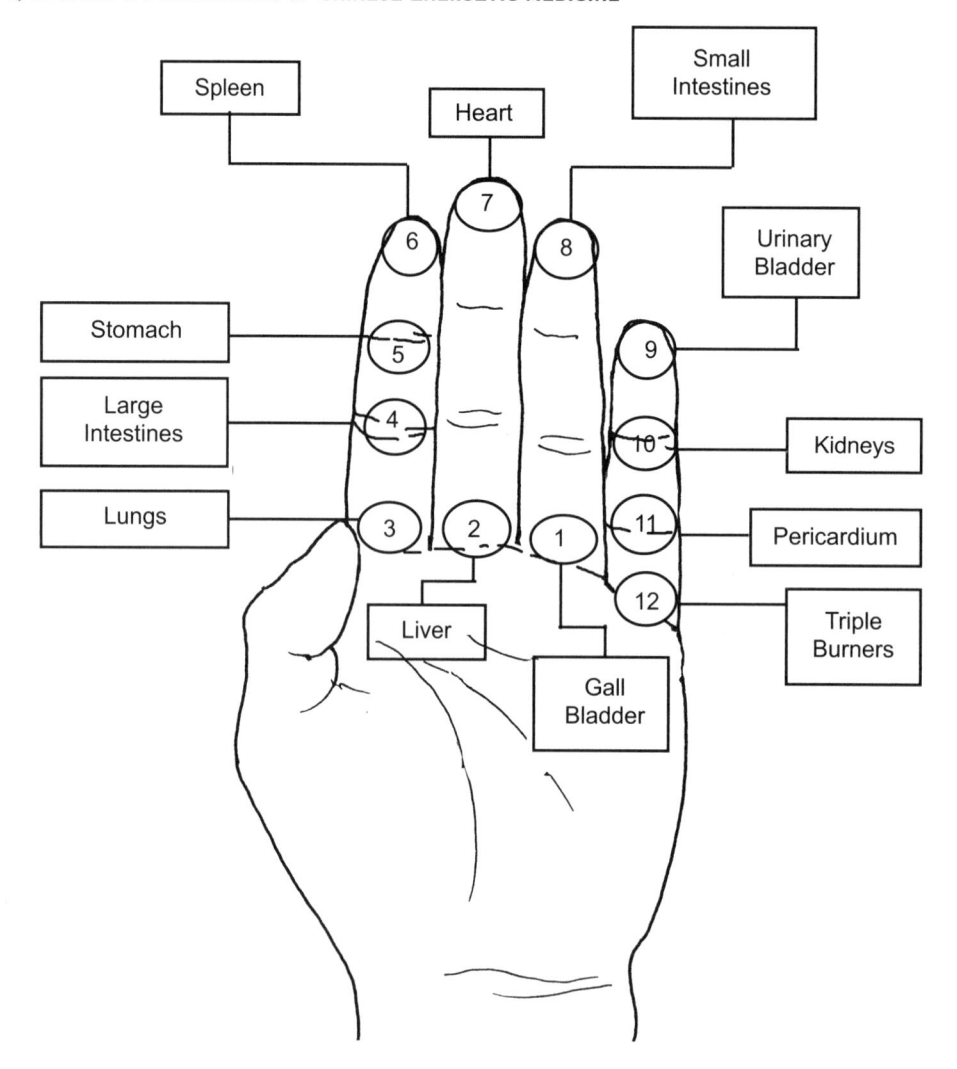

VOLUME 1, SECTION 1: FOUNDATIONS OF CHINESE ENERGETIC MEDICINE

Figure 8.157. The Compass Image was Imprinted as a Hand Seal (Mudra) on the Left Hand.

CHAPTER 9
THE CONNECTING VESSELS, DIVERGENT CHANNELS, MUSCLE AND TENDON CHANNELS AND SKIN ZONES

THE FIFTEEN CONNECTING VESSELS: LUO MAI

The Chinese word "Luo" denotes a net or a web, and is translated as "Connecting Vessel" or "Collateral." In Traditional Chinese Medicine this refers to the "passageways" for the circulation of energy through the body's primary channels. The energetic field of the Luo points extends deep into the tissues, beyond the level of the Muscle and Tendon Channels. The body's energy emerges from fifteen primary Luo "pathway" points, thirteen of which are located on the Twelve Primary Channels, while the two other Luo pathway points are located on the Governing and Conception Vessels. The majority of the body's Luo points are located below the elbows and knees and provide an additional energetic barrier to keep "Evil Winds" from affecting the primary channels. The Collaterals are the streams of energy that connect the paired primary channel rivers.

ORIGIN OF NAME

Though often translated as "Collaterals," the literal meaning of the Chinese term Luo Mai is "Connecting Vessels."

- The first character depicts the Chinese ideogram for Luo (connecting), which can also be translated as resembling a net, cord, a fibrous mesh or a fine silk thread. The character is composed of two radicals. Positioned to the left is the radical "Mi," used for silk, net or string-like objects; the right side of the character is the phonetic sound. The word Luo carries the meaning of energetically enveloping something in a net (Figure 9.1).

- The second character is the Chinese ideograph "Mai," which is generally translated as "vessel." It is composed of two characters: the character to the left, "Ji" depicts the Chinese ideogram for body tissue, muscle or flesh (all of which are forms of connective tissue). The character on the right "Mai" depicts a current of water, stream, or branch of a river. As a whole, the character can be translated as arteries, veins or pulse, representing a form of energetic circulation (Figure 9.2).

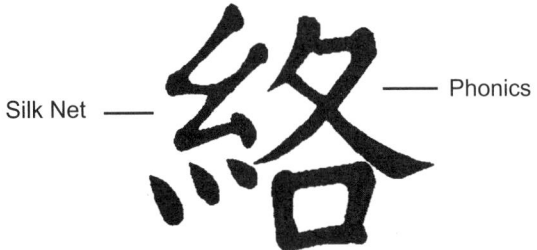

Figure 9.1. The Chinese character for "Luo," Connecting

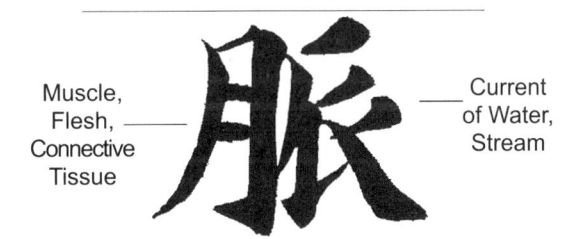

Figure 9.2. The Chinese character for "Mai," Vessel

ENERGETIC ANATOMY

The Luo distribute Qi and Blood to those areas not directly traversed by the Extraordinary Vessels and Twelve Primary Channels. The Luo Mai are known as the "interconnecting passageways" that branch out through the body. They appear in several forms, from deep to superficial, and are usually divided into three levels, described as follows:

- The Fifteen Connecting Vessels (Shi Wu Luo Mai) are also known as the Fifteen Major (or Great) Connecting Vessels (Shi Wu Da Luo Mai); they are the Luo of the Twelve Primary Channels, the Governing Vessel, and the Conception Vessel.
- The Secondary Branches or Minute Collaterals of the Fifteen Connecting Vessels are finer manifestations of the Luo, dispersed throughout the tissues.
- The Grandson Connecting Vessels (Sun Luo Mai), are sometimes called the Superficial Collaterals or the "floating" Luo, as they seem to float on the surface of the body. These are the smallest of the Luo, and spread-out into the countless terminal branches of the entire Luo system. The Superficial Collaterals are the subtlest sub-branches of the Luo system. They distribute Qi and Blood directly to the tissues of the body, similar in energetic function to the capillaries of the vascular system.

Both the secondary branches of the Fifteen Connecting Vessels and the Grandson Connecting Vessels, which can be seen beneath the surface as Blood Vessels, are sometimes called "Blood Luo Vessels."

EMBRYOLOGICAL FUNCTION

The Luo Mai have a functional relationship with the developmental aspects of ancestral and embryological energetic formation. The Luo Mai contain certain command points that allow access to the Eight Extraordinary Vessels, which are responsible for energetic embryological development.

In ancient China, the Fifteen Collaterals were believed to be the intersecting streams of energy existing between the body's Wai (External) Qi and Nei (Internal) Qi flow. The Qi of Heaven and Earth was believed to merge and interact with the body's Twelve Primary Channels via the intersecting energy of the Fifteen Collaterals.

To understand the energetic significance of the collaterals, it is helpful to think of the body's energy flowing like a river (primary channel) to the surface of the body, where it becomes a "marsh" (collaterals). The "marsh" absorbs the universal and environmental energy (sun, wind, rain, etc.) before reversing its course and flowing in the opposite direction back to its source.

TRANSVERSE AND LONGITUDINAL LUO

Flowing from each primary channel's Luo point are two Luo vessels, which are energetically counted as one. The transverse Luo vessel and the longitudinal Luo vessel are described as follows:

1. **The Transverse Luo Vessels** connect to the Source points on the Yin and Yang coupled primary channels. They act as energetic safety valves, maintaining balance between the Yin and the Yang channels by diverting the excess energy of one channel into the Orb (internal organ and energetic field) of its paired primary channel. When a channel is deficient (empty) and its paired channel is in excess (full), for example, the tonification of the Luo point on the deficient channel replenishes the deficiency, while simultaneously normalizing the excess energy of its paired channel.
2. **Longitudinal Luo Vessels** flow out from the Luo points but do not connect with the coupled primary channels. The Luo Vessels usually flow proximally toward the channel's organ.

ENERGETIC FUNCTION

Located on each primary channel are specific Luo points which act as the origins of the branching Luo vessels (Figures 9.3 through 9.8). The main function of the Luo Vessels is to transfer Qi and Blood from the primary channels to all parts of the body so as to nourish the tendons, the Bones, the skin, and the five sense organs (nose, eyes, ears, lips, and tongue). The Luo vessels also link the interior with the exterior of the body, connecting the internal channels with the superficial channels.

Pathology

The pathology of the Fifteen Major Collaterals is classified into syndromes of Excess and syndromes of Deficiency, described as follows:

1. **Excessive Conditions of the collaterals** arise from exogenous invasion if (1) the organ associated with the Luo is in excess or (2) the body's Wei Qi is weak. Evil Winds may enter the body the through Jing Well or Wind points and start moving up the channel. The Longitudinal Luo Vessels provide a route for the diversion of Evil Winds. The Longitudinal Luo Vessels have more Wei Qi than the primary channels and can thus fight pathogens more effectively. Sometimes in cases of Wind Cold invasion, a blue color is visible along the path of the Longitudinal Luo Vessel. If the invasion is due to Wind Heat, there may be a red color along the vessel.

2. **Deficient Conditions of the collaterals** are due to: (1) the organ associated with the Luo being deficient or (2) the patient's Qi is deficient due to exogenous factors.

Point Location of the Fifteen Major Collaterals

1. **The Foot Tai Yin (Greater Yin) Spleen-4 Point:** This point is located on the medial side of each foot, just posterior to the base of the first metatarsal bone. After energetically branching from the Spleen Channel, this Luo flows downward to connect with the Stomach Channel on each foot. A second branch of this Luo flows from the Sp-4 point upward along the medial aspect of the inner thigh, passing the abdomen and connecting with the Stomach and Small Intestine (Figure 9.3).
   - Symptoms of Excess in this Luo include sharp intestinal pain, vomiting, and diarrhea.
   - Symptoms of Deficiency in this Luo include abdominal swelling.

2. **The Foot Shao Yin (Lesser Yin) Kidney-4 Point:** This point is located on the Kidney Channel of each foot just posterior to the medial malleolus. The energy of this Luo flows downward, crossing the heel, to connect with the Urinary Bladder Channel by the ankle on each foot. A second branch of this Luo flows upward along the medial aspect of the inner thigh, following the Kidney Channel. It then ascends the abdomen to connect with the Pericardium of the Heart, before descending laterally to connect with the lumbar vertebrae (Figure 9.3).
   - Symptoms of Excess in this Luo include en-

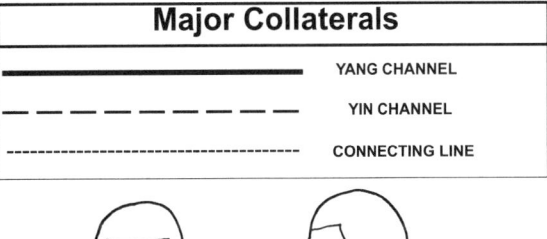

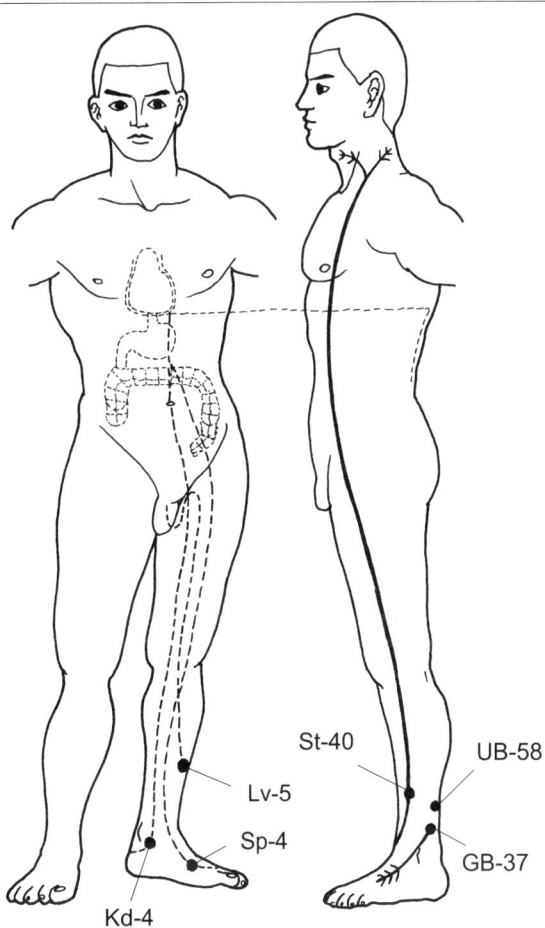

Figure 9.3. The figure at left illustrates the three Luo points of the Yin Collaterals on the left foot, which are located on the primary channels of the Kidneys, Spleen, and Liver. The figure on the right shows the three Luo points on the Yang Collaterals of the left foot located on the primary channels of the Stomach, Urinary Bladder, and Gall Bladder.

uresis, emotional irritability, and depression.
- Symptoms of Deficiency in this Luo include lower back pain.

3. **The Foot Jue Yin (Terminal Yin) Liver-5 Point:** This point is located on the medial side of each foot, several inches above the medial malleolus. After energetically branching from the Liver Channel, this Luo connects with the Gall Bladder Channel. It then flows upward along the medial aspect of the inner thigh, connecting with the genitals. It terminates at the tip of the penis in males, and the clitoris in women (Figure 9.3).
   - Symptoms of Excess in this Luo include swelling of the testicles.
   - Symptoms of Deficiency in this Luo include itching in the pubic region.

4. **The Foot Tai Yang (Greater Yang) Urinary Bladder-58 Point:** This point is located on the lateral side of each foot, several inches above the external malleolus. After energetically branching from the Urinary Bladder Channel, the energy of this Luo flows downward to connect with the Kidney Channel on each foot (Figure 9.3).
   - Symptoms of Excess in this Luo include nasal congestion, occipital headache, and back pain.
   - Symptoms of Deficiency in this Luo include clear mucus nasal discharge and nosebleed.

5. **The Foot Shao Yang (Lesser Yang) Gall Bladder-37 Point:** This point is located on the lateral side of each foot, several inches above the external malleolus. After energetically branching from the Gall Bladder Channel, this Luo flows downward to connect with the Liver Channel on each foot. It then continues downward to disperse over the dorsum on each foot (Figure 9.3).
   - Symptoms of Excess in this Luo include fainting.
   - Symptoms of Deficiency in this Luo include weak and flaccid muscles of the feet.

6. **The Foot Yang Ming (Bright Yang) Stomach-40 Point:** This point is located on the lateral side of each foot, several inches above the external malleolus. After energetically branching from the Stomach Channel, this Luo flows downward to connect with the Spleen Channel on each foot. A second branch of this Luo ascends along the lateral aspect of the tibia, flowing upwards to the top of the head. At the top of the head this Luo branch divides into two smaller branches, one branch connects with the throat, while the other branch converges with all the Yang Channels on the neck and head (Figure 9.3).
   - Symptoms of Excess in this Luo include epilepsy and insanity.
   - Symptoms of Deficiency in this Luo include pharyngitis, sudden aphasia, and flaccid or atrophied muscles in the legs or feet.

7. **The Hand Tai Yang (Greater Yang) Small Intestine-7 Point:** This point is located by the ulnar bone, on the dorsal side of each hand, several inches above the wrist. After energetically branching from the Small Intestine Channel, this Luo flows upward past the elbow and connects with the Large Intestine 6

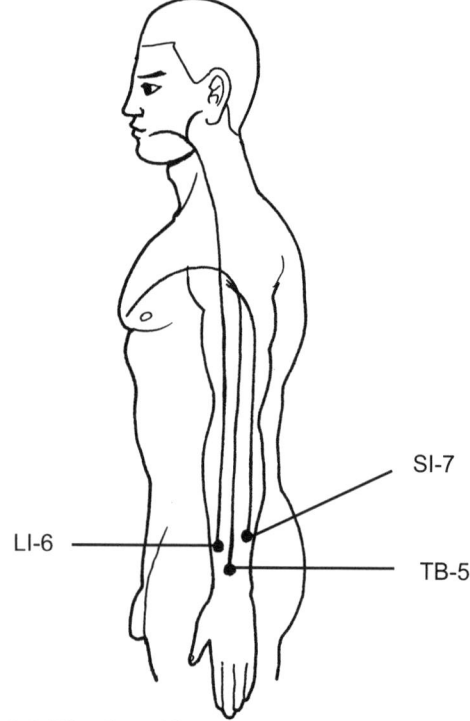

Figure 9.4. The three Yang collaterals and their Luo points, located on the hand and on the primary channels of the Large Intestine (LI), Triple Burners (TB), and Small Intestine (SI)

point (Figure 9.4).
- Symptoms of Excess in this Luo include fever, headaches, and blurred vision.
- Symptoms of Deficiency in this Luo include atrophy of the muscles in the elbow and arm and a looseness in the joints.

8. **The Hand Yang Ming (Bright Yang) Large Intestine-6 Point:** This point is located by the radial bone, on the dorsal side of each hand, several inches above the wrist. After energetically branching from the Large Intestine Channel, this Luo flows upward on each arm to the jaw and pours into the area of the teeth. Another branch of this Luo ascends into each ear, connecting with the Thrusting Vessels which supply energy to the head (Figure 9.4).
- Symptoms of Excess in this Luo include deafness and toothache in the lower jaw.
- Symptoms of Deficiency in this Luo include a sensation of coldness in the teeth, as well as fullness and congestion in the chest.

9. **The Hand Shao Yang (Lesser Yang) Triple Burner-5 Point:** This point is located just above the dorsal transverse crease of each wrist. After energetically branching from the Triple Burner Channel, this Luo flows upward past the arm and over the shoulder, dispersing into the chest and connecting with the Pericardium Channel (Figure 9.4).
- Symptoms of Excess in this Luo include muscle spasms around the elbow.
- Symptoms of Deficiency in this Luo include flaccid muscles around the arm and elbow joint.

10. **The Hand Tai Yin (Greater Yin) Lung-7 Point:** This point arises from the cleft of the tendons and bones on the radial side of each wrist. After energetically branching from the Lung Channel, this Luo flows down into the palm before spreading throughout the thenar eminence (Figure 9.5).
- Symptoms of Excess in this Luo include heat in the palms or wrists.
- Symptoms of Deficiency in this Luo include enuresis and shortness of breath.

11. **The Hand Shao Yin (Lesser Yin) Heart-5 Point:** This point is located on the Heart Channel of each hand, just above the transverse crease of the wrist. The energy of this Luo ascends along the Heart Channel, enters the Heart, and then continues up the chest into the head, where it flows into the root of the tongue, then finally ascends to connect with each eye (Figure 9.5).
- Symptoms of Excess in this Luo include fullness and pressure in the chest.
- Symptoms of Deficiency in this Luo include aphasia.

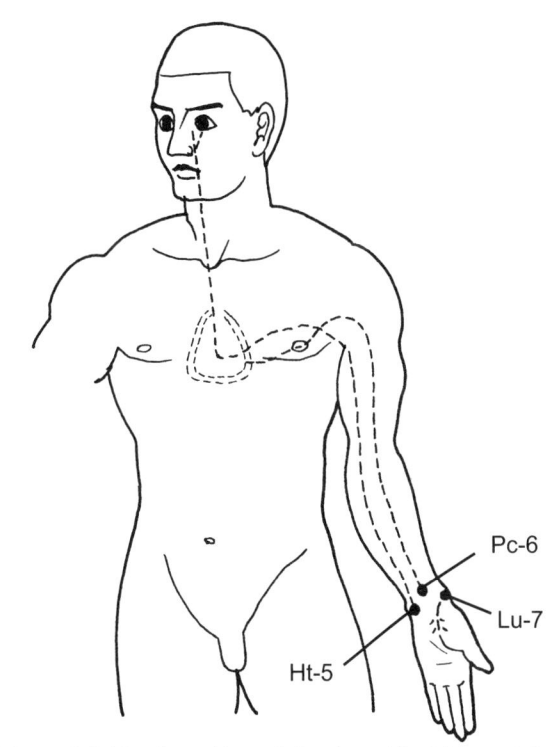

Figure 9.5. The three Yin collaterals and their Luo points located on the hand and on the primary channels of the Heart, Pericardium, and Lungs.

12. **The Hand Jue Yin (Terminal Yin) Pericardium-6 Point:** This point is located on the Pericardium Channel of each hand, just a few inches above the medial transverse crease of the wrist, between the two tendons. The energy of this Luo follows the Pericardium Channel, and eventually connects with the Heart (Figure 9.5).
- Symptoms of Excess in this Luo include chest pain.
- Symptoms of Deficiency in this Luo include irritability.

13. **The Governing Vessel-1 Point:** This point is located on the base of the Governing Vessel,

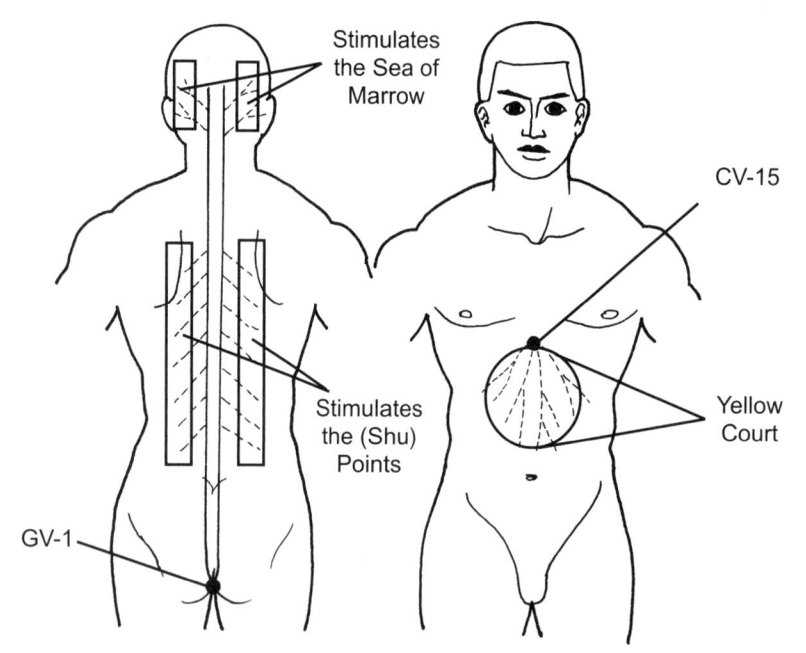

Figure 9.6. The main collateral of the Governing Vessel is located on the Governing Vessel (GV) 1 point.

Figure 9.7. The main collateral of the Conception Vessel is located on the Conception Vessel (CV) 15 point.

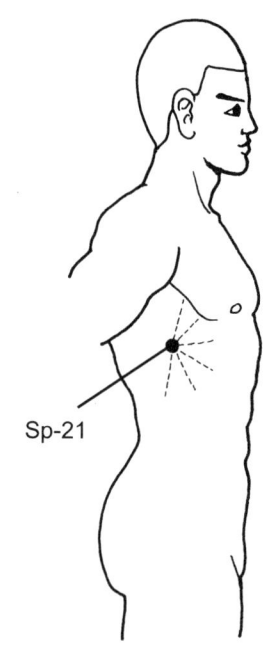

Figure 9.8. The major collateral and Luo point of the Spleen is located on the Spleen (Sp) 21 point.

at the perineum. The energy of this Luo flows upward along both sides of the spine, connecting with each of the body's correspondence (Shu) points before reaching the nape of the neck. From the nape of the neck, this Luo's energy spreads to the top of the head, stimulating the Sea of Marrow. From the top of the head, it continues flowing into the scalp regions on both sides of the head, eventually connecting with the Urinary Bladder Channel and merging with the spine (Figure 9.6).

- Symptoms of Excess in this Luo include stiffness along the spine.
- Symptoms of Deficiency in this Luo include dizziness or heaviness in the head.

14. **The Conception Vessel-15 Point:** This point is located on the Conception Vessel, just below the xiphoid process of the chest. The energy of this Luo flows into the Yellow Court and empties downward along the torso, pouring over the abdomen (Figure 9.7).

- Symptoms of Excess in this Luo include pain on the surface skin of the abdomen.
- Symptoms of Deficiency in this Luo include itching on the surface skin of the abdomen.

15. **The Major Luo of the Spleen-21 Point:** This point is located on the Spleen Channel of the chest, below the axillary fold of each arm. The energy of this Luo spreads through the chest and hypochondriac region, gathering the Blood like a net. In ancient Daoist training, this area is used as the energetic exit portal for the White Tiger (Po: Lung Qi released from the right side of the body) and Green Dragon (Hun: Liver Qi released from the left side of the body) during the Ren Wu Zang meditation (Figure 9.8).

- Symptoms of Excess in this Luo include general aches and pains throughout the entire body.
- Symptoms of Deficiency in this Luo include weakness in the muscles of the limbs and joints.

THE TWELVE DIVERGENT CHANNELS: JING BIE

The Twelve Divergent Channels comprise an important part of the body's channel system. These channels branch off from the Twelve Primary Channels and share the energetic function of circulating Qi throughout the body. The energetic field of the Twelve Divergent Channels forms an enormous web of complex interconnections within the network of the body's Twelve Primary Channels.

ORIGIN OF NAME

Also known as the "separate pathway channels," the literal translation of the Chinese term "Jing Bie" is "divergent channels."

- The first character depicts the Chinese ideogram for Jing (channel), which can also be translated as meridian, to pass through, and the wrapping of a silk fiber or net. The word Jing carries a multitude of meanings, reflected by the many components of the character. Positioned to the left is the radical "Mi," used for silk, net or string-like objects. The right side of the character is the phonetic "Jing," and is sometimes used to denote the flow of water underground (the top right character represents the ground, while the three curved lines beneath it represent the flow of water). Positioned to the bottom-right is a modification of the ancient phonetic "Ting," meaning to examine the underground veins. Together, the ideograph describes the deep aquatic passageways or subterranean rivers which energetically knit together the internal fabric of the human body (Figure 9.9).
- The second character depicts the Chinese ideogram for Bie (divergent) and can be translated as "to separate from, difference, and distinction." The character is composed of two separate ideographs: on the left is the ideograph "Ling," which translates as "another." On the right is an ideograph that describes the following of a straight line or pathway separate from the regular course (Figure 9.10).

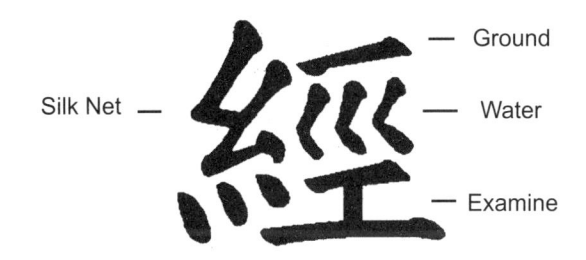

Figure 9.9. The Chinese character for "Jing," Channel, or Passageway

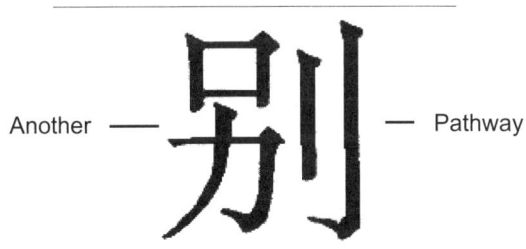

Figure 9.10. The Chinese character for "Bie," Divergent

ENERGETIC ANATOMY

Because the areas governed by the energy of the Twelve Divergent Channels are both detailed and extensive, they are considered to be a separate yet deeper component of the channel system. They are secondary streams that run parallel to the primary rivers, yet each has its own characteristic functions and unique clinical applications independent of the primary channels.

All of the Twelve Divergent Channels (except for the Pericardium Divergent Channel) begin somewhere on the four extremities. The energy runs shallowly at first, then flows deeper into the body before surfacing again at or near the channels' end points. Some Qigong masters believe that the body's Wei Qi also flows through the Twelve Divergent Channels, moving from the extremities inwards.

The Twelve Divergent Channels have no defined points of their own, although there are intersection points where they cross the major channels. All of the Twelve Divergent Channels separate from the body's main channels at the He-Sea points at the knees and elbows. The energy of the Twelve Divergent Channels travels through the Yellow Court (solar plexus), the Heart, and the throat (connecting through the "Windows of Heaven" points). Stimulation of these channels has a profound emotional and spiritual effect on the patient.

EMBRYOLOGICAL FUNCTION

In ancient China, the Twelve Divergent Channels were believed to be responsible for the prenatal formation of the body's internal organs and design and energetic imprinting of the postnatal Twelve Primary Channels. Some Qigong masters maintain that, due to their interconnection with the body's internal organs, the Twelve Divergent Channels have the deepest energetic flow of all the channels, penetrating deeper than even the Extraordinary Vessels, and are responsible for transporting Ying Qi and Yuan Qi.

Another essential action of the Twelve Divergent Channels appears to be the activation of the cerebral circulation, which serves to bring the body's ancestral (hereditary) energies and metabolic energies to the cranial level.

THE SIX CONFLUENCES

The Twelve Divergent Channels are paired into six confluences according to their internal and external relationships. In ancient China, it was believed that the six pairs of Divergent Channels (also known as the Liu He - Six Confluences) corresponded to the six directions of space (Heaven: up, Earth: down, North: back, South: front, East: left and West: right).

It was also believed that specific meditations could stimulate the energy within these six pairs of Divergent Channels, the overflow of which could then be used to stimulate the Taiji Pole. The stimulation of the Taiji Pole would in turn evoke a subtle type of heavenly resonance, allowing the individual to flow beyond the boundaries of both space and time.

The Twelve Divergent Channels are divided into six pairs, described as follows (Figure 9.11).
1. Urinary Bladder Divergent Channel (Foot Tai Yang) and Kidney Divergent Channel (Foot Shao Yin)
2. Stomach Divergent Channel (Foot Yang Ming) and Spleen Divergent Channel (Foot Tai Yin)

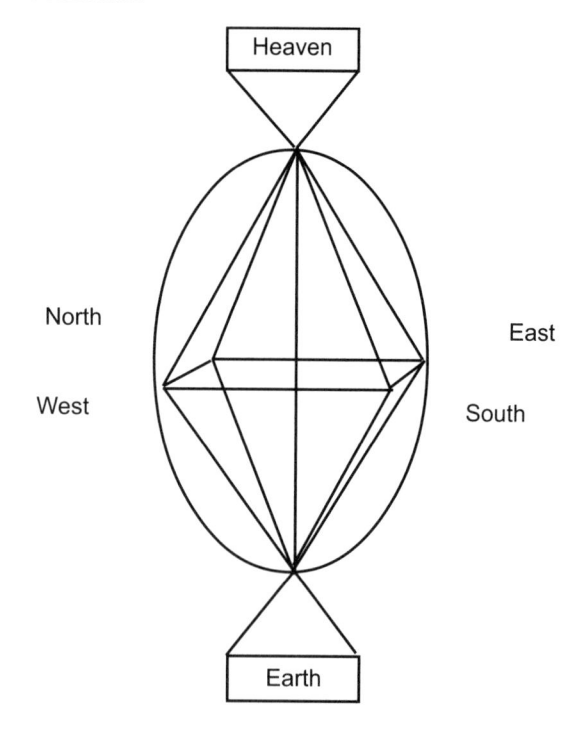

Figure 9.11. The Six Divergent Channel Pairs Correspond to the Six Directions of Space

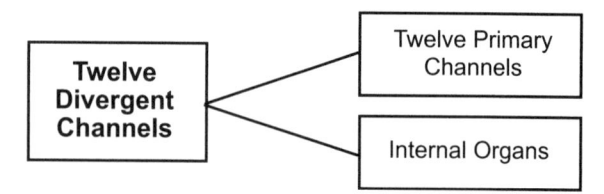

Figure 9.12. The Twelve Divergent Channels intersect with the Twelve Primary Channels and penetrate the internal organs.

3. Gall Bladder Divergent Channel (Foot Shao Yang) and Liver Divergent Channel (Foot Jue Yin)
4. Small Intestine Divergent Channel (Hand Tai Yang) and Heart Divergent Channel (Hand Shao Yin)
5. Large Intestine Divergent Channel (Hand Yang Ming) and Lung Divergent Channel (Hand Tai Yin)
6. Triple Burners Divergent Channel (Hand Shao Yang) and Pericardium Divergent Channel (Hand Jue Yin)

ENERGETIC FUNCTION

One of the primary functions of the Twelve Divergent Channels is to integrate all parts of the body with the Twelve Primary Channels, supplementing Qi and Blood to the areas of the body that are not directly traversed by the pathways of the Twelve Primary Channels. They also connect to those internal organs that are either unconnected or only remotely connected by the primary channels (Figure 9.12). These internal organ areas are more securely linked by the energetic flow of the Twelve Divergent Channels, which strengthen the bonds between the Twelve Primary Channels and the physical areas that are connected to, or adjoining, their pathways.

YIN AND YANG

Another important function of the Twelve Divergent Channels is to facilitate the connection between the linked pairs of Yin and Yang primary channels and organs. Therefore, all primary Yin and Yang organs are interconnected by the Divergent Channels. Both Yin and Yang Divergent Channels ultimately connect with the body's Yang Primary Channels (Figures 9.13 through 9.18), which are described as follows:

1. **The Yang Divergent Channels** complete a cycle of leaving the primary channels (e.g., Primary Gall Bladder Channel) and entering their associated internal organ (e.g., the Gall Bladder organ) before they resurface on the neck and head to reconnect with their original channels (e.g., the Primary Gall Bladder Channel).
2. **The Yin Divergent Channels** leave their primary channels (e.g., Primary Liver Channel), to join their associated Yang Divergent Channels (e.g., the Divergent Gall Bladder Channel), which then join with the Yang Primary Channels (e.g., the Primary Gall Bladder Channel). The Yin Divergent Channels influence and are influenced by the same areas on the body as their Yang Divergent Channel Confluent pair.

Similarly, within the body's cavities, most of the Twelve Divergent Channels first join with their primary Yin or Yang organ before connecting with the associated organ (through its associated channel) in the Yin/Yang pair. Through this interaction, the connection between paired Yin and Yang organs and channels is strengthened.

An understanding of the relationship between the paired Yin and Yang channels is important to the Qigong doctor, as sometimes a disease affecting a Yang channel can be treated by selecting certain areas on its associated Yin channel, and vice versa. The same theory holds true for the treatment of diseases of the internal organs.

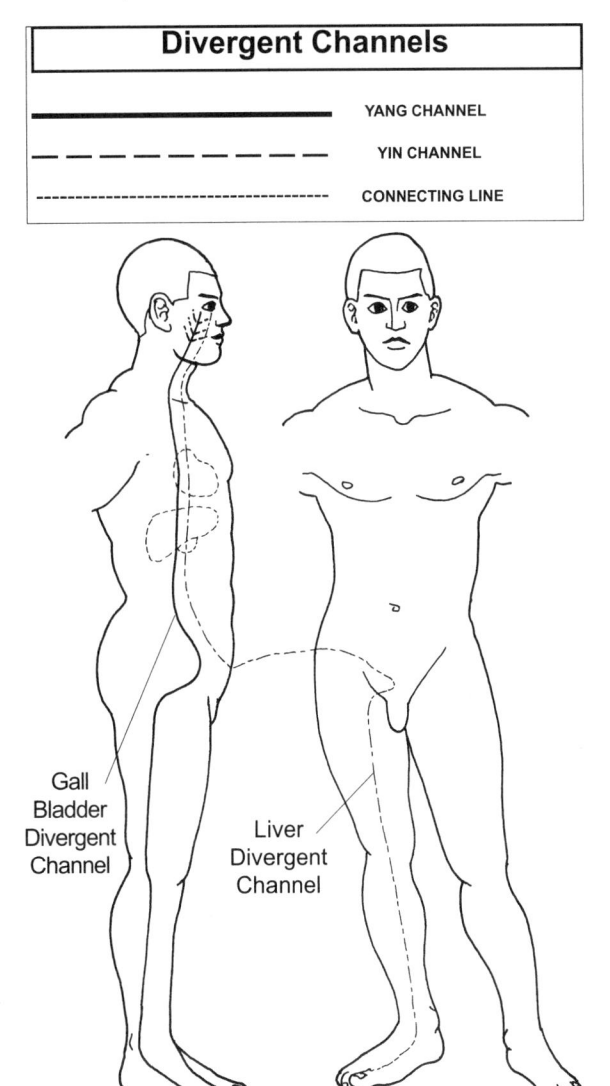

Figure 9.13. The Divergent Channels of the Gall Bladder and Liver

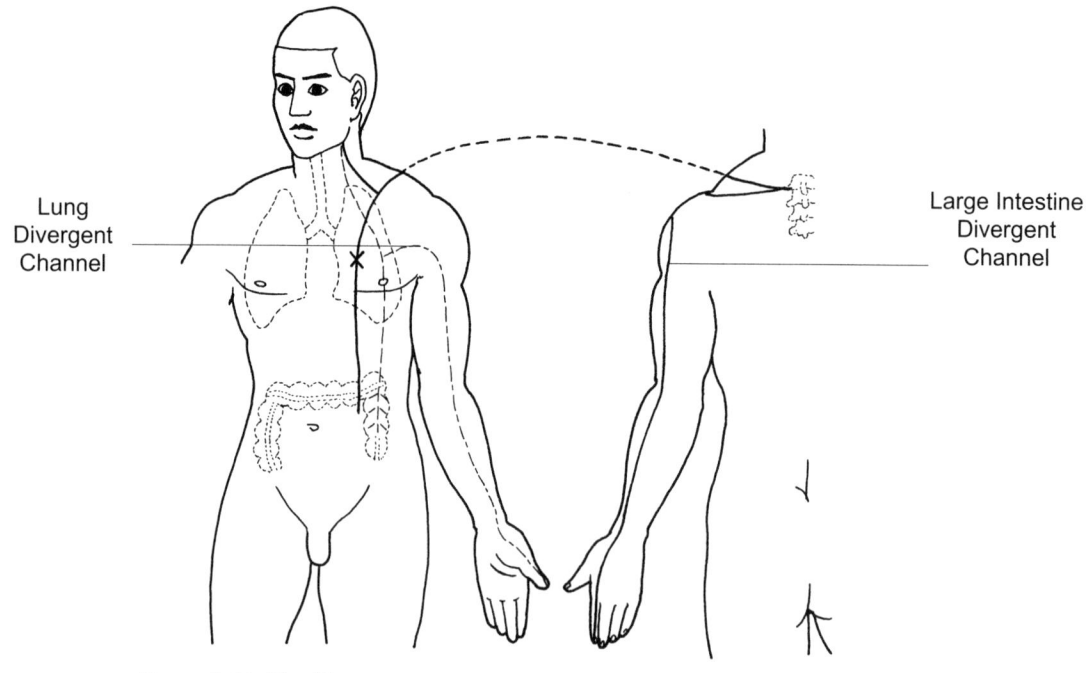

VOLUME 1, SECTION 1: FOUNDATIONS OF CHINESE ENERGETIC MEDICINE

Figure 9.14. The Divergent Channels of the Lungs and Large Intestine

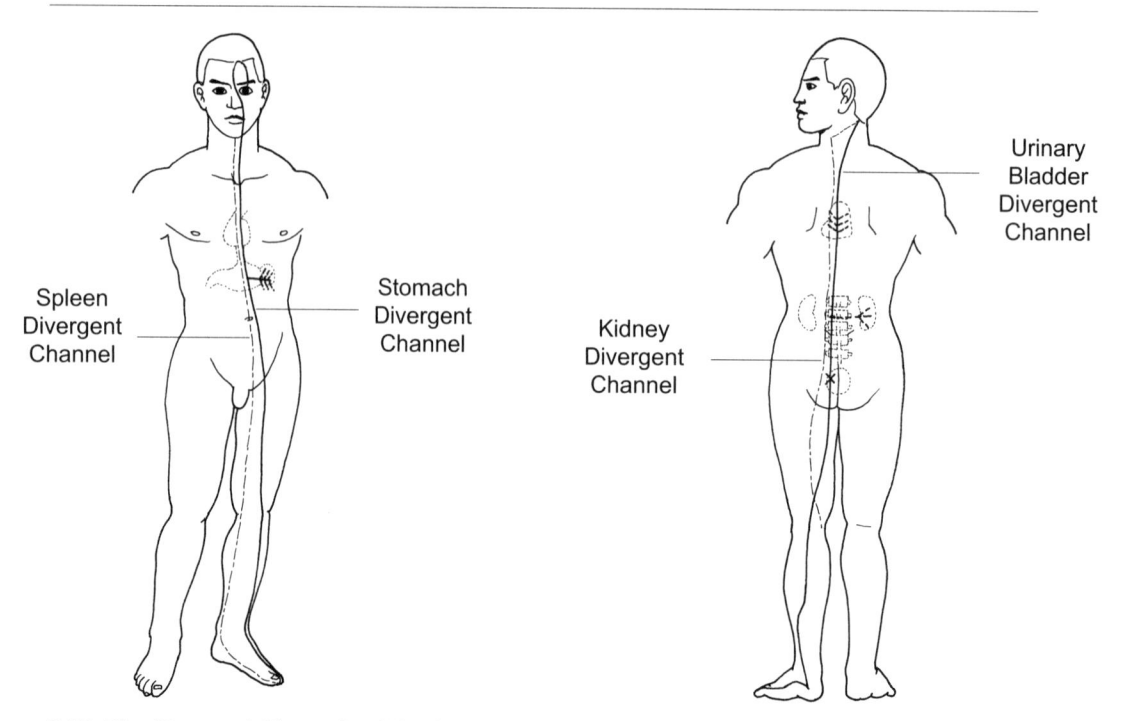

Figure 9.15. The Divergent Channels of the Stomach and Spleen

Figure 9.16. The Divergent Channels of the Urinary Bladder and Kidneys

CHAPTER 9: THE CONNECTING VESSELS, DIVERGENT CHANNELS, MUSCLE/TENDON CHANNELS AND SKIN ZONES

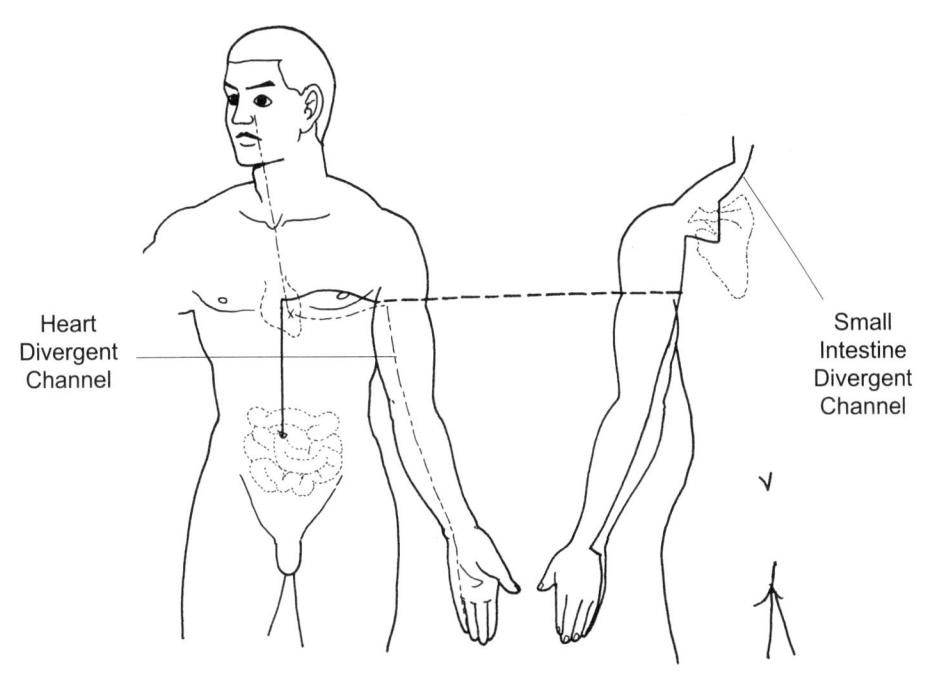

Figure 9.17. The Divergent Channels of the Heart and Small Intestine

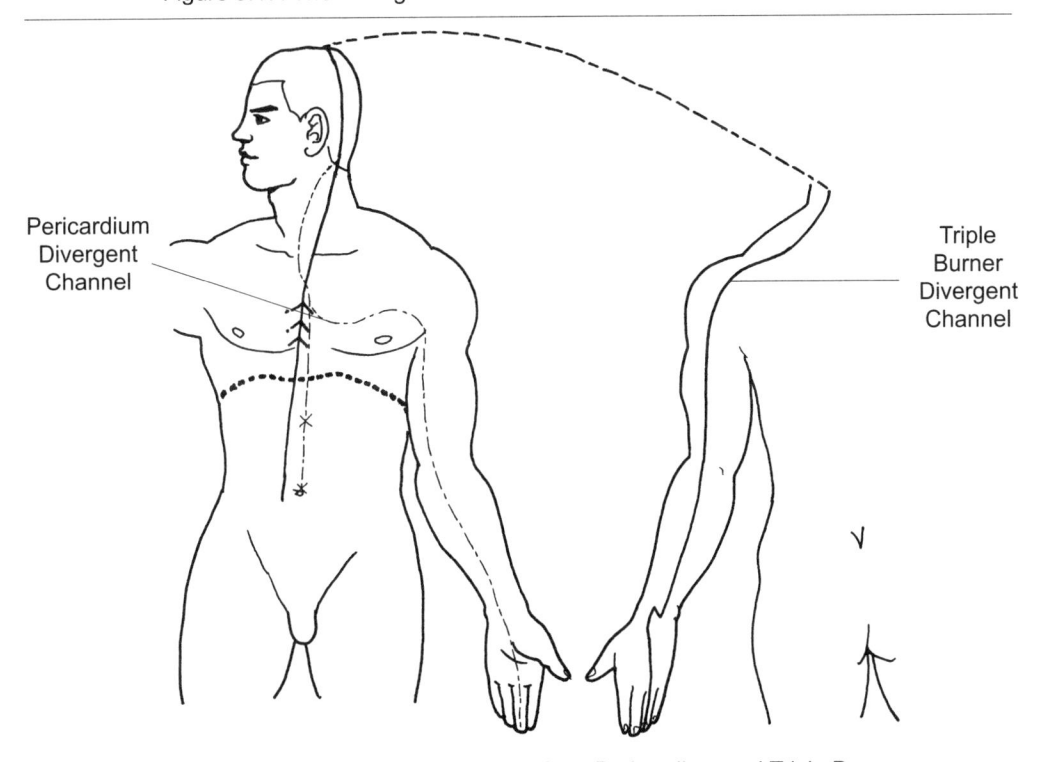

Figure 9.18. The Divergent Channels of the Pericardium and Triple Burner

The Twelve Muscle and Tendon Channels: Jing Jin

Skeletal muscles and tendons link together and mobilize the Bones of the body, acting on specific joints to provide movement. The Twelve Muscle and Tendon Channels are the muscle and soft tissue regions of the body where the Qi and Blood of the primary channels nourish the skin, muscles, and tendons. They are very superficial in relation to the primary channels, and they form a capillary network that travels in the depressions and planes between muscles and tendons. The Twelve Muscle and Tendon Channels subsequently spread over the whole of the epidermis, through their close connection with the cutaneous tissues.

Origin of Name

Long before the Zhou Dynasty (1028-221 B.C.), the ancient Chinese had already identified all of the body's muscles and their attachments to specific Bones. When observing the longitudinal organization of the muscular system, the ancient Chinese described its energetic flow as being similar to that of a valley (where the larger muscles gathered) or a stream (where the smaller muscles gathered). The spaces between the striated muscles were viewed as the "meeting of the valleys and streams".

Commonly known as "the Tendino-Muscular Meridians" and "the Ligamentous Meridians," the literal translation of the Chinese term "Jing Jin" is "the muscles of the channels" or "the muscles within the channels."

- The first character depicts the Chinese ideogram for Jing (channel), which can also be translated as meridian, to pass through, and the wrapping of a silk fiber or net. The word Jing carries a multitude of meanings, reflected by the many components of the character. Positioned to the left is the radical "Mi," used for silk, net or string-like objects. The right side of the character is the phonetic "Jing," and is sometimes used to denote the flow of water underground (the top right character represents the ground, while the three curved lines beneath it represent the flow of water). Positioned to the bottom-right is a modification of the ancient phonetic "Ting," meaning to examine underground veins. Together, the ideograph describes the deep aquatic passageways or subterranean rivers which energetically knit together the internal fabric of the human body (Figure 9.19).

- The second character depicts the Chinese ideogram for Jin (tendon). One of the earliest Chinese medical dictionaries, the *Shou Wen Jie Zi*, explains the term "Jin" (translated as sinew, tendon or ligament) as "the strength of the flesh," and explains that the ancient character is composed of the bamboo radical "Zhu" above two other radicals. The character to the left, "Ji" depicts the Chinese ideogram for body tissue, muscle or flesh (all of which are various forms of connective tissue), and on the right is the character "Li" meaning "strength" (Figure 9.20). With this description, we can understand the word "Jin" to mean that the resilient fibrous qualities of the tendons are similar to that of the flexible fibrous, intertwining quality of bamboo (Figure 9.21).

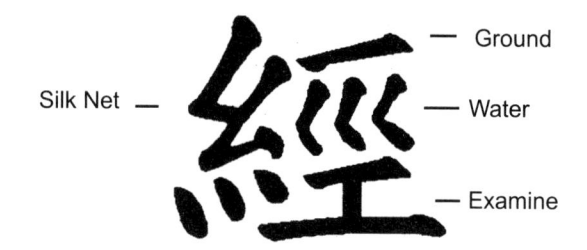

Figure 9.19. The Chinese character for "Jing," Channel, or Passageway

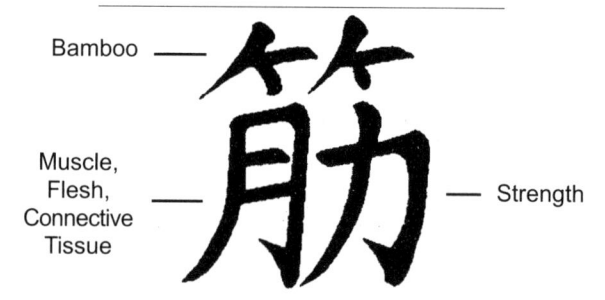

Figure 9.20. The Chinese character for "Jin," Sinew, Tendon, or Ligament

EMBRYOLOGICAL DEVELOPMENT

The Twelve Muscle and Tendon Channels have their embryological origin separate from the Twelve Primary Channels. Because of their connection to the Liver and the mesenchymal formations in the body, the Twelve Muscle and Tendon Channels are associated with the formation of the skeletal system, muscle-tendon system, and the early development of the limbs. The Twelve Muscle and Tendon Channels are also associated with the embryological formation of the diaphragm and the thoraco-abdominal serous membranes: specifically the pleura, the peritoneum and the Pericardium.

Each of the Twelve Muscle and Tendon Channels appears to regulate and govern a definite number of muscle fasciculi, with each muscle spindle covering a certain amount of the body's fibrous or membranous casings. The function of the Twelve Muscle and Tendon Channels is also associated with the body's Wei Qi, barring access to the deeper channels.

ENERGETIC FORMATION

Originating in the extremities, the Twelve Muscle and Tendon Channels ascend to the head and torso. They coordinate the movement of the Bones and limbs but do not enter into the internal organs. They are connected to the inner fascial structure of the body's muscles, tendons, and ligaments, as well as to the fascial structure of other connective tissues. The Twelve Muscle and Tendon Channels are affiliated with the network of primary channels and collaterals (Luo) on the exterior of the body and also serve as mediators between any energetic reactions (trauma, stress, etc.) that vibrate from the body's exterior into the deep internal organs.

These channels are found along the four extremities on the surface of the body, as well as along the head, neck, back, chest, and abdomen. The name of each Muscle and Tendon Channel comes from the Twelve Primary Channels whose external energy flow they follow. They also receive the Blood and Qi nourishment necessary for their proper functioning activity through the Twelve Primary Channels.

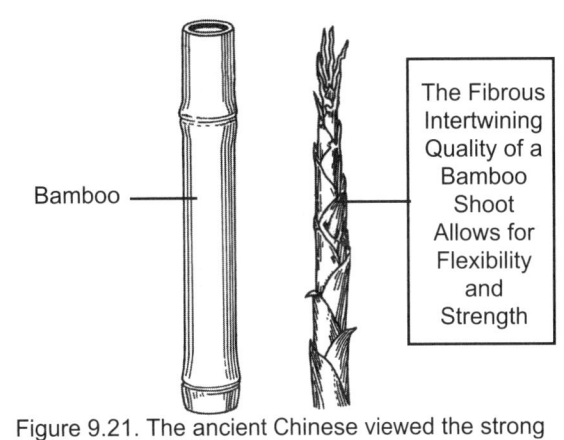

Figure 9.21. The ancient Chinese viewed the strong and resilient quality of the tendons as being similar to the fibrous and flexible structure of bamboo (Inspired from the original artwork of Lilian Lai Bensky).

YIN AND YANG

In Traditional Chinese Medicine the muscles and tendons are described in characteristics of Yin (flexion, contraction, internal rotation, etc.) and Yang (extension, expansion, external rotation, etc.) which balance each other. When the Yin and Yang actions of the muscles and tendons fail to balance and regulate each other, Muscle Channel Dysfunction results. For example, when exposed to cold, the muscles and tendons become tense and over-contract. Conversely, when exposed to heat, muscles and tendons become loose and overextend.

CLINICAL APPLICATION

There are connecting and intersecting points found all along the Twelve Muscle and Tendon Channels. Treatment of these points can create a favorable response, allowing for successful purgation and tonification techniques. Therefore, the Qigong doctor can effectively apply Jing Point therapy to specific areas and points along the Twelve Muscle and Tendon Channels in order to apply purging and tonifying tissue stimulation (Figure 9.22 through 9.33). Because these channels are also responsible for extending and flexing the muscles, tendons, ligaments and joints, their pathology is reflected in symptoms of impaired movement (i.e., pulled, twisted, strained, cramped or atrophied muscles, flaccid muscles, spasms, etc.).

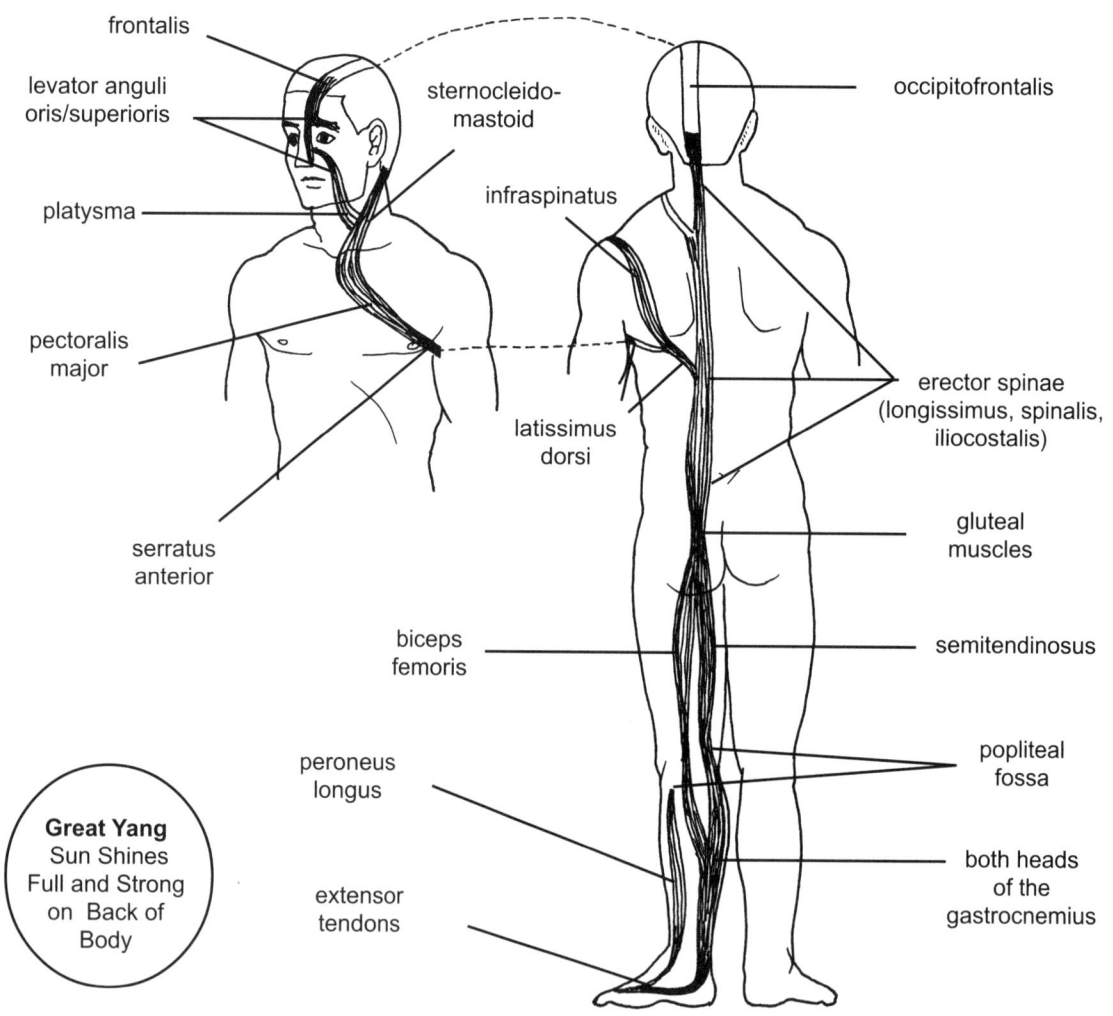

VOLUME 1, SECTION 1: FOUNDATIONS OF CHINESE ENERGETIC MEDICINE

Labels on figure: frontalis; levator anguli oris/superioris; platysma; pectoralis major; serratus anterior; sternocleidomastoid; infraspinatus; latissimus dorsi; biceps femoris; peroneus longus; extensor tendons; occipitofrontalis; erector spinae (longissimus, spinalis, iliocostalis); gluteal muscles; semitendinosus; popliteal fossa; both heads of the gastrocnemius.

Great Yang — Sun Shines Full and Strong on Back of Body

Figure 9.22. The Muscle Tendon Channel of the Urinary Bladder Channel (The Foot Tai Yang Muscle Tendon Channel). High Tide is 3 p.m. to 5 p.m. Pathological symptoms include the following: strained muscles of the small toe; swelling and pain in the heels; stiffness or spasms along the spine and back area; frozen shoulder; and stiffness or spasms in the axillary and clavicle regions.

The pathology of the Muscle and Tendon Channels is also reflected in symptoms of dysfunction in corresponding groups of muscles and other associated connective tissues. The connective tissues are divided into three groups: the large, the small, and the membranous connective tissues.

A local Muscle and Tendon Channel symptom can be treated by stimulating an area located next to the origin of the pain. For example, if the area is Yang (lateral) and overactive, then the Yin (medial) will be underactive, and vice versa. Treatment is thus directed towards restoring balance between the Yin and Yang Muscle and Tendon Channels.

The Twelve Muscle and Tendon Channels, being superficial, contain and circulate Wei Qi. They thus provide the body's third line of defense against any unfavorable exogenous influence. The body's first line of defense is the external Wei Qi field, and second line of defense is the Wei Qi stored within the skin. Only after overcoming the resistance of the body's Muscle and Tendon Wei

CHAPTER 9: THE CONNECTING VESSELS, DIVERGENT CHANNELS, MUSCLE/TENDON CHANNELS AND SKIN ZONES

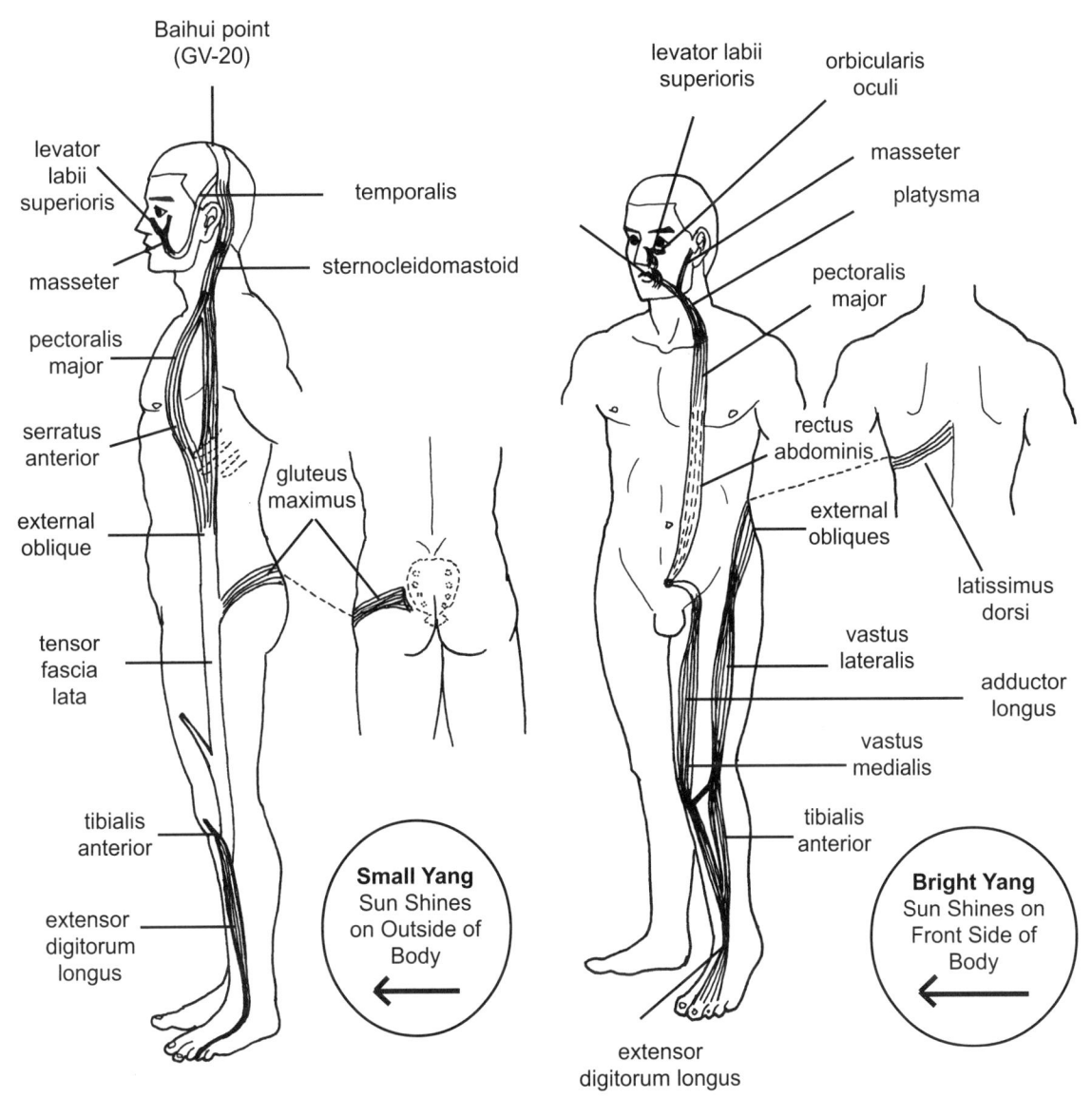

Figure 9.23. The Muscle Tendon Channel of the Gall Bladder Channel (The Foot Shao Yang Muscle and Tendon Channel). High Tide is 11p.m. to 1 a.m. Pathological symptoms include: strained muscles from the fourth toe to the knee upon lateral rotation, with an inability to bend the knee; muscle spasms or stiffness within the popliteal fossa; strained muscles of the sacrum, pelvis, and lower ribs; pain in the hypochondria, chest, and clavicle region; muscle spasms (fascial tics) occurring around the outer edges of the eyes, and an inability to turn the eyes to the left or right.

Figure 9.24. The Muscle Tendon Channel of the Stomach Channel (The Foot Yang Ming Muscle and Tendon Channel). High Tide is 7 a.m. to 9 a.m. Pathological symptoms include: strained muscles of the big toe; spasms or hardening of the muscles in the foot; knotted or twisted muscles in the lower leg and thigh; swelling in the anterior pelvis region; hernia; spasms of the abdominal muscles; spasms or stiffness of neck and cheek muscles; and eye spasms.

Small Yin
Sun Shines Deep on Inside of Thigh →

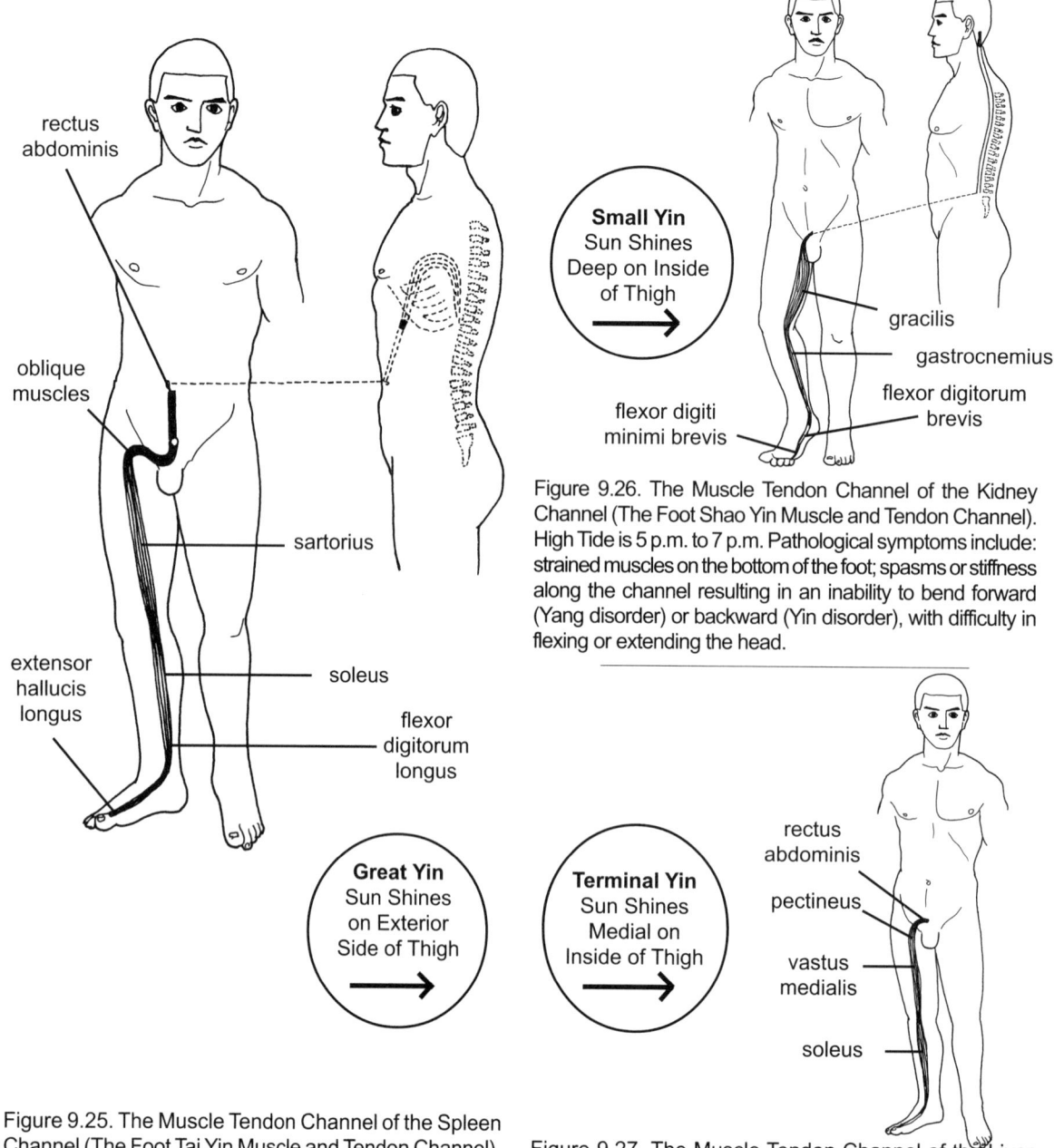

Figure 9.26. The Muscle Tendon Channel of the Kidney Channel (The Foot Shao Yin Muscle and Tendon Channel). High Tide is 5 p.m. to 7 p.m. Pathological symptoms include: strained muscles on the bottom of the foot; spasms or stiffness along the channel resulting in an inability to bend forward (Yang disorder) or backward (Yin disorder), with difficulty in flexing or extending the head.

Great Yin
Sun Shines on Exterior Side of Thigh →

Terminal Yin
Sun Shines Medial on Inside of Thigh →

Figure 9.25. The Muscle Tendon Channel of the Spleen Channel (The Foot Tai Yin Muscle and Tendon Channel). High Tide is 9 a.m. to 11 a.m. Pathological symptoms include: strained muscles of the big toe; pain in the internal malleolus of the ankle upon rotation; pain along the medial aspect of the knee and adductor muscles of the thigh; groin strain; and pain due to strained upper abdominal muscles and mid-thoracic vertebrae.

Figure 9.27. The Muscle Tendon Channel of the Liver Channel (The Foot Jue Yin Muscle and Tendon Channel). High Tide is 1 a.m. to 3 a.m. Pathological symptoms include: strained muscles of the big toe; pain in the anterior internal malleolus of the ankle; pain at the medial aspect of the knee and thigh; and dysfunction of the reproductive organs, i.e., impotence.

CHAPTER 9: THE CONNECTING VESSELS, DIVERGENT CHANNELS, MUSCLE/TENDON CHANNELS AND SKIN ZONES

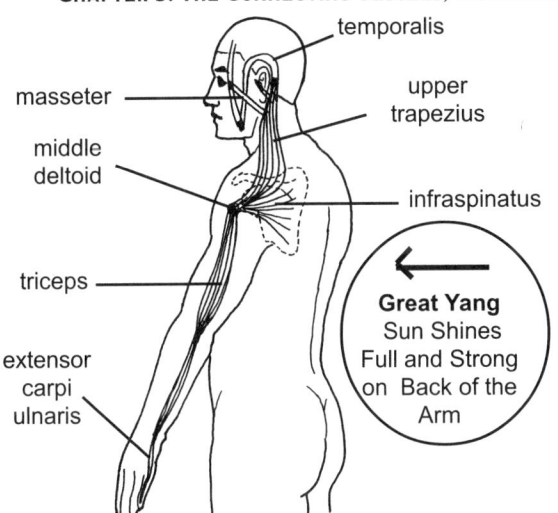

Figure 9.28. The Muscle Tendon Channel of the Small Intestine Channel (The Hand Tai Yang Muscle and Tendon Channel). High Tide is 1 p.m. to 3 p.m. Pathological symptoms include: strained muscles of the little finger; pain along the medial and posterior aspects of the elbow; pain in the posterior aspect of the axilla, neck, and scapula region; tinnitus related to ear ache; and poor vision.

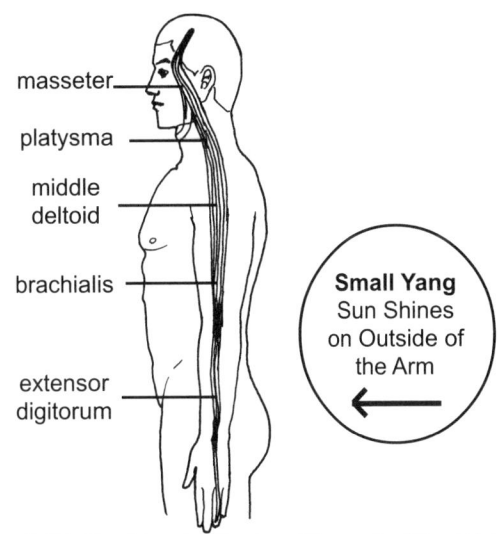

Figure 9.29. The Muscle Tendon Channel of the Triple Burner Channel (The Hand Shao Yang Muscle and Tendon Channel). High Tide is 9 p.m. to 11 p.m. Pathological symptoms include: strained muscles of the ring finger; stiff or strained muscles, or spasms and/or pain along the course of the channel.

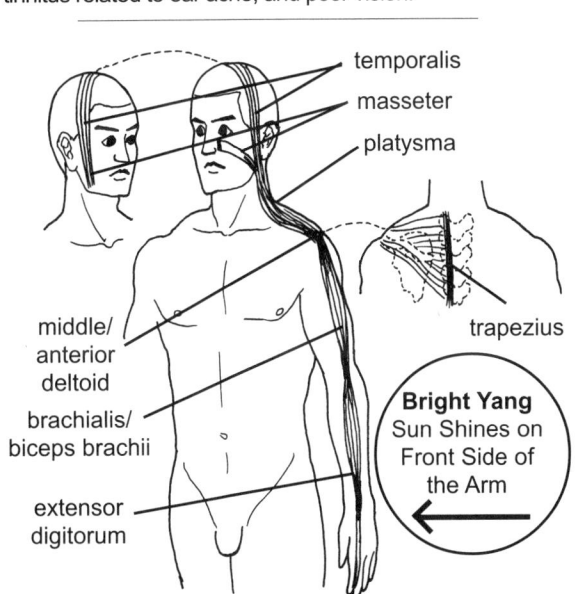

Figure 9.30. The Muscle Tendon Channel of the Large Intestine Channel (The Hand Yang Ming Muscle and Tendon Channel). High Tide is 5 a.m. to 7 a.m. Pathological symptoms include: strained muscles of the index finger; stiffness, strained, or muscle spasms along the course of the channel, resulting in frozen shoulder; and an inability to rotate the neck from side to side.

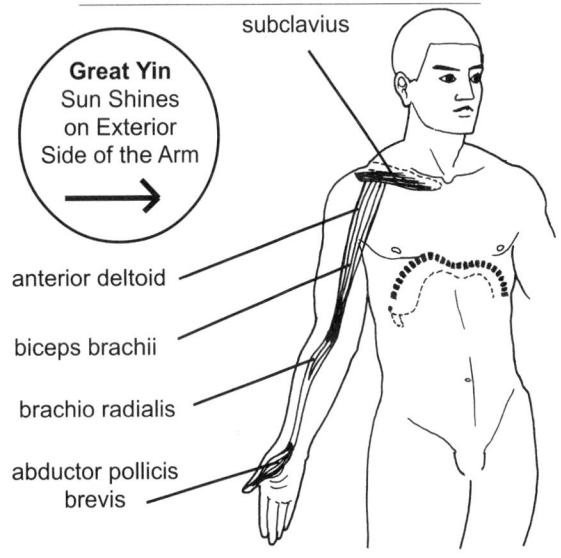

Figure 9.31. The Muscle Tendon Channel of the Lung Channel (The Hand Tai Yin Muscle and Tendon Channel). High Tide is 3 a.m. to 5 a.m. Pathological symptoms include: strained muscles of the thumb; stiff, strained or muscle spasms, and/or pain along the course of the Lung Channel. In more serious cases, there will be muscle spasms over the rib area and spitting of blood.

469

Small Yin
Sun Shines Deep on Inside of the Arm →

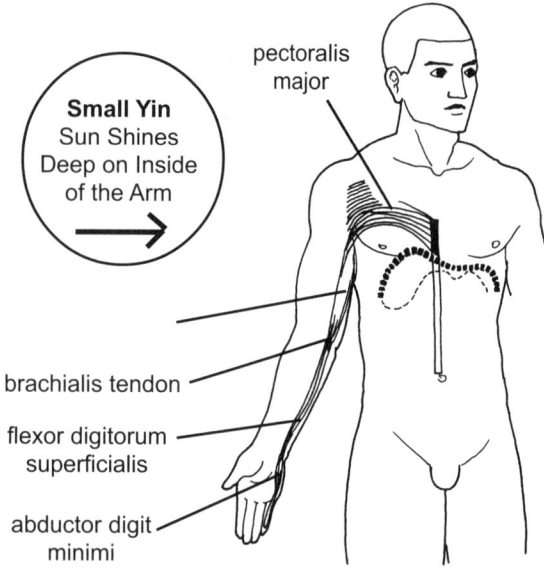

- pectoralis major
- brachialis tendon
- flexor digitorum superficialis
- abductor digit minimi

Figure 9.32. The Muscle Tendon Channel of the Heart Channel (The Hand Shao Yin Muscle and Tendon Channel). High Tide is 11 a.m. to 1 p.m. Pathological symptoms include: strained muscles of the little finger; stiff or strained muscles with spasm and/or pain along the course of the Heart Channel, including internal cramping within the diaphragm and upper abdominal area.

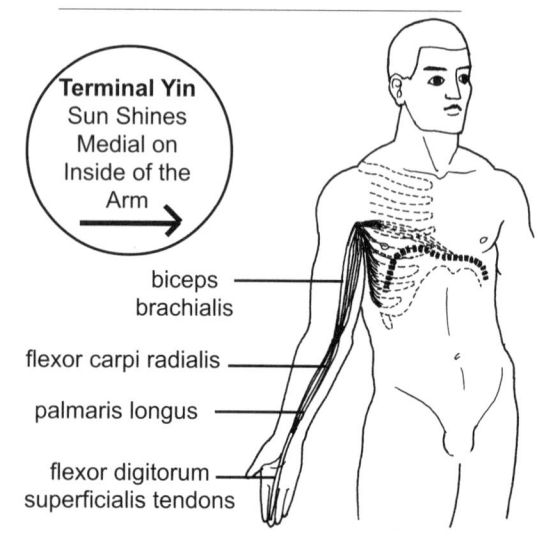

Terminal Yin
Sun Shines Medial on Inside of the Arm →

- biceps brachialis
- flexor carpi radialis
- palmaris longus
- flexor digitorum superficialis tendons

Figure 9.33. The Muscle Tendon Channel of the Pericardium Channel (The Hand Jue Yin Muscle and Tendon Channel). High Tide is 7 p.m. to 9 p.m. Pathological symptoms include: strained muscles of the middle finger; stiff or strained muscles, or spasms and/or pain along the course of the channel; and chest pain and spasms.

Qi can the Exogenous pathogens travel down the length of the channel to penetrate the corresponding primary channel at the Jing-Well point. Jing-Well points are points of energetic union, connecting primary channel points together with the points where the Muscle and Tendon Channels have their origin.

THE SKIN ZONES: PI FU

Based along the body's Twelve Primary Channels, Connecting Vessels, and Muscle and Tendon Channels, the body's outermost tissue is divided into Twelve Skin Zones (also known as the Twelve Cutaneous Regions). These skin zones are the surface contact areas for the body's channel and collateral systems.

The regions (or zones) of the skin (Pi Fu) are located in the superficial layers of the external derma and have continuous and direct contact with the external environment. They are, therefore, the areas of the body that are the most sensitive to climactic changes and must adapt to protect the body from external pathogenic factors.

ORIGIN OF NAME

The literal translation of the Chinese term "Pi Fu" is "skin."

- The first character "Pi," depicts the Chinese ideogram for skin.
- The second character "Fu," also depicts the Chinese ideogram for skin. It is composed of two radicals. The character to the left, "Ji" depicts the Chinese ideogram for body tissue, muscle or flesh (all of which are various forms of connective tissue). The right side of the character is the phonetic sound. Together the words Pi Fu translate as skin (Figure 9.34).

ENERGETIC FUNCTION

The Qi and the Blood of the Twelve Skin Zones receive their nourishment via the connecting vessels. The Twelve Skin Zones circulate Wei Qi, which in addition to having a defensive function, is also in charge of opening and closing the pores. The skin relies primarily upon the strength of the Wei Qi for its ability to resist the invasion of external patho-

CHAPTER 9: THE CONNECTING VESSELS, DIVERGENT CHANNELS, MUSCLE/TENDON CHANNELS AND SKIN ZONES

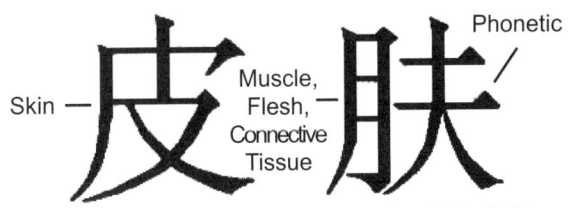

Figure 9.34. The Chinese character for "Pi Fu," Skin

genic influences. Any harmful influences must first penetrate the skin before they can affect the body's internal tissues and organs. Since the Lungs rule the skin, weak Lung Qi can allow pathogens to penetrate the skin and affect the Lungs.

PATHOLOGICAL SYMPTOMS

Pathological symptoms associated with the Twelve Primary Channels and Connecting Vessels manifest along the surface of the Twelve Skin Zones before progressing deeper into the body's connective tissue. The early stages of disease are called exterior conditions; if the exterior Wei Qi is strong enough, pathogens will be stopped at the external level. The progression of pathogenic invasion is described as follows (Figure 9.35).

1. **The Body's Wei Qi:** This is the body's first line of defense. A healthy body will project a strong, protective, external energetic field, which will maintain a capable defensive boundary. If the patient becomes weak, tired, or stressed, however, External pathogens may advance onto the patient's skin and begin attacking his or her health.

2. **The Skin:** This is the body's second line of defense. If the body's Wei Qi is not strong enough to resist an external attack and the skin is not capable of warding off the invading pathogens, then the pathogens will attack the skin, causing the sweat pores to open, thus allowing the pathogens to advance towards the patient's collaterals.

3. **The Collaterals (or Connecting Vessels):** This is the third line of defense. If the body's collaterals are unable to redirect or purge the advancing pathogens, the pathogens will then advance into the patient's channels.

4. **The Channels (including the Twelve Primary Channels, Eight Extraordinary Vessels, and Twelve Divergent Channels):** This is the body's last line of defense before the advancing external pathogens invade the patient's internal organs. If the body's channels are unable to redirect or purge the pathogens and the pathogens are allowed to continue their pro-

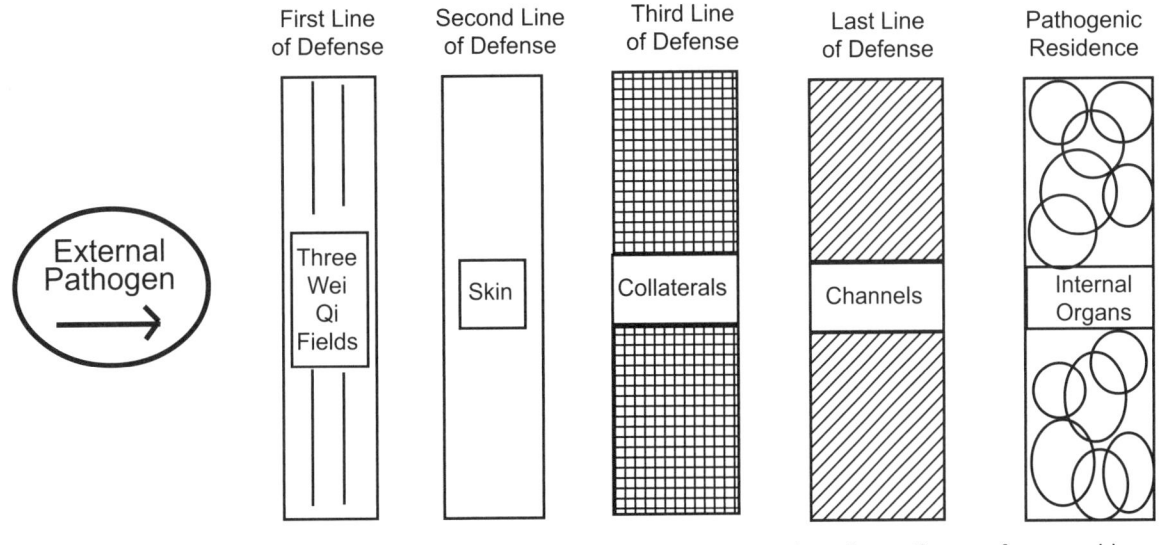

Figure 9.35. The body utilizes multiple lines of defense in order to prevent invading pathogens from reaching the internal organs.

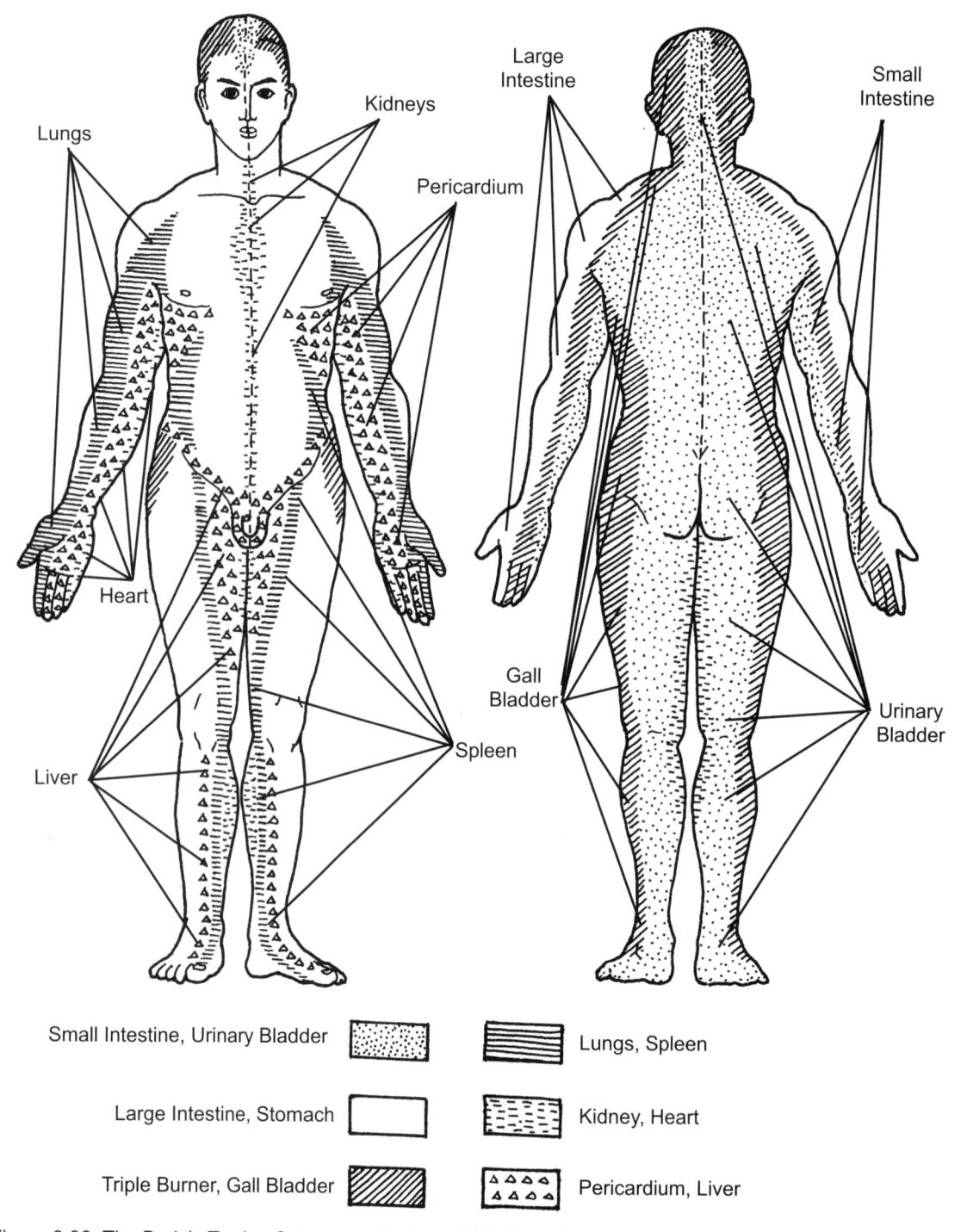

VOLUME 1, SECTION 1: FOUNDATIONS OF CHINESE ENERGETIC MEDICINE

Figure 9.36. The Body's Twelve Cutaneous Regions (Skin Zones), are based on the external flow of Qi from the Twelve Primary Channels and their Fifteen Collaterals

gression, they will advance further into the body's internal organs.

5. **The Internal Organs:** The internal organs are affected by pathogenic invasion only after the pathogens have penetrated all the outer defenses. Once the pathogens have reached the internal organs, they begin establishing a residence within the body's inner most tissues, causing and contributing to chronic disease.

Pathologies associated with the primary channels may manifest diagnostically through symptoms affecting the body's skin, channels, and points. Pimples, moles, skin discolorations, and changes in electro-conductivity are all signs of pathogens, or obstructions, invading the skin.

A disease of external origin that first lodges within the patient's skin can be treated by the Qigong doctor. The doctor stimulates the Wei Qi in the affected skin zone through external Qi projection in order to purge or disperse the pathogen before it progresses further into the body's connective tissue. Another common treatment used to stimulate the Wei Qi of the skin and disperse pathogens is the application of herbal ointments and/or moxa therapy.

THE CONNECTIVE TISSUE OF THE TWELVE SKIN ZONES

From a Traditional Chinese Medical perspective, the Qi circulating within the body's inner fascial connective tissue can be accessed with the external energy stimulation of the Twelve Skin Zones.

The body's underlying connective tissue always responds to the external stimulation of the Twelve Skin Zones. The body's vast network of connective tissue begins just below the skin and is regarded as one of the largest, most extensive tissue organs in the body. The connective tissue simultaneously fulfills the functions of supporting, connecting, containing, and transmitting Jing, Qi, Shen, Blood and Body Fluids. It is a continuous structural network that binds tissues into their organ shape. It also supplies the internal organ's with vessels and ducts, and securely fastens each organ within the body cavity. This connective tissue surrounds and anchors the vessels within the muscles, Bones, and organ tissue. Its fluid nature supports the entire body structurally by transmitting and absorbing hydrostatic pressure. Any stimulation of one of the body's Twelve Skin Zones will directly affect the body's connective tissue and will stimulate the corresponding internal organ associated with that particular zone (Figure 9.36).

The superficial fascia (the connective tissue just under the skin) divides into a top and bottom layer. The top layer is the fatty layer, which constitutes the main fatty tissue of the outer surface of the body and fascia. This fatty layer acts as an insulator, helping to maintain a constant body temperature. It is thus metabolically significant: storing fat as fuel, and releasing it in response to nerve and hormonal stimuli. It corresponds to the greasy layer where the Wei Qi circulates throughout the body's surface tissues. The deeper layer of the superficial fascia envelops the nerves, veins, arteries, lymph vessels, and nodes.

Heat and movement help maintain the health of the body's connective tissue's base fluids, increasing flexibility and further enabling the conduction of energy. Any obstruction occurring in or on the body's surface tissues can result in the binding or thickening of the connective tissue beneath it, thus causing adhesions. This obstruction decreases physical strength and range of motion, slows the metabolic process, and compromises the body's immunity.

If the integrity of the connective tissue is compromised, the health of the body's immune system declines. Compartments of connective tissue influence the spread of toxins, diseases, infections, and tumors. The fibrous walls of connective tissue, as well as chemicals present in the fluid of the connective tissue, help to prevent the spread of pathogens from one area of the body to another.

CLINICAL DIAGNOSIS AND THE TWELVE SKIN ZONES

Clinical diagnosis and treatment techniques relating to the use of the Twelve Skin Zones are quite extensive. The skin along these zones is examined for evidence of discoloration or tissue obstruction. Changes in skin color and tissue formations are ob-

served and categorized as follows (Figure 9.37):
- A darkish hue reflects obstruction of Qi and Blood.
- A bluish-purple color indicates local pain.
- Change in color from yellow to red shows evidence of Heat.
- A white or pallid skin tone signifies deficiency or Cold.
- Boils, pimples (especially on the back), hives, and eczema, as well as hard lumps or nodules beneath the surface of the skin, indicate diseases associated with the Twelve Primary Channels (manifesting through the Twelve Skin Zones).

A palpable lump can develop from a variety of sources, including congealed or stagnant Blood. There are generally eight types of lumps observed in the Medical Qigong clinic:

1. **The Shrimp Lump** is shaped in the form of a shrimp.
2. **The Turtle Lump** is named for its shape and often has multiple lump formations.
3. **The Green/Blue Lump** derives its name and color from the superficial Blood Vessels on which it forms.
4. **The Single Lump** appears in isolation and is differentiated from multiple lump formations.
5. **The Dry Lump** indicates an obstruction.
6. **The Blood Lump** relates to congealed Blood.
7. **The Abdominal Lump** is named for its physical location.
8. **The Yellow Lump** is named because of the yellow color in the specific region of the lump.

Palpating the Patient's Skin

Before palpating and diagnosing the skin, the Qigong doctor first scans the patient's body energetically to feel the temperature, moisture, and texture of the patient's tissues.

1. The doctor scans and palpates the patient to diagnose the condition according to temperature:
- If the skin feels hot to the touch it often indicates the presence of a Damp-Heat condition.
- When first touching the patient with light pressure, if the skin feels immediately hot and as the pressure is maintained the feeling of heat increases, this indicates an invasion of exterior Wind-Heat (with a pathogenic factor still present on the surface).
- If the skin over a blood vessel feels hot on medium pressure, it indicates interior Heat.
- If the skin feels hot on deep, heavy pressure, it indicates a Deficient Heat condition from a Yin Deficiency.
- If the skin feels cold to the touch, it often indicates a Cold condition. This condition is often manifested in the lower back and lower abdominal region, indicating a deficiency of the Kidney Yang.

2. The doctor scans and palpates the patient to diagnose the condition according to the amount of moisture present on the skin:
- A moist feeling of the skin may indicate an invasion of the exterior by Wind-Cold or Wind-Heat.
- If the skin feels moist due to spontaneous sweating, it indicates a deficiency of Lung Qi (in the absence of exterior symptoms).

3. The doctor scans and palpates the patient to diagnose the condition according to the texture of the skin:

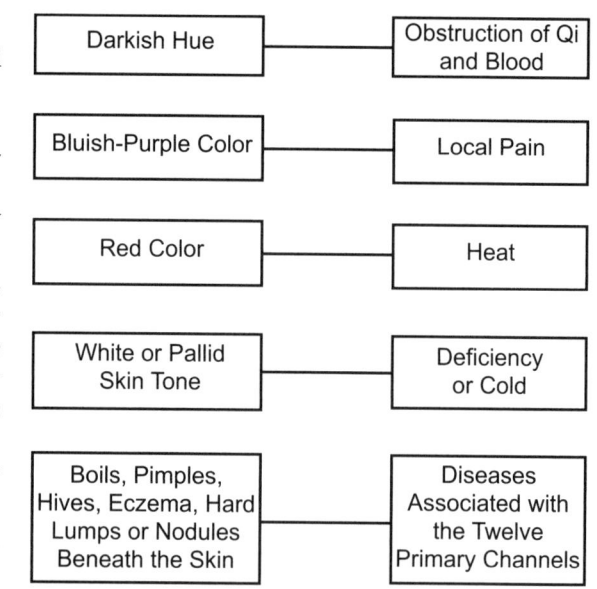

Figure 9.37. The Changes in skin color, shape, and texture are observed and categorized.

Darkish Hue	Obstruction of Qi and Blood
Bluish-Purple Color	Local Pain
Red Color	Heat
White or Pallid Skin Tone	Deficiency or Cold
Boils, Pimples, Hives, Eczema, Hard Lumps or Nodules Beneath the Skin	Diseases Associated with the Twelve Primary Channels

- If the skin feels dry, it indicates either a Yin condition of the Lungs or a Blood Deficiency.
- If the skin is scaly and dry, it indicates an exhaustion of the Body's Fluids.
- If the skin is swollen and visible indentation remains after applying pressure, it indicates edema (called water swelling).
- If the skin is swollen and no visible indentation remains after applying pressure, it indicates a retention of Dampness (called Qi swelling).

Channel And Collateral Therapy

Because the Qi of the Yin and Yang organs flows along the body's internal and external surfaces, all of the internal and external channels and collaterals, five tissues (tendons, blood vessels, muscles, skin, and Bones), and five sense organs (eyes, ears, nose, mouth, and tongue), link together to create an energetic network. Patients as well as Qigong practitioners can become aware of the circulation of Qi along the body's channels and collaterals by practicing sitting meditations. The awareness of what the Qi feels like enables the meditators to feel the flow and function of each channel, as well as the Blood and Heat cycles in each Skin Zone. This eventually makes it possible to control the Qi circulation through intention and imagination.

Balancing the Conception and Governing Vessels is of the utmost importance in the practice of any Qigong regulation. This balance is created through the discipline of the Microcosmic Orbit meditation, which connects the Governing and Conception Vessels. The Qigong practitioner draws the Yang Fire and Yin essences up and down the body along these two Vessels, thus fusing together the Water and Fire energies. This fusion is utilized by the doctor in every Qigong treatment, as it maintains proper balance of the patient's Yin and Yang energy.

The Qigong doctor's awareness of Qi flow in the body usually develops in three distinct stages, which are described as follows:
1. First, they begin to feel the energy flow along the surface channels of the body, especially within the areas of the extremities. Usually at this stage, Heat and tingling sensations within the body's surface muscles will be felt.
2. Next, they begin to feel the energy flow deeper within their tissues, especially along the tendons, deeper muscles, and visceral organs. Usually at this stage, they begin to feel mild electric shocks and vibrations within their muscles, Bones, and internal organs.
3. In the final stage, they feel the Earth and Heaven energy penetrate their bodies, outside channels, and internal organs, connecting into their Taiji Pole, and then turning outward again. Usually at this stage, they will feel their entire energized body vibrate. This vibration may be triggered through either universal or environmental changes, as the Medical Qigong practitioner becomes hypersensitive to any form of external energetic disturbance.

Controlling Qi Extension through the Channels

The Qigong doctor must first be able to control his or her own energy circulation, causing it to flow in or out, expand or contract at will, before beginning to extend energy for the treatment of any patient. This energetic control is gained through specific imagination and visualization techniques. The fundamental premise for these techniques is reflected in the Daoist saying, "the imagination leads the Mind, the Mind leads the Qi." The doctor must also be able to utilize energy from the natural environment (trees, waterfalls, ocean, desert, etc.) in order to replenish and facilitate his or her own energy.

By drawing in Heavenly Qi and combining it with already gathered Earthly Qi, the doctor uses powerful energies beyond himself or herself to mobilize and activate the Qi of the patient. This method of combining Heavenly and Earthly energies establishes a powerful healing field of Qi. This field of Qi then responds to the Qigong doctor's own Qi circulation, the energy of the natural environment, and the energy of the patient. This ability must be achieved in order to activate the patient's Qi and then regulate it by purging the excess Qi, dredging the channel Qi, replenishing the deficient Qi, and guiding the Qi back to its origin.

Figure 9.38

Superficial ↓ Deep	
	Twelve Skin Zones
	Muscle and Tendon Channels
	Collateral System
	Twelve Primary Channels
	Eight Extraordinary Vessels
	Twelve Divergent Channels
	The Internal Organs

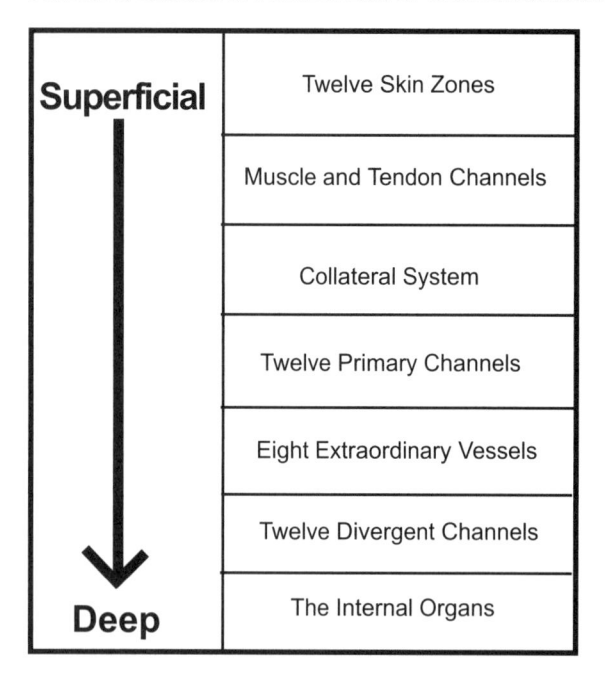

Figure 9.38. The Body's Energetic Flow According to Traditional Chinese Medicine

THE DEPTH OF THE BODY'S ENERGETIC CHANNEL FLOW

According to most modern acupuncture colleges of Traditional Chinese Medicine, the energetic flow of the body's channel system begins superficially along the Twelve Skin Zones of the body. Next, the energy flows deeper into the body along the Muscle and Tendon Channels. After the Muscle and Tendon Channels, the energy of the Collateral System is considered deeper still. Next is the flow of the Twelve Primary Channels, then the Eight Extraordinary Channels. Deeper than the Eight Extraordinary Channels is the network of the Twelve Divergent Channels. Deeper still is the energetic matrix of the Zang Fu Organs (the six viscera and five bowels) (Figure 9.38).

Figure 9.39

Superficial ↓ Deep		
	Three Wei Qi Fields	(3) (2) (1)
	Twelve Skin Zones	Twelve Chakras Gates
	Muscle and Tendon Channels	Internal Current of Ying Qi
	Collateral System	Sea of Blood
	Twelve Primary Channels	Sea of Marrow
	Eight Extraordinary Vessels	Twelve Divergent Channels
	The Three Dantians	
	The Five Thrusting Channels	
	The Seven Major Chakras	
	The Taiji Pole	

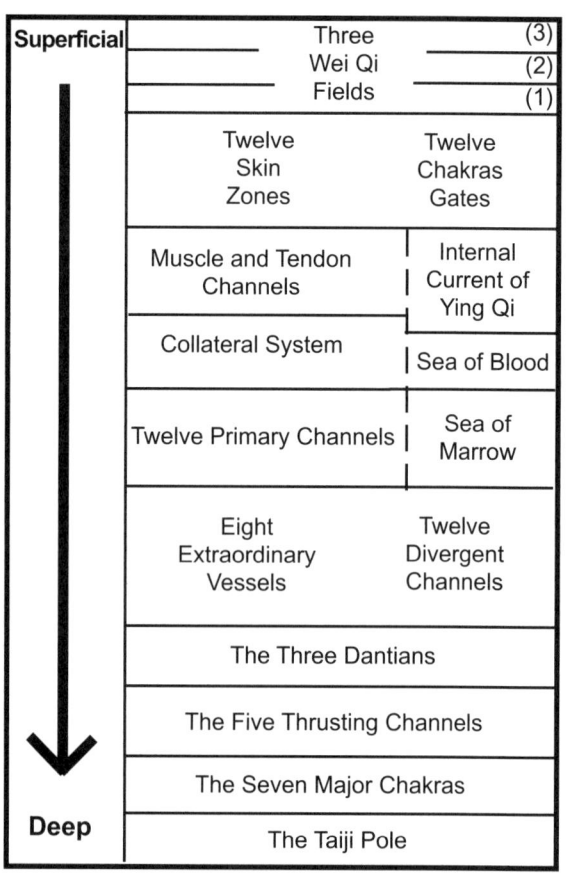

Figure 9.39. The Body's Energetic Structures According to Ancient Chinese Medicine

According to the ancient Chinese Medicine and various Medical Qigong colleges in China, the body's energetic flow also includes: the Three Wei Qi Fields, the Twelve Chakra Gates, the Internal Current of Ying Qi, Sea of Blood, the Sea of Marrow, the Eight Extraordinary Vessels, the Three Dantians, the Five Thrusting Channels, the Seven Major Chakras, and the Taiji Pole (Figure 9.39).

Chapter 10
The Body's Energetic Points

Introduction to Energetic Points

The Chinese ideograph for "point" ("Xue" or "Xue Wei") is translated as "cavity place, cave, den, hole, or hollow." The word Xue also implies a den or lair. Thus, it is not only a cave but a home for some type of powerful life form.

Chinese Characters for Point: Xue

The character for "Xue" is divided into two parts. The top of the character represents a "roof" or "covering." The bottom part of the character is the word "Ba," and in ancient times originally represented the "division of two parts." The character was later changed to mean "eight," referring to the "Eight Treasures" (Viscera, Bowels, Qi, Blood, Sinews, Vessels, Bone, and Marrow). Together, the translation reveals a hidden space which contains passage to the "Eight Treasures," accessible only after removing or uncovering its entry portal (Figure 10.1).

Although the Chinese word Xue is usually translated into English as "point" or "acupoint," it is valuable for the non-Chinese speaking student to understand the word's different connotations. The body's energetic points, over 1,000 of which have been identified and categorized in Traditional Chinese Medicine, are almost always located on prominent depressions or hollows in the patient's physical structure. These points lie all over the body, and many (but not all) of them are located along the major channels and vessels. Sometimes when touching a point, it feels as if one's fingertip has found the entrance of a small cave or opening that is hidden by the skin covering it.

In the human body, our living Qi gathers and pools within these protected hollows (Figure 10.2). For this reason, some writers have preferred to translate Xue as "vital hollow," rather than "point." Because of its popular acceptance, how-

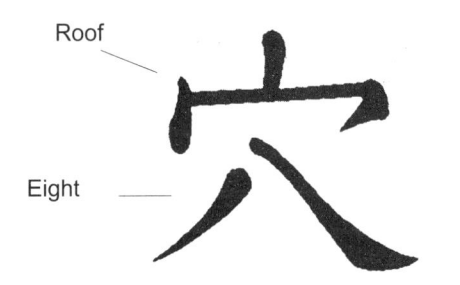

Figure 10.1. The Chinese character for "Xue," Cave

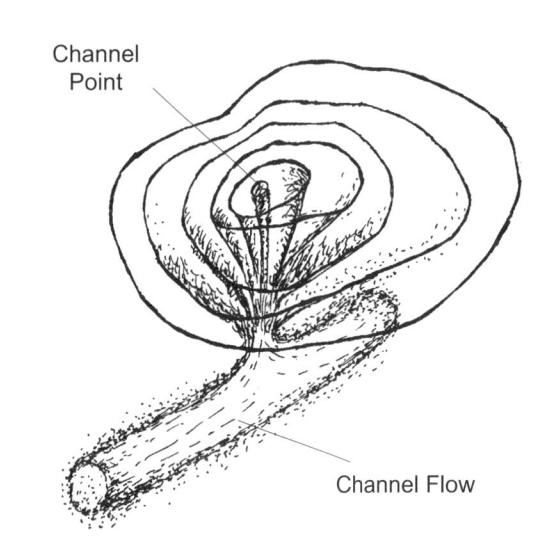

Figure 10.2. The energetic points can be seen as small energetic pools lying along the body's channels.

ever, the term "point" is used throughout this textbook series.

Historical Use of Energetic Points

Though the therapeutic use of point stimulation is most often associated with Traditional Chinese Medicine (acupuncture and massage), numerous other cultures around the world have been treating illness and disease with point therapy for many thousands of years.

The first references to point therapy in Chinese Medicine are from the Shang era (1600-1028 B.C.). It is quite possible, however, that the use of the human body's energetic points for healing arose at a much earlier time in human history, perhaps independently in different cultures around the globe. There is some debate as to the original discovery of the energetic points used in ancient (and modern) Chinese medicine. Some scholars claim that these points were first discovered through a trial and error process of random tissue stimulation by ancient Chinese shaman healers, while others believe that energetic points (and energetic channels) were first "seen" by shamans in altered states of consciousness.

The human body naturally seeks a state of health and balance (homeostasis), and the first discovery of point therapy may have been made by an individual - or individuals - unconsciously or inadvertently stimulating an area that felt tender or blocked. This principle can also be observed in the modern Medical Qigong clinic. When describing a headache, for example, a patient may be observed to touch the same energetic points that, when stimulated, can bring about a release of the very condition from which he or she is suffering. This kinesthetic observation is an important part of Medical Qigong diagnosis, as it can provide important clues as to the best strategy for point stimulation. However, this diagnostic observation must be integrated with the Qigong doctor's ability to see the patient's energetic field directly, a skill that is developed with diligent practice of Qigong self-regulation exercises.

Though it may be impossible to know for certain where point therapy first originated (if indeed there was a single place of origin), we can be fairly certain that acupuncture and other forms of point therapy were practiced throughout the ancient world. If extended to include the laying on of hands, the origins of point therapy would most certainly date back tens of thousands of years, if not more.

India's indigenous medical system of Ayurveda traditionally incorporates the stimulation of various energy points (called "marma" points) on the body through the use of therapeutic pressure, needling, and moxibustion, known as marmapuncture.

A marma is defined as "secret, hidden or vital energy" and therefore a marma point is a receptor or reflex point on the skin which has a high concentration of prana (Qi). A marma is also a junction where flesh, veins, arteries, tendons, Bones and joints meet. In India, there are thousands of marmas located all over the body, 365 of which are considered essential points.

The marma points and locations are measured in "anguli" which are finger units relative to the individual. Additionally, the marmas are located along the nadis (channels) which link the marmas to each other and to the organs.

Indian acupuncture stems from an ancient Indian branch of surgery, which used the knowledge of the marma points so as not to cause harm during surgical procedures, or when treating scar tissue. Knowledge of marma points is also drawn from Kalari, an ancient Indian martial art form used for self defense, which used 107 lethal marma points to cause extreme pain, unconsciousness or even death.

References (dating as far back as 4000 B.C.) to the use of Indian acupuncture as a healing modality have been found in the Vedic texts of ancient India, leading some scholars to believe that the knowledge of the healing use of the body's energetic points traveled to China from India along with the theory of the Five Elements (see Volume 3, Chapter 24).

Similar references to acupuncture have surfaced in the relics of the ancient Egyptian culture, also dating back several thousand years. Point therapy is also traditionally utilized by shamans and healers in such geographically separated locations as Sri Lanka, Africa, Peru, and the Amazon basin. Today, acupuncture and point therapy are widely practiced throughout Asia, though the systems that are utilized are almost exclusively derived from Chinese medicine. Examples of other modern derivatives of Chinese point therapy include: acupressure, shiatsu, auriculotherapy, Jin Shin Jyutsu, reflexology, and trigger point therapy.

CHAPTER 10: THE BODY'S ENERGETIC POINTS

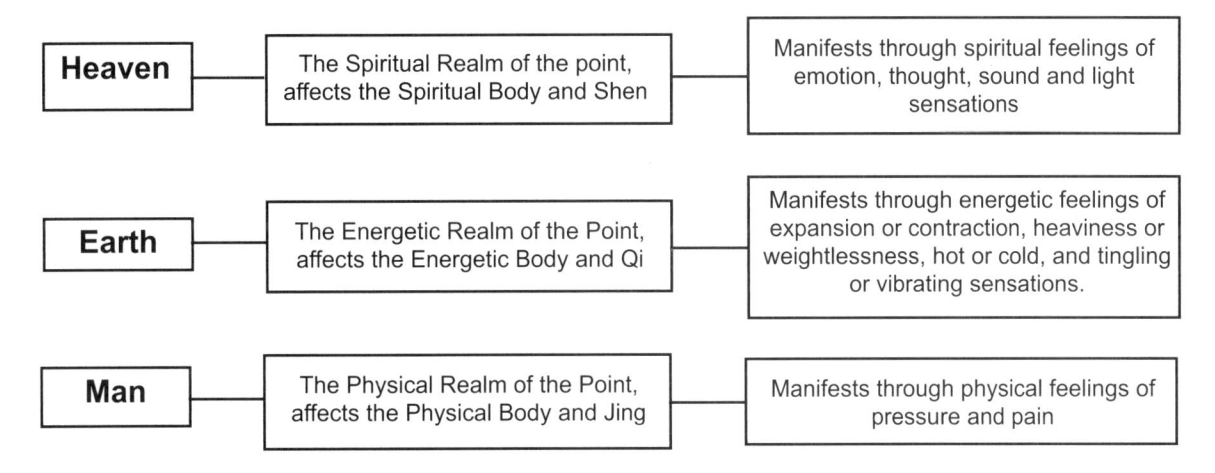

Heaven	The Spiritual Realm of the point, affects the Spiritual Body and Shen	Manifests through spiritual feelings of emotion, thought, sound and light sensations
Earth	The Energetic Realm of the Point, affects the Energetic Body and Qi	Manifests through energetic feelings of expansion or contraction, heaviness or weightlessness, hot or cold, and tingling or vibrating sensations.
Man	The Physical Realm of the Point, affects the Physical Body and Jing	Manifests through physical feelings of pressure and pain

Figure 10.3. The energetic points can be seen as small energetic pools lying along the body's channels.

THE THREE ENERGETIC LEVELS OF POINTS

In Traditional Chinese Medicine, studying the flow and energetic nature of the body's channel points is essential. The ancient Chinese believed that the points along the channels allowed the individual's spirit Qi to flow in and out of the body, unhampered by physical tissues such as skin, flesh, muscle, and bone.

In ancient times, the interior of the channel points were divided into three energetic levels: Heaven, Earth and Man. Each energetic point contains three progressively subtle aspects or dimensions, affecting an individual's physical, energetic and spiritual bodies. These subtle influences also correlate to the physical, energetic and spiritual realms, described as follows (Figure 10.3):

- **The physical nature of a point** is expressed through the individual's sensory perceptions, and manifests through feelings of pressure and pain.
- **The energetic nature of a point** is expressed through the individual's subtle sensory perceptions, manifesting through feelings of expansion or contraction, heaviness or weightlessness, hot or cold, and tingling or vibrating sensations.
- **The spiritual nature of a point** is expressed through the individual's subtlest sensory perceptions, manifesting through experiences of sound, light, thought, and emotion.

When diagnosing the conditions of the disease, the doctor was required to ascertain at which level the pathogen was residing. For example, sometimes the Righteous Qi is flowing within the Heavenly level, while Turbid Qi is subtly active within the patient's Earthly level. If these subtle energy flows are not clearly distinguished, then it is impossible to use the needle properly to balance the disharmony.

THE FORMATION OF ENERGETIC POINTS

Generally, points are formed in four ways. The first type of point occurs when two or more muscles, tendons, or ligaments intersect or overlap in a way that creates a small depression at the area of convergence. To form the depression, the two muscles either come together, separate, overlap, or run parallel to each other. Usually the channels lie under a protective layer of muscle, but at the aforementioned junctures the channels may be exposed, and thus lie closer to the surface. Examples of this type of point include:

- Liver 8 point
- Kidney 10 point
- Triple Burner 4 point

The second type of point occurs when a nerve is exposed in an area with relatively little muscle

479

tissue to cover and protect it. Because the nerve is exposed, such points are especially sensitive, and when stimulated may cause the patient to experience a sharp pain or a sensation like an electric shock. Examples of this type of point include:
- Large Intestine 4 point
- Pericardium 6 point
- Small Intestine 8 point

The third type of point lies under a protective superficial layer of muscle. It can however, still be stimulated due to its natural sensitivity and because the overlying layer of muscle is thin. Examples of this type of point include:
- Gall Bladder 1 point
- Urinary Bladder 16 point
- Urinary Bladder 46 point

The fourth type of point is located in the natural depressions on the surfaces of the bones and cartilage. These depressions may take the form of grooves, pits, hollows, indentations, fissures, or crevices. Examples of this type of point include:
- Governing Vessel 20 point
- Gall Bladder 20 point
- Kidney 1 point

Scientific Research of Acupoints

In the early 1970's, shortly after President Nixon's historic visit to China, Dr. Robert O. Becker, M.D., a Syracuse University orthopedist, received a grant from the National Institutes of Health to research how acupuncture works. Dr. Becker reasoned that the channels were electrical conductors that existed independent of the nervous system yet somehow communicated with it. He theorized that these channels carried an injury message to the brain, which then responded by sending back the appropriate level of direct current (DC) that would stimulate healing in the troubled area.

Becker also suggested, in his book *The Body Electric*, that "any current grows weaker with distance, due to resistance along the transmission cable. The smaller the amperage and voltage, the faster the current dies out. Electrical engineers solve this problem by building booster amplifiers every so often along a power line to get the signal back up to strength. For currents measured in nanoamperes and microvolts (such as those gen-

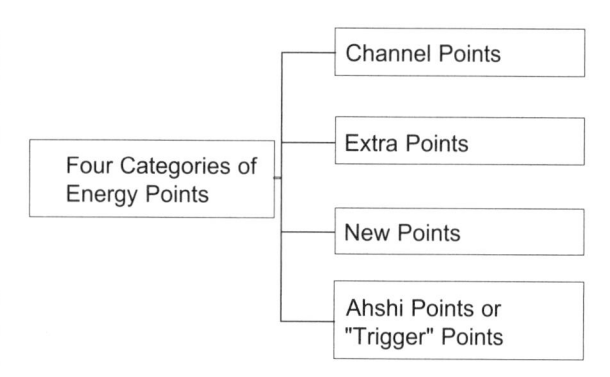

Figure 10.4. The Four Categories of Energetic Points

erated in the human body), the amplifiers would have to be no more than a few inches apart—just like the acupuncture points."

Dr. Becker and his assistant Maria Reichmanis, herself a biophysicist, designed special equipment to measure and map the electrical conductivity along the channels. They found the predicted electrical characteristics along the channels charted in Traditional Chinese Medicine and at half of the known points. These same points showed up consistently on all the people tested. Because they were able to measure only half of the traditionally charted points, Becker and Reichmanis suggested that the other points may simply be weaker, or of a different kind, than the ones that their instruments detected.

Each point that they found was electrically positive in comparison to its surrounding tissue, and each point had an electrical field surrounding it with its own characteristic shape.

Later research in China, France, and the United States has demonstrated that not only do these points and channels have electrical properties, but they also emit and absorb light and sound, both of which are vital to healthy biological functions.

The Four Categories of Energetic Points

Points are divided into four categories: Channel Points, Extra points, New points, and Ahshi Points, described as follows (Figure 10.4):

1. **Channel Points:** These points are the primary points that are distributed along the Twelve Primary Channels and the Conception and Gov-

erning Vessels. There are 365 channel points.
2. **Extra Points:** These points are not regarded as having a specific origin in the twelve main channels, although they are named and have definite locations. These points are also called "miscellaneous points."
3. **New Points:** This includes a fairly large group of points discovered since the Communist "Liberation" of 1949, in many cases through electric point detection. These points generally have no energetic description but do have indications. There are more than 700 new points, when counted to include the extra points.
4. **Ahshi Points:** These points are tender or painful spots near a diseased or injured area and can be anywhere on the body. They function like trigger points, as they are points of tension or pain. Ahshi points differ according to each patient and condition, and are often not given specific names or definite locations. They are most commonly used for pain syndromes.

THE TWO GATES OF ENERGETIC POINTS

It is useful to further categorize the points into two general types of points commonly used by Medical Qigong doctors. These two types of points (or gates) are specific areas where Qigong doctors concentrate their intention and focus their energy extension. Point locations have a greater amount of accumulated Qi than do the surrounding channels or tissues, and are thus used for purging or tonifying the body's organ energy to promote the balanced circulation of Qi and Blood. The two types of points, the Outer Qi Gates and the Inner Qi Gates are described as follows:

1. **The Outer Qi Gates:** These are points through which the patient's Shen and Qi enter and leave the body. The Qigong doctor or patient may gather healing Qi from the outer environment through these gates, and may also use them to purge the body of internal excesses or stagnations. These points are especially vulnerable to the Six External Pathogens (i.e., Cold, Hot, Wind, Damp, Dry, and Fire), which tend to enter the body through these gates (see Volume 3, Chapter 22). These same pathogens may also be expelled through these gates. For this reason, many of these outer Qi gates have the word Feng (Wind) in their names, such as Fengchi GB-20 (Wind Pool), Fengmen Bl-12 (Wind Gate) and Fengfu GV-16 (Wind Palace).

2. **The Inner Qi Gates:** These are points through which the Qi of the Yin and Yang organs and channels is transported back and forth internally and externally, from deep to superficial and back again. These points are more involved with the movement of Qi within the body and are less involved in the exchanging energy with the outer environment. In this way, the inner Qi gates enable the Qi to communicate between the different parts of the body.

When stimulating the patient's energetic tissues and treating either of the two gates, the Qigong doctor can initiate the healing potential of a specific point by using various modalities, such as Energy Projection, Energetic Point Therapy, Jing Point Therapy, or Invisible Needle Therapy.

THE THREE FUNCTIONS OF ENERGETIC POINTS

The use of energetic points has three important clinical functions: Diagnosis, The Manipulation of Qi and Blood, and To Serve as Pathways for the Elimination of Disease. These three clinical functions are described as follows (Figure 10.5):

1. **Diagnosis:** Diagnosis through point palpation and inspection is an important tool in all branches of Chinese medicine. If a point hurts when touched with light pressure, is hard or

Three Clinical Functions
- Diagnosis
- The Manipulation of Qi and Blood
- To Serve as Pathways for the Elimination of Disease

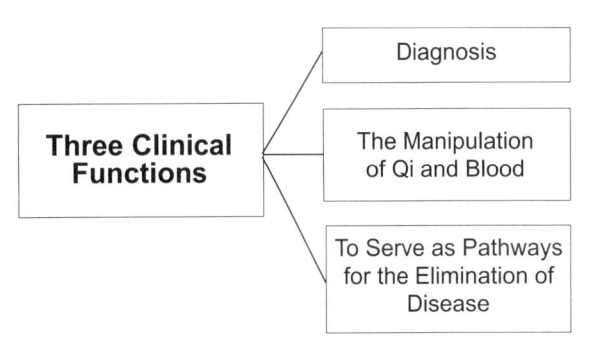

Figure 10.5. The Three Clinical Functions of Energetic Points

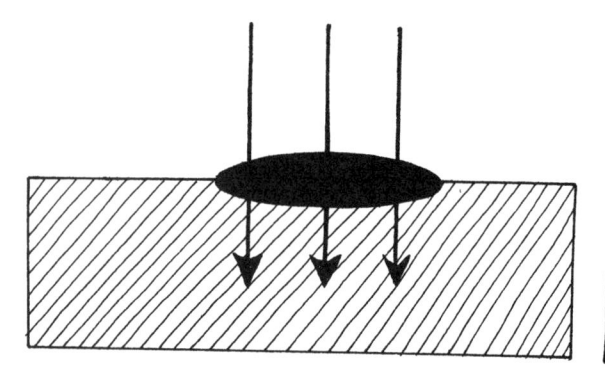

Figure 10.6. Weak or Deficient tissue will naturally pull and absorb Qi into the surrounding areas.

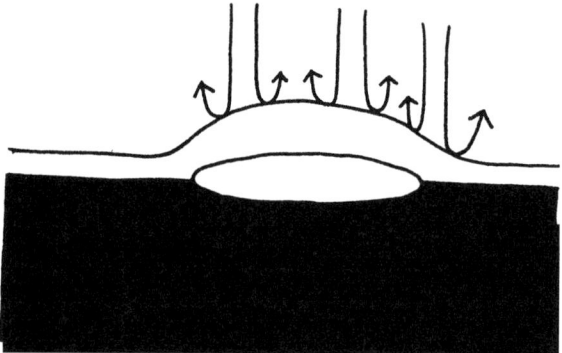

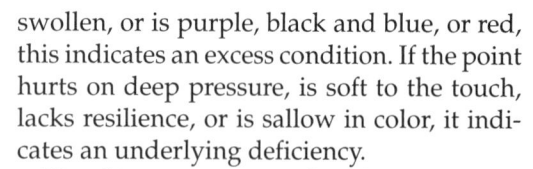

Figure 10.7. Strong, Excess, or Armored tissue will naturally repel Qi from the surrounding areas.

swollen, or is purple, black and blue, or red, this indicates an excess condition. If the point hurts on deep pressure, is soft to the touch, lacks resilience, or is sallow in color, it indicates an underlying deficiency.

The skin over points often feels sticky, in contrast to the slippery or smooth quality of the skin surrounding the point. When passing the fingers over a point, the doctor generally feels the energetic pulse of the channel. When touched, the point responds like an energetic echo, vibrating through the channel into the organ and then back again to the doctor's finger. The doctor can use this energetic response for diagnostic evaluation by sending a pulse into the organ itself along the flow of the channel (for those channels that flow inwards), or against it (for those channels that flow outwards). Once sufficient stimulation is applied to the point, its organ or region is "reminded" of its normal function. In this way, diagnosis and treatment are accomplished simultaneously.

Once the point and energy flow of the channel to be treated is diagnosed, the doctor must take into consideration that each patient will react differently according to the severity of the presenting symptoms, and the individual's basic constitutional type. Before beginning a treatment, the doctor should extend Qi into the point to the depth of the energetic space that exists between the Wei and Ying energy fields. Once contact is made, the doctor uses either the tips of his or her fingers or the palm of the hand like a barometer to detect if there is any soreness or distention at that particular point. This form of diagnosis determines the condition of the channel and the area needing treatment. Although the feelings and sensations will vary with each patient, correct diagnosis depends on recognizing energetic patterns that reveal the nature of the disharmony, for example:

- **Weak or deficient areas** will often feel like an empty hole or a deep well. Deficient Blood or Qi will actually pull energy into the deficient area and may feel something like a subtle vacuum suction (Figure 10.6). If the area attacks the doctor's Qi and begins to absorb it, the doctor should tonify that area immediately. This reaction is like that of a dry house plant that is starving for water. The minute the water touches the soil, the plant immediately absorbs it into its roots.
- **Strong or excess areas** will repel the doctor's Qi (Figure 10.7). If the diseased area repels the doctor's Qi, he or she must immediately dredge the excess energy from the tissues. First, the doctor should focus on the region surrounding the excess to drain the additional energy away from the damaged points. Once the excess is removed, the doctor then dredges the excess energy away from the original trauma area. This technique is excellent for treating damaged or sprained joints. When dredging, the doctor should focus on the

patient's breathing in order to maximize the efficacy of the treatment. As the patient inhales, the doctor exhales and vice-versa. As the patient exhales, he or she releases pathogenic factors; by inhaling when the patient exhales, the doctor facilitates this process, and prevents the depletion of his or her own Qi.

2. **Manipulate of Qi and Blood:** Qi and Blood can be manipulated through accessing the body's energetic points, in order to purge excess conditions, to tonify deficient conditions, or to regulate and balance internal harmony.

- **To Purge or disperse an Excess condition,** the Qigong doctor emits his or her Qi over a specific point (or points) and begins to purge, or disperse, the energy from the area. Purging involves the removal of toxins directly from the organ, whereas dispersing is to lead the toxins out of the tissue area via the channels. The goal of this treatment is to remove any excess, particularly stagnant Qi and Blood. A dull, moving pain is characteristic of Qi stagnation. If the blockage is primarily due to Blood stagnation, the patient will experience a sharper pain that does not move. This distinction, however, is more clinically significant in Chinese herbology than it is for Medical Qigong, acupuncture, or massage. It is stated in the Chinese medical classics that, "Qi is the commander of Blood," therefore, moving the Qi will also move stagnant Blood.

- **To Tonify a Deficient condition,** the Qigong doctor emits Qi over a specific point or points with the intention of tonifying or strengthening the patient's Qi, Blood, Yin, Yang, or specific organs and tissues. The Qigong doctor may use a variety of techniques according to the patient's needs. For example, in order to prevent discomfort, the doctor will tonify weak patients slowly by emitting Qi into his or her Kd-1 points and directing the Qi to flow up the Kidney Channels and fill the Lower Dantian, using the Sword Finger technique.

- **To Regulate,** the Qigong doctor emits Qi over a specific point or points and allows the body's natural homeostasis to take over and restore healthy function. This type of treatment may be used when a patient has a combined excess or deficiency syndrome (such as stagnant Qi in the chest due to Qi deficiency in the Lungs and Kidneys).

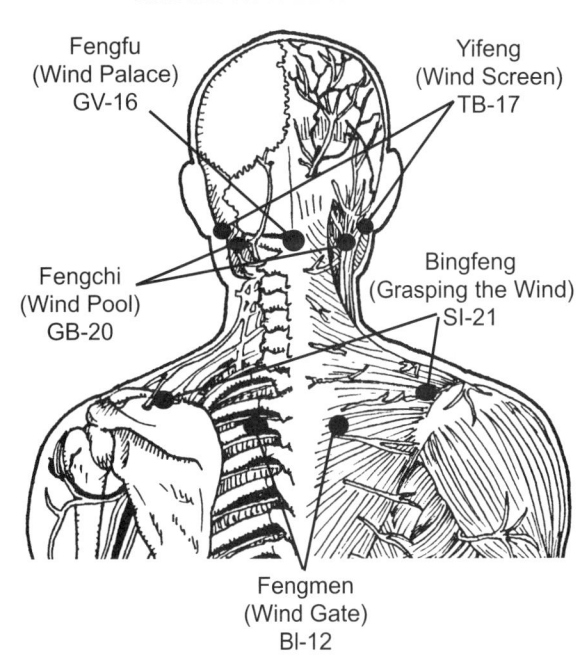

Figure 10.8. Points on the back of the neck that are especially vulnerable to external Wind invasion.

3. **Serve as Pathways for the Elimination of Disease:** Through the centrifugal and centripetal energetic flow of the energetic points, the Qigong doctor can effectively eliminate pathogens from the patient's tissues. Disease transmission may occur due to the invasion of external pathogenic Qi (Wind, Fire, Summer Heat, Damp, Dry and Cold). Some of the body's points are especially vulnerable to exogenous invasions, particularly the invasion of External Wind. Wind-susceptible points, for example, usually have the word Feng (Wind) in their names. Some examples of Wind susceptible points include (Figure 10.8): Bingfeng (Grasping the Wind) SI-12 , Fengchi (Wind Pool) GB-20, Fengmen (Wind Gate) Bl-12, Yifeng (Wind Screen) TB-17, and Fengfu (Wind Palace) GV-16. Due to their susceptibility to Wind penetration, these specific points may also be used to purge Wind inva-

sion, or used to release other types of toxic energy from the body.

CENTRIFUGAL AND CENTRIPETAL ENERGY FLOW

All of the body's points are capable of energetically spiraling in two opposite directions: centrifugally spiralling away from the body, or centripetally spiralling into the body. Each point's capacity to energetically spiral in either direction is independent of whether the primary flow of its associated channel is moving from the extremities into the center of the body, or moving away from the center of the body towards the extremities.

The energy of a channel normally flows in only one direction, while the polarity of the body's points normally alternates between Yang (centrifugal spirals) and Yin (centripetal spirals) movements. The polarity of these two energy currents are described as follows:

1. **The Point's Outward Centrifugal Flow of Qi:** Qi moves from the channel, to the point, to the external environment. This outward flow of energy is expressed or intensified during the exhalation. The outward centrifugal flow of energy manifests in points along the channel, or in other areas of the body where there are conditions of excess. These points have a positive polarity, and repel Qi from the surrounding tissue area.

2. **The Point's Inward Centripetal Flow of Qi:** Qi is drawn from the external environment, through the point, and into the channel. This inward flow of energy is expressed or intensified during the inhalation. The inward centripetal flow of energy manifests in points along the channel, or in other areas of the body where there are conditions of deficiency. These points have a negative polarity, pulling and absorbing Qi from the surrounding tissue area.

The stimulation of channel points has two important clinical results. Centrifugally, the stimulation of channel points informs the doctor of impending internal disorders by discharging excess energy. Centripetally, they transmit the energy and intention placed on them back to their source organ or tissue, absorbing energy to remedy and counteract the body's internal deficiencies.

POINT NAMES

Each point has a traditional name, which either describes its location, its energetic function, or both. In addition, modern acupuncture texts have assigned a name and a number for each point, according to the channel on which it is located and its order along the natural course of that channel.

Sometimes a point may have several different traditional names, varying according to whether they are being used by Medical Qigong doctors, acupuncturists, martial artists, or religious practitioners. For example, GV-1 is called Changqiang (Long Strength) in Traditional Chinese Medicine, and Weilu (Tail Gate) in Medical Qigong and Daoist inner alchemy.

The history of point naming and the different terminologies used can usually be traced back to different Buddhist and Daoist temples in ancient China. Each religious sect gave its own particular names to certain points, in accordance with the temple's spiritual and energetic needs. Giving different names to common points was used as a form of secret code to keep the system pure, and to prevent the knowledge from falling into the hands of the unscrupulous or uninitiated.

Sometimes the same name may refer to different points or areas on the body. For example, Yuzhen (Jade Pillow), located in the occipital region on the posterior base of the skull, is the name commonly used for UB-9 in Traditional Chinese Medicine. However, in medical Qigong and Daoist inner alchemy, Yuzhen instead refers to an entire area the size of one's fist placed between the bilateral UB-9 points.

CLASSIFICATION OF ENERGETIC POINTS

Points in similar locations (i.e., ankles and wrists) often have similar actions, thus many points are further classified into groups of similar energetic potential. This classification will assist the doctor of Traditional Chinese Medicine in choosing the right point or points to use in treatment. The following is a list of energetic point classifications.

Points	Yin Channel Elements (Ethereal Soul—Hun)	Yang Channel Elements (Corporeal Soul—Po)
Jing-Well Points	Wood	Metal
Ying-Spring Points	Fire	Water
Shu-Stream Points	Earth	Wood
Jing-River Points	Metal	Fire
He-Sea Points	Water	Earth

Figure 10.9. The Five Shu Points and their Correspondence to the Five Elements

THE FIVE SHU POINTS

Like the internal organs and channels, some points have a more powerful influence on the body than others. Each point has an action on the quality and quantity of energy of an organ. Along each of the Twelve Primary Channels lie five specific points below the elbow or the knee called Shu points (also called transporting points). These points belong to the oldest classification of points, and are described using water as a metaphor. Each section of the channel is compared to the course water takes as it emerges from the ground and makes its way to the ocean. In this system, points are identified as follows: Jing (Well), Ying (Spring), Shu (Stream), Jing (River), and He (Sea). These five points exist on each of the Twelve Primary Channels, and are located sequentially between the patients hands (or feet) and elbows (or knees). Flowing from distal to proximal, the point progression is as follows: Well, Spring, Stream, River, and Sea.

YIN AND YANG CHANNELS AND FIVE ELEMENTS

Each of the five Shu points also corresponds to one of the Five Elements, in the progression of the Creative Cycle. Each Yin channel begins with the Hun progression through the Five Elements, starting with Wood, then Fire, Earth, Metal, and Water. Each Yang channel begins with the Po progression through the Five Elements, starting with Metal, then Water, Wood, Fire, and Earth (Figure 10.9).

Similar to the eyes' relationship to Wood (Hun) and Metal (Po), the beginning points on the Twelve Primary Channels also have a relationship to either a Wood (Ethereal Soul) or Metal (Corporeal Soul). Hence, in meditation exercises, when specific finger tip points are connected, it facilitates a specific blending of the Hun and Po energies. The practice of connecting specific finger tip points is sometimes referred to as the connection (or fusion) of the body's Ethereal and Corporeal Souls.

The five Shu points energetically flow from superficial to deep and are susceptible to external pathogens and climatic changes. The distal points on the feet tend to be more powerful than those on the hands. After the manipulation of the patient's distal points, the local channel points are used according to their feeling of tenderness. The five Shu points, are described as follows (Figure 10.10 and 10.11):

1. **Jing-Well Points:** these are the first points along the extremities of the channels and are located at the tips of the fingers and toes. These pools of energy are where the channel is at its thinnest and most superficial.

   These are the points from which the energy of the channels leaves the body when moving outward centrifugally. At the end of the fingertips and toes, the channel's energetic polarity changes from Yin to Yang or vice versa. Due to this shift in polarity, the energy at the channel's extremities tends to be un-

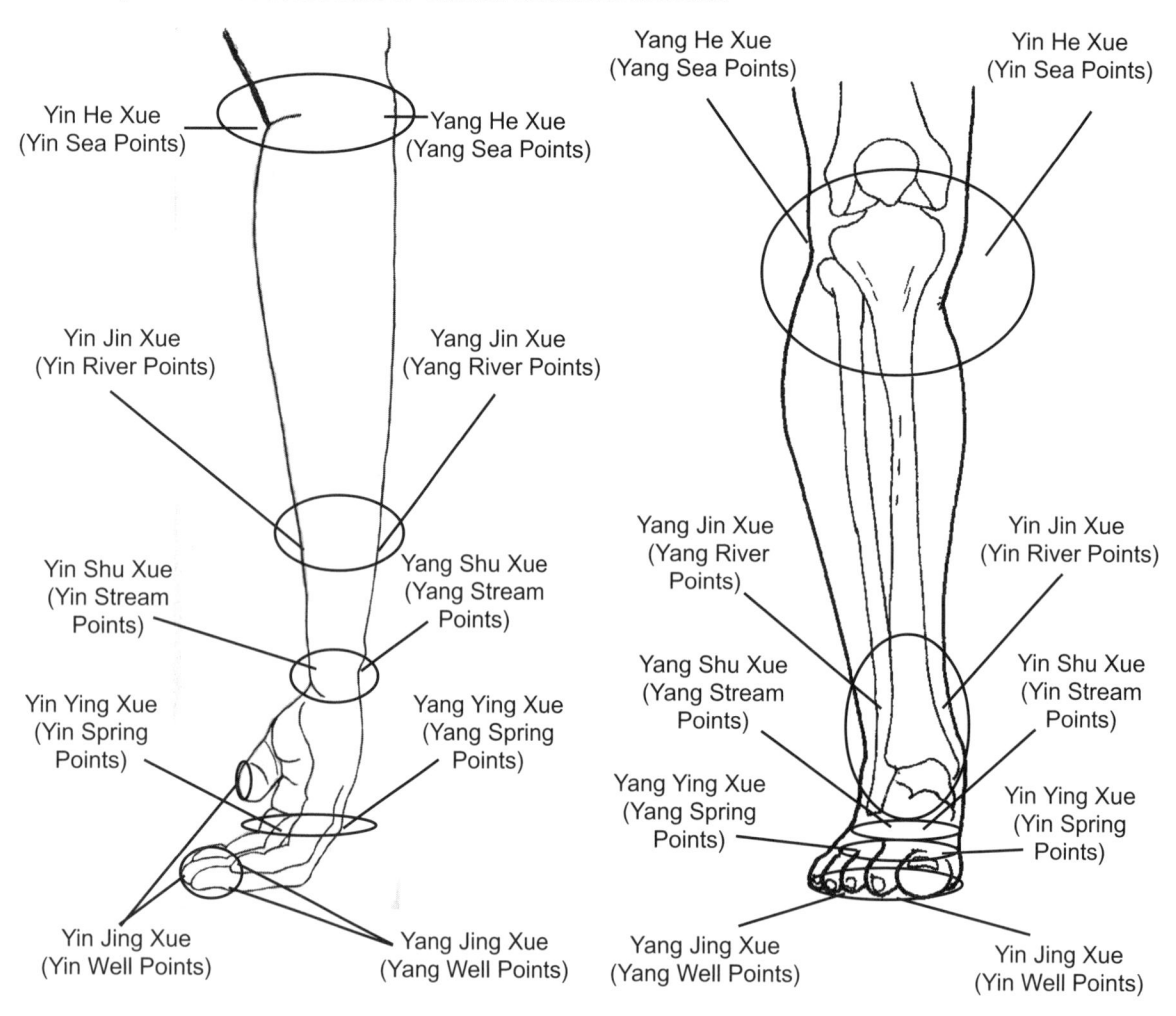

VOLUME 1, SECTION 1: FOUNDATIONS OF CHINESE ENERGETIC MEDICINE

Figure 10.10. The Five Shu Points and their Arm Channel Flow Correspondences

Figure 10.11. The Five Shu Points and their Leg Channel Flow Correspondences

stable, and is therefore more easily influenced.

Due to their outward movement of energy, the Well points can be used by the Qigong doctor to eliminate the patient's pathogenic factors quickly, especially when the Yin organs are affected. The Well points will also have a strong effect on the patient's mental state, and can be used to quickly change the patient's mood. These points are generally used for resolving acute disorders, expelling exogenous pathogens, and for relieving mental disorders. They are used as "revival" points for loss of consciousness due to fainting and heat stroke. They can also be used to treat convulsions, local neuropathy (tingling, numbness, burning pain), or a feeling of fullness below the Heart. In mental disorders, the Jing-Well points are commonly used for irritability, mental restlessness, anxiety, hysteria, mania, and insomnia.

2. **Ying-Spring Points:** these are the second set of points along the channels, and are located in the second position of the channels' energetic progression up the arms or legs just above the Well points. The Ying-Spring points are where the channel's energetic flow quick-

ens its progression of Qi into the body.

At the location of the Spring points, the Qi in the channels is very dynamic and powerful. The energy in these points can change quickly, slipping and gliding like the swirling movements of cascading water. The Spring points are generally used to eliminate both internal and external pathogenic factors (especially Heat) from the patient's body. They are also used when a disease effects a color change in the patient's complexion.

In the Yin channels, this point corresponds to the Fire Element. Purging the Spring point in the Yin channels reduces Heat and clears Fire. In the Yang channels, the Spring point is corresponds to the Water Element. The doctor can reduce Heat in the patient's Yang channels by tonifying this Water point.

3. **Shu-Stream Points:** these are the third set of points along the channels, and are located in the third position in the channels' energetic progression up the arms or legs, just above and next to the Spring point (except for the Gall Bladder Channel where it is located at the fourth point). The Shu-Stream points are where the channel's energy rapidly pours through and slightly deepens its flow into the body.

At the Shu-Stream points, the external pathogenic factors may penetrate deep into the channels and can then be "transported" into the body's interior. The Shu-Stream points are used to clear Wind and Dampness from the patient's channels, and are also used when a disease manifests intermittently.

4. **Jing-River Points:** these are the fourth set of the five transporting points; though they are not always located on the fourth point along the channel. The points are, however, always located between the wrist and elbow on the arms and between the ankle and knee on the legs. The Jing-River points are where the channels broaden, and the energy flow continues to increase.

At the Jing-River points, the energy current flows wider, deeper, and more irregularly, like a large river, directing the energy (or the invasion of external pathogenic factors) inwards towards the body's tendons, joints, and Bones. These points are generally used when there is stagnation of Qi and Blood in the patient's channels. They are also used for treating such symptoms as coughing, asthma, dyspnea, sore throat, and upper respiratory diseases.

5. **He-Sea Points:** these are the fifth set of points of the five transporting points and, in all cases, are located at the elbows and knees. These points are where the energy of the channels is vast and plunges deep into the body.

The Qi at the He-Sea points moves centripetally inward, flowing relatively slowly, while joining, collecting, and fusing with the general circulation of the body's energy the way a mighty river flows into the sea. The He-Sea points are generally used for all Stomach and intestinal diseases and for internal disorders of the organs.

THE FIVE ELEMENTAL POINTS

Each of the Five Element points corresponds to one of the five Shu points. The Five Elemental points are aligned in the progression of the Creative Cycle. Each Yin channel begins with the Hun progression through the Five Elements, starting with Wood, then Fire, Earth, Metal, and Water (Figure 10.12). Each Yang channel begins with the

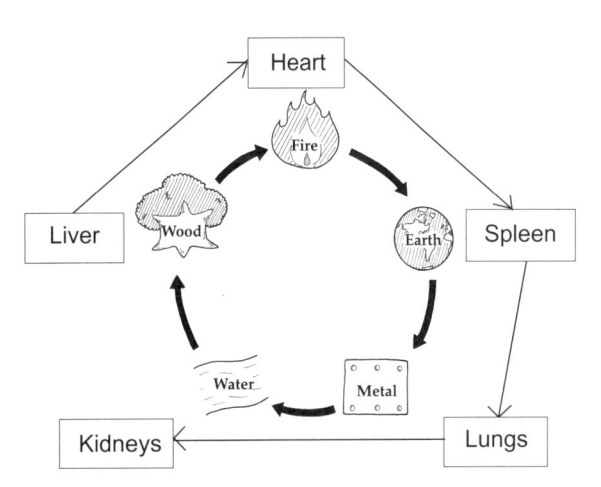

Figure 10.12. The Hun Progression of the Five Element Creative Cycle

Po progression through the Five Elements starting with Metal, then Water, Wood, Fire, and Earth (Figure 10.13).

THE SIXTEEN XI-CLEFT (ACCUMULATION) POINTS

The Sixteen Xi-Cleft points are where the Qi and Blood gather and plunge deeply into the body. They are used for purging acute conditions of excess in the channels and organs. There is one Xi-Cleft point on each of the Twelve Primary Channels, plus one point on each of the Yin and Yang Heel Vessels, and one point on each of the Yin and Yang Linking Vessels. The Yin Channel Accumulation points are Lu-6, Pc-4, Ht-6, Sp-8, Lv-6, Kd-5, Yin Heel Kd-8, and Yin Linking Kd-9. The Yang Channel Accumulation points are LI-7, TB-7, SI-6, St-34, GB-36, UB-63, Yang Heel UB-59, and Yang Linking GB-35.

THE TWELVE FRONT-MU (ALARM, COLLECTING) POINTS

The twelve Front-Mu points are located on the chest and abdomen. The energy of the internal organs collects at these points, and thus they can be used for both diagnosis and treatment. These points are palpated for diagnosis and may feel tender to the patient, either with light touch or with the application of pressure. If they respond to a light touch or feel tight or swollen, the patient has an excess condition. If the points respond to deep pressure, or feel hollow or deflated, the patient has a deficient condition. The Twelve Front Alarm points are: Lungs Lu-1, Pericardium CV-17, Liver Lv-14, Spleen Lv-13, Gall Bladder GB-24, Kidneys GB-25, Heart CV-14, Stomach CV-12, Large Intestine St-25, Triple Burners CV-5, Small Intestine CV-4, and Urinary Bladder CV-3.

THE EIGHTEEN BACK-SHU (ASSOCIATED, TRANSPORTING) POINTS

The eighteen Back-Shu points are all located on the back along the Urinary Bladder Channel. They correspond to the twelve Zang Fu organs and are used both for diagnosis and for treatment. These points transport Qi very effectively and directly to the internal organs. They can also be used for treating disorders of the corresponding sense organs. The Eighteen Back Transporting points

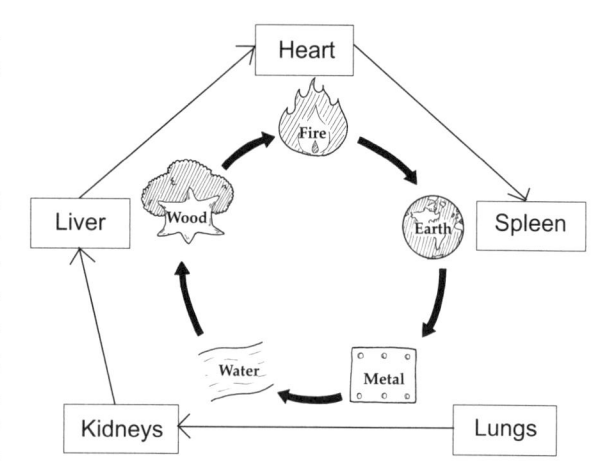

Figure 10.13. The Po Progression of the Five Element Creative Cycle

are: Lungs UB-13, Pericardium UB-14, Heart UB-15, Governing Vessel UB-16, Diaphragm UB-17, Liver UB-18, Gall Bladder UB-19, Spleen UB-20, Stomach UB-21, Triple Burners UB-22, Kidneys UB-23, Sea of Qi UB-24, Large Intestine UB-25, Gate to the Yuan Qi (Guan Yuan) UB-26, Small Intestine UB-27, Urinary Bladder UB-28, Sacrum UB-29, and Anus UB-30.

THE FIFTEEN LUO (CONNECTING, COLLATERAL) POINTS

The Fifteen Luo points are used in treating channel pathologies. There is a Luo-Connecting point located on each of the Twelve Primary Channels, as well as on the Governing and Conception Vessels. The Fifteenth Luo point is clinically known as the Great Luo point of the Spleen. The Fifteen Connecting points are divided into Yin and Yang channel points. Yin Channel points include: Lu-7, Pc-6, Ht-5, Sp-4, Lv-5, Kd-4, CV-15, and the Great Luo Channel Sp-21. The Yang Channel points include LI-6, TB-5, SI-7, St-40, GB-37, UB-58, and GV-1.

THE TWELVE ENTRY POINTS

The Twelve Entry points are where each Primary Channel connects with and receives energy from the channel immediately proceeding it in the 24 hour Blood-Heat cycle. The Entry point is the first point on each channel in all cases except for the Large Intestine Channel, which is LI-4. The Yin Channel Entry points include: Lu-1, Pc-1, Ht-1, Sp-

1, Lv-1, and Kd-1. The Yang Channel Entry points include: LI-4, TB-1, SI-1, St-1, GB-1, and UB-1.

THE TWELVE EXIT POINTS

The Twelve Exit points are where the energy of each primary channel exits to connect with the channel immediately following it in the 24 hour Blood-Heat cycle. The Yin Channel Exit points include: Lu-7, Pc-8, Ht-9, Sp-21, Lv-14, and Kd-22. The Yang Channel Exit points include: LI-20, TB-23, SI-19, St-42, GB-41, and UB-67.

THE EIGHT INFLUENTIAL POINTS

The Eight Influential points have specific effects on their respective organs, substances, and tissues. They affect the body's Qi, Blood, sinews, Blood Vessels, Bones, and Marrow, as well as the Yin and Yang organs. The Eight Influential points and their respective influences are listed as follows: Lv-13 Yin Organs; CV-12 Yang Organs; CV-17 Qi; UB-17 Blood; GB-34 Sinews; Lu-9 Blood Vessels; UB-11 Bones; and GB-39 Marrow.

THE EIGHT CONFLUENT POINTS

The Eight Confluent points communicate with the Eight Extraordinary Vessels. The Confluent points are divided into Master points and Coupled points. The Master point is the primary point chosen for treatment, and its Coupled point is the connecting or secondary point that is used in conjunction with the Master point to open the specific Vessel. Each of the Eight Extraordinary Vessels has both a Master and Coupled Confluent point on the upper or lower limbs.

All of the Eight Extraordinary Vessels can be treated in various combinations according to their specific Master and Coupled point locations. If, for example, the Qigong doctor causes Qi to flow from the patient's Master point on the hand (SI-3) to its Coupled point (UB-62) on the foot, the Governing Vessel will open. To complete the treatment, the doctor must first remove stimulation from the Coupled point then disconnect from the Master point (Figures 10.14 and 10.15).

The Eight Confluent points are as follows: Governing Vessel SI-3, Conception Vessel Lu-7, Belt Vessel GB-41, Thrusting Vessels Sp-4, Yang Heel Vessel UB-62, Yin Heel Vessel Kd-6, Yang Linking Vessel TB-5, and Yin Linking Vessel Pc-6.

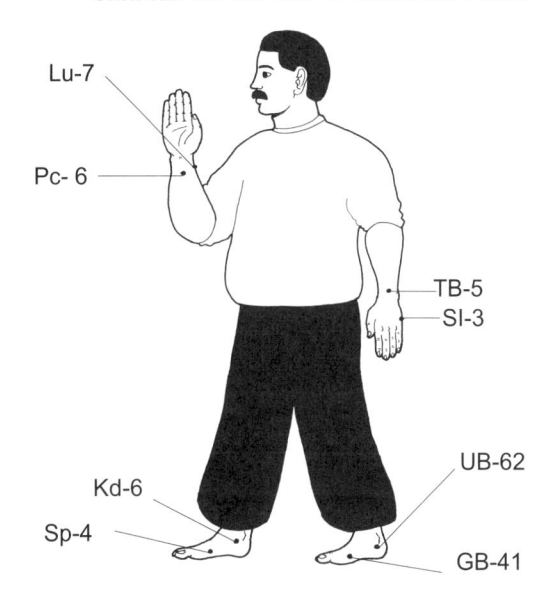

Figure 10.14. Locations of the Body's Master and Couple Points

Channel	Open with Master Point	Complete with Couple Point
Governing	Hand (SI-3)	Foot (UB-62)
Conception	Hand (Lu-7)	Foot (Kd-6)
Thrusting	Foot (Sp-4)	Hand (Pc-6)
Belt	Foot (GB-41)	Hand (TB-5)
Yin Linking	Hand (Pc-6)	Foot (Sp-4)
Yang Linking	Hand (TB-5)	Foot (GB-41)
Yin Heel	Foot (Kd-6)	Hand (Lu-7)
Yang Heel	Foot (UB-62)	Hand (SI-3)

Figure 10.15. The Vessels with their Associated Master Points and Couple Points

THE TWELVE YUAN-SOURCE POINTS

Each of the Twelve Primary Channels has a Yuan-Source point, where the body's Original Qi surfaces and pools. On the Yin channels, the Yuan-Source points are always the Shu-Stream points. On the Yang channels, however, the Yuan-Source points are separate points located between the Shu-Stream and the Jing-River points. These points are usually the fourth point from the distal end of the channel, except in the case of the Gall Bladder Channel where the Yuan-Source point is the fifth point.

The Yuan Qi originates and resides in the Lower Dantian area, and it is dispersed to the Yin and Yang organs and then to the limbs by the action of the Triple Burners.

The Yuan-Source points can be used for clinical diagnosis of the Yin organs. For this, the Qigong doctor examines the points by both palpation and visual diagnosis. The Yuan-Source points are the primary points on the Yin channels for tonifying and regulating their respective Yin organs.

The Yuan-Source points of the Yang channels have different energetic functions and clinical applications than do the Yin channels' Source points. These points generally have a small tonifying effect on their related Yang organs and comparatively little Qi regulating effect. Their main functions are to expel various pathogenic factors, and to treat disorders along their channel pathways. The Twelve Yuan points are as follows: Gall Bladder GB-40, Liver Lv-3, Lungs Lu-9, Large Intestine LI-4, Stomach St-42, Spleen Sp-3, Heart Ht-7, Small Intestine SI-4, Bladder UB-64, Pericardium Pc-7, and Triple Burners TB-4.

THE POINTS OF THE FOUR SEAS

In Chinese Medicine, the human body is seen to have four seas: the Sea of Qi, Sea of Blood, Sea of Marrow, and the Sea of Nourishment (literally Water and Grain). The Qigong doctor can access these seas by stimulating the following points:

1. **The points used for accessing the Sea of Qi:** These points include UB-10, St-9, CV-17, GV-14 and GV-15. Excess in the Sea of Qi manifests in symptoms such as fullness in the chest, flushed complexion, and dyspnea. Deficiency in the Sea of Qi manifests in symptoms such as fatigue, low energy, or an inability to speak.

2. **The points used for accessing the Sea of Blood:** These points include UB-11, St-37, and St-39. Excess in the Sea of Blood manifests in symptoms such as: anxiety, uneasiness, unrest, and a feeling of the body being too big. Deficiency in the Sea of Blood manifests in symptoms such a feeling that the body is too small for no apparent reason.

3. **The points used for accessing the Sea of Marrow:** These points include GV-15, GV-16, GV-17, and GV-20. Excess in the Sea of Marrow manifests in symptoms such as: sensations relating to that of excess energy (lightness, feelings of strength and vitality). Deficiency in the Sea of Marrow manifests in symptoms such as: fatigue, vertigo, dizziness, tinnitus, pain in the lower legs, impaired vision, and a desire to sleep.

4. **The points used for accessing the Sea of Nourishment:** These points include St-30 and St-36. Excess in the Sea of Nourishment manifests in symptoms such as abdominal distention. Deficiency in the Sea of Nourishment manifests in symptoms such as hunger with an inability to eat.

UPPER (UNITING) HE-SEA POINTS

There are three points on the upper arm that have a particularly powerful effect on certain Yang organs. The affected organs and their points include the Stomach LI-10, Large Intestine LI-9, and the Small Intestine LI-8.

LOWER (UNITING) HE-SEA POINTS

Each of the Yang organs has a uniting He-Sea point on the leg, which can be used to treat Yang organ problems. The three Yang channels of the feet also correspond to the three Yang channels of the hands. The Lower Six He-Sea points are as follows: Stomach St-36, Large Intestine St-37, Small Intestine St-39, Triple Burners UB-39, Urinary Bladder UB-40, and Gall Bladder GB-34.

THE THIRTEEN GHOST POINTS

In ancient times, the Thirteen Ghost points were used in the treatment of spirit possession, mania disorders, and epilepsy, as these points have a particularly strong effect on the patient's overall mental, emotional and spiritual balance.

CHAPTER 10: THE BODY'S ENERGETIC POINTS

Category	Points	Description
Five Shu Points	Jing-Well, Ying-Spring, Shu-Stream, Jing-River, He-Sea	Transporting and Command Points
Sixteen Xi Cleft Points	Yin: Lu-6, Pc-4: Ht-6, Sp-8, Lv-6, Kd-5, Yin Heel Kd-8, and Yin Linking Kd-9 Yang: LI-7, TB-7, SI-6, St-34, GB-36, UB-63, Yang Heel UB-59 and Yang Linking GB-35	Accumulation Points
Twelve Front Mu Points	Lungs Lu-1, Pericardium CV-17, Liver Lv-14, Spleen Lv-13, Gall Bladder GB-24, Kidneys GB-25, Heart CV-14, Stomach CV-12, Large Intestine St-25, Triple Burners CV-5, Small Intestine CV-4, and Urinary Bladder CV-3	Alarm, Collecting Points
Eighteen Back Shu Points	Lungs UB-13, Pericardium UB-14, Heart UB-15, Governing Vessel UB-16, Diaphragm UB-17, Liver UB-18, Gall Bladder UB-19, Spleen UB-20, Stomach UB-21, Triple Burners UB-22, Kidney UB-23, Sea of Qi UB-24, Large Intestine UB-25, Gate to the Original Qi (Guan Yuan) UB-26, Small Intestine UB-27, Urinary Bladder UB-28, Sacrum UB-29 and Anus UB-30	Associated, Transporting Points
Fifteen Luo Points	Yin: Lu-7, Pc-6, Ht-5, Sp-4, Lv-5, Kd-4, CV-15, the Great Luo Channel Sp-21 Yang: LI-6, TB-5, SI-7, St-40, GB-37, UB-58 and GV-1	Connecting Points
Twelve Entry Points	The first point on each channel except for the Large Intestine Channel in which it is LI-4	Qi enters Channel
Twelve Exit Points	Yin: Lu-7, P-8, Ht-9, Sp-21, Lv-14 and Kd-22 Yang: LI-20, TB-23, SI-19, St-42, GB-41 and UB-67	Qi exits Channel
Eight Influential Points	Yin Organs Lv-13, Yang Organs CV-12, Qi CV-17, Blood UB-17, Sinews GB-34, Blood Vessels Lu-9, Bones UB-11 and Marrow GB-39	Influence Internal Organ Function
Eight Confluent Points	Governing Vessel SI-3, Conception Vessel Lu-7, Belt Vessel GB-41, Thrusting Vessels Sp-4, Yang Heel Vessels UB-62, Yin Heel Vessels Kd-6, Yang Linking Vessels TB-5 and Yin Linking Vessels Pc-6	Master and Couple Points
Twelve Yuan-Source Points	Gall Bladder GB-40, Liver Lv-3, Lungs Lu-9, Large Intestine LI-4, Stomach St-42, Spleen- Sp-3, Heart Ht-7, Small Intestine SI-4, Urinary Bladder UB-64, Pericardium Pc-7, and Triple Burners TB-4	Source of Original Qi Points
Four Seas Points	Sea of Qi Points: UB-10, St-9, CV-17, GV-14 and 15 Sea of Blood Points: UB-11, St-37 and 39 Sea of Marrow Points: GV-15, GV-16, GV-17, and GV-20 Sea of Nourishment Points: St-30 and St-36	Give Access to the Four Seas
Upper He-Sea Points	Stomach LI-10, Large Intestine LI-9 and the Small Intestine LI-8	Affect the Yang Organs
Lower He-Sea Points	Stomach St-36, Large Intestine St-37, Small Intestine St-39, Triple Burners UB-39, Urinary Bladder UB-40, and Gall Bladder GB-34	Affect the Yang Organs
Thirteen Ghost Points	GV-26, Lu-11, Sp-1, Pc-7, UB-62, GV-16, St-6, CV-24, Pc-8, GV-23, LI-11, CV-1, and She Xia Feng	Affect the Mind, Emotion, and Spirit
Ten Windows of Heaven Points	Lung 3, Large Intestine 18, Triple Burners 16, Urinary Bladder 10, Stomach 9, Conception Vessel 22, Governing Vessel 16, Small Intestine 16, Small Intestine 17, and Pericardium 1	Affect the Mind, Emotion, and Spirit

Figure 10.16. Point Chart

These specific points were formulated by Sun Simiao during the 7th century and listed in the *Thousand Ducat Formulas*. In Traditional Chinese Medical clinics today, these points are commonly used to treat emotional disorders. The Thirteen Ghost points are as follows: GV-26, Lu-11, Sp-1, Pc-7, UB-62, GV-16, St-6, CV-24, Pc-8, GV-23, CV-1, LI-11 and She Xia Feng (two extra points located under the tongue).

THE TEN WINDOW OF HEAVEN POINTS

The Window of Heaven Points are ten points that have a specific effects on the mind's psychological functions, and thus are also commonly used to treat emotional disorders. The Ten Window of Heaven points are as follows: Lu-3, LI-18, TB-16, UB-10, St-9, CV-22, GV-16, SI-16, SI-17, and Pc-1.

SUMMARY OF POINTS

Understanding the origin and function of the body's energetic points, as well as the Qi flow along the energetic channels, allows the Qigong doctor to emit energy through these energetic cavities in order to easily and directly access the tissues and internal organs of the patients body. This understanding also enables the Qigong doctor to purge the toxic or pathogenic Qi (which has become stagnant or detrimentally active within the patient's body) away from the diseased organs, through specific channels, and out the body.

The preceding chart (Figure 10.16) is a basic categorization of the body's points and their descriptions.

Appendix 1
Chronology of Chinese Dynasties

Introduction

The following Appendix has been added in order to assist the reader in comprehending the chronology of the Chinese Dynasties. It is important to note that the years of the dynasties were not always the same in all regions of China. Some dynasties overlap in time and there were also various periods of political upheaval where no specific emperor or ruling family was in control.

China's Pre-Dynasty Myths

The Reign of Fu Xi:
Emperor of the East:
founder of home and family

The Reign of Shen Nong:
Emperor of the South:
founder of farming and fertility

The Reign of Huangdi:
Emperor of the Center:
founder of silk weaving and medicine

The Reign of Shaohao:
Emperor of the West:
founder of burial and afterlife rites

The Reign of Zhuanxu
Emperor of the North:
founder of martial arts and exorcism

The Three Rulers Period

The Reign of Yao:
Heaven appointed ruler because of human virtue

The Reign of Shun:
Appointed Yao's successor because of virtue

The Reign of Yu the Great:
Controlled the floods, Xia Dynasty begins

Dynasties of China

Xia Dynasty:	2205 - 1600 B.C.
Shang Dynasty:	1600 - 1028 B.C.
Zhou Dynasty:	1028 - 221 B.C.
Western Zhou Dynasty:	1028 - 771 B.C.
Eastern Zhou Dynasty:	1028 - 221 B.C.
Spring and Autumn Period	770 - 476 B.C.
Warring States Period	475 - 221 B.C.
Qin Dynasty:	**221 - 206 B.C.**
Han Dynasty:	**206 B.C. - 220 A.D.**
Western Han Dynasty:	206 B.C. - 8 A.D.
Xin Dynasty:	9 A.D. - 24 A.D.
Eastern Han Dynasty:	25 - 220 A.D.
Three Kingdoms Period:	**220 - 280 A.D.**
Wei Dynasty:	220 - 265 A.D.
Shu Dynasty:	221 - 263 A.D.
Wu Dynasty:	222 - 280 A.D.
Jin Dynasty:	**265 - 420 A.D.**
Western Jin Dynasty:	265 - 316 A.D.
Eastern Jin Dynasty:	317 - 420 A.D.
Northern Dynasties Period:	**386 - 588 A.D.**
Northern Wei Dynasty:	386 - 533 A.D.
Eastern Wei Dynasty:	534 - 549 A.D.
Western Wei Dynasty:	535 - 557 A.D.
Northern Qi Dynasty:	550 - 577 A.D.
Northern Zhou Dynasty:	557 - 588 A.D.
Southern Dynasties Period:	**420 - 588 A.D.**
Song Dynasty:	420 - 478 A.D.
Qi Dynasty:	479 - 501 A.D.
Liang Dynasty:	502 - 556 A.D.
Chen Dynasty:	557 - 588 A.D.
Sui Dynasty:	**581 - 618 A.D.**
Tang Dynasty:	**618 - 907 A.D.**
Five Dynasties Period:	**907 - 960 A.D.**
Later Liang Dynasty:	907 - 923 A.D.
Later Tang Dynasty:	923 - 936 A.D.
Later Jin Dynasty:	936 - 946 A.D.
Later Han Dynasty:	947 - 950 A.D.
Later Zhou Dynasty:	951 - 960 A.D.

VOLUME 1: APPENDIX # 1

TEN KINGDOMS PERIOD:	**907- 979 A.D.**
SONG DYNASTY:	**960 - 1279 A.D.**
Northern Song Dynasty:	960 - 1127 A.D.
Southern Song Dynasty:	1127 - 1279 A.D.
LIAO DYNASTY:	**907 -1125 A.D.**
WESTERN XIA DYNASTY:	**1032 -1227 A.D.**
JIN DYNASTY:	**1115 -1234 A.D.**
YUAN (MONGOL) DYNASTY:	**1279 -1368 A.D.**
MING DYNASTY:	**1368 -1644 A.D.**
QING (MANCHU) DYNASTY:	**1644 -1911 A.D.**
THE REPUBLIC OF CHINA (MAINLAND):	**1912 -1949 A.D.**
THE REPUBLIC OF CHINA (TAIWAN):	**1949 - PRESENT**
PEOPLE'S REPUBLIC OF CHINA:	**1949 - PRESENT**

Appendix 2
Medical Qigong Instruction

Introduction

Due to the overwhelmingly positive response to the academic standards and clinical qualifications established by the International Institute of Medical Qigong (I.I.M.Q.), the following appendix includes information on the current Medical Qigong programs offered by several U.S. colleges of Traditional Chinese Medicine.

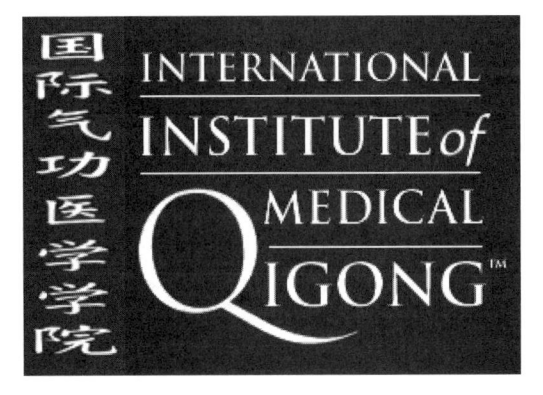

Founded by Dr. Jerry Alan Johnson in 1985, and currently overseeing branches in 10 countries and 23 states, the International Institute of Medical Qigong is known for maintaining the highest standards in Medical Qigong instruction and therapy. Because of the consistent high standards, in March of 2005 the Chinese Ministry of Health honored Professor Johnson and the International Institute of Medical Qigong as exceeding the Chinese academic and clinical standards for Chinese medical instruction and practice.

At the International Institute of Medical Qigong, it is our policy that all our Medical Qigong programs maintain the same teaching standards, syllabi, and clinical hours for certification. Therefore, prospective students may feel confident in attending the specific college or institute of their choice, knowing that each Medical Qigong educational facility will teach and maintain the same clinical format and strict standards as established by the International Institute of Medical Qigong.

Medical Qigong Classes

Classes entail two to six year programs in Medical Qigong therapy plus clinical internship. Programs include classes, labs, and seminars on Traditional Chinese Medical theory, the foundations of Chinese medicine for internal diseases according to the *Yellow Emperor's Inner Canon: Spiritual Pivot, Essential Questions,* and the *Canon of Perplexities.*

Classes also include energetic anatomy and physiology, diagnosis and symptomatology, energetic psychology, Qigong pathology and Medical Qigong therapy, as well as a survey of other related medical modalities. Other related modalities include: a basic understanding of herbal medicine, acupuncture therapy, and Chinese massage. Classes in Western anatomy and physiology, Western internal diseases, and health and recovery are also required

The certification programs offered by the I.I.M.Q. are based upon the curriculum that was originally established by the Medical Qigong College at the Hai Dian University, and implemented at the Xi Yuan Medical Qigong Hospital in Beijing, China.

Medical Qigong in T.C.M. Colleges

In the Spring of 1999, Professor Johnson accepted the position of Dean of Medical Qigong Science from the Five Branches Institute, College and Clinic of Traditional Chinese Medicine, in Santa Cruz, California. The Five Branches T.C.M. curriculum consists of a two year - 200 hour Medical Qigong Practitioner (M.Q.P.) certification program, and an ongoing Medical Qigong clinic.

In May of 2003, Professor Johnson accepted the position of Dean of Medical Qigong Science from The Academy For Five Element Acupuncture, in Hallandale, Florida. There are three programs offered at the Academy For Five Element Acupuncture. They include: A 200 hour Medical Qigong Practitioner (M.Q.P.) certification program; A 500 hour Medical Qigong Therapist (M.Q.T.) certification program; and an ongoing Medical Qigong clinic.

In January of 2005, Dr. Suzanne Friedman, L.Ac., D.M.Q. (China), one of Professor Johnson's senior students instituted a 200 hour Medical Qigong Practitioner (M.Q.P.) certification program and ongoing Medical Qigong Clinic at the Acupuncture and Integrative Medicine College, in Berkeley, California.

In August 2005, the He Nan University of Traditional Chinese Medicine, in Zheng Zhou China appointed Professor Jerry Alan Johnson as the Overseas Director of Medical Qigong. At that time the university invited Professor Johnson to join the facility as an Honorary Professor of Medical Qigong, and he was issued an official government seal authorizing his post as Overseas Director. Professor Johnson is the official representative of the He Nan University of Traditional Chinese Medicine for the United States.

Additionally, the He Nan University has recognized the International Institute of Medical Qigong (I.I.M.Q.) as a "sister school" of the university, and has adopted the I.I.M.Q.'s curriculum and the text authored by Professor Johnson titled, *Chinese Medical Qigong Therapy: A Comprehensive Clinical Text*.

The International Institute of Medical Qigong certificate programs are described as follows:

TWO YEAR - 200 HOUR MEDICAL QIGONG PRACTITIONER (M.Q.P.) COURSE

There are no prerequisites for this primary level certification. A 200 hour Medical Qigong Practitioner (M.Q.P.) certificate will be issued to students who have successfully completed Courses 1 through 4 (128 academic hours) in addition to 72 hours of clinical internship.

The final will include written, oral, and practical examinations plus clinical competencies. Successful completion of the examinations will enable the student to qualify for the more advanced 500-hour Medical Qigong Therapist (M.Q.T.) program.

INTRODUCTION TO MEDICAL QIGONG THERAPY: P1 (2-UNITS: 32 HRS.)

This first course is designed to introduce the student to Medical Qigong exercises to maintain health, heal their bodies, calm their minds, and reconnect with their spirit.

Medical Qigong exercises will also be taught that help the body correct any physical or energetic imbalances. These exercises strengthen and regulate the internal organs, nervous system and immune system, relieves pain, regulate hormones, and help release deep-seated emotions.

The course will introduce the student to the basic theories used in the energetic tonification, purgation, and regulation of the body's organ and channel systems. Other topics covered in this course include:
- Respiration, posture, and mental training
- Emotional detoxification
- Healing sound therapy
- Analyzing and categorizing Qigong exercises
- Introduction to Medical Qigong prescriptions
- Establish a personal Medical Qigong workout

Objective: Students will develop a basic understanding of the three regulations of Medical Qigong and be able to properly formulate a safe and productive Medical Qigong routine.

INTRODUCTION TO DIAGNOSIS AND TREATMENTS: P2 (2-UNITS: 32 HRS.)

This second course is designed to introduce the student to advance theories of energy purgation, tonification, regulation and cultivation. Techniques used to avoid absorbing Toxic Qi while in a clinical environment will be discussed, in addition to strengthening the body's protective energy field (Wei Qi).

Students are led through a progressive series of Shen Gong (Spirit Skill) meditations and exercises used to develop advanced intuitive diagnostic skills. Additionally, students will be introduced to the Medical Qigong treatment protocols used for treating patients. Other topics covered in this course will include:
- Developing Energetic Sensitivity and Perception Skills
- Energetic Projection Skills
- Advanced emotional detoxification therapy

The International Institute of Medical Qigong in Pacific Grove, CA.

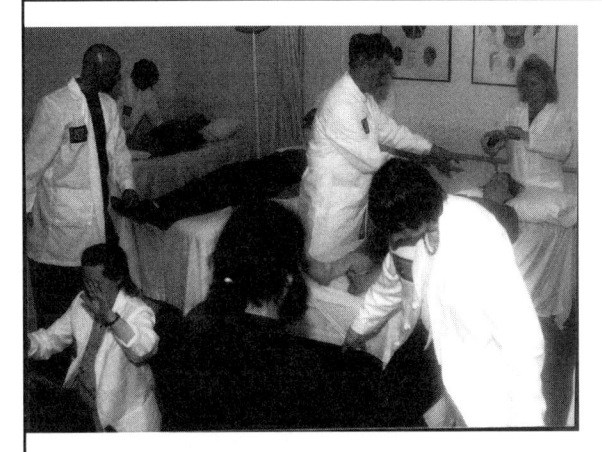

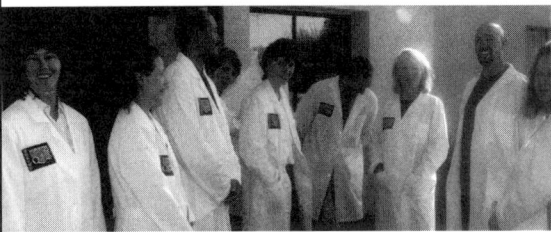

Right: The International Institute of Medical Qigong was founded by Professor Jerry Alan Johnson, Ph.D., D.T.C.M., D.M.Q. (China), in 1985.

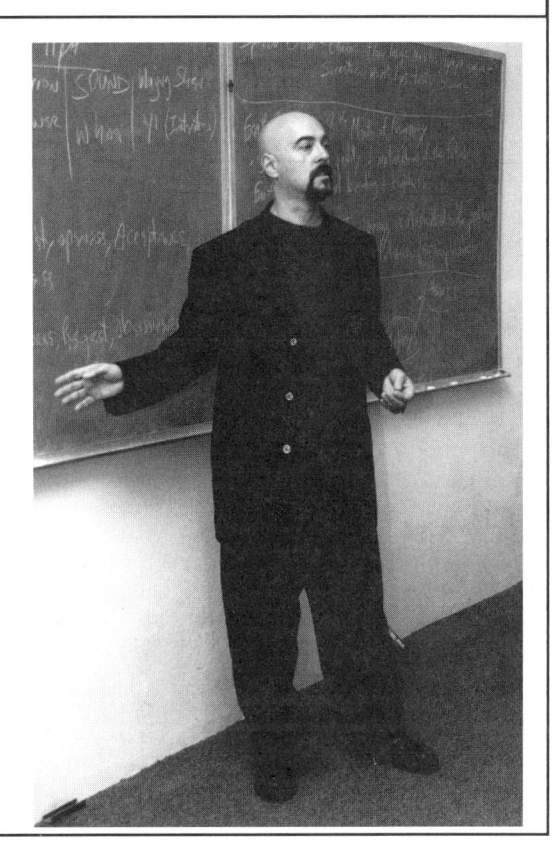

- Yi-Quan meditation exercises to develop focused intention of mind and energy
- Introduction to clinical energetic diagnostic techniques
- Introduction to prescriptions and clinical treatments

Objective: Students will develop energetic diagnostic and projection skills with a focus on Medical Qigong therapy and Traditional Chinese Medicine. Emphasis will be placed on the practical clinical applications of Medical Qigong therapy.

Clinical Foundations of Medical Qigong Therapy: P3 (2-units: 32 hrs.)

This third course is designed to offer the student an overview of the major principles and foundational structures that govern Chinese Medical Qigong therapy. Other topics covered include:

- Three levels of Ancient Daoist Mysticism
- Four Functional Properties of Energy
- Materializing and Dematerializing Energy
- Establishing a Medical Qigong Clinic
- Combining Medical Qigong with Other Healing Modalities
- Qi Emitting Methods (including Invisible Needle, Energetic Point Therapy, etc.)
- Internal Organ Prescriptions and Healing Sound Therapy

Objective: Students will develop a deeper comprehension of the body's energetic matrix as it pertains to Traditional Chinese Medicine, Disease, Diagnosis, and the Medical Qigong Clinic. The focus will be placed on integrating clinical Qigong modalities, advanced assessment, energetic modulation skills, case studies, and clinical exercises.

THE INTERNATIONAL INSTITUTE OF MEDICAL QIGONG IN PACIFIC GROVE, CA.

MASTER OF MEDICAL QIGONG GRADUATING CLASSES

The 1997 M.M.Q. Graduating Class of the International Institute of Medical Qigong

Shannon K. Brown, M.M.Q.
Anne Elderfield, M.M.Q.
Pamela Lee Espinoza, N.C.T.M.B., M.M.Q.
Carole Marie Kelly, Ed.D., M.M.Q.
Dr. Seth Lefkowitz, D.C., M.M.Q.
Shifu Arnold E. Tayam, C.M.T., M.M.Q.
Dr. Stephanie Taylor, M.D., Ph.D., M.M.Q.

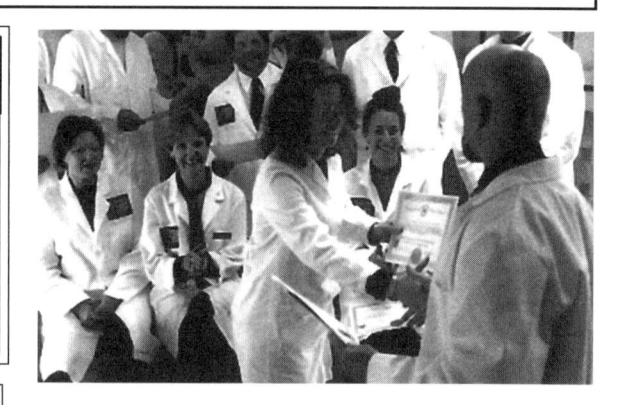

Graduation time at the
International Institute of Medical Qigong

The 1999 M.M.Q. Graduating Class of the International Institute of Medical Qigong

William H. De Groat, M.M.Q.
Diane De Terra, Ph.D., M.M.Q.
Dennis M. Earnest, M.M.Q.
Brooks M. Fiske, C.P.A., M.M.Q.
Michael J. Finch, M.M.Q.
Madeleine H. Howell, M.F.T., M.M.Q.
William H. Lewington, B.Sc., P.H.M., L.Ac., M.M.Q.
Paul E. Miller, M.M.Q.
Katy Reed, M.M.Q.
Shifu Matthew B. Weston, M.M.Q.
Jean R. Vlamynck, L.Ac., Dipl.Ac., M.T.C.M., M.M.Q.

The 2000 M.M.Q. Graduating Class of the International Institute of Medical Qigong

Adam Atman, L.Ac., Dipl.Ac., M.T.C.M., M.M.Q.
Louis Frizzell, C.P.A., M.M.Q.
Shifu Todd Mathew Gedryn, M.M.Q.
Geoffrey Greenspahn, M.M.Q.
Layth Hakim, M.M.Q.
Luc Arnauld Logan, M.M.Q.
Maria Pepe, L.Ac., Dipl.Ac., M.T.C.M., M.M.Q.
Rose Mary Stewart, M.M.Q.
Dr. Amos Ziv, L.Ac., Dipl.Ac., M.T.C.M., M.M.Q.

After a full day at the clinic, some of the Medical Qigong Doctors (China) and Internists relax and share encouraging experiences with each other.

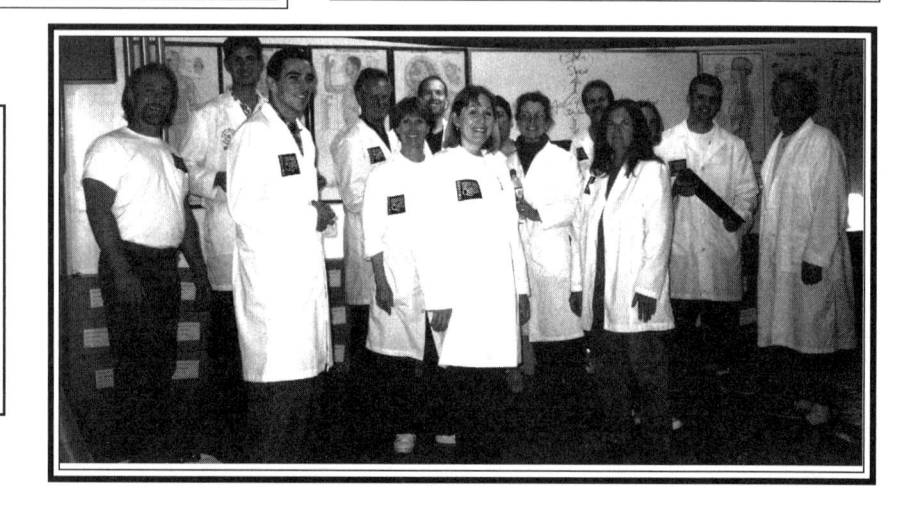

The 2001 M.M.Q. Graduating Class of the International Institute of Medical Qigong

Sue Angulo, M.M.Q.
Eddie L. Bates, M.M.Q.
Robert B. Bates, D.C., M.M.Q.
Robert C. Bawol, M.A., N.M.S.U., M.A., M.M.Q.
Shifu Reginald Cann, B.Sc., O.B.T., H.H.P., M.T.O.M., L.Ac., Dipl.Ac., M.M.Q.
Janette L. Carver, C.M.T., M.M.Q.
Ted J. Cibik, N.D., M.M.Q.
Francesca Ferrari, L.Ac., Dipl.Ac., M.T.C.M., M.M.Q.
Emma Deepa Gleason, R.N., L.Ac., Dipl.Ac., M.T.C.M., M.M.Q.
Robert C. Grant, M.M.Q.
Robert W. Haberkorn, D.C., M.M.Q.
Carla Hughett, L.Ac., Dipl.Ac., M.T.C.M., M.M.Q.
Harvey D. Jennell, M.M.Q.
Wendy A. Lang, M.M.Q.
Dia Lynn, B.A., L.M.T., M.M.Q.
Elizabeth M. Marcum, M.Ed., M.M.Q.
Celestine McMahan, Ph.D., M.M.Q.
Mark L. Rappaport, M.M.Q.
Ryan M. Rrusuelas, M.M.Q.
Deneen C. Seril, M.M.Q.

The 2003 M.M.Q. Graduating Class of the International Institute of Medical Qigong

Lois Brunner, M.M.Q.
Joy Li Duremdes, BA, M.M.Q.
Gideon B. Enz, M.M.Q.
Calvin Fahey, M.M.Q.
Anna Belle Fore. M.M.Q.
Bradley M. Gilbert, B.A., M.M.Q.
Harry Asoka Haryanto, M.S.C., M.M.Q.
Mark Frederick Herro, M.M.Q.
Michele Ann Katsabekis, M.M.Q.
Thomas Katsabekis, M.M.Q.
Rana C. A. De Keczer, O.T.R./L, L.C.M.T., A.A.M.T., M.M.Q.
Tomas C. Leichardt, C.M.T., N.C.B.T.M.B., M.M.Q.
Francesca Marie O'Dona, B.S., M.M.Q.
Dermot A. O'Connor, Dip. Ac., M.M.Q.
Lisa Van Ostrand, M.M.Q.
Keiko Pence, M.M.Q.
Paul Pheasey, B.A., M.M.Q.
Lucy M. Roberts, L.Ac., Dipl.Ac., M.T.C.M., M.M.Q.
James Bryant Seals, Jr., M.S., M.M.Q.
Jade Goldstein Stewart, M.M.Q.
J. Michael Wood, PBMC, OBDS, M.M.Q.

The 2002 M.M.Q. Graduating Class of the International Institute of Medical Qigong

Jeff Tukum Barnard, E.M.T., M.M.Q.
Donna Bell, R.N., M.M.Q.
Mitchell Blank, D.C., M.M.Q.
Alan C. Fischer, L.Ac., Dipl.Ac., M.T.C.M., M.M.Q.
Suzanne B. Friedman, L.Ac., Dipl.Ac., M.T.C.M., M.M.Q.
Myrt Hawkins, M.D., M.M.Q.
Ann-Sofie Gustavsson Hobbs, M.M.Q.
Leah Ann Johnson, M.M.Q.
Nora Kim, M.M.Q.
Kelly Loos, M.M.Q.
Stuart Loyd, M.M.Q.
Ti Pence, M.M.Q.
Judy Pruzinsky, L.Ac., Dipl.Ac., M.T.C.M., M.M.Q.
Ijaz Rasool, B.Sc., M.Sc., M.M.Q.
Eric W. Shaffer, M.M.Q.
Shifu Bernard Shannon, M.M.Q.
Joyce Thom, M.M.Q.
Camille Vardy, L.Ac., Dipl.Ac., M.T.C.M., M.M.Q.
Nadezhda Zoe Wein, C.M.T., M.M.Q.
Gary S. Weinstein, M.D., M.M.Q.
Catherine Zimmerman, D.C., M.M.Q.

The 2004 M.M.Q. Graduating Class of the International Institute of Medical Qigong

Stephen Armstrong, M.M.Q.
V. Daniel Azcarate, M.M.Q.
Caroline Deery, M.M.Q.
Denise Douglass-White, M.M.Q.
Eddie Dowd, M.M.Q.
Jan Eeckhout, D.O., Dipl.Ac., M.T.C.M., M.M.Q.
Jose E. Gonzalez, M.M.Q.
Allison L. Harter, M.M.Q.
Cathriona Hillery, Lic. Ac., Dipl.Ac., M.M.Q.
Matthew Jones, M.M.Q.
Brian McKenna, D.O.M., Lic. Ac., M.M.Q.
Stephen McNamee, Lic. Ac., Dipl.Ac., Dipl.Tuina, M.M.Q.
Paula S. Medler, D.V.M., M.M.Q.
Ted O'Brian, L.Ac., M.M.Q.
Edwin T. Pickett, Jr., M.M.Q.
Rodney G. Sasaki, M.M.Q.
Stephen D. Steidle, M.M.Q.
Sara R. Storm, L.Ac., M.M.Q
Allen Wentland, M.M.Q.
Catherine A. White, M.M.Q.
Vic Wouters, Lic. Fysio, Dipl.Ac., Tuina, M.T.C.M., M.M.Q.
Myles Wray, Lic. Ac., Dipl.Ac. & Tuina, M.M.Q.

The 2005 M.M.Q. Graduating Class of the International Institute of Medical Qigong

Maryann Allison, M.M.Q.
Christopher Michael Axelrad, L.Ac., M.M.Q.
Dr. Mona A. Boudreaux, M.M.Q.
Lou Eberle, M.S.O.M., M.M.Q.
Maria Sal Eberle, M.M.Q.
Layth Hakim, M.M.Q.
Mollie Kelleher, M.M.Q.
Zhanneta Raskin, M.M.Q.
Gregory D. Sparkman, M.M.Q.
Sifu William L. Welch Jr., M.M.Q.
Douglas K. Womack, J.D., M.M.Q.
Robert Youngs, R.M.T., Ac., M.M.Q.

In August 2005, the He Nan University of Traditional Chinese Medicine, in Zheng Zhou China, recognized the International Institute of Medical Qigong (IIMQ) as a "sister school" of the university, and adopted the I.I.M.Q.'s curriculum and textbooks as part of their Medical Qigong graduate program.

THE INTERNATIONAL INSTITUTE OF MEDICAL QIGONG IN PACIFIC GROVE, CA.
DOCTOR OF MEDICAL QIGONG GRADUATING CLASSES

- Seth Lefkowitz, D.C., D.M.Q. (China), 1997
- Arnold E. Tayam, D.M.Q. (China), 1997

- Lois Brunner, M.S., D.M.Q. (China), 2003
- Janette Lillian Carver, D.M.Q. (China), 2003
- Ted J. Cibik, N.D., D.M.Q. (China), 2003
- Dennis Martin Earnest, D.M.Q. (China), 2003
- Gideon B. Enz, D.M.Q. (China), 2003
- L. Francesca Ferrari, L.Ac., D.T.C.M., D.M.Q. (China), 2003
- Suzanne B. Friedman, L.Ac., D.M.Q. (China), 2003
- Louis B. Frizzell, D.M.Q. (China), 2003
- Thomas Katsabekis, D.M.Q. (China), 2003
- Michelle Ann Katsabekis, D.M.Q. (China), 2003
- Elizabeth M. Marcum, M.A., D.M.Q. (China), 2003
- Deneen C. Seril, D.M.Q. (China), 2003
- Eric W. Shaffer, B.A., D.M.Q. (China), 2003

- Shifu Bernard Shannon, D.M.Q. (China), 2004
- Jade Goldstein Stewart, D.M.Q. (China), 2004
- Lisa Van Ostrand, D.M.Q. (China), 2004

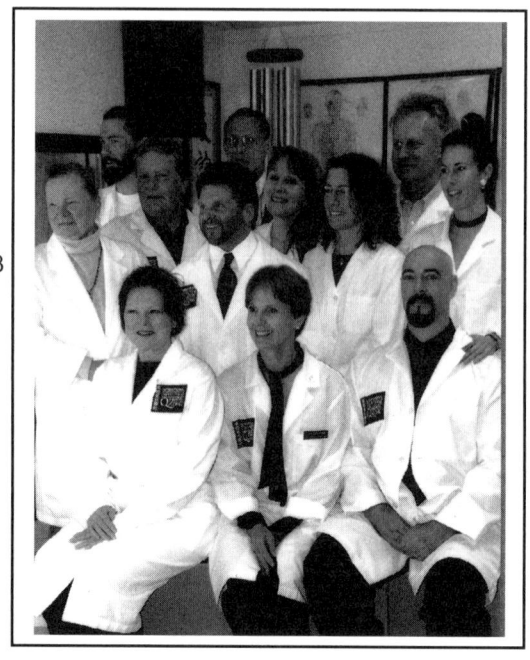

After completing a 4 year course and obtaining their Master of Medical Qigong (M.M.Q.), several students of the International Institute of Medical Qigong entered into an additional two-year Doctoral program and specialized in the treatment of cancer, receiving a D.M.Q. from China.

MEDICAL QIGONG INSTRUCTION

1999 - MEDICAL QIGONG PRACTITIONER CLASSES TAUGHT AT THE FIVE BRANCHES T.C.M. COLLEGE IN SANTA CRUZ, CALIFORNIA

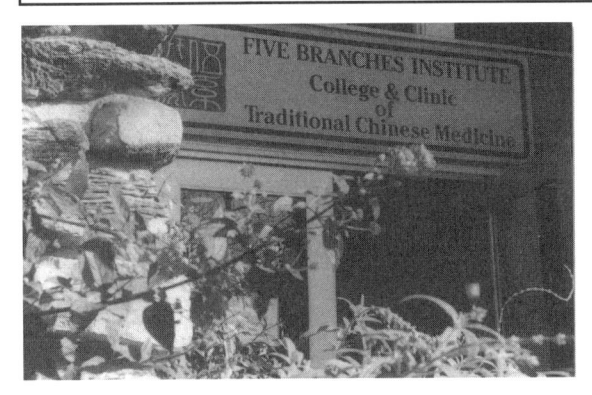

The Five Branches Institute: College and Clinic of Traditional Chinese Medicine

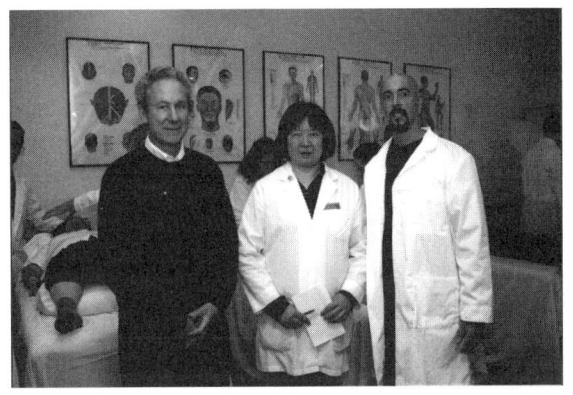

Pictured from left to right are the Five Branches President and CEO Ron Zaidman, M.B.A., M.T.C.M.; the Academic Dean and Clinical Medical Director Dr. Joanna Zhao L.Ac., Dipl. Ac (NCCA), D.T.C.M. (China); and the Dean of Medical Qigong Science and Director of the Medical Qigong Clinic Professor Jerry Alan Johnson, Ph.D., D.T.C.M., D.M.Q. (China).

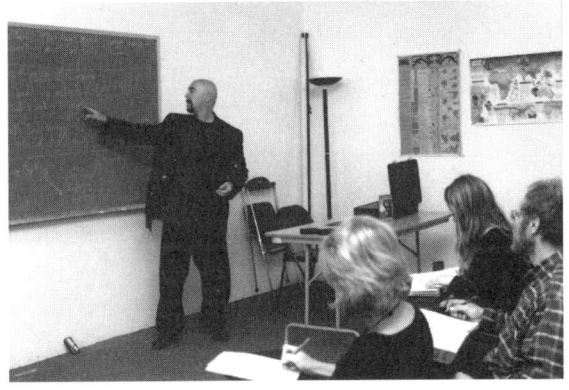

In addition to clinical modalities and energetic prescriptions, the Five Branches Medical Qigong students are also taught energetic psychology and how to handle the toxic emotional discharges released from their patients.

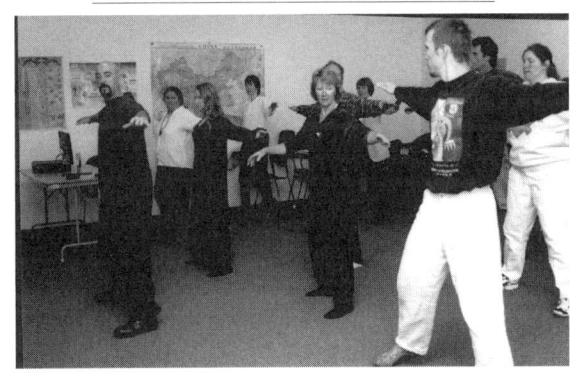

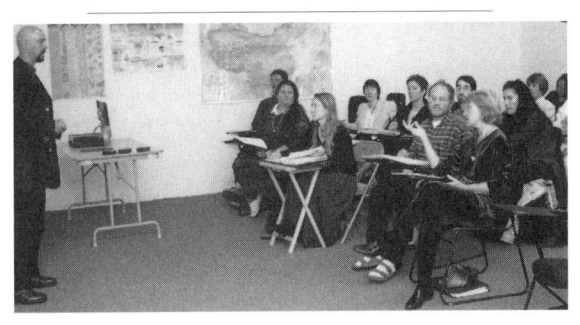

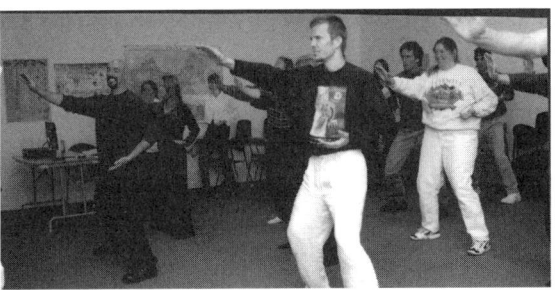

During the first semester, the Medical Qigong students at the Five Branches Institute learn and experience basic applications of Medical Qigong purgation, tonification and regulation exercises. They are also taught the underlying principles for each prescription exercise and its contraindications.

THE MEDICAL QIGONG CLINIC AT THE FIVE BRANCHES INSTITUTE T.C.M. COLLEGE IN SANTA CRUZ, CALIFORNIA

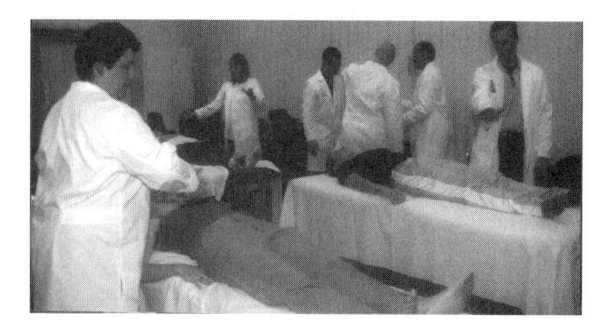

In the main treatment area, patients are categorized according to the severity of their condition.

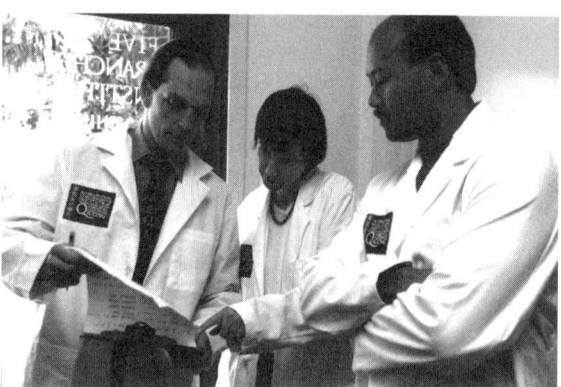

The resident Associate Dean, Jean Ruth Vlamynk, L.Ac, Dipl. Ac., M.T.C.M., M.M.Q. (in the middle) oversees the clinic's daily schedule.

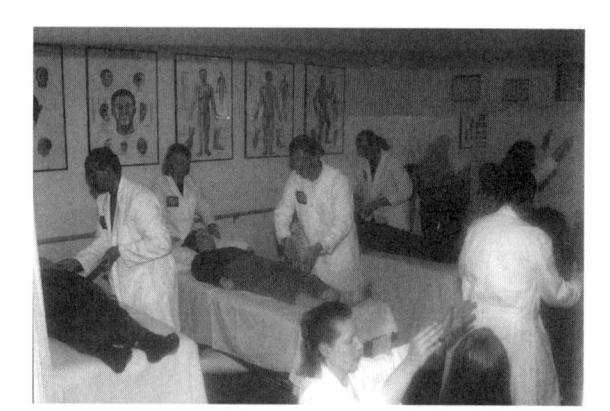

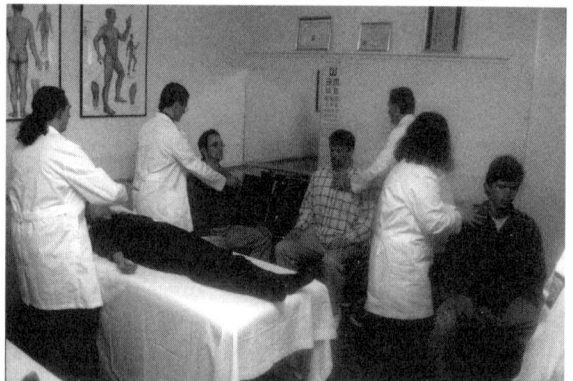

Students at the Five Branches Medical Qigong clinic

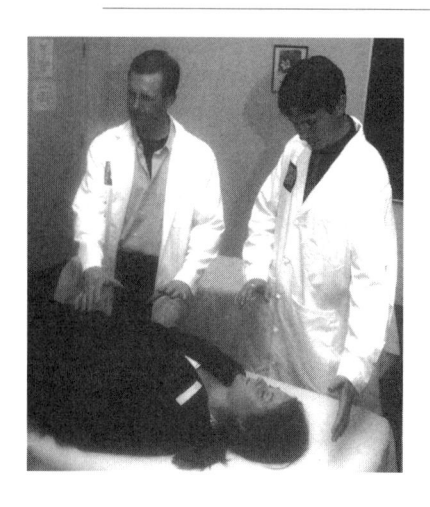

Doctors of the International Institute of Medical Qigong combine their energies to treat cancer patients.

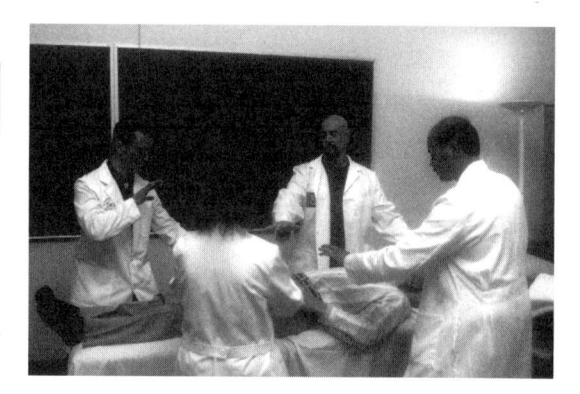

MEDICAL QIGONG INSTRUCTION

2003 - MEDICAL QIGONG THERAPIST CLASSES TAUGHT AT THE ACADEMY FOR FIVE ELEMENT ACUPUNCTURE, IN HALLANDALE, FLORIDA

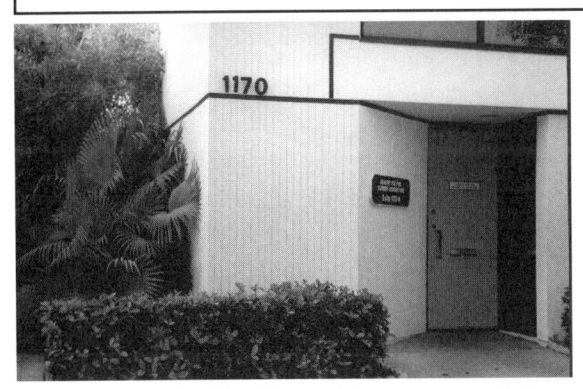

The Academy For Five Element Acupuncture: College and Clinic of Classical Chinese Medicine

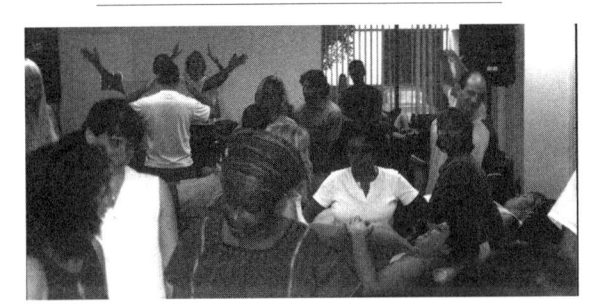

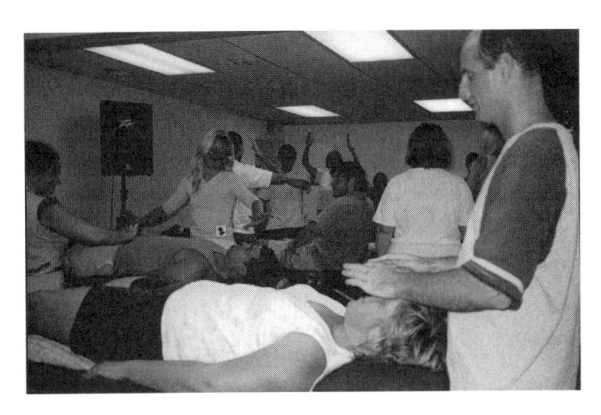

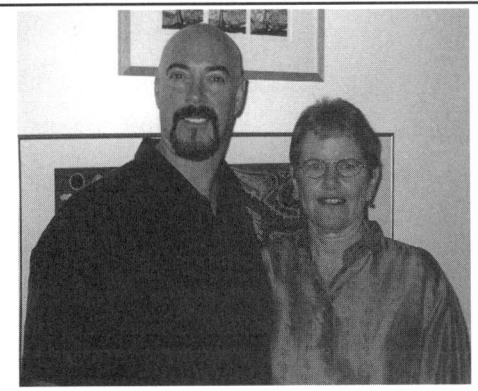

Pictured from left to right is the Dean of Medical Qigong Science and Director of the Medical Qigong Clinic Professor Jerry Alan Johnson, Ph.D., D.T.C.M., D.M.Q. (China) and The Academy For Five Element Acupuncture C.E.O. and President Dorit Reznek, M.Ac., A.P.

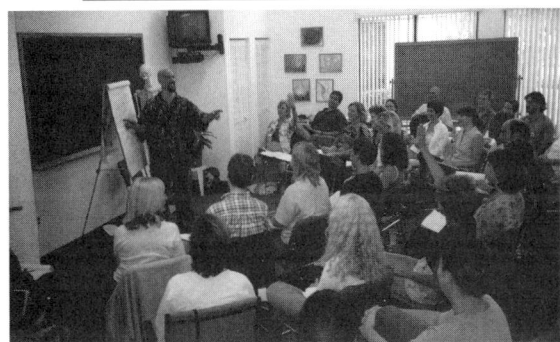

In addition to clinical modalities and energetic prescriptions, the Academy For Five Element Acupuncture students are also taught energetic psychology and how to handle the toxic emotional discharges released from their patients.

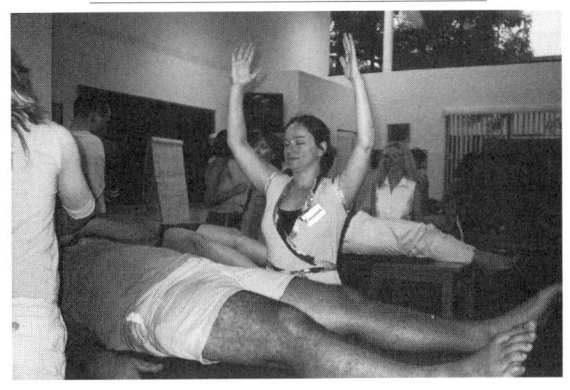

During the first semester, the Medical Qigong students at the Academy For Five Element Acupuncture have learned and experienced basic applications of Medical Qigong purgation, tonification and regulation exercises. They are taught the underlying principles for each Prescription exercise and its contraindications.

STUDENTS AT THE MEDICAL QIGONG CLINIC AT THE ACADEMY FOR FIVE ELEMENT ACUPUNCTURE, IN HALLANDALE, FLORIDA

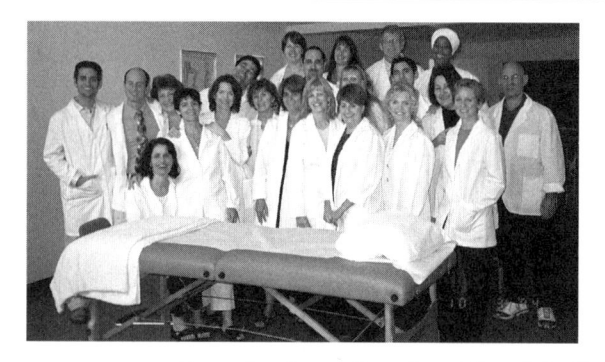

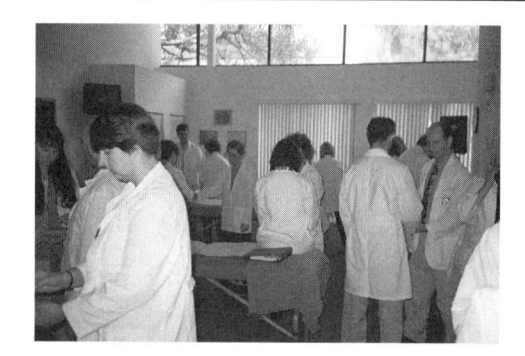

Preparing for another day at the clinic, the Five Element Medical Qigong students take time to share and support each other.

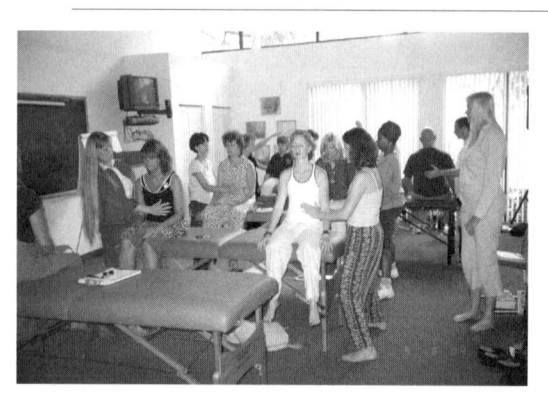

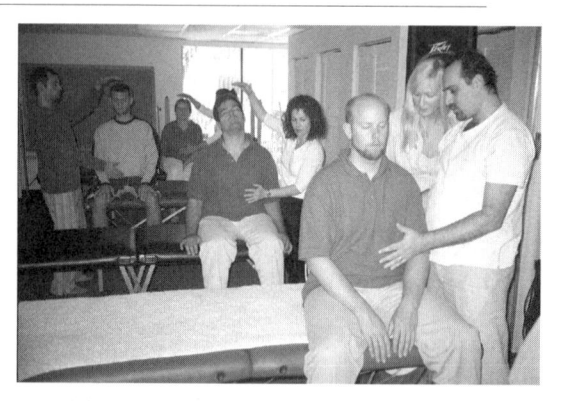

The Five Element Medical Qigong students take turns practicing the technique of treating hypertension.

TREATMENT OF ORGAN DISEASES AND PRESCRIPTION EXERCISES: P4 (2-UNITS: 32 HRS)

This fourth course offers the student an overview of the major principles and foundational structures that govern Traditional Chinese Medical Qigong therapy. This course is designed to introduce students to the advanced theories and clinical modalities of internal organ treatment, as well as the Medical Qigong exercises and meditations prescribed as homework in the clinic. Other topics covered include:

- Treatment of Liver diseases
- Treatment of Heart diseases
- Treatment of Spleen diseases
- Treatment of Stomach diseases
- Treatment of Lung diseases
- Treatment of Kidney diseases

Objective: Students will develop a deeper comprehension of specific organ diseases as they pertain to Traditional Chinese Medicine, Diagnosis, and Medical Qigong prescriptions. Emphasis will be placed on the practical clinical applications of Chinese Medical Qigong Therapy.

CLINICAL THEATER: CT (12 HRS.)

In the Clinical Theater, the academic and theoretical knowledge of various case studies are discussed, demonstrated and re-enacted. Conducted in a small class setting, Clinical Theatre gives the students exposure and first hand experience in the application of Medical Qigong diagnoses and treatments. This is a hands on experience where the different aspects of energetic dysfunctions and symp-

MEDICAL QIGONG INSTRUCTION

2005 - INTERNING STUDENTS AT THE MEDICAL QIGONG CLINIC AT THE ACUPUNCTURE AND INTEGRATIVE MEDICINE COLLEGE, IN BERKELEY, CA.

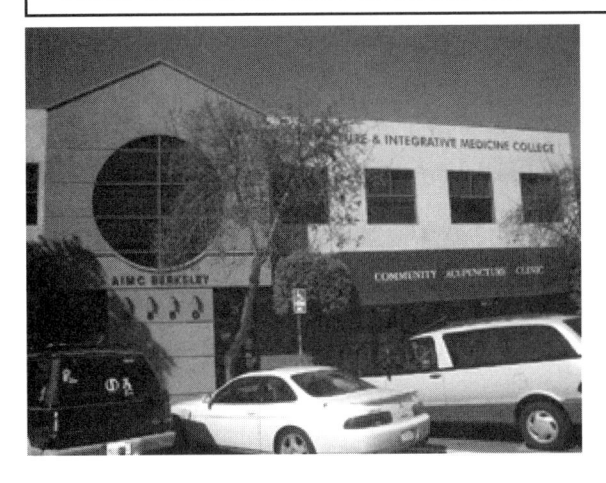

The Acupuncture and Integrative Medicine College, Berkeley, California. AIMC-Berkeley is the first Chinese medicine school in the Bay Area of California to offer the International Institute of Medical Qigong's Medical Qigong Practitioner Certification Program.

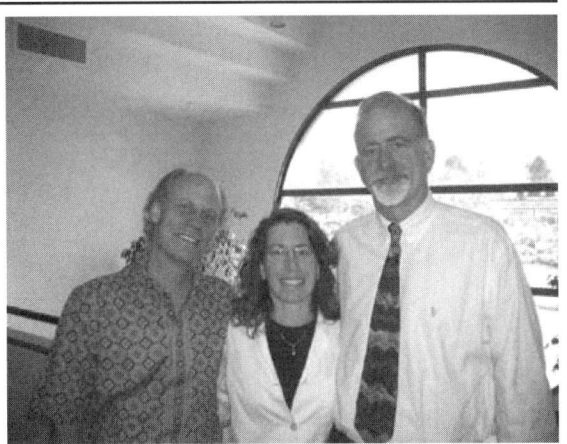

Pictured from left to right: AIMC Academic Dean Benjamin Dierauf, L.Ac., Dr. Suzanne B. Friedman, L.Ac., D.M.Q. (China), Director of the International Institute of Medical Qigong (San Francisco Branch) and Chair of the Medical Qigong Science Department at AIMC, and AIMC President Skye Sturgeon, DOM.

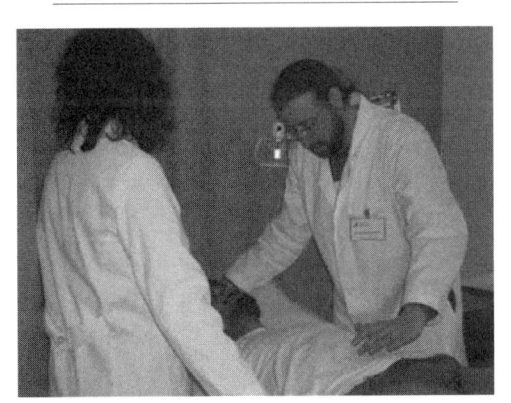

The Students pair up to treat a patient at the AIMC Medical Qigong Clinic. Each student is assigned a specific treatment technique depending on each patient's constitution.

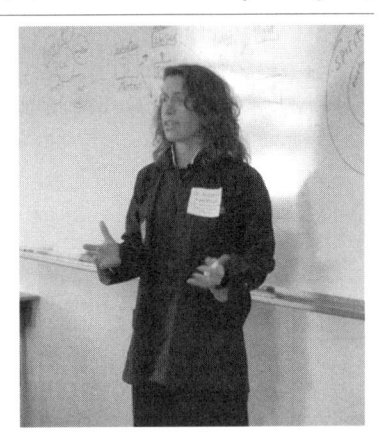

Dr. Suzanne B. Friedman lecturing on Energetic Anatomy and Physiology to a beginning Medical Qigong class

tom manifestations are studied and experienced by the Medical Qigong students. Under the careful guidance of the instructor, the Medical Qigong students will assist in all phases of diagnosis and treatment. After completing Clinical Theatre courses, Medical Qigong students will develop confidence in diagnosing and treating patients, as well as creating and maintaining accurate clinical records.

CLINICAL INTERNSHIP: C1 (60 HRS.)

In the clinical internship, the academic and theoretical knowledge gained in the Medical Qigong courses is placed into practical application. The objective is for the student to develop confidence in diagnosing and treating patients, as well as creating and maintaining accurate clinical records.

505

In the first phase of internship, the Medical Qigong student will work as part of a Qigong treatment team, assisting a senior intern. In the second phase of internship, the Medical Qigong student will work with their own patients while under the supervision of the instructor. After completing Clinical Internship, Medical Qigong students will have received their highest level of Medical Qigong patient care guidance prior to completing the M.Q.P. program.

The student is expected to keep complete records on each patient, including histories, diagnosis, treatments, and homework prescription exercises. After completing the "Introduction to Diagnosis and Treatments" (P2), the student should begin to treat patients on a consistent basis in order to gain additional clinical experience. As the student gains experience and attends more advanced courses their knowledge and abilities will increase as will their abilities to diagnose and treat more challenging cases.

Previous to completing certification for M.Q.P., M.Q.T., and M.M.Q., the student must provide copies of clinic log (verifying clinic hours).

THREE YEAR - 500 HOUR MEDICAL QIGONG THERAPIST (M.Q.T.) COURSE

This is a 500 hour Medical Qigong Therapist (M.Q.T.) certification program. This program will include oral and practical examinations plus clinical competencies. Successful completion of the examinations will enable the student to also qualify for the more advanced 1,000-hour Master of Medical Qigong (M.M.Q.) program.

Prerequisite for certification in the Medical Qigong Therapist program is the successful completion of the requirements for Medical Qigong Practitioner (M.Q.P.).

INTRODUCTION TO CHINESE ENERGETIC ALCHEMY: T5 (2-UNITS: 32 HRS.)

This fifth seminar offers the student an overview of the major principles and foundational structures that govern Medical Qigong Therapy. This course is designed to introduce students to the study of the Daoist Three Outer Forces (Heaven, Earth, and Man). Course content will include:

- The Influences of Energy, Food and Diet
- Prenatal and Postnatal Jing, Qi and Shen
- The Body's Energetic Internal Structures
- The Five Spiritual Aspects of the 5 Yin Organs
- Advanced Shen Gong Cultivation Methods
- The 6 Transportation's of Shen
- The 8 Supernatural Powers
- Soul Projection, Spirit Projection and Energy Projection.

Objective: Students will develop a deeper comprehension of the body's physical, emotional, mental, and energetic relationship to the universal and environmental energetic fields.

DAO YIN THERAPY AND RECTIFYING QI DEVIATIONS: T6 (2-UNITS: 32 HRS)

This sixth seminar offers the student an overview of the major principles and foundational structures that govern Chinese Medical Qigong therapy. This course is designed to introduce students to the study of proper Dao Yin training and rectifying Qi Deviations. Course content will include:

- The study of the internal principles and Medical Qigong functions of
- Postural Dao Yin Training,
- Respiratory Dao Yin Training,
- Mental Dao Yin Training,
- Rectifying Qi Deviations occurring from improper Qigong training.
- Dealing with Psychic Attacks using Mantras for protection
- Encounters with Ghosts and Spirit Entities
- Treating Shen Disturbances
- Using the Thirteen Ghost Points

Objective: After completing this course, students will develop a deeper comprehension of the body's energetic relationship to the physical structure and mental and emotional disorders and deviations of the psyche.

MEDICAL QIGONG THERAPY FOR PEDIATRICS, GERIATRICS, GYNECOLOGY, NEUROLOGY, AND PSYCHOLOGY: T7 (2-UNITS: 32 HRS.)

This seventh seminar offers the student an overview of the major principles and foundational structures that govern Chinese Medical Qigong therapy. This course is designed to introduce specialized clinical treatments in specialized areas. Course content will include:

- Early stages of child growth and development

- Prescriptions for children
- Prescriptions for senility
- Etiology and pathology of gynecological diseases
- Menstrual complications
- Treatment protocols for menopause
- Stroke (Wind-Stroke)
- Coma
- Facial paralysis (Bells Palsy)
- Multiple sclerosis (MS)
- Self treatment prescriptions for psycho-emotional disorders
- Treating emotional anxieties, phobias, and addictions
- Treating phobias and depression using the "Windows of the Heavens" points

Objective: Students will have an exposure to specialized clinical treatments of specific illnesses, and the management of the patient's emotional, mental, and spiritual states.

INTRODUCTION TO CANCER TREATMENT (1): T8 (2-UNITS: 32 HRS.)

This eighth seminar offers the student an overview of the major principles and foundational structures that govern Chinese Medical Qigong therapy. This course is designed to introduce students to the study of the treatment of various types of cancers and tumor formations. Course content will include:

- Etiology and Pathology of Cyst, Tumor and Cancer Formation
- The Multifaceted Causes of Cyst, Tumor and Cancer Formations
- Categorization of Cysts and Tumors According to Traditional Chinese Medicine
- Medical Qigong Approach to Cancer Prescriptions
- Emission Therapy for the treatment of Brain Tumors, Breast Cysts Tumors and Cancer, Uterine Tumors and Cancer, Cervical Cancer, Ovarian Cysts, Prostate Cancer, Lung Cancer, and Colon and Rectal Cancer.

Objective: Students will have an exposure to specialized clinical treatments of cancer and the management of the patient's emotional, mental and spiritual states surrounding the disease.

ADDITIONAL REQUIREMENTS:

Additional requirements for Medical Qigong Therapist certification include:

- Basic T.C.M. Theory (50 Hrs.)
- Western Anatomy and Physiology I (50 Hrs.)
- Western Anatomy and Physiology II (50 Hrs.)
- Clinical Internship II (60 Hrs.)

1000 HOUR MASTER OF MEDICAL QIGONG (M.M.Q.) COURSE

This is a 1000 hour Master of Medical Qigong (M.M.Q.) certification program. This program will include oral and practical examinations plus clinical competencies.

Prerequisite for enrollment is the successful completion of the requirements for Medical Qigong Therapist (M.Q.T.).

SENSORY, INTUITIVE, AND PERCEPTUAL DIAGNOSIS: M9 (2-UNITS: 32 HRS.)

This ninth seminar offers the student an overview of the major principles and foundational structures that govern Chinese Medical Qigong therapy. This course is designed to introduce students to the use of various sensory, intuitive, and perceptual skills used in the Medical Qigong clinic for the diagnosis and treatment of patients. Course content will include:

- Including Applications of Intuitive and Perceptual Qi Diagnosis
- Diagnosis Based on Flat Palm Detection (Hand Sensing)
- Diagnosis Based on Kinesthetic and Empathic Qi Absorption
- Hand Diagnosis Based on Body Association
- Diagnosis by Observing Aura Fields
- Diagnosis Based on Intention
- Long Distance Medical Qigong Therapy
- Faith Projection
- Negative Thought Projections and Medical Qigong Therapy
- Auxiliary Medical Qigong Healing Modalities

Objectives: Students will have an exposure to a variety of diagnosis methodologies and auxiliary Medical Qigong healing modalities.

ENERGETIC ANATOMY AND PHYSIOLOGY: M10 (2-UNITS: 32 HRS.)

This tenth seminar offers the student an overview of the major principles and foundational structures that govern Chinese Medical Qigong therapy.

This course is designed to introduce students

to the five dominions of energy, energetic embryology, and TCM theory from a Medical Qigong perspective. Course content will include:
- Understanding Fetal Toxins
- Energy, Matter and Spiritual Interactions
- Fascia Development and Energy Flow
- Classifications of the Body's Five Constitutions
- The Five Energies of the Human Body
- The Three Dantians
- Yin and Yang Divisions
- Nine Chambers and Center Taiji Pole
- The Twelve Primary Channels and Interacting Organs
- The Eight Extraordinary Vessels and their Functions
- The Fifteen Collaterals
- The Function of the Body's Energetic Points
- The Extraordinary Yang Organs
- Etiology of Medical Qigong Therapy
- The Eight Miscellaneous Causes of Disease
- The Differentiation of Syndromes and the Diagnosis and Treatment of Patients

Objective: Students will develop a deeper comprehension of the body's emotional, psychological and energetic matrix through an overview of the major principles and foundational structures that govern Medical Qigong therapy.

TREATMENT OF CANCER WITH MEDICAL QIGONG THERAPY (2): M11 (2-UNITS: 32 HRS.)

This eleventh seminar offers the student an overview of the major principles and foundational structures that govern Traditional Chinese Medical Qigong. This course is designed to further the students understanding of to the study of the treatment of various types of cancers and tumor formations. Course content will include:
- Emission Therapy for the treatment of bone cancer, myeloma, leukemia, lymphoma, and skin cancer
- Radiation and chemotherapy
- Medical Qigong and surgery
- Treatment of Scar Tissue
- Diet and nutrition
- Social Oncology

Objective: Students will have an exposure to specialized clinical treatments of cancer and the management of the patient's emotional, mental and spiritual states surrounding the disease.

MEDICAL QIGONG TREATMENT OF SPIRITUAL DISORDERS: M12 (2-UNITS: 32 HRS.)

This twelfth seminar offers the student an overview of the major principles and foundational structures that govern Traditional Chinese Medical Qigong. This course is designed to introduce students to Chinese spiritual dimensions and clinical interactions with the spirit world. Course content will include:
- Sorcery and Psychic Attacks
- Defending Against Psychic Attacks
- Encounters with Ghosts and Spirit Entities
- Dealing with Demonic and Evil Spirit Oppression and Possession

Objective: Students will have an exposure to specialized clinical treatments of spirit and demon oppression and possession.

ADDITIONAL REQUIREMENTS:

Additional requirements for Master of Medical Qigong certification include:
- Advanced T.C.M. Theory (32 Hrs.)
- First Aid and CPR (16 Hrs.)
- Taijiquan or Baguazhang training (48 Hrs.)
- Additional Qigong Treatment Modalities (32 Hrs.)
- Traumatology (32 Hrs.)
- Clinical Internship III (156 Hrs.)

CLINICAL THEATRE, INTERNSHIP, AND FINAL EXAMINATION: M13 (2-UNITS: 32 HRS.)

This thirteenth seminar offers the student exposure and first hand experience of Medical Qigong diagnoses and treatments. The student will study and experience different aspects of energetic dysfunctions and symptom manifestations.

In the first phase of internship, the senior Medical Qigong students will work as the leader of a Qigong treatment team, overseeing the beginning interns. In the second phase of final internship, the senior Medical Qigong interns will work as a supervising instructor, maintaining the responsibility of overseeing a productive Medical Qigong clinic.

After completing the senior Clinical Internship, the Medical Qigong students will have received their highest level of Medical Qigong patient care guidance prior to completing the program. The instructor will guide and assist the student in all

MEDICAL QIGONG INSTRUCTION

IN 1995, THE HAI DIAN UNIVERSITY OF TRADITIONAL CHINESE MEDICINE IN BEIJING, CHINA HAD AN ACTIVE MEDICAL QIGONG COLLEGE AND CLINIC

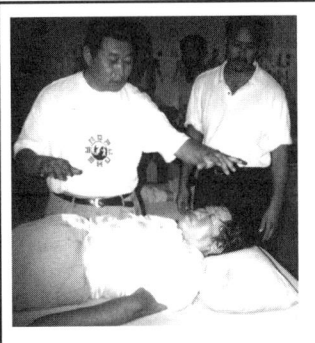

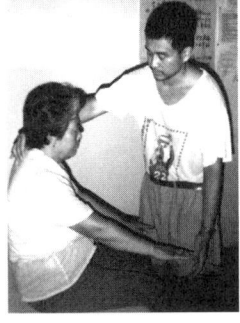

In 1995 Dr. Lu Guo Hong (Director) and Dr. Niu Yu Hua (Associate Director) of the Medical Qigong College at Hai Dian University.

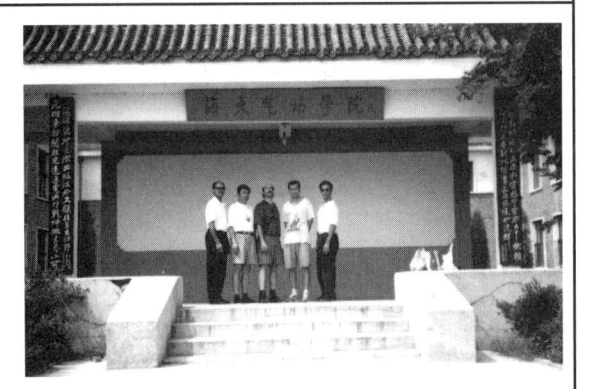

The front entrance of the Medical Qigong College at the Hai Dian T.C.M. University in Beijing, China.

Right: In 1995, the graduate students of the Medical Qigong College at Hai Dian University, interned at the Xi Yuan Hospital in Beijing, China, for a period of 6 months to a year before being licensed as Doctors of Traditional Chinese Medicine through the government's Ministry of Health, which monitored the student programs.

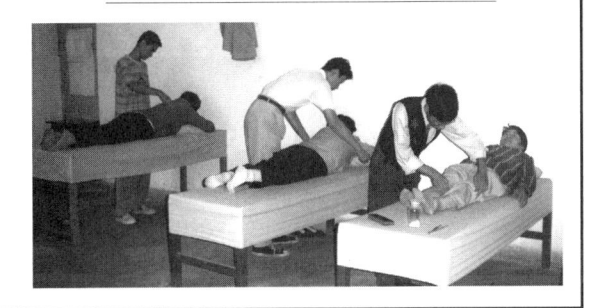

phases of diagnosis and treatment. Course content will include:
- Integrating advanced clinical modalities
- Advanced diagnosis and advanced energetic modulation skills
- Exploring case studies

Objective: Students will develop confidence in diagnosing and treating patients, as well as creating and maintaining accurate clinical records.

At the completion of this course if the student has successfully completed all requirements for the Master of Medical Qigong certificate program, an M.M.Q. certificate will be issued at that time.

CHANGING TIMES IN CHINA FOR MEDICAL QIGONG THERAPY

Contained within this five volume Medical Qigong textbook series is ancient knowledge and privileged information detailing how to effectively diagnose and energetically treat patients using Medical Qigong therapy, as set forth by the Hai Dian Medical Qigong College of Beijing. At one time in China's history, the Medical College at the Hai Dian University was recognized as one of the leading Medical Qigong colleges in Beijing (Hai Dian translates to "Sea of Elixir").

Graduating students from the Medical Qigong College at Hai Dian University interned at the Xi Yuan Hospital for a period of 6 months to a year before being licensed as Doctors of Traditional Chinese Medicine through the government's Ministry of Health, which monitored the student programs.

By the year 1999, the study of Qigong had taken a sudden change in formal development. Due to the political actions and activities of the Falun Gong Qigong Schools, the Chinese government put a sudden halt to any and all Qigong practices. In the middle of the night, armed guards entered the various Medical Qigong colleges, laboratories, and clinics and removed all of the scien-

509

The Medical Qigong Clinic at Xi Yuan Hospital in Beijing, China - 1995

The Xi Yuan Hospital in Beijing, China, was at one time the academic equivalent of the Stanford Medical Center in the United States. It specialized in training interning doctors from several medical universities, and focused on the various clinical protocols utilized in all four distinct branches of Traditional Chinese Medicine: Acupuncture, Herbs and Nutrition, Medical Qigong, and Massage Therapy. Up until 1999, the Medical Qigong Department at the Xi Yuan Hospital had their own wing, which extended throughout several floors, and included both inpatient and outpatient clinics. In addition, the Medical Qigong Department also maintained an active division of research scientists for clinical research. The scientists were specifically trained for gathering information on the healing effects of Qi Emission Therapy.

However, due to the extreme political actions of the Falun Gong Qigong Association, stern restraints on all Qigong activities were immediately applied throughout the country, especially to those Qigong Departments existing within the government hospitals and clinics in Beijing. As of 2004, the Medical Qigong departments of the Xi Yuan hospital have been extremely down-sized and reduced to only two small treatment rooms, one of which is currently being shared with the Massage Department.

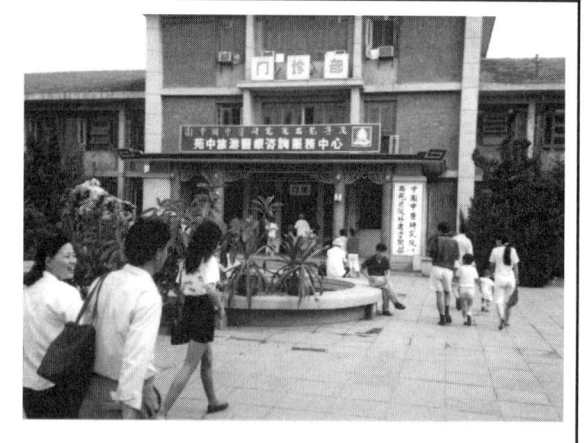

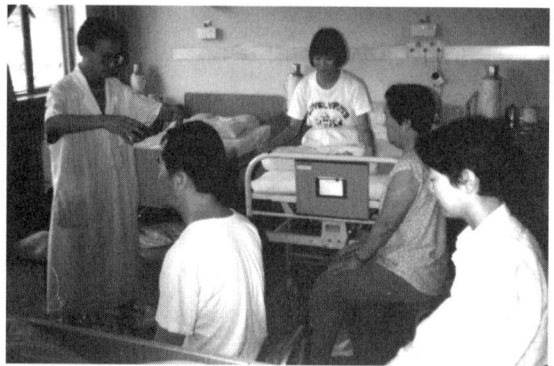

Doctor Xu Hongtao treating patients at the Xi Yuan Hospital in 1995.

tific equipment, chaining and padlocking the doors. Some Qigong doctors and instructors were held and interrogated, and several Medical Qigong hospitals and clinics throughout China were closed. All practice groups of Qigong were dispersed. Even small, individual groups practicing in the various parks were ordered to disband and the leaders were taken in for questioning. Sadly, this closure also included that of the Medical Qigong college at the Hai Dian University.

By the end of 2000, many of the Medical Qigong clinical application and prescription exercises that were considered to be common treatment protocols in the Medical Qigong hospitals were no longer being taught to the public, or utilized in the various clinics.

Even more shocking is that the Medical Qigong treatment protocols have dramatically changed, as doctors in Beijing are no longer allowed to purge, tonify, and regulate the patients' life-force energy. The new government treatment policy only allows them to emit Qi into the patient's body until they fall asleep.

The faculty and graduate students of the I.I.M.Q. have accepted the responsibility of teaching the same information and maintaining the same strict standards established by the former Hai Dian Medical Qigong College of Beijing, China. It is our hope that one day the Chinese government will loosen its restraint on Medical Qigong Therapy and actively return this great knowledge back to the Chinese people.

Glossary of Terms

A

Abdominal Breathing - to breathe from the abdomen (expand with inhalation, contract with exhalation).

Acupuncture - one of the Four branches of Traditional Chinese Medicine, which involves treating patients through the use of needling, cupping, Bloodletting, moxa and magnets in order to stimulate energy flow.

Acupuncturist - a doctor of acupuncture therapy.

Acquired Essence - also called Postnatal Jing, is acquired energetic tissue substance, developed after birth.

Acquired Force - energy pertaining to the earth and surrounding environment.

Acquired Qi - also called Postnatal Qi, is the body's energy derived from food, air and drink, acquired after birth.

Acquired Rational Mind - also called Postnatal Mind, are thoughts and feelings derived from the acquired experiences of one's environment.

Acute - a rapid onset and short duration of a particular condition.

Adenoma - a neoplasm (abnormal formation of tissue) of glandular epithelium.

Adenocarcinoma - a malignant tumor arising from a glandular organ.

Affirmation - a word, phrase or sentence that is repeated frequently to influence, or change, a belief held deeply within the unconscious mind.

Agoraphobia - fear of places or situations from which escape might be difficult or embarrassing. Symptoms include panic like symptoms and a precondition towards panic attacks.

Akashic Records - a Sanskrit term used to describe the detailed knowledge of all the historical events of the world recorded within the "all-pervasive space of the universe" or "Wuji," also called the "knowledge of the infinite Void."

Alchemy - internal transformation of body and energy brought about by: Nei Dan (inner alchemy) through internal Qigong training, and Wai Dan (external alchemy) using herbal formulas.

Amenorrhea - the absence or suppression of menstruation.

Ancestral Channel - a term used to describe one of the Eight Extraordinary Vessels.

Ancestral Qi - energy inherited from both parents at the time of conception, responsible for innate talents and skills.

Ancestral Traits - pertaining to the ancestral spiritual influence which affects the patient's body. Ancestral traits are developed according to the geographic location at the time of conception.

Anemia - a reduction in the number of circulating red Blood cells.

Angina Pectoris - severe pain and a sensation of constriction about the Heart.

An Jing - see Hidden Power.

Ankylosing Spondylitis - inflammation of the vertebrae, giving rise to stiffness of the back and neck.

An Mo Therapy - a tissue manipulation therapy that focuses primarily on the treatment of internal organ disorders.

Anorexia - loss of appetite.

An Sound Resonation - hidden or inaudible sound resonation.

Antibody - any of the numerous proteins produced by the immune system that defend against antigens.

Anxiety - emotional distress, resulting in Heart palpitations, inability to concentrate, muscle tension causing muscle aches.

Aphasia - the absence or impairment of the ability to communicate through speech, writing, or signs, due to a dysfunction within the Brain center.

Aplastic Anemia - anemia caused by deficient red cell production, due to Bone marrow disorders.

Apoptosis - the disintegration of cells into membrane-bound particles that are then phagocytosed by other cells.

Archetypes - a term coined by the psychiatrist Carl G. Jung to describe the collective unconscious images and motifs (e.g., warrior, healer, priest, etc.). An inherited idea or mode of thought derived from the experiences of the race which is present in the unconscious of the individual.

Arrhythmia - an irregularity or loss of rhythm pertaining to the Heart.

Arteriosclerosis - term pertaining to a number of pathological conditions in which there is a thickening, hardening, and loss of elasticity of the artery walls.

Arthralgia - pain in the joints.

Arthritis - pain and inflammation of the joints, followed by progressive stiffness.

Arthropathy - pertaining to any joint disease.

Ascariasis - infestation of ascaris lumbicoides parasite (pinworm).

Ascending Qi - the action and flow of energy moving upward.

Ashi Points - also called "Trigger Points" are places on the body which are tender spots or painful areas near diseased or injured tissue.

Asthma - a disease caused by increased responsiveness of the tracheobronchial tree within the Lungs, due to various stimuli, causing severe difficulty in breathing.

Astral Body - also called the soul body, describes the energetic vehicle in which the eternal soul can journey outside of the physical body. The astral body is connected to the Middle Dantian by a silver "cord of life."

Astral Matter - the energetic substance located within the second field of the body's external Wei Qi and attributed to the emotional energy body.

Astral Plane - an energetic and spiritual plane of existence parallel to the physical plane.

Astral Travel - also called soul travel (or astral projection) describes the condition of the eternal soul journeying outside of the physical body, connected to the Middle Dantian by a silver "cord of life."

Astringent - any substance or agent that causes tissues to contract or that inhibits secretion of Body Fluids such as mucus or Blood.

Antigens - any substance able to provoke an immune response in the human body.

Atelectasis - pulmonary collapse.

Atrophic - pertaining to atrophy.

Atrophy Syndrome - a disorder characterized by flaccidity and weakness of the limbs and a progressive loss of strength and muscle tone.

Attention Deficit Disorder - a learning disorder manifesting through the following symptoms: habitual failure to pay attention, easily distractible, inability to organize, extreme impulsiveness, difficulty in studying, often accompanied by hyperactivity.

Aura - the energetic field which radiates light and circulates around the second field of the body's external Wei Qi

Aura Colors - the body's energetic luminous colors ranging from red, orange, yellow, green, blue, violet to white.

Auspicious Powers - the energy potential contained within the Five Yin Organs.

B

Ba Gan - eight diagnostic principles used in Traditional Chinese Medicine in order to differentiate symptoms.

Bai Dai - leukorrhea or white vaginal discharge.

Baihui Point (One Hundred Meetings) - the Governing Vessel point at the top of the head (GV-20).

Bellows Palm Technique - a palm technique in which the thumb and little finger compress and release like a bellows.

Bells Palsy - unilateral facial paralysis of sudden onset.

Benign - gentle or kindly, not aggressive, the opposite of malignant.

Bile - a secretion stored in the gall bladder released into the duodenum as a digestive juice.

Bio-Rhythm - three distinct cycles and energy flow that pertain to the body's physical, emotional and intellectual rhythms.

Bipolar Personality Disorder - formerly known as manic depressive personality disorder, a state of extreme euphoria or pervasive irritability, with racing thoughts, inability to sleep, and impulsive behavior (that may last for days or months), that alternate with morbid depression with suicidal ideation or attempts at suicide (see depression). During the manic phase there may be hallucinations.

Bird's Bridge - pertaining to the energetic connection between the tongue and the upper "hard" palate, behind the teeth.

Birth Energetic Patterns - pertaining to the energetic patterns developed according to the influence of the time and geographic location of the patient's birth.

Blended Originals (Hun Yuan) - the body's "internal combined energy" fused into the Lower Dantian area.

Bloated and Expanded Stagnation - stagnation with a characteristically expansive or bloated appearance, can be caused from an accumulation of phlegm and Body Fluids (in addition to Qi and Blood) in the adjacent tissue areas of the body.

Blood (Xue) - the dense fluid which nourishes the body, transmits Qi, and provides the material for the mind and emotions.

Blood Heat - a condition categorized by Heat and Blood signs (retching of Blood, expectoration of Blood, Bloody stool or urine, nosebleeds, and menstrual irregularities).

Bloodletting - a technique used in acupuncture therapy which entails pricking the skin to release and remove Blood Heat and Blood stagnation.

Blood Stagnation - the impairment or cessation of normal Blood flow.

Blood Stasis - the impairment or cessation of normal Blood flow.

Blood Vessels - the body's transportation system for Qi and Blood nutrition and regeneration. The Blood Vessels are one of the Eight Extraordinary Organs, its function is to moisten the body's tissues.

Body Fluids (Ye) - these are clear, light, and watery. They originate from food and drink and are transformed and separated by the Spleen (aided by the Kidneys) and dispersed by the Lungs and Triple Burners. (i.e., perspiration, tears, saliva, and mucus.)

Body Liquids (Jin) - these are a heavier, denser form of Body Fluids, compared to the Body Fluids (Ye). Their function is to nourish the joints, spine, Brain, and Bone marrow. They lubricate the orifices of the sensory organs.

Bone - the body's skeletal material related in essence to the Kidneys. The Bones are one of the Eight Extraordinary Organs, its function is to store the body's Marrow.

Bone Marrow - sustains and nurtures the Bones, composed of Kidney Jing (Essence) and Marrow. The Marrow is one of the Eight Extraordinary Organs.

Book of Commentaries - consisting of ten commentaries from Confucius and his disciples, pertaining to the study of the eight Trigrams, sixty-four hexagrams, and the Yi-Jing.

Book of Oracles - written by King Wen and the Duke of Zhou, pertaining to the study of the eight Trigrams, sixty-four hexagrams, and the Yi-Jing.

Borborygmus - a gurgling, rumbling sound heard over the Large Intestine, caused by the passing of gas through the liquid contents of the intestines.

Borderline Personality Disorder - a psychological disorder characterized by a pervasive pattern of intense, unstable relationships, and an unstable self-image. Such patients suffer from chronic feelings of emptiness stemming from abandonment issues. They exhibit self-destructive behavior and transient paranoia, or dissociative symptoms.

Brain - pertaining to the Sea of Marrow issuing from the Kidneys that collects within the cranium. The Brain is one of the Eight Extraordinary Organs.

Brain Tumor Point - Shihmien Point located on the heel of each foot.

Bronchial Asthma - asthma caused by a hypersensitivity to an allergen.

Bronchiectasis - chronic dilatation of a bronchus or bronchi, with a secondary infection (usually involving the lower portion of the Lungs).

Bronchitis - inflammation of mucous membrane of the bronchial tubes.

C

Caduceus - medical insignia picturing double snakes wrapping a winged staff.

Calculi - the plural of calculus or stones, usually composed of mineral salts.

Cancer (Carcinoma) - an obstruction of Qi and Blood circulation resulting in stagnation and the formation of a malignant tumor that tends to spread.

Carbuncle - a circumscribed inflammation of the skin and deeper tissues.

Carcinogens - any substance or agent that produces or increases the risk of developing cancer.

Carcinoma (Cancer or Tumor) - a malignant growth or tumor that occurs in the epithelial tissue (the outer surface or first layer of tissue that lines the body's cavities, as well as the principal tubes and passageways leading to the exterior of the body)

Catatonic - totally withdrawn, almost unconscious, frozen and unable to move.

Celestial Stems - see Ten Celestial Stems.

Center Core - pertaining to either the core of light within the Taiji Pole which joins the body's three Dantians through the center of the body, or the True Self (the essence of a person's spirit).

Cerebral Embolism - a condition which occurs when an embolus (bubble of air, or piece of a thrombus) detaches from a thrombus and obstructs a cerebral artery.

Cerebral Hemorrhage - bleeding caused from a rupture of a sclerosed or diseased vessel in the Brain.

Cerebral Thrombosis - an obstruction of a cerebral artery by a thrombus (Blood clot).

Cerebro-Vascular Accident (CVA) - in the clinic, conditions referred to as stroke (or Windstroke) include cerebral hemorrhage, cerebral thrombosis, cerebral embolism, and cerebrovascular spasm. These four conditions are termed in Western Medicine as "Cerebro-Vascular Accident."

Cervical Spondylosis - a degenerative arthritis (osteoarthritis) of the cervical vertebrae and related tissues.

Chakra - an energetic vortex, spiraling out from the body's center Taiji Pole, and extending through the external field of Wei Qi.

Chakra Gates - the twelve major energy gates located on the center line of the anterior and posterior aspects of the body, as well as at the lower perineum and the top of the head.

Chakra System - the seven major Chakra or energy centers that connect to the Taiji Pole. Five Chakras extend to the front and back of the torso, with one located at the top of the head and the other located on the perineum.

Channels - the body's energetic rivers responsible for transporting Qi, also called "meridians."

Channel Points - areas or points (similar to small pools of Qi) found along the streams of a Channel, through which energy of the Yin and Yang (Zang/Fu) organs and channels are transported internally and externally.

Channel Qi - pertaining to the Qi found within the energetic flow of a channel.

Cholangioles - pertaining to small terminal portions of the bile duct.

Charts of the Hall of Light - ancient diagram depicting the body's internal organs and channels.

Chemotherapy - the application of chemical agents that have a specific and toxic effect upon the disease-causing microorganism, as well as the patient's tissues, energetic fields and immune system.

Chicken Pecking Palm Technique - a palm technique wherein the doctor's hand resembles the head of a chicken while manipulating the energy flow of the Invisible Needle.

Chi Dai - red vaginal discharge.

Child Element - pertaining to the Five Element Creative Cycle of Traditional Chinese Medical, the primary organ is considered the Mother and its sequential organ is considered the Child.

Chinese Massage - one of the four branches of Traditional Chinese Medicine, which involves treating patients through the use of tissue manipulation, including Jie Gu Therapy for Bone disorders, Tui Na Therapy for muscle disorders, Gua Sha Therapy for febrile diseases and Blood Stagnation, An Mo therapy for internal organ disorders, and Jing Point Therapy for channel and internal organ regulation.

Cholecystitis - inflammation of the Gall Bladder.

Cholelithiasis - formation of calcium, i.e., bile stones in the Gall Bladder.

Cholestasis - an infection of the biliary tract.

Chronic - the long duration of a specific disease or condition, showing slow or little improvement.

Chronic Fatigue Syndrome - debilitating fatigue that is not the result of physical or mental exertion, and is not relieved by resting.

Chrono-biology - the science that deals with the study of the body's biological clocks and fluctuations in accordance with the cycles of the sun, moon and nature's rhythms.

Chyluria - the passing of fat globules in the urine.

Circle of Willis - the union of the anterior and posterior cerebral arteries, forming an anastomosis at the base of the Brain.

Circulating Energy Technique - this method refers to rotating Qi in a circular pattern (clockwise or counterclockwise) to move Qi and Blood stagnation, or to gather energy for tonification.

Cirrhosis - Cirrhosis is a generalized Liver disease marked by hepatic lesions, characterized by the formation of dense lobular connective tissue, degenerative changes in the parenchymal cells, structural alterations in the Liver lobules, and sometimes fatty and cellular infiltration within the Liver.

Clairaudience - the ability to hear sounds, music, and voices not audible to normal hearing (for example, receiving Messages and/or inspirations from the divine).

Clairasentience - the ability to perceive smells, taste, touch, emotions and physical sensations that contribute to an overall psychic and intuitive impression.

Clairvoyance - the ability to perceive current objects, events and/or people that may not be discerned through the body's normal senses. Both time and space are perceived on a clairvoyant spiritual dimension.

Clean Qi - Energy which has been purified.

Clinical Ethics - the moral principles and standards governing the doctor's conduct with patients in or away from the clinic.

Coccyx Pass (Wei Lu Guan) - is located on the lowest segment of the spine just posterior to the anus, near the Chang Qiang (GV-1) point.

Colitis - the inflammation of the colon.

Cold - one of the Six Evils

Cold Constitution - pertaining to a physical body innately prone towards coldness.

Collapsed Qi - this is considered a subcategory of Deficient Qi, and is regarded as the third and most severe type of Deficiency.

Collaterals (Luo) - the body's energetic streams that branch off the Twelve Primary Channels and the Conceptional and Governing Vessels.

Collective Unconsciousness - concept of psychiatrist Carl G. Jung pertaining to the memories of mental patterns that are experienced and shared by all mankind.

Coma - an abnormal deep state of unconsciousness with some possible awareness of surroundings, but a total inability to communicate with the outside environment. Comas result from a Qi obstruction to the Brain caused by illness or injury.

Common People's Fire - pertaining to the generated Heat originating from the Urinary Bladder Fire, located in the perineal area of the body.

Compressed Stagnation - a type of stagnation caused by the patient's energy contracting (externally moving inward); Compressed Stagnation feels energetically armored and hollow.

Conception Vessel - one of the Eight Extraordinary Vessels, also known as the "Sea of Yin".

Concentrative Meditation - keeping the mind focused and under control.

Congealed - when Qi and/or Blood become thick and solid within the body's tissues, energetic fields, or both.

Congenital Qi (Prenatal Qi) - energy existing before the fetus is born, acquired from the mother's, father's energies, as well as from the environmental and universal energies. It is sustained through prayer, meditation and sleep.

Conscious Mind - acquired mental reasoning, created through learning via the five senses and interactions with other people.

Constipation - difficulty or infrequent defecation, with the passage of unduly hard and dry fecal material.

Constitutions - see Five Elemental Constitutions.

Contracted Stagnation - stagnation caused by the patient's energy pulling inward, feels armored and solid.

Contraindications - any symptom or circumstance indicating the inappropriateness of a form of treatment that would be otherwise advisable.

Controlling Cycle - pertaining to the Five Element Cycle, where one elemental organ controls the second elemental organ in the Five Elements' Circle.

Corporeal Soul - associated with the Lungs, see Po.

Coryza - the inflammation of the respiratory mucous membranes.

Cosmology - the study of the universe.

Countertransference - this is the process whereby a doctor loses objectivity and unconsciously projects feelings, thoughts, beliefs and patterns of behavior onto the patient.

Couple Point - the Master Point's secondary point of connection affecting the Eight Extraordinary Vessels.

Cranio-Sacral Rhythm - Western term given to the fluctuating rhythm of the Sea of Marrow flowing from the Kidneys.

Creative Cycle - pertaining to the Five Element Cycle, where one organ creates the energy for the next.

Creative Subconscious Mind - the part of the mind that maintains the patient's reality by making him or her act like the person they believe themselves to be.

Creative Visualization - the process of using visualization as a tool for transforming energy and spirit.

Crown Center - the name given to the Baihui Point (GV-20) and Upper Chakra Gate, at the top of the head.

Crystal Palace - the energetic field of Qi located within the third ventricle of the Brain.

Cupping - a technique used in acupuncture therapy in which wooden, clay, or glass cups adhere to the patient's skin by suction, to drain or remove pathogenic Qi from the body's pores.

Curious Organs - the body's Six Extraordinary Yang Organs which function like Yin Organs as they store Yin Essence (i.e., Blood, Marrow, or Kidney Essence), but look like Yang Organs (because they are hollow). These organs consist of the Uterus, Brain, Marrow, Bones, Blood Vessels and Gall Bladder.

Cycle of Disharmony - an emotional state which induces a vicious cycle of physical, mental, emotional, energetic and spiritual disharmony.

Cyst - a closed sac that forms in tissue or a body cavity.

Cystitis - inflammation of the Urinary Bladder, usually occurring secondary to ascending urinary tract infection.

Cytotoxic Treatments - treatment containing toxins which attack the cells of the body (for example: radiation, chemotherapy and toxic herbs).

D

Dacryorrhea - excess tear flow.

Damp - a internal pathogenic condition relating to the storage of Damp or Wet toxins; Damp is one of the Six Evils; long-term Dampness may lead to Phlegm.

Dantians - the body's three main energetic pools, or reservoirs of Qi located in the head, chest and lower abdominal areas.

Dantian Regulation - the principle of balancing the energy governing the body's Three Dantians.

Dao - pertaining to God or divine consciousness.

Daoist - a student of the "Dao" or way of life, pertaining to living in harmony with the universe and environment.

Dao Yin - energy regulation exercises consisting of training the body, mind, and breath.

De - pertaining to an individual's personal Virtue.

Defence Mechanisms - see Ego Defence Mechanisms.

Deficiency (Xu) - a condition relating to the inadequate degree of a particular substance, e.g., Qi, Blood, Yin, Yang, Heat, etc.

Delusions - refers to the occurrence of a mental derangement in the patient resulting in a false belief based on incorrect inference about external reality. Regardless of the evidence to the contrary, the belief is strongly maintained.

Demon or Spirit Oppression - the condition of having a foreign spirit attach to a patient's external Wei Qi field, resulting in emotional disharmony.

Demon or Spirit Possession - the condition of having a foreign spirit invade and inhabit the patient's body, mind, emotion, and spirit.

Denial - a conscious refusal of an impulse-evoking fact, feeling or memory.

Depersonalization Disorder - persistent, recurring episodes of depersonalization, characterized by a feeling of detachment, or estrangement from one's self.

Depression (Major) - a psychological disorder resulting in major sadness and pessimism, feelings of worthlessness, helplessness and hopelessness. Symptoms include overeating or under-eating, insomnia or hyper-insomnia, difficulty concentrating, and fatigue. In Traditional Chinese Medicine, depression often emanates from Liver Qi Stagnation.

Descending - the action of energy moving downward.

Diabetes - a general term used to describe diseases characterized by excessive urination and a sugar imbalance in the Blood.

Diaphoresis - profuse sweating.

Diastolic - the resting phase of the Heart.

Diathermy - the therapeutic use of a high-frequency current to generate Heat within a certain area of the body.

Di Qi - Earth (Environmental) Energy.

Disharmony - pertaining to a lack of adequate balance of energy.

Disorder - an abnormal state of physical, mental, emotional, energetic or spiritual disharmony.

Dispersing - the spreading of Qi to other parts of the body, or purging of pathogenic energy from the body.

Displacement - the shifting of impulses aroused by one person, or situation to a safe target.

Dissociated Identity Disorder - new terminology used for multiple personality disorder.

Distance Therapy - also called External Qi Therapy, Qi Emission and Outgoing Qi Therapy, is defined as extending or projecting energy into a patient from a distance.

Divergent Channels - twelve secondary channels that parallel the Twelve Primary Channels.

Divine - pertaining to God.

Divine Center - referring to the North Star's stable position in the sky.

Divine Hook-Up - the Qigong doctor's initial preparation for therapy, wherein he or she connects with the divine for guidance.

Divine Therapy - long distance Qigong healing.

D.M.Q. - a licensed Doctor of Medical Qigong Therapy, presently only obtainable in China.

Dong - the Yang method of dynamic Postural Dao Yin training.

Dragon's Mouth Palm Technique - hand technique wherein the thumb touches the other four fingers of the hand, forming an image of the head of a dragon. This hand manipulation is used for leading and pulling the Qi.

Draining Qi - drawing off or releasing pathogenic energy from a specific organ area or channel of the patient's body.

Dredging - a type of energetic purging, used to clean the patient's energetic fields and channels.

Drilling Energy Technique - this method refers to rotating Qi in a spiraling pattern (clockwise or counterclockwise) to access the energy deep inside the patient's body.

Dry - one of the Six Evils

Dryness - a internal pathogenic condition relating to the storage of Dry toxins (i.e., dry mucus membranes resulting from a lack of Body Fluids).

Dynamic Qigong - energy gathering which utilizes active movements of the body.

Dysmenorrhea - painful menstruation.

Dyspepsia - painful digestion.

Dyspeptic - one afflicted with dyspepsia.

Dysphagia - difficulty in swallowing.

Dysphoria - exaggerated feeling of depression, anxiety and unrest.

Dysplasia - the abnormal development of tissue.

Dyspnea - air hunger, resulting in difficult breathing, shortness of breath, sometimes accompanied by pain.

Dysthymia - a chronic, form of depression (lasting at least two years), for children and adolescents the mood can be irritable rather than sad.

E

Earth Element - one of the Five Elements, pertaining to the Spleen and the Stomach.

Earth Energy (Qi) - Energy pertaining to the Earth and surrounding environment.

Earth Jing - energy that supervises the maturation phase of the fetus's ability for emotional and spiritual bonding during the seventh month of pregnancy.

Earthly Branches - twelve energies of the Earth

GLOSSARY OF TERMS

represented in the human body as the Twelve Primary Channels.

Earth Transpersonal Point - pertaining to the body's energetic connection to the Earth, located several feet beneath the feet.

ECG (or EKG) Eletrocardiogram - a graphic record made by an instrument that measures the Heart's electrical activity; usually used to confirm a diagnosis of a Heart condition.

Eclampsia - coma and convulsive seizures (between the 20th week of pregnancy and first week postpartum). Symptoms result in edema of the legs and feet, puffiness of the face, hypertension, severe headaches, dizziness, epigastric pain, nausea, sudden convulsive seizures and coma.

Eczema - an acute or chronic inflammation of the skin.

Edema - an acute or chronic cutaneous inflammatory condition.

EEG Electroencephalogram - a graphic record made by an instrument that measures the brain's electrical activity and records it as patterns of fluctuating waves.

Ego - the ego is the mediator between the id and the superego. According to Dr. Sigmund Freud's psychoanalytical theory, the superego combines the critical inner parent aspect with the idealistic aspect of the individual's conscience; the id consists of unconscious drives and instincts. The ego as meditator is responsible for ensuring rational behavior.

Ego Defense Mechanisms - according to Dr. Sigmund Freud's psychoanalytical theory, the ego defence mechanisms include: Repression, Displacement, Projection, Intellectualization, Regression, Fixation, Denial, Reaction-Formation, and Sublimation.

Eight Confluential Points - the areas where the Eight Extraordinary Vessels and Twelve Primary Channels intersect with each other.

Eight Energetic Principles (Eight Principle Theory) - a system of differential diagnosis using four pairs of opposites (Yin and Yang, Cold and Hot, Deficient and Excess, Internal and External).

Eight Energetic Touches - pertaining to the somatic tissue response to energy stimulation (tingling, sensations of Heat, coldness, expansiveness, contracted, heaviness, lightness, and vibration).

Eight Extraordinary Vessels (Ancestral Channels) - the primary channels responsible for the formation of the fetus, which after birth, are considered the body's reservoirs for collecting the overflow energy from the Twelve Primary Channels.

Eight Miscellaneous Factors - eight factors that can off set the patient's Yin and Yang balance (diet, overexertion, excessive sex, child bearing, traumatic injuries, exposure to poisons, parasites, and iatrogenic disorders).

Eight Trigrams (Bagua) - eight cosmological patterns of three lines (solid and/or broken), called Yaos, used to diagnose as well as predict future transitions.

Emaciation - the state of being malnourished and extremely lean.

Embolus - a plug, composed of a thrombus or vegetation, mass of bacteria, or other foreign body obstructing a vessel.

Embolism - the obstruction of a Blood Vessel by foreign substances or a Blood clot.

EMG Electromyogram - a graphic record made by an instrument that measures the muscle's electrical activity and records its function.

Emitting Qi - the Qigong doctor extending energy outside the body for the purpose of treating a patient.

Emotional Energy Body - is the external energy existing in the body's second field of Wei Qi, which is attached to the internal organs.

Emotional Spirit - pertaining to the Emotional Energy Body.

Empathic Communication - the doctor's ability to experience the feelings and thoughts of his/her patients.

Empty Qi - a serious weakness or Deficiency of the body's Qi.

Encephalomyelitis - acute inflammation of the Brain and spinal cord.

Endrometrial Hyperplasia - excessive proliferation of the cells within the lining of the Uterus.

Energetic Armoring - a condition resulting from the patient protecting specific tissues, organs, or areas of the body. Energetic armoring is initiated when the patient freezes certain emotional feelings to maintain the denial system.

Energetic Barriers (Energetic Boundaries) - the protective barriers existing within and outside of the body's tissues.

Energetic Complications - pertaining to energetic imbalances within the patient's tissues (e.g., compressed energy stagnation, energetic armoring, migrating Qi deviations, etc.)

Energetic Cords - energetic bands of light and vibration which form an emotional attachment, connecting the patient to certain people, places, or things.

Energetic Grids - an energetic net covering the surface of Heaven, Earth or the human body.

Energetic Leakage - a condition resulting from the leaking of Qi from the joints, due to an injury or unconscious sabotage.

Energetic Medicine - any and all medicine having to do with the stimulation, cultivation, tonification, purgation, balance and maintenance of the body's Qi.

Energetic Point Therapy - Emitting Qi into specific channel points or vessels on the body.

Enteric Nervous System - pertaining to the nervous system of the Small Intestine.

Enuresis - the involuntary discharge of urine.

Environmental Energy (Qi) - Energy pertaining to the Earth and surrounding environment.

Environmental Force - energy pertaining to the Earth and surrounding environment.

Epigastric Pain - pain in the region over the pit of the Stomach.

Epileptiform - having the form of epilepsy.

Epistaxis - bleeding of the nose.

Epithelial Hyperplasia - excessive proliferation of the cells within the outer surface of the body, including the secreting portions of the glands and ducts.

Essence (Jing) - referring to either Prenatal and Postnatal energetic tissue mass.

Eternal Soul - the individual's True Self, which is always connected to the divine. It is absorbed into the mother's egg at the time of conception, and is rooted within the body's Taiji Pole.

Ethereal Souls - associated with the Liver, see Hun.

Etiology - the causes of a disease.

Eustachian Tubes - the auditory tube, extending from the middle ear to the pharynx.

Evil Embryo - pertaining to a toxic formation in the form of a tumor or cancer mass.

Evil Influences - pathogenic factors that can be either physical, mental, emotional, energetic or spiritual.

Evil Qi (Xie Qi) - also called Pathogenic Qi, Perverse Qi, Toxic Qi, and Heteropathic Qi, is energy that causes disease or harmful effects to the body.

Evil States - a condition wherein the patient experiences mental delusions, obsessions, infatuations with the doctor, spiritual oppression or possession.

Evil Wind - toxic Wind that invades the body, tissues or organs.

Excess - a condition relating to the over abundance of a particular substance. (e.g., Heat, Wind, Damp, Cold, etc.).

Exopathogenic - a disease or pathogen originating outside of the body.

Extended Fan Palm Technique - hand technique where the fingers separate like a Chinese fan, used for extending energy through the doctor's palm.

External Pathogenic Factors - an external invasion of Heat, Damp, Cold, Dryness, or Wind, or a combination thereof.

External Qi Therapy - a technique used in Medical Qigong therapy which pertains to Qi being emitted onto a patient.

Extraordinary Organs - also called Curious Organs, these six organs are shaped like Yang (Hollow) organs but function like Yin organs. The Brain stores Marrow, the Marrow stores Kidney Jing, the Bones store Marrow, the Blood vessels store the Blood, the Gall Bladder stores the bile, and the Uterus stores Kidney Jing, Blood, and Qi.

Extraordinary Vessels - secondary channels that flow in conjunction with the body's Twelve Primary Channels.

Extra Point - a point with a definite location, but not originating on the fourteen main channels.

F

False Cold (Pseudo Cold) - a clinical condition wherein Heat has become stagnated within the Interior of the body and the patient experiences symptoms of cold in the extremities.

False Heat (Pseudo Heat) - a clinical condition wherein an overabundance of Cold is transformed into Heat within the Interior of the body and the patient experiences symptoms of Heat in the extremities.

False Self - pertaining to the dark emotional side of the self, i.e., the masks and defence mechanisms that serve to protect the individual from dealing with his or her issues.

Fascia - a fibrous membrane covering, supporting, and separating the muscles, as well as uniting the skin with the body's underlying tissues.

Febrile Diseases - any and all diseases which cause the body to produce a fever.

Feng Shui (Wind and Water) - the study of harmonizing the energetic flow of Wind and Water, and the healing art of adjusting the person's environment to create improvements in the person's health and life.

Fetal Education - regulating the mother's behavior to improve her child's physical, emotional, and mental health is called "fetal education" in Traditional Chinese Medicine, and is important in the development of the child's Prenatal Essence, Energy, and Spirit.

Fetal Leakage - after conception, if a small amount of Bloody fluid discharges from a woman's vagina, it is known as Tai Lou or fetal leakage.

Fibroadenoma - a tumor with fibrous tissue, forming a dense covering.

Fire - one of the Five Elements, pertaining to the Heat and can be transformed into a pathogenic condition

Fire Element - one of the Five Elements, pertaining to the Heart, Small Intestine, Pericardium, and Triple Burners.

Fire Jing - energy that controls the development phase of the fetus's emotional and spiritual well-being during the fifth month of pregnancy.

Five Agents - the five energies that are linked to the moral qualities of a person's inner characteristics (the five virtues stored within the body's Wood, Fire, Earth, Metal and Water elements).

Five Elements - Wood, Fire, Earth, Metal and Water.

Five Element Animals - Green Dragon, Red Phoenix, White Tiger, Black (Indigo) Turtle, and Yellow Phoenix.

Five Elemental Constitutions - physical constitutions based upon the observation of the Five Elemental formations within the human body.

Five Element Organs - the organs related to the Five Elements, including: Wood - Liver and Gall Bladder; Fire - Heart and Small Intestine (Pericardium and Triple Burners); Earth - Spleen and Stomach; Metal - Lungs and Large Intestine; Water - Kidneys and Urinary Bladder.

Five Energetic Fields - pertaining to the body's five levels of energy, including: The External Wei Qi Fields, Internal Ying Qi Field, Sea of Blood, Sea of Marrow, and Center Core of Light (Taiji Pole).

Five Flavors (Five Tastes) - sour, bitter, sweet, pungent, and salty.

Five Major Yang (Fu) Organs - also called the Five Bowels, they are the body's five hollow organs: Gall Bladder, Small Intestine, Stomach, Large Intestine, and Urinary Bladder.

Five Major Yin (Zang) Organs - are the body's five solid organs: Liver, Heart, Spleen, Lungs and Kidneys.

Five Orbs - pertaining to the 5 Yin internal organs (Liver, Heart, Spleen, Lungs and Kidneys), their complete organ system, and the surrounding areas that they influence.

Five Palms Hot - a condition in which the patient feels a hot sensation in the palms and soles of the feet, accompanied by Heat and agitation of the chest and/or head area.

Five Passes - five important gates on the Governing Vessel located at the coccyx, Mingmen, Shendao, occiput and Baihui, where energy tends to stagnate.

Five Portals of the Earthly Yin Gate - pertaining to the five points at the bottom of the perineum through which the Qi of Earth enters into the body.

Five Portals of the Heavenly Yang Gate - pertaining to the five points at the top of the head through which the Qi of Heaven enters into the body.

Five Sense Organs - eyes, tongue, mouth, nose and ears.

Five Thunder Fingers Technique - hand manipulation technique wherein the fingers and thumb are rapidly extended from a closed soft fist, to strike with Qi for dispersing stagnations.

Five Thrusting Channels - see Thrusting Channels.

Five Tissues - tendons, Blood vessels, muscles, skin and Bones.

Five Zhi - in connection with the five mental aspects of the Mind, the Hun (Ethereal Soul), Po (Corporeal Soul), the Shen (Spirit), the Yi (Intellect), and the Zhi (willpower) are sometimes referred to as the Five Zhi.

Fixation - has the same result as regression, but the person becomes fixated at a particular stage of mental and emotional development.

Flat Palm Detection - an extended palm technique used for sensing and diagnosing.

Four Bigs - pertaining to severe excess of fever, sweating, thirst, and pulse.

Four Doors - the center of each palm and foot.

Four Winds - pertaining to the Energy of the four compass points. (North - back, South - front, West - right, and East - left.)

Fu Organs - Yang or hollow organs (Gall Bladder, Small Intestine, Stomach, Large Intestine, and Urinary Bladder). The Fu Organs operate primarily to relieve the Zang (Yin) Organs of toxic energies and wastes.

G

Gallow's Syndrome - laughing at a very painful experience instead of grieving or crying.

Gastritis - the inflammation of the Stomach.

Gastroptosis - the downward displacement of the Stomach.

Gate of Access - the passageway between life and death, believed to be related to the stars of the Big Dipper.

Gate of the Moon - the western energetic region, which the sun must pass through in order to create Autumn.

Gathering the Immortal's Water (Juice of Jade) - pertaining to the energetic production of the saliva used to create the "Immortal Pill."

Gathering Qi - also called Respiratory Qi, Collection Qi, Chest Qi, Pectoral Qi, and Big Qi of the Chest. It is derived from the conversion of the purest and most potent forms of the body's Jing (particularly sexual fluids, hormones, and neurochemicals).

Ghosts (Gui) - disembodied spirits.

Ghost Points - points used for the treatment of emotional and spiritual disorders.

Gland - an organ that produces a hormone or other secretion.

Golden Gate in the East - the Eastern energetic region, which the sun must pass through in order to create Spring.

Gong - meaning skill or study.

Gout - sudden intense pain in a joint, usually the big toe or ankle, followed by swelling, inflammation and Heat in the joint (in extreme cases alternating chills and fever are experienced).

Grandmother Element - pertaining to the Five Element Creative Cycle of Traditional Chinese Medical, the primary organ is considered the Mother and its previous organ is considered the Grandmother.

Grain Qi (Gu Qi, Nutritive Energy) - Energy derived from food and drink and processed by the Spleen and Stomach.

Grounding - see Rooting.

Gua Sha Therapy - an external "surface" tissue scraping technique commonly used to clear Excess Heat from the body and remove stagnation.

Guiding Qi - the technique of leading Qi.

Gu Qi (Grain Qi, Nutritive Energy) - Energy derived from food and drink and processed by the Spleen and Stomach.

Gui - ghosts or spirits.

H

Hai - means sea.

Healing Tones - resonant sounds used to purge the body of pathogens.

Heart Fire - pertaining to the energy of the Heart, which is responsible for transforming the body's Energy into Spirit. This occurs in the chamber of the Heart's courtyard (the Yellow Court).

Heaven Qi - also known as Heavenly Qi, this energy pertains to the Heavens, the divine and the celestial influences.

Heavenly Stems - the ten energies of Heaven represented in the human body as the Yin and Yang aspects of the Five Elements or ten major internal organs.

Heavenly Transpersonal Point - pertaining to the body's energetic connection to the Heavens, located two to five feet above the head.

Hei Xia - dark brown or black vaginal discharge.

Hematuria - Blood in the urine.

Hemiparalysis - paralysis on one side of the body

Hemiplegia - paralysis on only one side of the body.

Hemoptysis - the expectoration of Blood.

Hepatitis - inflammation of the Liver.

Hepatolithiasis - calculi or concretions in the Liver.

Hepatomegaly - enlargement of the Liver.

Hepatosplenomegaly - the enlargement of both the Spleen and Liver.

Herbal Therapy - one of the four branches of Traditional Chinese Medicine, which involves treating patients through the use of formulas created through teas, soups, tinctures, wines, oils, balms, liniments and pills to stimulate energy flow.

Herbalist - a doctor of Herbal Therapy.

Herpes Simplex I - an infectious disease caused by the herpes simplex virus. This disease is characterized by thin-walled vesicles that occur in the skin, usually at a site where the mucus membrane joins the skin, above the waist area.

Herpes Simplex 2 - an infectious disease caused by the herpes simplex virus. This disease is characterized by thin-walled vesicles that occur in the skin, usually at a site where the mucus membrane joins the skin, below the waist area.

Hexagram - a six line symbol representing the function and flow of Yin and Yang energy, formed by stacking two Trigrams on top of each other.

Hibernation Breathing - a breathing method which includes inhaling and exhaling through every pore on the body's surface, from the body's Center Core (Taiji Pole).

Hidden Power (An Jing) - techniques that emphasize stretching and twisting the tendons and ligaments (known as Reeling and Pulling the Silk) to cultivate resonant vibration within the body for striking and breaking up energetic stagnations or tissue masses.

Hollow Organs - the body's Yang organs, which consist of the Gall Bladder, Small Intestine, Stomach, Large Intestine, Urinary Bladder. Also included in this list are the Triple Burners.

Hologram - pertaining to the body's energetic three dimensional image.

Hook-Up - see divine Hook-Up.

Hostile Forces - dark spiritual forces which seek to influence the physical, mental, emotional, energetic and spiritual life of an individual.

Hot Constitution - pertaining to a physical body innately prone towards Heat.

Hot Evil - also known as Evil Heat, a pathogenic condition causing Excess patterns that are Hot and Yang in nature.

Hou Tian Zhi Qi (Postnatal Qi) - translates to mean "after the baby sees the Heavens."

Hua Jing - see Mysterious Power.

Huang - any membranous tissue.

Hua Sound Resonation - Mysterious or Spiritual Sound Resonation.

Huang Dai - yellow vaginal discharge.

Hui Yin Point (CV-1) - Conception Vessel point located between the scrotum (or vagina) and the anal sphincter.

Human Force - the energy or force manifesting from inside of the human body, as well as the within the human energetic field.

Humor - any fluid or semifluid substance in the body.

Hun (Ethereal Soul) - the Three Ethereal Souls which are the spiritual part of man that ascends to Heaven upon the death of the body. The Hun is stored in the Liver.

Hunter Killer Cells - the body's neutrophils and macrophages, as well as the interferons and antibodies.

Hun Yuan - the body's internal energies that has been combined and fused into the Lower Dantian area.

Hyperbilirubinemia - excessive amounts of bilirubin (the orange-colored or yellowish pigment in bile) in the Blood.

Hyperhidrosis - excessive sweating due to an over-activity of the sweat glands.

Hypertension - high Blood pressure.

Hyperthyroidism - a condition caused by excessive secretions of the thyroid glands, resulting in an increased metabolic rate and the consumption of food to support this increased metabolic activity.

Hypertrophy - the increase in the size of an organ or structure that does not involve tumor formation.

Hypochondriac Pain - pain in the upper lateral region on each side of the body below the thorax and beneath the ribs.

Hypomania - a milder form of mania and excitement with moderate change in behavior.

Hyposmia - a deficient sense to smell.

Hypotension - low Blood pressure.

I

Iatrogenic Disorders - any adverse mental or physical disorder induced in a patient from the treatment by a doctor or surgeon.

I-Ching - see Yi-Jing

Id - Dr. Sigmund Freud's terminology for one of the three divisions of the psyche in Psychoanalytic Theory that is the unconscious source of psychic energy responsible for the body's drives and instincts.

Immortal's Pill - pertaining to the energetic production of Heaven and Earth Qi, in conjunction with the saliva.

Immortal's Water - when meditating, another word for energized saliva.

Incontinence - an inability to control urination, involuntary urination when coughing, laughing, sneezing, running, or performing some other physical activity. This condition can also refer to involuntary defecation.

Indole - A solid, crystalline substance found in feces. It is the bases of many biologically active substances formed in degeneration of tryptophan and is largely responsible for the odor of feces.

Infatuations - refers to the patient feeling intensely amorous towards the doctor.

Influenza - an acute contagious respiratory infection, characterized by a sudden onset, with chills, fever and headache.

Inner-vision - the skill of observing images of the internal organs, and energetic fields relating to the body, mind, emotion and spirit, and their transition stages.

Insight Meditation - focusing on sensual stimuli (sounds, smells, colors, etc.) while meditating.

Insomnia - a sleeping disorder resulting in the inability to sleep.

Insulting Cycle - pertaining to the Five Elemental Cycle, wherein the Child Element counter attacks the Grandmother Element.

Intellectualization - an elaborate rationalization of a naked impulse, to justify it.

Interferons - a group of proteins released by the white Blood cells and fibroblasts, responsible for fighting infection.

Interjection - the insertion or interpose the energetic pattern.

Internal Dialogues - internal conversations, which are part of the patient's personal belief structure.

Internal Pathogenic Factors - pertaining to diseases originating from the body's internal organs and emotions (e.g., anger, fear, grief, worry, etc.).

Internal Viewing - technique used by the Qigong doctor to view the patient's internal organs.

Interpersonal Relationships - close personal relationships, relating to self and others.

Invading Cycle - pertaining to the Five Elemental Cycle, wherein the Grandmother Element overcontrols the Child Element.

Invisible Needle Therapy - the insertion of invisible energetic needles into the patient's body to stimulate energy flow.

Invisible Needle Palm Technique - Qi emission in which energy is emitted in a very fine line, to stimulate specific channel points.

J

Jaundice - a condition due to deposition of the bile, characterized by the yellowing of the skin, eyes, mucous membranes and Body Fluids.

Jia Ji Guan (Spinal Pass) - two points located on the lateral sides of the Mingmen (GV-4) where Qi can become stagnant.

Jie Gu Therapy - a tissue manipulation therapy that focuses on the adjustment of Bones and ligaments.

Jin - Body Fluids whose function is to moisten.

Jing - the human body's Essence, divided into Prenatal and Postnatal Essence.

Jing Luo - the body's channels and collaterals.

Jing Point Therapy - the original term for Channel Point Therapy or Acupressure.

Jing Shen Bing - pertains to all types of mental illness.

Jiu Wei (Yellow Court) - located in the center of the diaphragm, below the xiphoid process of the sternum. Its function is that of being the access point to release emotional memories from the body's internal organs. Its location is attributed to the 3rd Chakra.

Jue Yin (Reverting Yin) - associated with the most severe diseases, indicates Yin Qi developing its final stage and then reverting into Yang. Jue Yin is categorized with the Liver and Pericardium Channels.

Juice of Jade - Energized saliva produced in meditation practices.

K

Karma - the manifestation of consequences to our actions and beliefs: "As you sew, so shall you reap."

Karmic Related Illness - pertaining to spiritual illnesses, which can be either congenital or acquired.

Ketheric Matter or Substance - pertaining to the spiritual energy located within the third external field of Wei Qi.

Kidney Fire (Mingmen Fire) - the energy that heats the body's Essence (Jing), and dominates all Twelve Primary Channels. It is the motivating force of the body.

Kinetic Communication - the intuition of the physical body, felt by the Qigong doctor as a movement in or of his or her own body.

Kneading Tiger Palm Technique - hand manipulation technique resembling the movement of a tiger kneading the ground, used for dispersing Qi stagnations.

Kyphotic - the exaggeration or angulation of the normal posterior curve of the spine (humpback).

L

Laogong (Pc-8) - Pericardium Channel point located at the center of each palm.

Large Heaven Cycle (Macrocosmic Orbit) - Qigong Meditation which connects the Qi of the extremities to the Qi within the Governing and Conception Vessels.

Leading Qi - technique of manipulating the patient's Qi by using a guiding gesture with the hands.

Leukocyte - the body's white Blood corpuscles, which included lymphocytes and other immune system cells.

Leukorrhea - an acute or chronic disease caused by the unregulated clonal proliferation of stem cells within the Blood forming tissues.

Ley Lines - the energetic pathways that connect energy spots on the planet.

Life Force Energy - Qi.

Light Energy Therapy - color, light projection and visualization used for healing.

Light of the Dao - divine healing light energy.

Lipid Bilayers - the outer membrane of most cells, includes two layers of lipid molecules.

Lithotripsy - crushing of a calculus in the Urinary Bladder or urethra.

Liver Wind - terminology used to describe excess Heat generated from a toxic Liver condition which can cause pathogenic symptoms. Liver Wind often stems from Liver Blood and Yin Deficiency.

Lobular - composed of small lobes.

Lords of the Three Dantians - three spiritual energies used to describe the energetic aspects of the human soul (Tai Yi, Si Ming and Xia Tao Kang).

Lo Scroll (Magic Square) - a tool used for diagnosis and treatment of disorders through number configurations, which correspond to the Late-Heaven sequence of the Trigrams of the Yi-Jing (I-Ching).

Lower Burner - area of the body in the Lower Dantian, responsible for the separation of Clean and Dirty Fluids. It also facilitates the production of urine.

Lower Dantian - area in the center of the lower abdomen, attributed to the body's chamber of Heat and physical power. The Lower Dantian is also known as the Sea of Energy, Pill of Immortality, Root of life, Source of Generating Qi, Five Qi Collection Seat, Progenitor of Life, Stove of Spirit, Root of Heaven, and Cinnabar Field.

Lower Unconsciousness - pertaining to the acquired mind which is connected to the primal senses.

Lumbago - dull, aching pain in the lumbar region of the lower back.

Luo - translates as "a net or web," and in Traditional Chinese Medicine it refers to the Connecting Vessels (i.e., the Fifteen Collaterals).

These vessels are the major "passage ways" for the circulation of the body's channel energy, emerging out of the Luo (pathway) points on the Twelve Primary Channels (plus the Governing and Conception Vessels).

Luo Points - are the major intersecting points of the Fifteen Collaterals. The Luo points are located below the elbows and knees and provide an additional energetic barrier to keep Evil Winds from affecting the Twelve Primary Channels, being somewhat deeper then the Muscle/Tendon Channels.

Lymphocytes - immune cells present in the Blood and lymphatic tissue.

Lymphoma - a group of malignant solid tumors of the lymphoid tissue.

Lymphosarcoma - a sarcoma of the lymphatic system.

M

Macrocosmic Orbit - Qigong Meditation which connects the Qi of the Governing and Conception Vessels with the extremities of the body.

Macrophages - the major phagocytic cells of the immune system (also known as Hunter Killer Cells).

Magic Square - also known as the Lo Scroll, a tool used for diagnosis and treatment of disorders through number configurations corresponding to the Late-Heaven sequence of the Trigrams of the Yi-Jing (I-Ching).

Magnetic Energy Therapy - magnetic energy affecting the body's channels and points via electromagnetic field stimulation.

Malar Flushes - pertaining to flushed skin along the cheeks.

Malignant - detrimental; growing worse; threatening to produce death.

Man Qi - general term used to describe the energy relating to the body, mind, emotion, energy and spirit of both men and women. In the body, the area between the navel and the lower sternum correspond to "Man."

Manic Depressive Personality Disorder - see Bipolar Personality Disorder

Mantra - a Sanskrit word, meaning a spiritual phase or sound repeated internally or externally, used as a tool in meditation to induce an altered state of consciousness.

Marrow - derived from the Kidneys, nourishes the Brain, spinal cord and forms the Bone Marrow.

Master Point - the main point of energy interaction on a specific channel, used to affect another organ system or channel energy flow.

Mastitis - inflammation of the breast.

Medical Qigong - one of the four branches of Traditional Chinese Medicine.

Menorrhagia - excessive bleeding during the time of menstruation.

Menoxenia - the pathological changes of menstruation occurring in a woman's cycle, affecting the color, quantity and quality of Blood flow.

Mental Delusions - the occurrence of mental derangement in the patient resulting from a false belief based on an incorrect inference regarding external reality. This belief is firmly sustained despite incontrovertible evidence to the contrary.

Meridians - the body's channels or rivers of Energy.

Mesenchymal - a diffused network of cells forming the embryonic mesoderm, and eventually creating the connective tissues, Blood and Blood Vessels, lymphatic system and the cells of the reticuloendothelial system.

Message (Xin Xi) - knowledge stored within the Wuji or the Void.

Metal Element - one of the Five Elements, relating to the Lungs and Large Intestine.

Metal Jing - Energy that supervises the development phase of the fetus's ability for emotional attachment and bonding during the sixth month of pregnancy.

Metrorrhagia - bleeding from the Uterus.

Microcosmic Orbit - energetic orbits that circulate the Qi within the body's energetic channels; divided into Fire, Water and Wind pathways.

Micturition - discharging urine.

Middle Burner - area of the body pertaining to the body's digestive system, responsible for transporting Gu Qi (derived from food and drink).

Middle Dantian - area in the center of the chest, attributed to the body's chamber of emotional and vibrational power. The Qi of the Middle Dantian is called Zong Qi. Zong Qi is translated as Gathering Qi, Ancestral Qi, Genetic Qi, or Essential Qi. The Middle Dantian is also known as Middle Field of Elixir, Scarlet Palace, Central Altar, Middle Sea of Energy, Courtyard of the Heart, Opening of Suspended Gold, and the Seat of Emotion.

Middle Emotional/Mental Barrier - the second and middle energetic barrier of the Wei Qi fields.

Mind Regulation - the principles governing the conduct, action or functions of the mind.

Ming Jing - see Obvious Power.

Mingmen (Gate Of Life, GV-4) - area in the lower back responsible for heating the body, in particular the Kidneys and Lower Dantian.

Mingmen Fire (also known as Kidney Fire, Advisor Fire, or Ministerial Fire,) - the Energy that heats the body's Essence (Jing), and dominates all Twelve Primary Channels. It is the motivating force of the body.

Ming Sound Resonation - Obvious or Audible Sound Resonation.

Ministerial Fire - pertaining to the Energy responsible for heating the Middle Burner.

Monocytes - A mononuclear phagocyte white Blood cell derived from the myeloid stem cells.

Moon Essence - energy gathered during meditation from the moon's Essence in the form of cool light.

Morphogenic Field - pertaining to the form of the energetic field of Jing.

Mother and Child Therapy - the Traditional Chinese Medical description of the primary organ (Mother) and its sequential organ (Child) in the Five Elemental Creative Cycle.

Mother Element - pertaining to the Five Element Creative Cycle, the primary organ is considered the "mother."

Moxa Therapy (Mugwart, Ai Ye) - herb heated and applied in a clinical setting for tonification of Yang.

Multiple Personality Disorder - also called Identity Disorder, is a mental state in which the patient develops "alter" personalities as a coping mechanism in dealing with severe emotional traumas.

Multiple-Sclerosis (MS) - an inflammatory disease of the central nervous system in which infiltrating lymphocytes degrade the myelin sheath of nerves.

Muscle/Tendon Channels - channel connections to the body's muscles, tendons, ligaments and other connective tissues.

Myalgic Encephalomyelitis - acute inflammation of the Brain and spinal cord.

Myocarditis - the inflammation of the cardiac muscle (located in the middle layer of the walls of the Heart).

Myoma - a uterine tumor that is a solid benign growth in the myometrium, often called a fibroid, containing muscle tissue.

Myophagism - a condition where the macrophages destroy (eats) muscular tissue.

Mysterious Pass - the space between Yin and Yang where infinite space and time (Wuji) exists.

Mysterious Power (Hua Jing) - techniques which emphasize training and conditioning the mind's imagination and intention, to project and utilize the power of the individual's Shen (Spirit).

N

Nebula - a translucent fog-like opacity of the cornea.

Necrosis - part of an area of tissues or Bone that is dying or dead and may spread to healthy tissues or Bones.

Nei Dan Shu - internal elixir cultivation, that focuses on cultivating Qi from within the individual's body.

Nei Gong (Internal Skill) - the training of the body's tendons, Bone, breath, mind, emotion, and spirit to facilitate internal power.

Nei Guan (Internal Viewing) - see inner vision.

Nei Jing - the Yellow Emperor's classics on Chinese internal medicine.

Neoplasm - a new or abnormal formation of tissue, as in a tumor growth.

Nephritis - inflammation of the Kidneys.

Neurasthenia - unexplained chronic fatigue and lassitude.

Neutrophils - the most common type of granulocytic white Blood cell, responsible for fighting infection.

Nine Dantian Chambers - the nine internal cavities established within the energetic matrix of each Dantian.

Nine Palaces - the Later-Heaven sequence of the Trigrams of the Yi-Jing (I-Ching), represented in the human body as the Eight Extraordinary Vessels and the Taiji Pole.

Nine Star System - pertaining to the total development of the three periods of life and the three star developmental sequence.

Noxious Qi (Turbid Qi) - coarse, Toxic, Evil, unrefined, polluted, or dirty Energy.

O

Objective World - pertaining to the spiritual world existing outside an individual's thoughts or feelings.

Obstructed Qi - Energy that is immobile.

Obstruction - the inhibition of the flow of Qi or Blood, caused by Cold, Damp, Heat and Wind, etc.

Obvious Power (Ming Jing) - techniques that emphasize the training and conditioning of the muscles, strengthening the Bone structure, and increasing the individual's overall stamina. This school also includes such techniques as pounding the body (arms, hands, legs, and torso) to strengthen and toughen the tissues.

Occipital Pass (Yu Zhen Guan) - the area located just inferior to the occipital Bone where the Brain originates (according to energetic embryology), known as a specific point where Qi often stagnates.

Oliguria - diminished amount of urine formation.

Omniscient Sight - the ability to see 360 degrees simultaneously.

One Finger Skill Technique - clinical modality involving Energy extension employed through a single finger.

Ontology - the study of the historical development of an individual.

Opening and Closing - the method of leading Qi into and out of specific internal organs, the Triple Burners areas, or one of the Three Dantians, via the hands.

Opisthotonosis - a form of spasm in which the patient's head and heels are bent backwards, and the body is bowed forward.

Organ Dysfunction - the impaired or abnormal function of an internal organ.

Organ Regulation - technique for balancing the action or functional principles of the internal organs.

Organ Qi - Energy of the body's Yin and Yang organs.

Original Spirit (Yuan Shen) - see Prenatal Spirit.

Original Qi (Yuan Qi) - pertaining to the body's Prenatal Qi acquired from both parents at conception, and from the mother during gestation.

Original Force - pertaining to the Heavenly energy, manifesting as the energy of the entire cosmos.

Original Yang - pertaining to the body's Prenatal Kidney Yang.

Original Yin - pertaining to the body's Prenatal Kidney Yin.

Osteoarthritis - a chronic disease involving the joints and the deterioration of the articular cartilage.

Osteoporosis - a general term used for describing any disease process that results in the reduction of Bone mass.

Osteosarcoma - a sarcoma of the Bones.

Outer Spiritual Barrier - the third and furthermost energetic barrier of the Wei Qi fields.

Overcontrolling Cycle - pertaining to one of the Five Elemental Cycles, where one organ overcontrols the second elemental organ in the Five Elements' Circle.

P

Palace of Eternal Frost - the northern energetic region, which the sun must pass through in order to create Winter.

Palace of Universal Yang - the southern energetic region, which the sun must pass through in order to create Summer.

Palpitations - an abnormal rapid, throbbing, or fluttering of the Heart.

Pancreatitis - inflammation of the pancreas.

Panic Attack - overwhelming panic and sense of impending doom, resulting in hyperventilation (breathlessness), Heart palpitations and visual distortions.

Papillary Masses - small, nipple-like protuberances or elevated tissue masses.

Paraplegia - paralysis on both sides of the body.

Parenchymal Cells - the essential parts of an organ's cells that are concerned with the organ's function.

Parkinson's Disease - a chronic nervous disease characterized by muscular weakness, rigidity and a fine, slow tremor.

Past Life Regression - pertaining to the patient's exploration and experiences of previous lives.

Pathogenic (Evil) - disease-causing; see Internal Pathogenic Factors and External Pathogenic Factors.

Penetrating Wind - pertaining to the external pathogen of Wind invading the tissues.

Peptones - pertaining to the term applied to intermediate polypeptide products, formed in partial hydrolysis of proteins, that are soluble in water, diffusible, and not coagulable by Heat.

Peribronchial - surrounding the windpipe (bronchus).

Perineural Cells - the sheath of cells around a bundle of nerve fibers within the perineurium.

Peristalsis - a progressive wave like movement that occurs involuntarily in the hollow tubes of the body.

Peritonitis - inflammation of the abdominal cavity.

Pernicious Influences (Evil) - pertaining to the Six External Factors that cause disease.

Personal Subconscious Mind - part of the mind associated with the recording and storing of personal interpretations of reality.

Peyer's Patch - an aggregation of lymph nodes found chiefly in the ilium.

Phagocytes - cells that have the ability to destroy and ingest bacteria, protozoa, unhealthy cells and cell debris.

Phantom Embryo - an energetic thought form in the shape of an embryo created through the woman's feelings of grief, guilt or remorse after a surgical abortion.

Phantom Organ - the energy of a particular organ which still exists, even after surgical removal.

Phantom Pain - the feeling of pain relating to a particular organ which still energetically exists, even after surgical removal.

Phlegm - pathogenic factor responsible for the formation of diseases including tumors.

Physical Barrier - the first level and closest to the

body of the three Wei Qi energetic barriers.

Piezoelectric - pertaining to the electricity created from pressure, especially pressure on or within the Bones.

Po (Seven Corporeal Souls) - sometimes called the Seven Turbid Demon Natures, this spiritual energy manifests as the physical or material soul of the human body that returns to the Earth at death. The Po are associated with the Lungs.

Points - specific areas on the body where energy can intersect to travel externally to internally, or visa versa.

Point Respiration - exercise which requires breathing into a specific channel point, organ, or area of the body.

Polarity - opposite negative and positive qualities of power.

Polergeists - malevolent spiritual entities. Parapsychology research indicates that poltergeist activity is often the manifestation of a psychokinetic ability.

Polydipsia - excessive thirst.

Polyphagia - eating abnormally large amounts of food at a meal.

Polyuria - the excessive secretion and discharge of urine.

Portal Hypertension - the increased pressure in the portal vein resulting from an obstruction of the Blood flow through the Liver.

Postnatal Essence (Postheaven Jing) - sometimes called the Acquired Essence, it is the Essence acquired after birth from food, air and drink.

Postnatal Qi (Postheaven Qi) - sometimes called the Acquired Qi, it is the Energy acquired after birth from food, drink, and air.

Postnatal Spirit (Zhi Shen) - also called the body's Mental Spirit, Acquired Spirit, and Conscious Spirit. This spiritual essence is acquired after birth through the refinement of one's Qi.

Post Traumatic Stress Disorder - characterized by the reexperiencing of an extremely traumatic event or events, accompanied by symptoms of increased arousal, and by avoidance of stimuli associated with the traumas. This includes the general numbing of the patient's emotional responsiveness.

Prenatal Essence (Yuan Jing) - also called Preheavenly Essence, Original Essence, Inherited Essence, Congenital Essence, Primordial Essence, and Ancestral Essence. It is the Original Essence existing before the fetus is born, acquired from the mother and father.

Prenatal Qi (Yuan Qi) - sometimes referred to as Congenital Qi, Pre-Heaven Qi, Inherited Qi, Source Qi, Ancestral Qi, Primordial Qi, Genuine Qi, and Kidney Qi. It is energy existing before the fetus is born, acquired from the mother's, father's, environmental and universal energies, and sustained through prayer, meditation and sleep.

Prenatal Spirit (Yuan Shen) - also called the Intuitive Spirit, Perceptual Spirit, Primordial Spirit, Congenital Spirit, and the Original Subconscious. It is the Spirit essence existing before the fetus is born, acquired from fusing the mother's, father's, environmental and universal energies. The Prenatal Spirit also relates to the individual's ability to perceive and intuit information.

Prescriptions - directions given to the patient with regard to the manner of Medical Qigong exercises and meditations that must be practise after the initial Medical Qigong treatment.

Primal Senses - pertaining to the gross physical, animalistic survival senses (seeing, hearing, feeling, smelling, etc.).

Primary Channels - the body's twelve main channels, containing six Yin and six Yang rivers of Energy.

Primary Posture - the main posture, in a series of Medical Qigong prescriptions, that the patient focuses on.

**Primitive Unconsciousness (Lower Unconsciousness) - pertaining to the acquired mind and related to the primal senses.

Projection - the attribution of unacceptable impulses within oneself to other people.

Proliferative Arthritis - the rapid reproduction and growth of arthritis.

Prostatitis - the inflammation of the prostate.

Protective Qi (Wei Qi) - the body's external field of defensive, protective energy (divided into three external fields of Qi).

Pruritus - severe itching.

Psychogenic - a condition developed from the beliefs originating within the mind.

Psychogenic Polyuria - pertaining to the belief that one must frequently secrete and discharge urine.

Psychometry - the act of sensing the thoughts, images and so on, with which the object has been imprinted.

Psychoneurosis - emotional disfunction caused from unresolved unconscious conflicts.

Psychosexual Qi Deviation - a condition resulting from an immediate energetic tissue overstimulation of the sexual organs. Patients with this condition experience intense sexual undulations and orgasms when being treated in a safe clinical environment.

Psychosis - a term formerly applied to any mental disorder, but now generally restricted to those conditions resulting from personal disintegration and loss of contact with reality.

Psychosomatic - pertaining to the relationship between the physical tissues and the emotions.

Pulling Down the Heavens - an opening and closing meditation used to energize and clear the body from the top of the head to the bottom of the feet, with breath, mind and hand movements.

Pulmonary Emphysema - a chronic disease of the Lungs characterized by a destructive increase in the normal size of air spaces distal to the terminal bronchiole.

Purpura - a condition characterized by hemorrhages of the internal organs, skin, mucous membranes and other tissues, with various manifestations and diverse causes.

Purgation (Purging) - technique used in order to reduce Excess and expel pathogenic Evils located within the energetic fields and tissues of the body.

Pyelonephritis - the inflammation of the Kidneys and pelvis.

Q

Qi - the energetic medium existing between matter and spirit (also known as Life Force Energy, when pertaining to the physical body).

Qi Collapse - pertaining to the complete absence (void) of either Yin or Yang Qi.

Qi Compression - using the Qi to press the tissues.

Qi Deviations - an alteration of energetic patterns and flow of energy that affects the body, mind, emotion and spirit, resulting in disease.

Qi Dysfunction - the impaired or abnormal function of the body's energy.

Qi Extension - the emission of energy from the body.

Qigong (Energy Skill) - pertaining to exercises and meditations that cultivate Life Force Energy. There are three primary schools of Qigong training - Martial, Medical and Spiritual.

Qigong Clinic - a facility for diagnosis and treatment of outpatients with Medical Qigong therapy.

Qigong Doctor - in China, a person who medically treats patients for mental or physical disorders using Qi.

Qigong Massage - soft tissue regulation wherein the Doctor's hand lightly skims the patient's body. This gentle surface tissue stimulation is used to energize, stimulate or dredge the patient's Wei Qi fields. It is used with purging and tonifying techniques.

Qigong Therapy - one of the four branches of Traditional Chinese Medicine, which involves treating patients through the use of Energetic Point Therapy, Qigong Massage, Distance Therapy, Self-Regulation Therapy, and Invisible Needle Therapy, to stimulate energy flow.

Qigong Therapist - in North America, a person who medically treats patients for mental or physical disorders using Qi.

Qi Hai - Sea of Qi point (CV-6).

Qi Manipulations - techniques used to treat or influence the flow of energy in the body.

Qing Dai - green-blue vaginal discharge.

Qi Projection (Energy Extension) - the emission of energy from the body.

Qi Regulation - energetically balancing the action or functions of the body's Yin and Yang energies.

Qi Stasis - the total stagnation of energy.

Quiescent - a meditative state wherein the individual's mind and body becomes quiet and peaceful.

R

Rachialgia - spinal inflammation.

Reaction-Formation - the conversion of one feeling into its opposite, typically seen in love turning into hate, or vice versa.

Rebellious Qi - energy that does not follow the correct flow or current, acting recklessly.

Reconstructive Qi Therapy - pertaining to the reconstruction and energizing of the body's energetic fields and organ systems (especially after surgery).

Reducing Qi - to lessen or decrease an organ or channel's energy.

Reflexology - the skill of pressing specific areas of the body's hands and feet to initiate internal energetic movement.

Regression - the return to an earlier childhood stage of behavior to reduce the demands on the ego.

Regulating - pertaining to the balancing of the body's Yin and Yang Energies.

Reinforcing Qi - to strengthen and support the body's organ or channel Energy.

Repression - the pushing down of unwanted ideas and emotions into the unconscious.

Respiratory Qi - Energy of the chest.

Restrictive Cycle - pertaining to the Five Elemental Controlling Cycle, where one organ restricts the energy of another organ (as depicted in the pentagram drawing).

Retrobulbar Neuritis - inflammation of the nerves behind the eyeball.

Returning To The Origin - see Rooting the Lower Dantian.

Reverse Breathing - opposite of abdominal breathing, wherein the patient will contract the abdomen with the inhalation, and expand the abdomen with the exhalation.

Rhabdomyosarcoma - a sarcoma of the muscles.

Rheumatic - pertaining to a rheumatism (a general term used to describe an acute or chronic condition characterized by inflammation, soreness and stiffness of the muscles, and pain in the joints and associated structures.

Rheumatoid Arthritis - a form of arthritis, characterized by inflammation of the joints, swelling, stiffness, cartilaginous hypertrophy, and pain.

Rheumatoid Spondylitis - a chronic, progressive disease, characterized by inflammation of the joints between the articular processes, costovertebral joints, and sacroiliac joints.

Rheumatosis - an acute or chronic condition characterized by inflammation, soreness and stiffness of the muscles, and pain in the joints.

Rhinitis - the inflammation of the nasal mucosa.

Righteous Qi (Zheng Qi) - is also called Upright Qi and Correct Qi. It is energy that heals the body and fights disease.

Rigor - a sudden, chill with high temperature, followed by Heat and profuse perspiration.

Can also be referred to a state of hardness and stiffness, as in the muscles.

Root - the original cause of a disease; or to energetically secure into the Earth by extending the body's Energy deep into the ground, as if growing tree roots.

Rooting - the process of extending the body's Qi into the Earth to either establish a solid energetic foundation, or if need be, disperse Toxic Qi.

Rooting the Lower Dantian (Returning to the Origin) - returning the body's collected Qi back into the Lower Dantian.

S

San Bao (Three Treasures of Man) - pertaining to Jing (Essence), Qi (Energy) and Shen (Spirit).

San Jiao (Triple Burners) - corresponding to three main body cavities, responsible for heating the body and transporting the Body Fluids. The Triple Burner Channels are considered one of the Twelve Primary Channels.

Sarcoma - a malignant growth, or tumor, that occurs within the connective or mesenchymal tissue. It may affect the muscles, Bones, fat, Blood Vessels, lymph system, Kidneys, Bladder, Liver, Lungs, Spleen, and/or parotid glands.

Schizophrenia - a mental disorder, that induces hallucinations - usually auditory - through can also be visual, accompanied by very disordered thinking, delusions, disorganized speech, irrational or catatonic behavior, such as stupor, rigidity, or flaccid movement of the limbs. The ability to interact with others is greatly impaired.

Sclera - a tough white fibrous tissue that covers the white of the eyes.

Sea of Blood (Sea of the Twelve Channels) - pertaining to the Energy located in the Thrusting Vessel.

Sea of Energy - Energy located in the Lower Dantian, or Qi Hai area.

Sea of Grain and Water (Sea of Nourishment) - pertaining to the Energy located in the Stomach.

Sea of Marrow - pertaining to the Energy flowing in the spinal column and Brain, originating from the Kidneys.

Sea of Qi - the chest center. Some Medical Qigong schools maintain that there are two reservoirs of Qi: the Middle Dantian, being the Sea of Postnatal Qi, and the Lower Dantian, being the Sea of Prenatal Qi (which is regulated by the Qihai CV-6 point).

Sea of Yang Channels - pertaining to the Governing Vessel.

Sea of Yin Channels - pertaining to the Conception Vessel.

Secondary Gains of Disease - pertaining to the subconscious psychological empowerment of a patients disease and its sabotaging potential.

Self Regulation Therapy - pertaining to the patient's Qigong prescriptions (meditations and/or exercises).

Seven Emotions - see Seven Internal Factors.

Seven Essential Stars - the Sun, Moon, Mars, Venus, Mercury, Saturn and Jupiter, associated with the body's seven orifices.

Seven Internal Factors - pertaining to the seven emotional pathogenic factors that cause disease, when in an Excess condition (Joy, Sorrow, Worry, Grief, Fear, Fright, and Anger).

Seven Material Souls - pertaining to the seven Earthly spirits that reside in the body as the Po.

Seven Orifices - ears, eyes, nostrils, mouth, anus and urethra, which are considered the gates and windows of Essence, Energy and Spirit.

Seven Turbid Demon Natures - see Po.

Shaman - an ancient Tungus term meaning "between the worlds." A Shaman is a tribal priest or priestess who heals the physical, mental, emotional, energetic and spiritual aspects of the patient.

Shao Yang - Small Yang, also called Lesser Yang,

Minor Yang, or Young Yang, is affiliated with the sunrise and the waxing-moon phase. Modern physicists associate the Lesser Yang with a light force and electromagnetism.

Shao Yin (Small Yin) - also called Lesser Yin, Minor Yin, or Young Yin, is affiliated with the sunset and the waning-moon phase. Modern physicists associate the Lesser Yin with a heavy force, and gravity. Shao Yin is associated with the Kidney and Heart Channels.

Shen - meaning Spirit; when speaking about physical development, it is derived from Qi, and can be divided into both Prenatal and Postnatal Shen.

Shen Deviations - mental and emotional disorders which have caused the Three Ethereal Souls (Hun) to leave the patient's body.

Shengong - training of the spirit through meditation and visualization.

Shening Out - terminology used to describe the Ethereal Soul (Hun) wandering away from the body.

Shi Qi (Turbid Qi) - also known as Evil Qi, Toxic Qi, and Pathogenic Qi, it is coarse, unrefined, polluted or dirty energy.

Shou Zhen (Hand Diagnosis) - a form of diagnosis, wherein, the doctor assess the "energetic blueprint" of the patient's body transformed onto the doctor's left hand.

Shu Points - five specific points below the elbows and knees identified as the Well, Spring, Stream, River and Sea points. Each point has an affect on the quantity of the energy of an organ.

Sishencong (Four Spirit Hearings) Points - also known as the "Four Alert Spirit Points," they are a group of four points located at the top of the head (surrounding the Baihui point), used for absorbing Heavenly Qi into the body through the Taiji Pole.

Six Evils (Six External Factors) - also known as the Six Pernicious Influences, these factors pertain to the six climatic changes (Wind, Summer Heat, Heat, Damp, Dryness, Cold, and Fire).

Six Extraordinary Organs - also called Curious Organs, these six organs are shaped like Yang (Hollow) organs but function like Yin organs. The Brain stores Marrow, the Marrow stores Kidney Jing, the Bones store Marrow, the Blood vessels store the Blood, the Gall Bladder stores the bile, and the Uterus stores Kidney Jing, Blood, and Qi.

Six Storage Areas - the body's Yang organs constantly fill and empty, and include the Urinary Bladder, Gall Bladder, Stomach, Large Intestine, Small Intestine, and Triple Burners.

Skatol - Beta-methyl indole, formed in the intestine by the bacterial decomposition of L-tryptophan and found in fecal matter, to which it imparts its characteristic odor.

Skin Zones - twelve dermal-zones, based upon the surface location of the body's Twelve Primary Channels.

Soaring Dragon Technique - hand technique for Qi emission, where the energy is emitted through the middle finger bent and pointing downward, while the other fingers are extended straight outwards.

Solid Organs - the body's Yin organs, which include the Liver, Heart, Spleen, Lungs, and Kidneys (also included in this list is the Pericardium).

Soul - immaterial Spiritual Essence of an individual's life, stored within the Heart and Middle Dantian.

Soul Body - see Astral Body.

Soul Extensions - the Shen develops and contains Twelve Soul Extensions. These Twelve Soul Extensions contain the body's different personality characteristics.

Soul Loss - the loss of parts of the Eternal Soul.

Soul Retrieval - to spiritually search for and bring back one's forgotten memories (soul), which have been isolated from consciousness due to trauma and shock.

Soul Travel - see Astral Travel.

Sound Energy Therapy - sound projected as

audible and inaudible tone resonation, used for healing.

Sound Resonation - healing tones used for tonifying or dispersing the patient's Energy.

Spider Nevus - a branched growth of dilated capillaries on the skin, that resemble a spider.

Spinal Pass (Jia Ji Guan) - two points located on the lateral sides of the Mingmen (GV-4), where energy has a potential to stagnate.

Spinous Process - the single midline posterior projection arising at the junction of each vertebra.

Spiraling Energy Technique - hand manipulation, that extends and spirals the doctor's projected energy.

Spirit - the energetic manifestation of the Eternal Soul.

Spirit Body - the energetic vehicle in which the body's Shen can travel throughout the Astral Plane. The Spirit Body can manifest through many forms (Body of Light, animal forms, etc.).

Spirit Demons - see Demon Possession and Oppression.

Spirit Soul - the Three Ethereal Souls, accompanied by the individual's consciousness, acting as one unit for spirit travel.

Spirit Travel - the spirit (Hun) journeying outside of the physical body.

Splenomegaly - the enlargement of the Spleen.

Squamous Metaplasia - the conversion of tissue into a form of scalelike cells, that is abnormal for that tissue.

Stacking the Bones - allowing the Bones to stack upon each other from the bottom of the feet to the top of the head.

Stagnation (Yu - Stasis) - not moving, inactive; pertaining to Qi, Blood, or thought patterns.

Static Qigong - the process of stationary, quiescent Energy gathering.

Stroke (Wind Stroke) - caused by the buildup of Excess Liver Fire creating Internal Wind. This Internal Wind causes Qi and Blood to rebel upwards causing Phlegm to form and obstruct the cavities and vessels, creating Penetrating Wind or Stroke.

Subarachnoid Hemorrhage - bleeding internally, within the spaces at the base of the Brain, between the pia proper and arachnoid contain the cerebrospinal fluid.

Subconscious Mind - part of the mind associated with the recording and storing of personal interpretations of reality (not readily accessible to the conscious mind).

Sublimation - the channeling of unacceptable impulses into acceptable, refined social forms and is the only defence mechanism considered to be a healthy reaction.

Substances - pertaining to the body's essential parts of physical and energetic material.

Sui - Marrow.

Summer Heat - one of the Six Evils.

Super Ego - Dr. Sigmund Freud's terminology for the division of the psyche in psychoanalytic theory, responsible for the psychic reward and punishment system.

Sun's Essence - energy gathered from the sun, ingested as warm light.

Sword Fingers Technique - hand manipulation that emits Qi through the extended index and middle fingers.

Symptoms - a subjective manifestation of a pathological condition, reported by the patient.

Syndromes - a grouping of signs and symptoms, based on their frequent reoccurrence, that may suggest a common underlying pathogenesis.

Systemic - affecting the entire body.

Systolic - vascular Blood pressure relating to the contraction of the Heart.

T

Taiji Pole - the Center Core of light which joins the body's three Dantians and the Eternal Soul together originating at the Baihui at the top of the head and extending through the center of the body, terminating at the Huiyin, located at the base of the perineum.

Tai Yang - Great Yang, also called Strong Yang, Major Yang, or Old Yang, is affiliated with high noon and the full-moon phase. Modern physicists associate the Strong Yang with a strong nuclear force. Associated with the Urinary Bladder and the Small Intestine Channels.

Tai Yi - meaning Great Divinity or God.

Tai Yin - Great Yin, also called Strong Yin, Major Yin, or Old Yin, is affiliated with midnight and the new-moon phase. Modern physicists associate the Great Yin with a weak nuclear force. Associated with the Spleen and the Lung Channels.

Ten Heavenly Stems - the ten energies of Heaven that rule the changes of the Five Elemental seasonal transitions, and are represented in the human body as the Yin and Yang aspect of the Five Elements (represented in the human body as the ten major internal organs).

Ten Thousand Voices - pertaining to the state of open receptivity of the Qigong doctor's Heart, after rooting the mind.

Ten Wings - consisting of ten commentaries from Confucius and his disciples, pertaining to the study of the eight Trigrams, sixty-four hexagrams, and the Yi-Jing.

Tenesmus - spasmodic contraction of the anal or vesical sphincter combined with pain.

Third Eye Point (Yin Tang- Extraordinary Point) - located in the center of the forehead, between the eyebrows, responsible for spiritual intuition and communication.

Thought-forms - images of concentrated thought patterns that manifest on the vibrational resonance of the Astral Plane.

Three Ethereal Souls (Hun) - pertaining to the three heavenly spirits that reside in the body.

Three Fires - the Heat in the body, generated from the energy radiating from the Heart Fire, Kidney Fire, and Urinary Bladder Fire.

Three Outer Forces - pertaining to the three natural powers of Heaven, Earth and Man.

Three Parts Wisdom - knowledge obtained through the doctor's connection and communication with his or her Upper, Middle, and Lower Dantians.

Three Periods of Life - the developmental stages of the patient's Jing, Qi and Shen divided into the womb, childhood and adulthood.

Three Stars - pertaining to the three periods of life, each period is divided into three stages of development, known as the Three Stars.

Three Treasures of Earth - pertaining to the energy of Soil, Water and Wind, and the study of Feng Shui (Wind and Water).

Three Treasures of Heaven - pertaining to the energy of the sun, moon and stars, and the study of Chinese astrology.

Three Treasures of Man - pertaining to the energetic interaction of the body's Essence, Energy and Spirit, and the study of the Yi-Jing (I-Ching or Book of Changes).

Three Wonders - Clinical manifestations of Qi, categorized as Subtle, Mysterious and Incredible Wonders.

Thrombosis - the formation and development or existence of a Blood clot (thrombus) within the walls of the vascular system.

Thrusting Channels - the Five Energy Channels which surround and penetrate the body's center core via the Taiji Pole.

Thrusting Vessels (Chong Mai) - they are the Five Energy Vessels which originate from the center of the body and internally transverse the legs and torso. The Thrusting Vessels are responsible for the connection between the Conception and Governing Vessels.

Ti - referred to as the Divine Center.

Tian Qi (Heavenly Energy) - the transformed energy of the Yuan Qi and the divine.

Tian Shen (Heavenly Spirit) - the transformed energy of the Yuan Shen and the divine.

Tie Bi (Iron Wall) - the areas of the body where it is most difficult for the energy to pass through when circulating the Microcosmic Orbit.

Tinnitus - a ringing, tinkling, or buzzing sound in the ear. In Traditional Chinese Medicine, tinnitus can originate from either an Excess or Deficient condition.

Toe Raised Stepping - pertaining to energetic walking therapy, wherein the toes are stretched when stepping in order to facilitate the increase of Qi flowing into the body via the leg channels.

Tonification (Tonify) - to supplement the insufficiency and strengthen the body's resistance.

Traditional Chinese Medicine - Chinese Energetic Medicine, divided into four branches of healing modalities (Acupuncture, Herbal Therapy, Medical Qigong Therapy, and Tissue Regulation Therapy (Chinese Massage).

Transference - the process whereby a patient unconsciously transfers feelings, thoughts, beliefs and patterns of behavior that had been previously experienced with others onto the doctor.

Transient Ischemic Attacks (TIA) - temporary interference with the Blood supply to the Brain. Multiple TIA can lead to a stroke.

Treatment - the medical care given to a specific condition.

Trigger Points (Ashi Points) - places on the body which are tender spots, or painful areas near diseased or injured tissue.

Trigram - pertains to three Yao lines stacked upon one another forming a specific symbol, which represents certain characteristics.

Triple Burners (San Jiao) - also known as the Triple Heaters and Triple Warmers, they correspond to three main body cavities (perineum to navel, navel to base of solar plexus, solar plexus to throat), and are responsible for heating the body and transporting Body Fluids.

True Fire - the original Heat or Fire Energy that regulates the body's Yin and Yang Qi, created from the radiating energy of the Heart's Fire, Kidneys' Fire and Urinary Bladder's Fire.

True Nature - one's innate nature in harmony with life.

True Qi - the energy that circulates in the body's channels and collaterals which nourishes the Yin and Yang organs and fights disease.

True Self - one's true nature, connected to the subconscious mind.

True Spirit - pertains to the spiritual nature of the True Self. The Hun and Po are expressions of the body's True Spirit.

Tsou Hou Ru Mo ("the Spirit leaves and the Demon enters") - describes self induced psychosis, pertaining to improper Qigong training, wherein the patient's Hun leave the body and the Po take over.

Tui Na Therapy - a tissue manipulation therapy that focuses on the adjustment and/or stimulation of the muscles and tendons.

Tumor - an abnormal growth, either benign or malignant, caused by a retention of mass due to stasis of Qi, Blood and Phlegm, etc.

Turbid Qi - also called Evil Qi, is coarse, unrefined, polluted, and dirty energy.

Twelve Pi Hexagrams - the twelve symbols pertaining to the twelve time periods of the day and year.

Twelve Primary Channels - the body's twelve main energetic rivers (Liver, Lungs, Large Intestine, Stomach, Spleen, Heart, Small Intestine, Urinary Bladder, Kidneys, Pericardium, Triple Burners, and Gall Bladder).

Twelve Earthly Branches - twelve energies of the Earth that determine the six Qi factors of the seasonal transitions (represented in the human body as the Twelve Primary Channels).

Two Breathings - pertaining to the abdominal breathing method of holding the breath.

U

Umbilications - a depression resembling a navel.

Universal Qi - energy pertaining to the Heavens, the divine and the celestial influences.

Upper Burner - pertaining to the body's complex system of Fluid distribution via the Lungs and located within the upper chest cavity.

Upper Dantian - area within the center of the head, attributed as the body's chamber of light and door to psychic and intuitive powers. The Upper Dantian is also known as Seal Palace, Ancestral Opening, Calm Fountain, Heaven's Valley, Inner Source, and Clay Pill Palace.

Urinary Bladder Fire - also called Common Peoples' Fire, or Perineal Fire, is located in the lower abdomen by the perineum, and is responsible for evaporating water.

Urodynia - painful urination

Uterus - female reproductive organ, one of the Eight Extraordinary organs.

V

Vasculitis - the inflammation of a Blood or lymph vessel.

Vertigo - the sensation of moving in space, resulting in such symptoms as dizziness and light-headedness.

Virtue (De) - pertaining to the function of the divine in man.

Virtue of Dao - pertaining to the commendable quality of the divine.

Viscera - the body's internal organs.

Void - also called Wuji, it pertains to the infinite space between matter and energy.

W

Wai Dan Shu - external elixir cultivation, that focuses on cultivating Qi from outside the individual's body.

Wai Qi - external, extended energy.

Walking Therapy - Postoral Dao Yin walking exercises and dynamic "moving" meditations used for the treatment of organ Deficiencies.

Wandering Bi - migrating pain within the body's cavities.

Waning - to grow smaller.

Water Element - one of the Five Elements, pertaining to Kidneys and Urinary Bladder.

Water Jing - energy that controls the genetic development phase of the fourth fetal month.

Waxing - to grow larger.

Wei Lu Guan (Coccyx Pass) - located on the lowest segment of the spine just posterior to the anus, near the Chang Qiang (GV-1) point.

Wei Qi - the body's external field of Defensive and Protective energy, which is subdivided into three fields of Qi.

Wen Huo - pertaining to the gentle breathing method of Respiratory Dao Yin training.

White Blood Cell - any of a group of Blood cells that have no hemoglobin and migrate into tissues to fight infection and digest cell debris.

Wind - one of the Six Evils.

Wind Bi - pain in the body created by toxic Wind invasion.

Wind Stroke - Stroke caused by the buildup of Excess Liver Fire creating Internal Wind. This Internal Wind causes Qi and Blood to rebel upwards causing Phlegm to form and obstruct the cavities and vessels, thus creating Penetrating Wind or Stroke.

Windy Breathing Method - pertaining to the method of breathing through the nose.

Wood Element - one of the Five Elements, pertaining to the Liver and Gall Bladder.

Wood Jing - energy that controls the development phase of the direction of the fetus's emotional and spiritual aspects during the seventh month of pregnancy.

Wu Guan (Five Passes) - five important gates on the Governing Vessel located at the coccyx, Mingmen, Shendao, occiput, and Baihui areas where energy tends to stagnate.

Wu Huo - pertaining to the vigorous breathing method of Respiratory Dao Yin training.

Wuji - pertaining to infinite space or the formless Void.

Wuji Posture - a quiet standing posture used in

meditation to allow the practitioner to return to a state of tranquility.

Wu Jing Shen (Five Essence Spirits) - the spiritual energy radiating from the core of the Five Yin Organs. Combined, these energies create the foundation of the body's Shen (Spirit).

Wu Se Dai - pertaining to the five colors of vaginal discharge - white, yellow, red, green-blue, and dark brown or black.

Wu Wei - a state of "no mind," i.e., no thoughts.

Wu Zang - the Five Yin Organs. Wu translates to mean "five," Zang translates to mean "to store or hold."

X

Xie Qi (Evil Qi) - energy that causes disease or harmful effects to the body.

Xin Xi (The Message) - knowledge stored within the Wuji or the Void.

Xiphoid Process - the lowest part of the sternum Bone (sometimes referred to as the Doves Tail).

Xue - Blood.

Y

Yang - the positive charged energetic polarity, opposite of its companion Yin, pertaining to man, hard, light, hot, etc.

Yang Channels - the body's Yang energetic rivers, consisting of the Governing Vessel, Belt Vessel, Yang Linking Vessels, Yang Heel Vessels, Large Intestine Channels, Triple Burner Channels, Small Intestine Channels, Stomach Channels, Gall Bladder Channels, and Urinary Bladder Channels.

Yang Fire - also called Emperor's Fire, energy of the Heart Fire.

Yang (Fu) Organs - also known as Hollow Organs, that consist of the Gall Bladder, Small Intestine, Stomach, Large Intestine, Urinary Bladder. Also included is this category are the Triple Burners.

Yang Shen Disturbances - an emotional Yang state of energetic dysfunction.

Yang Ming (Yang Brightness) - indicates Yang Qi developing its final stage and then reverting into Yin. Associated with the Stomach and Large Intestine Channels.

Yao - a solid or broken line which is representative of either Yang or Yin energy, used in combination of three as Trigrams or six as Hexagrams.

Yao Cycles - the progression of twelve hexagrams (six Yang and six Yin) flowing in a waxing and waning cycle.

Ye (humor) - thick, turbid Body Fluids; its function is to nourish the tissues.

Yellow Court - located in the center of the diaphragm, just below the xiphoid process of the sternum. Its function is that of being the access point to releasing the body's internal organ emotional memories. Its location is also attributed to the 3rd Chakra.

Yi - the intention or thought (the cognitive mind).

Yi Jing - Chinese "Book of Changes," pertaining to the natural transitions of life.

Yin - the negative charged energetic polarity, opposite of its companion Yang, pertaining to woman, soft, dark, cold, etc.

Yin Channels - Yin energetic rivers, consisting of the Conception Vessel, Thrusting Vessel, Yin Linking Vessels, Yin Heel Vessels, Lung Channels, Pericardium Channels, Heart Channels, Spleen Channels, Liver Channels, and Kidney Channels.

Yin (Zang) Organs - also known as the Solid Organs, that consist of the Liver, Heart, Spleen, Lungs and Kidneys. Also included in this category is the Pericardium.

Yin Shen Disturbances - an emotional Yin state of energetic dysfunction.

Yin Tang (Third Eye Point) - located in the center of the forehead between the eyebrows, responsible for projecting the Spirit for psychic intuition and communication.

Yu (Stagnation) - an obstruction.

Ying Qi (Nutritive Qi) - the body's nourishing energy.

Yu (Surplus) Vessels - secondary vessels that branch away from the energetic flow of the major Linking Vessels (at the chest and back), connecting the Linking Vessels energetic flow to the hands.

Yuan Jing (Original Essence) - the Original Kidney or Prenatal Essence.

Yuan Shen (Original Spirit) - the Original Prenatal Spirit.

Yuan Qi (Original Energy) - the Original Kidney or Prenatal Qi.

Yun - the Yin method of dynamic postural Dao Yin training.

Yu Zhen Guan (Occipital Pass) - the area located just inferior to the occipital Bone where the Brain originates, known as a specific point where Qi often stagnates.

Z

Zang Organs - Yin or solid organs (Liver, Heart, Spleen, Lungs, Kidneys and Pericardium).

Zang/Fu Organs - the body's Yin and Yang organs.

Zhang Xiang Xue Shou - in Chinese medical science, the study of energetic physiology.

Zhen Qi - see True Qi

Zheng Qi - Righteous Qi, pathogenic fighting Energy.

Zhi - the Will power, mental drive and determination.

Zhong Qi - Center Qi, Energy of the chest.

Zhou Qi - Turbid Qi, Evil Qi, Impure Qi

Zong Qi - Gathering Qi, and/or Respiratory Qi.

Zygomatic Facial Regions - pertaining to the sides of the cheeks below the eyes.

BIBLIOGRAPHY

A Barefoot Doctor's Manual
    A Guide To Traditional Chinese and
    Modern Medicine
    A Cloudburst Press Book
    Madrona Publishers, 1977
    Seattle, Washington

Agrippa, Henry Cornelius
    Occult Philosophy or Magic
    Ernest Loomis and Company, 1897
    New York City, New York

Allen, James
    As a Man Thinketh
    Grosset and Dunlap, 1940
    New York City, New York

Ames, T. Roger and David L. Hall
    Daodejing "Making This Life Significant"
    Ballantine Books 2003
    New York, New York

Anodea, Judith
    Wheels of Life
    Liewellyn Publications, 1990
    St. Paul, Minnesota 55164-0383

Atteshlis, Dr. Stylianos
    The Esoteric Teachings
    A Christian Approach to Truth
    The Stoa Series, 1992
    Strovolos, Cyprus

Bai, Jingfeng
    Episodes in Traditional Chinese Medicine
    Panda Books
    Beijing, China 1998

Bao, Fei et al.
    Application of Acupuncture in the
    Treatment of malignant Tumors
    Medical Research Bulletin
    Beijing, China 1997

Bandler, Richard, and John Grinder
    The Structure of Magic
    A Book About Language and Therapy
    Science and Behavior Books, Inc. 1975
    Palo Alto, California 94306

Bardon, Franz
    Initiation into Hermetics
    The Path of the True Adept
    Merkur Publishing, Inc.
    Madrona Publishers, 2001
    Salt Lake City, Utah

Bardon, Franz
    The Practice of Magical Evocation
    A Complete Course in Instruction in
    Planetary Spheric Magic
    Merkur Publishing, Inc.
    Madrona Publishers, 2001
    Salt Lake City, Utah

Beaulieu, John
    Music and Sound in the Healing Arts
    An Energy Approach,
    Station Hill Press 1987
    Barrytown, New York

Becker, Robert O., M.D. and Gary Selden
    The Body Electric
    Electromagnetism and the Foundation of Life
    Quill - William Morrow and Co., 1985
    New York City, New York 10016

Becker, Robert O., M.D
    Cross Currents
    The Perils of Electropollution
    The Promise of Electromedicine
    Jeremy P. Tarcher, Inc., 1990
    Los Angeles, Ca. 90036

Beer, Robert
    The Encyclopedia of Tibetan Symbols and Motifs
    Shambhala, 1999
    Boston, Mass. 02115

Beinfield, Harriet, L.Ac. and
   Efrem Korngold, L.Ac., O.M.D.
   Between Heaven And Earth
   A Guide To Chinese Medicine,
   Ballantine Books, 1991
   New York, New York

Bensky, Dan and Andrew Gamble
   with Ted Kaptchuck
   Illustrations Adapted by Lilian Lai Bensky
   Chinese Herbal Medicine
   Materia Medica - Revised Edition
   Eastland Press, Inc., 1993
   Seattle, Washington

Berkow, Robert, M.D., Andrew J. Fletcher M.B.
   The Merck Manual of Diagnosis and Therapy
   17th Edition, Merck Research Laboratories
   Merck & Co. Inc., 2000
   Rahway, N.J.

Blofeld, John
   The Secret and Sublime
   Taoist Mysteries and Magic
   E.P. Dutton & Co., Inc
   George Allen & Unwin Ltd., 1973
   New York, New York

Bokenkamp, Stephen R.
   Early Daoist Scriptures
   E.P. Dutton & Co., Inc
   University of California Press, 1997
   Berkely, California

The Brain Workshop Handbook
   The Brain Company, Inc., 1984
   Burlington, Mass. 01803

Brennan, Barbara Ann
   Hands of Light
   A Guide to Healing Through the
   Human Energy Field
   Bantam Books Publishing, 1988
   New York, New York

Bryant, Darren A.
   Ancestors and Ghosts:
   The Philosophic and Religious Origins
   of the Hungry Ghost Festival
   Asian Studies, 2003
   Hong Kong

Burnham, Sophy
   A Book of Angels
   Ballantine Books
   New York City, New York

Carlo, George and Martin Schram
   Cell Phones
   Invisible Hazards in the Wireless Age
   Carroll & Graf Publishers, 2001
   New York City, New York

Carus, Paul
   Chinese Astrology
   Early Chinese Occultism
   Open Court Publishing, 1989
   La Salle, Illinois

Cao, Guangwen et al.
   Current Biological Treatment of Cancer
   People's Military Press
   Beijing, China 1995

Castleman, Michael
   The New Healing Herbs
   Rodale Press, Inc., 2001
   Emmaus, Pennsylvania.

Ce, Jin and Hu Zhanggui, with Jin Zhenghua
   Practical Chinese Qigong for Home Health Care
   Foreign Languages Press, 1996
   Beijing, China

Chang, Stephen T., Dr.
   The Complete System of Self-healing
   Internal Exercises
   Tao Publishing, 1986
   San Francisco, Ca. 94132

Chang, Minyi
   Anticancer Medical Herbs
   Hunan Science and Technology Pub. House
   Beijing, China 1992

Charles, George
   Le Rituel du Dragon
   ILes sources et les racines des Arts Martiaux
   Editions, Chariot d'Or, 2003
   France

Chen, Kaiguo and Zheng Shunchao
Opening the Dragon Gate
The Making of a Modern Taoist Wizard
Translated by Thomas Cleary
Charles E. Tuttle Co., Inc., 1998
North Clarendon, VT, 05759

Chen, Yan-Feng, Dr.
Pre-Natal Energy, Mobilizing Qigong
China Taoist Ancient Qigong
Chinese Kung Fu Series, 1992
Guandong Xin hua Printing House

Chen, Yaoting
Origin of the Big Dipper
Translated by Luo Tongbing 2002
Taoist Culture and Information Center
www.eng.taoism.org.hk/

Chen, Zeming
Complete Effective Prescriptions for
Women's Diseases
Jin Dynasty, China 1237

Chinese Qigong
Publishing House of Shanghai, 1990
College of Traditional Chinese Medicine
Shanghai, China

Chinese Qigong, Outgoing - Qi Therapy
Shandong Science and
Technology Press, 1992
Shandong, China

Chinese Qigong Therapy
Shandong Science and
Technology Press, 1995
Shandong, China

Choa, Kok Sui, Dr.
Pranic Healing
Samuel Weiser, Inc., 1990
York Beach, Maine

Chogyal, Namkhai Norbu
Dream Yoga and the practice of Natural Light
Snow Lion Publications, 1992
Ithaca, New York

Cleary, Thomas
Immortal Sisters
Secret Teachings of Taoist Women
North Atlantic Books, 1996
Berkeley, Ca.

Cleary, Thomas
The Inner Teachings of Taoism
Chang Po-Tuan,
Commentary by Liu I-Ming
Shambhala Press, 2001
Boston & London

Cleary, Thomas
The Secret of the Golden Flower
Harper Collins Publishers 1991
New York City, New York

Cleary, Thomas
Understanding Reality
A Taoist Alchemical Classic
by Chang Po-tuan with a Concise
Commentary by Liu I-ming
University of Hawaii Press 1987
Honolulu, Hi

Cleary, Thomas
The Taoist Classics Volume Two
The Collected Translations of Thomas Cleary
Shambhala Publications, Inc. 2003
Boston, Massachusetts

Cohen, Kenneth S.
The Way of Qigong
Ballantine Books 1997
Random House, New York

Concise
English-Chinese,
Chinese-English Dictionary
Second Edition
Oxford University Press, 1999
Oxford, New York

Cooper, Primrose
The Healing Power of Light
A Comprehensive Guide to Healing and the
Transformative Powers of Light
Weiser Books, Inc. 2001
York Beach, ME

Cunningham, David Michael
Creating Magickal Entities
Egregore Publishing 2003
Perrysburg, OH

Davis, Edward L.
Society and the Supernatural in Song China
University of Hawaii Press 2001
Honolulu, Hawaii

Deadman, Peter
Selected Articles from the
Journal of Chinese Medicine
England

Deadman, Peter & Maazin Al-Khafaji
with Kevin Baker
A Manual of Acupuncture
Journal of Chinese Medicine
Publications 1998
England

DeGroot, J.J.M., Ph.D., LL.D.
Religion in China:
Universalism: A Key To The Study of
Taoism and Confucianism
G.P. Putnam's Sons
The Knickerbocker Press, 1912
New York and London

DeGroot, J.J.M., Ph.D., LL.D.
The Religious System of China:
Book 1, Volume I
Its Ancient Forms, Evolution, History and
Present Aspect Manners, Customs and Social
institutions Connected Therein
Disposal of the Dead,
Part 1 - Funeral Rites
Part 2 - The Ideas of Resurrection
Ch'eng Wen Publishing Co., 1976
Taipei, Taiwan

DeGroot, J.J.M., Ph.D., LL.D.
The Religious System of China:
Book 1, Volume II
Its Ancient Forms, Evolution, History and
Present Aspect Manners, Customs and Social
institutions Connected Therein
Disposal of the Dead,
Part 3 - The Grave (First Half)
Ch'eng Wen Publishing Co., 1976
Taipei, Taiwan

DeGroot, J.J.M., Ph.D., LL.D.
The Religious System of China:
Book 1, Volume III
Its Ancient Forms, Evolution, History and
Present Aspect Manners, Customs and Social
institutions Connected Therein
Disposal of the Dead,
Part 3 - The Grave (Second Half)
Ch'eng Wen Publishing Co., 1976
Taipei, Taiwan

DeGroot, J.J.M., Ph.D., LL.D.
The Religious System of China:
Book 2, Volume IV
Its Ancient Forms, Evolution, History and
Present Aspect Manners, Customs and Social
institutions Connected Therein
On the Soul and Ancestral Worship
Part 1 - The Soul in Philosophy
Ch'eng Wen Publishing Co., 1976
Taipei, Taiwan

DeGroot, J.J.M., Ph.D., LL.D.
The Religious System of China:
Book 2, Volume V
Its Ancient Forms, Evolution, History and
Present Aspect Manners, Customs and Social
institutions Connected Therein
Disposal of the Dead,
Part 2 - Demonology
Part 3 - Sorcery
Ch'eng Wen Publishing Co., 1976
Taipei, Taiwan

DeGroot, J.J.M., Ph.D., LL.D.
The Religious System of China:
Book 2, Volume VI
Its Ancient Forms, Evolution, History and
Present Aspect Manners, Customs and Social
institutions Connected Therein
Disposal of the Dead,
Part 4 - The War against Spectres
Part 5 - The Priesthood of Animism
Ch'eng Wen Publishing Co., 1976
Taipei, Taiwan

DeSchepper, Luc, M.D., Ph.D., C.Ac.
Acupuncture for the Practitioner
Santa Monica, California 91403

BIBLIOGRAPHY

DeVita, Vincent T., Jr., Samuel Hellman, and Steven A. Rosenberg
Cancer Principles and Practice of Oncology
Fifth Edition - Vol 1
Lippincott - Raven Publishers, 1997
Philadelphia - New York

DeVita, Vincent T., Jr., Samuel Hellman, and Steven A. Rosenberg
Cancer Principles and Practice of Oncology
Fifth Edition - Vol 2
Lippincott - Raven Publishers, 1997
Philadelphia - New York

Diagnostics of Traditional Chinese Medicine
Publishing House of Shanghai, 1990
College of Traditional Chinese Medicine
Shanghai, China

Ding, Li, Professor
Acupuncture, Meridian Theory, and Acupuncture Points
China Books & Periodicals, Inc., 1992
Foreign languages Press, Beijing

Dong Paul and Thomas Raffill
Empty Force
Element Books, Inc., 1996
Rockport, Mass. 01966

Duan, Shizhen
A Modern Chinese-English Dictionary
Hai Feng Publishing Co., Ltd.
Oxford University Press

Eberhard, Wolfram
A Dictionary of Chinese Symbols
Hidden Symbols in Chinese Life and Thought
Routledge, 2003
New York City, New York

Eckman, Peter, M.D., Ph.D., M.Ac. (UK)
In the Footsteps of the Yellow Emperor
Tracing the History of Traditional Acupuncture
Cypress Book Company, Inc. 1996
San Francisco, California

Ellis, Andrew, Nigel Wiseman, Ken Boss
Grasping the Wind
An exploration into the meaning of Chinese acupuncture point names
Paradigm Publications, 1989
Brookline, Massachusetts

Essentials of Chinese Acupuncture
Beijing College of Traditional Chinese Medicine
Foreign Languages Press, 1980
Beijing, China

Evola, Julius
The Yoga of Power
Tantra, Shakti, and The Secret Way
Inner Traditions International, 1992
Rochester, Vermont

Feit, Richard and Paul Zmiewski
Acumoxa Therapy
A Reference and Study Guide
Volume II The Treatment of Diseases
Paradigm Publications, 1990
Brooklyn, Massachusetts

Flaws, Bob and James Lake, M.D.
Chinese Medical Psychiatry
A Textbook and Clinical Manual
Blue Poppy Press, 2001
Boulder, Colorado

Flaws, Bob
Curing Headaches Naturally with Chinese Medicine
Blue Poppy Press, 1998
Boulder, Colorado

Gao, Bingjun
A Collection of Expieriences in the Treatment of Sores
Qing Dynasty, China 1808

Gao, Qiyun
Questions and Answers in External Diseases
Ming Dynasty, China 1517

Gerber, Richard, M.D.
Vibrational Medicine
Bear and Company, 1988
Santa Fe, New Mexico 87504-2860

Goldman, Jonathan
Healing Sounds
The Power of Harmonics
Healing Arts Press, 2002
Rochester, Vermont

Gordon, James S., M.D. and Sharon Curtin
Comprehensive Cancer Care
Integrating Alternative, Complementary,
and Conventional Therapies
Perseus Publishing, 2000
Cambridge, Massachusetts

Gore, Belinda
Ecstatic Body Postures
An Alternate Reality Workbook
Bear and Company Publishing, 1995
Santa Fe, New Mexico

Govinda, Anagarika, Lama
The Inner Structure of the I-Ching
The Book of Transformations
A Wheelwright Press Book, 1981
Tokyo, Weatherhill, New York

Graham, Donald H, Jr.
Bronze Mirrors From Ancient China
Techpearl Printing, Ltd., 1994
Hong Kong

Graves, Tom
Needles of Stone Revisited
Gothic Image Publications, 1986
Glastonbury, Somerset, England

Gray, Henry F.R.S.
Gray's Anatomy
Barnes & Noble Books, 1995
The United States of America

Grof, Stanislav, M.D. with Hal Zina Bennett
The Holotropic Mind
Harper Collins Publishers, Inc., 1993
New York City, New York

Guiley, Rosemary Ellen
Harper's Encyclopedia of
Mystical and Paranormal Experiences
Harper Collins Publishers Inc., 1991
New York City, New York

Guo, Liang Cao, Dr.
Essentials Of Tuinaology
Chinese Medical Massage and
Manipulation
Cao's Fire Dragon, 1983
Hilo, Hawaii

Guo, Shuping, Dr.
Selections from Gao's Medical Works on Tumor
Treatment using Traditional Chinese Medicine
China Press of Traditional Chinese
Medicine, 1997
Beijing, China

Hai Dian University, Medical Qigong Textbook
The Cultivation of the Innate and the Destines
White Cloud Monastery, 1988
Beijing, China

Hall, Manly P.
Magic
A Treatise on Esoteric Ethics
Philosophical Research Society, 1998
Los Angeles, Ca.

Hammer, Leon, M.D.
Dragon Rises and Red Bird Flies
Psychology and Chinese Medicine
Staton Hills Press, Inc., 1990
Barrytown, New York

Han, Rui
Chemical Drugs and Preparations in the
Treatment of Tumors
Beijing Medical University and Peking
Union Medical University Joint Press
Beijing, China 1992

Harper, Donald
Early Chinese Medical Literature
The Mawangdui Medical Manuscripts
Kegan Paul International, 1998
London and New York

Hawk, Ambrose
Exploring Scrying
New Page Books, 2001
Franklin Lakes, N.J.

Ho, P.Y. and F.P.Lisowski
A Brief History of Chinese Medicine,
2nd Edition
World Scientific Publishing Co., 1997
Singapore

Holmes, Peter
The Energetics of Western Herbs Volume 1
Snow Lotus Press, Inc., 1997
Boulder, Colorado

BIBLIOGRAPHY

Holmes, Peter
The Energetics of Western Herbs Volume 2
Snow Lotus Press, Inc., 1997
Boulder, Colorado

Huang, Jane and Wurmbrand, Michael
The Primordial Breath, Volume 1
Original Books Inc., 1998
Torrance, Ca. 90509

Huang, Jane and Wurmbrand, Michael
The Primordial Breath, Volume 2
Original Books Inc., 1990
Torrance, Ca. 90509

Illustration of Channels and Points For Acupuncture and Moxibustion and Qigong
Hunan Science and Technology Press, 1992
Hunan, China

Jahnke, Roger, D.O.M.
The Healer Within
Harper Publishing, 1997
San Francisco, Ca.

Jarrett, Lonny S.
Nourishing Destiny
The Inner Traditions of Chinese Medicine
Spirit Path Press, 2000
Stockbridge, Mass.

Jarrett, Lonny S.
The Clinical Practice of Chinese Medicine
Spirit Path Press, 2003
Stockbridge, Mass.

Jiao, Guo Rui, Dr.
Qigong Essentials for Health Promotion
China Reconstruction Press, 1990

Johnson, Jerry Alan, C.Ac., Master Instructor
Chi Kung Correspondence Course, Vol. 1-6
Ching Lung Martial Arts Association, 1988
Pacific Grove, CA

Johnson, Jerry Alan, C.Ac., C.M.T., Master Instructor
The Essence of Internal Martial Arts, Vol. 1
Esoteric Fighting Techniques and Healing Methods
Ching Lien Healing Arts Center, 1994
Pacific Grove, CA

Johnson, Jerry Alan, C.Ac., C.M.T., Master Instructor
The Essence of Internal Martial Arts, Vol. 2
Energy Theory and Cultivation
Ching Lien Healing Arts Center, 1994
Pacific Grove, CA

Johnson, Jerry Alan, Ph.D., D.M.Q. (China)
The Emotional Components of Tumor Formations
Doctoral Theses - Beijing Western District Qigong Research Institute, 1995
Beijing, China

Johnson, Jerry Alan, Ph.D., D.T.C.M., D.M.Q. (China)
Chinese Medical Qigong Therapy: A Comprehensive Clinical Text
The International Institute of Medical Qigong, 2000, Pacific Grove, CA

Johnson, Jerry Alan, Ph.D., D.T.C.M., D.M.Q. (China)
The Treatment of Cancer With Chinese Medical Qigong Therapy
The International Institute of Medical Qigong, 2001, Pacific Grove, CA

Johnson, Jerry Alan, Ph.D., D.T.C.M., D.M.Q. (China)
Chinese Medical Qigong Therapy Vol 1: Energetic Anatomy and Physiology,
The International Institute of Medical Qigong, 2002, Pacific Grove, CA

Johnson, Jerry Alan, Ph.D., D.T.C.M., D.M.Q. (China)
Chinese Medical Qigong Therapy Vol 2: Energetic Alchemy, Dao Yin Therapy and Qi Deviations
The International Institute of Medical Qigong, 2002, Pacific Grove, CA

Johnson, Jerry Alan, Ph.D., D.T.C.M., D.M.Q. (China)
Chinese Medical Qigong Therapy Vol 3: Differential Diagnosis, Clinical Foundations, Treatment Principles and Clinical Protocols
The International Institute of Medical Qigong, 2002, Pacific Grove, CA

Johnson, Jerry Alan, Ph.D., D.T.C.M., D.M.Q. (China)
Chinese Medical Qigong Therapy Vol 4: Prescription Exercises and Meditations, Treatment of Internal Organ Diseases, Pediatrics, Geriatrics, Gynecology, Neurology and Energetic Psychology
The International Institute of Medical Qigong, 2002, Pacific Grove, CA

Johnson, Jerry Alan, Ph.D., D.T.C.M., D.M.Q. (China)
Chinese Medical Qigong Therapy Vol 5:
An Energetic Approach to Oncology
The International Institute of Medical Qigong,
2002, Pacific Grove, CA

Johnson, Yanling Lee
A Woman's Qigong Guide
Empowerment Through Movement, Diet, and Herbs
Y.M.A.A. Publication Center, 2001
Boston, Mass 02130

Jou, Tsung Hwa
The Tao of Meditation
Way to Enlightenment
Tai Chi Farm, 1986
Warwick, New York 10990

Jurasunas, Serge, Dr.
Orthomolecular Treatment of Cancer
Townsend Letter for Doctors and Patients
The Examiner of Medical Alternatives 2002
February/March 1999

Kapit, Wynn and Lawrence M. Elson
The Anatomy Coloring Book
Harper Collins Publishers, 1977
New York, New York, 10022

Kaplan, Aryeh
Meditation and Kabbalah
Samuel Weiser, Inc., 1982
York Beach, ME 03910

Kaptchuk, Ted J., O.M.D.
The Web That Has No Weaver
Congdon and Weed, Inc., 1983
New York, New York, 10001

Kendall, Donald E.
Dao of Chinese Medicine
Understanding An Ancient Healing Art
Oxford University Press, Inc. 2002
New York, New York, 10001

Keville, Kathi, with Peter Korn,
Herbs for Health and Healing
Rodale Press, Inc., 1996
Emmaus Pennsylania, p. 109

Kohn, Livia and Harold D. Roth
Daoist Identity
History, Lineage and Ritual
University of Hawaii Press, 2002
Honolulu, Hawaii

Kohn, Livia & Yoshinobu Sakade
Taoist Meditation and
Longevity Techniques
Center for Chinese Studies, 1989
University of Michigan

Komjathy, Louis
Scripture on the Hidden Talisman
Wandering Cloud Press, 2003
Seattle, Washington

Komjathy, Louis
Book of Master Celestial Seclusion
Wandering Cloud Press, 2003
Seattle, Washington

Konstantinos
Summoning Spirits
The Art of Magical Evocation
Liewellyn Publications, 2001
St. Paul. MN 55164-0383

Lade, Arnie, Dr., D.O.M.
Acupuncture Points
Images & Functions
Eastland Press, 1989
Seattle, Washington, 98111

Larre, Claude and Elisabeth Rochat de la Vallee
The Seven Emotions
Psychology and Health in Ancient China
Monkey Press, 1996
Cambridge, CB4 3PU

Larre, Claude and Elisabeth Rochat de la Vallee
The Eight Extraordinary Meridians
Monkey Press, 1997
Spider Web, London N7

Larre, Claude and Elisabeth Rochat de la Vallee
Essence Spirit Blood and Qi
Monkey Press, 1999
Spider Web, London N7

Larre, Claude and Elisabeth Rochat de la Vallee
The Extraordinary Fu
Monkey Press, 2003
Spider Web, London N7

Larre, Claude and Elisabeth Rochat de la Vallee
Heart Master - Triple Heater
Monkey Press, 1998
Spider Web, London N7

Larre, Claude and Elisabeth Rochat de la Vallee
The Lung
Monkey Press, 2001
Spider Web, London N7

Larre, Claude and Elisabeth Rochat de la Vallee
The Liver
Monkey Press, 1999
Spider Web, London N7

Larre, Claude and Elisabeth Rochat de la Vallee
The Kidneys
Monkey Press, 2001
Spider Web, London N7

Larre, Claude and Elisabeth Rochat de la Vallee
Essence Spirit Blood and Qi
Monkey Press, 1999
Spider Web, London N7

Larre, Claude and Elisabeth Rochat de la Vallee
Rooted in the Spirit
The Heart of Chinese Medicine
Station Hill Press, Inc., 1992
Barrytown, New York,

Larre, Claude, Jean Schatz, and
   Elisabeth Rochat de la Vallee
Survey of Traditional Chinese Medicine
Institut Ricci, Paris
and Traditional Acupuncture Institute, 1986
Columbia, Maryland

Lee, John R., M.D., David Zava, Ph.D., and
   Virginia Hopkins
What Your Doctor May Not Tell You
About Breast Cancer
Warner Books, 2002
New York City, New York,

Lee, Mariam, Dr., D.O.M.
Insights of a Senior Acupuncturist
Blue Poppy Press, 1992
Boulder, Colorado

Lee, Richard H.
Qi and Kirlian Photography
China Healthways Institute, 1996
San Clemente, Ca 92672

Legeza, Laszlo
Tao Magic
The Secret Language of Diagrams
and Calligraphy
Thames and Hudson, 1975
New York, New York 10110

Li, Gang
Ancient Shamanism
Translated by David Palmer 2002
Taoist Culture and Information Center
www.eng.taoism.org.hk/

Li, Yan
Essentials of Clinical Pattern Identification
of Tumors
People's Medical Publishing House
Beijing, China 1998

Li, Zhongzi
Required Readings for Medical Professionals
Ming Dynasty, China 1637

Liang, Shou-Yu, Master and Wen-Ching Wu
Qigong Empowerment, A Guide to Medical, Taoist,
Buddhist and Wushu energy Cultivation
The Way of Dragon Publishing, 1997
East Providence, Rhode Island 02914-0561

Lieberman, S.
Maitake, King of Mushrooms
Keats Publishing, 1991
Los Angeles, Ca., p. 16-19.

Lin, Henry B.
The Art & Science of Feng Shui
The Ancient Chinese Tradition of Shaping Fate
Llewellyn Publications, 2000
St. Paul, Min.

Lin, Huo Sheng, Dr. & Dr. Luo Pei Yu
Three Hundred Questions on Qigong Exercises
Guandong Science and Technology Press, 1994
Guandong, China

Liu, Hong, Dr. with Paul Perry
Mastering Miracles
Warner Books Inc., 1997
New York, New York, 10020

Liu, Zheng-Cai and Hua Ka
A Study of Daoist Acupuncture
Blue Poppy Press, 1999
Boulder, Colorado

Liu, Zhongyu
Divine Incantations
Translated by Ginny Yue 2002
Taoist Culture and Information Center
www.eng.taoism.org.hk/

Liu, Zhongyu
The Origin of Talismans
Translated by Ginny Yue 2002
Taoist Culture and Information Center
www.eng.taoism.org.hk/

Liu, Zhongyu
The Structure of Talismans
Translated by Ginny Yue 2002
Taoist Culture and Information Center
www.eng.taoism.org.hk/

Liu, Zhongyu
The Underworlds (of Chinese Mythology)
Translated by David Palmer 2002
Taoist Culture and Information Center
www.eng.taoism.org.hk/

Loo, May
Pediatric Acupuncture
Churchill Livingston, 2002
Printed in China

Lu, Ke Yun
The Essence of Qigong
A Handbook of Qigong Therapy and Practice
Abode of the Eternal Tao, 1998
Eugene, Oregon

Lu, K'uan Yu
Taoist Yoga
Alchemy & Immortality
Weiser Books, 1973
Boston, Ma 02210

Maciocia, Giovanni
Tongue Diagnosis in Chinese Medicine
Eastland Press Inc., 1987
Seattle, Washington 98111

Maciocia, Giovanni
Obstetrics & Gynecology in Chinese Medicine
Churchill Livingstone Inc., 1998
New York City, New York, 10011

Maciocia, Giovanni
The Foundations of Chinese Medicine
Churchill Livingstone Inc., 1989
New York City, New York, 10011

Maciocia, Giovanni
Diagnosis in Chinese Medicine
A Comprehensive guide
Churchill Livingstone Inc., 2004
New York City, New York, 10011

Maclean, Will with Kathryn Taylor
The Clinical Manual of Chinese Herbal Patent Medicines: A guide to ethical and pure patent medicines
Pangolin Press, 2000
Sydney, Australia

MacGregor, Mathers, S.L.
The Book of the Sacred Magic of Abramelin the Mage
Dover Publications, Inc. 1975
New York City, New York

MacRitchie, James
Alive With Energy
The Chi Kung Way
Harper-Collins Publishers, 1997
San Francisco, Ca. 94111-1213

Marieb, Elaine N., R.N., Ph.D.
Human Anatomy and Physiology
Second Edition
The Benjamin/Cummings Pub. Co., Inc., 1992
Redwood City, California, 94065

Markides, Kyriacos C.
   Homage to the Sun
   The Wisdom of the Magus of Strovolos
   Arkana: Penguin Books, 1987
   New York City, New York, 10014

Markides, Kyriacos C.
   Fire in the Heart
   Healers, Sages and Mystics
   Arkana: Penguin Books, 1990
   New York City, New York, 10014

Matsumoto, Kiiko & Stephen Birch
   Extraordinary Vessels
   Paradigm Publications, 1986
   Brookline, Massachusetts

Matsumoto, Kiiko and Stephen Birch
   Hara Diagnosis: Reflections on the Sea
   Paradigm Publications, 1988
   Brookline, Massachusetts 02146

Melchizedek, Drunvalo
   The Ancient Secret of the Flower of Life, Vol.1
   Light Technology Publishing, 1998
   Flagstaff, Az 86003

McAfee, John
   Beyond the Siddhis
   Supernatural Powers and the Sutras
   of Patanjali
   Woodland Publications, 2001
   Woodland Park, Co.

McTaggart, Lynne
   The Field
   The Quest For The Secret Force Of The Universe
   Harper-Collins Publishers, 2002
   New York, New York 10022

McTaggart, Lynne
   The Cancer Handbook
   Vital-Health Publishing, 1997
   Bloomingdale, Ill 60108

Moss, Ralph W., Ph.D.
   The Cancer Industry
   New Update Edition
   The Classic Expose on the Cancer Establishment
   Equinox Press, 1999
   Brooklyn, New York, 11217

Milne, Hugh
   The Heart of Listening
   A Visionary Approach to Craniosacral Work
   North Atlantic Books, 1995
   Berkeley, California

Needham, Joseph, F.R.S., F.B.A.
   Science and Civilization in China
   Volume 5 Chemistry and
   Chemical Technology
   Part V: Spagyrical Discovery and Invention:
   Physiological Alchemy
   Cambridge University Press, 1986
   Cambridge, London

Netter, Frank H., M.D.
   The CIBA Collection of Medical Illustrations
   Volume 1 Nervous System
   Part II - Neurologic and
   Neuromuscular Disorders
   CIBA Pharmaceutical Co., 1986
   West Caldwell N.J.

Netter, Frank H., M.D.
   The CIBA Collection of Medical Illustrations
   Volume 2 Reproductive System
   CIBA Pharmaceutical Co., 1965
   West Caldwell N.J.

Netter, Frank H., M.D.
   The CIBA Collection of Medical Illustrations
   Volume 3 Digestive System
   Part I Upper Digestive Tract
   CIBA Pharmaceutical Co., 1989
   West Caldwell N.J.

Netter, Frank H., M.D.
   The CIBA Collection of Medical Illustrations
   Volume 3 Digestive System
   Part II Lower Digestive Tract
   CIBA Pharmaceutical Co., 1959
   West Caldwell N.J.

Netter, Frank H., M.D.
   The CIBA Collection of Medical Illustrations
   Volume 3 Digestive System
   Part III Liver, Biliary Tract and Pancreas
   CIBA Pharmaceutical Co., 1964
   West Caldwell N.J.

Netter, Frank H., M.D.
    The CIBA Collection of Medical Illustrations
    Volume 5 Heart
    CIBA Pharmaceutical Co., 1978
    West Caldwell N.J.

Netter, Frank H., M.D.
    The CIBA Collection of Medical Illustrations
    Volume 6 - Kidneys, Ureters, and
    Urinary Bladder
    CIBA Pharmaceutical Co., 1979
    West Caldwell N.J.

Netter, Frank H., M.D.
    The CIBA Collection of Medical Illustrations
    Volume 7 Respiratory System
    CIBA Pharmaceutical Co., 1980
    West Caldwell N.J.

Ni, Hua Ching, Master
    The Book of Changes and
    the Unchanging Truth
    The Shrine of the Eternal Breath of Tao, 1983
    Malibu, CA

Ni, Hua Ching, Master
    Mysticism
    Empowering the Spirit Within
    The Shrine of the Eternal Breath of Tao, 1992
    Malibu, CA

Niranjanananda, Saraswati Swami
    Prana Pranayama
    Prana Vida
    Shi Panchdashnam Paramahamsa
    Alakh Bara, 2002
    Deoghar, Bihar, India

Niranjanananda, Paramahamsa
    Dharana Darshan
    Empowering the Spirit Within
    Shi Panchdashnam Paramahamsa
    Alakh Bara, 1993
    Deoghar, Bihar, India

O'Connor, John and Dan Bensky
    Acupuncture, A Comprehensive Text
    Shanghai College of Traditional Medicine
    Eastland Press, 1981
    Chicago, Illinois

Olsen, Cynthia
    Essiac A Native Herbal Cancer Remedy
    Kali Press, 1996
    Pagosa Springs, Colorado

Omura, Yoshiaki, Sc.D., M.D.
    Acupuncture Medicine
    Japan Publications, Inc., 1982
    Tokyo, Japan

Panchadas, Swami
    Clairvoyance and Occult Powers
    Fujian Science and Technology
    Yogi Publication Society, 1916
    Chicago, Illinois U.S.A.

Pan, Mingji, M.D. (China)
    How to Discover Cancer Through
    Self-Examination
    Fujian Science and Technology
    Publishing House, 1992
    Beijing, China

Pan, Mingji, M.D. (China)
    Cancer Treatment with Fu Zheng Pei
    Ben Principle
    Fujian Science and Technology
    Publishing House, 1992
    Beijing, China

A Modern Chinese-English Dictionary
    Hai Feng Publishing Co., Ltd.
    Oxford University Press, 1997
    Oxford, New York

Pearsall, Paul, Ph.D.
    The Heart's Code
    Tapping the Wisdom and Power of
    Our Heart Energy
    Broadway Books, 1998
    New York City, New York,

Peoples Republic of China
    The Cultivation of the Innate and the Destined
    White Cloud Monastery 1988
    Beijing, China

Pereira, M. A., et al
> *Effects of the Phytochemicals, Curcumin and Quercitin, upon Azoxymenthane-Induced Colon Cancer and 7, 12-Dimenthybenz A Chinese Traditional Therapeutic Skill*
> Shandong Science and
> Technology Press, 1990
> Shandong, China

Pidwirny, Michael, Dr.
> *Introduction to the Hydrosphere*
> Department of Geography
> Okanagan University College, 2004

Rago, D. Scott
> *Leaving the Body*
> *A Complete Guide to Astral Projection*
> Prentice-Hall, Inc., 1983
> Englewood Cliffs, New Jersey

Ramacharaka, Yogi
> *Fourteen Lessons in Yogi Philosophy and Oriental Occultism*
> Yogi Publication Society, 1903
> Chicago, Illinois U.S.A.

Ramacharaka, Yogi
> *Science of Breath A Complete Manual of The Oriental Breathing Philosophy of Physical, Mental, Phychic and Spiritual Development*
> Yogi Publication Society, 1904
> Chicago, Illinois U.S.A.

Ramacharaka, Yogi
> *Raja Yoga or Mental Development*
> Yogi Publication Society, 1906
> Chicago, Illinois U.S.A.

Ramacharaka, Yogi
> *The Science of Phychic Healing*
> Yogi Publication Society, 1909
> Chicago, U.S.A.

Ramacharaka, Yogi
> *The Life Beyond Death*
> Yogi Publication Society, 1909
> Chicago, Illinois U.S.A.

Ramacharaka, Yogi
> *The Hindu Yogi Practical Water Cure*
> Yogi Publication Society, 1909
> Chicago, Illinois U.S.A.

Reid, Daniel
> *The Complete Book of Chinese Health and Healing*
> Shambhala Publications, Inc., 1994
> Boston, Massachusetts

Reid, Daniel
> *A Complete Guide to Chi-Gung Harnessing the Power of the Universe*
> Shambhala Publications, Inc., 2000
> Boston, Massachusetts

Requena, Yves
> *Character and Health*
> *The Relationship of Acupuncture and Psychology*
> Paradigm Publications, Inc., 1989
> Brookline, Massachusetts

Rinpoche, Tenzin Wangyal
> *Healing with Form, Energy and Light*
> *The Five Elements in Tibetan Shamanism, Tantra and Dzogchen*
> Snow Lion Publications, 2002
> Ithaca, New York,

Robinet, Isabelle
> *Taoist Meditation*
> *The Mao-shan Tradition of Great Purity*
> State University of New York Press, 1993
> Albany, New York

Ros, Frank, Dr.
> *The Lost Secrets of Ayurvedic Acupuncture*
> Lotus Press, 1994
> Twin Lakes, Wisconsin

Ross, Elisabeth Kubler, M.D.
> *On Death and Dying*
> Collier Books, 1969
> Macmillan Pub. Co., New York

Ross, Jeremy, C.Ac. (Nanjing), B.Ac. (M.B.Ac.A.), C.Ed.
> *Zang Fu, The Organ Systems of Traditional Chinese Medicine Functions, Interrelationships and Patterns of Disharmony in Theory and Practice*
> Churchill Livingstone, 1985
> Edinburgh, London, Melbourne and New York

Sabetti, Stephano
The Wholeness Principle
Exploring Life Energy Process
Life Energy Media, 1986
Sherman Oaks, California

Sagar, Stephen M., M.D.
Restored Harmony
An Evidence Based Approach for
Menlo Park, California

Sancier, Kenneth M., Ph.D.
Anti-Aging Benefits of Qigong
Qigong Institute, 1986
Menlo Park, California

Sankey, Mikio, Ph.D., L.Ac.
Esoteric Acupuncture
Gateway to Expanded Healing Vol.1
Mountain Castle Publishing, 1999
Los Angeles, Ca.

Saso, Michael
The Gold Pavilion
Taoist Ways to Peace, Healing and Long Life
Charles E. Tuttle Co., 1995
Boston, Mass. 02109

Saso, Michael
Taoist Master Chuang
Sacred Mountain Press, 2000
Eldorado Springs, Co. 80025

Satyananda Saraswati, Swami
Sure Ways to Self Realization
Yoga Publications Trust, 1980
Bihar, India

Satyananda Saraswati, Swami
Taming the Kundalini
Yoga Publications Trust, 1982
Bihar, India

Satyananda Saraswati, Swami
Yoga Nidra
Yoga Publications Trust, 1998
Bihar, India

Satyananda Saraswati, Swami and
Muktibodhananda Saraswati, Swami
Swara Yoga
Tantric Science of Brain Breathing
Satyananda Ashram, 1983
Australia

Satyasangananda, Swami
Tattwa Shuddhi
Yoga Publications Trust, 2000
Bihar, India

Scambia, G., et al
Antiproliferative Effects of Silybin on
Gynaecological Malignancies: Synergism
with Cisplatin and Dororubien
European Journal of Cancer, 1996.
32A (5): 877-882

Scanlan, Michael T.O.R., Randall J. Cirner
Deliverance From Evil Spirits
A Weapon for Spiritual Warfare
Servant Books, 1980
Ann Arbor, Michigan

Schneider, Michael S.
A Beginner's Guide to Constructing the Universe
The Mathematical Archetypes of Nature,
Art and Science
Harper Collins Publishers, 1994
New York City, New York

Schwark, Jack
Human Energy Systems
The Aletheia Foundation, 1980
New York, New York

Sheldrake, Rupert
The Presence of the Past
Morphic Resonance &the Habits of Nature
Park Street Press, 1995
Rochester, Vermont 05767

Sha, Zhi Gang (Xiao Gang Guo)
Zhi Neng Medicine Revolutionary Self-Healing
Methods from China
Zhi Neng Press, 1997
Vancouver, B.C. Canada

Sha, Zhi Gang, Dr.
> *Power Healing: The Four Keys to Energizing Your Body, Mind and Spirit*
> Harper Collins Publishers Inc., 2002
> New York City, New York

Shi, Lanling
> *Experience In Treating Cancers with Traditional Chinese Medicine*
> Shandong Science and Technology Press, 1992
> Shandong, China

Shih, Tzu Kuo, Dr.
> *Qigong Therapy*
> *The Chinese Art of Healing With Energy*
> Station Hill Press, 1994
> Barrytown, New York 12507

Sivapriyananda, Swami
> *Secret Power of Tantrik Breathing*
> Abhinav Publications, 1996
> New Delhi, India

Small, Eric, et al.
> *Journal of Clinical Oncology*
> Vol 18, November 2000

Smith, Jia Yin
> *The Application of Talisman in Feng Shui*
> Translated by K.C. Goh 2002
> Taoist Culture and Information Center
> www.universalfengshui.com/

Stedman's Medical Dictionary.
> Vol 18, 2000

Stewart, Goldstein Jade, D.M.Q. (China)
> *Oncology, Traditional Chinese Medicine and Clinical case Studies*
> International Institute of Medical Qigong, September, 2004
> Monterey, Ca.

Strickmann, Michel
> *Chinese Magical medicine*
> Stanford University Press, 2002
> Stanford, Ca.

Sun, Jiyuan
> *A Probing into the Treatment of leukemia with Traditional Chinese Medicine*
> Hai Feng Publishing Co., 1990
> Hong Kong

Svoboda, Robert E.
> *The Art of Sacred Speech*
> Yoga International
> Vol. No.69, January 2003

Svoboda, Robert, and Arnie Lade
> *Chinese Medicine and Ayurveda*
> Motilal Banarsidass Publishers, 1998
> Delhi, India

Svoboda, Robert E.
> *Aghora: At the Left Hand of God*
> Brotherhood of Life, Inc., 1986
> Albuquerque, New Mexico

Svoboda, Robert E.
> *Aghora II: Kundalini*
> Brotherhood of Life, Inc., 1993
> Albuquerque, New Mexico

Svoboda, Robert E.
> *Aghora III: The Law of Karma*
> Brotherhood of Life, Inc., 1997
> Albuquerque, New Mexico

Talbot, Michael
> *The Holographic Universe*
> Harper Collins Publishers, 1991
> New York City, New York, 10022

Taylor, Kylea
> *The Ethics of Caring*
> Hanford Mead Publishers, 1995
> Santa Cruz, California

Tayson, Donald
> *The Power of the Word*
> *The Secret Code of Creation*
> Llewellyn Publications, 2004
> Saint Paul, MN 55164-0383

Textbook of Medical Qigong Therapy
> Haidian Qigong University
> Medical Qigong College
> White Cloud Monastery, 1988
> Beijing, China

Thomas, Clayton L., M.D., M.P.H.
> *Taber's Cyclopedic Medical Dictionary*
> F.A. Davis Company, 1993
> Philadelphia, Pa., 19103

Thornes, D., et al
  *Prevention of Early Recurrence of High
  Risk Malignant Melanoma by Coumarin.*
  Irish Melanoma Group, 1989
  European Journal of Surgical Oncology
  15 (5): 431- 435.

Tierra, Michael, L.Ac., N.D., A.H.G.
  East West Master Course In Herbology , 1981
  Santa Cruz, California

Tierra, Michael, L.Ac., N.D., A.H.G.
  *Treating Cancer with Herbs
  An Integrative Approach,*
  Lotus Press 2003
  Twin Lakes, Wi

Torisu, M., et al
  "*Significant Prolongation of Disease-free
  Period Gained by Oral Polysaccharide K
  (PSK) Administration after Curative
  Surgical Operation of Colorectal Cancer*"
  Cancer Immunology and
  Immunotherapy, 1990
  31 (5): 261-268.

Tortora, Gerard J. and Sandra R. Grabowski
  "*Principles of Anatomy and Physiology
  Seventh Edition*
  Harper Collins College Publishers, 1993
  New York City, New York 10022

Tyson, Donald
  Scrying for Beginners
  Liewellyn Publishers, 2004
  St. Paul, Minnesota 55164-0383

Tyson, Donald
  Familiar Spirits
  Liewellyn Publishers, 2004
  St. Paul, Minnesota 55164-0383

The University of Rochester
  School of Medicine
  *Clinical Oncology
  A multidisciplinary approach,* 1978
  Rochester, New York

Unschuld, Paul U.
  *Medicine in China
  Nan-Ching
  The Classic of Difficult Issues*
  University of California Press 1986
  Berkeley, California

Unschuld, Paul U.
  *Forgotten Traditions of Ancient Chinese Medicine
  A Chinese View of the Eighteenth Century*
  Paradigm Publications 1998
  Brookline, Massachusetts

Van Ostrand, Lisa, D.M.Q.
  *Treating Cysts, Tumors and Cancer Using
  a Medical Qigong Approach*
  International Institute of Medical Qigong,
  Florida Branch, 2004

Van Buskirk, Patricia, L.Ac.
  Anatomy of a Stroke
  Journal of Oriental Medicine in America,
  Summer 1997, Volume 1, Number 4, Ca.

Veith, Ilza
  *The Yellow Emperor's Classic of
  Internal Medicine*
  University of California Press, 1966
  Berkeley and Los Angeles, Ca.

Vieira, Waldo, M.D.
  *Projections of the Consciousness
  A Diary of Out-of-Body Experiences*
  International Institute of Projectiology
  and Conscientiology, 1997
  Rio De Janerio, Brazil

Walker, Martin J.
  *Dirty Medicine
  Science, big business and the assault on
  natural health care*
  Slingshot Publishing, 1993
  London, England

Walters, Derek
  The Complete Guide to Chinese Astrology
  Watkins Publishing, 2005
  London, England

Walters, Derek
Ming Shu
The Art and practice of Chinese Astrology
Kim Hup Lee Printing Co. 1989
Singapore

Weed, Susan S.
Breast Cancer? Beast Health!
The Wise Woman Way
Ash Tree Publishing, 1996
Woodstock, New York.

Welch, Holmes
Taoism: The Parting of the Way
Beacon Press, 1972
Boston, Mass.

Weil, Andrew, M.D.
Spontaneous Healing
Fawcett Columbine
Published by Ballantine Books, 1995
New York City, New York

Whitcomb, Bill
The Magician's Companion A Practical & Encyclopedic Guide to Magical & Religious Symbolism
Llewellyn Publications, 2002
St. Paul, MN

Wieger, L. Dr., S.J.
Chinese Characters
Their origin, etymology, history, classification and signification
Dover Publications, Inc., 1965
New York City, New York

Wilber, Ken, Carol McCormick, Alex Grey
Sacred Mirrors
The Visionary Art of Alex Grey
Inner Traditions International, 1990
Rochester, Vermont

Willmont, Dennis
The Twelve Spirit Points of Acupuncture
Willmountain Press, 1999
Roslindale, Massachusetts

Wing, R. L.
The I Ching Workbook
Doubleday Dell Publishing Group, 1979
New York, New York

Wiseman, Nigel and Feng Ye
A Practical Dictionary of Chinese Medicine
Second Edition
Paradigm Publications, 1998
Brooklyn, Massachusetts

Wiseman, Nigel and Feng Ye
Chinese Medical Chinese
Grammar and Vocabulary
Paradigm Publications, 2002
Brooklyn, Massachusetts

Wong, Eva
Teachings of the Tao
Shambhala Press, 1997
Boston & London

Wong, Eva
The Shambhala Guide to Taoism
A complete introduction to the history, philosophy, and practice of an ancient Chinese spiritual tradition
Shambhala Press, 1997
Boston & London

Wu, Baolin, Dr. and Jessica Eckstein
Lighting the Eye of the Dragon
Inner Secrets of Taoist Feng Shui
St. Martin's Press, 2000
New York, New York

Wu, Henry S., D.C.
Differentiation of Syndromes
California Acupuncture College, 1982
Los Angeles, Ca.

Wu, Jing-Nuan
Ling Shu or The Spiritual Pivot
Asian Spirituality, Taoist Studies Series
The Taoist Center
University of Hawaii Press, 1993
Honolulu, Hawaii

Wu, Qian
The Goldem Mirror of Medicine
Qing Dynasty, China 1742

Wu, Zhongxian
Ba Zi - Chinese Astrology
Qi The Journal of Health and Fitness
Volume 14, No. 2 Summer 2004

Xiao, Qian
Observations on the Therapeutic Efficacy of the Treatment of 38 cases of Acute Leukemia with a Combination of Chinese Medicines and Chemotherapy, 1998
Zhong Yi Za Zhi (Journal of Chinese Medicine), #5, p.283-285.

Xie, Wenwei
Cancer = Death
New World Press
Beijing, China 1997

Xu, Rui-rong et al.
The Treatment of 50 Cases of Acute Nonlymphocytic Leukemia with a combination of Chinese Medicine Pattern Discrimination & the HA Program,
Zhong Guo Zhong Xi Yi Jie He Za Zhi (Chinese National Journal of Integrated Chinese-Western Medicine), 1995, #5, p 302-303.

Yan, De-Xin
Aging & Blood Stasis
A New TCM Approach to Geriatrics
translated by Tang Guo-shun & Bob Flaws
Blue Poppy Press, 1995
Boulder, Co.

Yance, Donald R., Jr. with Arlene Valentine
Herbal Medicine, Healing & Cancer
Keats Publishing, 1999
Los Angeles, Ca. p.116

Yang, D. A., S. Q. Li, X. T. Li,
Chinese Journal of Surgery
Hua Wei Ko Tsa Chih
July 1994, p. 434.

Yang, Jwing Ming, Ph.D.
The Root of Chinese Qigong
The Secrets of Qigong Training
Yang Martial Arts Association, 1989
Jamaica Plain, Mass. 02130

Yang, Li
Book of Changes and Traditional Chinese Medicine
Beijing Science and Technology Press, 1998
Beijing, China

Yang, Qiyuan
Chinese Yuanbao Qigong
New World Press, 1998
Beijing, China

Yeung, Him-che, L.Ac, O.M.D., Ph.D.
Diseases of the Colon and Rectum
Institute of Chinese medicine, 1993
Rosemead, Ca. 91770

Yin, Hui He
Fundamentals of
Traditional Chinese Medicine
Foreign Languages Press, 1995
Beijing, China

Yu, Gong Bao
Chinese Qigong Illustrated
New World Press, 1995
Beijing, China

Zhao, Ruan Jin, Dr.
The Origin of Cancer and Phlegm
Traditional Chinese Medicine World
March 2002 - Vol.3. No. 4
New York City, New York 10013

Zhang, Enqin
Basic Theory of Traditional Chinese Medicine
Publishing House of Shanghai College of Traditional Chinese Medicine, 1988
Shanghai, China

Zhang, Yu Huan & Ken Rose
A Brief History of Qi
Paradigm Publications, 2001
Brookline, Massachusetts

Zhang, Yu Huan & Ken Rose
Who Can Ride the Dragon?
An Exploration of the Cultural Roots of Traditional Chinese Medicine
Paradigm Publications, 1999
Brookline, Massachusetts

Zhu, Danxi
Danxi's Experiential Therapy
Revised by Cheng Yun
Ming Dynasty, China 1481

Clinic References

American Cancer Society
  Cancer Facts and Figures
  www.cancer.org. 2002

American Cancer Society
  Melanoma Skin Cancer
  www.cancer.org. 2002

Fey, John, Master
  Clinical Notes from Lectures
  Medical Qigong Therapy
  Reference: Differential Healing Modalities
  Los Angeles, CA 1984 to 1987

Gershon, Michael, M.D.
  Professor of Anatomy and Cell Biology
  Columbia Presbyterian Medical Center
  Research presented by Sandra Blakeslee
  New York Times, New York   1996

Gill, Jason L.Ac.
  Lectures on Traditional Chinese Medicine
  Clinical Notes on Differential Diagnosis
  Pacific Grove, CA 1994 to 1997

Gill, Jason L.Ac.
  Clinical notes and Lectures
  Reference: Dr. Jeremy Ross Lectures
  on Traditional Chinese Medicine
  Pacific Grove, CA. 1994 to 1997

Guo Xian He, Dr., Dr. Zhou Jun Jie
  Clinical notes from Orthopedic Traumatology
  Clinic of the Hu Guo Si Hospital of T.C.M.
  on Medical Qigong Therapy and Anmo
  Therapy: Internship specializing in Chinese
  bone-setting, traumatology, and tissue
  manipulation Sept. 1993

Hong, Lu Guo, Dr., Dr. Niu Yu Hua, Dr. Li Fu Dong
  Clinical notes from Hai Dian Medical
  University on Medical Qigong Therapy and
  Differential Healing Modalities
  Beijing, China 1993 - 1996

Integrative Medicine Communications
  Skin Cancer
  www.ivillagehealth.com. 2001

Johnson, Jerry Alan, Ph.D., D.T.C.M., D.M.Q. (China)
  Clinical notes from the First World
  Conference on Medical Qigong
  Medical Qigong Therapy and Differential
  Healing Modalities
  Reference Conference No. 1, Sept. 1988

Johnson, Jerry Alan, Ph.D., D.T.C.M., D.M.Q. (China)
  Clinical notes from the International
  Symposium on Chinese Qigong Health
  Preservation and Qigong Techniques
  Medical Qigong Therapy and Differential
  Healing Modalities
  Reference Symposium, Nov. 1990

Johnson, Jerry Alan, Ph.D., D.T.C.M., D.M.Q. (China)
  Clinical notes from the Second World
  Conference on Medical Qigong
  Medical Qigong Therapy and Differential
  Healing Modalities
  Reference Conference No. 2, Sept. 1993

Johnson, Jerry Alan, Ph.D., D.T.C.M., D.M.Q. (China)
  Clinical notes from Xi Yuan Hospital
  on Medical Qigong Therapy and
  Differential Healing Modalities
  Internship July 1993 through Sept. 1995

Johnson, Jerry Alan, Ph.D., D.T.C.M., D.M.Q. (China)
  Clinical notes from Orthopedic Traumatology
  Clinic of the Hu Guo Si Hospital of T.C.M.
  on Medical Qigong Therapy and Anmo
  Therapy: Internship specializing in Chinese
  bone-setting, traumatology, and tissue
  manipulation Sept. 1993

Johnson, Jerry Alan, Ph.D., D.T.C.M., D.M.Q. (China)
Clinical notes from Hai Dian Medical University on Medical Qigong Therapy and Differential Healing Modalities
July 1993 through Sept. 1995

Johnson, Jerry Alan, Ph.D., D.T.C.M., D.M.Q. (China)
Clinical notes from the Third World Conference on Medical Qigong
Medical Qigong Therapy and Differential Healing Modalities
Reference Conference No. 3, Sept. 1996

Johnson, Jerry Alan, Ph.D., D.T.C.M., D.M.Q. (China)
Clinical notes from the Second World Congress on Medical Qigong
Medical Qigong Therapy and Differential Healing Modalities
San Francisco, California Nov. 1997

Johnson, Jerry Alan, Ph.D., D.T.C.M., D.M.Q. (China)
Clinical notes from the Fourth World Conference on Medical Qigong
Medical Qigong Therapy and Differential Healing Modalities
Reference Conference No. 4, Sept. 1998

Johnson, Jerry Alan, Ph.D., D.T.C.M., D.M.Q. (China)
Clinical Notes from International Institute of Medical Qigong
Medical Qigong Clinical Therapy and Differential Healing Modalities
Pacific Grove, CA 1988 - 2004

Johnson, Jerry Alan, Ph.D., D.T.C.M., D.M.Q. (China)
Clinical Notes from The Five Branches Acupuncture and Medical Qigong Clinic
Santa Cruz, CA 2000 - 2004

Johnson, Jerry Alan, Ph.D., D.T.C.M., D.M.Q. (China)
Clinical Notes from The Academy of Five Element Acupuncture and Medical Qigong Clinic, Hallandale, Fl 2003 - 2004

Johnson, Mark, Sifu
Clinical Notes in Geriatric Medical Qigong Therapy and Esoteric Daoist Studies of the Yi-Jing and Feng Shui
Mill Valley, CA 1998 - 1999

Krieger, Lisa M.
Full-body X-ray scans boost cancer risk
San Jose Mercury News
Tuesday, August 31, 2004

Li, Fudong, D.M.Q., Lu Guohong D.M.Q., Niu Yuhua D.M.Q.
Clinical notes from Hai Dian Medical University on Medical Qigong Therapy and Differential Healing Modalities
July 1993 through Sept. 1995

Lu, Dr. and Dr. Xu Zong Wei
Clinical Notes from Xi Yuan Hospital
Medical Qigong Therapy and Differential Healing Modalities
Beijing, China 1993

Meng, Xiantong, D.T.C.M., and Tara Peng, D.M.Q.
Clinical notes from the Beijing Chengjian Clinic of Integrated T.C.M. and Western Medicine Sept. 1998

Milne, Hugh, Dr.
Clinical Notes from Cranial-Sacral Therapy
Level 1 through 6, 1990-1995
Monterey, Calif.

National Cancer Institute
What You need To Know About Skin Cancer
www.nci.org. 1998

National Women's Health Resource Center
Skin Cancer
www.ivillagehealth.com 2000

Pang, Jeffrey, L.Ac., M.D. (China)
Clinical Notes from class on Traditional Chinese Medical Treatment for Oncology
Five Branches Institute Feb. -June 2003
Santa Cruz, California

Pang, Jeffrey, L.Ac., M.D. (China)
Clinical Notes from class on Traditional Chinese Medicine: Dietetics
Five Branches Institute Feb. -June 2002
Santa Cruz, California

Pereira, M. A., et al
> Effects of the Phytochemicals, Curcumin and Quercitin, upon Azoxymenthane-Induced Colon Cancer and 7,12-Dimenthybenz (a) anthracene-Induced Mammary Cancer in Rats Carcinogenesis 17 (6): 130 5-11 1996.

Ren, Shun Tu, Dr. & Dr. Xu Hong Tao
> Clinical Notes from Xi Yuan Hospital Medical Qigong Therapy and Differential Healing Modalities
> Beijing, China 1995

Sun, Dr., and Dr. Tu
> Clinical notes from Xi Yuan Hospital on Medical Qigong Therapy and Differential Healing Modalities Internship July 1993 through Sept. 1995

Sun, Shuchun, D.T.C.M., Dr. Fan
> Clinical notes from Orthopedic Traumatology Clinic of the Hu Guo Si Hospital of T.C.M. on Medical Qigong Therapy and Anmo Therapy: Internship specializing in Chinese bone-setting, traumatology, and tissue manipulation Sept. 1993

Turk, Michael, L.Ac.
> Clinical Notes from CSOMA International Expo & Comvention 2002 Seminar Healing Chronic Pain and Disability
> San Francisco, California 2002

Teng, Ying Bo, Dr.
> Clinical Notes from Beijing Medical Qigong Science and Research Institute Medical Qigong Therapy and Differential Healing Modalities
> Beijing, China 1995

Xu, Hongtao, D.M.Q., Ren Shuntu, D.M.Q., and Xu Zongwei
> Clinical Notes from Xi Yuan Hospital Medical Qigong Therapy and Differential Healing Modalities
> Beijing, China 1995

Zheng, Zhan Ding, Master
> Clinical Notes on Medical Qigong Diagnosis, Therapy and Differential Healing Modalities
> Beijing, China 1993 - 1998

Zhong, Jiang Gui, Dr. and Dr. Cai Chang Rong
> Clinical Notes from Hu Guo Hospital Medical Qigong Therapy, An Mo Therapy and Differential Healing Modalities
> Beijing, China 1993

Zhou, Fang, D.M.Q.
> Clinical Notes on Medical Qigong Therapy, An Mo Therapy and Differential Healing Modalities, Hai Dian University Clinic
> Beijing, China 1993

INDEX

A
abdominal pain 42, 256, 341, 368, 409, 410
abnormal qi circulation 40
absorbing qi 179
acquired cellular patterns 150
acupuncture **34-36**, 184
acupuncture points 35, 315, 491
acupuncture therapy 35
    blood letting 36
    cupping 36
    magnetic 36
    moxa burning 36
    needle insertion 35
aeromancy 20
affirmation 149
agents of shang ling 102
    earth agent 103
    fire agent 102
    metal agent 103
    prenatal wu jing shen 102
    water agent 103
    wood agent 102
ahshi points 481
akasha 50
alchemy 484
alternating current 182
Alzheimer's disease 184
amenorrhea 260, 261, 332, 340
amniotic fluid 79, 83, 92
an mo visceral manipulation 40, **41**, 50
anemia 221
anger 126, 333
anal canal 370
anal sphincter 248, 371
ancestral channel 239
ancestral qi 220
ancestral traits 96-97
ancient Chinese medicine college 24
anesthesia 184
anxiety 399, 486
aphasia 341, 399, 457
apnea 363
archetypes **99**, 333
arteriosclerosis 398, 404
arthritis 42
ascending qi 248
asthma 340, 355, 356, 363, 428, 487

astrology 127
atria 225
atrophy 355, 449
attention deficit disorder (A.D.D.) 75, 85, 226, 420, 427
augury 19
aura seeing 236, 171-172
awakening 189

B
back pain 264, 456
bagua 8, 52, 64, 217
    earth (kun) 52, 54, 57
    fire (li) 52, 54, 57
    heaven (quan) 52, 54, 57
    lake (dui) 52, 54, 57
    mountain (gen) 52, 54, 57
    thunder (zhen) 52, 54, 57
    water (kan) 52, 54, 57
    wind (sun) 52, 54, 57
bagua eight trigrams 7, 8, 40, **52-72**
Bai Yuan 99
baihui (one hundred meetings) 186, 207, 208, **229**, 231, 467
bao (uterus) 72, 73, 80, **81-82**, 248, 256, **282-285**, 331, 382
Bao Pu Zi (he who embraces the uncarved block) 11
belt vessel (dai mai) 77, 78, 240-241, 243, 245-248, 257, **261-264**, 278, 330, 489
Bian Que 9
bile 332, **343-344**, 345, 411
biochemical 221
biophotons 165
biorhytms 98, 99
blastomere 72
blastula 73
blazing heart fire 400, 409
blazing liver fire 340-341
blood 260, 299, 311, 331-332, 381-382, 389-390, 394, 397
blood deficiency 475
blood heat cycle 311, 315, 320
blood stasis 398
blood vessels (xue mai) 83, 85, 103, **299-306**, 350, 385, 392, 401
bloodletting 36
body alignment 40
body fluids (jin and ye) 37, 310, 311, 349, 381, 385, **394, 421**, 446
bone 85, **296-299**

brain 76, 84-85, 184, 226, 243, 248, **285-292**, 391
breast cyst 140
bronchi 359
bronchitis 363

C

Cade, Maxwell C. 289
carbohydrates 344
carcinoma 256
cardia 377-378
cardiac cycle 403-404
cecum 369-370
celestial divination 22-23
center core **188**, 316
cerebellum 226, 227
cerebral hemispheres 286-288
chakra 185, 208, 229
    chakra one 195-197
    charka two 197-198
    charka three 198-199
    charka four 199-200
    charka five 200-201
    charka six 201-202
    charka seven 202-203
    charka eight 203-204
    charka nine 505
chakra gates 63
chakra gate reconstructing 209
channel and collateral therapy 475
channel function 321
channel pathology 448-451, 488
channel points 470, 480-481
channels 314
Chao Yuanfang 12
chaotic resonance 160
charts of halls of light 307, 308
Chen Menglei 12
China Healthways Institute 183
Chinese massage therapy 39-41
cholera 40
chong mai (thrusting vessel) 47, 78, 185, 240-241, 242, 243, 244, 245, 246, 247, 248, 247, 248, 256, **257- 261**, 278, 330
chong qi 47, 185
chronic obstructive pulmonary disease (C.O.P.D.) 363
chyme 328, 370, 411
clairaudience 236, 394
clairvoyance 236, 394
classification of energetic points 484
clean qi 444
climate 276
cold phlegm misting the heart 398-399

collaterals 315
colon 369, 370
color imagery 172-176
color vibration 171
coma 236, 399, 400, 401, 437
common cold 356, 357
compassion 333
conception 46, 351
conception vessel (ren mai) 74, 77, 94, 240-241, 245-248, **253-257**, 278
confluent points 489-490, 491
congealed blood 474
congenital cellular patterns 149-150
congenital constitution 127
congenital jing 149
congenital qi 74, 76, 85
conjuring spirits 17-18
constipation 196, 339, 340, 366, 376, 377, 409, 428
constitutions 35, 53, 94, **127-142**
    earth constitution 133-134
    fire constitution 131-132
    metal constitution 135-136
    water constitution 137-138
    wood constitution 128-130
    combined constitution 139-142
controlling cycle 128
coronary artery disease (C.A.D.) 397
corporeal soul (po) 67, 74, 79, 84, 89, 93, 100, 101, **107-113**, 215, 221, **323**, 333, **351-353**, 485
cough 355, 356, 357
creative cycle (generating cycle) 128, 485, 487, 488
crystal room or palace 226
cultural revolution 13
cupping 36
cystic fibrosis 363
cysts 42, 140, 388

D

Da Nan Yang Sheng Lun (on difficulties of health preservation) 10
dazhui (big vertebae) 224-225
dai mai (belt vessel) 77, 78, 240-241, 243, 245-248, 257, **261-264**, 278, 330, 489
damp cold 368, 387, 416
damp heat 263, 341, 366, 368, 385, 388, 415, 416, 446
dantian (field of cinnabar) 63, 91, 92, 185, 189, 211, 237
dantian
    lower dantian 81, 91, 93, 94, 99, 103, 119, 135, 167, 178, 180, 185, 197, 207, 211, 212, **213- 219**, 221, 223, 226, 233, 235, 236, 243, 249, 250, 253, 254, 258, 272, 274, 296, 316, 490, 509

middle dantian 61, 93, 167, 185, 200, 207, 211, 212, 213, **219-225**, 233, 235, 236, 243, 316, 441
upper dantian 93, 99, 101, 102, 119, 167, 178, 185, 202, 207, 211, 212, 213, 219, 220, 223, **225-233**, 235, 236, 244, 316
dantian energetic functions 233
dantian nine chambers 91
dao 4, 7, **46-48**, 61, 64, 185, 187, 188, 189, 212, 224, 226, 227, 244, 310
Daodejing (the way and its power) 9
daoist 92-93, 127, 159, 484
daoist alchemy 12, 212-213, 484
daoist mysticism 285, 286, 295, 296, 298, 302
daoyin 7, **9-10**, 12
de (virtue) 60, 94, 113-116, 218, 224, 423
death 98, 106, 108, **116-118**
dementia 437
depression 184, 203, 252, 253, 260, 273, 332-333, 338-339, 340, 341, 399, 400, 456, 479
diabetes 42
diarrhea 256, 339, 368, 376, 387, 410, 428
diet 5, 37, 53, 121, 127, 149, 375
digestion 325, 378, 381, 385, 440, 444
diphtheria 363
distance qigong emission 42
divergent channels 317-318, **459-463**
divine energy 5, 27, 212, 291
dizziness 399, 340, 341, 427
DNA 71
DNA and light 165-166
doctor of
    acupuncture therapy 30
    herbal medicine 30
    massage therapy 30
    medical qigong therapy 30
down syndrome 75, 85, 420, 427
dream interpretation 18-19
dreams 104, 105, 119, 334, 335, 423
du mai (governing vessel) 74, 77, 94, 240-241, 243, 245-248, **248-253**, 278
duodenum 410
dynasty **3, 493-494**
    Eastern Han 9, 51
    Han 8, 9, 10, 15, 39, 261, 262, 307
    Jin 11, 12, 25
    Ming 12, 25, 71, 181, 144, 419, 422, 439
    Northern Wei 23
    Qin 9, 14, 39
    Qing 12, 25
    Shang 3
    Song 7, 12, 23-24
    Southern Liang 11

Spring and Autumn 46, 59
Sui 11, 79
Tang 11, 23, 299
Three Kingdoms Period 11
Warring States 8, 9, 34
Wei 10
Western Han 9
Western Zhou 4
Xia 113
Yuan 12, 25, 117
Zhou 3, 8-9, 15, 23, 308
dynasty
    chronological chart 493-494
dysmenorrhea 256, 332, 339
dyspnea 243, 355, 363, 487, 490

E

ears 422, 427
earth element 125-126, 128, **133-134**, 372, 339
earth jing 74, 76, 90, 380
earth qi 70, 92, 213, 215
earthly branches 208-209, 316
eczema 474
edema 355, 385, 387, 388, 398, 428, 475
ego 115, 187, 227, 228, 422
eight confluent points **245-247**, 489, 491
eight extraordinary vessels 77-78, 79, 93, 95, 139, 186, 187, 213, **239-247**, 281, 315, 317
eight influential points 489, 491
eight trigrams **53-55**, 217
eigth lunar month 90
electricity 151, 152, 177, 182, 183, 226
elements 34, 102, 125, 126, 127, 139, 158, 176, 323, 485, 487, 488
embryo 73, **116**, 185, 282
embryological development **70-79**, 248, 261
empathic communication 221-222
emphysema 363
endorphins 184
energetic body 58
energetic grids 113
energetic medicine 208
energetic point therapy 481
energetic projection 158, 172
energetic special cavities (internal organ chambers) 91, 93
energy 151-153
enteric nervous systems 216
entrainment 160
enuresis 355, 415, 455, 457
environmental energy 27, 70, 112, 179, 186, 187, 316
environmental qi 100, 206, 231

esophagus 377, 383, 384, 406
essence palace (jing gong) 214
eternal soul **60-63**, 95, **116-117**
ethereal soul (hun) 67, 74, 79, 84, 86-87, 89, 94, **100-106**, 108, **112-113**, 118, 215, 221, **323**, **333-336**, 393, 423, 485
excess qi 35, 38, 139, 140, 141, 184, 225, 242
external pathogenic factors 28, 470, 487
external wei qi fields 42, 206, 235, 237
extra points 481
extraordinary organs 226, 242-243, 279, **281-306**
    blood vessels 242, 279, **299-305**
    bone 242, 279, **296-299**
    brain 76, 242, 279, **285-292**
    gall bladder 242, 279, **293-295**
    marrow 76, 242, 279, **295-296**
    uterus 242, 279, **282-285**
eye 332-333, 335, 340, 341

F

fa men (dharma gates) 35
Fang, Chao Yuan 79
fascia 39, 70, 85, **121-122**, 315, 322, 467, 473
fatigue 385, 387, 398, 400
fear 41, 42, 103, 110, 126, 133, 135, 137, 142, 184, 188, 198, 228, 365, 413, 422
febrile conditions 36, 40
fengfu (wind palace) 228-229
feng shui (wind water) **8**, 19, 164
fetal toxins **73**, 75, 85, 419, 427
fetus 50, 71, 73, 76, 78, 80-92, 97, 111, 127, 239, 254, 258, 305
fifteen connecting vessels (luo mai) 453
        collateral point location 455
        energetic anatomy 454
        du (governing vessel) 457-458
        foot jue yin (terminal yin, liver) 456
        foot shao yang (lesser yang, gallbladder) 456
        foot shao yin (lesser yin, kidney) 455
        foot tai yin (greater yin, spleen) 455
        foot yang ming (bright yang, stomach) 456
        hand jue yin (terminal yin, pericardium) 457
        hand shao yang (lesser yang, triple burner) 457
        hand shao yin (lesser yin, heart) 457
        hand tai yang (greater yang, small intestine) 456-457
        hand tai yin (greater yin, lung) 457
        hand yang ming (bright yang, large intestine) 457
        ren (conception vessel) 458
        pathology 455
fifth lunar month 86-87
fire cycle 94, 209, 296
fire element 125-126, **131-132**, 391, 405, 433, 439
first lunar month 80-82

five agents 86, 100, **102-103**, 119, 126, 158, 220, 221
five element
    earth 96, 125, 220
    fire 88, 96, 125, 128, 220
    metal 96, 125, 220
    water 96, 125, 220
    wood 96, 125, 220
five element constitutions 93, 122, 127, 128, 139, 149, 150
five element theory 310
five essence spirit (wu jing shen) 27, 45, 65, 85, 89, 92, **102-103**, 120, 226
five sense organs 454, 475
five shu points 485
five virtues 221
five viscera (wu zang) 308-309
five yin organs 89, 254
flu 40, 363
fluids 37, 63, 84, 103, 220, 311, 321, 350, 372, 413, 440, 443, 473
fontanel 95
fourth lunar month 85
fu (hollow) organs 285, **310**
fundus 378

G

gall bladder (dan) 83, 87, **293-295**, 317, **324-329**, 331, 336, 342, 343, 380, 406, 421, 434, 443, 449
    anatomy 328-329
    channels 325
    in Chinese medicine 324-325
    in western medicine 328-329
    patterns of disharmony 327-328
gallstones 165, 329
Ge Hong 11
Gershon, Dr. Michael 216
ghost points 490, 491
ghosts (gui) 107, 117, 351
golden fetus 285
governing vessel (du mai) 74, 77, 94, 240-241, 243, 245-248, **248-253**, 256, 260, 263, 267, 269, 278, 296, 457-458, 489
grief 28, 41, 103, 108, 110, 126, 135, 136, 140, 184, 351, 365
Gu Jin Shu Ji Cheng (collected ancient and modern books) 12
gu qi 93, 321, 349, **380-381**, 392, 444
gua sha (tissue scraping) 30, 33, **40**
gui (ghosts) 107, 117, 351
gui men (ghost gate) 350

H

Hai Dian University 73, 509
harmful effects of chaotic resonance sounds 163
harmful effects of entrainment sounds 162-163

he sea points 487, 490, 491
headaches 42, 150, 253, 267, 268, 270, 273, 340, 341, 357, 399, 457
healing by wuji shaman 21-22
healing sound therapy 43, 88
heart (xin) 90, 99, 206, **221**, 223, 272, 283, 383, **391-404**, 423, 457
    anatomy 402-403
    channels 395-397
    fire jing 391
    four chambers 402-403
    heartbeat 403-404
    in Chinese medicine 392-394
    in western medicine 400-402
    patterns of disharmony 398-400
    shen 393, **394-395**
heart fire 180, 206, 220, 398, 444, 445, 445
heaven qi 70, 178, 213, 224, 225
heavenly stems 96, 316
hemothorax 363
herbology 28, 32, 37-39, 322, 495
hertz (hz) 164, 288, 289
hexagram 143, **144-147**
hidden power 25, 296
high blood pressure 42, 126, 272, 340, 397, 398, 404, 509
hormones 345
Hua Tuo 9-10
Huang Di **7-8**
Huang Hua Jing (cultivation of the sea of essence) 11
Huangdi Neijing (yellow emperor's cannon of internal medicine) **8, 9,** 34, **70,** 308, 448
huiyin (meeting of yin) 93, 207, **216-217**, 233, 248, 254, **255**, 258
hun (ethereal soul) 67, 74, 79, 84, 86-87, 89, 94, **100-106**, 108, **112-113**, 118, 215, 221, **323**, **333-336**, 393, 423, 485
    tai suan 101, 227
    shang ling 102, 221
    yu jing 103
    shen 394
    sleeping and dreaming 334
    spirit travel 335
hypertension 42, 126, 272, 340, 397, 398, 404, 509
hypochondriac pain 276, 340, 341
hypotension 273, 404
hypothalamus 226

I

i-ching **7-8**, 20
ileum 411
immune system 4, 197, 219, 242, 296, 389-390, 473

impotence 197, 252, 253, 427, 428, 468
infertility 427
inhalation 422
insomnia 42, 104, 221, 256, 268, 273, 327, 334, 340, 341, 398, 399, 400, 437, 486
intent 28, 88, 89, 215, 381, 382, 441
internal palaces 91
internal wind 252, 253, **341**
intuition 105, 129, 130, 199, 202, 215, 225, 229, 231, 235, 236, 249, 355
intuitive female energy 86
invisible needle 33, 42, 43-44

J

Jacobs, Greg 289-290
jaundice 341, 345, 346, 388
jejunum 410-411
Ji Kang 10
jie gu (bone setting) 30, 40
jin ye (body fluids) 37, 349, 381, **394**, **421**, 446
jing (essence) 4, 74, 91, 93, 96, 226, 281, 338, **420**
jing formation 74
    earth jing 76, **380**
    fire jing 76, **391**
    metal jing 76, **347**
    water jing 75, **419-420**
    wood jing 76, **330**
jing mai 301
jing point therapy 30, **40**
jing river point 487
jing shen 186, 225
jing well point 485-486
jinsuo (sinew contraction) 224
joy 126, 184, 441

K

karma 98
kidney (shen) 91, 94, 140, 242, 248, 258, 264, 266, 281, **418-432**, 449, 455, 456
    anatomy 429-431
    channels 424-426
    in Chinese medicine 420-423
    in western medicine 428
    jing 282, 338
    kidney fire 445
    patterns of disharmony 427-428
kinesthetic 215
kinetic communication 99, 119, 215, 216
knees 144, 146, 276, 277, 420, 427, 428, 453, 487
knowing without knowing 227

L

Laozi **9**, 14
large intestine (da chang) 78, 87, 88, 89, 90, 92, 109, 125, 219, 274, 316, 317, 347, 353, **364-371**, 415, 444, 449, 456, 462, 472, 488, 490
   anatomy 369-370
   channels 366-367
   in Chinese medicine 364-366
   in western medicine 369-370
   patterns of disharmony 366-369
laryngitis 363
larynx 359
Lee, Richard 159, 178, 183
left atrium 403
left ventricle 403
leukorrhea 388-389, 341
li (cosmic and organic patterning) 126-127
life force energy 45
life purpose 94
ligamentum teres 91
light and cancer 166
light and energetic fields 165
light and food 165
ling qi 113, 285
ling hun 113
ling shen 113, 285
Ling Shu 28, 32, 76, 85, 223, 243, 259, 303, 349, 382, 449
ling zi 116
lipids 344-345
liver (gan) 79, 81, 83, 86, 88, 89, 91, 92, 104, 112, 119, 125, 127, 128, 140, 174, 175, 176, 195, 216, 244, 260, 263 264, 272, 283, 292, 316, 317, 321, 325, 326, **330-346**, 393, 415, 426, 444, 449, 455, 456, 472, 487, 488, 490
   anatomy 342-343
   channels 336-337
   hun 333-334
   in Chinese medicine 331-333
   in western medicine 341-346
   patterns of disharmony 338-341
   wind 337, 341
Loiu Guizhen 13
loop of henle 431
lotus flower 185
lower burner 226, 267, 413, 443, **444**, 446, 447
lower dantian 81, 91, 93, 99, 103, 119, 135, 167, 178, 180, 197, 207, 211, 212, **213-219**, 221, 223, 226, 235, 236, 243, 249, 250, 253, 254, 258, 272, 274, 296, 316, 490, 509
Lu Buwei 9
Lu Guo Hong 509
lungs (fei) 199, 219, 220, 224, 242, 316, 336, **347-363**, 365, 366, 385, 395, 426, 442, 443, 444, 446
   anatomy 357-359
   blood supply 361
   channels 353
   common disorders 363
   in Chinese medicine 347-350
   in western medicine 360-363
   patterns of disharmony 355-357
   po 351-353
   respiration 361-362
   respiratory capacities 362-363
luo points 455, 456, 457, 491

M

Maciocia, Giovanni 449
macrocosmic orbit 221, 441
magic square 72, **246-247**
Magical Pivot 28, 32, 76, 85, 223, 243, 258, 303, 349, 382, 449
magnetic energy 177
magnetic fields and the body 177-178
magnetic therapy 36, 179, 180
malaria 40
Mao Zedong 13
marrow 74, 76, 85, 226, 243, 250, 252, 281, 282, 285, **295-296**, 302, 390, 419, **420-421**, 427, 490
martial qigong
   ming jing 26
   an jing 26
   hua jing 26
master and couple points 245, 489
master points 246, 276, 489
material body 58
medical intuitive 226
medical qigong 26-34
   defined 27-28
   distance qi emission 42
   examinations 30-32
   healing sound therapy 43
   history 7-14
   introduction 3-4
   invisible needle 43
   qi (energy) 26
   qigong massage 42-43
   self regulation prescriptions 42
   therapy 41-43
   traditional Chinese medicine 34-36
   training in China 28-29,
   training in T.C.M. colleges 32-33,
   training in United States 32
   jing (essence) 26
meditation 5, 25, 27, 113, 127, 149, 175, 180, 183, 187, 188, 212, 214, 227, 231-233, 276, 277, 296, 445, 475, 485

medium 18
medullae oblongata 226, 227
memory 148, 188, 225, 226, 252, 286, 382, 383, 393, 423, 427, 423
menopause 256
menstruation 254, 256, 283, 331-332
meridians 315
mesenteric membrane 79, 83
metal element 125-126, **135-136**, 347, 364
microcosmic orbit fire cycle **94-95**, 208, 210, 221, 241, 244, 249, 296
microcosmic orbit water cycle 249, 336
middle burner 353, 386, **443-444**, 446, 447-448
middle dantian 61, 198, 199, 200, 207, 211, 212, 213, **219-225**, 235, 236, 243, 316, 441
migraine 42
minerals 345
mingmen (gate of destiny) 47, 71, 93, **207**, **218**, 296
mingmen fire 81, 181, 214, 262, 284, 422, 426, **445**
ming shu 96
moxa 33, 35, **36**, 182, 270, 473
mu points 488, 491
music in ancient China 163-164
myocardiac infarction 398, 404
myocarditis, 397-398, 404
myofacial 148
Myss, Caroline 226
mysterious power 25

N

nausea 339, 357, 388
necromancy 18
needle insertion 35
neidan 212
nephrons 431
new points 481
ni wan (mud pill) palace 231
nine chambers 81, 205, 216, 219, 222, 225, **230-233**
nine chambers of lower dantian 81, 219
nine chambers of middle dantian 225
nine palaces of the upper dantian 230-233
    palace of mysterious cinnabar 230
    palace of the jade emperor 230
    palace of flowering pearls 230
    palace of the supreme august 230
    palace of ni wan or cinnabar field 230
    palace of the ultimate truth 231
    palace of the celestial court 231
    palace of the grotto chamber 231
    hall of light (mingtang) 231
ninth lunar month 91

Niu Yu Hua 509
Nordenstrom, Bjorn 183
nose 358

O

obvious power 25
omens 19-21
opening and closing 207, 350, 470
orbs 86, 153, 185, 314
orifices 89, 315, 427
organ regulation 41
organs
    acquired emotions 312
    climate 312
    color 314
    congenital emotions 312
    odors 350
    sensory openings 312
    sounds 313
    spiritual aspects 312
    taste 313
ovarian cyst 42

P

palpitations 398, 399, 400
Pang Dong 509
People's Republic of China **12-13**, 25, 39
perineum 93, 144, 145, 178, 182, 185, 186, 187, 196, 206, 207, 213, 214, 216, 233, 248, 255, 413, 444, 445, 458
pericardium (xin zhu) 79, 84, 88, 222, 223, 225, 272, 316, 317, 394, 395, 400, 415, **433-438**, 441, 442, 443, 446, 451, 455, 457, 463, 472, 488, 490
    anatomy 438
    channels 435-437
    in Chinese medicine
    in western medicine 438
    patterns of disharmony 437
phagocytosis 345
pharynx 358-359
phlegm 355, 357, 386
phlegm fire agitating the heart 376, 400
phlegm misting the heart 398-399
photosynthesis 165
physiology of visual perception 171
pi fu (cutaneous skin region) 319
piezoelectric qualities **183**, 298
pineal gland 203, 226, 229
pitches (elemental sounds) 88
    gong (earth) 88
    jue (wood) 88
    shang (metal) 88

yu (water) 88
zhi (fire) 88
pituitary 226
placenta 83, 91
planetary influence on sense organs 89
pleural cavities 225
pleurisy 363
plum pit stagnation 339
pneumonia 363
pneumothorax 363
po (corporeal soul) 67, 74, 79, 84, 89, 93, 99, 100, 101, 103, 105, 106, **107-113**, 118, 119, 215, 221, 225, 226, 235, 236, **323**, 333, 351, 352, 353, 383, 423, 485
po men (gate of po) 353
polarity 183, 184, 193, 194, 245, 248, 485
pole star 186
postnatal 92
postnatal jing 127, 220, 280
postnatal qi 214, 243, 383
postnatal shen 105
pregnancy 73, 80, 83, 84, 91, 97, 127, 253, 258, 283, 331
prenatal jing 226
prenatal qi 92, 167, 220, 243, 296
prenatal wu jing shen 55, 56,74, 94-95
primary channels 78, 81, 93, 95, 186, 187, 215, 239, 240, 242, 244, 257, 284, 307, **315-320**, 441, 451, 453, 459, 460, 461, 464, 465, 470, 472, 474, 480, 485, 488, 490
projecting colored light 172
prolapse 387
pronucleus 72
protective qi 274, 443
psyche 225
psychological disorders 75, 85
psychology 28
psychosis 398
pulmonary edema 363
pulmonary embolism 363
pulse 173, 187, 206, 207, 482
purgation 95
pyelitis 431
pylorus 378
pyromancy 21

Q

qi **3-4**, 200, 208, 220, 239, 300, 397
qi blood cycle 315
Qi Bo **7**
qi deficiency 74, 76, 85, 387, 419, 427
qi deviations 12, 215, 219
qi flow 332
Qi Jing Ba Mai (eight extraordinary vessels) 239

qi of earth 279
qi of heaven 279
qi, sea of qi 81, 214, 219, 243 , 281
qigong 7, 25
qigong clinic 497, 501, 502
Qigong Liao Fa Shi Jian (application of qigong to medical practice) 13
qigong massage **33,** 42-43
qing 74
Quan Zhen (complete reality) 12

R

radiation 170, 171, 183
rainmaking 21
rational male energy 86
rebellious qi 260
reflexology 39, 40, 146
regulation 95, 314
ren mai (conception vessel) 74, 77, 94, 240-241, 245-248, **253-257**, 278
renal cortex 430
renal medulla 430
renal pelvis 430
Republic of China **12-13**, 25, 39
respiration 361-362
rheumtic heart disease 398
rhinitis 355, 356, 363
rhythm 160
right atrium 403-404
right ventricle 404

S

sadness 108, 110, 126, 221, 351, 365
san (powders) 37
scrotum 90
sea of blood 78, 243, 244, 257, 259, 281, 490
sea of marrow sea of marrow 74, 76, 85, 226, 243, 250, 252, 281, 282, 285, **295-296**, 302, 390, 419, **420-421**, 427, 490
sea of nourishment 243, 281
sea of qi 81, 214, 219, 220, 243 , 281, 415, 488, 490
second lunar month 83
self regulation therapy 33, 42, 43
seven corporeal souls seven corporeal souls 67, 74, 84, 89, 93, 100, 101, **107-113**, 215, 221, **323**, 333, **351-353**, 485
seven emotions 126
seven essential stars 88
seventh lunar month 88
shaman 14-16, 17-23
shanzhong (central altar) 224
shang ling (hun) 101,102, 119

shao yang 142, 143, 317
shao yin 142, 143, 317
Shealy, C. Norman 226
shen (spirit) 4, 27, 74, 93, 101, 221, **226-227, 334-335,** 393-394, **394-395**
shen dao (way of the spirit) 206, 207, 208, **224**
shen gong 231
shen ling (supernatural spirit) 45, **59-60,** 86
shen ming (bright spirit) 27, 117, 434
shen que (spirit's watch tower) 217-218
shen xian 27, 45, 48, 59-60, **60-62,** 81, 96, 189, 392
shen zhi 45, 63-65, 92-93, 114-115, **393-395**
shu points 246, 488, 491
shu stream points 487
si ming (administrator of destiny) 99-100, 117, 118
Simple Questions 381
sinusitis 355, 363
sishencong (four spirits hearing) 186
six energetic pitches 88
six storage areas 87, 88
six transportations of shen 395
sixth lunar month 87, 88
skin zones (pi fu) 316, 318, **319, 470-475**
sleep 103, 104, 105, 127, 266, 267, 270, 327, 334, 426, 490
small intestine (xiao chang) 88, 125, 173, 219, 365, 395, **405-411,** 444, 449, 455, 456, 463, 469
    anatomy 410-411
    channels 406-408
    in Chinese medicine 405-406
    in western medicine 410-411
    patterns of disharmony 408-410
solid organs 315
sore throat 363
soul body 62
soul travel 285
soul retrieval 19
sound modalities 159
    characteristic sound therapy 159
    extraordinary sound therapy 159
    infrasonic sound therapy 159, 160
sound therapy 157
    audible toning 158
    slightly audible toning 158
    inaudible toning 158
    combined toning 158-159
sound vibration 157, 158
sounds 88
    heart "ha" 391
                "ke" 391
                "zheng" 391
                "zhi" 88

    kidneys "chree" 420
                   "fu" 420
                   "yu" 88
    liver "guo" 337
           "shu" 337
           "jue" 88
    lungs "shang" 88
             "shh" 347
             "sss" 347
    spleen "gong" 88
              "who" 385
spirit possession 229
spirit travel **18**, 94, 113, **335-336**
spiritual awakening 189
spiritual body 58
spiritual path 115
    desire 115
    renunciation 115
    service 116
    realization of immortality 116
spiritual qigong 27
spleen (pi) 86, 88, 89, 92, 93, 174, 318, 321, 372, 373, **379-390,** 426, 443, 449
    anatomy 388-389
    channels 383-385
    in Chinese medicine 380-383
    in western medicine 388-390
    patterns of disharmony 385-388
    yi 382-383
stagnant heart blood 398
sternum 224, 254, 296, 297
stomach (wei) 87, 92, 93, 243, **372-378,** 381, 383, 384, 406, 443, 444, 446, 449
    anatomy 377-378
    channels 373-375
    in Chinese medicine 372-373
    in western medicine 377-378
    patterns of disharmony 376-377
stream points 487, 490
stroke 42, 486
Su Wen 28, 279, 285, 291, 302, 350, 381
subconscious mind 105, 159, 215, 335
sudden infant death syndrome (S.I.D.S.) 363
Sun Simao **8, 11-12,** 229, 299
surgery 121, 177

T

Tao Hongjing 11
Tai Ji Tu Shuo (teaching of the taiji symbol) 12
tai yang 142, 143, 317
tai yi 99, 117, 118

tai yin 142, 317
taiji 45, **51-52**, 53, 64
taiji pole 61, 63, 64, 76, **77**, 78, 93, 94, 96, 101, 109, 110, 118, 119, 158, 167, 172, 173, 178, **185-186**, 187-188, 189, **191-193**, 195, 196, 206, 207, 209, 213, 217, 229, 233, 234, 236, 239, 242, 286, 316, 392, 475
    charka system 191-192
    energy within 189
taiji within human body 53
talisman 71, 295
tang (soups and teas) 37
ten heavenly systems 96
tenth lunar month 92
testes 90, 409
thalamus 226, 286, 287, 290
The Secret of Opening the Passes 12
The Four Hundred Character Treatise on the Golden Elixer 12
therapeutic effect of sound 160, 161
therapeutic uses of chaotic resonances 161, 162
therapeutic uses of entrainment 161
third eye 118, 231
third lunar month 84, 100
three fires 180, 182, 446
three treasures 65, 212
thrusting vessel (chong mai) 47, 78, 185, 240-241, 242, 243, 244, 245, 246, 247, 248, 247, 248, 254, 256, **257- 261**, 278, 282, 330, 332, 457
thymus 219, 220
tiantu (heaven's chimney) 224
timbre 160
tinnitus 252, 253, 276, 341, 420, 469, 490
tongue 394
tone or pitch 160
tonification 96
traditional Chinese medicine (T.C.M.) 3, 6, 27, 28, 30, 32-33, 45, 68, 72, 73, 121, 123, 128, 159, 166, 220, 314, 315, 320, 448, 465, 484
trachea 359
transference 43, 71, 383
transformation 27, 56, 62, 67, 122, 126, 160, 182, 183, 212, 214, 220, 234, 244, 257, 300, 381, 383, 397, 413, 443, 444
Trappier, Dr. Arthur 180
tremors 341
triple burner (san jiao) 85, 88, 182, 214, 218, 275, 435, **439-447**, 451, 463, 469
    anatomy energetic 442
    channels 441
true fire 180, 181, 218
true-self 228
tui na (massage) 30, 33, **40**, 42

turbid qi 444
twelve charka gates 206, 208, 209
twelve divergent channels (jing bie) 315, 317, 459, 461
twelve earthly branches 96, 208, 209
twelve entry points 488
twelve exit points 489
twelve primary channels (jing jin) 78, 93, 95, 166, 167, 186, 215, 239, 240, 242, 244, 257, 307, 315, 317, 318, 319, 320, 441, 451, 459, 461, 465, 472, 474, 490
twelve skin zones 319, 470, 472, 473, 474, 476

U

umbilical cord 83, **91**, 306
Understanding Reality 12
upper burner **443**, 444, 446
upper dantian 99, 101, 102, 119, 167, 178, 202, 207, 211, 212, 213, 219, 220, 223, **225-233**, 235, 236, 244, 316
urinary bladder (pang guang) 88, **412-417**
    anatomy 416-417
    channels 413-415
    in Chinese medicine 412-413
    in western medicine 416-417
    patterns of disharmony 415-416
urinary bladder fire 413, 445
uterus (bao) 72, 73, 80, **81-82**, 84, 85, 86, 88, 90, 91, 142, 248, 253, 254, 256, **282-285**, 331, 382

V

vaginal discharge 264
vascular system 92
vasculitis 397
ventricles 225
vertigo 399, 428, 490
vessels foundational four 240
    belt vessel 240
    conception vessel 240, 242
    governing vessel 240, 242
    thrusting vessel 240, 242
vessels secondary eight 241
    left and right yang linking 241
    left and right yin linking 241
    left and right yang heel 241
    left and right yin heel 241
virtues 86, 102, 108, 112, 126, 221, 235, **310**, 352, 423
    prenatal five agents 86
        integrity to the lungs 86
        kindness to the liver 86
        order to the heart 86
        truth to the spleen 86
        wisdom to the kidneys 86
visceral manipulation 41

visualization 28, 43, 106, 475
vomiting 339, 376, 377, 387, 388, 411

W

wai dan (outer alchemy) 212
wan (pills) 37
Wan Jin 12
Wan Mi Zhai Yi Shu Zhong (Wan Mi Zhong's ten medical books) 12
Wang Lu 12
water cycle 94
water element 125-126, **137-138**, 412-418
weather 177, 276
Wei Boyang 10
wei qi (defensive energy) 27, 28, 42, **188**, 206. 213, 220, 225, 226, 233, 234, 234, 237, **242**, 248, 322, 349, **441**, 471
wei qi field 27, 197, 199, 206, 233
will power 206, 383, 423
wind cold 356, 446, 455
wind damp 356-357
wind heat 356, 446, 455
wind stroke 337, 398
window of heaven points 491, **492**
wood element 125-126, **128-130**, 330, 324
worry 41, 42, 110, 126, 129, 133, 141, 142, 184, 221, 365, 382
wu (magician) **14-16**, 48
wu cai (five materials) 127
wu jing shen (five essence spirits) 27, 45, 65, 85, 89, 92, 100, **102-103**, 120, 226
wu xing (five phases) 45, **55**, 64, 125
wu yi (shaman) 14-16, 17-23
wu zang (five viscera) 308-309
wuji (infinite space) 4, 46, **48-51**, 61, 64, 186, 187, 188, 200, 212, 226, 227

X

Xi Yuan Hospital 45, 507, 509
xi cleft points 488, 491
xia tao kang (below healthy peach) 99, 100, 117, 118
xin xi (the message) **49-50**
xing 126, 127
Xing Qi Yu Pei Ming (jade pendant inscriptions of qigong) 9
xiphoid process 144, 146
xue mai (blood vessels) 83, 85, 103, **299-306**, 350, 385, 392, 401

Y

yang 6, 51-57, 62, 72, 74, 81, 83, 86, 90, 95, 122-123, 125, 142, 185, 208, 219, 317, 325, 366, 373, 406, 413, 441
    tai yang 142
    shao yang 142
    yang ming 317

Yang Li 8
yang organs 87, 90, 92, 279, 242, 279, 461, 475, 481, 489, 490
    gall bladder 87, 88, 92, 242, 279
    large intestine 87, 88, 92, 243, 279
    small intestine 87, 88, 92, 242, 279
    stomach 87, 92, 240, 279
    urinary bladder 87, 88, 92, 243, 279
    triple burners 87, 88, 243, 279
yang heel vessel (yang qiao mai) 241, 243, 245-248, 264-265, **268-271**, 278
yang linking vessel (yang wei mai) 241, 245-248, **274-278**
yang qiao mai (yang heel vessel) 241, 243, 245-248, 264-265, **268-271**, 278
Yang Shen Lun (on health preservation) 10
Yang Xing Yan Ming Lu (record of cultivating one's nature and longevity) **11**
yang wei mai (yang linking vessel) 241, 245-248, **274-278**
yao 53, 142-148
ye (body fluids) 325, 349, 405
yellow court (huang ting) 193, 194, 198, 219, **223-224**, 254, 256, 258, 435, 458, 459
yellow emperor (huang di) **7-8**, 127, 242, 379, 448
yi 26, 88, 89, 99, 101, 103, 114, 117, 118, 119, 143, 218, 225, 226, 333, 381, **382-383**, 394, 423
yi jing **7-8**, 20, 73, 143, 217, 233
Yi Jing Su Hui Ji (recall of medical text) **12**
yin 6, 51-57, 62, 72, 74, 81, 83, 86, 90, 95, 122, 123, 125, 142, 185, 208, 219
yin heel vessel (yin qiao mai) 241, 243, 245-248, **264-268**, 278
yin linking vessel (yin wei mai) 241, 245-248, **271-274**, 278
yin organs 86, 90, 92, 279, 283, 309, 486, 490
yin qiao mai (yin heel vessel) 241, 243, 245-248, **264-268**, 278
yin tang (hall of impression) **228**, 230, 231-233
yin wei mai (yin linking vessel) 241, 245-248, **271-274**, 278
ying qi 198, 218, 349
ying spring points 486-487
Yuan Fang 79
yuan jing (original essence) 81, 82, 214, 285
yuan qi (original energy) 71, 77, 80, **81**, 82, 83, 214, 218, 219, 220, 225, 242, 249, 253, 254, 284, 285, 289, 392, 415, 441, 488, 490
yuan shen (original spirit) 27, 45, 48, 60, 63, 64, **82**, 93, 94, 100, 112, 113, 116, 119, 159, 202, 204, 205, 221, 227, 249, 286, 383, 393, **394-395**
yuan source points 490-491
yuan yang 71, 284
yuan yin 71, 221

Z

Zan Dong Ji (union of three equations) 10
zang (yin organs) 285, 309, **310**, **312-314**

zang fu (yin and yang organs) 310
Zhang Boduan 12
Zhang Jieban 439
Zhang Lu 12
Zhang Shiyi Tong (Zhang's medical experience) 12
Zhang Zhongjing 9
zhi 26, 74, 88, 89, 103, 119, 132, 206, 218, 225, 226, 311, 383, **422-423**
zhi yi tian 45, 61, 63, 114, 117, 218

zhen qi 90, 349
zhong dantian 219
Zhou Dunyi 12
Zhou Qianchuan 28, 127
Zhu Bing Yuan Hou Lum (general treatise on cause and symptoms of disease) 12
Zhuangzi 9
zong qi 76, 90, 199, **220**, 349, 380, 442
zygote 54, 70, 71, 72

About the Author

PROFESSOR OF MEDICAL QIGONG:
- He Nan University of Traditional Chinese Medicine, Zheng Zhou, China

OVERSEAS DIRECTOR OF MEDICAL QIGONG:
- He Nan University of Traditional Chinese Medicine, Zheng Zhou, China

DEAN OF MEDICAL QIGONG SCIENCE:
- Academy For Five Element Acupuncture, Inc. Hallandale, Florida (U.S.A.)
- Five Branches Institute, College and Clinic of Traditional Chinese Medicine, Santa Cruz, California (U.S.A.)

DIRECTOR OF MEDICAL QIGONG CLINIC:
- Academy For Five Element Acupuncture, Inc. Hallandale, Florida (U.S.A.)
- Five Branches Institute, College and Clinic of Traditional Chinese Medicine, Santa Cruz, California (U.S.A.)

FOUNDER AND EXECUTIVE DIRECTOR OF THE INTERNATIONAL INSTITUTE OF MEDICAL QIGONG:
- Belgium, Bermuda, Bosnia, Canada, Central America, England, France, Ireland, Israel, South Africa, Sweden, and the Unites States

PROFESSOR OF MEDICAL QIGONG SCIENCE AND PHILOSOPHY (PH.D.):
- Academic License from the Beijing Western District Medical Qigong Science and Traditional Chinese Medicine Research Institute (China)

DOCTOR OF TRADITIONAL CHINESE MEDICINE (D.T.C.M.):
- Clinical License from the People's Republic of China, Ministry of Health

LICENSE OF ACADEMIC QUALIFICATIONS TO PRACTICE CHINESE MEDICINE:
- Issued by The Beijing Bureau of Public Health and The People's Republic of China, Ministry of Health

LICENSE OF CLINICAL QUALIFICATIONS TO PRACTICE CHINESE MEDICINE:
- Issued by The Beijing Bureau of Public Health and The People's Republic of China, Ministry of Health

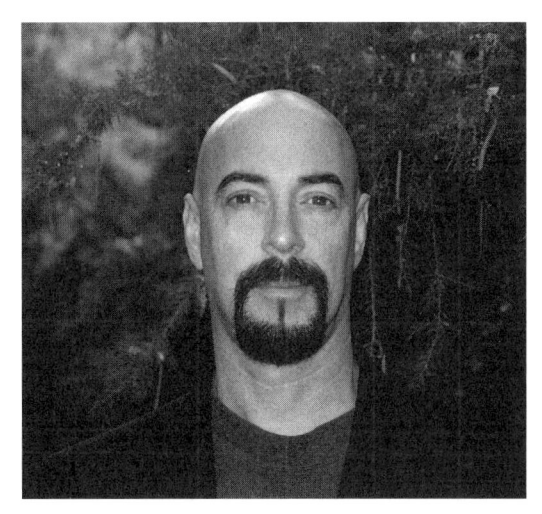

Professor Jerry Alan Johnson, Ph.D., D.T.C.M., D.M.Q.

MASTERS DEGREE IN MEDICAL QIGONG & ANMO THERAPY:
- Graduated from the Hai Dian University, Medical Qigong College of Beijing, China

W.H.O. AMBASSADOR OF CHINESE MEDICAL QIGONG THERAPY TO NORTH AMERICA:
- Commissioned by The World Health Organization (W.H.O.) Collaborating Center for Traditional Chinese Medicine, Beijing, China

W.A.S.O.M.Q. COUNCIL BOARD MEMBER (U.S. REPRESENTATIVE):
- World Academic Society of Medical Qigong (W.A.S.O.M.Q.) - Beijing, China

EXTERNAL ADVISORY COMMITTEE FOR CLINICAL ONCOLOGY: M.D. ANDERSON CANCER CENTER
- M.D. Anderson Cancer Center, Department of Palliative Care & Rehabilitation Medicine, Houston, Texan - (U.S.A.)

N.Q.A. COUNCIL BOARD MEMBER (CHAIRMAN OF THE MEDICAL QIGONG STANDARDS COMMITTEE):
- National Qigong Association (N.Q.A.) - (U.S.A.)

A.O.B.T.A. NATIONAL MEDICAL QIGONG CERTIFICATION INSTRUCTOR-EXAMINER:
- The American Organization for Bodywork Therapies of Asia - (U.S.A.)

MEDICAL BACKGROUND

Professor Jerry Alan Johnson is one of the few internationally recognized non-Chinese Grand Masters, practicing doctors, and Director/Professors of Medical Qigong Therapy. Having studied for more than thirty-two years, he is recognized both in China and the West as America's leading authority on Medical Qigong Therapy. Professor Johnson is licensed as a Doctor of Traditional Chinese Medicine (D.T.C.M.) in Beijing, China, and has served with national and international committees to promote and encourage the practice of Medical Qigong Therapy.

Professor Johnson is the Founder and Executive Director of the International Institute of Medical Qigong, in Pacific Grove, California, and has designed several Medical Qigong programs which have been implemented into various T.C.M. colleges and Medical Qigong Institutes throughout the United States, Belgium, Bermuda, Bosnia, Canada, Central America, England, France, Ireland, Israel, South Africa and Sweden.

HISTORY

Professor Johnson began his initial training in energetic medicine in 1972. In 1974, he started his formal clinical studies of Traditional Chinese Medicine (T.C.M.) in Monterey, California, where he focused his studies on acupuncture, herbology, Medical Qigong therapy, traumatology, and Chinese massage. After receiving certification in acupuncture and herbology from an 1978-81 internship, Professor Johnson operated clinics in Colorado Springs, Colorado (1981-84), working as a consultant and associate in acupuncture and Medical Qigong therapy to Western medical doctors, naturopaths, and chiropractors.

In 1993, Professor Johnson furthered his clinical studies at the China Beijing International Acupuncture Training Center and at the Acupuncture Institute of China, Academy of T.C.M. He was the first foreigner from the Acupuncture Institute of China invited to treat patients in the Medical Qigong Clinic at the Xi Yuan Hospital of T.C.M. (featured in Bill Moyer's special "Healing and the Mind"). There he interned as a Doctor of Medical Qigong Therapy, specializing in the treatment of cysts, tumors, and kidney dysfunctions.

In 1993, Professor Johnson also interned as a Doctor of Anmo Therapy at the Orthopedic Traumatology Clinic of the Hu Guo Si Hospital of T.C.M. (in Beijing, China) specializing in Chinese bone-setting, traumatology, and tissue manipulation. His training in somatic regulation also includes Neuromuscular Therapy, Psychophysical Integrational Therapy, Advanced Visceral Manipulation, and Advanced Cranio-Sacral Therapy.

In 1995, Professor Johnson obtained his Masters Degree in Medical Qigong Therapy from the Medical Qigong College at the Hai Dian University in Beijing, China. He then received his clinical license as a "Doctor of Traditional Chinese Medicine" specializing in Medical Qigong therapy and massage.

Professor Johnson received his "License of Academic Qualifications to Practice Chinese Medicine," and "License of Clinical Qualifications to Practice Chinese Medicine" from The Beijing Bureau of Public Health and The People's Republic of China, Ministry of Health.

After completion of both academic doctoral thesis and numerous clinical field studies, the Beijing Western District Medical Qigong Science and Traditional Chinese Medicine Research Institute (China) awarded Doctor Johnson an academic license as "Professor of Medical Qigong Science and Philosophy."

1996

An active member of the World Academic Society of Medical Qigong, Professor Johnson was a key speaker at the 1996 Third World Conference on Medical Qigong held in Beijing, China, lecturing on "The Psychophysical Components Associated With Tumor Formation."

In 1996, Professor Johnson lectured on "Traumatology, Chinese Massage and Herbal Healing" at the Emerge International Tai Chi Chuan and Qigong Meditation Arts in Toronto, Canada.

In 1996, Professor Johnson lectured on "The Healing Benefits of Medical Qigong" at the Monterey Institute of International Studies, in Monterey California.

In 1996, Professor Johnson lectured on "Healing Emotional Traumas With Medical Qigong" at the Psychology Department at the Monterey Peninsula College, in Monterey California.

1997

In 1997, Professor Johnson became the first Qigong doctor allowed to assist in surgery at the Community Hospital of the Monterey Peninsula in Carmel, California, where he continues to work closely with Western doctors.

In 1997, Professor Johnson lectured and taught a seminar on "Treating Patient with Medical Qigong" to Nurses, Acupuncturists, faculty and students of the University of California San Francisco and the American College of Traditional Chinese Medicine, in San Francisco, California.

In 1997, Professor Johnson lectured at the Second World Congress on Medical Qigong and the First American Qigong Association Conference held in San Francisco, California.

In 1997, Professor Johnson was elected to the Board of Directors of the National Qigong Association-U.S.A.

In 1997, Professor Johnson was interviewed in Newsweek Magazine, and the Discovery Channel on the use of Medical Qigong Therapy for the treatment of internal organ diseases.

1998

In 1998, Professor Johnson lectured at the Northern California Society of Radiation Therapists on "The Use of Medical Qigong to Rectify the Side Affects of Radiation Therapy" at the Queen of the Valley Hospital in Napa, California.

In 1998, Professor Johnson was appointed the National Qigong Association's Chairman of the Medical Qigong Committee, responsible for establishing the guidelines and national standards for Medical Qigong practitioners working in clinical settings.

In 1998, Professor Johnson lectured on the "Utilization of Medical Qigong Therapy and Surgery" at the Fourth World Conference on Medical Qigong held in Beijing, China, and was elected to the Board of Directors of the World Academic Society of Medical Qigong (W.A.S.O.M.Q.) centered in Beijing, China. He serves as one of four Council Board Members that represent the United States at the W.A.S.O.M.Q. Conferences.

Additionally, in 1998, the status of Professor Johnson's Clinical License was elevated to the position of "Physician in Charge" (Clinical Director) and he was licensed as a "Doctor of Traditional Chinese Medicine" from the Beijing Bureau of Medical Science and Technology in Beijing, China.

1999

In 1999, Professor Johnson was interviewed in Health and Fitness Magazine on "The Healing Power of Medical Qigong."

In 1999, Professor Johnson lectured on "Correcting Qi Deviations with Medical Qigong Therapy" at the National Qigong Gathering held in Baltimore, Maryland.

In the Spring of 1999, Professor Johnson accepted the position of Dean of Medical Qigong Science from the Five Branches Institute, College and Clinic of Traditional Chinese Medicine, in Santa Cruz, California. Professor Johnson developed two programs: a 200 hour Medical Qigong Practitioner (M.Q.P.) program and a 500 hour Medical Qigong Therapist (M.Q.T.) program. Both programs include specific instruction and training gathered from his textbook entitled: *Chinese Medical Qigong Therapy, A Comprehensive Clinical Text*. The courses also include the specialization of specific Medical Qigong Therapies such as Pediatrics, Geriatrics, Gynecology, Neurology, Psychology, Oncology, and Surgery.

2000

In 2000, Professor Johnson lectured on "Healing Qi Deviations" at the National Qigong Gathering held in Portland, Oregon; and the Fourth World Congress on Medical Qigong and Fourth American Qigong Association Conference, held in San Francisco, California.

In 2000, Professor Johnson was interviewed in a film documentary featured by the Seoul Broadcasting System (SBS) of Korea, on "The Effects of Medical Qigong and the Treatment of Patients."

In the Spring of 2000, Professor Johnson implemented within the Five Branches Institute the first Medical Qigong Clinic at a T.C.M. College in North America, facilitating the combined use of acupuncture, herbs, and Medical Qigong therapies to the general public.

2001

In May 2001, Professor Johnson presented to the White House Commission on Complementary and Alternative Medicine Policy (W.H.C.C.A.M.P.) the governmental standards established by The Peoples Republic of China. These strict standards have currently been implemented into several T.C.M. colleges in the U.S. through his own International Institute of Medical Qigong (I.I.M.Q.) organization. These standards were presented to the W.H.C.C.A.M.P. to be incorporated in the future, integrating Complementary and Alternative Medical (CAM) policies for health care for the U.S.

In August 2001, Professor Johnson joined with colleagues to establish the Educational Competency of Medical Qigong Therapy for the California State Acupuncture Board. At that meeting the Educational Competency and Outcomes Task-force of the California State Acupuncture Board was formed.

In September 2001, Professor Johnson was approved as a Continuing Education Provider for the Board of Behavioral Sciences (PCE 2272), authorized to issue C.E.U.s for Marriage Family Therapist (M.F.T.) and License Clinical Social Workers (L.C.S.W.).

Also in September 2001, Professor Johnson began teaching a two year 250-hour intensive study course on Chinese Medical Qigong Therapy and Chinese Clinical Oncology. The focus of this course entailed several Medical Qigong therapeutic modalities for the treatment of various types of cancer, as well as primary Medical Qigong prescription exercises and meditations used in China for the treatment of cancer and the side effects of radiation and chemotherapy. This course was offered through the International Institute of Medical Qigong of Pacific Grove, California.

In October 2001, Professor Johnson lectured on "The Healing practice of Medical Qigong" at the California State Oriental Medicine Association's International Expo and Convention, held in San Francisco, California.

In November 2001, Professor Johnson was approved as a Continuing Education Provider for the California State Acupuncture Board (CEP 369), authorized to issue C.E.U.s for Licensed Acupuncturist (L.Ac.).

2002

In February 2002, Professor Johnson was included in the "Who's Who in the 21st Century" for his "Outstanding Contribution in the Field of Chinese Medicine - Medical Qigong Therapy," through the International Biographical Center in Cambridge, England.

In May 2002, Professor Johnson was approved as a A.O.B.T.A. Certified Instructor in Medical Qigong by the American Organization for Bodywork Therapies of Asia, allowing graduate students from the I.I.M.Q. and several T.C.M. colleges to qualify in taking the 500 hour National Certification Examination developed for graduate students of Medical Qigong Therapy, by the National Certification Commission for Acupuncture and Oriental Medicine (NCCAOM).

In 2002, Professor Johnson lectured on "Treating Cancer with Chinese Medical Qigong Therapy," at the Academy of oriental Medicine at Austin, in Austin Texas.

In 2002, Professor Johnson lectured on "Chinese Medical Qigong Therapy and the Treatment of Cancer," at the International Healing Center, in Carracas, Venezuela.

In 2002, Professor Johnson lectured on "Medical Qigong Therapy and the Treatment of Breast Cancer," at the California State Oriental Medicine Association's International Expo and Convention, held in San Francisco, California.

2003

In January 2003, Professor Johnson began reviewing case reports and providing editorial reports on research articles on Medical Qigong for the Journal of Alternative and Complementary Medicine.

In March 2003, Professor Johnson was nominated as the "2003 International Health Professional of the Year." He was also honored for his outstanding achievements and leadership in the International Medical Community, by the International Biographical Center, Cambridge, England.

In April 2003, Professor Johnson met with the Accreditation Commission for Acupuncture and Oriental Medicine (ACAOM) to secure Educational Competency of Medical Qigong Therapy standards as taught at the Five Branches T.C.M.

College for the California State Board of Education, as well as other T.C.M. Colleges throughout North America.

In May of 2003, Professor Johnson became the Academic Dean of Medical Qigong Science in two existing Acupuncture Colleges; accepted the additional position of Dean of Medical Qigong Science from The Academy For Five Element Acupuncture, Inc., in Hallandale, Florida. At the Florida acupuncture college, Professor Johnson developed two Medical Qigong programs: a 200 hour Medical Qigong Practitioner (M.Q.P.) and a 500 hour Medical Qigong Therapist (M.Q.T.) program.

In 2003, Professor Johnson lectured on "The Effective Treatment of Migraine Headaches using Medical Qigong Therapy," at the Asian Organization for Bodywork Therapist of America (AOBTA) National Convention, Boston, Massachusetts.

In 2003, Professor Johnson was interviewed by the Nirvana Magazine in Paris, France, and lectured on "The Treatment of Emotional Disorders with Chinese Medical Qigong Therapy."

He was also honored for his outstanding contributions to the American way of life and his leadership role in implementing Traditional Chinese Medicine with Allopathic (Western) Medicine, nominated in the 2003 American Biography Profile, by the American Biographical Institute, Raleigh, North Carolina, USA.

2004

In February of 2004, Professor Johnson implemented within the Academy For Five Element Acupuncture, Inc., in Hallandale, Florida, an active Medical Qigong Clinic. This is the second T.C.M. College in North America to facilitate the combined use of acupuncture, herbs, and Medical Qigong therapies to the general public.

In February of 2004, Professor Johnson began teaching a six month 186-hour intensive study course on Chinese Medical Qigong Therapy and Chinese Clinical Oncology. The focus of this course entailed several Medical Qigong therapeutic modalities for the treatment of various types of cancer, as well as primary Medical Qigong prescription exercises and meditations used in China for the treatment of cancer and the side effects of radiation and chemotherapy. This course was made possible to the public by a grant from the Fant Foundation, and offered through the International Institute of Medical Qigong, sponsored by the Institute for Regenerative Medicine in Houston, Texas.

In August of 2004, Professor Johnson implemented within the Belgium College of Traditional Chinese Medicine an active 200 hour Medical Qigong Practitioner program.

2005

In January of 2005, Professor Johnson was invited to serve on the External Advisory Committee for the Department of Palliative Care & Rehabilitation Medicine at the M.D. Anderson Cancer Center, in Houston, Texas. His responsibility included advising the specific research using Medical Qigong Therapy for the treatment of various types of cancer.

Also in January of 2005, another 200 hour Medical Qigong Practitioner (M.Q.P.) certification program and ongoing Medical Qigong Clinic was started at the Acupuncture and Integrative Medicine College, in Berkeley, California.

Founded in 1985 and currently having branches in 10 countries and 23 states, the International Institute of Medical Qigong is known for maintaining the highest standards in Medical Qigong instruction and therapy. Because of the consistent high standards, in March of 2005 the Chinese Ministry of Health honored Dr. Johnson and the International Institute of Medical Qigong as exceeding the Chinese academic and clinical standards for clinical instruction and practice.

In July 2005, Professor Johnson's Biography was included in the "Great Minds of the 21st Century," by the American Biographical Institute, Raleigh, North Carolina.

In August 2005, the He Nan University of Traditional Chinese Medicine, in Zheng Zhou China appointed Professor Jerry Alan Johnson as the Overseas Director of Medical Qigong. At that time the university invited Professor Johnson to join the facility as an Honorary Professor of Medical Qigong, and he was issued a government seal authorizing his post. Professor Johnson is the official representative of the He Nan University of Traditional Chinese Medicine for the United States.

Additionally, the He Nan University has recognized the International Institute of Medical Qigong (IIMQ) as a "sister school" of the university, and has adopted the IIMQ's curriculum and the text authored by Professor Johnson titled, *Chinese Medical Qigong Therapy: A Comprehensive Clinical Text*.

Martial Arts Background

Professor Johnson is also internationally renowned as a Shifu (Master Instructor) of several Chinese Martial Arts Systems, having studied the martial arts for over 39 years.

History

Professor Johnson began his initial training in martial arts at a very young age, inspired by his father's boxing skill and training. He continued learning combative skills in western boxing and wrestling and in 1965 began formal training under Sense John Brown at a Kodokan Judo club in Jacksonville, Florida. Throughout the years he continued his studies in western boxing, grappling, wrestling, and several styles of Karate.

While teaching Okinawan Goju Ryu Karate for the Philippine-American Karate Association (P.A.K.A.) in 1974, he was introduced to the Chinese Martial Arts system of Northern Praying Mantis, and immediately began studying Tang Lang Shaolin under the stern private tutelage of Shifu (Master Instructor) John Staples. While studying Northern Praying Mantis, he became intrigued with the fighting techniques used in the Northern Shaolin system of Mizongquan, and for the next several years focused his attention on training in Mizong combat. He completed his training in 1978, earning the Shaolin name "Shao Ying" ("Little Eagle") and becoming a certified Shifu through the Mi Tsung-I Northern Shaolin Federation of Taiwan, and the Ching Wu Kung Fu Association in Hong Kong. In 1978 he also began teaching Shaolin fighting to an elite special forces unit at the Fort Ord Military Base, in Seaside, California. There, along with two Hung Gar Shaolin Masters, he formed the Fort Ord Shaolin Federation.

During the mid 1970's he began training in Yang Style Taijiquan. After several years of training, he become a certified Shifu in Yang Style Taijiquan through the Tai Chi Chuan Federation of Taiwan.

From 1978 to 1980 Professor Johnson began training in Baguazhang and Xingyiquan from Shifu Michael Alan Brown, becoming certified as an instructor in Baguazhang through the Ching Yi Kung Fu Association. Throughout the years, Professor Johnson continued training in several Northern and Southern Shaolin and Wudang styles of combat.

Shaolin

In Shaolin, he has studied Northern and Southern Praying Mantis, Hung Gar, Wing Chung, and Mizongquan Shaolin styles of fighting, weapons, and Martial Qigong, Shengong, and Neigong training. He is a certified Master Instructor in Mizongquan Shaolin, teaching through the authority of the Mi Tsung-I Northern Shaolin Federation of Taiwan, and the Ching Wu Kung Fu Association in Hong Kong.

Baguazhang

In Baguazhang, he has studied several schools of fighting, including the Yin Fu, Cheng Ting-Hua, Liu De Kuan, Fu Zhen-Song, and the Chang Zhao-Dong Styles of combat, weapons, and Martial Qigong, Shengong, and Neigong training. He is a certified Shifu in Chang Zhao-Dung Baguazhang, teaching through the authority of the Ching Yi Baguazhang Association, the Hsiao Mien Hu Martial Arts Association, and The Canadian Martial Arts Society.

He was elected to the International Baguazhang Research and Teachers Exchange Council, and served as a judging official and member of the Executive Committee of the U.S. Chinese Kuo Shu Federation. He became a coaching official, national certifier, and council board member of the Amateur Athletic Union (A.A.U.) affiliated with the U.S. Olympics.

Professor Johnson also participated on the Board of Advisors for the United States of America Wushu-Kung Fu Federation, and is a member of the International Congress of Oriental Medicine and

Martial Arts. He is also a standing member of the North American Chinese Martial Arts Federation.

TAIJIQUAN

In Taijiquan, Professor Johnson has studied several schools of fighting, including the Yang Pan-Hou, Yang Chien-Hou, and Chen Fa Ke styles of combat, weapons, and Martial Qigong, Shengong, and Neigong training.

In 1993, Professor Johnson traveled to China and continued extensive training in the Yin Fu style of Baguazhang. At that time period he additionally began training in the Chen Fa Ke style of Chen Taijiquan. He eventually became accepted as a "Tudi," earning the linage name "Yuan Long" ("Dragon in the Clouds") and accepting the position of 20th generation disciple of Chen Family Taijiquan from the Beijing Martial Arts Association, as well as the Beijing Chen Style Taijiquan Association of China.

He is currently certified as a Master Instructor from Feng Zhi Qiang's "Hun Yuan" Chen Style Taijiquan; and is also a certified Master Instructor in the Yang Style Taijiquan, teaching through the authority of the Tai Chi Chuan Federation of Taiwan.

XINGYIQUAN

In Xingyiquan, Professor Johnson has studied several schools of fighting, including the Hebei and Henan styles of combat, weapons, and Martial Qigong, Shengong, and Neigong training.

YIQUAN AND DACHENGQUAN

In Yiquan and Dachengquan, Professor Johnson has studied under several excellent masters from both Taiwan and mainland China. He has received training in several variations of Yiquan and Dachengquan combat, Martial Qigong, Shengong and Neigong.

CHAMPIONSHIP COMPETITIONS

Excelling in "Empty Hand," as well as "Weapons Fighting" from both the Shaolin and Wudang Martial Arts Systems, Professor Johnson competed regularly in the tournament circuit and was titled:
- 1980 Southbay National Champion
- 1982 Tournament of Fighters Champion
- 1982 Universal Tae Kwon Do/Tang Soo Do Invitational Grand Champion
- 1983 Colorado National Kung Fu Champion
- 1983 Tournament of Fighters Grand Champion
- 1984 Colorado National Kung Fu Champion
- 1984 Tournament of Fighters Kung Fu Champion

In 1984 Professor Johnson retired from competition. In addition to his own success in championship competitions, many of Professor Johnson's students have also gone on to compete at the national level, bringing several first place championship titles to the school. Like their teacher, Professor Johnson's students excelled in free-form fighting, Taiji Push-hands, and Chinese Gongfu forms, as well as weapon competitions.

In May of 2004, Professor Johnson was inducted into the U.S.A. "Martial Arts Hall of Fame."

DAOIST BACKGROUND

Professor Johnson is also internationally renowned as a Shifu in ancient Daoist Mysticism, having studied several esoteric systems for over 31 years.

HISTORY

In the early 1970's, Professor Johnson's was introduced to the Wu Dang Shan Monastery - Pole Star School of Daoist Mysticism (Quan Zhen branch) from his Taijiquan instructor. Through this esoteric Daoist training, he was taught beginning, intermediate, and advanced levels of Qigong and Shengong skills.

In the early 1980's, Professor Johnson was introduced to the Mao Shan Monastery - Highest Purity School of Daoist Mysticism (Zheng Yi branch), from one of his Baguazhang instructors. Because of his prior training, he was taught advanced levels of Daoist Qigong and Shengong skills.

The advantage of having trained in both schools of Daoist Mysticism opened the doors for him to also train with several Jesuit priests and Daosit monks schooled in the Celestial Master, Complete Reality, and Red Hat Schools of Daoist Mysticism.

2004

In September of 2004, Professor Johnson returned to China to continue extensive training in Daoist Mysticism. While training in the Jiang Su province, he became accepted as a disciple (Dizi) from Daoist master Min Xian, and was given the Daoist lineage name "Chi Fu" (meaning to grasp and keep good fortune, blessings and happiness). Professor Johnson was then indoctrinated into the Zheng Yi sect of Daoism, becoming an 80th Generation Disciple of the Mao Shan Monastery, from the Shang Qing (Highest Clarity) branch. He is the first non-Chinese to ever be accepted as a Disciple of Thunder Magic at the Mao Shan Daoist Monastery.

2005

In March of 2005, Professor Johnson returned to China to continue extensive training in Daoist Mysticism. However, while training at the Mao Shan Monastery, and sharing advanced training methods in Daoist spiritual skills and exorcistic techniques, Professor Johnson inquired about receiving his "Lu" (the spiritual register of talismans, hand seals, and incantations used for controlling spirits). Abbot Feng stated that the resident Mao Shan priests were not capable of initiating him into the most advanced levels of esoteric Daoist mysticism. This was because many of the sacred texts had been destroyed during the Sino-Japanese War and by the Red Guard.

In order to continue training in advanced Daoist mysticism, Abbot Feng suggested that Professor Johnson travel to the other Zheng Yi branch located in the Long Hu Shan region. It was at the Celestial Masters Mansion, in the Jiangxi Province, where the Abbot had personally received his "Lu" and other advanced levels of spiritual training.

After thanking the Abbot, Professor Johnson made route to the Long Hu Shan Monastery. Upon arriving at the monastery, he was greeted by the resident Abbot and gave him a letter of introduction that Professor Johnson's teacher had prepared for this occasion. Upon reading the letter of introduction and hearing his formal request, the Abbot immediately took him to meet the senior Abbot Zhang Jing Tao, the 65th Celestial Master, whose Daoist name is "Da Ming."

After subsequent examinations, Professor Johnson was invited to become a Dizi (disciple) of the 65th Celestial Master and receive his "Lu." In doing so, he became the first non-Chinese descendent to ever be accepted as a disciple of the Celestial Masters Mansion in the Jiangxi Province. Professor Johnson was given the Daoist lineage name "Lou Sheng" ("Luo" is the generation name, and "Sheng" means "to bring forth life").

Immediately upon completion of the ceremony Professor Johnson was introduced to his new Daoist Master, Qiu Yu Song. Master Qiu Yu Song is the senior most Fa Shi (Master of the laws of Heaven, Earth, and Man) in the Long Hu Shan sect, and his expertise in Shengong is well known in both the Zheng Yi (Orthodox Daoism) and Quan Zhen (Complete Reality) branches of Daoism. At that time, the Fa Shi taught Professor Johnson the skill of creating talismans and invocations to bind evil spirits.

AUTHOR AND PUBLISHER:

Professor Johnson was a contributing author, selected to write the Medical Chi Kung section for the book *The Complete Illustrated Guide to Chi Kung*, a cooperative project between Element Books (UK) and author James MacRitchie. Professor Johnson was also one of the selected contributing authors for the book *Qigong-Essence of the Healing Dance*, a cooperative project between P.B.S. and Documentary Producer/Director Garri Garripoli.

Professor Johnson has been interviewed many times on local radio programs and has been featured in numerous local and international newspapers and magazines, including: *Newsweek Magazine* "The International Addition," *The World Medical Qigong Quarterly, Qi-The Journal of Traditional Eastern Health & Fitness, The Empty Vessel Magazine, Penthouse Magazine, Self Magazine, Billboard Magazine, The Mystical World of Chinese Martial Arts, Inside Kung Fu Magazine, Combat Karate Magazine, Internal Arts Magazine, Black Belt Magazine, The Pa Kua Chang Journal,* and *Inside Karate's Master Series Magazine*.

Televised specials include: *NBC News* "Dateline," *CBS/Channel 46* "Eye on America," featured in a documentary on Medical Qigong filmed for the *"Discovery Channel,"* featured in a documentary on Medical Qigong filmed for SBS "Qi-into the world of the unknown," and *K.P.B.S.* "Managing Health and Productivity; New Approaches In Technology," as well as *The David Letterman Show.*

In 1988, Professor Johnson created and published a six level "Pa Kua Chang Chi Kung Correspondence Course," and in 1989, founded the "Pa Kua Chang News Letter," which later became known as the "Pa Kua Chang Journal," and was distributed worldwide. Professor Johnson has written and published five books on martial arts entitled:

- *The Secrets of the Eight Animals,*
- *The Masters Manual of Pa Kua Chang,*
- *Classical Pa Kua Chang Fighting Systems and Weapons,*
- *The Essence of Internal Martial Arts Vol. 1: Esoteric Fighting Techniques and Healing Methods, and*
- *The Essence of Internal Martial Arts Vol. 2: Energy Theory and Cultivation.*

From 1984 to 1986, Professor Johnson produced and directed six Baguazhang instructional videos entitled:

- *The Eight Animal School of Pa Kua Chang*
- *The Original Form of Pa Kua Chang*
- *The Eight Circular Pa Kua Staff*
- *The Eight Circular Pa Kua Broadsword*
- *The Dragon School of Pa Kua Chang, and*
- *The Fighting Techniques of Pa Kua Chang.*

In 1994, he was featured in two videos on Taijiquan, as well as one Qigong video narrated by movie-star John Saxon, entitled:

- *Tai Chi-The Empowering Workout,*
- *Power Tai Chi- Total Body Workout, and*
- *Chi Kung-The Healing Workout.*

In 1994, Professor Johnson additionally created two Meditation CD/cassette tapes with composer John Serri entitled:

- *Tai Chi Meditation - [1] Life Force Breathing, and*
- *Tai Chi Meditation - [2] Eight Direction Perception.*

In 1999, Professor Johnson produced 10 Medical Qigong Instructional Videos and DVD's as a compendium to his textbook *Chinese Medical Qigong Therapy, A Comprehensive Clinical Text*, entitled:

- *Gathering Energy from Heaven and Earth,*
- *Stationary and Dynamic Medical Qigong Posture Training,*
- *Treating Patients with Medical Qigong Therapy (Vol.1),*
- *Treating Patients with Medical Qigong Therapy (Vol.2),*
- *Medical Qigong Energy Techniques and Qi Emitting Methods,*
- *Medical Qigong Invisible Needle Technique, Five Element Qigong Massage, and Energetic Point Therapy,*
- *Medical Qigong Healing Sound Therapy and Prescriptions,*
- *Treatment of Internal Organ Diseases with Medical Qigong,*
- *Treatment of Cysts, Tumors, and Cancer with Medical Qigong Therapy, and*
- *Soul Retrieval.*

In May 2000, Professor Johnson released his sixth book entitled:

- *Chinese Medical Qigong Therapy, A Comprehensive Clinical Text.*

In September 2000, Professor Johnson produced the first in a series of new Medical Qigong videos and Interactive CD-ROMs. The featured topic for the first CD-ROM was entitled:

- *Medical Qigong for Understanding, Prevention & Treatment of Breast Disease (CD-ROM).*
- *Medical Qigong for Treating Breast Disease (Instructional Video).*

In August 2001, Professor Johnson composed and published a series of five new books based on the previous work in his Medical Qigong Textbook. The names of the five new books are entitled:

- *Chinese Medical Qigong Therapy Vol 1: Energetic Anatomy and Physiology,*
- *Chinese Medical Qigong Therapy Vol 2. Energetic Alchemy, Dao Yin Therapy and Qi Deviations*
- *Chinese Medical Qigong Therapy Vol 3: Differential Diagnosis, Clinical Foundations, Treatment Principles and Clinical Protocols*
- *Chinese Medical Qigong Therapy Vol 4: Prescription Exercises and Meditations, Treatment of Internal Organ Diseases, Pediatrics, Geriatrics, Gynecology, Neurology and Energetic Psychology*
- *Chinese Medical Qigong Therapy Vol 5: An Energetic Approach to Oncology*

In September 2004, Professor Johnson began

producing a new series of six Medical Qigong Oncology DVD sets. This new series accompanies the clinical textbook entitled: *Chinese Medical Qigong Therapy Vol 5: An Energetic Approach to Oncology,* and contains four to five DVDs in each set. The name of the six new DVD sets are entitled:
- *Houston Cancer Seminar #1 - Introduction to Medical Qigong Therapy and Cancer Treatment:*
- *Houston Cancer Seminar #2 - An Energetic Approach to Oncology*
- *Houston Cancer Seminar #3 - Medical Qigong Treatment Protocols Used for Breast, Cervical, Prostate, Ovarian, and Uterine Cancer*
- *Houston Cancer Seminar #4 - Medical Qigong Treatment Protocols used for Brain, Skin, and Bone Cancer, Leukemia, Malignant Lymphoma, and Multiple Myelomas*
- *Houston Cancer Seminar #5 - Medical Qigong Cancer Prescription Exercises and Meditations*
- *Houston Cancer Seminar #6 - Medical Qigong Treatment Protocols Used For Radiation and Chemotherapy*

In May 2005, Professor Johnson composed and published a series of 2 new books based on his extensive training in ancient Chinese Daoist Mysticism. The names of the two new books are entitled:
- *Introduction to Daoist Mysticism #1: Lighting the Eyes of the Dragon*
- *Introduction to Daoist Mysticism #2: Journey into the Infinite Void*

Professor Johnson's books, video tapes, meditation C.D.'s and cassette tapes have been translated into other languages and are currently being sold around the world.

For more information about the author, the reader can connect to his web site at:
www.qigongmedicine.com

The International Institute of Medical Qigong

Academic Directory

At the International Institute of Medical Qigong, it is our policy that all our Medical Qigong programs maintain the exact same teaching standards, syllabi and clinical hours for certification. Therefore, the following "Academic Directory" has been established so that perspective students may feel confident in attending the specific college or institute of their choice, knowing that each Medical Qigong educational facility member will teach and maintain the exact same clinical format and strict standards as established by the International Institute of Medical Qigong.

The following list of Traditional Chinese Medical colleges and institutions teach the I.I.M.Q. qualifications for the Introduction to Medical Qigong Course; the 200-hour Medical Qigong Practitioner Certification Course (M.Q.P.); the 500-hour Medical Qigong Therapist Certification Course (M.Q.T.); or the 1,000-hour Master of Medical Qigong Certification Course (M.M.Q.).

Faculty of the International Institute of Medical Qigong

Name	Contact Information	Intro. to M.Q.	M.Q.P.	M.Q.T.	M.M.Q.
Professor Jerry Alan Johnson, Ph.D., D.T.C.M., D.M.Q. (China) • Executive Director and Founder of the International Institute of Medical Qigong • Dean of Medical Qigong Science and Director of Medical Qigong Clinic of Academy of Five Element TCM College (Hallandale, FL) • Dean of Medical Qigong Science and Director of Medical Qigong Clinic of Five Branches TCM College (Santa Cruz, CA)	P.O. Box 52144 Pacific Grove, California 93950 Phone: (831) 646-9399 Fax: (831) 646-0535 E-Mail: drjerryalanjohnson@earthlink.net Web Page: www.qigongmedicine.com	X	X	X	X
Dr. L. Francesca Ferrari, L.Ac., D.T.C.M., D.M.Q. (China) • Medical Qigong Faculty and Clinical Supervisor - Five Branches Institute, College & Clinic of TCM (Santa Cruz, California) • Dean of Traditional Chinese Medicine - International Institute of Medical Qigong • Director of the International Institute of Medical Qigong (Carmel Branch)	Ferrari Center of Chinese Medicine 222 Forest Avenue Pacific Grove Ca. 93950 Phone: (831) 818-3993 E-Mail: francescaferrari@earthlink.net Web Page: www.francescaferrari.com	X	X	X	X
Dr. Bernard Shannon, D.M.Q. (China) • Director of International Clinical Studies • Director of the International Institute of Medical Qigong (Palm Desert, California)	P.O. Box 1435 Palm Desert, California 92261 Phone: (760) 485-0169 Fax: (760) 341-4166 E-Mail: Bernard@MedicalQigong.org Web Page: www.medicalqigong.org	X	X	X	X

FACULTY OF THE INTERNATIONAL INSTITUTE OF MEDICAL QIGONG					
Name	Contact Information	Intro. to M.Q.	M.Q.P.	M.Q.T.	M.M.Q.
Dr. Suzanne B. Friedman, L.Ac., Dipl.Ac., M.S.T.C.M., D.M.Q. (China) • Chair of Medical Qigong Science and Director of Medical Qigong Clinic at the Acupuncture and Integrative Medicine College (Berkeley, California) • Director of Nutrition & Herbal Medicine • Director of the International Institute of Medical Qigong (San Francisco Branch)	650 Chenery Street, San Francisco, Ca 94131 USA Phone: (415) 505-8855 Fax: (415) 285-8868 E-Mail: suzannefriedman@earthlink.net Web Page: www.daoclinic.org	X	X	X	X
Dr. Seth Lefkowitz, D.C., D.M.Q. (China) • Director of An Mo and Jie Gu Therapy • Director of the International Institute of Medical Qigong (North San Jose Branch)	Natures Path Center 351 South Baywood Avenue, San Jose, California 95128 Phone: (408) 243-1565 Fax: (408) 243-1568 E-Mail: seth@naturespathcenter.com Web Page: www.naturespathcenter.com	X	X	X	X
Dia Lynn, M.M.Q. • Director of Western Anatomy and Physiology	Equilibrium Center for Integrative Bodywork 2560 Garden Road Suite 211, Monterey, California 93940 Phone: (831) 373-4042 Fax: (831) 372-1788 E-Mail: dia@dialynn.com Web Page: www.dialynn.com	X	X	X	X
Dr. Lisa Van Ostrand, D.M.Q. (China) • Associate Dean of Medical Qigong Science and Associate Clinical Director of Academy of Five Element TCM College (Hallandale, FL) • Director of the International Institute of Medical Qigong (S.E. Florida Branch)	751 Euclid Ave. Apt 1 Miami Beach, Florida 33139 USA Phone: (786) 512-7096 E-Mail: lisa@lisavanostrand.com Web Page: www.lisavanostrand.com	X	X	X	X
Jean Ruth Vlamynck, L.Ac., Dipl.Ac., M.T.C.M., M.M.Q. • Associate Dean of Medical Qigong Science, Five Branches TCM College (Santa Cruz, CA) • Associate Clinical Director, Five Branches TCM College (Santa Cruz, CA)	257 B Center Ave. Aptos, California 95003 Phone: (831) 689-9093 Fax: (831) 689-9094 E-Mail: jeanhere@bigplanet.com	X	X	X	X

THE INTERNATIONAL INSTITUTE OF MEDICAL QIGONG - CALIFORNIA					
Name	Contact Information	Intro. to M.Q.	M.Q.P.	M.Q.T.	M.M.Q.
Shifu Matthew B. Weston, M.M.Q. • Director of the International Institute of Medical Qigong (Big Sur Branch)	South Coast Qigong Center P.O. Box 223373 Carmel, California 93922 Phone: (831) 626-3347 Fax: (831) 626-3347 E-Mail: qigongr@hotmail.com	X	X	X	X
Jose E. Gonzalez, M.M.Q. • Director of the International Institute of Medical Qigong (Los Angeles Branch)	Healing Qi Institute P.O. Box 251558 Glendale, California 91225 Phone: (323) 664-8241 E-Mail: info@healingqiinstitute.com Web Page: www.healingqiinstitute.com	X	X	X	X
Calvin Fahey, M.M.Q. • Director of the International Institute of Medical Qigong (Monterey Branch)	1406 B Yosemite Street Seaside, Ca 93955 USA Phone: (831) 393-0663 Fax: (603) 375-6203 E-Mail: calvinfahey@yahoo.com Web Page: www.iimq.org	X	X	X	X
Robert W. Haberkorn, D.C., M.M.Q., HHP • Director of the International Institute of Medical Qigong (Palm Springs Branch)	1276 N. Palm Canyon Dr., Suite 105 Palm Springs, CA 92262 Phone: (760) 285-8894 E-Mail: rwhdc@juno.com	X	X	X	
Dr. Eric Shaffer, M.M.Q., D.M.Q. (China) • Director of the International Institute of Medical Qigong (Asilomar Branch)	775 Asilomar Blvd. Pacific Grove, California 93950 Phone: 831.375.0593 E-Mail: ericwshaff@aol.com	X	X		

THE INTERNATIONAL INSTITUTE OF MEDICAL QIGONG - CALIFORNIA					
Name	Contact Information	Intro.to M.Q.	M.Q.P.	M.Q.T.	M.M.Q.
Bradley Gilbert, B.A., M.M.Q. • Director of the International Institute of Medical Qigong (Sacramento Branch)	PO Box 255761 Sacramento, Ca. 95865 Phone: 916.616.5227 E-Mail: bradfinity@aol.com Web Page: www.diamond-integration.com	X	X		
Five Branches Institute, College and Clinic of Traditional Chinese Medicine	200 Seventh Avenue Santa Cruz, Ca. 95062 Phone: 831.476.9424 Fax: 831.476.8928 E-Mail: tcm@fivebranches.edu Web Page: www.fivebranches.edu	X	X		
Acupuncture and Integrative Medicine College	2550 Shattuck Ave. Berkeley, Ca. 94704 College: 510.666.8248 Clinic: 510.666.8234 Fax: 510.666.0111 Email: info@aimc.edu Web Page: www.aimc.edu	X	X		
Wendy Lang, M.M.Q. • Director of the International Institute of Medical Qigong (Marin County Branch)	12 Skylark Dr. Apt 33 Larkspur, California 94939 Phone: (415) 924-7883 E-Mail: wendyandphillip@netzero.net	X	X		

THE INTERNATIONAL INSTITUTE OF MEDICAL QIGONG - FLORIDA

Name	Contact Information	Intro. to M.Q.	M.Q.P.	M.Q.T.	M.M.Q.
Academy for Five Element Acupuncture, College of Traditional Chinese Medicine	1170-A East Hallandale Beach Blvd. Hallandale, Florida 33009 Phone: 954.456.6336 Fax: 954.456.3944 E-Mail: afea@compuserve.com Web Page: www.acupuncturist.org	X	X	X	
Anna Belle Fore, M.M.Q. • Director of the International Institute of Medical Qigong(S.W. Florida Branch)	P.O. Box 770485 Naples, Florida 34107 Phone: (239) 398-0291 E-Mail: anabel4@angelfire.com	X	X		

THE INTERNATIONAL INSTITUTE OF MEDICAL QIGONG - PENNSYLVANIA

Name	Contact Information	Intro. to M.Q.	M.Q.P.	M.Q.T.	M.M.Q.
Dr. Ted Cibik, N.D., D.M.Q. (China) • Director of the International Institute of Medical Qigong (Pennsylvania Branch)	Inner Strength Inc. 825 Lovers Leep Rd. Leechburg, Pa 15656 USA Phone: (724) 845-1041 Fax: (724) 845-7739 E-Mail: ted@inner-strength.com Web Page: www.inner-strength.com	X	X	X	X

THE INTERNATIONAL INSTITUTE OF MEDICAL QIGONG - TENNESSEE

Name	Contact Information	Intro. to M.Q.	M.Q.P.	M.Q.T.	M.M.Q.
J. Michael Wood, PMBC, OBDS, M.M.Q. • Director of the International Institute of Medical Qigong (Central Tennessee Branch)	500 Castlegate Dr. Nashville, Tn. 37217 Phone: (615) 366-8940 Fax: (615) 399-8479 E-Mail: jmichaelwood@comcast.net	X	X	X	X
Bryant Seals, M.M.Q. • Director of the International Institute of Medical Qigong (East Tennessee Branch)	P.O. Box 51604 Knoxville, Tn. 37950 Phone: (865) 691-0622 E-Mail: astro320@msn.com	X	X	X	X

THE INTERNATIONAL INSTITUTE OF MEDICAL QIGONG - TEXAS (EAST)

Name	Contact Information	Intro. to M.Q.	M.Q.P.	M.Q.T.	M.M.Q.
Lucy M. Roberts, L.Ac., Dipl.Ac., M.T.C.M., M.M.Q. • Director of the International Institute of Medical Qigong (East Texas Branch)	P.O. Box 1060 Friendswood, Tx 77546 Phone: (281) 648-3102 Fax: (281) 648-3384 E-Mail: tianearthqi@aol.com Web Page: www.balanceyourenergy.com	X	X		

THE INTERNATIONAL INSTITUTE OF MEDICAL QIGONG - TEXAS (CENTRAL)

Name	Contact Information	Intro. to M.Q.	M.Q.P.	M.Q.T.	M.M.Q.
Lou and Maria Eberle, M.S.O.M., M.M.Q. • Director of the International Institute of Medical Qigong (Central Texas Branch)	600 Hart Lane Dripping Springs, Texas 78620 Tel: 512-894-0337 Cell: 512-684-1274 Email: qigong@centexfamily.org	X	X	X	X

THE INTERNATIONAL INSTITUTE OF MEDICAL QIGONG - WASHINGTON

Name	Contact Information	Intro. to M.Q.	M.Q.P.	M.Q.T.	M.M.Q.
Robert B. Bates, D.C., M.M.Q. • Director of the International Institute of Medical Qigong (NW Washington Branch)	Bellingham Institute of Healing 1095 E. Axton Road Bellingham, WA 98226 Phone: (360) 398-7466 E-Mail: RBbatesDC@aol.com	X	X	X	
Sara Storm, L.Ac., M.M.Q. • Director of the International Institute of Medical Qigong (NE Washington Branch)	11512 32nd Ave. N.E. Seattle, WA 98125 Phone: (206) 363-0909 E-Mail: sara@sarastorm.com Web Page: www.sarastorm.com	X	X		

International Branches of the International Institute of Medical Qigong - Belgium

Name	Contact Information	Intro. to M.Q.	M.Q.P.	M.Q.T.	M.M.Q.
Belgium College of Traditional Chinese Medicine	OTCG vzw - Kerkgate 89 B-9700 Oudenaarde, Belgie Phone: 0032.5545.6120 Fax: 0032.5545.6576 E-Mail: otcg@skynet.be Web Page: otcg.be	X	X	X	

The International Institute of Medical Qigong - Bosnia

Name	Contact Information	Intro. to M.Q.	M.Q.P.	M.Q.T.	M.M.Q.
Calvin Fahey, M.M.Q. • Director of the International Institute of Medical Qigong (Bosnia Branch)	Londza 92/2/8 Zenica Bih 72000 Phone: +387.061.825.084 c/o 1406 B Yosemite Street Seaside, Ca 93955 USA Phone: (831) 393-0663 Fax: (603) 375-6202 E-Mail: calvinfahey@yahoo.com Web Page: www.iimq.org	X	X	X	X

The International Institute of Medical Qigong - Canada

Name	Contact Information	Intro. to M.Q.	M.Q.P.	M.Q.T.	M.M.Q.
Paul Pheasey, B.A., M.M.Q. • Director of the International Institute of Medical Qigong (Vancouver Branch)	2586 Kitchener Street Vancouver, B.C. Canada V5K3C6 Phone: (604) 255-0856 Fax: (604) 255-0856 E-Mail: paulpheasey@telus.net	X	X	X	X
Shifu Andy James, B.Sc., F.C.A., M.Q.T. • Director of the International Institute of Medical Qigong (Ontario Branch)	Tai Chi and Meditation Centre 800 Baxter Rd. Hastings Ontario, Canada KOL 1YO Phone: (705) 696-2066 E-Mail: emerge@powerofbalance.com Web Page: www.harmonydawn.com	X	X	X	
Robert A. Youngs, M.Q.T. • Director of the International Institute of Medical Qigong (Pickering Branch)	Pickering, Ontario Canada L1X 2P4 Phone: (905) 420-2662 Fax: (905) 420-2662 E-Mail: robert.youngs@sympatico.ca Web Page: www.medicalqigongcanada.org	X	X	X	

THE INTERNATIONAL INSTITUTE OF MEDICAL QIGONG - CENTRAL AMERICA

Name	Contact Information	Intro. to M.Q.	M.Q.P.	M.Q.T.	M.M.Q.
Lou and Maria Eberle, M.S.O.M., M.M.Q. • Director of the International Institute of Medical Qigong (Guatemala Branch)	Panajachel, Solola, Guatemala Email: qigong@centexfamily.org Tel: 502-77-622030 Tel: 502-77-620059	X	X	X	X

THE INTERNATIONAL INSTITUTE OF MEDICAL QIGONG - IRELAND

| Dermot A. O'Connor, Dip. Ac., M.M.Q.
• European Headquarters of the International Institute of Medical Qigong | 33 Haddington Road
Ballsbridge
Dublin 4
Ireland
Phone: ++ 353.1.667.2222
E-Mail:
dermot@acupunctureireland.com
Web Page:
www.acupunctureireland.com | X | X | X | X |

THE INTERNATIONAL INSTITUTE OF MEDICAL QIGONG - ISREAL

Name	Contact Information	Intro. to M.Q.	M.Q.P.	M.Q.T.	M.M.Q.
Amos Ziv, L.Ac., M.M.Q. • Director of the International Institute of Medical Qigong (Middle East Branch)	7 Rupin St., Rehovot 76353 Israel Tel/Fax: 972-8-9361-916 Cell: 972-64-419-884 E-Mail: aaziv@hotmail.com	X	X	X	X

THE INTERNATIONAL INSTITUTE OF MEDICAL QIGONG - SWEDEN

| Fia G. Hobbs, M.M.Q.
• Director of the International Institute of Medical Qigong (Sweden Branch) | Bjulevagen 40
122 41 Enskede
Sweden
Phone: 46.8.508.64101
Phone: (Mobile) 46 070.658.6865
E-Mail:
fiahobbs@hotmail.com
Web Page:
www.qigongmedicine.se | X | X | X | X |

THE INTERNATIONAL INSTITUTE OF MEDICAL QIGONG - UNITED KINGDOM

Name	Contact Information	Intro. to M.Q.	M.Q.P.	M.Q.T.	M.M.Q.
Jazz Rasool, B.Sc., M.Sc., M. M.Q. • Director of the International Institute of Medical Qigong (United Kingdom Branch)	20 Greensword Bushey Hertfordshire United Kingdom Phone: +44 (0) 208.950.2720 E-Mail: jazras@bodymind.co.uk Web Page: www.medicalqigong.info	X	X	X	X

The International Institute of Medical Qigong

Clinical Directory

At the International Institute of Medical Qigong, it is our policy that all our Medical Qigong graduates maintain the exact same clinical standards and health healing practices. Although the various personalities and different medical histories will slightly alter each individual's approach the energetic healing, the following "Clinical Directory" has been established so that perspective patients may feel confident in attending the specific I.I.M.Q. graduates of their choice. Each energetic healer has been trained to maintain the exact same clinical format and strict standards as established by the International Institute of Medical Qigong.

The following list of Medical Qigong healers have establish their healing clinics according to the strict qualifications established by the I.I.M.Q. Master of Medical Qigong (M.M.Q.) certification program, or Doctor of Medical Qigong (D.M.Q.) certification program, certified by the Beijing Western District Medical Qigong Science and Traditional Chinese Medicine Institute from Beijing, China.

U.S. Clinical Directory

Arizona

Paula Medler, D.V.M., M.M.Q
2626 N. Campbell Avenue
Tucson, AZ. 85719
Phone: (520) 327-5763
E-mail: docpsm@aol.com

California

Sue Angulo, M.M.Q., Louis Frizzell, D.M.Q., and Leela Marcum, M.Ed., D.M.Q.
Energetic Health at the Healing
Collaborative Center
222 Forest Avenue,
Pacific Grove, California 93923
Phone: (831) 783 -1387
Toll Free: (866) 701-4445

MaryAnn Allison
Highway 111
301
Palm Desert, Ca. 92260
Phone: (760) 641-3456
E-Mail: Ma_A@EarthLink.net
Web Page: www.QigongHealthPartners.com

Jeff Tukum Barnard, E.M.T.-P., M.M.Q.
North Star Education
445 Elm Avenue
Seaside, Ca. 93955
Phone: (831) 393-9690
E-Mail: barneyphil@hotmail.com

Eddy L. Bates, M.M.Q.
1373 Elm Avenue
Seaside, Ca. 93955
Phone: (831) 393-1850
E-Mail: eddylight@aol.com

Dennis Earnest, D.M.Q. (China)
154 Junco Dr.
Santa Cruz, Ca. 95060
Phone: (831) 469-41

Pamela Espinoza, N.C.T.M.B., M.M.Q.
P.O. Box 104
Big Sur, Ca. 93920
Offices in Pacific Grove and
the Esalen Institute (Big Sur, Ca.)
Phone: (831) 667-2446
Voice Mail: (831) 644-8096

Five Branches Institute Medical Qigong Clinic
200 Seventh Avenue
Santa Cruz, California 95062
Phone: (831) 476-9424
Fax: (831) 476-8928
E-Mail: tcm@fivebranches.edu
Web Page: www.fivebranches.edu

Calvin. Fahey, M.M.Q.
1406 B Yosemite Street
Seaside, Ca 93955 USA
Phone: (831) 393-0663
Fax: (603) 375-6203
E-Mail: calvinfahey@yahoo.com
Web Page: www.iimq.org

L. Francesca Ferrari, L.Ac., D.T.C.M., D.M.Q. (China)
Ferrari Center of Chinese Medicine
222 Forest Avenue
Pacific Grove Ca. 93950 USA
Phone: (831) 818-3993
E-Mail: francescaferrari@earthlink.net
Web Page: www.francescaferrari.com

Suzanne B. Friedman, L.Ac., D.M.Q. (China)
Director of the International Institute of Medical Qigong (San Francisco Branch)
650 Chenery Street
San Francisco, Ca 94131 USA
Phone: (415) 505-8855
Fax: (415) 285-8868
E-Mail: suzannefriedman@earthlink.net
Web Page: www.daoclinic.org

Bradley Gilbert, B.A., M.M.Q.
Director of the International Institute of Medical Qigong (Sacramento Branch)
PO Box 255761
Sacramento, California 95865
Phone: 916.616.5227
E-Mail: bradfinity@aol.com
Web Page: www.diamond-integration.com

Emma Deepa Gleason, R.N., M.M.Q.
Deepa Health
1 West Campbell Ave. J-70
Campbell, Ca. 95008
Phone: (408) 370-3007
Fax: (408) 370-5007
E-Mail: deepahealth@yahoo.com
Web Page: www.deepahealth.com

Jose E. Gonzalez, M.M.Q.
Healing Qi Institute
P.O. Box 251558
Glendale, California 91225 USA
Phone: (323) 664-8241
E-Mail: info@healingqiinstitute.com
Web Page: www.healingqiinstitute.com

Geoffery Greenspahn, M.M.Q.
Director of the International Institute of Medical Qigong (Los Angeles Branch)
Los Angeles, California
Phone: 310-621-8787
E-Mail: rumblej@hotmail.com

Robert W. Haberkorn, D.C., M.M.Q., HHP,
Director of the International Institute of Medical Qigong (Palm Springs Branch)
1276 N. Palm Canyon Dr., Suite 105
Palm Springs, CA 92262
Phone: (760) 285-8894
E-Mail: rwhdc@juno.com

Layth Hakim, M.M.Q.
11755 Dorothy St., Apt #1
Los Angeles, Ca. 90049
Phone: (310) 571-1963
E-Mail: lhakim@rpa.com

Madeleine Howell, M.F.T., M.M.Q.
63 Montsalas Dr.
Monterey, Ca. 93940
Phone: (831) 646-0888

Prof. Jerry Alan Johnson, Ph.D., D.T.C.M., (China)
Executive Director and Founder of the
International Institute of Medical Qigong
P.O. Box 52144
Pacific Grove, California 93950 USA
Phone: (831) 646-9399
Fax: (831) 646-0535
E-Mail: drjerryalanjohnson@earthlink.net
Web Page: www.qigongmedicine.com

Matthew B. Jones MMQ, LMT
3886 State St. #J
Santa Barbara, CA 93105
Phone: (805) 680-9032
E-Mail: mateotec@yahoo.com

Dr. Carole Kelly, Ed.D., M.M.Q.
P.O. Box 222843
Carmel, Ca. 93922
Phone: (831) 622-9522
E-Mail: scmkelly@cs.com

Wendy Lang, M.M.Q.
Director of the International Institute of
Medical Qigong (Marin County Branch)
12 Skylark Dr. Apt 33
Larkspur, California 94939
Phone: (415) 924-7883
E-Mail: wendyandphillip@netzero.net

Dr. Seth Lefkowitz, D.C., D.M.Q. (China)
Director of the International Institute of
Medical Qigong (North San Jose Branch)
c/o Natures Path Center
351 South Baywood Avenue,
San Jose, California 95128 USA
Phone: (408) 243-1565
Fax: (408) 243-1568
E-Mail: seth@naturespathcenter.com
Web Page: www.naturespathcenter.com

Bill Lewington, L.Ac., B.Sc. P.H.M., M.M.Q.
572 Pearl St.
Monterey, Ca. 93940
Clinic: 230 Fountain Avenue Pacific Grove, Ca.
Phone: (831) 375-1719
E-Mail: aculew@aol.com

Dia Lynn, B.A., L.M.T., M.M.Q.
Directors of the International Institute of
Medical Qigong (Carmel Valley Branch)
27820 Dorris Dr., Suite 201
Carmel, California 93923
Phone: (831) 625-1752
Cell Phone: (831) 915-6640
E-Mail: dia.lynn@att.net
E-Mail: lmarcumpg@aol.com.

Paul Miller, M.M.Q.
3310 Kirk Rd.
San Jose, Ca. 95124
Phone: (408) 265-5892
Fax: (408) 267-3917
E-Mail: paulmiller@mindspring.com

Katy Reed, M.M.Q.
1145 Clementine Avenue
Seaside, Ca. 93955
Phone: (831) 394-2088

Deneen C. Seril, D.M.Q. (China)
Director of the International Institute of
Medical Qigong (Marina Branch)
P.O. Box 77
Pacific Grove, Ca. 93950
Phone: (831) 601-0652
E-Mail: deneen@montereyisp.com

Eric Shaffer, M.M.Q., D.M.Q. (China)
Director of the International Institute of
Medical Qigong (Asilomar Branch)
775 Asilomar Blvd.
Pacific Grove, California 93950
Phone: 831.375.0593
E-Mail: ericwshaff@aol.com

Shifu Bernard Shannon, D.M.Q. (China)
Rivers of Qi
P.O. Box 9365
San Bernardino, California 92427 USA
Phone: 909.228.4752
Fax: 909.887.3738
E-Mail: bshannon@riversofqi.com
Web Page: www.riversofqi.co

Dr. Arnold Tayam, D.M.Q. (China)
The Longevity Center
P.O. Box 26712
San Jose, California 95159-6712   USA
Phone: (408) 246-4166
E-Mail: chi@longevity-center.com
Web Page: www.longevity-center.com

Dr. Stephanie Taylor, M.D., Ph.D., M.M.Q.
40 Dormody Ct. (office)
Monterey, Ca. 93940
Phone: (831) 655-1995
E-Mail: sst@redshift.com

Jean Ruth Vlamynck, L.Ac., Dipl.Ac., M.T.C.M., M.M.Q.
Director of the International Institute of Medical Qigong (Santa Cruz Branch)
257 B Center Avenue
Aptos, California 95003 USA
Phone: (831) 689-9093
Fax: (831) 689-9094
E-Mail: jeanhere@bigplanet.com
Web Page: www.relaxationresources.com/assoc/jeanv.html

Shifu Matthew B. Weston, M.M.Q.
South Coast Qigong Center
P.O. Box 223373
Carmel, California 93922 USA
Phone: (831) 626-3347
Fax: (831) 626-3347
E-Mail: qigongr@hotmail.com

FLORIDA

Academy for Five Element Acupuncture, Medical Qigong Clinic
1170-A East Hallandale Beach Blvd.
Hallandale, Florida 33009
Phone: 954.456.6336
Fax: 954.456.3944
E-Mail: afea@compuserve.com
Web Page: www.acupuncturist.org

Anna Belle Fore, M.M.Q.
Director of the International Institute of Medical Qigong (S.W. Florida Branch)
P.O. Box 770485
Naples, Florida 34107
Phone: (239) 398-0291
E-Mail: anabel4@angelfire.com

Lisa Van Ostrand, D.M.Q. (China)
Director of the International Institute of Medical Qigong (S.E. Florida Branch)
Miami Beach, Florida 33139 USA
Phone: (786) 512-7096
E-Mail: lisa@lisavanostrand.com
Web Page: www.lisavanostrand.com

ILLINOIS

Catherine White, Dipl. ABT, R.I., M.M.Q.
Director, MI ZAI Shiatsu - Chicago
379 W. Hamilton Lane
Palatine, IL 60067
Phone: (847) 358-8968
E-Mail: cwmizai@sbcglobal.net
Web: www.mizai-shiatsu.org

PENNSYLVANIA

Ted Cibik, N.D., D.M.Q. (China)
c/o Inner Strength Inc.
825 Lovers Leep Rd.
Leechburg, Pa 15656 USA
Phone: (724) 845-1041
Fax: (724) 845-7739
E-Mail: ted@inner-strength.com
Web Page: www.inner-strength.com

TENNESSEE

J. Michael Wood, PMBC, OBDS, M.M.Q.
Director of the International Institute of Medical Qigong (Middle Tennessee Branch)
500 Castlegate Dr.
Nashville, Tn. 37217
Phone: (615) 366-8940
Fax: (615) 399-8479
E-Mail: jmichaelwood@comcast.net

Bryant Seals, M.M.Q.
Director of the International Institute of Medical Qigong (East Tennessee Branch)
P.O. Box 51604
Knoxville, Tn. 37950
Phone: (865) 691-0622
E-Mail: medqigong@ataoistway.com
Web Page: www.ataoistway.com

TEXAS

Chris Axelrad, L.Ac., M.S.O.M., M.M.Q.
The Center for Healing Energetics
2203 San Felipe St
Houston, TX 77019
Phone: 713-527-9555
E-Mail: chris@healingenergetics.com
Web Page: www.healingenergetics.com

Dr. Brian McKenna, D.O.M., Lic. Ac., M.M.Q.
Acupuncture Medical Services
716 Chelsea Place
Houston, Texas 77006
Phone: (713) 942-9688
E-Mail: acupuncturemedical@sbcglobal.net

Lucy M. Roberts, L.Ac., Dipl.Ac., M.T.C.M., M.M.Q.
Director of the International Institute of Medical Qigong (Texas Branch)
P.O. Box 1060
Friendswood, Tx 77546
Phone: (281) 648-3102
Fax: (281) 648-3384
E-Mail: tianearthqi@aol.com
Web Page: www.balanceyourenergy.com

Lou and Maria Eberle, M.S.O.M., M.M.Q.
Director of the International Institute of Medical Qigong (Central Texas Branch)
600 Hart Lane
Dripping Springs, Texas 78620
Tel: 512-894-0337
Cell: 512-684-1274
Email: qigong@centexfamily.org

NEW YORK

Edwin Pickett, M.M.Q.
Lock Box 30926
New York, NY 10011
Phone: 718.510.0364
E-mail: edwin.pickett@dreamcarp.com
Web Page: www.dreamcarp.com

WASHINGTON

Robert B. Bates, D.C., M.M.Q.
Director of the International Institute of Medical Qigong (NW Washington Branch)
c/o Bellingham Institute of Healing
1095 E. Axton Road
Bellingham, WA 98226
Phone: (360) 398-7466
E-Mail: RBbatesDC@aol.com.

Sara Storm, L.Ac., M.M.Q.
Director of the International Institute of Medical Qigong (NE Washington Branch)
11512 32nd Avenue N.E.
Seattle, WA 98125
Phone: (206) 363-0909
E-Mail: sara@sarastorm.com.
Web Page: www.sarastorm.com

WISCONSIN

Denise Douglass-White, M.M.Q.
31 North Star Lane
St. Croix Falls, WI 54024
Phone: 715-483-9886
E-mail: nstar4@centurytel.net.

International Clinical Directory

Bermuda

Sifu Reginald Cann, B.Sc., O.B.T., H.H.P., M.T.O.M., L.A.c., Dipl.Ac., M.M.Q.
Director of the International Institute of Medical Qigong (Bermuda Branch)
c/o "Edville Cottage"
2 Bat-N-Ball-Lane
Sandys, MA-03
Bermuda
Phone: (441) 234-0669
Phone: (441) 799-8643
E-Mail: sifug@yahoo.com

Canada

Paul Pheasey, B.A., M.M.Q.
Director of the International Institute of Medical Qigong (Vancouver Branch)
2586 Kitchener Street
Vancouver, B.C.
Canada V5K3C6
Phone: (604) 255-0856
Fax: (604) 255-0856
E-Mail: paulpheasey@telus.net

Ireland

Dermot A. O'Connor, , Dip. Ac., M.M.Q.
Director of the International Institute of Medical Qigong (Ireland Branch)
33 Haddington Road
Ballsbridge
Dublin 4
Ireland
Phone: ++ 353.1.667.2222
E-Mail: dermot@acupunctureireland.com
Web Page: www.acupunctureireland.com

Israel

Amos Ziv, L.Ac., M.M.Q.
Director of the International Institute of Medical Qigong (Middle East Branch)
7 Rupin St., Rehovot 76353
Israel
Tel/Fax: 972-8-9361-916
Cell: 972-64-419-884
E-Mail: aaziv@hotmail.com

Sweden

Fia G. Hobbs, M.M.Q.
Director of the International Institute of Medical Qigong (Sweden Branch)
Bjulevagen 40
122 41 Enskede
Sweden
Phone: 46.8.508.64101
Phone: (Mobile) 46 070.658.6865
E-Mail: fiahobbs@hotmail.com
Web Page: www.qigongmedicine.se

Also Available By The Author
Chinese Medical Qigong Companion Video or DVD-R Series

This detailed Video or DVD-R series was developed to supplement the information contained in the *Chinese Medical Qigong Therapy Volumes 1 through 5*, written by Professor Jerry Alan Johnson. Each video or DVD-R sells for $50.00, and targets a specific area of training, corresponding to detailed instruction from the Medical Qigong textbook series.

VIDEO OR DVD-R #1:
GATHERING ENERGY FROM HEAVEN AND EARTH

This information is found in *Chinese Medical Qigong Therapy, Volume 2: Energetic Alchemy, Dao Yin Therapy and Qi Deviations* (Chapters 11 through 13).

This first in a series of ten videos/DVDs was developed in order to teach Medical Qigong students how to strengthen their energetic fields, as well as how to replenish energetic depletion which can incur during Qi emission therapy.

This video/DVD contains the following exercises and meditations: Gathering Energy of the Sun's Essence, Gathering Energy of the Moon's Cream, Gathering Energy from the Four Constellations, Gathering Energy from the Five Planets, Gathering Energy from the Earth's Environment, and Gathering Energy from Trees, Bushes, Flowers, Mountains and Oceans.

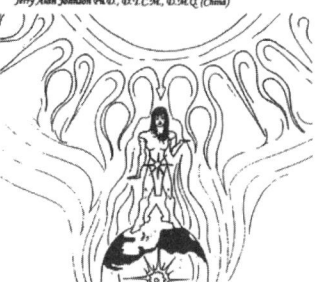

VIDEO OR DVD-R #2:
STATIONARY AND DYNAMIC MEDICAL QIGONG POSTURE TRAINING

This information is found in *Chinese Medical Qigong Therapy, Volume 2: Energetic Alchemy, Dao Yin Therapy and Qi Deviations* (Chapters 15 and 16).

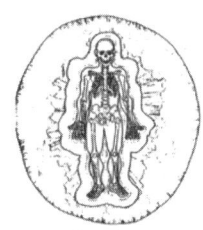

This second in a series of ten videos/DVDs was developed in order to teach Medical Qigong students the proper physical, respiratory and mental training needed for prescribing Self-Regulation Therapy.

This video/DVD contains the following exercises and prescriptions: The 18 Rules of Proper Body Structure, Static and Dynamic Posture Training: Proper Use of the Hands to Lead Qi, Medical Qigong Prescriptions using Dynamic Postures: Treating Patients with Hypertension, Yin and Yang Imbalance, Chronic Fatigue Syndrome, Hypotension, Prolapsed Internal Viscera. Also included are Medical Qigong Walking Therapy used for Regulation, Lung, Kidney, Liver, Spleen and Heart Tonification, as well as the Three Stepping Methods used to treat cancer.

VIDEO OR DVD-R #3: TREATING PATIENTS WITH MEDICAL QIGONG THERAPY (#1)

This information is found in *Chinese Medical Qigong Therapy, Volume 3: Differential Diagnosis, Clinical Foundations, Treatment Principles and Clinical Protocols* (Chapters 27 and 28).

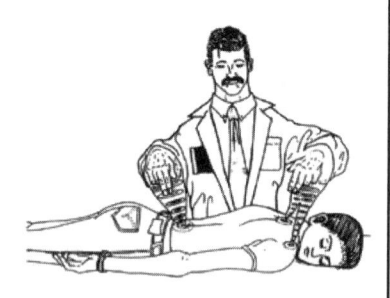

This third in a series of ten videos/DVDs was developed in order to teach Medical Qigong students how to properly and safely establish and operate a Medical Qigong clinic.

This video/DVD contains the following meditations and clinical procedures: Preparing the Clinical Environment, Energetic Grounding and Establishing a Safe Healing Environment (1-10 Meditation), The Divine Hook-Up and Three Invocations, Preparation for Clinical Treatment, The Energetic Circle Drawing Pattern, Dredging and Purging the Patient, Examples of Medical Qigong Therapeutic Tonification Techniques, and Disposing the Patient's Toxic Qi.

VIDEO OR DVD-R #4: TREATING PATIENTS WITH MEDICAL QIGONG THERAPY (#2)

This information is found in *Chinese Medical Qigong Therapy, Volume 3: Differential Diagnosis, Clinical Foundations, Treatment Principles and Clinical Protocols* (Chapters 28, 30 and 32).

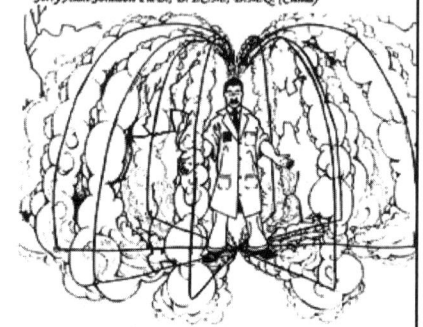

This forth in a series of ten videos/DVDs was developed in order to teach Medical Qigong students how to avoid Energetic Depletion and the Toxic Invasion of the patient's pathogenic Qi when operating a Medical Qigong clinic, as well as how and when to properly and safely Purge, Tonify and Balance the patient's internal organs and energetic fields.

This video/DVD contains the following meditations and clinical procedures: How to create an Energetic Force Field in order to prevent the invasion of the patient's Toxic Qi, The Ren Wu Zang Meditation, Energetic Boundary Invasion, Examples of Purging, Tonification and Regulation Therapeutic Techniques, Ending the Treatment, The Doctor/Patient Intake, Homework and Medical Qigong Prescriptions.

VIDEO OR DVD-R #5:
MEDICAL QIGONG ENERGY TECHNIQUES AND QI EMITTING METHODS

This information is found in *Chinese Medical Qigong Therapy, Volume 3: Differential Diagnosis, Clinical Foundations, Treatment Principles and Clinical Protocols* (Chapters 35 and 36).

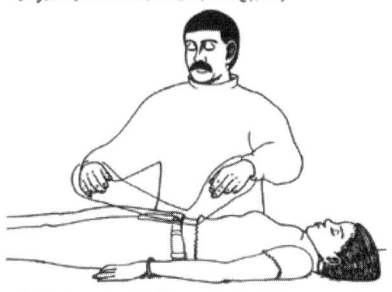

This fifth in a series of ten videos/DVDs was developed in order to teach the Medical Qigong students the various hand postures and Qi emitting methods effectively used for Qi manipulation in the Medical Qigong clinic.

This video/DVD contains the following Medical Qigong treatment techniques and Qi emitting methods: Controlling Energy Projection, Hand Postures for Energy Extension and Qi Manipulation, the Extended Fan Palm, the Sword Fingers Technique, One Finger Skill, the Invisible Needle Technique, the Five Thunder Fingers Technique, the Dragon's Mouth Palm, the Kneading Tiger Palm, Energy Extension, Guidance and Regulation Techniques, Guiding Linear Flow of Energy, Pushing, Pulling and Leading Energy, Circling and Spiraling Energy, Energetic Cupping, Guiding the Flow of Stationary Qi, Shaking and Vibrating Energy, Emitting Hot and Cold Energy, Emitting Qi of the Five Element Organs, and Five Element Channels.

VIDEO OR DVD-R #6:
MEDICAL QIGONG INVISIBLE NEEDLE TECHNIQUE, FIVE ELEMENT QIGONG MASSAGE AND ENERGETIC POINT THERAPY

This information is found in *Chinese Medical Qigong Therapy, Volume 3: Differential Diagnosis, Clinical Foundations, Treatment Principles and Clinical Protocols* (Chapters 37 and 38).

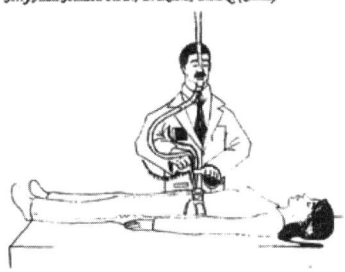

This sixth in a series of ten videos/DVDs was developed in order to teach Medical Qigong students the various hand postures and Qi emitting methods effectively used when applying the Invisible Needle Technique, Five Element Qigong Massage and Energetic Point Therapies.

This video/DVD contains the following Medical Qigong treatment techniques: Preparation for Invisible Needle Therapy, Hand Postures for the Invisible Needle Technique, Tonification and Sedation Techniques, Removing and Disposing of Invisible Needles, Five Element Qigong Massage Techniques, the Circle Compression Method, the Compression Release Method, Thrusting Method, Grasping and Shaking Method, Tapping Method, and Point Therapy Treatments.

VIDEO OR DVD-R #7:
MEDICAL QIGONG HEALING SOUND THERAPY AND PRESCRIPTIONS

This information is found in *Chinese Medical Qigong Therapy, Volume 3: Differential Diagnosis, Clinical Foundations, Treatment Principles and Clinical Protocols* (Chapters 39) and the clinical text found in Chinese Medical Qigong Therapy, Volume 4: Prescription Exercises and Meditations, Treatment of Internal Diseases, Pediatrics, Geriatrics, Gynecology, Neurology, and Energetic Psychology (Chapters 42).

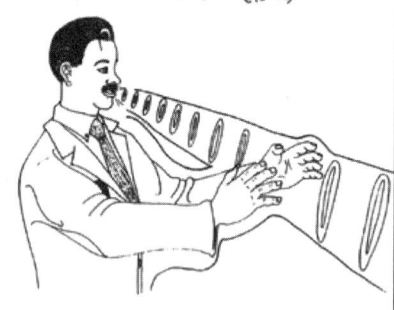

This seventh in a series of ten videos/DVDs was developed in order to teach Medical Qigong students the various Healing Sound Therapies and Prescriptions, as well as when to prescribe them and when they are contraindicated.

This video/DVD contains the following Medical Qigong treatment therapies: Preparation for the Six Healing Sounds, the Six Healing Sound Therapies, Combining Multiple Organ Sounds, Contraindications for the Six Healing Sound Therapy, Specialized Sound Therapy for Treating Internal Organ Diseases, Cysts, Tumor and Cancer, Tones for Treating Radiation and Chemotherapy Patients, and Contraindications for Internal Organ Disease, Tumor and Cancer Sound Therapy.

VIDEO OR DVD-R #8:
TREATMENT OF INTERNAL ORGAN DISEASES WITH MEDICAL QIGONG

This information is found in *Chinese Medical Qigong Therapy, Volume 4: Prescription Exercises and Meditations, Treatment of Internal Diseases, Pediatrics, Geriatrics, Gynecology, Neurology, and Energetic Psychology* (Chapters 50 and 54).

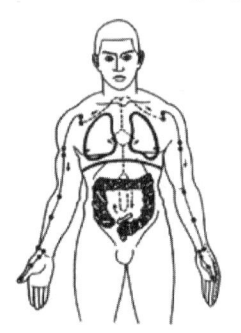

This eighth in a series of ten videos/DVDs was developed in order to teach Medical Qigong students the various hand postures and Qi emitting methods that are effectively used in China when treating specific Internal Organ Diseases with Medical Qigong Therapy.

This video/DVD contains the following treatment therapies: Medical Qigong Therapy and Prescriptions used for the treatment of Migraine Headaches, Chronic Fatigue Syndrome, Multiple Sclerosis and Fibromyalgia. Also included is the Emotional Detoxifying Prescription, "Old Man Searching For The Reflection Of The Moon At The Bottom Of The Tide Pool."

VIDEO OR DVD-R #9:
TREATMENT OF CYSTS, TUMORS AND CANCER WITH MEDICAL QIGONG THERAPY

This information is found in *Chinese Medical Qigong Therapy, Volume 5: An Energetic Approach to Oncology* (Chapters 56, 57, 58, 60, 61, 66, 67, and 68).

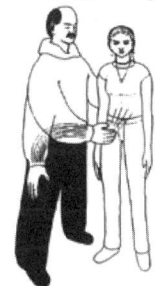

This ninth in a series of ten videos/DVDs was developed in order to teach Medical Qigong students the various hand postures and Qi emitting methods effectively used in treating cysts, tumors and cancer with Medical Qigong Therapy.

This video/DVD contains the following information and treatment therapies: Introduction to Medical Qigong Therapy and Oncology, Treating Brain Tumors, Breast Cysts, Tumors and Cancer, Treating Lung Cancer, Treating Uterine and Cervical Cysts Tumors and Cancer, Treating Prostate Cancer, Homework and Prescriptions. Also included are defining the difference between Healing and Curing.

VIDEO OR DVD-R #10:
SOUL RETRIEVAL

This information is found in *Chinese Medical Qigong Therapy, Volume 2: Energetic Alchemy, Dao Yin Therapy and Qi Deviations* (Chapters 20), and in *Chinese Medical Qigong Therapy, Volume 4: Prescription Exercises and Meditations, Treatment of Internal Diseases, Pediatrics, Geriatrics, Gynecology, Neurology, and Energetic Psychology* (Chapters 55).

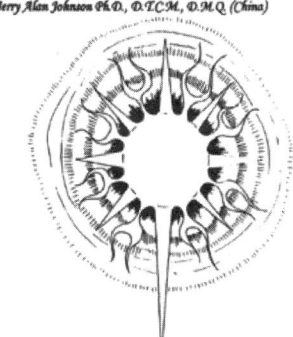

This tenth and final video/DVD was developed in order to teach Medical Qigong students how to assist patients in addressing and overcoming the suppressed emotional traumas which are responsible for creating and sustaining their disease (if the disease is emotionally induced).

This video/DVD contains the following information: Introduction to Soul Retrieval, The Five Levels of Feelings, Physiological Affects of Benign and Malignant Emotional Patterns, Wounding and Closing the Spirit, Soul Retrieval Stage #1: Finding the Storage Chambers of the Body's Past, Present and Future Emotions, Soul Retrieval Stage #2: Pulling Out the Pain Meditation, Soul Retrieval Stage #3: Finding, Healing and Reprogramming Past Emotional Patterns, as well as Facing the Transitions of Life and Death.

CHI KUNG: THE HEALING WORKOUT VIDEO - $19.95

The sharpness of the mind, the strength of the body and the clarity of the spirit are all essential for health and vitality. Chi Kung exercises work on all three. Chi Kung combines the power of meditation with Tai Chi Chuan-like individual movements in order to form energy building exercises. So effective are these exercises that today in China, Chi Kung is prescribed for ailments and illnesses as readily as medicine is administered in the West. So powerful are these exercises that for centuries martial artists have used Chi Kung to empower their fighting and athletic abilities. These exercises are simple, gentle, easy to learn and are for all ages and levels of fitness and coordination.

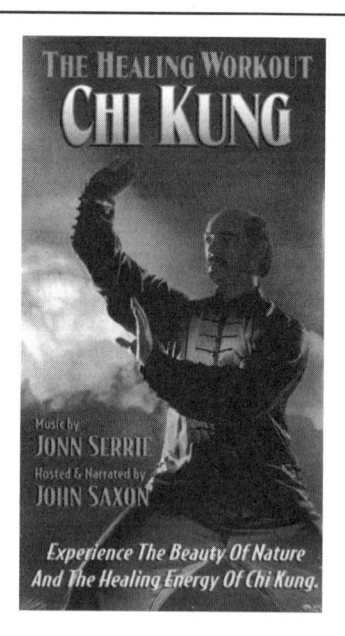

TAI CHI: THE EMPOWERING WORKOUT VIDEO - $19.95

The beauty and power of Tai Chi Chuan is created in the "way" one moves. In essence, the mastery of one move is superior to the learning of a hundred moves. The purpose of this program is not to learn a series of complicated moves, but to simplify and clarify the mental and physical dynamics that empower Tai Chi Chuan. The first section explores the structural mechanics universal to all Tai Chi Chuan movements and styles. Section two focuses the attention on loosening and lubricating all of the joints of the body. Section three integrates the structural mechanics into ten Tai Chi Chuan movements. The final section combines mind intent and inner body skill to maximize strength, energy and power.

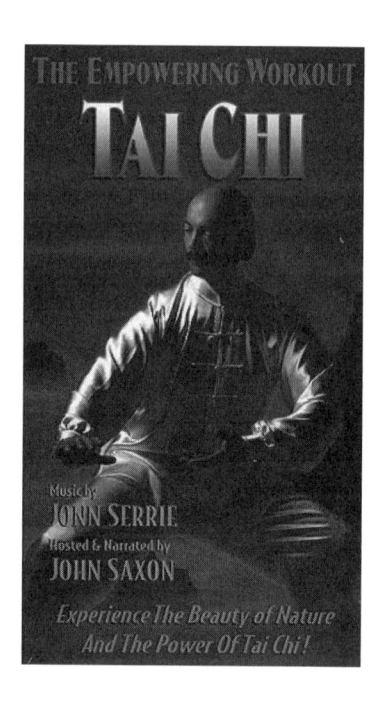

TAI CHI MEDITATION CASSETTE #1: LIFE FORCE BREATHING - $15.95

The ancient masters of Tai Chi Chuan believed that health and self empowerment were dependent upon one's "Life Force Energy." They found that "meditation" proved to be one of the most effective and concise ways of developing internal energy. They created the "Life Force Breathing" meditation, which is designed to mentally touch and energize every cell of the body. This meditation begins by liberating the body of energy obstructions that cause stagnation in the tissues and channels (meridians). The body is then reconstructed energetically, thereby cleansing and rejuvenating the viscera, circulatory, digestive, respiratory, nervous, muscular, and reproductive systems of the body. Finally, the "Wei" Qi (body's protective energy) is expanded and strengthened.

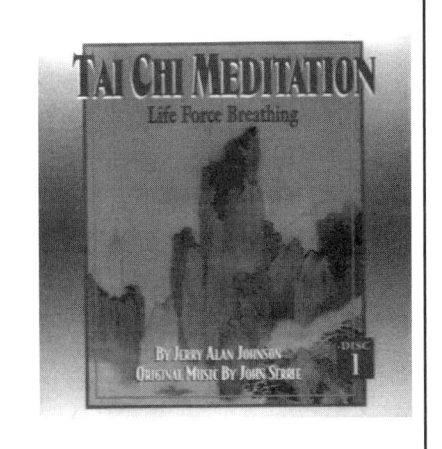

TAI CHI MEDITATION CASSETTE #2: EIGHT DIRECTION PERCEPTION - $15.95

The ancient masters of Tai Chi discovered that powerful meditations were required to enhance and deepen their training. The "Eight Direction Perception" meditation, adopted from the Buddhist Monks, was practiced in order to expand awareness, perception, and psychic ability. Through the complexities of modern society, many people have numbed their abilities to feel their own emotions, internal energies and the subtle powers and intentions that permeate our existence. This meditation releases the trapped emotional memory and stagnant energy lodged in the body's tissues, which inhibit sensory functioning.

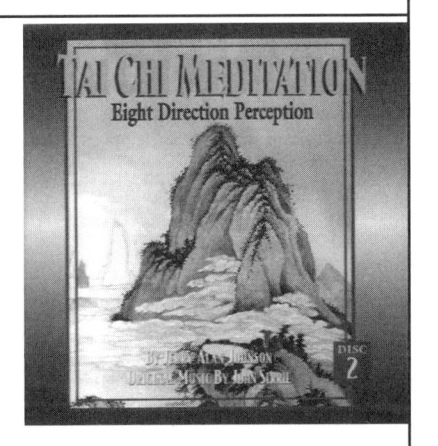

MEDICAL QIGONG VIDEO OR DVD-R #11: MEDICAL QIGONG FOR UNDERSTANDING, PREVENTING AND TREATING BREAST DISEASE - $24.95

The ancient masters of Chinese Energetic Medicine discovered powerful exercises and meditations that can be used in modern times to not only enhance the body's immune system but also treat specific disease conditions. This VHS video tape is an informative, instructional powerhouse of knowledge, providing needed information concerning the energetic cause, formation and treatment of breast cysts, tumors and cancer.

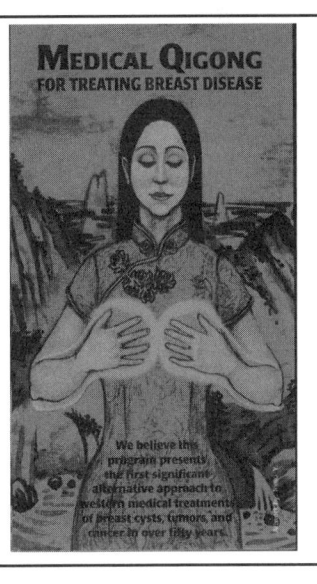

THE INTERNATIONAL INSTITUTE OF MEDICAL QIGONG PRESENTS

MEDICAL QIGONG THERAPY FOR CANCER DVD-R SERIES

This DVD-R series was filmed during a six month intensive training program on Medical Qigong Therapy for the treatment of cancer. Professor Johnson taught 45 professionals and guest participants specific Medical Qigong clinical protocols used for the treatment of various types of cancer, as taught in various hospitals and clinics throughout Beijing China. Included in this six month seminar series are specific Medical Qigong prescription exercises and meditations used for enhancing Medical Qigong treatments. Also included are Medical Qigong treatment protocols specifically used for addressing the side effects caused from radiation and chemotherapy.

The initial goal of this six month oncology seminar series is to assist professionals in establishing an "alternative" and "complimentary" approach to Western cancer treatment protocols using Chinese Medical Qigong Therapy and herbal formulas; as well as to work in conjunction with the programs already established at other Western Medical cancer centers.

This detailed DVD-R series was developed to supplement the information contained in *Chinese Medical Qigong Therapy Volume 5: An Energetic Approach to Oncology*, by Professor Jerry Alan Johnson. Each DVD-R targets a specific area of training, corresponding with detailed instruction from the oncology textbook.

DVD-R #12: HOUSTON CANCER SEMINAR #1 - INTRODUCTION TO MEDICAL QIGONG THERAPY AND CANCER TREATMENT: SETTING A CLINICAL FOUNDATION

This first DVD set was developed in order to teach Medical Qigong students, as well as other health professionals, the foundational knowledge needed to operate a safe and effective Medical Qigong clinic, as established by the Hai Dian University and the Xi Yuan Hospital in Beijing China.

This 5 DVD set contains the following information: An Introduction to Medical Qigong Therapy, The Five Energies of the Human Body; Building an Energetic Boundary; Clinical Safety (understanding toxic energetic pathogens); Contraindication and Improper Qigong Training; Building an Energetic Boundary; Introduction to Energy Blockages; Understanding the Structural Matrix of an Energetic Cluster; Combining Medical Qigong Therapy with Sound and Color; Treating Phantom Pains and Rebuilding The patient's Energetic Fields; Qi Emitting Methods; An Introduction to Cancer Prescription Exercises; The Basic Clinical Protocol; and Treating the Patient.

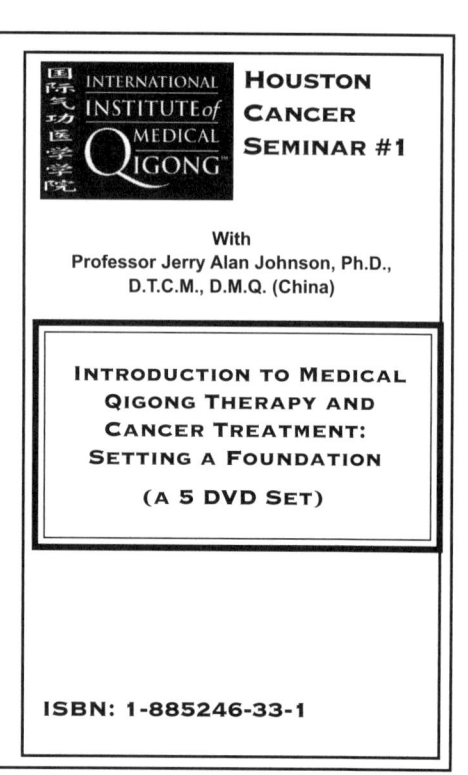

HOUSTON CANCER SEMINAR #1

With
Professor Jerry Alan Johnson, Ph.D.,
D.T.C.M., D.M.Q. (China)

INTRODUCTION TO MEDICAL QIGONG THERAPY AND CANCER TREATMENT: SETTING A FOUNDATION

(A 5 DVD SET)

ISBN: 1-885246-33-1

DVD-R #13: HOUSTON CANCER SEMINAR #2 - AN ENERGETIC APPROACH TO ONCOLOGY

This second DVD set was developed in order to teach Medical Qigong students, as well as other health professionals, the foundational knowledge needed to diagnose and treat cyst, tumor and cancer formations from a Chinese Medical Qigong perspective.

This 4 DVD set contains the following information: An Introduction to History of Cancer Treatments and Medical Qigong; Introduction to Cancer Treatments; The Five Primary Causes of Cancer; Categorization of Benign and Malignant Tumors; Three Types of Cancer; Three Types of Cancer Growth; Theories of Cancer Metastases; Cancer Staging Systems; T.C.M. Theory on Cancer Etiology; Four Approaches to Cancer Therapy; Energy Protection Meditations Used Before Treating Cancer Patients; How to Release Qi from the Body; An Introduction to Cancer Treatments; Introduction to Cancer Healing Sounds; Creating an Energy Ball; Introduction to Cleaning the Chakra Gate Filters; and An Introduction to Invisible Needle Therapy.

HOUSTON CANCER SEMINAR #2

With
Professor Jerry Alan Johnson, Ph.D., D.T.C.M., D.M.Q. (China)

CHINESE MEDICAL QIGONG THERAPY AND AN ENERGETIC APPROACH TO CANCER ONCOLOGY

(A 4 DVD SET)

ISBN: 1-885246-34-X

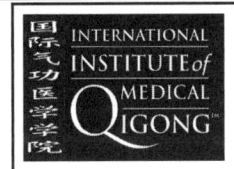

DVD-R #14: HOUSTON CANCER SEMINAR #3 - MEDICAL QIGONG TREATMENT PROTOCOLS USED FOR BREAST, CERVICAL, PROSTATE, OVARIAN, AND UTERINE CANCER

This third DVD set was developed in order to teach Medical Qigong students, as well as other health professionals, the foundational knowledge needed to treat specific types of tumors and cancer, as well as how to facilitate the patient's needs in providing the specific Medical Qigong prescriptions needed to augment the Medical Qigong treatment protocols.

This 4 DVD set contains the following information: Introduction to Treating Tumors; Energetic Imprinting; Clinical Diagnosis; Type and location of Stagnation; Origin of tumor formation; Energetic patterning, how the tumor is being fed; Secondary factors of tumor growth; Medical Qigong Treatment Protocols and Prescription Homework for the treatment of Breast Cancer, The Treatment of Cervical Cancer; The Treatment of Prostate Cancer; The Treatment of Ovarian Cancer; The Treatment of Uterine Cancer; Understanding Death and Dying; What Happens When a Tumor Energetically Unwinds; and Testimony from an Acupuncturist who, after the last month, applied the Medical Qigong Treatment Protocol to a patient in his clinic and dissolved her Breast Tumors.

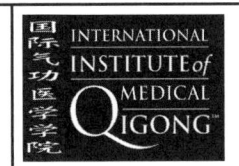

HOUSTON CANCER SEMINAR #3

With
Professor Jerry Alan Johnson, Ph.D., D.T.C.M., D.M.Q. (China)

MEDICAL QIGONG TREATMENT PROTOCOLS USED FOR BREAST, CERVICAL, PROSTATE, OVARIAN, AND UTERINE CANCER

(A 4 DVD SET)

ISBN: 1-885246-35-8

DVD-R #15: HOUSTON CANCER SEMINAR #4 - MEDICAL QIGONG TREATMENT PROTOCOLS USED FOR BRAIN, SKIN, AND BONE CANCER, LEUKEMIA, MALIGNANT LYMPHOMA, AND MULTIPLE MYELOMAS

This fourth DVD set was developed in order to teach Medical Qigong students, as well as other health professionals, the foundational knowledge needed to treat specific types of tumors and cancer, as well as how to provide specific Medical Qigong prescriptions needed to augment the Medical Qigong treatment protocols.

This 4 DVD set contains the following information: Three Medical Qigong Treatment Protocols for the Treatment of Brain Tumors and Cancer; How Cancer Metastasizes to the Brain; Prescription Homework for the Treatment of Brain Tumors and Cancer; Two Medical Qigong Treatment Protocols for the Treatment of Skin Cancer; Using Hand Seals (Mudras) in the Clinic; Introduction to Bone Cancer Treatment Protocols; The Treatment of Leukemia; Introduction to the Treatment of Malignant Lymphoma; Treating Multiple Myelomas; Specific Medical Qigong Prescription Exercises for the Treatment of Skin Cancer, Bone Cancer, Leukemia, Malignant Lymphoma, and Multiple Myelomas; and Student Examination.

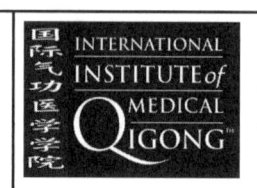

HOUSTON CANCER SEMINAR #4

With Professor Jerry Alan Johnson, Ph.D., D.T.C.M., D.M.Q. (China)

MEDICAL QIGONG TREATMENT PROTOCOLS USED FOR BRAIN, SKIN, AND BONE CANCER, LEUKEMIA, MALIGNANT LYMPHOMA, AND MULTIPLE MYELOMAS

(A 4 DVD SET)

ISBN: 1-885246-36-6

DVD-R #16: HOUSTON CANCER SEMINAR #5 - MEDICAL QIGONG CANCER PRESCRIPTION EXERCISES AND MEDITATIONS

This fifth DVD set was developed in order to teach Medical Qigong students, as well as other health professionals, the foundational knowledge needed to effectively provide the Medical Qigong prescription homework exercises and meditations needed to augment the Medical Qigong treatment protocol, as well as their contraindications.

This 4 DVD set contains the following information: Establishing a Cancer Support Group; Establishing an Instant Relationship Exercise; The Psycho-Physical Aspects of the Emotions; The Splintering of the Spirit and Body; Stages of Emotional Reactions; The Need for Emotional Security; Finding the Chambers of the Past, Present, and Future Meditation; Pulling Out the Pain Meditation; Dissolving Emotional Blockages Meditation; Stages of Emotional Healing; The Great Illuminating Pearl Meditation; The Sun and Moon Meditation; Energy Ball Meditation; Overview of the Dry Crying and Beating the Bag Exercises; Treating Scar Tissue; Disease Patterns and Energy Flow; and Student Examination.

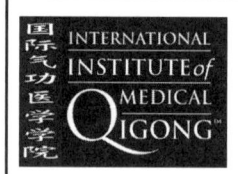

HOUSTON CANCER SEMINAR #5

With Professor Jerry Alan Johnson, Ph.D., D.T.C.M., D.M.Q. (China)

MEDICAL QIGONG CANCER PRESCRIPTION EXERCISES AND MEDITATIONS

(A 4 DVD SET)

ISBN: 1-885246-37-4

DVD-R #17: Houston Cancer Seminar #6 - Medical Qigong Treatment Protocols Used For Radiation and Chemotherapy

This sixth DVD set was developed in order to teach Medical Qigong students, as well as other health professionals, the foundational knowledge needed to effectively treat patients who are currently receiving radiation therapy and chemotherapy, as well as how to effectively treat the side effects of such treatments.

This 4 DVD set contains the following information: Overview of Tissue Damage Caused From Cytotoxic Treatments; Introduction to Radiation Therapy; Questioning Radiation Therapy; How to Treat Patients Who Have Undergone Radiation Therapy; Student Examination; Introduction to Chemotherapy; Clinical Protocol for Chemotherapy Patients; How to Energetically Seal the Wrists to Prevent Toxic Qi Invasion; Treating the Side Effects of Chemotherapy; Cautions of Treating Patients Who Are Pregnant; Treating Urinary Bladder Infections; Treatment for Diminished White Blood Cell Count; Juice Formulas that Nourish The Body's Yin; Lecture on Nutritional Therapy for Cancer Treatment; Lecture on Fu Zheng Herbs and for Cancer Treatment; The 2004 Graduating Class of Medical Qigong Clinical Oncology; and a Group Photo of Graduating Students.

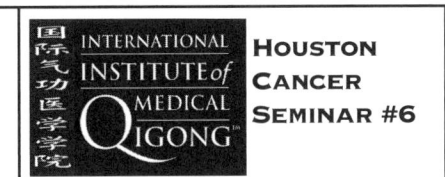

HOUSTON CANCER SEMINAR #6

With
Professor Jerry Alan Johnson, Ph.D.,
D.T.C.M., D.M.Q. (China)

MEDICAL QIGONG TREATMENT PROTOCOLS USED FOR RADIATION AND CHEMOTHERAPY

(A 4 DVD SET)

ISBN: 1-885246-38-2

TO ORDER THESE EXCITING NEW DVD-R SERIES CONTACT

The International Institute of Medical Qigong
P.O. Box 52144
Pacific Grove, California
93950   U.S.A.
Fax (831) 646-0535
E-Mail: drjerryalanjohnson@earthlink.net
Web Page: www.qigongmedicine.com

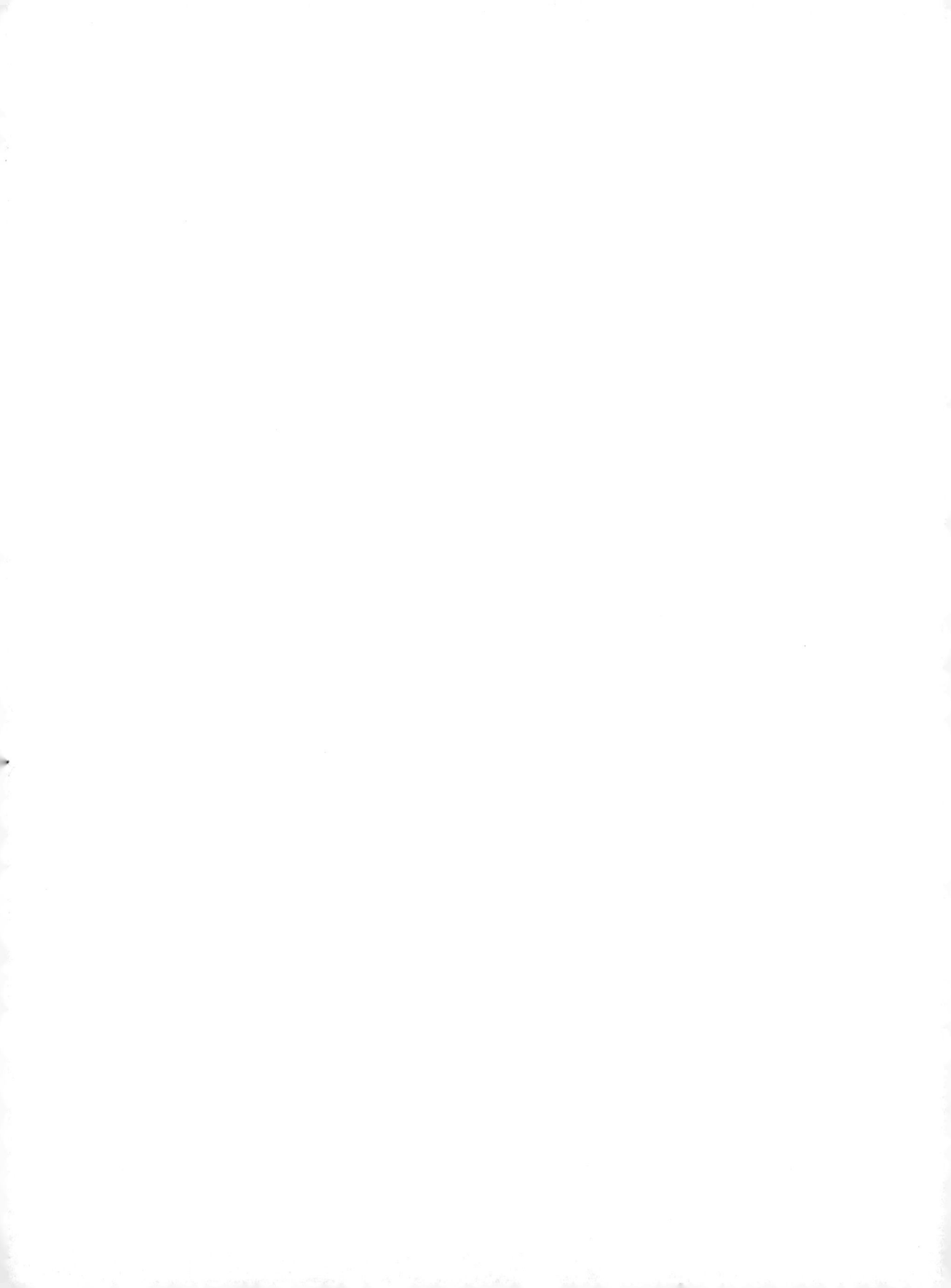